Essentials of Psychiatric Mental Health Nursing

THIRD EDITION

Essentials of Psychiatric Mental Health Nursing

THIRD EDITION

A Communication Approach to Evidence-Based Care

Elizabeth M. Varcarolis, RN, MA

Professor Emeritus
Formerly Deputy Chairperson and Psychiatric Nursing Coordinator
Department of Nursing
Borough of Manhattan Community College;
Associate Fellow
Albert Ellis Institute for Rational Emotional Behavioral Therapy
(REBT);
Former Major, Army Nurse Corps Reserve
New York, New York

ELSEVIER

ELSEVIER

3251 Riverport Lane
St. Louis, Missouri 63043

ESSENTIALS OF PSYCHIATRIC MENTAL HEALTH NURSING:
A COMMUNICATION APPROACH TO EVIDENCE-BASED CARE, THIRD EDITION   ISBN: 978-0-323-38965-5

Notices

Knowledge and best practice in this field are constantly changing. As new research and experience broaden our understanding, changes in research methods, professional practices, or medical treatment may become necessary.

Practitioners and researchers must always rely on their own experience and knowledge in evaluating and using any information, methods, compounds, or experiments described herein. In using such information or methods they should be mindful of their own safety and the safety of others, including parties for whom they have a professional responsibility.

With respect to any drug or pharmaceutical products identified, readers are advised to check the most current information provided (i) on procedures featured or (ii) by the manufacturer of each product to be administered, to verify the recommended dose or formula, the method and duration of administration, and contraindications. It is the responsibility of practitioners, relying on their own experience and knowledge of their patients, to make diagnoses, to determine dosages and the best treatment for each individual patient, and to take all appropriate safety precautions.

To the fullest extent of the law, neither the Publisher nor the authors, contributors, or editors, assume any liability for any injury and/or damage to persons or property as a matter of products liability, negligence or otherwise, or from any use or operation of any methods, products, instructions, or ideas contained in the material herein.

Library of Congress Cataloging-in-Publication Data
Names: Varcarolis, Elizabeth M., author.
Title: Essentials of psychiatric mental health nursing : a communication
    approach to evidence-based care / Elizabeth M. Varcarolis.
Description: Third edition. | New York, New York : Elsevier, [2017] |
    Includes bibliographical references and index.
Identifiers: LCCN 2016022588 | ISBN 9780323389655 (pbk. : alk. paper)
Subjects: | MESH: Mental Disorders--nursing | Psychiatric Nursing--methods
    | Evidence-Based Nursing
Classification: LCC RC440 | NLM WY 160 | DDC 616.89/0231--dc23 LC record
available at https://lccn.loc.gov/2016022588

Senior Content Strategist: Yvonne Alexopoulos
Content Development Manager: Laurie Gower
Senior Content Developmental Specialist: Lisa P. Newton
Publishing Services Manager: Jeff Patterson
Senior Project Manager: Tracey Schriefer
Interior Designer: Paula Catalano
Cover Designer: Patrick Ferguson

Printed in Canada

Last digit is the print number: 9 8 7 6 5 4 3 2

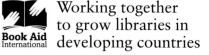

Working together
to grow libraries in
developing countries

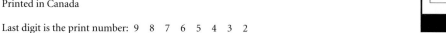

www.elsevier.com • www.bookaid.org

ACKNOWLEDGMENTS

As is always the case, I owe a huge debt of gratitude to many for their contributions and support.

First, I would like to thank my consultants, Susan Frost and Chyllia Dixon, for their contributions to the new format for "Applying Evidence-Based Practice (EBP)" in the clinical chapters and to revising seven chapters. Susan and Chyllia contributed many creative ideas and suggestions during the planning phase for this third edition of *Essentials*.

I am also indebted to Dawn Scheick for the "Applying the Art" boxes found in all of the clinical chapters (Chapters 10 to 19). Dawn offered excellent examples of how a nurse can incorporate effective and insightful communication while working with patients who possess a variety of needs and display a wide range of behaviors.

Communication is one of the arts taught to all nursing students, and effective communication strategies are the cornerstone of psychiatric mental health nursing. This text offers many pedagogical features that will benefit both the cognitive learner and the visual learner. It is hoped that the reader will gain fresh insights, attain a broader understanding, and learn effective tools in interactions with vulnerable individuals during their treatment toward a more mentally healthy quality of life.

I want to offer special thanks to the amazing authors who have contributed to this edition of *Essentials of Psychiatric Mental Health Nursing* for their expertise and hard work. Sincere and profound thanks go to Peggy Halter, Dorothy Varchol, Penny Brooke, Kathleen Ibrahim, Carol O. Long, and Ed Herzog, in order of the appearance of their chapters.

A very special thanks to Teresa Burckhalter, Marie Messier, and Linda Turchin for their creative work on the instructor and student ancillaries that accompany this text.

I have been fortunate to be part of a hard-working team. Those who work behind the scenes are always pivotal to the production of any successful text. These are the people who have provided support, kept the project on track, and solved a myriad of problems that are inherent to any production:

- Yvonne Alexopoulos, Senior Content Strategist, always provided support and everything needed to make the third edition of *Essentials* a success.
- Lisa P. Newton, Senior Content Developmental Specialist, pulled together resources, provided support, and untangled dilemmas during the publication process.
- Tracey Schriefer, Senior Project Manager, managed consistency to the minutest detail and has made me look good throughout the process.
- Paula Catalano, Book Designer, created a vivid, exciting, and reader-friendly design.

CONTRIBUTORS

Penny Simpson Brooke, APRN, MS, JD
University of Utah
College of Nursing
Salt Lake City, Utah

Ann Wolbert Burgess, DNSc, APRN, BC, FAAN
Professor of Psychiatric Nursing
William F. Connell School of Nursing
Boston College
Chestnut Hill, Massachusetts

Chyllia D. Fosbre, MSN, PMHNP-BC, LMT
Psychiatric Nurse Practitioner
West Yavapai Guidance Clinic
Prescott Valley, Arizona

Susan L. Frost, DNP, MC, MS, FPMHNP-BC
Psychiatric Nurse Practitioner
Psychiatric Nursing Professor
West Yavapai Guidance Clinic
Prescott Valley, Arizona;
GateWay Community College (retired)
Phoenix, Arizona

Margaret Jordan Halter, PhD, PMH-APRN
Editor, *Foundations of Psychiatric Mental Health Nursing*;
Adjunct Faculty
Ohio State University
Columbus, Ohio;
Clinical Nurse Specialist
Cleveland Clinic Akron General
Akron, Ohio

Edward A. Herzog, MSN, APRN-CNS
Senior Lecturer
Kent State University College of Nursing
Kent, Ohio

Kathleen Ibrahim, MA, PMHCNS-BC
Private Practice, Psychotherapy
Tenafly, New Jersey

Carol O. Long, PhD, RN, FPCN, FAAN
Principal, Capstone Healthcare;
Founder, Palliative Care Essentials;
Adjunct Faculty, Arizona State University
College of Nursing and Health Innovation
Phoenix, Arizona

Dawn M. Scheick, EdD RN, PMHCNS, BC
Chair and Professor of Nursing
Alderson-Broaddus College;
Therapist
Barbour County Health Department
Philippi, West Virginia
Applying the Art boxes

Shirley A. Smoyak, RN, PhD, FAAN
Professor II (distinguished)
Rutgers University
New Brunswick, New Jersey

Dorothy A. Varchol, MSN, MA, RN-BC
Professor of Psychiatric Nursing
Cincinnati State Technical and Community
College
Cincinnati, Ohio

Ancillary Writers

Teresa S. Burckhalter, MSN, RN, BC
Nursing Faculty
Technical College of the Lowcountry
Beaufort, South Carolina
Chapter Review Questions and Test Bank

Marie Messier, MSN, RN
Associate Professor of Nursing
Germanna Community College
Locust Grove, Virginia
Case Studies and Nursing Care Plans

Linda Turchin, RN, MSN, CNE
Associate Professor of Nursing
Fairmont State University
Fairmont, West Virginia
NCLEX Review Questions

Sheila Rouslin Welt, MS, APN
Private Practice, Psychotherapy
Morristown, New Jersey;
Educational Consultation
The Pingry School
Short Hills, New Jersey

Linda Wendling, MS, MFA
Learning Theory Consultant
University of Missouri – St. Louis
St. Louis, Missouri
TEACH for Nurses

REVIEWERS

Lorraine Chiappetta, RN, MSN, CNE
Professional Faculty
Washtenaw Community College
Nursing Department
Ann Arbor, Michigan

Marnita Jo Guinn, PhD, RN
Dean of Associate Degree Nursing
Ranger College
Ranger, Texas;
Brown County Campus
Early, Texas

Tammy Hostetler, MS-Ned, RN-BC
Assistant Professor (Lead)
Grand Canyon University
College of Nursing and Health Care Professionals
Phoenix, Arizona

Katherine Howard, MS, RN-BC, CNE
Nursing Instructor
Middlesex County College
Nursing Department
Edison, New Jersey

Phyllis Jacobs, RN, MSN
Assistant Professor Emeritus
Wichita State University
School of Nursing
Wichita, Kansas

Renee Menkens, RN, MS
Clinical Assistant Professor
Oregon Health & Science University
School of Nursing
Portland, Oregon;
Staff RN
Bay Area Hospital
Coos Bay, Oregon

Kesha Marie Nelson, MSN/Ed, RN, CPN
Assistant Professor
Department of Nursing
Northern Kentucky University
Highland Heights, Kentucky

Cristina M. Perez, PhD, RN
Assistant Professor of Nursing
Ramapo College of New Jersey
Nursing Programs Department
Mahwah, New Jersey

Nancee Wozney, PhD, RN
Dean of Nursing and Allied Health
Minnesota State College – Southeast Technical
Department of Nursing
Winona, Minnesota

Dawn Wright, PhD, PMHNP, CNE
Associate Professor
Western Kentucky University
School of Nursing
Bowling Green, Kentucky

The *Diagnostic and Statistical Manual of Mental Disorders*, Fifth Edition (*DSM-5*) is well represented in this third edition of *Essentials of Psychiatric Mental Health Nursing: A Communication Approach to Evidence-Based Care*, as are medications recently approved by the U.S. Food and Drug Administration at this writing. Color plates depicting "The Neurobiology of Specific Disorders" is also new to this edition. They come alive through animations on the Evolve website. Most of the clinical chapters are totally revised, in particular, Chapter 19, *Substance-Related and Addictive Disorders* and Chapter 25, *Care for the Dying and Those Who Grieve*, which has been completely updated and revamped by a new expert in the field. This edition continues to provide the essential content for a shorter course without sacrificing either the current research or the nursing and psychotherapeutic interventions necessary for sound practice. In fact, all efforts have been made to ensure that research and psychotherapeutic interventions reflect current knowledge.

Essentials of Psychiatric Mental Health Nursing, Third Edition, continues to provide a comprehensive but concise review of the prominent theorists and all therapeutic modalities in use today, including milieu, group, and family therapies (Chapter 3, "Theories and Therapies"). Within each of the clinical chapters (Chapters 10 to 19), chapters that examine various psychiatric emergencies (Chapters 20 to 25), and chapters that address discrete patient populations across the life span (Chapters 26 to 28), specific therapeutic modalities that have proven effective for each topic are covered thoroughly.

In addition to the overview of medication groups provided in Chapter 4 ("Biological Basis for Understanding Psychopharmacology"), specific medications are covered in full for each of the discrete clinical disorders and include patient and family teaching guidelines. Integrative therapies are also included in each of the clinical chapters where they have proven effective.

To present the most essential base of knowledge for a shorter course, the pertinent information on some topics has been incorporated in the clinical chapters where applicable rather than discussed in a separate chapter. For example, rather than include a general chapter on culture, each of the clinical chapters incorporates relevant information on cultural aspects of the various clinical disorders, which can also help to give the reader a broader cultural perspective.

Forensic issues related to the nursing care of patients are included in specific chapters, especially Chapters 21 ("Child, Partner, and Elder Violence") and 22 ("Sexual Violence"). This discussion is in addition to Chapter 6 ("Legal and Ethical Basis for Practice").

THE SCIENCE AND ART OF PSYCHIATRIC MENTAL HEALTH NURSING

The American Nurses Association's *Psychiatric–Mental Health Nursing: Scope and Standards of Practice* begins with the following statement that stresses the importance of both the art and the science employed by nurses caring for patients with mental health problems and psychiatric disorders:

> *Psychiatric–mental health nursing, a core mental health profession, employs a purposeful use of self as its art and a wide range of nursing, psychosocial, and neurobiological theories and research evidence as its science.*

In *Essentials of Psychiatric Mental Health Nursing: A Communication Approach to Evidence-Based Care*, Third Edition, there is an effort to integrate and balance these two aspects of nursing care and to present all essential information on each so that students will be prepared to offer the best possible care when they enter practice.

The Science

Over the past few decades, we have seen remarkable scientific progress in our understanding of the workings of the brain and how abnormalities in the functioning of the brain are related to mental illness. As confidence in this research grew, the focus on scientific research expanded and led to more scientifically based treatment approaches, and the concept of *evidence-based practice* (EBP) became a dominant focus of mental health treatment.

While writing this text, great effort was made to provide the most current evidence-based information in the field while still keeping the material comprehensible and reader-friendly. Relevant information drawn from science is woven throughout the text.

Chapter 1 ("Practicing the Science and the Art of Psychiatric Nursing") introduces the student to the evolution of EBP and its mechanics and provides guidelines for where and how to gather information for applying EBP in psychiatric nursing practice.

One of the two unique features of this text is **Applying Evidence-Based Practice (EBP)**, which is introduced in Chapter 1 and runs throughout the clinical chapters. Each box poses a question, walks the readers through the process of gathering evidence-based data from a variety of sources, and presents a plan of care based on the evidence.

The Art

In comparison with the medical model, the **recovery model** is a more social, relationship-based model of care. The focus of the recovery model is a nurse-physician partner relationship. The recovery model began in the addiction field, in which the goal was for individuals to recover from substance abuse and addictions. Today the recovery model is gaining momentum in the larger mental health community. Its focus is on empowering patients by supporting hope, strengthening social ties, developing more effective coping skills, fostering the use of spiritual strength, and more.

By definition, nurses are primed to incorporate the biopsychosocial and cultural/spiritual approaches to care. Some nursing leaders express concern that the "art" of nursing is becoming marginalized by the emphasis on EBP. Chapter 1 covers some of these often minimized and uncharted interventions, such as the art of caring, the skill of attending, and patient advocacy. However, what also might be minimized and deemphasized are the tools that make nurses unique. Some of these tools include possessing effective communication skills, forming therapeutic relationships, and understanding ways of interviewing and assessing patients' needs. These areas are stressed in Chapters 8 ("Communication Skills: Medium for All Nursing Practice") and 9 ("Therapeutic Relationships and the Clinical Interview"). There is also a section in each of the clinical chapters on useful communications techniques for a specific disorder or situation.

The second unique feature that is included in the clinical chapters is **Applying the Art**, which depicts a clinical scenario demonstrating the interaction (both therapeutic and nontherapeutic) between a student and a patient, the student's perception of the interaction, and the identification of the mental health nursing concepts in play.

ORGANIZATION

Organized into five units, the chapters in the text have been grouped to emphasize the clinical perspective and to facilitate locating information. All clinical chapters are organized in a clear, logical, and consistent format with the nursing process as the strong, visible framework. The basic outline for the clinical chapters is as follows.

- Prevalence and Comorbidity
  Knowing the comorbid disorders that are often part of the clinical picture of specific disorders helps students as well as clinicians to understand how to better assess and treat their patients.
- Theory
- Cultural Considerations
- Clinical Picture
- *Application of the Nursing Process*
  - Assessment
    Presents appropriate assessment for a specific disorder, including assessment tools and rating scales. The rating scales included help to highlight important areas in the assessment of a variety of behaviors or mental conditions. Because many of the answers are subjective, experienced clinicians use these tools in addition to their knowledge of their patients as a guide when planning care.
  - Diagnosis
    Includes the latest NANDA-I (2015–2017) terminology.
  - Outcomes Identification
  - Planning
  - Implementation
    Interventions follow the categories set by the American Nurses Association's Psychiatric–Mental Health Nursing: Scope and Standards of Practice *(2014). Various interventions for each of the clinical disorders are chosen based on which most fit specific patient needs and include communication guidelines; health teaching and health promotion; milieu therapy; psychotherapy; and pharmacological, biological, and integrative therapies.*
  - Evaluation

FEATURES

In addition to the **Applying Evidence-Based Practice (EBP)** and **Applying the Art** boxes described above, the following features are included in the text to inform, heighten understanding, and engage the reader.

- Chapters open with **Objectives** and **Key Terms and Concepts** to orient the reader.
- Numerous **Vignettes** describing psychiatric patients and their disorders attract and hold the reader's interest.
- **Assessment Guidelines** are included in clinical chapters to familiarize readers with methods of assessing patients; these also can be used in the clinical setting.
- **Potential Nursing Diagnoses** tables list several possible nursing diagnoses for a particular disorder along with the associated signs and symptoms.

- **Nursing Interventions** tables list interventions for a given disorder or clinical situation, along with rationales for each intervention.
- *DSM-5 criteria boxes for selected mental health disorders.*
- **Neurobiology illustrations of selected mental health disorders and how medications help to mitigate classic symptoms.** Also provided on the Student Resources of Evolve as Animations. See the Animation icon ▶ in the textbook.
- **Key Points to Remember** present the main concepts of each chapter in an easy to comprehend and concise bulleted list.
- **Critical Thinking** questions at the end of all chapters introduce clinical situations in psychiatric nursing and encourage critical thinking processes essential for nursing practice.
- **NEW! Chapter Review Questions** at the end of each chapter reinforce key concepts. Answers are provided in Appendix C.
- Appendixes provide the *DSM-5 Classification* list, **NANDA-I Nursing Diagnoses**, and **Answers to Chapter Review Questions**.

LEARNING AND TEACHING AIDS

For Students

The Evolve Student Resources for this text include the following.

- *Animations* of the neurobiology illustrations for selected mental health disorders and how medications help to mitigate classic symptoms. You can also find these illustrations in the textbook with the ▶ icon next to them.
- *Case Studies* and *Nursing Care Plans* for clinical disorders.
- *Student Review Questions* for each chapter.

For Instructors

The Evolve Instructor Resources for this text include the following.

- *TEACH for Nurses lesson plans*, based on chapter Learning Objectives, serve as ready-made, modifiable lesson plans and a complete roadmap to link all parts of the educational package. These concise and straightforward lesson plans can be modified or combined to meet your particular scheduling and teaching needs.
- *Test Bank* in ExamView format, featuring approximately 800 test items, complete with correct answer, rationale, cognitive level, nursing process step, appropriate NCLEX® label, and corresponding text page reference. The ExamView program allows instructors to create new tests; edit, add, and delete test questions; sort questions by NCLEX category, cognitive level, and nursing process step; and administer and grade tests online.
- *PowerPoint Presentations* with more than 600 customizable lecture slides.
- *Audience Response Questions* for i>clicker and other systems, with 2 to 5 multiple-answer questions per chapter to stimulate class discussion and assess student understanding of key concepts.

I hope you all find that *Essentials of Psychiatric Mental Health Nursing: A Communication Approach to Evidence-Based Care,* Third Edition, provides you with the information you need to be successful in your practice of nursing. Good luck to you all.

Betsy M. Varcarolis

CONTENTS

Essential Theoretical Concepts for Practice

Dr. Hildegard E. Peplau (1909–1999)
"Mother of Psychiatric Nursing"

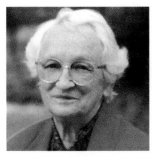

Hildegard Peplau, known as the mother of psychiatric nursing, has had the most profound effect on the practice of nursing since Florence Nightingale. As a child, Peplau witnessed a devastating influenza epidemic that influenced her perceptions. She worked as a staff nurse and school nurse, then received bachelor's, master's, and doctoral degrees in psychology and went on to become a certified psychoanalyst. She was later an Army Corps nurse, and at a psychiatric nursing faculty at Rutgers University she developed the first program specifically for psychiatric nursing. She later worked with the World Health Organization (WHO), published extensively, served as executive director and president of the American Nurses Association, and was a visiting faculty and lecturer around the world (D'Antonio et al., 2014).

Peplau's Theory of Interpersonal Relations, also known as psychodynamic nursing, was strongly influenced by Harry Stack Sullivan's Interpersonal Relationship Theory and was the first to integrate concepts from other psychological and scientific fields into a nursing theory. Her interpersonal theory led to a paradigm shift in the nature of the nurse-patient relationship, now referred to as patient-centered relationship or patient-centered care. According to Peplau, the nurse holds many roles, including teacher, counselor, advocate, and leader, and works collaboratively with the patient toward creative and productive community living and independence. The therapeutic use of self positively affects patient outcomes. The nurse-patient relationship moves through stages from identifying the problem, to selecting and using all available resources, to terminating the therapeutic relationship (D'Antonio et al., 2014; Nursing Theory, 2013). Peplau's theory has been used as a framework for a plethora of research topics, including patient education, depression, survivors of sexual violence, and research subject retention (Penckofer et al., 2011).

As you read through this textbook you will learn about levels of anxiety, phases of the nurse-patient relationship, and the importance of observing your own thoughts and feelings within the context of the nurse-patient interaction. These indispensible tools used by competent nurses today are all contributions from Hildegard Peplau, and her theory continues to serve as a foundation for development of therapeutic nursing interventions. Peplau's influence goes beyond psychiatric nursing. She was a determined advocate of advanced practice nursing and expansion of nursing from a job to a profession, which was key in the development of standards and credentialing. Every nurse is profoundly affected by the art and science that Peplau brought to nursing (Tomey, 2006).

Practicing the Science and the Art of Psychiatric Nursing

Susan L. Frost, Chyllia D. Fosbre, Elizabeth M. Varcarolis

ⓔ http://evolve.elsevier.com/Varcarolis/essentials

KEY TERMS AND CONCEPTS

5 A's, p. 3
attending, p. 6
caring, p. 6
clinical algorithms, p. 4
clinical/critical pathways, p. 4

clinical practice guidelines, p. 4
evidence-based practice (EBP), p. 3
nurse-patient partnership, p. 5
patient advocate, p. 7
psychiatric mental health nursing, p. 3

Quality and Safety Education for Nurses (QSEN), p. 3
recovery model, p. 5
trauma-informed care, p. 5

SELECTED CONCEPT: PATIENT ADVOCACY

Patient advocacy can occur on many levels including providing direct patient care, pleading for a course of action, and supporting change in institutional, global, and legislative arenas. The following are examples of patient advocacy activities:

- Providing informed consent, including refusal of treatment
- Respecting patient decisions, even those with whom we disagree
- Protecting against threats to well-being
- Being informed about best practices

Patients are afforded protection through providing privacy and confidentiality during participation in research, using standards and reviews, and taking action against questionable or impaired practice. Ethics is such an important concept that the American Nurses Association (ANA) designated 2015 "The Year of Ethics."

(ANA, 2015; Long, 2015)

SELECTED CONCEPT: EVIDENCE-BASED PRACTICE (EBP)

Evidence-based practice is a concept that will arise throughout this text and in the clinical setting. Rather than doing things "the way we have always done them," the standard of care is now an integrated approach. Three basic aspects (or prongs) of EBP are the following:

- Evidence gleaned in review of the literature
- Clinical knowledge of the nurse from training and experience
- The desires of patients and the values for their care

Case study examples of **Applying Evidence-Based Practice** will be highlighted in boxes throughout the clinical chapters in the textbook.

(ANA, 2015; Laibhen-Parkes, 2014; Melnyk & Fineout-Overholt, 2014)

OBJECTIVES

1. Recognize the evidence-based practice (EBP), recovery, and trauma-informed care models.
2. Identify the 5 A's used in the process of integrating EBP into the clinical setting.
3. Discuss at least three dilemmas nurses face when attempting to utilize EBP.
4. Identify four resources that nurses can use as guidelines for best-evidence interventions.
5. Defend why the concept of "caring" should be a basic ingredient to the practice of nursing and how it is expressed while giving patient care.
6. Discuss what is meant by being a patient advocate.

INTRODUCTION

Psychiatric mental health nursing is a specialized area of nursing practice focusing on the treatment of individuals with psychiatric and substance abuse disorders. Like all nursing specialties, psychiatric mental health nursing employs both the *science* and the *art* of nursing. Included in the *science* of nursing are the major concepts of evidence-based practice (EBP), the recovery model, trauma-informed care, and Quality and Safety Education for Nurses (QSEN), as well as incorporating theory from a range of nursing, psychological, and neurobiological research. Concepts related to the *art* of nursing include caring, attending, and advocacy (ANA, 2015). The *art* of nursing also includes the implementation of evidence, theories, and therapy models. These concepts will be discussed as this chapter progresses.

EVIDENCE-BASED PRACTICE

With the increased understanding of the biology of psychiatric illnesses beginning in the 1990s ("Decade of the Brain"), treatment approaches rapidly evolved into more scientifically grounded methods, now known as evidence-based practice. In psychiatry, the evidence-based focus extends to treatment approaches in which there is scientific evidence for psychological and sociological modalities, as well as evidence related to the neurobiology of psychiatric disorders and psychopharmacology. The emergence of evidence-based nursing in the United States originated from the EBP movement in the medical community in England and Canada during the 1980s and 1990s (Sur & Dahm, 2011). A noteworthy concept differentiating EBP in nursing from medicine is that the approach utilized in nursing incorporates more than clinical research. Evidence is not limited to what is found in research studies, but also incorporates the nurse's clinical knowledge and experience, as well as the patient's preferences and desires in the three-basic aspects mentioned above (Disch, 2014; Melnyk & Fineout-Overholt, 2014).

Basing nursing practice on a systematic approach to care is not new. McDonald (2001) states that Florence Nightingale (1820 to 1910), the founder of modern nursing, had a philosophy reflecting an evidence-based framework, advocating for the "best possible research, access to the best available governmental statistics and expertise" (p. 2). In 1860, Nightingale made a proposal that resulted in "the first model for systematic collection of hospital data using a uniform classification of diseases and operations," eventually forming the basis of the coding system used worldwide, the *International Statistical Classification of Diseases and Related Health Problems (ICD)* (Centers for Disease Control and Prevention, 2011). Mental health professionals in the United States have used the *Diagnostic and Statistical Manual of Mental Disorders (DSM)* classifications rather than the ICD system. This has recently changed with implementation of the *DSM-5* and *ICD-10* versions, where the mental health coding systems are now the same.

Hildegard Peplau (1909 to 1999), considered the mother of psychiatric nursing, had a passion for clarifying and developing the art and science of professional nursing practice and believed that a scientific approach was essential to the practice of psychiatric nursing (D'Antonio et al., 2014). Her contributions went far beyond what she brought to the field of psychiatric nursing. She introduced the concept of advanced nursing practice and promoted professional standards and regulation through credentialing among a multitude of other foundational contributions to nursing (D'Antonio et al., 2014).

It should be noted that psychiatry was one of the first medical specialties to extensively use randomized controlled trials. One of the founding principles of clinical psychology in the 1950s was that practice should be based on the results of experimental comparisons of treatment methods (Jackson, 2011). However, with limited scientific evidence for practice at that time, much of nursing care has been based on tradition, personal experience, unsystematic trial and error, and the earlier experiences of nurses and others in the health care profession (Jackson, 2011). During that time, there was an increase in the publication of research-related journals; the most relevant for nurses was the development of the *Evidence-Based Nursing* journal in 1998.

The University of Minnesota defines EBP as "the process by which the best available research evidence (from well-designed studies), clinical expertise, and patient preferences are used for making clinical decisions." Melnyk (Melnyk & Fineout-Overholt, 2014) states there is no magic bullet that provides a formula describing the weight of evidence that patient values and preferences and clinical expertise should take in making clinical decisions. Although EBP is equated with effective decision making, avoidance of habitual practice, and enhanced clinical performance, there may be a tendency to overlook practical knowledge that can provide useful information for individualized and effective practice.

Numerous definitions delineate the multistep process of integrating EBP into clinical practice. One that is simply stated and apt is referred to as the 5 A's (Shaw-Kokot & Philpotts, 2015):

1. *Ask* a question. Identify a problem or need for change for a specific patient or situation.
2. *Acquire* literature. Search the literature for scientific studies and articles that address the issue(s) of concern.
3. *Appraise* the literature. Evaluate and synthesize the research evidence regarding its validity, relevance, and applicability using criteria of scientific merit.
4. *Apply* the evidence. Choose interventions that are based on the best available evidence with the understanding of the patient's preference and needs.
5. *Assess* the performance. Evaluate the outcomes, using clearly defined criteria and reports, and document results.

Evaluating the evidence is done through a hierarchical rating system (Figure 1-1). Systematic reviews or meta-analysis of randomized controlled studies and evidence-based clinical practice guidelines provide the strongest evidence on which to base clinical practice. In a randomized controlled trial (RCT), patients are chosen at random (by chance) to receive one of the different clinical interventions or be in a control group with no treatment. One intervention would be the intervention under study, and another intervention might be the usual standard of care or placebo. The weakest level of evidence includes expert committee reports, opinions, clinical experience, or descriptive studies. Although scientific evidence is ranked hierarchically, it is important to note the value of all types of evidence in clinical decision making.

The first Surgeon General's report published on the topic of mental health was in 1999 (U.S. Department of Health and Human Services [USDHHS], 1999). This landmark document was based on an extensive review of the scientific literature and in consultation with mental health providers and consumers. The document concluded that there are numerous effective psychopharmacological and psychosocial treatments for most mental disorders. However, it raised some questions for psychiatric nurses, including the following:

- Are psychiatric nurses aware of the efficacy of the treatment and interventions they provide?
- Are they truly practicing evidence-based care?
- Is there documentation of the nature and outcomes of the care they provide?

There is no question that emphasis on EBP in medicine and mental health is expanding. However, this approach does not provide easy answers. For example, consider the following points:

- Who interprets "best evidence"?

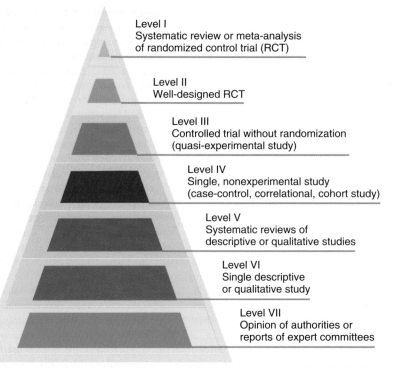

FIGURE 1-1 Hierarchy of evidence. (From Melnyk, B. M., & Fineout-Overholt, E. [2014]. *Evidence-based practice in nursing & healthcare: a guide to best practice*. [3rd ed.]. Philadelphia: Lippincott Williams & Wilkins; and from Newhouse, R. P., Dearholt, S. L., Poe, S. S., et al. [2007]. *Johns Hopkins nursing: evidence-based practice model and guidelines*. Indianapolis, Ind: Sigma Theta Tau International.)

- Not all nursing problems can be reduced to a clear issue, solvable by scientific experiments.
- Relatively little higher-level nursing research addressing psychiatric nursing intervention and practice has been available.
- Despite the expectation to use EBP, little education is provided in undergraduate programs or in the workplace to prepare nurses for this process.
- How do nurses who are practicing in complex environments of reduced staffing and budgetary constraints find time to research and evaluate the literature and make decisions on "best evidence"?

Resources for Clinical Practice

1. *Internet resources.* A number of websites provide mental health resources for information, treatment provisions, and the results of recent clinical studies. Some of the most extensive databases for psychiatric and medical resources include Cumulative Index to Nursing and Allied Health Literature (CINAHL), PubMed, and Cochrane reviews. There are self-tests for people to see if they may be experiencing symptoms of a specific disorder, such as depression, anxiety, or attention-deficit/hyperactivity disorder (ADHD). There are also resources for acquiring support and treatment. It is best to focus on sites that are maintained by professional societies, librarians, textbook publishers, or well-known organizations with a reputation for quality, evidence-based information.
2. *Clinical practice guidelines.* Clinical practice guidelines are systematically developed statements based on literature review that appraise and summarize the best evidence to guide clinicians in making informed decisions about specific health problems (Institute of Medicine, 2011). The use of practice guidelines can increase quality and consistency of care and facilitate outcome

research. Essentially, they (1) identify practice questions and explicitly identify all the decision options and outcomes; (2) identify the "best evidence" about prevention, diagnosis, prognosis, therapy, harm, and cost-effectiveness; and (3) provide decision points for deciding on a course of action. The American Psychiatric Association's (APA) *Clinical Practice Guidelines* and the National Quality Measures Clearinghouse offer such guidelines. The U.S. Department of Health and Human Services sponsors a National Guidelines Clearinghouse of evidence-based guidelines pertaining to a wide range of medical and mental health conditions (www.guidelines.gov).

3. *Clinical algorithms.* Clinical algorithms are step-by-step guidelines prepared in a flowchart or decision-tree format. Alternative diagnostic and treatment approaches are described based on decisional points using a large database relevant for the symptoms, diagnosis, or treatment modalities. Figure 1-2 depicts a clinical algorithm for the suspicion of suicide risk.

4. *Clinical/critical pathways.* Clinical/critical pathways are specific to the institution using them. These clinical pathways serve as a "map" for specified treatments and interventions to occur within specific time frames that have been shown to improve clinical outcomes. The interventions can include tests, health teaching, and medications. Each pathway lists the expected outcome using a measureable, time-specific format, and documentation is ongoing. Clinical pathways are one way EBP can be integrated into clinical care.

The Research-Practice Gap

Unfortunately, there is a wide gap between the best evidence treatments and their effective translation into practice. The need for continued research on how best to apply the findings of clinically relevant

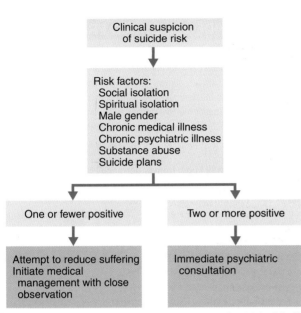

FIGURE 1-2 Clinical algorithm for the suspicion of suicide risk. (Modified from Goldman, L., & Ausiello, D. [2008]. *Cecil medicine*. [23rd ed.]. Philadelphia: Saunders.)

issues and their delivery into clinical practice has been the emphasis of the Institute of Medicine (2006):

> research that has identified the efficacy of specific treatments under rigorously controlled conditions has been accompanied by almost no research identifying how to make these same treatments effective when delivered in usual settings of care ... when administered by service providers without specialized education in the therapy (p. 350).

Effective research is reported in language that is understandable and free of statistical and research jargon, and appropriate dissemination of findings needs to reach nursing practitioners (Agency for Healthcare Research and Quality [AHRQ], 2012). Despite the complexities and concerns that demand to be addressed, evidence-based nursing is becoming a foundation for nursing practice. Eventually the use of scientific evidence-based practice will reduce the use of unwarranted nursing practices and alleviate the severity of nursing errors. Furthermore, the use of evidence-based practice optimizes the process of evaluation and facilitates the nurse's development and professional advancement (Jasmine, 2009).

To help the reader understand how best evidence is identified and applied to nursing interventions, this textbook contains a feature box titled **Applying Evidence-Based Practice.** It is hoped that this feature, presented in each of the clinical chapters, will underscore the importance of sound scientific inquiry and ignite the reader's interest in research.

Recovery Model

The mental health recovery model is more of a social model of disability than a medical model of disability. Therefore the focus shifts from one of illness and disease to an emphasis on rehabilitation and recovery (Caldwell et al., 2010). The recovery model originated from the 12-step program of Alcoholics Anonymous, and a grassroots advocacy initiative called the Consumer/Survivor/Ex-patient Movement during the 1980s and 1990s. It is now one of the leading models promoted by the Substance Abuse and Mental Health Services Administration (SAMHSA, 2014), a federal agency charged with improvement of mental health and substance abuse treatment. The concept of recovery

refers primarily to managing symptoms, reducing psychosocial disability, and improving role performance (SAMHSA, 2012, 2014). Holistic interventions such as encouraging supportive relationships are designed to promote recovery as evidenced by functioning in work, engagement in community/social life, and a reduction of symptoms (SAMHSA, 2014). Empowering patients to realize their full potential and independence within the limitations of their illness is the main goal of this model. Recovering from a mental illness is viewed as a personal journey of healing.

The focus of the recovery model has the following mandates (Caldwell et al., 2010, p. 43):
- Mental health care is to be consumer and family driven, with patients being partners in all aspects of care.
- Care must focus on increasing consumer success in coping with life's challenges and building resilience, not just managing symptoms.
- An individualized care plan is to be at the core of consumer-centered recovery.

In contrast to past hierarchical relationships in health care, the emphasis today is on the nurse-patient partnership, which is more in line with the recovery model (Stuart, 2011).

Trauma-Informed Care

A third model that is gaining momentum and legitimacy is trauma-informed care, a framework developed by the National Center for Trauma-Informed Care (NCTIC), a division of SAMHSA. Trauma-informed care recognizes that trauma is almost universally found in the histories of mental health patients and is a contributor to mental health issues, substance abuse, chronic health conditions, and contact with the criminal justice system. Trauma occurs in many forms, including physical, sexual, and emotional abuse; war; natural disasters; and other harmful experiences. Trauma-informed care provides guidelines for integrating an understanding of how trauma affects patients into clinical programming. A main concept of this approach is a change in paradigm from one that asks "What's wrong with you?" to one that asks "What has happened to you?" Key principles also include avoiding retraumatizing through restraints or coercive practices, an open collaborative relationship between patient and provider, empowerment, and cultural respect.

The American Nurses Association (2007), the Institute of Medicine (IOM, 2011, 2006), and QSEN (2014) all support patient-centered care as best practice. Nurses are increasingly expected to understand and synthesize best practice from the literature, care models and theories, neurobiology of psychiatric disorders and medications, and other professional domains into clinical practice.

Quality and Safety Education for Nurses (QSEN)

There is now a national initiative toward patient safety and quality, known as QSEN. The overall goal of QSEN is to prepare future nurses who will have the knowledge, skills, and attitudes (KSAs) necessary to continuously improve quality and safety of the health care systems in which they work (QSEN, 2014; Sullivan, 2010). QSEN defines KSAs in each of the following six standards:
- Patient-centered care
- Teamwork and collaboration
- Evidence-based practice
- Quality improvement
- Safety
- Informatics

These standards will be discussed in detail in Chapter 7. Relevant standards or KSAs will be referenced in the **Applying Evidence-Based Practice** boxes in the clinical chapters and woven throughout the text.

THE ART OF NURSING: DEVELOPING THE SKILLS FOR THE PRACTICE

Contemporary nursing relies on a scientific foundation and critical thinking. However, the art of nursing is equally important in comprehensive and holistic care. Even the best evidence-based guidelines may not encompass the entire complexity of an individual patient, disorder, or situation. As Williams and Garner (2002, p. 8) conclude, "Too great an emphasis on evidence-based medicine oversimplifies the complex and interpersonal nature of clinical care." The arts of intuition, interpersonal skills, therapeutic use of self, and cultural competence are indispensable for effective treatment.

Benner (2004) suggests that many of the attributes that fall under the "art of nursing" are invisible, intangible, rarely charted, and almost never suggested in a nursing care plan. Consequently, these attributes are often marginalized, undervalued, and demeaned. Three areas inherent in the "art" of nursing addressed here are (1) caring, (2) attending, and (3) patient advocacy.

Caring

Caring is the most natural and the most fundamental aspect of human existence (Smith et al., 2013). A survey by Schoenhofer and colleagues (1998) used a group process method to synthesize what was meant by caring to the participants. The following three themes emerged from the narratives:

1. Caring is evidenced by empathic understanding, actions, and patience on another's behalf.
2. Caring for another through actions, words, and being present leads to happiness and touches the heart.
3. Caring is giving of self while preserving the importance of self.

The caring nurse is first and foremost a competent nurse. Without knowledge and competence, the demonstration of compassion and caring alone is powerless to help those under our care. Without a base of knowledge and skills, care alone cannot eliminate another person's confusion, grief, or pain, but a response of care can transform fear, pain, and suffering into a tolerable, shared experience (Smith et al., 2013).

Dr. Jean Watson founded the Watson Caring Science Institute and has written more than 20 books on the concept of caring. Watson's Caring Theory has a spiritual and existential underpinning (Watson Caring Science Institute, 2015). The theory integrates *Ten Caritas* (loving principles) that encourage altruism, loving kindness toward self and others, faith and hope, honor, nurturing individual beliefs, helping and trusting relationships, accepting feelings while authentically listening, creative scientific problem-solving, teaching and learning using individual styles, physical and spiritual healing environment, and assisting with basic human needs and openness to mystery and miracles.

Comforting as a part of caring includes providing social, emotional, physical, and spiritual support for a patient consistent with holistic nursing care. The provision of comfort measures can even be lifesaving, and comfort measures are basic components to good care. Economic strain and nursing shortages are barriers to the practice of caring and comforting, because nurses are burdened with greater workloads and higher acuity patients. However, caring is both an attitude that one communicates (a way of being with a patient) and also a set of skills that can be learned and developed. Listening to patients takes time but with practice and experience, nurses can develop the ability to attend to emotional and spiritual needs and get to know their patients while completing an assessment or other tasks.

Attending

Attending refers to an *intensity of presence*, being there for and in tune with the patient. The experience of emotional or physical

APPLYING EVIDENCE-BASED PRACTICE (EBP)

Problem A 63-year-old female patient was discharged from a psychiatric hospital. She was homeless and not enrolled in insurance or outpatient mental health services. The message number in the electronic health record (EHR) was no longer valid, so follow-up appointments were not scheduled. A week after discharge, the patient's medication was stolen and she became suicidal and confused and called the crisis line at her community mental health clinic.

EBP Assessment

A. **What do you already know from experience?** Homeless patients have limited contact information and multiple health concerns.

B. **What does the literature say?** Some of the reasons cited for not attending follow-up appointments are illness, inadequate transportation, forgetting the appointment, and not feeling engaged with providers. Nurses can advocate for patients by addressing gaps in care.

C. **What does the patient want?** The patient wanted her medications and assistance with obtaining resources.

Plan The crisis team assisted the patient in obtaining medications, finding transportation to a shelter, and enrolling in outpatient mental health services. The nurse practitioner (NP) developed a demographic page in the EHR designed to capture complex contact information for homeless patients, such as where they sleep and eat meals on specific days.

QSEN **QSEN Prelicensure Knowledge, Skills, and Attitudes (KSAs) Addressed:**

Safety by minimizing the patient's risk through individual and system performance

Informatics by using technology to manage patient information and prevent error

                                  Susan L. Frost, Chyllia D. Fosbre, 2015

From Batscha, C., McDevitt, J., Weiden, P., et al. (2011). The effect of an inpatient transition intervention on attendance at the first appointment post-discharge from a psychiatric hospitalization. *Journal of the American Psychiatric Nurses Association, 17*(5), 330–337; Cronenwett, L., Sherwood, G., Barnsteiner, J., et al. (2007). Quality and safety education for nurses. *Nursing Outlook, 55*(3), 122–131; Lamb, V., & Joels, C. (2014). Improving access to health care for homeless people. *Nursing Standard, 29*(6), 45–51; and National Healthcare for the Homeless Council (HCH). (2014). *Health reform & homelessness: twelve key advocacy areas for the HCH community.* Retrieved from www.nhchc.org/wp-content/uploads/2011/10/2014-health-reform-policy-statement.pdf.

suffering can be isolating. When patients perceive that the nurse is there for them, a human connection is made and the patient's sense of isolation is minimized or eliminated (Dossey & Keegan, 2013). Being present requires entering the patient's experience. Attending behaviors include active listening skills such as body posture and eye contact, touching, or giving attentive physical care (Dossey & Keegan, 2013). It is through effective communication that we can fully understand another person's immediate experience, fears, perceptions, and concerns. Attending behaviors are learned and are inherent in a true therapeutic relationship. Chapter 9 discusses attending behaviors in more detail within the context of the nurse-patient relationship.

Patient Advocacy

A patient advocate is one who speaks up for another's cause, who helps others by defensive actions, especially when the other person lacks knowledge, skills, ability, or status to speak for himself/herself (Marcus, 2011). Lawyers are often viewed as advocates for their clients; however, in nursing, being a patient advocate is not a legal role but rather an ethical one. Ethics is an integral part of the foundation of nursing and you will undoubtedly discuss ethical concepts and dilemmas during your nursing education. The term *patient advocate* was first placed in the 1976 American Nurses Association (ANA) *Code of Ethics for Nurses, revision,* and remains essentially unchanged up to the present. It reads:

> *The nurse must be alert to and take appropriate action regarding any instances of incompetent, unethical, illegal, or impaired practices(s) by any member of the health team or the health care system itself, or any action on the part of others that places the rights or best interest of the patient in jeopardy (ANA, 2015, 3.5).*

It can take a great deal of courage to advocate for patients when we witness behaviors or actions of health care professionals that could have serious consequences.

Advocacy in nursing includes a commitment to patients' health, well-being, and safety across the life span and the alleviation of suffering and promotion of a peaceful, comfortable, and dignified death (ANA, 2015). Nurses advocate when they advise patients of their rights (including the right to refuse treatment), provide accurate and current information so patients can make informed decisions, and support those decisions (Walker et al., 2015). Advocating demonstrates respect and value for human life while saving lives or bringing comfort to those who are dying. Psychiatric mental health nurses also function as advocates when they engage in public speaking, write articles, and lobby congressional representatives to help improve and expand mental health care (ANA, 2007).

Throughout the text a special feature titled **Applying the Art** gives the reader a glimpse of a nurse-patient interaction and the nurse's thought processes, while attending to the patient's concerns.

KEY POINTS TO REMEMBER

- Nursing integrates both scientific knowledge and caring arts into a holistic practice.
- Evidence-based practice (EBP) is a process by which the best available research evidence, clinical expertise, and patient preferences are synthesized while making clinical decisions.
- The 5 A's process of integrating best evidence into clinical practice includes (1) asking, (2) acquiring, (3) appraising, (4) applying, and (5) assessing.
- Application of the recovery model assists people with psychiatric disabilities to effectively manage symptoms, reduce psychosocial disability, and find a meaningful life in a community of their choosing.
- Trauma-informed care recognizes that various traumas contribute to mental illness and substance abuse. Awareness of trauma can assist health care providers in giving appropriate care and avoiding retraumatization of patients.
- Some sources for obtaining research findings are (1) Internet resources, (2) clinical practice guidelines, (3) clinical algorithms, and (4) clinical/critical pathways.
- Three specific areas are inherent within the art of nursing: (1) caring, (2) attending, and (3) patient advocacy.

APPLYING CRITICAL JUDGMENT

1. A friend of yours has recently returned from military service. You are startled when you encounter him on the street in a disheveled state. He appears frightened, seems to be talking to himself, and jumps when a car backfires nearby. You are astounded because there is such a change in demeanor from the last time you saw him. When you approach him, he seems wary and guarded.
   - A. How would the contribution of evidence-based practice (EBP) be helpful to learn about your friend's symptoms of posttraumatic stress disorder?
   - B. What might be some specific needs that could be met under the recovery model?
   - C. What insight could the trauma-informed care model provide to what your friend is experiencing?
   - D. Discuss how nurses can incorporate EBP and care models in their practice.
2. A friend of yours says that he heard about a new practitioner in the area who is going to teach alcoholics how to safely drink in moderation. You state that from all you have read, and from what you know from your friends' experiences, that controlled drinking is not thought to be an acceptable practice. Your friend contends that the practitioner has stories and testimonials from people who are alcoholics and are able to drink in a controlled manner. You tell him that there is no strong evidence for this practice.
   - A. How would you, as a nurse, evaluate this claim? Explain the five steps you would take to find the strength of this claim.
   - B. Using Table 1-1, what would you say about the quality of the evidence given above?
   - C. If your friend was in recovery and thinking of trying this treatment, what would you say to him that would make a strong argument against such a decision?
3. You are a new nursing student and a friend of yours says, "What on earth is the 'art of nursing'? Isn't that some weird new-age stuff?"
   - A. Discuss three components that might be considered under the art of nursing.
   - B. Give your friend an example of how nurses demonstrate comfort or caring in the clinical area.
   - C. Explain why patients need to have nurses act as their advocate. Can you think of an example from your clinical experience?
4. Go to the Centre for Evidence-Based Mental Health at www.cebmh.com and review at least one available clinical trial.

CHAPTER REVIEW QUESTIONS

1. In which scenario is it most urgent for the nurse to act as a patient advocate?
   - a. An adult cries and experiences anxiety after a near-miss automobile accident on the way to work.
   - b. A homeless adult diagnosed with schizophrenia lives in a community expecting a category 5 hurricane.
   - c. A 14-year-old girl's grades decline because she consistently focuses on her appearance and social networking.
   - d. A parent allows the prescription to lapse for 1 day for their 8-year-old child's medication for attention-deficit/hyperactivity disorder.
2. The nurse interacts with a veteran of World War II. The veteran says, "Veterans of modern wars whine and complain all the time. Back when I was in service, you kept your feelings to yourself." Select the nurse's best response.
   - a. "American society in the 1940s expected World War II soldiers to be strong."

TABLE 1-1   Hierarchy of Evidence and Grading of Recommendations*

HIERARCHY OF EVIDENCE		GRADING OF RECOMMENDATIONS	
Level	Type of Evidence	Level	Type of Evidence
Ia	Evidence from systematic reviews or meta-analyses of randomized controlled trials	A	Based on hierarchy I evidence
Ib	Evidence from at least one randomized controlled trial		
IIa	Evidence from at least one controlled study without randomization	B	Based on hierarchy II evidence or extrapolated from hierarchy I evidence
IIb	Evidence from at least one other type of quasi-experimental study		
III	Evidence from nonexperimental descriptive studies, such as comparative studies, correlation studies, and case control studies	C	Based on hierarchy III evidence or extrapolated from hierarchy I or II evidence
IV	Evidence from expert committee reports or opinions and/or clinical experience of respected authorities	D	Directly based on hierarchy IV evidence or extrapolated from hierarchy I, II, or III evidence

*Each recommendation has been allocated a grading that directly reflects the hierarchy of evidence on which it has been based. Please note that the hierarchy of evidence and the recommendation gradings relate the strength of the literature, not the clinical importance.
From Hierarchy of evidence and grading of recommendations. (2004). *Thorax,59*(Suppl 1), i13–i14.

b. "World War II was fought in a traditional way but the enemy is more difficult to identify in today's wars."

c. "We now have a better understanding of how trauma affects people and the importance of research-based, compassionate care."

d. "Intermittent explosive devices (IEDs), which were not in use during World War II, produce traumatic brain injuries that must be treated."

3. A patient reports to a primary care provider about sleeplessness, constant fatigue, and sadness. In our current health care climate, what is the most likely treatment approach that will be offered to the patient?
   a. Group therapy
   b. Individual psychotherapy
   c. Complementary therapy
   d. Psychopharmacological treatment

4. The nurse prepares outcomes to the plan of care for an adult diagnosed with mental illness. Which strategy recognizes the current focus of treatment services for this population?
   a. The patient's diagnoses are confirmed using advanced neuroimaging techniques.
   b. The nurse confers with the treatment team to verify the patient's most significant disability.
   c. The nurse prioritizes the patient's problems in accordance with Maslow's hierarchy of needs.
   d. The patient and family participate actively in establishing priorities and selecting interventions.

5. Which scenario best demonstrates empathetic caring?
   a. A nurse provides comfort to a colleague after an error of medication administration.
   b. A nurse works a fourth extra shift in 1 week to maintain adequate unit staffing.
   c. A nurse identifies a violation of confidentiality and makes a report to an agency's privacy officer.
   d. A nurse conscientiously reads current literature to stay aware of new evidence-based practices.

REFERENCES

Agency for Healthcare Research and Quality. (2012). *Communication and dissemination strategies to facilitate the use of health and health care evidence.* Retrieved from http://effectivehealthcare.ahrq.gov/index.cfm/search-for-guides-reviews-and-reports/?productid=1208&pageaction=displayproduct.

American Nurses Association (ANA). (2007). *Psychiatric–mental health nursing: scope and standards of practice.* Silver Spring, Md: The Association.

American Nurses Association (ANA). (2015). Code of ethics for nurses with interpretive statements. Silver Spring, Md. Nursebooks.org. Retrieved from www.nursingworld.org/MainMenuCategories/EthicsStandards/Revision-of-Code-of-Ethics-Panel.

Benner, P. (2004). Relational ethics of comfort, touch, and solace endangered arts? *American Journal of Critical Care, 13,* 346–349.

Caldwell, B. A., Sclasani, M., Swarbrick, M., et al. (2010). Psychiatric nursing practice & the recovery model of care. *Journal of PSN, 48*(7), 42–48.

Centers for Disease Control and Prevention. (2011). *History of the statistical classification of diseases and causes of death.* Retrieved from www.cdc.gov/nchs/data/misc/classification_diseases2011.pdf.

D'Antonio, P., Beeber, L., Sills, G., et al. (2014). The future in the past: Hildegard Peplau and interpersonal relations in nursing. *Nursing Inquiry, 21*(4), 311–317.

Disch, J. (2014). Using evidence-based advocacy to improve the nation's health. *Nurse Leader, 12*(4), 2831.

Dossey, B. M., & Keegan, L. (2013). *Holistic nursing: a handbook for practice* (6th ed.). Burlington, Mass: Jones & Bartlett Learning.

Institute of Medicine (IOM). (2006). *Improving the quality of health care for mental and substance-use conditions.* Washington, DC: Institute of Medicine of the National Academies, National Academies Press.

Institute of Medicine (IOM). (2011). *Clinical practice guidelines we can trust.* Retrieved Sept 12, 2015, from http://iom.national academies.org/Reports/2011/Clinical-Practice-Guidelines-We-Can-Trust.aspx.

Jackson, M. (2011). *The Oxford handbook of the history of medicine.* New York: Oxford University Press.

Jasmine, T. (2009). Art, science, or both? Keeping the care in nursing. *Nursing Clinics of North America, 44,* 415–421.

Laibhen-Parkes, N. (2014). Evidence-based practice competence: a concept analysis. *International Journal of Nursing Knowledge, 25*(3), 173–182.

Long, B. (2015). What would Florence do? Nurses as patient advocates. *Nurse Leader, 13*(1), 37–39.

Marcus, K. (2011). The nurse as patient advocate: is there a conflict of interest? In P. S. Cowen & S. Moorehead (Eds.), *Current issues in nursing* (8th ed.) (pp. 609–674). St. Louis: Mosby/Elsevier.

McDonald, L. (2001). Florence Nightingale and the early origins of evidence-based nursing. *Evidence-Based Nursing, 4,* 68–69.

Melnyk, B. M., & Fineout-Overholt, E. (2014). *Evidence-based practice in nursing and healthcare: a guide to best practice* (3rd ed.). Philadelphia: Lippincott Williams & Wilkins.

Quality and Safety Education for Nurses (QSEN). (2014). *Competencies*. Retrieved from http://qsen.org/competencies/.

Schoenhofer, S., Bingham, V., & Hutchins, G. (1998). Giving of oneself on another's behalf: the phenomenology of everyday caring. *International Journal of Human Caring, 2*(2), 23–39.

Shaw-Kokot, J., & Philpotts, L. (2015). Using evidence based nursing in practice. Retrieved from http://guides.lib.unc.edu/ebn_practice.

Smith, M. C., Turkel, M. C., & Wolf, Z. R. (2013). *Caring in nursing classics: an essential resource.* New York: Springer Publishing Co.

Stuart, G. W. (2011). Psychiatric mental health nursing: recent changes in current issues. In P. S. Cowen & S. Moorehead (Eds.), *Current issues in nursing.* St. Louis: Mosby/Elsevier.

Substance Abuse and Mental Health Services Administration (SAMHSA). (2012). *SAMHSA's working definition of recovery: Ten guiding principles of recovery.* Retrieved from http://store.samhsa.gov/product/SAMHSA-s-Working-Definition-of-Recovery/PEP12-RECDEF.

Substance Abuse and Mental Health Services Administration (SAMHSA). (2014). *Recovery and recovery support.* Retrieved Sept 12, 2015, from www.samhsa.gov/recovery.

Sullivan, D. T. (2010). Connecting nursing education and practice: A focus on shared goals for quality and safety. *Creative Nursing, 16,* 37–43.

Sur, R. L., & Dahm, P. (2011). History of evidence-based practice. *Indian Journal of Urology, 27*(4), 487–489.

U.S. Department of Health and Human Services (USDHHS). (1999). *Mental health: a report from the surgeon general.* Rockville, Md: National Institute of Mental Health.

Walker, D. K., Barton-Burke, M., Saria, M. G., et al. (2015). Everyday advocates: nursing advocacy is a full-time job. *American Journal of Nursing, 115*(8), 66–70.

Watson Caring Science Institute (WCSI). (2015). *Global translations-10 Caritas processes [website].* Retrieved from www.watsoncaringscience.org.

Williams, D. D. R., & Garner, J. (2002). The case against "the evidence": a different perspective on evidence-based medicine. *British Journal of Psychiatry, 180,* 8–12.

Mental Health and Mental Illness

Susan L. Frost, Chyllia D. Fosbre, Elizabeth M. Varcarolis

ⓔ http://evolve.elsevier.com/Varcarolis/essentials

KEY TERMS AND CONCEPTS

biologically based mental illness, p. 13

culture-bound syndromes (or culture-related syndromes), p. 15

Diagnostic and Statistical Manual of Mental Disorders (DSM-5), p. 11

epidemiology, p. 12

mental disorders, p. 12

mental health, p. 10

mental illness, p. 10

myths and misconceptions, p. 12

prevalence rate, p. 12

psychiatry's definition of mental health, p. 12

psychobiological disorder, p. 13

resiliency, p. 12

stigma/stigmatizing, p. 16

SELECTED CONCEPT: STIGMA AND MENTAL HEALTH

False beliefs, myths, and lack of understanding of mental illness can cause tremendous pain and negative consequences for individuals or groups who develop mental health problems. Stigma may be obvious and direct or expressed in more subtle behaviors.

Some of the harmful effects of stigma toward those with mental health issues include:

- Discrimination at work or school
- Difficulty finding housing
- Bullying, physical violence, or harassment
- Health insurance that does not adequately cover a person's mental health disorder
- Instilling self-doubt regarding ability to succeed and feeling that nothing can help
- Isolation from friends, family, and colleagues

(Mayo, 2014 Stigma: www.stepuponsecond.org)

OBJECTIVES

1. Summarize factors that can affect the mental health of an individual and explain how they influence the conduction of a holistic nursing assessment.
2. Discuss some dynamic factors (including social climate, politics, cultural beliefs, myths, and biases) that make it difficult to formulate a clear-cut definition of mental health.
3. Identify the processes leading to stigmatization of an individual or group, and discuss some of the effects stigma can have on medical and psychological well-being.
4. Compare and contrast a *DSM-5* diagnosis with a nursing diagnosis.
5. Give examples of how cultural influences and norms can affect making an accurate *DSM-5* diagnosis.

INTRODUCTION

Mental health and mental illness are not specific entities but rather they exist on a continuum. The mental health continuum is dynamic and shifting, ranging from mild to moderate to severe (Figure 2-1). The diagnosis is an important factor; for example, schizophrenia is generally considered more impairing than anxiety. However, this is not always the case. An individual with schizophrenia with a good support system and treatment plan may be functioning at a higher level than someone with generalized anxiety who is in an abusive relationship with no mental health treatment. In addition, the same individual may function at different levels from week to week or year to year. Many biological and environmental factors influence mental health.

The groundbreaking *Report of the Surgeon General* (USDHHS, 1999) defines mental health as successful performance of mental functions, resulting in the ability to engage in productive activities, enjoy fulfilling relationships, adapt to change, and cope with adversity. Mental health is the foundation of thinking, communication skills, learning, emotional growth, resilience, and self-esteem throughout the life span (USDHHS, 1999). It is a state of well-being in which individuals are able to realize their abilities as well as contribute to their community within the context of life stressors (WHO, 2010).

According to the National Alliance on Mental Illness (NAMI, 2011) mental illnesses are medical conditions (dysfunctions of the brain and neurotransmitters) that affect a person's thinking, feeling, mood, ability to relate to others, and daily functioning. Basically, mental illness can be seen as the result of flawed biological, psychological, or social processes, which will be expanded as the text unfolds. Fortunately mental illnesses are treatable, and individuals can experience symptom relief, and complete cure in some cases, with treatment and support (NAMI, 2011).

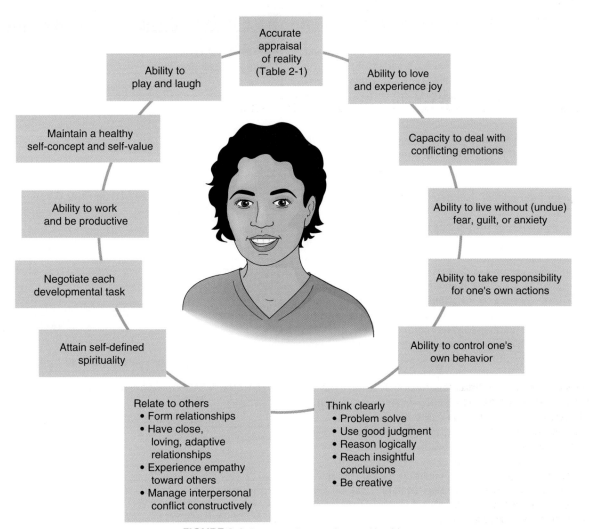

FIGURE 2-1 Some attributes of mental health.

In this chapter, the reader will be introduced to the concepts of mental health and mental illness, the idea of mental disorders as medical conditions, and the categorization of mental illness using the *DSM-5* and cultural beliefs to determine the factors that constitute normal and abnormal behavior.

THE *DIAGNOSTIC AND STATISTICAL MANUAL OF MENTAL DISORDERS, DSM-5*

The *Diagnostic and Statistical Manual of Mental Disorders, edition 5 (DSM-5)* is the current official guidebook for categorizing and diagnosing psychiatric mental health disorders in the United States (American Psychiatric Association [APA], 2013). *The DSM-5 provides clinicians, researchers, regulatory agencies, health insurance companies, pharmacological companies, and policy makers with a standard language and criteria for the classification of mental disorders.* The DSM-5 is used by psychiatrists, psychiatric nurse practitioners, and other clinicians as a guide for assessing, diagnosing, and planning care. The DSM-5 lists specific diagnostic criteria for each mental disorder, which were developed using research and clinical observation. This chapter also addresses the importance of considering an individual's cultural background in making a valid diagnosis and treatment plan. The DSM-5 is the most recent edition, being published in 2013 after 10 years of professional discussion and debate, and some notable changes were made in this edition. One of these changes was the deletion of the five-axis

system of diagnosis utilized in prior versions of the *DSM*. The intent of the axis system was to provide a global picture of an individual's functioning. The information previously organized in the axes will still be addressed in an unstructured, narrative form by the clinician. Another significant change is that the coding system now mirrors *ICD-10* codes. As of 2015, the *DSM-IV-TR* is still in use as clinicians and institutions transition into full use of the *DSM-5*, so the *DSM-IV-TR* axis system will be discussed here.

Axis I lists the psychiatric diagnosis or diagnoses (for example, major depressive disorder and alcohol dependence) that are generally considered biological in nature. All psychiatric disorders are listed on Axis I with the exception of personality disorders and mental retardation, which are listed on Axis II.

Axis II lists personality disorders and mental retardation to ensure long-standing issues that may co-occur with the Axis I disorders are considered, such as borderline personality disorder.

Axis III lists any medical conditions the patient may have, which may or may not influence the mental health diagnosis (for example, coronary artery disease and hypothyroidism).

Axis IV lists psychosocial stressors in a brief narrative form, such as homeless, going through divorce, or job loss.

Axis V, the Global Assessment of Functioning (GAF) score, is noted on this axis. The GAF is rated on a scale of 1 to 100 and indicates the patient's level of functioning. The higher the score, the higher the level of functioning.

CONCEPTS OF MENTAL HEALTH AND ILLNESS

The World Health Organization (WHO, 2010) declared that 4 of the 10 leading causes of disability in the United States and other developed countries are mental health disorders (NAMI, 2011). Unfortunately, our understanding of mental illness is plagued by various myths and misconceptions. One myth is that to be mentally ill is to be different and odd. Another misconception is that to be mentally healthy, a person must be logical and rational at all times. All of us dream "irrational" dreams at night, and "irrational" emotions are universal human experiences and essential to a fulfilling life. There is no obvious and consistent line between mental illness and mental health, and as humans we are far more similar than different despite any diagnosis or label.

Psychiatry's definition of mental health evolves over time and reflects changes in cultural norms, society's expectations and values, professional biases, individual differences, and even the political climate of the time. For example, criticisms have arisen from various groups who believe that they have been stereotyped in the psychiatric community with emphasis on the group's psychopathology rather than on health attributes. At points in history, women who worked outside of the home and homosexuals were considered to be mentally ill, while in today's society these groups are considered completely normal. You will find many attributes of mental health in your patients with mental illness. It is important to develop and encourage these strengths. Additionally, persons who are "normal" may also experience dysfunction during their lives. We are all different and reflect different cultural influences, even within the same culture. We grow at different rates intellectually, emotionally, and spiritually. Understandably, then, there can be no one definition of mental health that fits all. The continuum is depicted in Table 2-1.

An important characteristic of mental health is the concept of resiliency. Resiliency is the ability to recover from or adjust successfully to trauma or change (Ovans, 2015). Research has demonstrated that this ability to recover from painful experiences is not an unusual quality, but is a trait possessed by many people and can be developed in almost everyone. Disasters occur all too frequently, such as terrorist attacks, natural disasters, or senseless shootings. Being resilient does not mean that people are unaffected by stressors. Rather than becoming paralyzed by the negative emotions, resilient people recognize the feelings, readily deal with them, and learn from the experience. A successful transition through a crisis builds resiliency for the next difficult trial.

EPIDEMIOLOGY AND PREVALENCE OF MENTAL DISORDERS

Epidemiology studies the distribution (numbers of cases) of disorders in human populations. Epidemiologists can use this quantitative information to identify high-risk groups and factors, as well as learn about the etiology of mental disorders. In the field of *clinical* epidemiology, studies are conducted using groups of individuals with particular mental illnesses, symptoms, or treatments. Results of these studies are included in the *DSM-5* to help clinicians understand the frequency and factors associated with a particular diagnosis. For example, epidemiological studies have demonstrated that depression is a significant risk factor for death in patients with cardiovascular disease and breast cancer.

The prevalence rate is the proportion of a population with a mental disorder at a given time. About half of Americans will meet the criteria for a *DSM-5* disorder sometime in their lives, with the first onset in childhood or adolescence (National Institute of Mental Health, 2012).

TABLE 2-1 Continuum of Mental Health and Mental Illness

Ability to Function ⟷ Disability/Dysfunction

HAPPINESS	
Finds life enjoyable	Loss of interest or pleasure
Optimistic about needs being met	Discouraged or hopeless mood

CONTROL OVER BEHAVIOR	
Ability to recognize cues and act appropriately	Aggressive or violent behaviors

APPRAISAL OF REALITY	
Sees environment accurately	Inaccurate perceptions of environment
Understands consequences	Hallucinations or delusions

EFFECTIVENESS IN WORK	
Performs within abilities	Deterioration in work performance
Recovery from minor failures	Inability to maintain steady employment

HEALTHY SELF-CONCEPT	
Reasonable self-confidence	Lacks self-confidence
Resourcefulness	Inability to function independently

SATISFYING RELATIONSHIPS	
Stable, strong relationships	Unstable or intense relationships
Variety of social supports	Lack of support

EFFECTIVE COPING STRATEGIES	
Ability to problem solve and cope in ways that are not harmful (deep breathing, meditation)	Poor coping that creates further dysfunction (substance abuse, self-harm)

Modified from Redl, F., & Wattenberg, W. (1959). *Mental hygiene in teaching* (pp. 198–201). New York: Harcourt, Brace & World; Pierre, J. M. (2012). Mental illness and mental health: is the glass half empty or half full? *Canadian Journal of Psychiatry, 57*(11), 651–658; and Winzer R, Lindblad F, Sorjonen K, et al. (2014). Positive versus negative mental health in emerging adulthood: a national cross-sectional survey. *BioMed Central Public Health, (14)*, 1238.

Many individuals have more than one mental disorder at a time, known as dual diagnoses or co-occurring disorders.

Table 2-2 shows the epidemiology and prevalence rates of selected psychiatric disorders. Supported by the National Institute of Mental Health (NIMH), the study of epidemiology in mental health has progressed over the past 2 decades from simply counting the number of cases to delineating and understanding comorbidities, disease burden, and effective treatment. Kessler and colleagues (2007) found a lifetime history of a mental disorder in 46.4% of their sample, with half of all cases reporting onset by age 14. Nearly 60% of those diagnosed with a disorder in the previous 12 months were rated as "serious" rather than "moderate" or "mild," and reported a mean of 88.3 days when they were unable to function in their daily routines due to mental illness or substance abuse symptoms. "Serious" ratings were most common in patients with bipolar and other mood disorders, obsessive-compulsive disorder, and drug dependence, with almost half meeting criteria for two or more disorders.

Over a 12-month period, 60% of those with a mental illness received no treatment (American Psychological Association, 2015). Delay to first treatment ranged from 6 to 23 years. Patients are more likely to receive help from a general medical professional or spiritual

TABLE 2-2 Prevalence and Epidemiology of Psychiatric Disorders in the United States

Disorder	Prevalence over 12 Months (%)	Estimated Number of People Affected by Disorder in the United States	Epidemiology
Schizophrenia	1.1	3.5 million	Affects men and women equally; appears earlier in men
Any affective (mood) disorder; includes major depression, dysthymic disorder, and bipolar disorder	9.5	30.0 million	Women affected at twice the rate as men; often co-occurs with anxiety and substance abuse
Major depressive disorder	6.7	21.1 million	Leading cause of disability in the United States; nearly twice as many women
Bipolar affective disorder	2.6	8.2 million	Affects men and women equally
Anxiety disorders; includes panic disorder, obsessive-compulsive disorder, posttraumatic stress disorder (PTSD), generalized anxiety disorder, and phobias	18.1	57.0 million	Frequently co-occurs with depressive disorders, eating disorders, and/or substance abuse
Panic disorder	2.7	8.5 million	Typically develops in adolescence or early adulthood; about one in three people develops agoraphobia
Obsessive-compulsive disorder	1.0	3.2 million	First symptoms begin in childhood or adolescence
PTSD	3.5	11.0 million	Can develop immediately or be delayed onset; approximately 30% of Vietnam veterans experienced PTSD; common after 9/11/01 terrorist attacks
Generalized anxiety disorder	3.1	9.8 million	Risk is highest between childhood and middle age
Social phobia	6.8	21.4 million	Typically begins in childhood or adolescence
Agoraphobia	0.8	2.5 million	
Specific phobia	8.7	27.4 million	
Any substance abuse	9.4	24.6 million	
Alcohol dependence	6.3	16.5 million	
Serious thoughts of suicide	3.8	8.7 million	

National Institute of Mental Health. (2012). *The numbers count: mental disorder in America.* Retrieved from www.namigc.org/documents/numberscount.pdf; Substance Abuse and Mental Health Services Administration. (2014). *Results from the 2013 National Survey on Drug Use and Health: Summary of National Findings, NSDUH Series H-48, HHS Publication No. (SMA) 14-4863.* Retrieved May 30, 2015, from www.samhsa.gov/data/sites/default/files/NSDUHresultsPDFWHTML2013/Web/NSDUHresults2013.pdf; Substance Abuse and Mental Health Services Administration. (2012). *Results from the 2010 National Survey on Drug Use and Health: Mental Health Findings, NSDUH Series H-42, HHS Publication No. (SMA) 11-4667.* Retrieved May 5, 2015, from www.samhsa.gov/data/sites/default/files/NSDUHmhfr2010/NSDUHmhfr2010.pdf.

advisor than a psychiatrist because of already established relationships, and a shortage of psychiatric professionals, although the quality of treatment provided by psychiatric professionals is rated much higher. This illustrates that, as nurses, you will encounter psychiatric components in your career regardless of the specialty area or clinical setting.

MENTAL ILLNESS POLICY AND PARITY

In 1996 the Mental Health Parity Act was passed by Congress, and a series of legislation and commissions supporting parity followed over the next decade. This legislation required insurers to offer mental health benefits at the same level provided for medical coverage. In 2000 the Government Accounting Office found that although 86% of health plans complied with the 1996 law, they also imposed limits on mental health coverage. This has since improved with the implementation of the Affordable Care Act (ACA), which banned annual dollar limits on medical and mental health care and eliminated the preexisting conditions that had been in effect by insurance companies for this time (NMHA, 2004; USDHHS, 2015).

One method many states use to continue to limit coverage is by making a distinction of whether the problem is a biologically based mental illness, also called a psychobiological disorder (caused by

neurotransmitter dysfunction, abnormal brain structure, or genetic factors). These biologically influenced illnesses include the following:

- Schizophrenia
- Bipolar disorder
- Major depression
- Obsessive-compulsive and panic disorders
- Posttraumatic stress disorder
- Autism
- Anorexia nervosa
- Attention-deficit/hyperactivity disorder

Many of the most prevalent and disabling mental disorders have been found to have strong biological influences; therefore we can look at these disorders as "diseases." However, this interpretation overlooks many other influences that affect the severity and progress of a mental illness and can affect a "normal" person's mental status as well. Some of these factors include support systems, family influences, developmental events, cultural beliefs and values, health practices, and negative influences impinging on an individual's life (Figure 2-2).

The 1999 USDHHS report titled *Mental Health: A Report of the Surgeon General* stated the following:

- Mental health is fundamental to health.
- Mental disorders are real health conditions that have an immense impact on individuals and families.

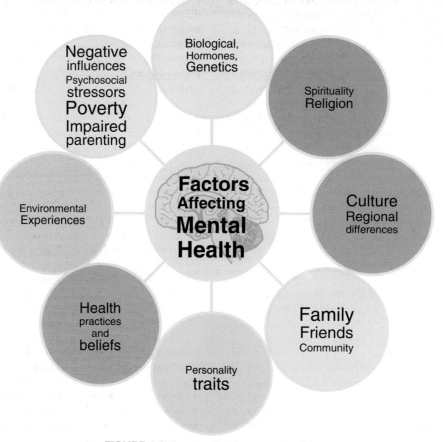

FIGURE 2-2 Factors affecting mental health.

- The efficacy of mental health treatment is well documented.
- A range of treatments exists for most mental disorders.

The *DSM-5* cautions that the emphasis on the term *mental disorder* implies a distinction between "mental" disorder and "physical" disorder, which is an outdated concept, and stresses mind-body dualism: "There is much 'physical' in 'mental' disorders and much 'mental' in 'physical' disorders" (American Psychiatric Association, 2013).

MEDICAL DIAGNOSIS AND NURSING DIAGNOSIS IN MENTAL ILLNESS

To perform their professional responsibilities, clinicians and researchers need clear and accurate guidelines for identifying and categorizing mental illness. Such guidelines help clinicians plan and evaluate treatment for their patients. A necessary element for categorization includes agreement regarding which behaviors constitute a mental illness.

Medical Diagnoses and the *DSM-5*

In the *DSM-5* the mental disorders are conceptualized as clinically significant behavioral or psychological syndromes or patterns that occur in an individual and that are associated with **distress** (a painful symptom), with **disability** (impairment in one or more important areas of functioning), or with a significantly increased risk of suffering death, pain, disability, or an important loss of freedom. This syndrome or pattern must not be merely an expected and culturally sanctioned response to a particular event, such as the death of a loved one, but rather a manifestation of a behavioral, psychological, or biological dysfunction in the individual as identified within the individual's cultural boundaries. Deviant behavior (political, religious, or sexual) and conflicts between the individual and society are not considered mental disorders according to the *DSM-5* unless the deviance or conflict is a symptom of a dysfunction in the individual.

It is important to stress that the *DSM-5* classifies disorders that people have, not the person. For this reason, the text of the *DSM-5* avoids the use of expressions such as "a schizophrenic" or "an alcoholic" and instead uses the more accurate terms "an individual with schizophrenia" or "an individual with alcohol dependence." The *DSM* system began with the *DSM-I* in 1952 and included descriptions of 106 disorders called "reactions." The publication has progressed through extensive collaboration among experts to arrive at the current version, the *DSM-5* published in 2013. The revision process from the *DSM-IV* and *DSM-5* took a decade and brought together hundreds of international scientists during conferences supported by the National Institutes of Health (NIH). This current version delineates almost 300 diagnoses with well-organized listings of diagnostic criteria and is used for clinical assessment, teaching, and research purposes.

The *DSM-5* in Culturally Diverse Populations

Special efforts have been made in the *DSM-5* to incorporate an awareness that the manual is used in culturally diverse populations in the United States and internationally. Most anthropologists agree that culture includes traditions of thought, behavior, knowledge, and practices that are socially acquired, shared, and passed on to new generations (APA, 2013; Hays, 2008). The concept of culture is most often considered with racial or ethnic minority groups. However, the concept of culture also includes sexual orientation, age groups, physical abilities or disabilities, gender, religion, or socioeconomic status. Almost any group of persons with some type of shared belief can be included in the definition of culture (Hays, 2008). Therefore clinicians are urged to consider these varying influences when evaluating individuals. Assessment can be especially challenging when a clinician from one ethnic/cultural or minority group evaluates an individual from a different group. The *DSM-5* and prior versions are strongly biased toward a Western view of what is acceptable behavior. Some criteria considered as mental illness could, in fact, be considered normal in another culture. One way the *DSM-5* attempts to correct for this is through inclusion of the Cultural Formulation Interview (CFI). The CFI assesses the client's cultural perception of distress, social supports such as family and religion, and relationship factors between the patient and provider including language and discrimination experiences in the societal majority. The *DSM-5* also provides a brief glossary of cultural concepts of distress, which includes culture-bound symptoms such as *ataque de nervios* ("attack of the nerves") or *sustos* ("fright") in Latino cultures and *shenjing shuairuo* ("weakness of the nervous system") in Mandarin Chinese culture.

Nursing Diagnoses and NANDA International

Psychiatric mental health nursing includes the diagnosis and treatment of human responses to actual or potential mental health problems. NANDA International (NANDA-I) describes a nursing diagnosis as a clinical judgment about individual, family, or community responses to actual or potential health problems and life processes. Therefore the *DSM-5* is used to diagnose a psychiatric disorder, whereas a well-defined nursing diagnosis provides the framework for identifying appropriate nursing interventions for dealing with the phenomena a patient with a mental health disorder is experiencing (e.g., hallucinations, self-esteem issues, impaired ability to function). See Chapter 7 for more on the formulation of nursing diagnoses in psychiatric nursing.

Appendix B lists NANDA-I (2015-2017) approved nursing diagnoses. The individual clinical chapters offer suggestions for potential nursing diagnoses for the behaviors and phenomena often encountered in association with specific disorders.

INTRODUCTION TO CULTURE AND MENTAL ILLNESS

As previously discussed, the *DSM-5* includes information related to culture in the discussion of each individual disorder, in the *Glossary of Cultural Concepts of Distress,* and by providing the Cultural Formulation Interview (CFI).

Health care providers must consider the norms and influence of culture in determining the mental health or mental illness of the individual. Throughout history, people have interpreted health or sickness according to their own cultural views. People in the Middle Ages, for example, regarded bizarre behavior as a sign that the person was possessed by a demon. To exorcise the demon, priests resorted to prescribed religious rituals. During the 1880s, when the "germ theory" of illness was popular, physicians interpreted bizarre behavior as stemming from attacks by biological agents. In Western culture before "the decade of the brain" and increased biological understanding, mental illness was perceived as a lack in character or spiritual flaw.

Cultures differ not only in the way they view mental illness but also in the expression of the symptoms. For example, the content of delusions, hallucinations, obsessional thoughts, and phobias often reflect what is important in the person's culture.

A number of culture-bound syndromes (or culture-related syndromes) appear only in particular cultures and do not appear globally in all societies or parts of the world. For example, one form of mental illness recognized in parts of Southeast Asia is ***running amok,*** in which someone (usually a male) runs around engaging in furious, almost indiscriminate violent behavior. ***Pibloktoq*** is an uncontrollable desire to tear off one's clothing and expose oneself to severe winter weather; it is a recognized form of psychological disorder in parts of Greenland, Alaska, and the Arctic regions of Canada. In our own society, we recognize ***anorexia nervosa*** as a psychobiological disorder that entails voluntary starvation. This disorder is well known in Europe, North America, and Australia, but unheard of in many other societies.

What is to be made of the fact that certain disorders occur in some cultures but are absent in others? One interpretation is that the conditions necessary for causing a particular disorder occur in some places but are absent in others. Another interpretation is that people learn certain kinds of abnormal behavior by imitation. However, the fact that some disorders may be culturally determined does not prove that all mental illnesses are so determined. The best evidence suggests that schizophrenia and bipolar affective disorders are found throughout the world. The symptom patterns of schizophrenia have been observed among indigenous Greenlanders and West African villagers, as well as in our own Western culture. Schizophrenia could be interpreted as possession or even a positive spiritual connection rather than a physical disorder in non-Western societies.

Each culture has identified preferred psychiatric practitioners, or healers, and therapeutic methods. In Western cultures these are often academically trained clinicians such as psychiatric nurse practitioners and therapists. One example would be *curanderos* (male healers) or *curanderas* (female healers) found in Latin cultures. These healers are sought for treatment of psychological conditions such as *susto* (fright) and *mal de ojo* (evil eye), and they incorporate a mixture of Catholicism, ancient Mayan and Aztec beliefs, and herbology (Hays, 2008).

A traditional helping strategy used in American mainstream therapies, especially with children, is that of storytelling. It is also one that is common to many indigenous tribal cultures. The therapist uses a metaphor in the form of a story that offers a social message, but does not directly give advice or tell the person what to do. The listeners are then left to draw their own conclusions and make changes if they are ready to do so (Swinomish Tribal Community, 1991).

Western-style psychotherapy would be considered the treatment of last resort in many cultures because it is unavailable, shame is attached to seeking help for mental health concerns, or there are more effective or preferred treatments in their own culture (Hays, 2008; Yeh et al., 2006). The most effective psychiatric professionals will be eclectic in their knowledge and skill-set, have experience working with different cultures, and be flexible in their approach (Hays, 2008).

PSYCHIATRY AND SPIRITUALITY/RELIGION

An important part of any culture is their religious or spiritual beliefs. Historically, Western psychiatry tended to respect the medical approach while largely ignoring the importance that religion or spirituality played in an individual's mental health. The profession of nursing has traditionally held a more holistic focus, which included recognizing religious and/or spiritual needs of patients. Nursing leaders have contributed significantly to the research body surrounding this concept. In more recent years, psychiatry has acknowledged and integrated the importance of religious and spiritual beliefs/staff in the philosophy of health and healing.

Spirituality can include but is not limited to religion. Spirituality can be defined as a belief in a higher power, connection to the universe or universal energy, feeling "one" with nature, or calling on ancestors for wisdom; and can include practices such as meditation, prayer, and helping others. Spirituality "provides an essential core, enriching experience, and a reason to live for many people" (Favazza, 2009, p. 2633). There are many ways to achieve a spiritual connection that must be considered during assessment and diagnosis. For example, among certain cultural groups, hearing or seeing a deceased relative during bereavement is common and accepted, yet may be misdiagnosed as a psychotic disorder by an unknowing clinician. These types of cultural misunderstandings have contributed to the distrust minority or immigrant groups can hold toward psychiatric professionals.

Altered states of consciousness such as those achieved through mysticism, meditation, and mindfulness can be spiritually enriching and bring peace and serenity into people's lives, but should not be confused with dissociative states caused through trauma. Variations of meditation include Dhyana, concentrated meditation passed down from Buddha; Zen Buddhism, a Japanese meditation guided by a spiritual master; and transcendental meditation, a Hindu process and mindfulness meditation derived from Buddhist practice. Meditation has many health benefits, is a valuable tool for dealing with chronic pain and stress, and is a component of dialectic behavioral therapy (DBT), stress reduction programs, and some forms of cognitive therapy (Favazza, 2009).

Prayer is a widely used religious/spiritual ritual. Individuals pray for comfort, to make requests, and to offer praise; and may incorporate singing, dancing, jumping, reciting prescribed words, and praying at certain locations or times. Prayer represents a way to connect with God or a supreme spiritual being or natural energy and to find support and meaning in life (Favazza, 2009).

Stigma

Closely related to culture and spirituality is the concept of stigma. *Stigma* has been acknowledged as a major barrier to mental health treatment and recovery (Pinto-Foltz et al., 2009). Stigma is defined as a collection of negative attitudes, beliefs, and thoughts that influence public perception of the mentally ill. Stigma contributes to fear, rejection, and discrimination against the mentally ill that taint and discount the individual. Stereotyping, labeling, and separating can occur on an individual or institutional level, resulting in an imbalance of power. Stigmatizing attitudes toward the mentally ill can have harmful effects on an individual and family and result in social isolation and reduced opportunities. For example, stigmatizing interferes with the person's ability to establish and maintain friendships, employment, and housing. It also impacts the person's ability to obtain psychological and general medical treatment, known as health care disparity (Sadow & Ryder, 2008). Stigmatizing results in feelings of shame and a negative sense of self, which can directly impact recovery (NAMI, 2011).

An example of the cultural influence of stigmatizing in psychiatry is the inclusion of homosexuality as a disorder in earlier versions of the *DSM*. Although research consistently failed to demonstrate that people with a homosexual orientation were any more maladjusted than heterosexuals, change occurred in the medical community only through the efforts of gay rights' activists. Stigma and bias also affect minority groups, the elderly, children, and women.

Biases are often reflected in our organizational structures and political systems. Awareness of the dangers inherent in stereotyping and stigmatizing attitudes has enormous implications for nursing practice, especially in the field of mental health. It is important to remember that a patient is first and foremost a human being, and not the patient's diagnosis. Although diagnoses are utilized to structure treatment and for billing purposes, labeling should be avoided whenever possible.

APPLYING EVIDENCE-BASED PRACTICE (EBP)

Problem An elementary school child is having difficulty focusing in class and turning in homework and is disruptive. The child was evaluated and diagnosed with ADHD. The parents are refusing to have the child treated because they do not want the child to "be labeled or on medications that will cause him to be addicted."

EBP Assessment

A. **What do you already know from experience?** Parents can be reluctant to admit problems with their children because of embarrassment, fear, and lack of knowledge. Errors can occur both in overmedicating and in undermedicating patients. When needed, medications can make a remarkable difference.

B. **What does the literature say?** Stigma and discrimination against people with mental illness are major barriers to success in relationships, treatment, and employment. Patients often avoid treatment as a result of stigma. Health care providers are not immune and can hold negative and inaccurate views of patients with mental illness. Research shows properly treated patients with ADHD are *less* likely to have addiction problems.

C. **What does the patient want?** The child in this case study wanted treatment because of decreasing self-esteem and performance at school. The parents are reluctant and refusing.

Plan Educate the parents in a nonjudgmental fashion about the benefits of medication and therapy, including preserving the child's self-esteem, social functioning, and school performance. Ultimately, the parents understood the need to help their child and accepted treatment. Medication times were scheduled so the child did not have to take medication at school, maintaining confidentiality. Unfortunately, stigma remains a concern for anyone receiving mental health treatment.

QSEN QSEN Prelicensure Knowledge, Skills, and Attitudes (KSAs) Addressed:

Patient-centered care by seeing the situation through both the child's and parents' perspectives, and maintaining confidentiality

Evidence-based care by using current research to help educate the parents and develop a plan of care that addresses their concerns

Susan L. Frost, Chyllia D. Fosbre, 2015

Chang, Z., Lichtenstein, P., Halldner, L., et al. (2013). Stimulant ADHD medication and risk for substance abuse. *Journal of Child Psychology and Psychiatry, 55*(8), 878–885; Gill, K. J. (2008, Winter). The persistence of stigma and discrimination. *Psychiatric Rehabilitation Journal*, 183–184; and Ross, C. A., & Goldner, E. M. (2009). Stigma, negative attitudes and discrimination towards mental illness within the nursing profession: a review of the literature. *Journal of Psychiatric and Mental Health Nursing, 16*(6), 558–567.

KEY POINTS TO REMEMBER

- Mental illness can be difficult to define. The *DSM-5* and cultural norms must be considered in evaluating mental health and illness. There are many myths surrounding mental illness, which contribute to stigmatization of individuals. The stereotyping, discrimination, and rejection accompanying stigma contribute to poor self-image, isolation, and mental anguish. Stigma erects barriers to obtaining employment, housing, and health services. Nurses can use sensitivity and compassion to bridge the shame patients feel and encourage them to seek care.

- Mental health can be conceptualized along a continuum, from mild to moderate to severe to a profound degree of impairment in functioning.
- There are various components and influences that contribute to mental health, which are identified in Figure 2-1.
- The study of epidemiology can help identify high-risk groups and behaviors and lead to enhanced understanding of causes and best treatment. Prevalence rates help us identify the proportion of a population with a mental disorder at a given time.
- With the current knowledge that many common mental disorders are biologically based, they are now recognized as medical diseases.
- Nursing diagnoses help to systematically target symptoms patients may experience.
- The way symptoms are expressed may reflect a person's cultural patterns and should be evaluated in this context.

APPLYING CRITICAL JUDGMENT

1. A 23-year-old male was brought to the emergency department by ambulance after a suicide attempt. He has been extremely depressed since the death of his girlfriend 5 months previously in a motor vehicle accident in which he was the driver. Since the accident, he has not been attending college although he was an honor student. He has also not shown up for his tutoring job. The patient's existing seizure disorder has worsened since the accident, but he refuses treatment. He states he deserves to be punished for "killing my girlfriend."
   A. What evidence can you identify indicating a decline in the patient's level of functioning?
   B. How might the patient's religious beliefs hinder and/or help his recovery?
   C. Formulate one nursing diagnosis and two interventions reflective of his mental health needs.
   D. Identify a concept from this chapter such as stigma, support system, or culture and relate it to this scenario.
   E. Using the mental health continuum, would you rate this patient's symptoms as mild, moderate, or severe?
2. Reflect on an encounter you had with someone from an unfamiliar background in your personal or work life. What did you learn from the experience? How was the person's background similar to or different from your own? How could this affect the therapeutic nursing relationship?
3. Before your first day of clinical in the mental health setting, briefly describe in writing your current thoughts and attitudes about people with mental illnesses and working with them. Where or how do you think you developed these perceptions? After the clinical day, reflect upon the experience. Have your perceptions changed, and if so in what way?

CHAPTER REVIEW QUESTIONS

1. A mentally ill gunman opens fire in a crowded movie theater, killing six people and injuring others. Which comment about this event by a member of the community most clearly shows the stigma of mental illness?
   a. "Gun control laws are inadequate in our country."
   b. "It's frightening to feel that it is not safe to go to a movie theater."
   c. "All these people with mental illness are violent and should be locked up."
   d. "These events happen because American families no longer go to church together."

2. The nurse presents a class about mental health and mental illness to a group of fourth graders. One student asks, "Why do people get mentally ill?" Select the nurse's best response.
   a. "There are many reasons why mental illness occurs."
   b. "The cause of mental illness is complicated and very hard to understand."
   c. "Sometimes a person's brain does not work correctly because something bad happens or they inherit a brain problem."
   d. "Most mental illnesses result from genetically transmitted abnormalities in cerebral structure; however, some are a consequence of traumatic life experiences."

3. An adult experienced a spinal cord injury resulting in quadriplegia 3 years ago and now lives permanently in a skilled care facility. Which comment by this person best demonstrates resiliency?
   a. "I often pray for a miracle that will heal my paralysis so I will be whole again."
   b. "I don't know what I did to deserve this fate or whether I am tough enough to endure it."
   c. "My accident was a twist of fate. I suppose there are worse things than being paralyzed."
   d. "Being paralyzed has taken things from me but it hasn't kept me from being mentally involved in life."

4. A nursing assistant says to the nurse, "The schizophrenic in room 226 has been rambling all day." When considering the nurse's responsibility to manage the ancillary staff, which response should the nurse provide?
   a. "It is more respectful to refer to the patient by name than by diagnosis."
   b. "Thank you for informing me about that. I will document the behavior."
   c. "It is not unusual for schizophrenics to do that. It's just part of their illness."
   d. "You have a difficult job. I'm glad you are so accepting of our patients' behaviors."

5. Which scenario meets the criteria for "normal" behavior?
   a. An 8-year-old child's only verbalization is "No no no."
   b. A 16-year-old girl usually sleeps for 3 or 4 hours per night.
   c. A 43-year-old man cries privately for 1 month after the death of his wife.
   d. A 64-year-old woman has difficulty remembering the names of her grandchildren.

REFERENCES

American Psychiatric Association. (2013). *Diagnostic and statistical manual of mental disorders (DSM-5)* (5th ed.). Washington, DC: APA.

American Psychological Association. (2015). Data on behavioral health in the United States. Retrieved from www.apa.org/helpcenter/data-behavioral-health.aspx.

Favazza, A. (2009). Psychiatry and spirituality. In B. J. Sadock, V. A. Sadock, & P. Ruiz (Eds.), *Kaplan and Sadock's comprehensive textbook of psychiatry* (9th ed.) *Vol. 11.* (pp. 2033–2049). Philadelphia: Williams & Wilkins.

Hays, P. A. (2008). *Addressing cultural complexities in practice: assessment, diagnosis, and therapy* (2nd ed.). Washington, DC: American Psychological Association.

Kessler, R. C., Berglund, P., Demler, O. L., et al. (2007). Lifetime prevalence and age-of-onset distribution of *DSM-IV* disorders in the national comorbidity survey replication. *World Psychiatry, 6*(3), 168–176.

Mayo Clinic. (2014). Mental health: Overcoming the stigma of mental health. Retrieved from. http://www.mayoclinic.org/diseases-conditions/mental-illness/in-depth/mental-health/art-20046477.

National Alliance on Mental Illness (NAMI). (2011). What is mental illness? Mental illness facts. Retrieved from www.nami.org/PrinterTemplate.cfm?section=about_mental_illness.

National Institute of Mental Health. (2012). The numbers count: mental disorder in America. Retrieved from www.namigc.org/documents/numberscount.pdf.

National Mental Health Association. (2004). Congress must pass mental health parity now. Retrieved from www.nmha.org/federal/parity/parityfactsheet.cfm.

Ovans, A. (2015). What resilience means, and why it matters. *Harvard Business Review*. Retrieved from https://hbr.org/2015/01/what-resilience-means-and-why-it-matters.

Pinto-Foltz, M., Space, D., & Logsdon, M. C. (2009). Reducing stigma related to mental disorders: initiatives, interventions, and recommendations for nursing. *Archives of Psychiatric Nursing, 23*(1), 32–40.

Sadow, D., & Ryder, M. (2008). Reducing stigmatizing attitudes held by future health professionals: the person is the message. *Psychological Services, 5*(4), 362–372.

Swinomish Tribal Community. (1991). *A gathering of wisdom: tribal mental health: a cultural perspective*. LaConnor, Wash.

U.S. Department of Health and Human Services (USDHHS). (2015). Key concepts of the Affordable Care Act. Retrieved from http://www.hhs.gov/healthcare/facts-and-features/key-features-of-aca-by-year/index.html#.

U.S. Department of Health and Human Services (USDHHS). (1999). *Mental health: a report of the Surgeon General*. Rockville, Md: USDHHS, Center for Mental Health Services, National Institutes of Health.

World Health Organization (WHO). (2010). Mental health: strengthening our response. Retrieved from www.who.int/mediacenter.

Yeh, C. J., Innan, A. G., Kim, A. B., et al. (2006). Asian American families collective coping strategies in response to 9/11. *Cultural Diversity and Ethnic Minority Psychology, 12*, 134–148.

Theories and Therapies

Margaret Jordan Halter

e http://evolve.elsevier.com/Varcarolis/essentials

KEY TERMS AND CONCEPTS

automatic thoughts, p. 24

boundaries, p. 31

cognitive distortions, p. 24

conscious, p. 20

countertransference, p. 20

curative factors, p. 30

ego, p. 20

group content, p. 29

group process, p. 29

id, p. 20

preconscious, p. 20

recovery model, p. 28

schemata, p. 24

self-actualization, p. 23

self-transcendence, p. 24

superego, p. 20

transference, p. 20

unconscious, p. 20

SELECTED CONCEPT: RECOVERY MODEL OF CARE

The Mental Health Recovery Model is not a focus on a cure, but instead emphasizes living adaptively with chronic mental illness. It is viewed both as an overarching philosophy of life for people with mental illness and as an approach to care for use by those who treat, finance, and support mental health care.

The recovery model switches the focus from nurse-patient relationship to nurse-patient partnership and had its initial success with those struggling with substances of abuse.

(Halter, the Text)

OBJECTIVES

1. Discuss the contributions of theories and therapies from a variety of disciplines and areas of expertise.
2. Choose two of the major theories that you believe are among the most relevant to psychiatric and mental health nursing care and defend your choice, giving examples.
3. Identify the origins and progression of dominant theories and treatment modalities.
4. Discuss the relevance of these theories and treatments to the provision of psychiatric and mental health care.

5. Demonstrate comprehensive understanding of Peplau's theoretical base for practice that is beneficial to all settings.
6. Identify three different theoretical models of mental health care and demonstrate how each could be used in specific circumstances.
7. Distinguish models of care used in clinical settings, and cite benefits and limitations of these models.

INTRODUCTION

We expect others (and ourselves) to behave in certain ways, and we seek explanations for behavior that deviates from what we believe to be normal. What causes excessive sadness or extreme happiness? How do we explain mistrust, anxiety, confusion, or apathy—degrees of which may range from mildly disturbing to incapacitating? It is by understanding a problem that we can begin to devise solutions to treat or eradicate it. Mental illness has long defied explanation, even as other so-called physical illnesses were being quantified and often controlled.

It was not until the late 1800s that psychological models and theories were conceived, developed, and disseminated into mainstream thinking. They provided structure for considering developmental processes and possible explanations for our thoughts, feelings, and behaviors. The theorists believed if complex workings of the mind could be

understood they also could be treated, and from these models and theories therapies evolved.

Early practitioners used various forms of talk therapy, or **psychotherapy,** focusing on the complexity and inner workings of the mind and emphasizing environmental influences on its development and its stability. Beginning in the early twentieth century, biological explanations for mental alterations began to gain acceptance. Currently the dominant and common belief is that mental health and mental illness are made up of both psychological and biological factors.

Mental health professionals continue to rely on theoretical models as a basis for understanding and treating psychiatric alterations and mental health issues. This chapter provides an overview of therapeutic models and related treatments and discusses the potential connection between them and the provision of psychiatric nursing care. Table 3-1 provides a snapshot of the major theories.

TABLE 3-1	Major Theories of Psychiatric Care		
Theory	**Theorist**	**Tenets**	**Therapeutic Model**
Psychoanalytic	Freud	Unconscious thoughts; psychosexual development	Psychoanalysis to learn unconscious thoughts; therapist is nondirective and interprets meaning
Interpersonal	Sullivan	Relationships as basis for mental health or illness	Therapy focuses on here and now and emphasizes relationships; therapist is an active participant
Behavioral	Pavlov, Watson-Skinner	Behavior is learned through conditioning	Behavioral modification addresses maladaptive behaviors by rewarding adaptive behavior
Cognitive	Beck	Negative and self-critical thinking causes depression	Cognitive behavioral therapists assist in identifying negative thought patterns and replacing them with rational ones, and often involves homework.
Biological	Many	Psychiatric disorders are heavily influenced by and/or cause changes to the brain and/or neurotransmitter(s) resulting in changes in thinking and behavior.	Neurochemical imbalances are corrected through medication and talk therapy (e.g., cognitive behavioral therapy)

PROMINENT THEORIES AND THERAPEUTIC MODELS

Psychoanalytic Theory

Sigmund Freud (1856 to 1939), an Austrian neurologist, is considered the "father of psychiatry." His work was based on psychoanalytic theory, in which Freud claims that most psychological disturbances are the result of early trauma or incidents that are often not remembered or recognized.

Freud (1961) identified three layers of mental activity: the conscious, the preconscious, and the unconscious mind. The conscious mind is your current awareness—thoughts, beliefs, and feelings. However, most of the mind's activity occurs outside of this conscious awareness, like an iceberg with its bulk hidden under the water. The preconscious mind contains what is lying immediately below the surface, not currently the subject of our attention, but accessible. The biggest chunk of the iceberg is made up of the unconscious mind. The unconscious is where our most primitive feelings, drives, and memories reside, especially those that are unbearable and traumatic. The conscious mind is then influenced by the preconscious and unconscious mind (Figure 3-1).

One of Freud's later and widely known constructs concerns the intrapsychic struggle that occurs within the brain among the id, the ego, and the superego. The id is the primitive, pleasure-seeking part (according to Freud, predominantly sexual pleasure) of our personalities that lurks in the unconscious mind.

The ego is our sense of self and acts as an intermediary between the id and the world by using ego defense mechanisms, such as repression, denial, and rationalization (see Chapter 11).

The superego is assigned to those processes that Freud referred to as our conscience (our sense of what is right or wrong) and is greatly influenced by our parents' or caregivers' moral and ethical stances. The assumption is made that in healthy individuals, the ego is able to realistically evaluate situations, limit the id's primitive impulses, and keep the superego from becoming too rigid and obsessive.

Freud believed that personality development is based on stages. During these stages, the id focuses on an erogenous zone of the body. These zones are oral, anal, and phallic. Fixation through overindulgence or frustration results in pathologic conditions and personality disorders. Freud's work has been criticized for a variety of reasons. One of the harshest criticism stems from the concept of penis envy in which females suffer from feelings of inferiority for not having male genitalia. Table 3-2 provides a comparison of Freud's, Sullivan's, and Erikson's developmental stages.

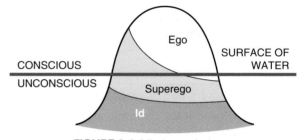

FIGURE 3-1 Mind as an iceberg.

Therapeutic Model

Psychoanalytic therapy was Freud's answer for a scientific method to relieve emotional disturbances by knowing the unconscious mind. An often time-consuming (sometimes daily), expensive, and emotionally painful process, the goal of this therapy is to know and understand what is happening at the unconscious level in order to uncover the truth. The analyst uses *free association* to search for forgotten and repressed memories by encouraging the patient to say anything that comes to mind. For example, "What do you think of when I say 'water'?" A patient may respond, "Warm … June … darkness … can't breathe," revealing a long forgotten, but traumatic near-drowning incident.

The analyst is nondirective, but does make interpretations of symbols, thoughts, and dreams. **Psychodynamic therapy** is theoretically related to psychoanalytic therapy and views the mind in essentially the same way. It tends to be shorter, about 10 to 12 sessions. The therapist takes a more active role since the therapeutic relationship is part of the healing process. Transference occurs as the patient projects intense feelings onto the therapist related to unfinished work from previous relationships; safe expression of these feelings is crucial to successful therapy. Psychodynamic therapists recognize that they, too, have unconscious emotional responses to the patient, or countertransference, which must be scrutinized in order to prevent damage to the therapeutic relationship.

Interpersonal Theory

Interpersonal theory focuses on what occurs between people, as opposed to psychoanalytic theory that is rooted in what occurs in the mind. Harry Stack Sullivan (1892 to 1949), an American psychiatrist, believed that personality dynamics and disorders were caused primarily by social forces and interpersonal situations. Human beings are driven by the need for interaction. In fact Sullivan (1953) viewed loneliness as the most painful human experience. He emphasized the

TABLE 3-2 Development of Personality According to Freud, Sullivan, and Erikson*

Freud	Sullivan *Piplean*	Erikson
Oral—birth to 1½ years	**Infancy**—birth to 1½ years	**Infancy**—birth to 1½ years
Pleasure-pain principle	Mothering object relieves tension through empathic intervention and tenderness, leading to decreased anxiety and increased satisfaction and security; mother becomes symbolized "good mother"	**Trust vs. mistrust**
Id, the instinctive and primitive mind, is dominant		Egocentric
Demanding, impulsive, irrational, asocial, selfish, trustful, omnipotent, and dependent	Goal is biological satisfaction and psychological security	**Danger**—during second half of first year, an abrupt and prolonged separation may intensify the natural sense of loss and may lead to a sense of mistrust that may last throughout life
Primary thought processes	Denial of tension relief creates anxiety, and mother becomes symbolized as "bad mother"	
Unconscious instincts—source-energy-aim-object	Anxiety in mother yields anxiety and fear in child via empathy	**Task**—develop a basic sense of trust that leads to hope
Mouth—primary source of pleasure	These states are experienced by the child in diffuse-undifferentiated manner	Trust requires a feeling of physical comfort and a minimal experience of fear or uncertainty; if this occurs, the child will extend trust to the world and self
Immediate release of tension/anxiety and immediate gratification through oral gratification	**Task**—learn to count on others for satisfaction and security to trust	
Task—develop a sense of trust that needs will be met		
Anal—1½ to 3 years	**Childhood**—1½ to 6 years	**Early childhood**—1½ to 3 years
Reality principle—postpone immediate discharge of energy and seek actual object to satisfy needs	Muscular maturation and learning to communicate verbally	**Autonomy vs. shame/doubt**
Learning to defer pleasure	Learning social skills through consensual validation	Develop confidence in physical and mental abilities that leads to the development of an autonomous will
Gaining satisfaction from tolerating some tension-mastering impulses	Beginning to develop self-esteem via reflected appraisals:	**Danger**—development of a deep sense of shame/doubt if child is deprived of the opportunity to rebel; learns to expect defeat in any battle of wills with those who are bigger and stronger
Focus on toilet training—retaining/letting go; power struggle	Good me Bad me Not me	
Ego development—functions of the ego include problem-solving skills, perception, ability to mediate id impulses	Levels of awareness Awareness Selective inattention Dissociation	**Task**—gain self-control of and independence within the environment
Task—delay immediate gratification	**Task**—learn to delay satisfaction of wishes with relative comfort	
Phallic—3 to 7 years		**Play**—3 to 6 years
Superego develops via incorporating moral values, ideals, and judgments of right and wrong that are held by parents; superego is primarily unconscious and functions on the **reward and punishment principle** (sexual identity attained via resolving oedipal conflict)		**Initiative vs. guilt**
		Interest in socially appropriate goals leads to a sense of purpose
		Imagination is greatly expanded because of increased ability to move around freely and increased ability to communicate
Conflict differs for boy and girl masturbatory activity		Intrusive activity and curiosity and consuming fantasies, which lead to feelings of guilt and anxiety
		Establishment of conscience
Task—develop sexual identity through identification with same-sex parent		**Danger**—may develop a deep-seated conviction that he or she is essentially bad, with a resultant stifling of initiative or a conversion of moralism to vindictiveness
		Task—achieve a sense of purpose and develop a sense of mastery over tasks
Latency—7 to 12 years	**Juvenile**—6 to 9 years	**School age**—6 to 12 years
Desexualization; libido diffused	Absorbed in learning to deal with ever-widening outside world, peers, and other adults	**Industry vs. inferiority**
Involved in learning social skills, exploring, building, collecting, accomplishing, and hero worship	Reflections and revisions of self-image and parental images	Develops a healthy competitive drive that leads to confidence
Peer group loyalty begins	**Task**—develops satisfying interpersonal relationships with peers that involve competition and compromise	In learning to accept instruction and to win recognition by producing "things," the child opens the way for the capacity of work enjoyment
Gang and scout behavior	**Preadolescence**—9 to 12 years	**Danger**—the development of a sense of inadequacy and inferiority in a child who does not receive recognition
Growing independence from family	Develop intimate interpersonal relationship with person of same sex who is perceived to be much like oneself in interests, feelings, and mutual collaboration	
Task—sexuality is repressed during this time; learn to form close relationship(s) with same-sex peers	**Task**—learn to care for others of same sex who are outside the family; Sullivan called this the "normal homosexual phase"	**Task**—gain a sense of self-confidence and recognition through learning, competing, and performing successfully

Continued

TABLE 3-2 Development of Personality According to Freud, Sullivan, and Erikson*—cont'd

Freud	Sullivan	Erikson
Genital phase (adolescence)—13 to 20 years	**Adolescence**—12 to 20 years	**Adolescence**—12 to 20 years
Fluctuation regarding emotion stability and physical maturation	*Early adolescence*—*12 to 14 years*	*Identity vs. role confusion*
Very ambivalent and labile, seeking life goals and emancipation from parents	Establishing satisfying relationships with opposite sex	Diffusion
Dependence vs. independence	*Late adolescence*—*14 to 20 years*	Differentiation from parents leads to fidelity (sense of self)
Reappraisal of parents and self; intense peer loyalty	Interdependent and establishing durable sexual relations with a select member of the opposite sex	Physiological revolution that accompanies puberty (rapid body growth and sexual maturity) forces the young person to question beliefs and to refight many of the earlier battles
Task—form close relationships with members of the opposite sex based on genuine caring and pleasure in the interaction	**Task**—form intimate and long-lasting relationships with the opposite sex and develop a sense of identity	**Danger**—temporary identity diffusion (instability) may result in a permanent inability to integrate a personal identity
		Task—integrate all the tasks previously mastered into a secure sense of self
		Young adulthood—20 to 30 years
		Intimacy and solidarity vs. isolation
		Maturity and social responsibility result in the ability to love and be loved
		As people feel more secure in their identity, they are able to establish intimacy with themselves (their inner life) and with others, eventually in a love-based satisfying sexual relationship with a member of the opposite sex
		Danger—fear of losing identity may prevent intimate relationship and result in a deep sense of isolation
		Task—form intense long-term relationships and commit to another person, cause, institution, or creative effort
		Adulthood—30 to 65 years
		Generativity vs. self-absorption
		Interest in nurturing subsequent generations creates a sense of caring, contributing, and generativity
		Danger—lack of generativity results in self-absorption and stagnation
		Task—achieve life goals and obtain concern and awareness of future generations
		Senescence—65 years to death
		Integrity vs. despair
		Acceptance of mortality and satisfaction with life leads to wisdom
		Satisfying intimacy with other human beings and adaptive response to triumphs and disappointments
		Marked by a sense of what life is, was, and its place in the flow of history
		Danger—without this "accrued ego integration," there is despair, usually marked by a display of displeasure and distrust
		Task—derive meaning from one's whole life and obtain/maintain a sense of self-worth

*Developed from original sources by Freud, Sullivan, and Erikson.

early relationship with the *significant other* (primary parenting figure) as crucial for personality development, and believed that healthy relationships were necessary for a healthy personality.

Another important concept in interpersonal theory is anxiety. Sullivan believed that anxiety is an interpersonal phenomenon brought about by interaction. In the earliest relationship anxiety is transmitted from the significant other to the child. The child's anxiety is also based on perceived degrees of approval or disapproval of the primary caregiver. According to Sullivan, all behavior is aimed at avoiding anxiety and threats to self-esteem.

One of the ways that we avoid anxiety is by focusing on positive attributes, or the *good me* ("I'm a good skier"), and by hiding the negative aspects, or the *bad me* ("I failed an exam"), of ourselves from others and maybe even from ourselves. The *not me* is used to separate us from parts of ourselves that we cannot bear to acknowledge that are pushed deeply into the unconscious and disassociated from one's own sense of self. An example is a female adolescent from a strict and conservative family who begins to have stirrings of attraction toward girls, yet firmly maintains (and believes) that she has feelings and interest in boys.

Sullivan's theory of development echoes that of Freud's in that personalities are influenced by the social environment as children, particularly as adolescents. He believed that personality is most influenced by the mother, but that personality could be molded even as adults. Stages occur in a stepwise fashion that is environmentally influenced (see Table 3-2).

Therapeutic Model

Interpersonal therapy (IPT) is a hands-on system in which therapists actively guide and challenge maladaptive behaviors and distorted views. The premise for this work is that if people are aware of their dysfunctional patterns and unrealistic expectations, they can modify them. The focus is on the "here and now" with an emphasis on the patient's life and relationships at home, at work, and in the social realm. The therapist becomes a "participant observer" and reflects the patient's interpersonal behavior, including responses to the therapist.

Behavioral Theories

As the psychoanalytic movement was developing in the twentieth century, so too was the behaviorist school of thought. Ivan Pavlov (1927) is famous for investigating *classical conditioning,* in which involuntary behavior or reflexes could be conditioned to respond to neutral stimuli. Pavlov's experimental dogs became accustomed to receiving food after a bell was rung. Later these dogs salivated in response to the ring alone. For human beings, classical conditioning can occur under such circumstances as when a baby's crying induces a milk let-down reflex or when a rape victim begins to hyperventilate and sweat when she hears footsteps behind her.

John B. Watson (1930) rejected psychoanalysis and sought an objective therapy that did not focus on unconscious motivations. He contended that personality traits and responses, adaptive and maladaptive, were learned. In a famous (but awful from an ethical standpoint) experiment, Watson conditioned Little Albert, a 9-month-old child, to be terrified at the sight of white fur or hair. He concluded that through behavioral techniques anyone could be trained to be anything, from a beggar to a merchant.

B. F. Skinner (1938) conducted research on operant conditioning in which voluntary behaviors are learned through consequences of positive reinforcement (a consequence that causes the behavior to occur more frequently) or negative reinforcement or punishment (a consequence that causes the behavior to occur less frequently). Studying hard results in good grades and increases the chances that studying will continue to occur. Driving too fast may result in a speeding ticket and in most individuals will decrease the chances that speeding will occur in the future.

Therapeutic Models

Behavioral therapy, or **behavior modification,** uses basic tenets from each of the behaviorists described previously. It attempts to correct or eliminate maladaptive behaviors or responses by rewarding and reinforcing adaptive behavior.

Systematic desensitization is based on classical conditioning. The premise is that learned responses can be reversed by first promoting relaxation and then gradually facing a particular anxiety-provoking stimulus. This method has been particularly successful in extinguishing phobias. Agoraphobia, the fear of open places, can be treated initially by visualizing trips outdoors while using relaxation techniques. Later, the individual can practice more challenging excursions, which should result in eliminating or reducing agoraphobia.

Aversion therapy is based on both classical and operant conditioning and is used to eradicate unwanted habits by associating unpleasant consequences with them. A pharmacologically based aversion therapy is a regimen of disulfiram (Antabuse). People who take this medication and then ingest alcohol become extremely ill with nausea, vomiting, and dizziness. Aversion therapy also has been used with sex offenders, who may, for example, receive electric shocks in response to arousal from child pornography.

Biofeedback is a technique in which individuals learn to control physiological responses such as breathing rates, heart rates, blood pressure, brain waves, and skin temperature. This control is achieved by providing visual or auditory biofeedback of the physiological response and then using relaxation techniques such as slow, deep breathing or meditation.

Humanistic Theory

Humanists rejected the psychoanalysts' focus on unconscious conflicts, which they considered overpessimistic. They also rejected the behaviorists' focus on learning, which they considered overscientific. The humanists developed a psychological science concerned with the human potential for development, knowledge attainment, motivation, and understanding.

Maslow's hierarchy of needs theory was developed in 1954 by an American psychologist, Abraham Maslow (1970). Needs are placed conceptually on a pyramid, with the most basic and important needs on the lower level (Figure 3-2). The higher levels, the more distinctly human needs, occupy the top sections of the pyramid. According to Maslow, when lower level needs are met, higher level needs are able to emerge.

- *Physiological needs.* The most basic needs are the physiological drives, including the need for food, oxygen, water, sleep, sex, and a constant body temperature. If all levels in the pyramid were deprived, this level would take priority.
- *Safety needs.* Once physiological needs are met, the safety needs take precedence. The safety needs include security; protection; freedom from fear, anxiety, and chaos; and the need for law, order, and limits.
- *Belongingness and love needs.* People have a need for intimate relationships, love, affection, and belonging and work to overcome loneliness and alienation. Maslow stresses the importance of having a family and a home and being part of identifiable groups.
- *Esteem needs.* People need to have a high self-regard and have it reflected to them from others. If self-esteem needs are met, we feel confident, valued, and valuable. When self-esteem is compromised, we feel inferior, worthless, and helpless.
- *Self-actualization.* According to Maslow, we are hard-wired to be everything that we are capable of becoming. He said, "What a man *can* be, he *must* be." What we are capable of becoming is highly individual—an artist must paint, a writer must write, and a healer must heal. The drive to satisfy this need is felt as a sort of restlessness, a sense that something is missing. It is up to each person to choose a path that will result in inner peace and fulfillment.

Although Maslow's early work included only five levels of needs, he later took into account two additional factors: (1) cognitive needs (the desire to know and understand) and (2) aesthetic needs (Maslow, 1970). The acquisition of knowledge and the need to understand are inborn and essential. Aesthetic needs result in a craving for beauty and symmetry. Maslow named the sixth level *Self-Transcendence.*

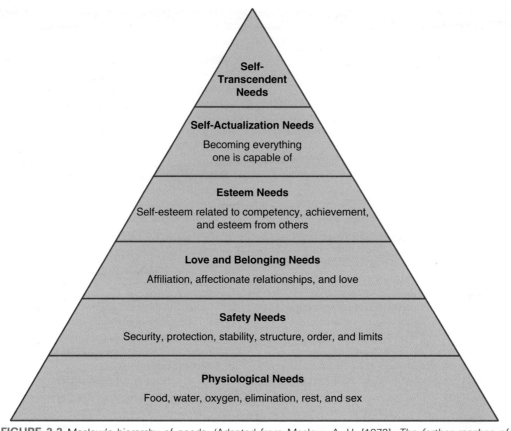

FIGURE 3-2 Maslow's hierarchy of needs. (Adapted from Maslow, A. H. [1972]. *The farther reaches of human nature.* New York: Viking.)

• *Self-transcendence* is when an individual "seeks to further a cause beyond the self and to experience a communion beyond the boundaries of the self through peak experiences" (Koltko-Rivera, 2006). Self-transcendent experiences are those in which a person experiences a sense of identity that transcends or extends beyond the personal self.

Therapeutic Model

Carl Rogers, an American psychologist, popularized **person-centered therapy** in the 1940s. Rogers, unlike Freud, saw people as basically healthy and good. He identified people and all living organisms as having innate self-actualizing tendencies to grow, to develop, and to realize their full potential (Rogers, 1986). He believed that clients (he did not call them patients) were in the best position to explore, understand, and identify solutions to their own problems. He uses the analogy of teaching a child to ride a bicycle. It is not enough to tell the child how to ride, but is imperative that the child tries to ride the bike. (See Chapter 9 for further discussion on Rogers's use of therapeutic relationships.)

Patient-centered therapy is an existentially based therapy. The emphasis is on self-awareness and on the present, because the past has already happened and the future has not yet occurred. The role of the therapist is that of a nondirective facilitator who seeks clarification and provides encouragement in this process. Three essential qualities in the therapist are congruence (genuineness), empathy, and respect. If these three qualities are present, the patient will improve; without them, there is little chance that the therapy will be successful.

Cognitive Theory

Aaron T. Beck was convinced that depressed people generally had standard patterns of negative and self-critical thinking (Beck, 1963).

Cognitive appraisals of events therefore lead to emotional responses—it is not the stimulus itself that causes the response, but instead one's evaluation of the stimulus. An example of the stimulus-appraisal-response relationship would be a woman whose sister had been depressed since their tumultuous and unsteady childhoods. In response to a question about how she and her sibling handled their parents' divorce and subsequent move to a small apartment, one of the siblings observed: "My sister fell apart. She retreated, barely talked. Mom asked me how I was doing. I told her I was excited to get a new bedroom and make new friends. And I was telling the truth."

Therapeutic Model

Cognitive behavioral therapy (CBT) is a popular and commonly used effective and well-researched therapeutic tool. It is based on both cognitive and behavioral theory and seeks to modify negative thoughts that lead to dysfunctional emotions and actions. Several concepts underlie this therapy. One is that we all have schemata, or unique assumptions about ourselves, others, and the world around us. For example, if someone has a schema that no one can be trusted, this person will question everyone's motives and expect deception and eventual pain in relationships. Other dominant forms of negative schemata include incompetence, abandonment, evilness, and vulnerability.

Typically, people are unaware of their basic assumptions. However, their beliefs and attitudes will make the assumptions apparent. Rapid, unthinking responses based on these schemata are known as automatic thoughts. These responses are particularly intense and frequent in psychiatric disorders such as depression and anxiety. Often these automatic thoughts, or cognitive distortions, are irrational because people make false assumptions and misinterpretations. Common cognitive distortions are listed in Table 3-3.

TABLE 3-3   Examples of Cognitive Distortions

Distortion	Definition	Example
All-or-nothing thinking	Thinking in black and white, reducing complex outcomes into absolutes	Cheryl got second-highest score in the cheerleading competition. She considers herself a loser.
Overgeneralization	Using a bad outcome (or a few bad outcomes) as evidence that nothing will ever go right again	Marty had a traffic accident. She refuses to drive and says, "I shouldn't be allowed on the road."
Labeling	A form of generalization where a characteristic or event becomes definitive and results in an overly harsh label for self or others	"Because I failed the advanced statistics exam, I am a failure. I might as well give up."
Mental filter	Focusing on a negative detail or bad event and allowing it to taint everything else	Anne's boss evaluated her work as exemplary and gave her a few suggestions for improvement. Anne obsessed about the suggestions and ignored the rest.
Disqualifying the positive	Maintaining a negative view by rejecting information that supports a positive view as being irrelevant, inaccurate, or accidental	"I've just been offered the job I've always wanted. No one else must have applied."
Jumping to conclusions	Making a negative interpretation despite the fact that there is little or no supporting evidence	"My fiancé, Mike, didn't call me for 3 hours; therefore, he doesn't love me."
a. Mind reading	Inferring negative thoughts, responses, and motives of others	The grocery store clerk was grouchy and barely made eye contact. "I must have done something wrong."
b. Fortune-telling error	Anticipating that things will turn out badly as an established fact	"I'll ask her out, but I know she won't have a good time."
Magnification or minimization	Exaggerating the importance of something (such as a personal failure or the success of others) or reducing the importance of something (such as a personal success or the failure of others)	"I'm alone on a Saturday night because no one likes me. When other people are alone, it's because they want to be."
a. Catastrophizing	An extreme form of magnification in which the very worst is assumed to be a probable outcome	"If I don't make a good impression on the boss at the company picnic, she will fire me."
Emotional reasoning	Drawing a conclusion based on an emotional state	"I'm nervous about the exam. I must not be prepared. If I were, I wouldn't be afraid."
"Should" and "must" statements	Rigid self-directives that presume an unrealistic amount of control over external events	"My patient is worse today. I should give better care so that she will get better."
Personalization	Assuming responsibility for an external event or situation that was likely out of personal control	"I'm sorry that your party wasn't more fun. It's probably because I was there."

Adapted from Burns, D. D. (1980). *Feeling good: the new mood therapy*. New York: William Morrow.

The goal of CBT is to identify the negative patterns of thought that lead to negative emotions. Once the maladaptive patterns are identified, they can be replaced with rational thoughts. A particularly useful technique in CBT is to use a four-column format to record the precipitating event or situation, the resulting automatic thought, the ensuing feeling(s) and behavior(s), and, finally, a challenge to the negative thoughts based on rational evidence and thoughts. This is sometimes referred to as the *ABCs of irrational beliefs* and is a good exercise for you to try for yourself (Box 3-1).

Biological Model

Psychiatric care is dominated by the biological model, in which mental disorders are believed to have physical causes. If mental disorders have physical causes then they will respond to physical treatment. Sigmund Freud himself researched neurological causes for mental illness and considered cocaine a possible treatment.

In the 1950s a surgeon noticed that surgical patients were calmed by the administration of chlorpromazine (Thorazine). It soon became widely used for the treatment of schizophrenia and dramatically reduced the use of restraint and seclusion. This discovery spurred the development of other drug-based treatments and the adoption of a chemical imbalance theory of mental disorders.

If chemical imbalances exist, how do they develop? Twin studies have been useful to support the genetic transmission of certain disorders. Whereas only 1% of the population has schizophrenia, among identical twins the concordance rate (the percentage of the time that both twins will be affected) is about 50% (Sadock et al., 2015). Although this indicates genetic involvement, it cannot be the whole story. If it were, the concordance rate of schizophrenia in

BOX 3-1   Example of ABCs of Irrational Beliefs

Activating Event
Jack has been in counseling for depression. His therapist's secretary called and canceled this week's appointment.

Belief
My therapist is disgusted with me and wants to avoid me.

Consequence
Sadness, rejection, and hopelessness. Decides to call off work and return to bed.

Reframing
There is no evidence to believe that I disgust my therapist. Why would he have rescheduled if he really didn't want to see me?

identical twins would be 100%. It is likely that the environment exerts an influence on the developing embryo or child. Research has shown that toxins, viruses, hostile environments, and brain traumas have been proposed as catalysts for the development of psychiatric disorders (see Chapter 4).

Biological Therapy

Psychopharmacology is the primary biological treatment for mental disorders. (Refer to Chapter 4 for a full discussion of the biological basis for understanding psychopharmacology.) Major classifications of medications are antidepressants, antipsychotics, antianxiety agents, mood stabilizers, and psychostimulants. Clinicians recognize the importance of optimizing other biological variables, such as correcting hormone levels (as in hypothyroidism), regulating nutritionally deficient diets, and balancing inadequate sleep patterns. (Refer to Chapters 10 through 19 for relevant uses of psychopharmacology.)

Electroconvulsive therapy (ECT) has proven to be an effective treatment for severe depression and other psychiatric conditions. ECT is a procedure that uses electrical current to induce a seizure, and is thought to work by affecting neurotransmitters and neuroreceptors (see Chapter 15 for more discussion regarding ECT).

Most mental health professionals combine biological approaches with talk therapy. Research indicates that using medication and cognitive behavioral therapy is an extremely effective treatment for many psychiatric disorders, especially major depression (Sadock et al., 2015). If a hostile environment can trigger negative brain chemistry or transmission, then a positive environment may reverse and improve the process.

A Note on How Psychotherapy Changes the Brain

Numerous studies have indicated that all mental processes are derived from the brain. Therefore psychotherapeutic outcomes, such as changes in symptoms, psychological abilities, personality, or social functioning, are generally accepted to be attributed to brain changes brought about either by medication or by psychotherapy. Numerous studies compiled by Karlsson (2011) substantiate positive treatment responses with various psychotherapies resulting in brain changes for the following disorders: major depressive disorder (MDD), anxiety disorders (panic disorder, social anxiety disorder, specific phobias), posttraumatic stress disorder (PTSD), borderline personality disorder, and obsessive-compulsive disorder (OCD). These studies suggest that currently the most effective therapies for treating the aforementioned disorders resulting in brain changes are cognitive behavioral therapy (CBT), dialectic behavior therapy (DBT), psychodynamic psychotherapy, and interpersonal psychotherapy (IP).

OTHER MAJOR THEORIES

Cognitive Development

Jean Piaget (1896 to 1980) was a Swiss psychologist and researcher. Piaget noticed that children consistently gave wrong answers on intelligence tests that revealed a pattern of cognitive processing. He concluded that cognitive development was a progression from primitive awareness to complex thought and responses (Piaget & Inhelder, 1969).

An understanding of cognitive development assists nurses in tailoring care to suit the cognitive level of the patient. For example, the concept of dying is difficult to grasp for the 5-year-old child who has lost a parent. Support for this child will require different skills than those required for a 10-year-old child, who can understand the permanence of death. A summary of stages are listed in Table 3-4.

Theory of Psychosocial Development

German-born American Erik Erikson (1902 to 1994) was a child psychoanalyst who described development as occurring in eight predetermined life stages, stages whose levels of success are related to the preceding stage (see Table 3-2).

Developmental tasks during these stages ideally result in a successful resolution. For example, from the ages of 7 to 12 the child's task is to understand her own abilities and competence, and expand relationships beyond the immediate. The attainment of this task *(industry)* brings about confidence. The inability to gain a mastery of age-appropriate tasks and make connections with peers results in failure *(inferiority)*.

TABLE 3-4	Stages of Cognitive Development
Stage	**Features**
Sensorimotor (birth to 2 years)	Begins with basic reflexes and culminates with purposeful movement, spatial abilities, and hand-eye coordination. Around 9 months, **object permanence** is achieved and the child can conceptualize objects that are no longer visible.
Preoperational (2 to 7 years)	Language develops, yet children think in a concrete fashion. Expecting others to view the world as they do is called **egocentric thinking.** Children begin to think in images and symbols and engage in such activities as playing house.
Concrete operational (7 to 11 years)	The child is able to think logically and use abstract problem solving. He/she is able to see another's point of view and is able to see a variety of solutions to a problem. **Conservation** is possible. For example, 2 small cups of liquid can be seen to equal a tall glass. The child is able to classify by characteristics, order objects in a pattern, and understand the concept of reversibility.
Formal operational (11 years to adulthood)	Conceptual reasoning begins at approximately the same time as puberty. At this stage the child's basic abilities to think abstractly and problem solve are similar to those of an adult.

Each stage does not depend completely on integrating the positive characteristic and completing abandoning the negative. Ideally, harmony is achieved between the two characteristics. For example, we would not want a person to be 100% trusting—a degree of mistrust is essential for safety.

Theory of Object Relations

The theory of object relations was developed by interpersonal theorists who emphasize past relationships in influencing a person's sense of self as well as the nature and quality of relationships in the present. The term *object* refers to another person, particularly a significant person.

Margaret Mahler (1895 to 1985) was a Hungarian-born child psychologist who developed a framework for studying how an infant transitions from complete self-absorption, with an inability to separate from its mother, to a physically and psychologically differentiated toddler. Mahler believed that psychological problems were largely the result of a disruption of this separation.

During the first 3 years, the significant other (e.g., the mother) provides a secure base of support that promotes enough confidence for the child to separate. This is achieved by a balance of holding (emotionally and physically) enough for the child to feel safe, while encouraging independence and natural exploration.

Problems may arise in this process. If a toddler leaves his or her mother on the park bench and wanders off to the sandbox, the child should be encouraged with smiles and reassurance, "Go on honey, it's safe to go away a little." The mother should be reliably present when the toddler returns, thereby rewarding his or her efforts. Mahler notes that raising healthy children does not require that parents never make mistakes, and that "good enough parenting" will promote successful separation-individuation.

Theories of Moral Development

Stages of Moral Development

Lawrence Kohlberg (1927 to 1987) was an American psychologist who applied Piaget's theory to moral development. Based on interviews with youths, Kohlberg developed a theory of how people progressively develop a sense of morality (Kohlberg & Turiel, 1971). His theory helps us understand the progression from black-and-white thinking to a context-dependent decision-making process regarding the rightness or wrongness of action.

Carol Gilligan (born in 1936) is an American psychologist, ethicist, and feminist who worked with Kohlberg. She later criticized his work for being male based. Gilligan also believed that the scoring method favored males' methods of reasoning. Based on Gilligan's critique, Kohlberg revised his scoring methods, which resulted in greater similarity between girls' and boys' scores.

Gilligan's ethics of care theory emphasizes the importance of forming relationships and putting the needs of those for whom we care above the needs of strangers. Like Kohlberg, Gilligan asserts that moral development progresses through three major divisions: pre-conventional, conventional, and post-conventional. These transitions are dictated by personal development and changes in a sense of self. Kolberg's and Gilligan's stages of moral development are summarized in Table 3-5.

NURSING MODELS

We have been examining theories and therapies developed by professionals from a variety of disciplines that date back to the late 1800s. It was not until the 1950s that the profession of nursing began to develop, record, and test theories (Alligood, 2013). The drive to create these theories began as a result of nursing education being moved from hospital-based programs to college- and university-based programs where nurses became involved in research. This research became the impetus for nurses to develop theories and a strong scientific body of knowledge.

Hildegard Peplau's work in the early 1950s is most often associated with psychiatric nursing, and her work will be presented in the following section. However, most nursing theories are applicable and of value to psychiatric nursing because interpersonal relations, caring, and communication are keys to the foundation of nursing. A summary of selected nursing theorists, the focus of their theoretical works, and examples of how their contributions could be utilized in psychiatric nursing is provided in Table 3-6. It is worth noting that among nurse theorists, psychiatric nurses are well represented.

Interpersonal Relations in Nursing

Hildegard Peplau's (1909 to 1999) seminal work, *Interpersonal Relations in Nursing*, was first published in 1952 and has served as a foundation for understanding and conducting therapeutic nursing relationships ever since. Peplau based her work on Sullivan's interpersonal theory and emphasized that the nature of the nurse-patient relationship strongly influenced the outcome for the patient.

Peplau made an extremely useful contribution to understanding anxiety by conceptualizing the four levels still in use today:

1. Mild anxiety is day-to-day, "I'm awake and taking care of business" alertness. Stimuli in the environment are perceived and understood, and learning can easily take place.
2. Moderate anxiety is felt as a heightened sense of awareness, such as when you are about to take an exam. The perceptual field is narrowed and an individual hears, sees, and understands less. Learning can still take place, although it may require more direction.
3. Severe anxiety interferes with clear thinking and the perceptual field is greatly diminished. Nearly all behavior is directed at reducing the

Level	Kolberg's Stages	Gilligan's Stages
Pre-conventional	Stage 1: Obedience and punishment—a focus on rules and listening to authority to avoid punishment. Stage 2: Individualism and exchange—growing awareness that not everyone thinks the same. Breaking rules is a personal choice.	The goal is individual survival. Characterized by selfishness.
Conventional	Stage 3: Good interpersonal relationships—rightness or wrongness is based on individual motivations, personality, or the goodness or badness of the person. People should get along and have similar values. Stage 4: Maintaining the social order—rules are rules. Listening to authority maintains the social order.	Self-sacrifice is good. A responsibility for others develops.
Post-conventional	Stage 5: Social contract and individual rights—social order is important, but it also must be *good*. A corrupt social order should be changed. Stage 6: Universal ethical principles—actions should create unbiased results for everyone. We are obliged to break unjust laws.	The principle of nonviolence and not hurting others or self is essential. A balance of caring for self with caring for others emerges.

TABLE 3-5 Stages of Moral Development according to Kolberg and Gilligan

anxiety. An example of this is your response to skidding your car on wet pavement.
4. Panic anxiety is overwhelming and results in either paralysis or dangerous hyperactivity. An individual cannot communicate, function, or follow direction. This is the sort of anxiety that is associated with the terror of panic attacks.

Refer to Chapter 11 for application of these levels to the nursing process.

One of the most useful constructs of Peplau's theory is in providing structure for how we view the therapeutic relationship, which she divided into four phases. Each of these overlapping and interlocking phases includes tasks, the expression of needs by the patient, and the interventions facilitated by the nurse. Refer to Chapter 9 for more information on the phases of the nurse-patient relationship.

Influence of Theories and Therapies on Nursing Care

Other theories and therapies presented earlier in this chapter also are relevant to nursing care. Nurses constantly borrow concepts and carry out interventions that are supported by these models. Some examples of how they may be used are as follows:

- **Behavioral:** Promoting adaptive behaviors through reinforcement can be valuable and important in working with patients, especially when working with a pediatric population. These patients look

TABLE 3-6   Nursing Theoretical Works Relevant to Psychiatric Nursing

Theorist	Model/Theory	Focus of Nursing	Example
Dorothy Johnson	Behavioral system	Helping a patient return to a state of equilibrium when exposed to stressors by reducing or removing them and by supporting adaptive processes (Johnson, 1980)	Providing prn antianxiety medication and encouraging slow, deep breathing for a patient who is experiencing panic attacks
Imogene King	Goal attainment	Developing an interpersonal relationship and helping the patient to achieve his/her goals based on the patient's roles and social contexts (King, 1981)	Sitting with a new mother who is experiencing depression and developing a discharge plan in the context of childcare and financial deficits
Madeleine Leininger*	Culture care	Promoting health and helping people to cope with illness while recognizing cultural issues and their importance to health (Leininger, 1995)	Including the family in the plan of care for an Amish man who has recently attempted suicide
Betty Neuman*	System model	Developing a nurse-patient relationship; assessing and intervening with the person's response to stress (Neuman, 1982)	Considering the impact of shingles and graduate school stressors on a person diagnosed with generalized anxiety disorder
Dorothea Orem	Self-care deficit	Addressing self-care deficits and encouraging patients to be actively involved in their own care (Orem, 2001)	Temporarily helping a person with an exacerbation of paranoia to meet his/her hygiene needs
Ida Orlando*	Dynamic nurse-patient relationship	Addressing the patient's immediate need for help; the longer the unmet need, the more stress will be experienced (Orlando, 1990)	Asking, "Would you like to talk?" to a man who has begun pacing in the hallway and shaking his head
Hildegard Peplau*	Interpersonal relations	Using the interpersonal environment as a therapeutic tool for healing and in reduction of anxiety (Peplau, 1992)	Sitting quietly beside a new father who has recently lost his job and attempted suicide and does not want to talk
Jean Watson*	Transpersonal caring	Caring is as important as procedures and tasks; developing a nurse-patient relationship that results in a therapeutic outcome (Watson, 2007)	Taking time from a busy assignment to meet a patient's husband

*Psychiatric nursing background.

forward to positive reinforcement for good behavior and will work hard for gold stars or other privileges.

- **Cognitive:** Helping patients identify negative thought patterns is a worthwhile intervention in promoting healthy functioning and improving neurochemistry. Workbooks are available to aid in the process of identifying these cognitive distortions.
- **Psychosocial development:** Erikson's theory provides structure for understanding critical junctures in development. The older adult gentleman who has suffered a stroke may be depressed and despairing because he can no longer take care of his house. In this case the nurse and patient could explore ways of optimizing the patient's remaining strengths and talents, such as by nurturing and tutoring young people or by developing attainable and progressive goals such as getting the mail, taking out the trash, and so forth.
- **Hierarchy of needs:** Maslow's work is useful in prioritizing nursing care. When working with an actively suicidal patient, students sometimes think it is rude to ask if the patients are thinking about killing themselves. However, safety supersedes this potential threat to self esteem. Although the "must do's" in nursing begin with physical care (such as providing medication and hydration through IV fluids), the goal should also include higher level needs, which can be obtained by listening, observing, and collaborating with the patient in the development of the plan of care.

The Mental Health Recovery Model in Psychiatric Nursing

Although we tend think of recovery as regaining health or being cured from an episode of illness, the term recovery in this model has a different meaning. The mental health recovery model is not a focus on a cure, but instead emphasizes living adaptively with chronic mental illness. It is viewed both as an overarching philosophy of life for people

with mental illness and as an approach to care for use by those who treat, finance, and support mental health care. It is also an effective approach to dealing with substance abuse.

A diagnosis of mental illness once meant that you listened to health care professionals and relied upon them to chart your course in treatment. This medical model approach often results in apathy and discouragement: "They want me to take medication for the rest of my life; I don't like it and won't take it." The recovery model shifts the responsibility for care from the provider to the individual: "I will discuss the medication side effects with my friends who have similar problems and then talk to my nurse practitioner about my options and preferences."

This model emphasizes hope, social connection, empowerment, coping strategies, and meaning in life. A recovery approach to care has been embraced by the American Psychiatric Association from a service perspective. The U.S. Department of Health and Human Services uses recovery concepts to guide federal and state initiatives, particularly as they relate to empowering mental health consumers (people with mental illness) and in campaigns to reduce mental illness stigma. Illness Management and Recovery (IMR) programs are becoming popular and are increasingly supported by research (McGuire et al., 2014).

The use of the recovery model in psychiatric nursing is a natural extension of what we have traditionally done. Peplau (1952) set the standard by urging nurses to develop therapeutic interpersonal relationships. The recovery model moves this relationship from nurse-patient to nurse-patient-partnership. It is crucial to increase individual and family roles in recovery.

Caldwell and colleagues (2010) assert that psychiatric nurses should educate other health care professionals about recovery concepts and suggest methods to empower consumers and promote recovery:

- Advocate for self-administration of medications when possible, with appropriate supports in the community.

- Encourage the development of medication records to schedule dosing and to share with other health care providers.
- Develop a personal relapse prevention program by knowing the symptoms of relapse, by realizing the effects of environmental and internal triggers on emotional well-being, and by enlisting others for support.
- Recommend supported employment in regular community settings to reduce isolation and improve confidence.
- Utilize psychiatric advance directives to enable consumers to plan for mental health treatment in the event that a crisis should render them incompetent.

Therapies for Specific Populations
Group Therapy

This therapeutic method is commonly derived from interpersonal theory and operates under the assumption that interaction among participants can provide support or bring about desired change among individual participants.

A **group** is defined as (a) "a gathering of two or more individuals (b) who share a common purpose and (c) meet over a substantial time period (d) in face-to-face interaction (e) to achieve an identifiable goal" (Arnold & Boggs, 2016, p. 525). Experts disagree on the ideal size of the group, but it is usually somewhere from 6 to 10 members. A group that is too small will limit diversity of opinion and put pressure on members to participate. Overly large groups reduce the members' ability to share, especially if some members dominate the group.

Setting. Settings for groups are important. The room should be private, and the seating should be comfortable and arranged so that people can see one another. Using tables is discouraged because they can be psychological barriers between group members. One of the worst arrangements for discussion is the traditional "classroom seating" with everyone facing a central speaker, thereby limiting free interaction among participants.

Groups possess both content and process dimensions. Group content refers to the actual dialogue between members or the type of information that can be transcribed (written or recorded) in minutes of meetings. Group process includes all the other elements of human interaction, such as nonverbal communication, adaptive and maladaptive roles, energy flow, power plays, conflict, hidden agendas, and silences. Although the content is essential to the group's work, it is the process that becomes the real challenge for leaders as well as participants.

Group development tends to follow a sequential pattern of growth and requires less leadership with time. Understanding this pattern is especially helpful to the leader in order to anticipate distinct phases and provide guidance and interventions that are most effective. Tuckman's (1965) model of group development has four stages: forming, storming, norming, and performing. A fifth stage, adjourning (mourning), was later added (Tuckman & Jensen, 1977). These stages are comparable to human development from infancy into old age, accompanied by varying levels of maturity, confidence, and need for direction (Table 3-7).

Roles of group members. Studies of group dynamics have identified informal roles of members that are necessary to develop a successful group. The most common descriptive categories for these roles are task, maintenance, and individual roles (Benne & Sheats, 1948). Task roles serve to keep the group focused and attend to the business at hand. Maintenance roles function to keep the group together and provide interpersonal support. There are also individual roles that can interfere with the group's functioning because they are not related to the group goals, but rather to specific personalities. Table 3-8 describes roles of group members.

TABLE 3-7 Tuckman's Stages of Group Development and Comparable Life Phase

Stage	Comparable Life Phase	Description
Forming	Infancy	The task and/or purpose of the group is defined. Connecting with others, desiring acceptance, and avoiding conflict define early groups. Members gather commonalities and differences as they attempt to know one another. The leader is the main connection and necessary for direction.
Storming	Adolescence	Important issues are being addressed, and conflict begins to surface. Personal relations may interfere with the task at hand. Some members will dominate, and some will be silent. Rules and structure are helpful. Members may challenge the role of the leader, who has the opportunity to model adaptive behavior.
Norming	Early adulthood	Members know one another, and rules of engagement (norms) are evident. There is a sense of group identity and cohesion. Members resist change, which could lead to a group breakup or a return to the discomfort of storming. Leadership is shared.
Performing	Mature adulthood	Groups who reach this stage are characterized by loyalty, flexibility, interdependence, and productivity. There is a balance between focus on work and focus on the welfare of group members.
Adjourning (mourning)	Older adult years	Groups in this stage are ready to disband, tasks are terminated, and relationships are disengaged. Accomplishments are recognized and members are pleased to have been part of the group. A sense of loss is an inevitable consequence.

From Tuckman, B. W., & Jensen, M. A. (1977). Stages of small-group development revisited. *Group & Organization Management, 2*, 419–427.

Roles of the group leader. The group leader has multiple responsibilities in starting, maintaining, and terminating a group. In the initial forming phase, the leader defines the structure, size, composition, purpose, and timing for the group. The leader facilitates communication and ensures that meetings start and end on time. In the adjourning phase, the leader ensures that each member summarizes individual accomplishments and gives positive and negative feedback regarding the group experience.

Leadership style depends on group type (Jacobs et al., 2012). A leader selects the style that is best suited to the therapeutic needs of a particular group. The **autocratic leader** exerts control over the group and does not encourage much interaction among members. In contrast, the **democratic leader** supports extensive group interaction

TABLE 3-8 Roles of Group Members

Role	Function
Task Roles	
Coordinator	Connects various ideas and suggestions
Initiator-contributor	Offers new ideas or a new outlook on an issue
Elaborator	Gives examples and follows up meaning of ideas
Energizer	Encourages group to make decisions or take action
Evaluator	Measures group's work against a standard
Information/ opinion-giver	Shares opinions, especially to influence group values
Orienter	Notes progress of the group toward goals
Maintenance Roles	
Compromiser	In a conflict, yields to preserve group harmony
Encourager	Praises and seeks input from others; warm and accepting
Follower	Attentive listener and integral to the group
Gatekeeper	Ensures participation, encourages participation, points out commonality of thought
Harmonizer	Mediates conflicts constructively among members
Standard setter	Assesses explicit and implicit standards for group
Individual Roles	
Aggressor	Criticizes and attacks others' ideas and feelings
Blocker	Disagrees with group issues, opposes others, stalls the process
Help seeker	Asks for sympathy of group excessively, self-deprecating
Playboy/playgirl	Distracts others from the task; jokes, introduces irrelevant topics
Recognition seeker	Seeks attention by boasting and discussing achievements
Monopolizer	Dominates conversation, thereby preventing equal input
Special interest pleader	Advocates for a special group, usually with own prejudice or bias

Data from Benne, K. D., & Sheats, F. (1948). Functional roles of group members. *Journal of Social Issues, 4*(2), 41.

in the process of problem solving. A **laissez-faire leader** allows the group members to behave in any way that they choose and does not attempt to control the direction of the group. For example, staff leading a community meeting with a fixed, time-limited agenda may tend to be more autocratic. In a psychoeducational group, the leader may be more democratic to encourage members to share their experiences. In a creative group such as an art or horticulture group, the leader may choose a laissez-faire style, giving minimal direction to allow for a variety of responses.

Types of groups. Education groups form for the purpose of imparting information and require active expert leadership and careful planning. Task groups are typically time limited and have a common goal, and the role of the leader is to facilitate team building and cooperation. Support groups bring together people with common concerns and may be facilitated by a supportive leader or by group members. Therapy groups are led by professional group therapists whose styles may range from a directive and confrontational approach to a more hands-off, let the group members learn from one another, approach.

Benefits of Group Therapy

One of the commonly cited benefits of group therapy is that it is more efficient, both pragmatically and financially, because many people can engage in therapy at once. However, it is the nature of the interaction between people with common concerns and frames of references that seems to provide the greatest benefit. Yalom (1985) identified 11 benefits, or curative factors, of group membership (Table 3-9).

Roles of Nurses

Psychiatric mental health nurses are involved in a variety of therapeutic groups in acute care and long-term treatment settings. For all group leaders, a clear theoretical framework is necessary to provide a structure to understand the group interaction. Co-leadership of groups is a common practice and has several benefits: it provides training for less experienced staff; it allows for immediate feedback between the leaders after each session; and it gives two role models for teaching communication skills to members.

TABLE 3-9 Yalom's Curative Factors of Group Membership

Curative Factor	Definition	Example
Altruism	Giving appropriate help to other members	"We've spent all this time talking about me. Lou needs to talk about his visit with his dad. Let's focus on him."
Cohesiveness	Feeling connected to other members and belonging to the group	"People in our group always listen to each other. We've been polite since the first day."
Interpersonal learning	Learning from other members	"Sammi said it takes 2 weeks for Prozac to really work. I should give it more time."
Guidance	Receiving help and advice	"I've also had that feeling where I just had to have a drink, Don. Just pick up the phone and call me next time it happens."
Catharsis	Releasing feelings and emotions	A new mother of twins begins to cry and says, "It sounds terrible, but sometimes I wish I'd never had children."
Identification	Modeling after member or leader	David notices that the leader projects confidence by speaking clearly, making good eye contact, and sitting up straight. David does the same.
Family reenactment	Testing new behaviors in a safe environment	"I learned to always smile and agree so Dad wouldn't go off on me. I don't have to be cheery and I can speak my mind here."
Self-understanding	Gaining personal insights	Dale realizes that his negativity has kept him from getting the friends he wants.
Instillation of hope	Feeling hopeful about one's life	"Sue has managed to stay sober for 2 years. I think I can do this."
Universality	Feeling that one is not alone	Aaron, a quiet group member, finally comments, "My son has schizophrenia, too, and it helps to hear that other people have the same worries I do."
Existential factors	Coming to understand what life is about	"I guess I've been obsessing about being a perfect housekeeper and haven't noticed that my children are growing up without me."

From Yalom, I. D. (1985). *The theory and practice of group psychotherapy.* New York: Basic Books.

BOX 3-2 Central Concepts to Family Therapy

- **Boundaries:** **Clear boundaries** maintain distinctions between individuals within the family and between the family and the outside world. Clear boundaries allow for balanced flow of energy between members. **Diffuse** or **enmeshed boundaries** are those in which there is a blending of the roles, thoughts, and feelings of the individuals so that clear distinctions among family members fail to emerge. **Rigid** or **disengaged boundaries** are those in which the rules and roles are followed in spite of the consequences.
- **Triangulation:** The tendency, when two-person relationships are stressful and unstable, to engage a third person to stabilize the system through formation of a coalition in which two members are pitted against the third.
- **Scapegoating:** A form of displacement in which a family member (usually the least powerful) is blamed for another family member's distress. The purpose is to keep the focus off the painful issues and the problems of the blamers.
- **Double bind:** A double bind is a no-win situation in which you are "darned if you do, darned if you don't."
- **Hierarchy:** The function of power and its structures in families, differentiating parental and sibling roles and generational boundaries.
- **Differentiation:** The ability to develop a strong identity and sense of self while maintaining an emotional connectedness with one's family of origin.
- **Sociocultural context:** The framework for viewing the family in terms of the influence of gender, race, ethnicity, religion, economic class, and sexual orientation.
- **Multigenerational issues:** The continuation and persistence from generation to generation of certain emotional interactive family patterns (e.g., reenactment of fairly predictable patterns; repetition of themes or toxic issues; and repetition of reciprocal patterns such as those of overfunctioner and underfunctioner).

Basic level registered nurses have biopsychosocial educational backgrounds. Psychiatric mental health registered nurses (PMH-RNs) gain experience and expertise in caring for individuals who have physical, psychological, mental, and spiritual distress (American Psychiatric Nurses Association et al., 2014). PMH-RNs are ideally suited to teach a variety of health subjects. *Psychoeducational groups* are established to support and teach patients and families ways to help prevent relapse. These groups may be time limited or may be supportive for long-term treatment. Generally, written handouts or audiovisual aids are used to focus on specific teaching points. Psychiatric mental health nurses commonly lead the following psychoeducational groups:

- **Medication education groups** allow patients to hear the experiences of others who have taken medication and to have an opportunity to ask questions without the fear of being judged; these groups also allow patients to learn to take the medications correctly.
- **Dual-diagnosis groups** focus on co-occurring psychiatric illness and substance abuse. The PMH-RN may co-lead this group with a dual-diagnosis specialist (master's level clinician).
- **Symptom management groups** are designed for patients to share coping skills regarding a common problem, such as anger or psychosis. New and alternate skills can be learned to enhance self-control in order to help patients develop more effective strategies for reducing relapse.
- **Stress management groups** teach members about various relaxation techniques, including deep breathing, exercise, music, and spirituality.
- **Self-care groups** focus on basic hygiene issues such as bathing and grooming.

Psychiatric mental health advanced practice registered nurses (PMH-APRNs) may lead any of the groups described earlier as well as psychotherapy groups. Psychotherapy groups require specialized training in techniques that allow for deep disclosure, sharing, confrontation, and healing among participants.

Therapeutic Milieu

A therapeutic milieu, or healthy environment, combined with a healthy social structure within an inpatient setting or structured outpatient clinic is essential to supporting and treating those with mental illness. Within these small versions of society, people are safe to test new behaviors and increase their ability to interact adaptively within the outside community.

Community meetings usually include all patients and the treatment team. Functions include orienting new members to the unit, encouraging patients to engage in treatment, and evaluating the treatment program. Nursing staff are the largest group of providers and give valuable feedback to the team about group interactions. Goal-setting meetings may be conducted in inpatient settings and partial hospitalization programs to plan daily goals for each patient.

Other therapeutic milieu groups aim to help increase patients' self-esteem, decrease social isolation, encourage appropriate social behaviors, and educate patients in basic living skills. These groups are often led by occupational or recreational therapists, although nurses frequently co-lead them. Examples of therapeutic milieu groups are recreational groups, physical activity groups, creative arts groups, and storytelling groups.

Family Therapy

Family therapy developed around the mid-twentieth century as an adjunct to individual treatment and refers to the treatment of the family as a whole. Family therapists use a variety of theoretical philosophies to effect change in dysfunctional patterns of behavior and interaction. Some therapists may focus on the present, whereas others may rely more heavily on the family's history and reports of interactions between sessions. Terms related to family therapy are listed in Box 3-2.

Although different therapists may adhere to different theories and use a wide variety of methods, the goals of family therapy are basically the same. These goals include the following (Nichols, 2012):

- To reduce dysfunctional behavior of individual family members
- To resolve or reduce intrafamily relationship conflicts
- To mobilize family resources and encourage adaptive family problem-solving behaviors
- To improve family communication skills
- To heighten awareness and sensitivity to other family members' emotional needs and help family members meet their needs
- To strengthen the family's ability to cope with major life stressors and traumatic events, including chronic physical or psychiatric illness
- To improve integration of the family system into the societal system (e.g., school, medical facilities, workplace, and especially the extended family)

KEY POINTS TO REMEMBER

- Theoretical models and therapeutic strategies provide a useful framework for the delivery of psychiatric nursing care.
- The psychoanalytic model is based on unconscious motivations and the dynamic interplay between the primitive brain (id), the sense of self (ego), and the conscience (superego). The focus of psychoanalytic theory is on understanding the unconscious mind.
- The interpersonal model maintains that the personality and disorders are created by social forces and interpersonal experiences. Interpersonal therapy aims to provide positive and repairing interpersonal experiences.

- The behavioral model suggests that because behavior is learned, behavioral therapy should improve behavior through rewards and reinforcement of adaptive behavior.
- The humanist model is based on human potential, and therapy is aimed at maximizing this potential. Maslow developed a theory of personality that is based on the hierarchical satisfaction of needs. Rogers's person-centered theory uses self-actualizing tendencies to promote growth and healing.
- The cognitive model posits that disorders, especially depression, are the result of faulty thinking. Cognitive behavioral therapy is empirically supported and focuses on the recognition of distorted thinking and the replacement with more accurate and positive thoughts.
- The biological model is currently the dominant model and focuses on physical causation for personality problems and psychiatric disorders. Medication is the primary biological therapy.
- A variety of nursing theories are useful to psychiatric nursing. Hildegard Peplau developed an important interpersonal theory for the provision of psychiatric nursing care.
- Group therapy offers the patient significant interpersonal feedback from multiple people.
- Groups transition through predictable stages, benefit from therapeutic factors, and are characterized by members filling specific roles.
- Family therapy is based on various theoretical models and aims to decrease emotional reactivity among family members and encourage differentiation among individual family members.

APPLYING CRITICAL JUDGMENT

1. How could the theorists discussed in this chapter impact your nursing care? Specifically:
   A. How do Freud's concepts of the conscious, preconscious, and unconscious affect your understanding of patients' behaviors?
   B. What are the implications of Sullivan's focus on the importance of interpersonal relationships for your interactions with patients?
   C. Can you think of anyone who seems to be self-actualized? What is your reason for this conclusion?
   D. How do you utilize Maslow's hierarchy of needs in your nursing practice?
   E. What do you think about the behaviorist point of view that to change behaviors is to change personality?
2. Which of the therapies described here do you think can be the most helpful to you in your nursing practice? What are your reasons for this choice?

CHAPTER REVIEW QUESTIONS

1. A nurse plans a group meeting for adult patients in a therapeutic milieu. Which topic should the nurse include?
   a. Coping with grief and loss
   b. The importance of hand washing
   c. Strategies for money management
   d. Staffing shortages expected over the next 3 days
2. Considering Maslow's pyramid, which comment indicates an individual is motivated by the highest level of need?
   a. "Even though I'm 40 years old, I have returned to college so I can get a better job."
   b. "I help my community by volunteering at a thrift shop that raises money for the poor."
   c. "I recently applied for public assistance in order to feed my family, but I hope it's not forever."

d. "My children tell me I'm a good parent. I feel happy being part of a family that appreciates me."
3. Which patient is likely to achieve maximum benefit from cognitive behavioral therapy (CBT)?
   a. Older adult diagnosed with stage 3 Alzheimer's disease
   b. Adult diagnosed with schizophrenia and experiencing delusions
   c. Adult experiencing feelings of failure after losing the fourth job in 2 years
   d. School-age child diagnosed with attention-deficit/hyperactivity disorder (ADHD)
4. An adult plans to attend an upcoming tenth high school reunion. This person says to the nurse, "I am embarrassed to go. I will not look as good as my classmates. I haven't been successful in my career." Which comment by the nurse addresses this cognitive distortion?
   a. "You look fine to me. Do think you will have fun at your reunion?"
   b. "Everyone ages. Other classmates have had more problems than you."
   c. "Do you think you are the only person who has aged and faced difficulties in life?"
   d. "I think you are doing well in the face of the numerous problems you have endured."
5. A distraught 8-year-old girl tells the nurse, "I had a horrible nightmare and was so scared. I tried to get in bed with my parents but they said, 'No.' I think I could have gone back to sleep if I had been with them." Which family dynamic is likely the basis of this child's comment?
   a. Boundaries in the family are rigid.
   b. The family has poor differentiation of roles.
   c. The girl is enmeshed in part of a family triangle.
   d. Generational boundaries in the family are diffuse.

REFERENCES

Alligood, M. R. (2013). *Nursing theorists and their work* (8th ed.). Maryland Heights, Mo: Mosby/Elsevier.

American Psychiatric Nurses Association, International Society of Psychiatric-Mental Health Nurses, & American Nurses Association. (2014). *Psychiatric-mental health nursing: scope and standards of practice* (3rd ed.). Silver Spring, Md: American Nurses Association.

Arnold, E., & Boggs, K. U. (2016). *Interpersonal relationships: professional communication skills for nurses* (7th ed.). St. Louis: Saunders.

Beck, A. T. (1963). Thinking and depression. *Archives of General Psychiatry*, 9, 324–333.

Benne, K. D., & Sheats, F. (1948). Functional roles of group members. *Journal of Social Issues*, 4(2), 41–49.

Caldwell, B. A., Sclafani, M., Swarbrick, M., et al. (2010). Psychiatric nursing practice and the recovery model of care. *Journal of Psychosocial Nursing*, 48(7), 42–48.

Freud, S. (1961). The ego and id. In J. Strachey (Ed.), *The standard edition of the complete psychological works of Sigmund Freud vol. 19.* (pp. 3–66). London: Hogarth Press. (Original work published 1923.)

Jacobs, E. E., Masson, R. L., Harvill, R. L., et al. (2012). *Group counseling: strategies and skills* (7th ed.). Pacific Grove, Calif: Brooks/Cole.

Johnson, D. E. (1980). The behavioral system model for nursing. In J. P. Riehl & C. Roy (Eds.), *Conceptual models for nursing practice* (2nd ed.). New York: Appleton-Century-Crofts.

Karlsson, H. (2011). How psychotherapy changes the brain. *Psychiatric Times*, 28(8). Retrieved from www.nwmedicalhypnosis.com/documents/How%20Psychotherapy%20Changes%20the%20Brain.pdf.

King, I. M. (1981). *A theory for nursing: systems, concepts, process*. New York: Wiley.

Kohlberg, L., & Turiel, E. (1971). Moral development and moral education. In G. Lesser (Ed.), *Psychology and educational practice*. Scott, Foresman and Company.

Koltko-Rivera, M. E. (2006). Rediscovering the later version of Maslow's hierarchy of needs: self-transcendence and opportunities for theory, research, and unification. *Review of General Psychology by the American Psychological Association, 10* (4), 302–317.

Leininger, M. (1995). Culture care theory, research, and practice. *Nursing Science Quarterly, 9*(2), 71–78.

Maslow, A. H. (1970). *Motivation and personality* (2nd ed.). New York: Harper and Row.

McGuire, A. B., Kukla, M., Green, A., et al. (2014). Illness management and recovery: a review of the literature. *Psychiatric Services, 65*(2), 171–179.

Nichols, M. P. (2012). *Family therapy: concepts and methods* (10th ed.). Upper Saddle River, NJ: Prentice Hall.

Orem, D. E. (2001). *Nursing: concepts of practice* (6th ed.). St. Louis, Mo: Mosby.

Orlando, I. J. (1990). *The dynamic nurse-patient relationship: function, process, and principles* (Pub. No. 15–2341). New York: National League for Nursing.

Pavlov, I. P. (1927). *Conditioned reflexes*. London: Routledge and Kegan Paul.

Peplau, H. E. (1952). *Interpersonal relations in nursing: a conceptual frame of reference for psychodynamic nursing*. New York: Putnam.

Peplau, H. E. (1992). *Interpersonal relations in nursing*. New York: Putnam.

Piaget, J., & Inhelder, B. (1969). *The psychology of the child*. New York: Basic Books.

Rogers, C. R. (1986). Carl Rogers on the development of the person-centered approach. *Person-Centered Review, 1*(3), 257–259.

Sadock, B. J., Sadock, V. A., & Ruiz, P. (2015). *Synopsis of psychiatry* (11th ed.). Philadelphia: Walters Kluwer.

Skinner, B. F. (1938). *The behavior of organisms*. New York: Appleton-Century-Crofts.

Sullivan, H. S. (1953). *The interpersonal theory of psychiatry*. New York: Norton.

Tuckman, B. W. (1965). Developmental sequence in small groups. *Psychological Bulletin, 63*, 384–399.

Tuckman, B. W., & Jensen, M. A. (1977). Stages of small-group development revisited. *Group & Organization Management, 2*, 419–427.

Watson, J. (2007). Watson Caring Science Institute. Retrieved April 13, 2011, from www.watsoncaringscience.org/caring_science/index.html.

Watson, J. B. (1930). *Behaviorism* (rev. ed.). Chicago, Ill: University of Chicago Press.

Yalom, I. D. (1985). *The theory and practice of group psychotherapy*. New York: Basic Books.

Biological Basis for Understanding Psychopharmacology

Dorothy A. Varchol

ⓔ http://evolve.elsevier.com/Varcarolis/essentials

KEY TERMS AND CONCEPTS

SELECTED CONCEPT: PHARMACOGENETICS

Pharmacology and genetics have merged into a new field called pharmacogenetics.

Genetic factors play a role in how individuals respond to drugs (if it works on them or not) and the side effects experienced (toxicity or tolerates well). How a drug is used in the body is determined by genetically mediated patterns of protein structures, receptor sensitivities, enzyme activity, and drug metabolism. These differences not only are present through individual genetic factors but also are greatly determined by ethnic associations as well.

Psychogenetics may one day lead to personalized medications, safer drugs, and targeted pharmacological therapies determined by genetically inherited factors.

(Preston et al., 2013)

OBJECTIVES

1. Identify at least three major brain structures and eight major brain functions that can be altered by mental illness and psychotropic medications.
2. Describe how **evidence-based neuroimaging** is helpful in understanding abnormalities of brain function, structure, and receptor pharmacology.
3. Explain the basic process of neurotransmission and synaptic transmission using Figures 4-5, 4-6, and 4-7.
4. Identify the main neurotransmitter systems affected by the following psychotropic drugs:
   a. Antidepressants
   b. Antianxiety agents
   c. Sedative-hypnotics
   d. Mood stabilizers
   e. Antipsychotic agents
   f. Anticholinesterase drugs
5. **QSEN** Explain the relevance of psychodynamic and psychokinetic drug interactions in the delivery of **safe, effective nursing care.**
6. **QSEN** Discuss safety concerns related to dietary and drug restrictions with monoamine oxidase inhibitors (MAOIs).
7. Compare and contrast typical and atypical antipsychotic drugs with regard to their side effect profile and quality of life.
8. Discuss the relationship between the immune system and the nervous system in mental health and mental illness.
9. Describe how genes and culture affect an individual's response to psychotropic medication.

INTRODUCTION

A primary goal of psychiatric mental health nursing is to understand the evidence underlying the neurobiology of psychiatric disorders and how psychotropic medications help manage a constellation of symptoms and reduce the risk of relapse. Because all brain functions are carried out by similar mechanisms (interactions of neurons), often in similar locations, it is not surprising that mental disturbances are frequently associated with alterations in other brain functions and that the drugs used to treat mental disturbances can also interfere with other activities of the brain. Box 4-1 summarizes some of the major brain functions.

BRAIN STRUCTURES AND FUNCTIONS

Cerebrum

Basic neural architecture is genetically programmed, but plasticity is evident throughout life as gray matter shrinks or thickens and synaptic connections are pruned or forged. Loss of cortical tissue has been associated with schizophrenia as well as with treatment involving haloperidol and typical antipsychotics. In contrast, some newer atypical antipsychotics and antidepressants have been found to increase brain volume and structural synaptic/neuronal plasticity (Paulzen et al., 2014).

Each hemisphere of the cerebral cortex is divided into four lobes (Figure 4-1) that control sensory and motor function as well as higher mental activities. The **prefrontal cortex (PFC)** coordinates complex cognitive functions and enables us to plan and execute goals. When circuitry in the PFC is impaired by a mental disorder (e.g., schizophrenia, major depression, addiction), there is a decrease in executive function, attention, impulse control, socialization, regulation of drives (such as libido), and emotions. Drugs targeting specific molecules within PFC circuits are being developed to normalize disrupted PFC activity.

In addition to the gray matter forming the cortex, there are pockets of integrating gray matter lying deep within the cerebrum: the hippocampus, the amygdala, and the basal ganglia. The **hippocampus** interacts with the PFC in making new memories. The **amygdala** plays a major role in processing fear and anxiety. The hippocampus and amygdala, along with the hypothalamus and thalamus, are part of a circle of structures called the limbic system or "emotional brain." Chronic stress triggers shrinkage of the hippocampus and gray matter in the PFC. These changes may mediate vulnerability to depression, addiction, and other stress-related disorders (Ansell et al., 2012). Experimental medication for major depressive disorder (MDD) is being investigated to increase the size of the hippocampus and the density of healthy neurons (Neuralstem Inc., 2015). Structural plasticity of both the hippocampus and the amygdala is induced by electroconvulsive therapy in MDD, especially in individuals with smaller hippocampal volumes at baseline (Joshi et al., 2016). Amygdala hyperactivity is common in trauma and may underlie paranoia in schizophrenia (Pinkham et al., 2015). Amygdala hypoactivity predicts a general capacity to respond to antidepressants (Williams et al., 2015).

Linking the frontal cortex, basal ganglia, and upper brainstem, the limbic system mediates thought and feeling through complex, bidirectional connections. Antianxiety drugs (**anxiolytics**) slow the limbic system. Subcortical basal ganglia play a major role in motor responses via the extrapyramidal motor system, which relies on the neurotransmitter dopamine to maintain proper muscle tone and motor stability. Neuroimaging shows that haloperidol can reduce striatal volume within hours, temporarily changing brain structure and producing abnormal involuntary motor symptoms (extrapyramidal symptoms [EPS]). In the basal ganglia, two types of movement disturbances may occur: (1) acute EPS, which develops early in treatment; and (2) tardive

---

dyskinesia (TD), which usually occurs much later. First-generation antipsychotics (FGAs) (typical agents) and high doses of second-generation antipsychotics (SGAs) (atypical agents) such as risperidone are most likely to cause EPS.

It is important to remember that movement is regulated by the basal ganglia, including the diaphragm—essential for breathing—and the muscles of the throat, tongue, and mouth—essential for speech. Thus drugs that affect brain function can stimulate or depress respiration or affect speech patterns (e.g., slurred speech).

Brainstem

Basic vital life functions occur through the brainstem, composed of the midbrain, pons, and medulla (Figure 4-2).

Through projections called the reticular activating system (RAS), the brainstem sets the level of consciousness and regulates the cycle of sleep and wakefulness. Unfortunately, drugs used to treat psychiatric problems may interfere with the regulation of sleep and alertness, thus the warning to take sedating drugs at bedtime and to use caution while driving.

Cerebellum

The cerebellum (see Figure 4-2) contributes to both motor control and cognitive processing. Alterations in cerebello-thalamo-cortical circuits may manifest as disturbances of coordination, balance, and gait as well as impaired attentional and emotional control in schizophrenia (Parker et al., 2014). Although it is believed that lithium targets an abnormally functioning cerebellum in bipolar disorder, a combination of antipsychotic drugs and lithium may cause cerebellar damage (Johnson et al., 2015).

Thalamus

The thalamus filters sensory information before it reaches the cerebral cortex. Disrupted sensory filtering in schizophrenia is associated with altered connections between the thalamus and prefrontal cortex (PFC). Deep brain stimulation (DBS) changes electrical impulses in the cortico-basal ganglia-thalamic loops and is being investigated in treating chronic, severe depression, obsessive-compulsive disorder, anorexia nervosa, and other psychiatric disorders (Karas et al., 2013).

Hypothalamus

The **hypothalamus** maintains homeostasis. It regulates temperature, blood pressure, perspiration, libido, hunger, thirst, and circadian rhythms, such as sleep and wakefulness. Hypothalamic **neurohormones**, often called releasing hormones, direct the secretion of hormones from the anterior pituitary gland. For example, **corticotropin-releasing hormone (CRH)** is secreted in response to stress.

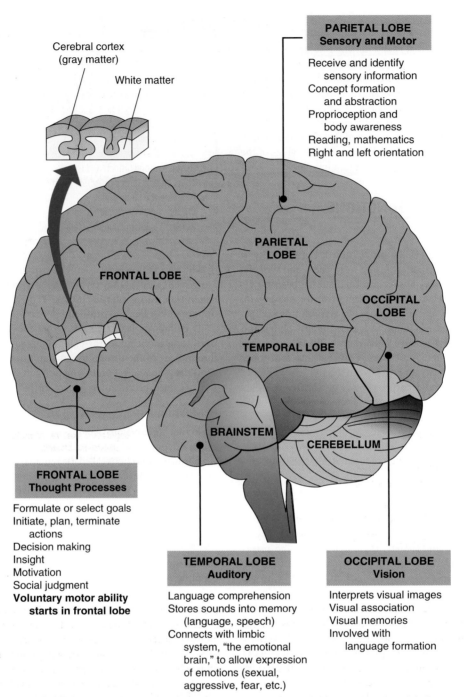

Cerebral cortex (gray matter)

White matter

PARIETAL LOBE
Sensory and Motor

Receive and identify
    sensory information
Concept formation
    and abstraction
Proprioception and
    body awareness
Reading, mathematics
Right and left orientation

PARIETAL LOBE

FRONTAL LOBE

OCCIPITAL LOBE

TEMPORAL LOBE

BRAINSTEM

CEREBELLUM

FRONTAL LOBE
Thought Processes

Formulate or select goals
Initiate, plan, terminate
    actions
Decision making
Insight
Motivation
Social judgment
Voluntary motor ability
starts in frontal lobe

TEMPORAL LOBE
Auditory

Language comprehension
Stores sounds into memory
    (language, speech)
Connects with limbic
    system, "the emotional
    brain," to allow expression
    of emotions (sexual,
    aggressive, fear, etc.)

OCCIPITAL LOBE
Vision

Interprets visual images
Visual association
Visual memories
Involved with
    language formation

FIGURE 4-1 Functions of the cerebral lobes: frontal, parietal, temporal, and occipital.

It stimulates the pituitary to release corticotropin, which in turn stimulates the cortex of each adrenal gland to secrete cortisol. This system is disrupted in depression, anxiety, insomnia, substance use disorder, and Alzheimer's dementia, but abnormalities in the system may someday be reversed by CRH antagonists (Beyer & Stahl, 2010).

The hypothalamic-pituitary-thyroid axis is involved in the regulation of nearly every organ system because all major hormones and catecholamines (e.g., cortisol, gonadal hormones, insulin) depend on thyroid status. Thyroid hormones are used to treat people with depression or rapid-cycling bipolar I disorder. They are also used as replacement therapy for people who develop a hypothyroid state from lithium treatment (Sadock et al., 2015).

The hypothalamic neurohormone dopamine inhibits the release of prolactin. When excess dopamine is blocked by the first-generation

(typical) antipsychotic drugs, blood prolactin levels increase (hyperprolactinemia) with subsequent amenorrhea, galactorrhea (milk flow), gynecomastia (development of breast tissue), or sexual dysfunction. Among antipsychotics, FGAs and the SGA (atypical) drug risperidone are the most frequent offenders whereas most SGAs (atypicals) are prolactin sparing.

In addition to working with the endocrine system, the hypothalamus sends instructions to the **autonomic nervous system,** which is divided into the **sympathetic and parasympathetic systems** (Figure 4-3).

The sympathetic system is highly activated by sympathomimetic drugs, such as amphetamine and cocaine, as well as by withdrawal from sedating drugs, such as alcohol, benzodiazepines, and opioids (Sadock et al., 2015). Sympathomimetics are first-line drugs for treating attention-deficit/hyperactivity disorder (ADHD). In low doses,

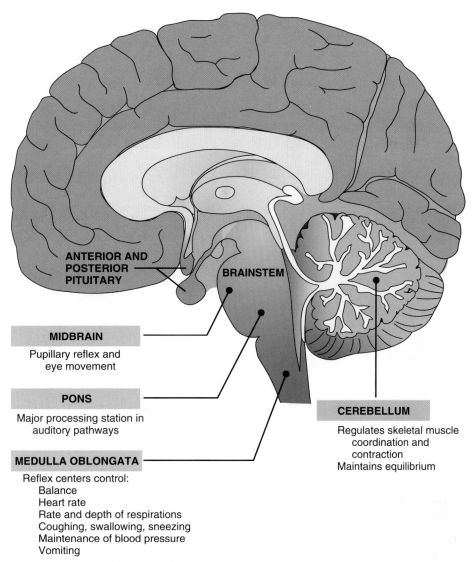

FIGURE 4-2 Functions of the brainstem and cerebellum.

stimulants improve focus and thinking by increasing synaptic levels of neurotransmitters, dopamine and norepinephrine. Higher doses cause cognitive impairment and locomotor activation. Both methylphenidates (e.g., Ritalin and Concerti) and amphetamines (e.g., Adderall) have the potential for abuse when taken in excessive doses or through routes other than oral (Brown, 2013). Lisdexamfetamine (Vyvanse) is a unique extended-release formulation that has been designated a "prodrug" to prevent abuse because its active ingredient is bound to an amino acid that has to be removed by an enzyme in the intestine before it works. A common side effect of stimulants is loss of appetite and loss of weight, which can often be managed by giving medications with meals and by maximizing caloric intake with snacks when "off" medications (e.g., at breakfast or for a bedtime snack).

Visualizing the Brain

Neuroimaging visualizes a brain that is structurally and functionally interconnected. Some common brain imaging techniques that measure structure and function are identified in Table 4-1.

Functional neuroimaging with positron emission tomography (PET) and single photon emission computed tomography (SPECT) use ionizing radiation to localize brain regions associated with perceptual, cognitive, emotional, and behavioral functions. Based on the increase in blood flow to the local vasculature that accompanies neural

activity, PET scans have provided evidence of decreased metabolism in unmedicated individuals with depression or schizophrenia and increased metabolism in obsessive-compulsive disorder (Figure 4-4). PET and SPECT have also shown dopamine system dysregulation in schizophrenia and loss of monoamines in depression.

Functional magnetic resonance imaging (fMRI) measures how well two regions of the brain communicate with each other. In patients suffering from first-episode schizophrenia, fMRI demonstrates that individual differences in striatal functional connectivity predict response to antipsychotic drug treatment. Researchers hope that this Striatal Connectivity Index (SCI) will eventually predict who will respond to medications and who will not (Sarpal et al., 2016).

CELLULAR COMPOSITION OF THE BRAIN

Neurons

The brain is composed of a vast network of more than 100 billion interconnected nerve cells (neurons) and supporting cells. An essential feature of neurons is their ability to initiate signals and conduct an electrical impulse from one end of the cell to the other, called neurotransmission (Figure 4-5). Electrical signals within neurons are then converted at synapses into chemical signals through the release of

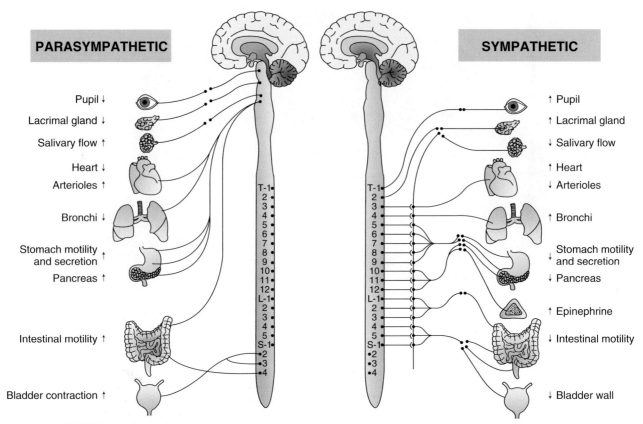

FIGURE 4-3 Autonomic nervous system has two divisions: sympathetic and parasympathetic. The sympathetic division is dominant in stress situations, such as fear and anger—known as the fight-or-flight response.

TABLE 4-1 Common Brain Imaging Techniques

Technique	Description	Uses	Clinical Research Examples
Structural: Show Gross Anatomical Details of Brain Structures			
Computed tomography (CT)	Series of x-ray images are taken of brain, and computer analysis produces "slices," providing a 3D-like reconstruction of each segment	Can detect lesions, abrasions, areas of infarct, aneurysm	**Schizophrenia** Gray matter reduction Ventricle abnormalities
Magnetic resonance imaging (MRI)	Uses a magnetic field and radio waves to produce cross-sectional images	Used to exclude neurological disorders in those presenting with mental illness	**Schizophrenia** Same as CT (but higher resolution)
Functional magnetic resonance imaging (fMRI)	Relies on magnetic properties to see images of blood flow in brain as it occurs; avoids exposure to radioactive isotopes	Can detect edema, ischemia, infection, neoplasm, trauma Detects blood flow to functionally active brain regions	
Functional: Show Some Activity of the Brain			
Positron emission tomography (PET)	Radioactive substance is injected, travels to brain, and appears as bright spots on scan; data collected by detectors are relayed to a computer, which produces images of activity and 3D visualization of central nervous system	Can detect oxygen utilization, glucose metabolism, blood flow, neurotransmitter receptor interaction	**Schizophrenia** Decreased metabolic activity in frontal lobes Dopamine system dysregulation Blockade of dopamine receptors with antipsychotic medications **Depression** Blockade of serotonin transporter receptors with antidepressant medications **Alzheimer's disease** Reduction in nicotinic receptor subtype
Single photon emission computed tomography (SPECT)	Similar to PET but uses γ-radiation (photons) SPECT is less costly, but resolution is poorer	Similar to PET	See PET

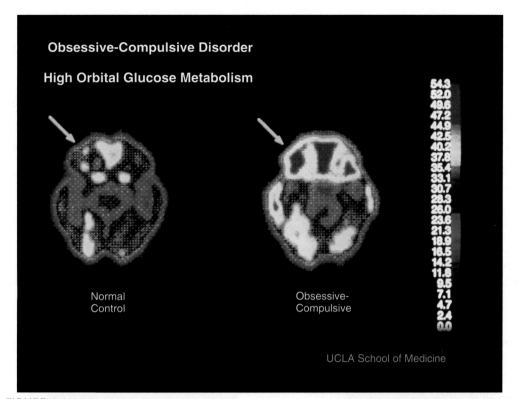

FIGURE 4-4 Positron emission tomographic scans show increased brain metabolism *(brighter colors),* particularly in the frontal cortex, in a patient with obsessive-compulsive disorder (OCD), compared with a normal control. This suggests altered brain function in OCD. (From Lewis Baxter, MD, University of Alabama, courtesy National Institute of Mental Health.)

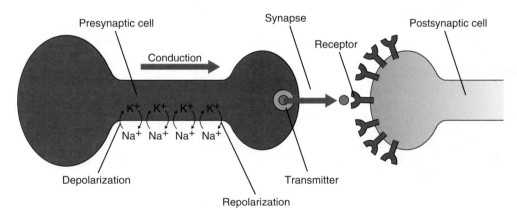

FIGURE 4-5 Activities of neurons. Conduction along a neuron involves the inward movement of sodium ions (Na+) followed by the outward movement of potassium ions (K+). When the current reaches the end of the cell, a neurotransmitter is released. The transmitter crosses the synapse and attaches to a receptor on the postsynaptic cell. The attachment of a transmitter to a receptor either stimulates or inhibits the postsynaptic cell.

molecules called **neurotransmitters,** which then elicit electrical signals on the other side of the synapse.

Synaptic Transmission

Once an electrical impulse reaches the end of a neuron, the neurotransmitter is released from the axon terminal at the presynaptic neuron and diffuses across a **synapse** to a postsynaptic neuron. Here it attaches to specialized **receptors** on the cell surface and either inhibits or excites the postsynaptic neuron. It is the interaction between neurotransmitter and receptor that is a major target of psychotropic drugs. Figure 4-6

shows how an insufficient degree of transmission may be caused by a deficient release of neurotransmitters from the presynaptic cell or by a decrease in receptors. Figure 4-7 illustrates how excessive transmission may be due to excessive release of a transmitter or to increased receptor responsiveness, as occurs in schizophrenia.

After attaching to a receptor and exerting its influence on the postsynaptic cell, the transmitter separates from the receptor and is destroyed. Some transmitters (e.g., acetylcholine) are destroyed by specific enzymes (e.g., acetylcholinesterase). In the case of monoamine transmitters, the destructive enzyme is monoamine oxidase (MAO).

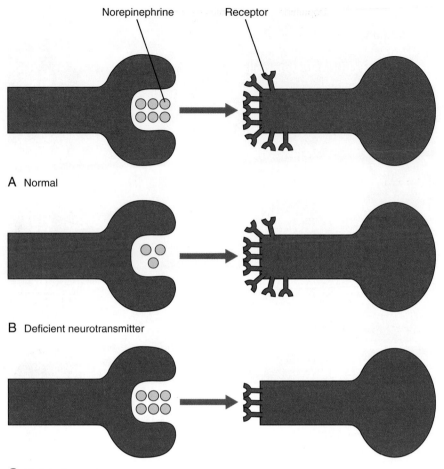

Norepinephrine   Receptor

A Normal

B Deficient neurotransmitter

C Deficient receptor

FIGURE 4-6 Normal transmission of neurotransmitters **(A).** Deficiency in transmission may be caused by a deficient release of transmitter, as shown in **B,** or by a reduction in receptors, as shown in **C.**

Other transmitters are taken back into the cell from which they were originally released by a process called cellular reuptake. The transmitters are then either reused or destroyed by intracellular enzymes. The two basic mechanisms of destruction are described in Box 4-2.

Neurotransmitters

A **neurotransmitter** is a chemical messenger between neurons by which one neuron triggers another. Four major groups of neurotransmitters in the brain are monoamines (biogenic amines), amino acids, peptides, and cholinergics (e.g., acetylcholine). Monoamine neurotransmitters (**dopamine, norepinephrine, serotonin**) and acetylcholine are implicated in a variety of neuropsychiatric disorders.

Amino acid neurotransmitters, such as the inhibitory γ-aminobutyric acid (GABA) and the excitatory **glutamate,** balance brain activity. Peptide neurotransmitters such as hypothalamic CRH modulate or adjust general brain function. Table 4-2 lists important neurotransmitters, types of receptors to which they attach, and mental disorders that are associated with an increase or decrease in the levels of neurotransmitters.

Interaction of Neurons, Neurotransmitters, and Receptors

Most psychotropic drugs produce effects by altering synaptic concentrations of dopamine, acetylcholine, norepinephrine, serotonin, histamine, GABA, or glutamate. These changes are thought to result from activation of receptor antagonists (blocking neurotransmitter activity)

or agonists (promoting neurotransmitter activity), interference with neurotransmitter reuptake, enhancement of neurotransmitter release, or inhibition of enzymes.

Dopamine

The monoamine **dopamine** is an important neurotransmitter involved in cognition, motivation, and movement. It controls emotional responses and the brain's reward and pleasure centers, stimulates the heart, and increases blood flow to vital organs.

Drugs such as cocaine interfere with reuptake of dopamine, thereby allowing more of the neurotransmitter to stay active in the synapse for a longer time. The dopamine hypothesis of schizophrenia originated from the observation that drugs (e.g., amphetamines) that stimulate dopamine activity can induce psychotic symptoms, whereas drugs that block dopamine receptors (e.g., haloperidol) have antipsychotic activity.

Acetylcholine

Dopamine is balanced by acetylcholine, which is released by cholinergic neurons. Acetylcholine plays a role in skeletal muscle movement, arousal, memory, and the sleep/wake cycle. Because acetylcholine is deficient in Alzheimer's disease, drugs have been developed to inhibit the enzyme that degrades acetylcholine (i.e., acetylcholinesterase). **Acetylcholinesterase (AChE) inhibitors** such as donepezil (Aricept), galantamine (Razadyne), and rivastigmine (Exelon) are prescribed to delay cognitive decline in Alzheimer's disease.

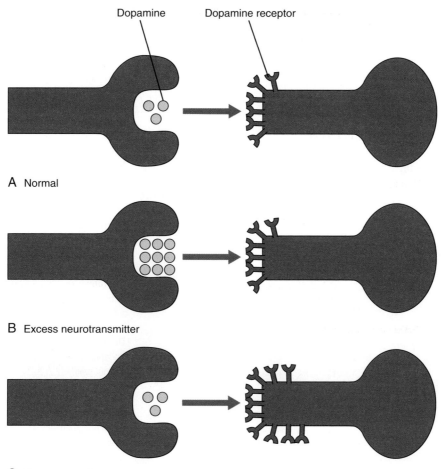

Dopamine   Dopamine receptor

A Normal

B Excess neurotransmitter

C Excess receptors

FIGURE 4-7 Causes of excess transmission of neurotransmitters **(A)**. Excess transmission may be caused by excess release of transmitter, as shown in **B,** or excess responsiveness of receptors, as shown in **C.**

BOX 4-2   Destruction of Neurotransmitters

A full explanation of the various ways in which psychotropic drugs alter neuronal activity requires a brief review of the manner in which neurotransmitters are destroyed after attaching to the receptors. To avoid continuous and prolonged action on the postsynaptic cell, the neurotransmitter is released shortly after attaching to the postsynaptic receptor. Once released, the transmitter is destroyed in one of two ways.

One way is the immediate inactivation of the transmitter at the postsynaptic membrane. An example of this method of destruction is the action of the enzyme acetylcholinesterase on the neurotransmitter acetylcholine. Acetylcholinesterase is present at the postsynaptic membrane and destroys acetylcholine shortly after it attaches to nicotinic or muscarinic receptors on the postsynaptic cell.

A *second* method of neurotransmitter inactivation is a little more complex. After interacting with the postsynaptic receptor, the transmitter is released and taken back into the presynaptic cell, the cell from which it was released. This process, referred to as the reuptake of neurotransmitter, is a common target for drug action. Once inside the presynaptic cell, the transmitter is either recycled or inactivated by an enzyme within the cell. The monoamine neurotransmitters norepinephrine, dopamine, and serotonin are all inactivated in this manner by the enzyme monoamine oxidase.

In looking at this second method, one might naturally ask what prevents the enzyme from destroying the transmitter before its release. The answer is that before release the transmitter is stored within a membrane and is thus protected from the degradative enzyme. After release and reuptake, the transmitter is either destroyed by the enzyme or reenters the membrane to be reused.

Although all acetylcholine receptors respond to acetylcholine, they also respond to other molecules. For example, nicotinic acetylcholine receptors are particularly responsive to nicotine. People with schizophrenia and attention problems may be more likely to smoke as a way of normalizing cognitive and sensory deficits. Because these individuals are also more likely to suffer adverse effects, scientists are trying to develop drugs that target nicotine receptors without the carcinogenic, cardiovascular, and addictive effects.

Norepinephrine

Norepinephrine (NE) is released from noradrenergic neurons. Low levels of NE are linked to low arousal (e.g., sedation) and depression. High levels can create a feeling of hyperarousal. NE is primarily an activator of α-receptors, subdivided into $\alpha 1$- and $\alpha 2$-receptors. Prazosin, an antihypertensive drug, blocks excessive responsiveness to NE at postsynaptic α_1-adrenergic receptors and shows promise for treating nightmares in posttraumatic stress disorder (Koola et al., 2014). Many FGA (conventional) antipsychotic drugs act as antagonists at the α_1-receptor for NE. Blockage of these receptors can cause vasodilation and a consequent drop in blood pressure, or orthostatic hypotension. Blockage of α_1-receptors on the vas deferens can lead to a failure to ejaculate.

Serotonin

Serotonin (5-HT), found in the brain and spinal cord, helps regulate mood, arousal, attention, behavior, and body temperature. When some antidepressants are combined with other drugs or supplements that

TABLE 4-2 Transmitters and Receptors

Transmitters	Receptors	Functions	Clinical Relevance
Monoamines			
Dopamine (DA)	D_1, D_2, D_3, D_4, D_5	Fine muscle movement Integration of emotions and thoughts Decision making Stimulates hypothalamus to release hormones (sex, thyroid, adrenal)	**Increase:** Schizophrenia Mania **Decrease:** Parkinson's disease Depression
Norepinephrine (NE) (noradrenaline)	α_1, α_2, β_1, β_2	Mood Attention and arousal Stimulates sympathetic branch of autonomic nervous system for "fight or flight" in response to stress	**Increase:** Mania Anxiety Schizophrenia **Decrease:** Depression
Serotonin (5-HT)	5-HT, 5-HT_2, 5-HT_3, 5-HT_4	Mood Sleep regulation Hunger Pain perception Aggression and libido Hormonal activity	**Increase:** Anxiety states **Decrease:** Depression
Histamine	H_1, H_2	Alertness Inflammatory response Stimulates gastric secretion	**Decrease:** Sedation Weight gain
Amino Acids			
γ-Aminobutyric acid (GABA)	$GABA_A$, $GABA_B$	**Inhibitory neurotransmitter:** Reduces anxiety, excitation, aggression May play a role in pain perception Anticonvulsant and muscle-relaxing properties May impair cognition and psychomotor functioning	**Increase:** Reduction of anxiety **Decrease:** Mania Anxiety Schizophrenia
Glutamate	NMDA, AMPA	**Excitatory neurotransmitter:** AMPA plays a role in learning and memory	**Increase NMDA:** Prolonged increase can kill neurons (neurotoxicity) Neurodegeneration in Alzheimer's disease **Decrease NMDA:** Psychosis **Increase AMPA:** Improvement of cognitive performance in behavioral tasks
Cholinergics			
Acetylcholine (ACh)	Nicotinic, muscarinic (M_1, M_2, M_3)	Plays a role in learning, memory Regulates mood: mania, sexual aggression Affects sexual and aggressive behavior Stimulates parasympathetic nervous system	**Decrease:** Alzheimer's disease Huntington's chorea Parkinson's disease **Increase:** Depression
Peptides (Neuromodulators)			
Substance P (SP)	SP	Centrally active SP antagonist has antidepressant and antianxiety effects in depression Promotes and reinforces memory Enhances sensitivity to pain receptors to activate	Involved in regulation of mood and anxiety Role in pain management
Somatostatin (SRIF)	SRIF	Altered levels associated with cognitive disease	**Decrease:** Alzheimer's disease Decreased levels of SRIF in spinal fluid of some depressed patients **Increase:** Huntington's chorea
Neurotensin (NT)	NT	Endogenous antipsychotic-like properties	Decreased levels in spinal fluid of schizophrenic patients

AMPA, α-Amino-3-hydroxy-5-methyl-4-isoxazolepropionic acid; NMDA, N-methyl-D-aspartate; SRIF, somatotropin release-inhibiting factor.

increase serotonin production (e.g., St. John's wort or over-the-counter cough and cold medications containing dextromethorphan), serotonin syndrome may occur. Symptoms of high levels of serotonin range from mild (restlessness, shivering, and diarrhea) to severe (muscle rigidity, fever, and seizures). These symptoms can be alleviated by muscle relaxants and drugs that block serotonin production. Research is shifting from antidepressants that elevate serotonin levels to new drugs that strengthen serotonergic signaling.

Regulation of the serotonin transporter (SERT), a protein that facilitates transport of serotonin into the cell, is a key action for major antidepressants. Blockade of SERT by a selective serotonin reuptake inhibitor leads to a decreased concentration of serotonin within platelets and a slight inhibition of platelet aggregation. Therefore, the risk of bleeding should be mentioned to patients taking nonsteroidal anti-inflammatory drugs (NSAIDs), aspirin, warfarin, or antiplatelet drugs.

Histamine

Many FGA's (conventional) antipsychotic agents, as well as a variety of other psychiatric drugs, block the H_1 receptors for **histamine.** Two significant side effects of blocking these receptors are sedation and substantial weight gain. Sedation may be beneficial in severely agitated patients, but weight gain can lead to disturbances in glucose and lipid metabolism and insulin resistance.

γ-Aminobutyric Acid (GABA)

The major inhibitory neurotransmitter γ-aminobutyric acid (GABA) modulates neuronal excitability and is associated with the regulation of anxiety. Most antianxiety (anxiolytic) drugs act by increasing the effectiveness of GABA primarily by increasing receptor responsiveness. Selective serotonin reuptake inhibitors augmentation of antipsychotics produces synergistic changes in $GABA_A$ receptors and related signaling systems that may ameliorate core features of schizophrenia (Silver et al., 2013). Since GABA neurons suppress dopamine release, a novel antipsychotic drug targeting dopamine hyperactivity and GABA hypoactivity might lead to a new and better option for treating schizophrenia.

Glutamate

Glutamate, a potent excitatory neurotransmitter, activates the N-methyl-D-aspartate (NMDA) receptor. Any disruption in this pathway leading to either enhanced or decreased activity may result in neuropsychiatric symptoms. High concentrations of glutamate or overly sensitive receptors can lead to cell death, as occurs in neurodegenerative conditions such as Alzheimer's disease. As a corollary, NMDA receptor antagonists, such as the drug memantine, decrease excitability and neurotoxicity. Glutamate acts at several receptor types in addition to NMDA, and it is the balance between these receptors as well as the balance between glutamate and GABA that may be critical in slowing the progression of psychosis (Kantrowitz & Javitt, 2011). An investigational drug, ITI-007, has a unique serotonergic-dopaminergic-glutamatergic profile that represents a new approach to treating schizophrenia (Melville, 2015). Both NMDA and α-amino-3-hydroxy-5-methyl-4-isoxazolepropionic acid (AMPA) receptors are binding sites for glutamate, and the interplay of the two receptors is being explored in developing ketamine-like drugs to rapidly reverse depressive symptoms.

PSYCHOTROPIC DRUGS AND INTERACTIONS

Psychotropic drugs work by mechanisms not yet fully understood, and understanding their action has become more challenging when drug interactions alter or modify their effects.

Pharmacokinetic interactions occur when one drug alters the absorption, distribution, metabolism, or elimination of another, thereby affecting plasma concentrations. Most pharmacokinetic interactions result from inhibition or induction of cytochrome P450 (CYP450) enzymes. Potent CYP450 inhibitors added to drugs metabolized by CYP450 enzymes increase drug concentrations and the risk for toxicity. CYP450 inducers decrease concentrations and result in decreased efficacy unless the dose is increased. With the exception of paliperidone, all SGA (atypical) antipsychotics undergo extensive hepatic metabolism and can be altered by CYP450 inducers or inhibitors.

Genomic tests provide information on which medications each individual can metabolize properly, primarily focusing on pharmacokinetic genes from the CYP450 family and pharmacodynamic genes related to the regulation of neurotransmitters. For example, GeneSight pharmacogenomics technology covers Food and Drug Administration (FDA)-approved medications for people diagnosed with behavioral health conditions such as schizophrenia, depression, anxiety, bipolar disorder, PTSD, and ADHD (GeneSight website, 2015).

Pharmacodynamic interactions occur when drugs act at the same or interrelated receptor sites, resulting in synergistic or antagonistic effects (Demler, 2012). For example, coadministration of higher dosages of a dopamine receptor antagonist (DRA) and lithium may result in a synergistic increase in neurological side effects and EPS (Sadock et al., 2015). Managing drug interactions is complicated by comorbid conditions and polypharmacy, especially in older adults.

ANTIDEPRESSANT DRUGS

Several hypotheses of depression have been proposed for the action of antidepressants:

1. The monoamine hypothesis suggests a lack of three monoamines (dopamine, norepinephrine, or serotonin) in various brain regions. However, there is no clear evidence that monoamine deficiency accounts for depression.
2. The monoamine receptor hypothesis suggests that low levels of neurotransmitters cause increased receptor sensitivity (up-regulation) over time; thus it may take several weeks for patients to feel better when they are taking antidepressants.
3. More recent hypotheses focus on "downstream molecular events" that the receptors trigger, including the regulation of genes. For example, one hypothesis is that the gene for brain-derived neurotrophic factor (BDNF) is repressed in depression and may be activated by antidepressants.

Monoamine Oxidase Inhibitors (MAOIs)

To understand the action of these drugs, keep in mind the following definitions:

- Monoamines: a type of organic compound, including the neurotransmitters, that are further divided into subgroups called catecholamines (e.g., norepinephrine, epinephrine, dopamine) and indolamines (e.g., serotonin) and many different drugs and food substances
- Monoamine oxidase (MAO): an enzyme that destroys monoamines
- Monoamine oxidase inhibitors (MAOIs): drugs that increase concentrations of monoamines by inhibiting the action of MAO (Figure 4-8)

Because MAOIs block the enzyme that metabolizes monoamines, they may occasionally be used to increase the levels of serotonin and norepinephrine in intractable depression. However, selective serotonin reuptake inhibitors (SSRIs) and serotonin-norepinephrine reuptake inhibitors (SNRIs) are the more commonly used antidepressants because of the vasopressor effects that occur when MAOIs are combined with other sympathomimetics (amines that stimulate the sympathetic nervous system). The most feared vasopressor effect is the **hypertensive crisis** that can result if a patient takes over-the-counter

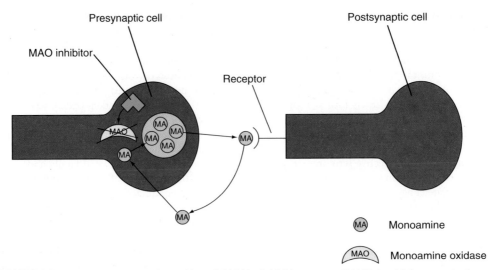

FIGURE 4-8 Blocking of monoamine oxidase (MAO) by inhibiting agents (MAOIs), which prevents the breakdown of monoamine by MAO.

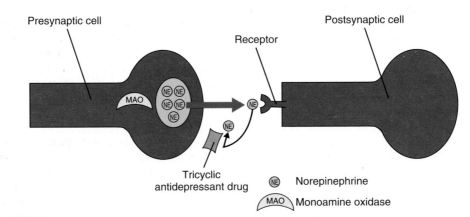

FIGURE 4-9 Mechanism by which tricyclic antidepressant drugs block the reuptake of norepinephrine.

medications with pseudoephedrine or consumes the adrenergic mono-amine tyramine, commonly found in aged foods, fermented foods, and certain beverages. Dietary restriction of tyramine must be maintained for 2 weeks after stopping MAOIs to allow the body to resynthesize the MAO enzyme. The EMSAM patch delivers the MAOI selegiline through the skin and has diminished hypertensive effects compared with the oral preparations phenelzine (Nardil) and tranylcypromine (Parnate). However, dietary precautions are still required. Chapter 15 contains a list of foods and beverages to avoid while taking MAOIs and gives nursing measures and instructions for teaching patients who are taking MAOIs. For a more detailed description of how MAOIs work, visit the Evolve website at http://evolve.elsevier.com/Varcarolis/essentials.

Tricyclic Antidepressants (TCAs)

Originally termed tricyclic antidepressants (TCAs), these agents are more accurately called *cyclic antidepressants (CAs)* because newer members of this class have a four-ring structure. TCAs, such as ami-triptyline (Elavil) and nortriptyline (Pamelor), act primarily by block-ing the presynaptic transporter protein receptors for norepinephrine and, to a lesser degree, serotonin (Figure 4-9). This blocking prevents norepinephrine from coming into contact with its degrading enzyme, MAO, and thus increases the level of norepinephrine at the synapse.

Multiple pharmacological mechanisms of TCAs have proven beneficial in treating difficult cases of depression and chronic pain. However, multiple actions on several receptors also earned TCAs the name "dirty drugs" because of their many side effects. For example, to varying degrees TCAs block muscarinic receptors that normally bind acetylcholine, leading to anticholinergic effects. Again to varying degrees, TCAs block H_1 receptors, causing sedation and weight gain. Strong binding at adrenergic receptors causes dizziness and hypoten-sion, thereby increasing the risk for falls. Pharmacokinetics must be considered in TCA overdose fatalities because TCAs are highly lipid soluble and rapidly absorbed. This may result in cardiotoxicity and death before the patient can reach a hospital, especially if the patient is an older adult with a slower rate of drug elimination. For a more detailed description of how TCAs work, visit the Evolve website at http://evolve.elsevier.com/Varcarolis/essentials.

Selective Serotonin Reuptake Inhibitors (SSRIs)

As the name implies, SSRIs inhibit reuptake of serotonin, making it stay longer in the synapse. Examples include fluoxetine (Prozac), ser-traline (Zoloft), paroxetine (Paxil), citalopram (Celexa), and escitalo-pram (Lexapro). Vilazodone *(Viibryd Medication Guide, 2015)* offers a novel combination of selective serotonin reuptake inhibition and sero-tonergic (5-HT$_{1A}$) receptor partial agonist activity. The idea behind a partial agonist is that it will effectively block the negative feedback caused by higher levels of serotonin and increase serotonin level release even more.

The new SSRI vortioxetine (Brintellix) displays agonist activity at the 5-HT$_{1A}$ receptor as well as partial agonist activity at 5-HT$_{1B}$, and

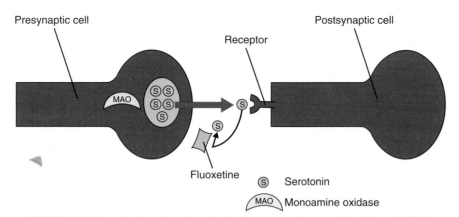

Presynaptic cell

Postsynaptic cell

Receptor

Fluoxetine

ⓈSerotonin

MAO Monoamine oxidase

FIGURE 4-10 Mechanism of action of selective serotonin reuptake inhibitors (SSRIs).

antagonist activity at 5-HT$_3$, 5-HT$_{1D}$, and 5-HT$_7$ receptors. These multimodal actions may benefit patients who failed first-line therapy (Alvidrez, 2014). Refer to Figure 4-10 for an explanation of the mechanism of action of SSRIs. For a more detailed description of how SSRIs work, visit the Evolve website at http://evolve.elsevier.com/Varcarolis/essentials.

Selectivity results in fewer side effects because SSRIs do not inhibit receptors for other neurotransmitters (e.g., acetylcholine, histamine, norepinephrine). However, too much serotonergic activity can result in *anxiety, insomnia, sexual dysfunction,* and *gastrointestinal disturbances.* Serotonin toxicity may occur with coadministration of other serotonergic drugs (e.g., MAOIs, SSRIs, SNRIs, lithium, triptan, buspirone, tramadol, over-the-counter cough and cold medications containing dextromethorphan) or antidopaminergic drugs. Similarly, the risk of serotonin toxicity may be increased by pharmacokinetic interactions because serotonergic antidepressants are metabolized by CYP450 enzymes, and any drug that inhibits a CYP450 enzyme increases serotonin levels. For example, metabolism by CYP3A4 is a major elimination pathway for SSRIs, so doses should be reduced with coadministered CYP3A4 inhibitors (e.g., ketoconazole). On the other hand, CYP34A inducers (e.g., rifampin) can result in inadequate plasma concentrations and diminished effectiveness.

Adverse events can occur upon discontinuation of serotonergic antidepressants, particularly when discontinuation is abrupt. The discontinuation syndrome is most likely to occur with SSRIs or SNRIs having a short half-life. Thus it is more common with paroxetine (Paxil) than with fluoxetine (Prozac).

Serotonin-Norepinephrine Reuptake Inhibitors (SNRIs)

SNRIs block reuptake of both serotonin and norepinephrine, but it remains controversial whether the dual action of SNRIs such as **venlafaxine** (Effexor), duloxetine (Cymbalta), and desvenlafaxine (Pristq) results in greater efficacy than SSRIs. SNRIs are also used to treat other conditions such as anxiety and neuropathic pain.

Serotonin-Norepinephrine Disinhibitors (SNDIs)

SNDIs, represented by only mirtazapine (Remeron), increase norepinephrine and serotonin transmission by blocking presynaptic α$_2$-noradrenergic receptors. Mirtazapine is often combined with SSRIs to augment antidepressant response or counteract serotonergic side effects of nausea, anxiety, or insomnia.

OTHER ANTIDEPRESSANTS

Norepinephrine-Dopamine Reuptake Inhibitors (NDRIs)

Unlike other currently used antidepressants, **bupropion** (Wellbutrin) does not act on the serotonin system. It inhibits dopamine-norepinephrine reuptake, and it also inhibits nicotinic acetylcholine receptors to reduce the addictive action of nicotine. Thus the bupropion preparation Zyban is also prescribed for smoking cessation.

Serotonin Antagonist/Reuptake Inhibitors (SARIs)

High doses are required for the serotonergic action of the SARI **trazodone** (Desyrel). At lower doses, it loses its antidepressant action while retaining hypnotic effects through histamine receptor antagonism (Stahl, 2013). Although useful for insomnia, trazodone's potent α-adrenergic blocking properties can cause priapism (painful prolonged penile erections).

Selective Norepinephrine Reuptake Inhibitors (NRIs)

NRIs block presynaptic norepinephrine transporters (NETs), thereby inhibiting reuptake of norepinephrine. The first truly selective noradrenergic reuptake inhibitor marketed in the United States was atomoxetine (Straterra). It is used to treat ADHD when stimulants cannot be tolerated, but it does not show a significant benefit for depression. Refer to Chapter 15 for more information on the antidepressant medications, nursing considerations, and patient and family teaching.

TREATING ANXIETY DISORDERS WITH ANTIDEPRESSANTS

Antidepressants have been found effective in treating anxiety disorders because of many shared symptoms, neurotransmitters, and circuits. SSRIs are commonly used to treat panic disorder, generalized anxiety disorder (GAD), OCD, PTSD, and social phobia. The SNRIs venlafaxine (Effexor) and duloxetine (Cymbalta) are also used to treat GAD.

ANTIANXIETY OR ANXIOLYTIC DRUGS

Benzodiazepines

The most commonly used antianxiety agents are **benzodiazepines,** which promote the activity of GABA by binding to a specific receptor on the GABA$_A$ receptor complex. Figure 4-11 shows that benzodiazepines such as diazepam (Valium), clonazepam (Klonopin), and alprazolam (Xanax) bind to GABA$_A$ receptors with different α-subunits.

The fact that benzodiazepines do not inhibit neurons in the absence of GABA limits their potential toxicity. However, sedative/hypnotic effects put patients at risk for developing tolerance and withdrawal. Some benzodiazepines, such as flurazepam (Dalmane) and triazolam (Halcion), have a predominantly hypnotic (sleep-inducing) effect, whereas others, such as lorazepam (Ativan) and alprazolam (Xanax), reduce anxiety without being as **soporific** (sleep-producing).

The ability of benzodiazepines to potentiate GABA could account for their ability to reduce neuronal excitement in seizures and alcohol withdrawal. When used alone, benzodiazepines rarely inhibit the brain to the degree that respiratory depression, coma, and death result. However, when combined with other central nervous system (CNS) depressants, such as alcohol, opiates, or TCAs, the inhibitory actions of the benzodiazepines can lead to life-threatening respiratory depression.

Any drug that inhibits electrical activity in the brain can interfere with motor ability and judgment. Therefore, patients must be cautioned about engaging in activities that could be dangerous if reflexes and attention are impaired (e.g., driving). Ataxia is a common side effect secondary to the abundance of GABA receptors in the cerebellum.

Non-Benzodiazepines
Buspirone (BuSpar)

Buspirone (BuSpar) reduces anxiety without causing the immediate sedative and mildly euphoric effects of benzodiazepines. Its mechanism of action is unknown, but it has a high affinity for serotonin 5-HT$_{1A}$ receptors, which mediate its antidepressant effects. Concomitant use of higher doses of buspirone and alcohol should be avoided, but the potential for addiction that exists with benzodiazepines does not exist for buspirone.

Short-Acting Sedative-Hypnotic Sleep Agents

Non-benzodiazepine hypnotic agents, such as zolpidem (Ambien), zaleplon (Sonata), and eszopiclone (Lunesta), demonstrate selectivity for GABA$_A$ receptors containing α_1-subunits. Termed the "Z-hypnotics," they have sedative effects without the antianxiety, anticonvulsant, or muscle relaxant effects of benzodiazepines.

Melatonin Receptor Agonists

Ramelteon (Rozerem), a hypnotic, acts much the same way as endogenous melatonin. It has a high selectivity at the melatonin-1 receptor site—thought to regulate sleepiness—and at the melatonin-2 receptor site—thought to regulate circadian rhythms.

MOOD STABILIZERS

Lithium

The precise action of lithium as a mood stabilizer has not been established, but a common theme is that lithium affects multiple steps in cellular signaling. It appears to exert therapeutic actions through second messenger systems, causing alterations in calcium and protein kinase C–mediated processes.

Primarily because of its effects on electrical conductivity, lithium has a low therapeutic index (the ratio of the lethal dose to the effective dose); therefore it is important to monitor blood lithium levels, which are dependent on kidney function. Changes in sodium and hydration can affect the amount of lithium salts excreted. When sodium is depleted, the kidneys attempt to retain lithium and this may result in toxicity. Conversely, excessive sodium lowers lithium. Long-term use of lithium increases the risk of both kidney and thyroid disease. Chapter 16 considers lithium treatment in more detail.

Anticonvulsant Mood Stabilizers

Valproate, available as **divalproex sodium** (Depakote) and **valproic acid** (Depakene), is helpful in bipolar patients unresponsive to lithium. It possibly works by inhibiting enzymes involved in GABA catabolism, thereby inhibiting neuronal excitability. Black Box warnings include hepatotoxicity, tetratogenicity, and pancreatitis.

Valproate increases the concentrations of another mood stabilizer, **lamotrigine (Lamictal).** Effective in bipolar depression, lamotrigine inhibits the release of glutamate and aspartate. Lamotrigine may trigger a severe allergic skin reaction called Stevens-Johnson syndrome (SJS).

Carbamazepine (Tegretol) is less effective than lithium and causes more side effects than valproate, but it may be better in rapid cycling bipolar disorder. It makes neurons less excitable in acute mania by stabilizing the inactive state of sodium channels in neurons (Stanford School of Medicine, 2015). A complete blood count (CBC) must be done periodically because of rare but serious blood dyscrasias (e.g., aplastic anemia and agranulocytosis).

Other Agents

Off-label mood stabilizers include oxcarbazepine (Trileptal), gabapentin (Neurontin), and topiramate (Topamax). Benzodiazepines may be used for their calming effects during mania, and sometimes antipsychotics and antidepressants are used along with a mood stabilizer. Refer to Chapter 16 for nursing considerations and patient and family teaching for the mood stabilizing drugs.

ANTIPSYCHOTIC DRUGS

First-Generation Antipsychotic (FGAs)/Conventional Antipsychotics

FGAs were once called **neuroleptics** because they caused significant neurological effects. They are also referred to as **dopamine receptor**

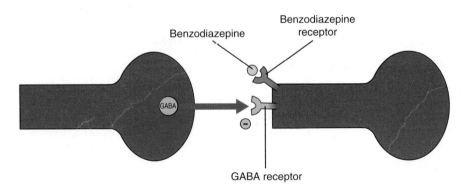

FIGURE 4-11 Action of the benzodiazepines. Drugs in this group attach to receptors adjacent to the receptors for the neurotransmitter γ-aminobutyric acid (GABA). Drug attachment to these receptors results in a strengthening of the inhibitory effects of GABA. In the absence of GABA, there is no inhibitory effect of benzodiazepines.

agonists (DRAs) because they bind to dopamine type 2 (D$_2$) receptors and reduce dopamine transmission, as illustrated in Figure 4-12.

D$_2$ blockade achieves the therapeutic effect of decreasing positive symptoms in schizophrenia, but it also can lead to extrapyramidal side effects such as dystonia (muscle stiffness), akathisia (restlessness), tardive dyskinesia (TD), and drug-induced parkinsonism. Anticholinergic agents such as benztropine (Cogentin) may be used to manage drug-induced parkinsonism, but anticholinergic therapy is itself linked to confusion, memory problems, and dementia in older adults (Gray et al., 2015).

D$_2$ blockade also may lead to a rare but life-threatening complication called neuroleptic malignant syndrome (NMS) involving autonomic, motor, and behavioral symptoms. The antipsychotic agent should be stopped immediately if the patient develops signs of NMS such as severe muscle rigidity, confusion, agitation, and increased temperature, pulse, and blood pressure.

In addition to adverse effects occurring with D$_2$ blockade, unpleasant effects also result from antipsychotics blocking other receptors, such as those identified in Figure 4-13. For example, blocking **muscarinic cholinergic** receptors can result in blurred vision, dry mouth, constipation, and urinary hesitancy. Antagonism of the **H$_1$** receptors causes sedation

and weight gain. Blockage at the **α$_1$-receptors for norepinephrine** can affect vasodilation and a consequent drop in blood pressure, or orthostatic hypotension. Antagonism of either **α$_1$-receptors** or **5-HT$_2$** receptors may result in ejaculatory dysfunction. For a more detailed description of how the antipsychotic drugs block specific receptors, visit the Evolve website at http://evolve.elsevier.comVarcarolis/essentials.

FGA uses are further classified as high potency or low potency to indicate the drug's affinity for the D$_2$ receptor, which, in turn, influences the adverse effect profile of the drug. Although high-potency haloperidol (Haldol) and **fluphenazine** (Prolixin) have less sedation and fewer anticholinergic effects than low-potency chlorpromazine (Thorazine), they cause more extrapyramidal symptoms (EPS). An acute dystonic reaction (ADR) is more likely to occur early in treatment with a high-potency neuroleptic, especially if the patient uses cocaine.

In a large government-sponsored trial called "The CATIE Project," the moderate-potency conventional antipsychotic perphenazine (Trilafon) was found to be comparable in efficacy to newer atypical agents. This finding, as well as the cost-effectiveness of FGA, has renewed interest in their use.

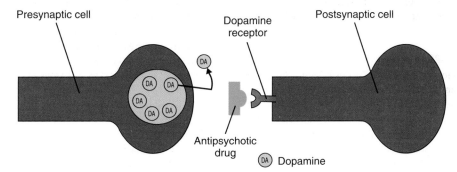

FIGURE 4-12 Mechanism by which antipsychotics block dopamine receptors.

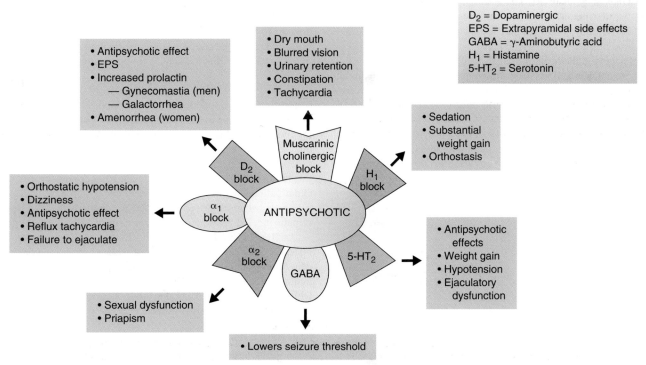

FIGURE 4-13 Adverse effects of receptor blockage of antipsychotic agents. (From Varcarolis, E. [2015]. *Manual of psychiatric nursing care plans* [5th ed.]. St. Louis: Saunders Elsevier.)

Second-Generation (SGA) or Atypical Antipsychotic Agents

Atypicals are known as serotonin-dopamine antagonists (SDAs) because they have a higher ratio of serotonin (5-HT_2) to dopamine D_2-receptor blockade than first-generation DRAs. They are prescribed more frequently because their different receptor-binding profile accounts for fewer EPS. Abnormal functioning of brain circuits involving serotonin is believed to be linked to bipolar disorder and depression. Therefore, several SGAs are FDA approved for treating these disorders.

In addition to being potent 5-HT_{2A} receptor antagonists, some SGAs have significant anticholinergic and antihistaminic activity.

Clozapine (Clozaril)

Clozapine, the first of the atypicals, is several times more potent in blocking 5-HT_2 receptors than D_2 receptors. It also has binding activity at a variety of other receptors, which may account for its advantages in treating patients who respond poorly to other antipsychotics. Clozapine is not a first-line treatment because it may suppress bone marrow, resulting in agranulocytosis, a rare but serious decrease in granulated white blood cells (WBCs). Seizures are a dose-related side effect of clozapine, so caution should be used with coadministration of drugs such as SSRIs that elevate clozapine concentrations. Drooling, a paradoxical side effect, can cause social discomfort or speech problems. Hypersalivation may be relieved by sublingual drops of atropine ophthalmic solution.

Orally disintegrating clozapine tablets (FazaClo) and an oral suspension of clozapine (Versalcloz) are useful formulations for individuals who have problems with swallowing.

Olanzapine (Zyprexa)

Olanzapine, a derivative of clozapine, has comparable receptor occupancies and similar metabolic side effects, such as weight gain. Metabolic monitoring for all patients receiving SGA (atypicals) is recommended, although risperidone (Risperdal) and quetiapine (Seroquel) have a lower weight gain and ziprasidone (Geodon) and aripiprazole (Abilify) are considered weight neutral. Metabolic monitoring usually includes measurements of body weight, body mass index (BMI), waist circumference, fasting plasma glucose level, and fasting lipid profile.

Metformin—a medication used to regulate blood glucose level—reduces weight gain and waist circumference when used as an adjunct to SGAs. Although metabolic effects are unhealthy, these adverse effects are often more tolerable than the neurological adverse effects of conventional antipsychotics.

Olanzapine is sedating because of its antagonism of H_1 receptors, so it is common practice to administer the medication at bedtime. It was the first antipsychotic available as orally disintegrating tablets. Olanzapine pamoate (Zyprexa Relprevv) is an extended release injectable suspension that carries a warning for postinjection delirium/sedation. Thus it requires at least 3 hours of continuous observation in a certified health care facility.

Risperidone (Risperdal)

Risperidone exhibits high levels of D_2-receptor blockade and a very high affinity for 5-HT_2 receptors. EPS may occur if the dosage is only slightly higher than the effective dose. Therefore, the patient should be carefully monitored for motor difficulties if the dosage exceeds 4 to 6 mg/day. Because risperidone blocks α_1 and H_1 receptors, it can cause orthostatic hypotension and sedation, which can lead to falls—a serious problem for older adults. Weight gain and sexual dysfunction also are adverse effects that may affect medication adherence.

Risperidone (Risperdal Consta) was the first atypical antipsychotic available as a long-acting injectable (LAI). It is useful with nonadherent patients when it is necessary to keep the dosage regimen constant, particularly in patients with schizophrenia incarcerated for violent acts (Nasrallah, 2011). Further research is needed to compare the more costly atypical LAI Risperdal Consta with the typical LAIs, haloperidol and fluphenazine decanoate.

Paliperidone is the principal active metabolite of risperidone in INVEGA extended-release tablets. Paliperidone is used in schizophrenia and schizoaffective disorder and as an adjunct to mood stabilizers or antidepressants. Unlike its parent compound, paliperidone is eliminated almost independently of the CYP2D6 pathway and is cleared through the kidneys. Due to the Osmotic Release Oral System (OROS) providing 24-hour release, morning administration is recommended. Paliperidone palmitate (Invega Sustenna) is offered as a once-monthly deltoid or gluteal injection.

Quetiapine (Seroquel)

Quetiapine has a broad receptor-binding profile with low binding at D_2 receptors and a low risk of EPS. Its strong blockage of histamine-1 receptors accounts for somnolence, making the immediate-release (IR) formulation an ideal hypnotic. The extended-release (XR) formulation is associated with milder sedation than quetiapine IR and is well tolerated in schizophrenia and bipolar disorder (El-Khalili, 2012). The combination of histamine-1 and serotonin receptor blockage leads to weight gain and moderate risk for metabolic syndrome. Orthostatic hypotension is explained by antagonism of adrenergic α_1 receptors.

Ziprasidone (Geodon)

Ziprasidone is a serotonin-norepinephrine reuptake inhibitor that also binds to multiple receptors. The main side effects are dizziness and sedation. One major safety concern with ziprasidone, as with other atypicals, is prolongation of the QT_c interval, which can be fatal if the patient has a history of cardiac dysrhythmias. Thus a baseline electrocardiogram is recommended before treatment. Another concern is a rare but serious skin reaction known as Drug Reaction with Eosinophilia and Systemic Symptoms (DRESS). Food increases its absorption up to twofold; therefore ziprasidone is always taken with food. Ziprasidone may be given intramuscularly for acute agitation, but it is important to note that it is not a long-acting preparation.

Aripiprazole (Abilify)

Aripiprazole is a dopamine-serotonin stabilizer that lowers dopaminergic neurotransmission in the mesolimbic pathway through partial D_2 agonism, thereby reducing positive symptoms of schizophrenia, but increasing dopaminergic activity in the hypofunctioning mesocortical pathway (Guzman, 2015). Partial agonist activity at 5-HT_{1A} receptors has been associated with improvement of depression and anxiety. Older patients with treatment-resistant depression have higher remission rates when aripiprazole is used to augment the antidepressant venlafaxine, but akathisia is a common adverse effect.

Aripiprazole is available in a ready-to-use vial for intramuscular injection and control of agitation in schizophrenia or bipolar disorder. Abilify Maintena is a once-monthly intramuscular injection for maintenance treatment of schizophrenia in adult patients stabilized with oral aripiprazole. An oral solution and oral disintegrating tablets (Abilify Discmelt) are also available.

Iloperidone (Fanapt)

Although iloperidone is like the other SGAs in having a high affinity for both D_2 and 5-HT_{2A} receptors, it also has a high affinity for the D_3

receptor and noradrenergic receptor. Although orthostatic hypotension related to noradrenergic A1 antagonism is problematic, it tends to abate with time.

Lurasidone Hydrochloride (Latuda)

Lurasidone HCl has a high affinity for D_2 and 5-HT_{2A} receptors in addition to other serotonergic receptors. It exerts its effect in bipolar depression through agonistic activity at 5-HT_{1A} and antagonism at $alpha_1$-noreadrenergic and 5-HT_{2A} receptors (Fountoulakis et al., 2015). It is indicated as monotherapy for major depressive episodes associated with bipolar I disorder and as adjunctive therapy with lithium or valproate.

The bioavailability of lurasidone is greatly enhanced when taken with food (at least 350 calories). However, grapefruit and grapefruit juice should be avoided since these may inhibit CYP3A4 and increase lurasidone concentrations. Refer to Chapter 17 for more information on adverse and toxic effects, nursing considerations, and patient and family teaching of the antipsychotics.

Cariprazine (Vraylar)

Cariprazine is a potent D_3/D_2 receptor partial agonist. Acting primarily on D_3 receptors, it has the potential of ameliorating negative symptoms of schizophrenia. Taken once a day, it is approved for schizophrenia and bipolar disorder in adults. Like other drugs in this class, cariprazine carries a boxed warning about increased death in older people with dementia-related psychosis. Cariprazine is the second atypical after brexpiprazole (Rexulti) to get FDA approval in 2015. Brexpiprazole treats schizophrenia and is used as an add-on in MDD (FDA News Release, 2015).

Psychoneuroimmunology (PNI)

Psychoneuroimmunology (PNI) is a research field that focuses on the interaction between the immune system and the nervous system and the relationship between behavior and health. Scientists investigate molecular, cellular, and neuronal events to determine their role in psychiatric disorders. For example, recent studies have suggested microglial activation in the brains of patients with neuropsychiatric disorders such as schizophrenia, depression, and autism (Kato et al., 2013). Activation of microglia, the brain's primary immune cells, and proinflammatory cytokines in bipolar disorder suggests an important link with inflammation (Maletic & Raison, 2014). Mood stabilizers, the primary treatment for bipolar disorder, have been shown to dampen the proinflammatory response (Watkins et al., 2014). Neuroimmunopharmacology focuses on drugs modulating neuroimmune processes and is beginning to explore highly advanced technologies such as nanotechnology to develop approved nanodrugs.

CONSIDERING CULTURE

Cross-cultural psychopharmacology explores different responses that exist among ethnic groups and the reasons for these effects. Ethnic variations are influenced by genetic predisposition as well as cultural beliefs surrounding mental illness and pharmacotherapy. A patient's perception of the need for treatment, aversion to certain side effects, and preference for alternative or complementary therapies must be considered.

Genes are considered "plastic" because the dynamic pattern of gene regulation is a response to internal cues (e.g., neurotransmitters) as well as external cues (e.g., psychotropic drugs, psychotherapies). Monitoring the effects of integrated methods of treatment and empowering

patients to make informed treatment decisions are at the heart of psychiatric nursing.

At present, psychotropic medications target "symptoms" and are classified by broad indications such as antipsychotics or antidepressants. *In the future, these medications will be reclassified from symptom-based to pharmacology-based actions (Zohar et al., 2013). A new neuroscience-based drug nomenclature will reflect evidence-based practice and allow patients to make informed decisions in an era of patient-centered care.*

KEY POINTS TO REMEMBER

- All actions of the brain—sensory, motor, intellectual—are carried out through the interactions of nerve cells involving impulse conduction, transmitter release, and receptor response. Alterations in these basic processes can lead to mental disturbances and physical manifestations.

- In particular, it seems that excess activity of dopamine, among other factors, is involved in the thought disturbances of schizophrenia, and deficiencies of norepinephrine, serotonin, or both underlie depression and anxiety. Insufficient activity of GABA also plays a role in anxiety.

- Pharmacological treatment of mental disturbances is directed at the suspected transmitter-receptor problem. Antipsychotic drugs decrease dopamine levels, antidepressant drugs increase synaptic levels of norepinephrine and/or serotonin, and antianxiety drugs increase the effectiveness of GABA or increase 5-HT and/or norepinephrine levels.

- Because the immediate target activity of a drug can result in many downstream alterations in neuronal activity, drugs with a variety of chemical actions may show efficacy in treating the same clinical condition. Thus, newer drugs with novel mechanisms of action are being used in the treatment of schizophrenia, depression, and anxiety.

- Unfortunately, agents used to treat mental disease can cause various undesired effects. Prominent among these can be sedation or excitement, motor disturbances, muscarinic blockage, α-adrenergic antagonism, sexual dysfunction, and weight gain. There is a continuing effort to develop new drugs that are effective, safe, and well tolerated.

APPLYING CRITICAL JUDGMENT

1. No matter where you practice nursing, individuals under your care will be taking psychotropic drugs. Consider the importance of understanding normal brain structure and function as they relate to mental disturbances and psychotropic drugs by addressing the following questions:
   A. How can you use your knowledge of normal brain function (control of peripheral nerves, skeletal muscles, the autonomic nervous system, hormones, and circadian rhythms) to better understand how a patient can be affected by psychotropic drugs or psychiatric illness?
   B. What information from the various brain imaging techniques can you use to understand and treat patients with mental disorders and provide support to their families? How might you use that information for patient and family teaching?
2. Based on your understanding of symptoms that may occur when the following neurotransmitters are altered, what specific information would you include in medication teaching?
   A. Dopamine D_2 (as with use of antipsychotic drugs)

B. Blockage of muscarinic receptors (as with use of phenothiazines and other drugs)

C. α_1-receptors (as with use of phenothiazines and other drugs)

D. Histamine (as with use of phenothiazines and other drugs)

E. Monoamine oxidase (MAO) (as with use of a monoamine oxidase inhibitor [MAOI])

F. γ-Aminobutyric acid (GABA) (as with the use of benzodiazepines)

G. Serotonin (as with the use of selective serotonin reuptake inhibitors [SSRIs] and other drugs)

H. Norepinephrine (as with the use of serotonin-norepinephrine reuptake inhibitors [SNRIs])

CHAPTER REVIEW QUESTIONS

1. A patient is diagnosed with an abscess in the cerebellum. Which nursing diagnosis has priority for the plan of care?
   a. Risk for falls related to loss of balance and equilibrium
   b. Unilateral neglect related to impairments to perception
   c. Impaired physical mobility related to spasticity and changes in muscle tone
   d. Risk for impaired cerebral tissue perfusion related to obstruction secondary to infection

2. A patient begins a new prescription for risperidone (Risperdal). Which intervention should the nurse include in the plan of care?
   a. Monitor intake and output daily.
   b. Educate patient about foods that contain tyramines.
   c. Assess sitting, standing, and lying blood pressure daily.
   d. Administer with food to reduce gastrointestinal irritation.

3. Systematic measurement of body weight, body mass index (BMI), waist circumference, and glucose levels would be most important for a patient beginning a new prescription for which medication?
   a. Aripiprazole (Abilify)
   b. Olanzapine (Zyprexa)
   c. Ziprasidone (Geodon)
   d. Quetiapine (Seroquel)

4. A patient tells the community mental health nurse, "I told my health care provider I was having trouble sleeping and he prescribed trazodone 50 mg every night. I read on the internet that drug is an antidepressant, but I'm not depressed. What should I do?" Which response by the nurse is correct?
   a. "I will help you contact your health care provider for clarification regarding this new prescription."
   b. "Insomnia and depression usually go hand-in-hand. If your depression is relieved, your sleep will improve."
   c. "In low doses, trazodone helps relieve insomnia. Higher doses are needed for antidepressant effects to occur."
   d. "Information on the internet is often misleading and incorrect. It's more important to trust the judgment of your health care provider."

5. Which patient would the nurse expect to have the most difficulty with problem solving and decision making?
   a. An 18-year-old diagnosed with bulimia nervosa at age 14; has taken oral doses of fluoxetine (Prozac) daily for 3 years
   b. A 46-year-old diagnosed with schizophrenia at age 24; has taken oral doses of clozapine (Clozaril) daily for 18 years
   c. A 62-year-old diagnosed with bipolar disorder at age 28; has taken oral divalproex sodium (Depakote) daily for 16 years
   d. A 52-year-old diagnosed with schizophrenia at age 21; has taken monthly injections of haloperidol (haldol decanoate) for 12 years

REFERENCES

Alvidrez, A. (2014, January). Drugs in perspective: Takeda's and Lundbeck's Brintellix. *Modern Medicine Network.* Retrieved March 28, 2014, from http://formularyjournal.modernmedicine.com/formulary-journal/content/tags/depression/drugs-context-takedas-and-lundbeck-s-brintellix?page=full.

Ansell, E. B., Rando, K., Tuit, K., et al. (2012, July). Cumulative adversity and smaller gray matter volume in medial prefrontal, anterior cingulate, and insula regions. *Biological Psychiatry, 72*(1), 2012. Retrieved September 27, 2015, from www.biologicalpsychiatryjournal.com/article/S0006-3223%2811%2901193-0/abstract.

Beyer, C. E., & Stahl, S. M. (2010). *Next generation antidepressants: moving beyond monoamines to discover novel treatment strategies for mood disorders.* London: Cambridge University Press.

Brown, T. E. (2013). *A new understanding of ADHD in children and adults: executive function impairments.* New York: Routledge.

Demler, T. L. (2012). Psychiatric drug-drug interactions. *U.S. Pharmacist, 37*(11). Retrieved March 29, 2015, from www.medscape.com/viewarticle/775394_3.

El-Khalili, N. (2012). Update on extended release quetiapine fumarate in schizophrenia and bipolar disorders. *Neuropsychiatric Disease and Treatment, 8,* 523–536.

FDA News Release July 13, 2015: *FDA approves new drug to treat schizophrenia and as an add on to an antidepressant to treat major depressive disorder.* Retrieved September 24, 2015, from www.fda.gov/NewsEvents/Newsroom/PressAnnouncements/ucm454647.htm.

Fountoulakis, K. N., Gazouli, M., Kelsoe, J., et al. (2014, November). The pharmacodynamics properties of lurasidone and their role in its antidepressant efficacy in bipolar disorder. Retrieved April 29, 2015, from www.ncbi.nlm.nih.gov/pubmed/25596883.

GeneSight AssureRx Health, Inc. (2015). Finding the right medications for your patients just got easier. Retrieved March 28, 2015, from http://genesight.com/clinicians/.

Gray, S. L., Anderson, M. L., Dublin, S., et al. (2015, March). Cumulative use of strong anticholinergics and incident dementia. *JAMA Internal Medicine.* Retrieved April 28, 2015, from www.ncbi.nlm.nih.gov/pubmed/25621434.

Guzman, F. (2015). Mechanism of action of aripiprazole. *Psychopharmacology Institute.* Retrieved April 21, 2015, from http://psychopharmacologyinstitute.com/antipsychotics/aripiprazole/mechanism-of-action-aripiprazole/.

Johnson, C. P., Follmer, R. L., Ogus, I., et al. (2015, February). Quantitative T1$_p$ mapping links the cerebellum and lithium use in bipolar disorder. *Molecular Psychiatry, 20,* 149.

Joshi, S. H., Espinoza, R. T., Pirnia, T., et al. (2016). Structural plasticity of the hippocampus and amygdala induced by electroconvulsive therapy in major depression. *Biological Psychiatry, 79*(4), 282–292.

Kantrowitz, J. T., & Javitt, D. C. (2011). Glutamate: new hope for schizophrenia treatment. *Current Psychiatry, 10*(4).

Karas, P. J., Mikell, C. B., Christian, E., et al. (2013, November). Deep brain stimulation: a mechanistic and clinical update. *Journal of Neurosurgery, 35*(5).

Kato, T. A., Hayakawa, K., Monji, A., et al. (2013). Missing and possible link between neuroendocrine factors, neuropsychiatric disorders, and microglia. Retrieved April 23, 2015, from *Frontiers in Integrated Neuroscience, 2013,* 7–53.

Koola, M. M., Vargese, S. P., & Fawcett, J. A. (2014, February). High-dose prazosin for the treatment of post-traumatic stress disorder. *Therapeutic Advances in Psychopharmacology, 4*(1), 43–47. Retrieved April 3, 2015, from www.ncbi.nlm.nih.gov/pmc/articles/PMC3896131/.

Maletic, V., & Raison, C. (2014). Integrated neurobiology of bipolar disorder. *Frontiers of Psychiatry, 5,* 98. Retrieved March 29, 2015, from www.ncbi.nlm.nih.gov/pmc/articles/PMC4142322/.

Melville, N. A. (2015). Novel drug promising for schizophrenia. *15th International Congress on Schizophrenia Research (ICOSR)*. Retrieved April 28, 2015, from www.medscape.com/viewarticle/842591.

Nasrallah, H. A. (2011, February). Two vastly underutilized interventions can improve schizophrenia outcomes. *Current Psychiatry Online*, 10(2). Retrieved April 29, 2015, from www.current-psychiatry.com/?id=22161&;tx_ttnews[tt_news]=175754&-cHash=b85589700229b44f619e34d868f36517.

Neuralstem Pharmaceuticals for Major Depressive Disorder. (2015). Retrieved September 23, 2015, from www.neuralstem.com/pharmaceuticals-for-depression.

Parker, K. L., Narayan, N. S., & Andreasen, N. C. (2014, September). The therapeutic potential of the cerebellum in schizophrenia. *Frontiers in Systems Neuroscience*, 8, 163. Retrieved March 28, 2015, from www.ncbi.nlm.nih.gov/pmc/articles/PMC4163988/.

Paulzen, M., Veselinovic, T., & Grunder, G. (2014). Effects of psychotropic drugs on brain plasticity in humans. *Restorative Neurology and Neuroscience*, 32(1), 163–181.

Pinkham, A. E., Liu, P., Lu, H., et al. (2015, August). Amygdala hyperactivity at rest in paranoid individuals with schizophrenia. *American Journal of Psychiatry*, 172(8), 784–792.

Preston, J. D., O'Neal, J. H., & Talaga, M. C. (2013). *Handbook of clinical psychopharmacology for therapists* (7th ed.). Oakland, Calif: New Harbinger.RxList The Internet Drug Index. Retrieved March 28, 2015, from www.rxlist.com/strattera-drug.htm.

Sadock, B. J., Sadock, V. A., & Ruiz, P. (2015). *Kaplan & Sadock's synopsis of psychiatry: behavioral sciences/clinical psychiatry* (11th ed.). Philadelphia: Wolters Kluwer.

Sarpal, D. K., Argyelan, M., Robinson, D. G., et al. (2016). Baseline striatal functional connectivity as a predictor of response to antipsychotic drug treatment. *American Journal of Psychiatry*, 173(1), 69–77.

Silver, H., Einoch, R., Youdim, M., et al. (2013). The role of GABA-A receptor in the synergism between SSRI and antipsychotic in schizophrenia; implications for antipsychotic modes of actions. *Current Medicinal Chemistry*, 20(3), 363–370. Retrieved April 4, 2015, from www.ncbi.nlm.nih.gov/pubmed/23157628.

Stahl, S. M. (2013). Mood disorders and antidepressants. In *Stahl's essential psychopharmacology*. New York: Cambridge University Press.

Stanford School of Medicine. Psychiatric medications. Retrieved April 8, 2015, from http://whatmeds.stanford.edu/medications/tegretol.html.

Viibryd Medication Guide. Retrieved March 28, 2015, from www.viibrydhcp.com/ssri-mechanism-of-action.aspx.

Watkins, C. C., Sawa, A., & Pomper, M. G. (2014). *Glia and immune cell signaling in bipolar disorder: insights from neuropharmacology and molecular imaging to clinical application*. Retrieved March 29, 2015, from www.nature.com/tp/journal/v4/n1/full/tp2013119a.html.

Williams, L. M., Korgaonkar, M. S., Song, Y. C., et al. (2015, September). Amygdala reactivity to emotional faces in the prediction of general and medication-specific responses to antidepressant treatment in the randomized iSPOT-D Trial. *Neuropsychopharmacology*, 40(10), 2398–2408.

Zohar, J., Nutt, D. J., Kupfer, D. J., et al. (2013). *A proposal for an updated nueropyshopharmacological nomenclature*. Retrieved April 2, 2015, from www.ecnp.eu/~/media/Files/ecnp/Projects %20and%20initiatives/Nomenclature/Review%20articleNE-UPSY_10717v2%20pdf.pdf.

Settings for Psychiatric Care

Margaret Jordan Halter

KEY TERMS AND CONCEPTS

co-occurring/comorbid conditions, p. 56

elopement, p. 54

least restrictive environment, p. 52

mental health parity, p. 59

patient-centered medical homes
(PCMHs), p. 53

primary care providers (PCPs), p. 53

stigma, p. 52

therapeutic milieu, p. 54

SELECTED CONCEPT: PATIENT-CENTERED MEDICAL HOMES (PCMHS)

Patient-centered medical homes received strong support from the Affordable Care Act of 2010. These health homes were developed in response to fragmented care that resulted in some services never being delivered while others were duplicated. The focus of care is patient centered and provides access to physical health, behavioral health, and supportive community and social services.

Electronic communication (e.g., follow-up e-mails and reminders) and record keeping are viewed as essential to this process.

(Halter, the Text)

OBJECTIVES

1. Describe the evolution of treatment settings for psychiatric care.
2. Compare and contrast inpatient and outpatient treatment environments in which psychiatric care is provided.
3. Discuss the role of mental health professionals in assisting people with mental illness symptoms or mental illnesses.
4. Explain methods for financing psychiatric care.

INTRODUCTION

Obtaining traditional health care is fairly straightforward. For example, if you wake up with a sore throat, you know what to do and basically what will happen. It is likely that if you feel bad enough, you will see your primary care provider (PCP), be examined, and maybe get a throat culture to diagnose the problem. If the cause is bacterial, you will probably be prescribed an antibiotic. If you do not improve in a certain length of time, your PCP may order more tests or recommend that you see an ear, nose, and throat specialist.

Compared to obtaining treatment for physical disorders, entry into the health care system for the treatment of psychiatric problems can be a mystery. Challenges in accessing and navigating this care system exist for several reasons. One reason is that we just do not have much of a frame of reference. We are unlikely to benefit from the experience of others because having a psychiatric illness is often hidden as a result of embarrassment or concern over the stigma, or a sense of responsibility, shame, and being flawed associated with these disorders (refer to Chapter 2 for more on stigma). You may know that when your grandmother had heart disease, she saw a cardiac specialist and had coronary artery bypass surgery, but you may be unaware that she was also treated for depression by a psychiatrist.

Seeking treatment for mental health problems is also complicated by the very nature of mental illness. At the most extreme, disorders with a psychotic component may disorganize thoughts and impede a person's ability to recognize the need for care. There is even a word for this inability: anosognosia (uh-no-sog-NOH-zee-uh). Major depression, a common psychiatric disorder, may interfere with motivation to seek care because the illness often causes feelings of apathy, hopelessness, and anergia (lack of energy).

Mental health symptoms are also confused with other problems. For example, anxiety disorders often manifest in somatic symptoms such as racing heartbeat, sweaty palms, and dizziness, which could be symptoms of cardiac problems. Prudence would dictate ruling out other causes, such as physical illness, particularly because diagnosing psychiatric illness is largely based on symptoms and not on objective measurements such as electrocardiograms (ECGs) and blood counts. This necessary process of ruling out other illnesses often results in an often-troublesome treatment delay.

Further complicating treatment for mental illness is the unique nature of the system of care, which is rooted in the public as well as private sectors. The purpose of this chapter is to provide an overview of this system, briefly examine the evolution of mental health care, and explore different venues by which people receive treatment for mental health problems. Treatment options are presented in order of acuteness, beginning with those in the least restrictive environment—the setting that provides the necessary care while allowing the greatest personal freedom. This chapter also explores how mental health care is funded and describes the challenges in securing adequate funding.

BACKGROUND

Although people with financial resources have a variety of psychiatric treatment options, state or county governments coordinate a separate care system for uninsured individuals, often for those with the most serious and persistent illnesses. This separate system of care has its roots in asylums that were created in most existing states before the Civil War. These asylums were created with good intentions in an environment of optimism about recovery and belief that states had a special responsibility to care for the "insane." Effective treatments were not yet developed and community care was virtually nonexistent. By the early 1950s, there were only two real options for psychiatric care—a private psychiatrist's office or a mental hospital. At that time, there were 550,000 patients in state hospitals. A majority were individuals with disabling conditions who had become "stuck" in the asylums.

The number of people in state-managed psychiatric hospitals began to decrease with the creation of Medicare and Medicaid during the 1960s Great Society reform period. Medicaid had an especially potent effect because it paid for short-term hospitalization in general hospitals and medical centers, and for long-term care in nursing homes; however, it did not cover care for most patients in psychiatric hospitals. These incentives stimulated development of general hospital psychiatric units, and also led states to transfer geriatric patients from 100% state-paid psychiatric hospitals to Medicaid-reimbursed nursing facilities.

In the 1999 Olmstead decision, the Supreme Court decreed that keeping people in psychiatric hospitals was considered "unjustified isolation." The opinion of the court was that mental illness is a disability and institutionalization is in violation of the Americans with Disabilities Act, and that all people with disabilities have a right to live in the community.

These forces combined to lead to the gradual and incomplete creation of state- and county-financed community care systems to complement, and largely replace, functions of the state hospitals. The number of state psychiatric hospitals continues to be cut and has been reduced from 322 in 1950 to 207 in 2012 (National Association of State Mental Health Program Directors, 2014). In Ohio, a state agency—the Ohio Department of Mental Health and Addictions Services—certifies, monitors, and funds agencies that provide services. These agencies may be for profit or nonprofit. County boards (depending on whether the alcohol or substance abuse and mental health boards are combined) provide more local oversight and management of these agencies.

Related to the shift from hospital to community care were the pharmacological breakthroughs in the latter half of the twentieth century that led to dramatic changes in the provision of psychiatric care. The introduction of chlorpromazine (Thorazine), the first antipsychotic medication, in the early 1950s contributed to hospital discharges. Gradually, more psychopharmacological agents were added to treat psychosis, depression, anxiety, and other disorders, and treatment could be provided not only from specialists in psychiatry but also from general practitioners.

Our current system of psychiatric care includes outpatient and inpatient settings. Decisions for level of care tend to be based on the condition being treated and the acuteness of the problem. However, these are not the only criteria. Levels of care may be influenced by such factors as a concurrent psychiatric or substance abuse problem, medical problems, acceptance of treatment, social supports, and disease chronicity or potential for relapse.

OUTPATIENT CARE SETTINGS

Primary care providers (PCPs) are the first choice for most people when they are ill, but what do people do when they suspect they may have a mental health problem? Imagine that you are feeling depressed, so depressed in fact that you are miserable and cannot carry out your normal activities. You recall that a friend who was depressed saw a psychiatrist (or was that a psychologist?), but that seems too drastic. You

do not feel *that* bad. Perhaps you are coming down with something. After all, you have been tired and you are not eating very well. You decide to visit your PCP, a general health care provider who may be a physician, an advanced practice nurse, or a physician assistant in an office, hospital, or clinic.

This is not an unusual choice. Seeking help for mental health problems from PCPs rather than from mental health specialists is common and similar to seeking help for other medical disorders. This is especially true because most psychiatric disorders are accompanied by unexplained physical symptoms. Most people treated for psychiatric disorders will not go beyond this level of care and may feel more comfortable being treated in a familiar setting. Furthermore, being treated in primary care rather than in the mental health system may lessen the degree of stigma, self-perceived or societally, attached to getting psychiatric care.

Disadvantages to being treated by PCPs include time constraints, because a 15-minute appointment is usually inadequate for a mental and physical assessment. Because PCPs typically have limited training in psychiatry, they may lack the expertise in the diagnosis and treatment of psychiatric disorders. Whereas this may be the only source many people use for receiving mental health services, sometimes PCPs refer people into specialty mental health care.

Patient-centered medical homes (PCMHs) or **primary care medical homes** received strong support from the Affordable Care Act of 2010 under President Barack Obama. These health homes were developed in response to fragmented care that resulted in some services never being delivered while others were duplicated. The focus of care is patient centered and provides access to physical health, behavioral health, and supportive community and social services. Services range from preventive care and acute medical problems to chronic conditions and end-of-life issues. According to the Agency for Healthcare Research and Quality (2015), these homes have five key characteristics:

1. **Patient centered**—Care is relationship based with the patient (family) and takes into account the unique needs of the whole person. The patient is a core member of the team who manages and organizes the care.
2. **Comprehensive care**—All levels (preventive, acute, and chronic) of mental and physical care are addressed. Physicians or advanced practice nurses lead teams that include nurses, physician assistants, pharmacists, nutritionists, social workers, educators, and care coordinators.
3. **Coordination of care**—Care is coordinated with the broader health system such as hospitals, specialty care, and home health.
4. **Improved access**—Patients do not wait until Monday through Friday from 9 AM to 5 PM to get the care they need. In addition to extended hours of service, these homes provide e-mail and phone support.
5. **Systems approach**—Evidence-based care is provided with a continuous feedback loop of evaluation and quality improvement.

The treatment of psychiatric disorders and mental health alterations can be addressed as part of a comprehensive approach to care. Electronic communication (e.g., follow-up e-mails and reminders) and record keeping are viewed as essential to this process.

Community mental health centers (CMHCs) developed from President John F. Kennedy's Community Mental Health Centers Act of 1963, signaling a new policy preference for community care as opposed to institutionalization. Although only about 700 of the anticipated 2800 CMHCs were funded, the legislation marked a change in direction and led to state laws and budgets favoring community care. CMHCs are regulated through state mental health departments and funded by the state. Some areas may provide local funding. Because of this limited government funding, financial support services may be restricted to those whose income and medical expenses make them eligible. Typically, fees are determined using a sliding scale based on income and ability to pay.

Community-based facilities provide comprehensive services to prevent and treat mental illness. These services include assessment, diagnosis, individual and group counseling, case management, medication management, education, rehabilitation, and vocational or employment services. Some centers may provide an array of services across the life span, whereas others may be population specific, such as adult, geriatric, or children.

People with serious mental illness are often isolated, impoverished, and regressed. They may benefit from **psychiatric rehabilitation services** that are provided through the community mental health system or other organizations. Psychiatric rehabilitation is a social model that emphasizes and supports recovery and integration into society rather than accepting a medical model of dysfunction. The development of social skills, the ability to access resources, and the acquisition of optimal social, working, living, and learning environments are the focus of this treatment method.

Psychiatric home care can be provided by any mental health professional, but it is typically nurses with previous inpatient experience who are able to provide biologically based and psychotherapeutic care. This care may be organized by the community mental health system or through other agencies such as Visiting Nurse Services. Home care may reduce the need for costly and disruptive hospitalizations and may provide a more comfortable and safe alternative to clinical settings.

To qualify for reimbursement, patients must have a psychiatric diagnosis, be under the care of a PCP, and be homebound. The designation of homebound generally is given when patients cannot safely leave home, if leaving home causes undue stress, if the nature of the illness results in a refusal to leave home, or if they cannot leave home unaided. However, one major insurer, Medicare, does allow the covered person to leave home once a week for religious services and once a week for hair care.

Intensive outpatient programs (IOPs) and **partial hospitalization programs (PHPs)** function as intermediate steps between inpatient and outpatient care. The primary difference between the two groups is the amount of time that patients spend in them. Both groups tend to operate Monday through Friday, but IOPs are usually half a day while PHPs are longer (about 6 hours since they are "partially hospitalized"). They provide structured activities with nursing and medical supervision, intervention, and treatment. These programs tend to be located within general hospitals, in psychiatric hospitals, and as part of community mental health. A multidisciplinary team facilitates group therapy, individual therapy, other therapies (e.g., art and occupational), and pharmacological management. Coping strategies that are learned during the program can be applied and practiced in the outside world, and then later explored and discussed. Patients who are admitted to IOPs and PHPs are closely monitored in case of need for readmission to inpatient care.

Role of Nurses in Outpatient Care Settings

Psychiatric-mental health registered nurses who work in outpatient settings provide nursing care for individuals with psychiatric disorders, substance use disorders, and intellectual disabilities, along with their families or caretakers. These community mental health nurses work to develop and implement a plan of care along with the multidisciplinary treatment team. They may choose to be certified in psychiatric mental health nursing.

Community mental health nurses need to be very knowledgeable about community resources such as shelters for abused women, food banks for people with severe financial limitations, and agencies that provide employment options for people with mental illness. Nurses may also assess the patient and living arrangements in the home, provide teaching, refer to community supports, and supervise unlicensed care staff. An important concept for community mental health nurses is viewing the entire community as a patient. This perspective promotes community interventions such as conducting stress reduction classes and facilitating grief support groups.

Psychiatric-mental health advanced practice registered nurses are valuable outpatient care providers. These master's or doctoral level prepared nurse practitioners and clinical nurse specialists provide assessment, diagnosis, and treatment in all outpatient treatment settings (ANA et al., 2014). In fact, in many community health centers, psychiatric-mental health advanced practice registered nurses far outnumber their medically prepared colleagues, psychiatrists. They are also instrumental in providing preventive care to the individuals in the community. The focus of this care is on teaching patients to pay attention to symptoms, seek help when necessary, and to be mindful of overall health.

INPATIENT CARE SETTINGS

Inpatient care has undergone significant change over the past 25 years. During the 1980s, inpatient stays were at their peak as private and nonfederal general hospital psychiatric units proliferated. During the mid-1990s, the number of patient days, psychiatric beds, and psychiatric facilities dipped sharply (Table 5-1). This decline was caused by improvements brought about by managed care, tougher limitations of covered days by insurance plans, and alternatives to inpatient hospitalization such as partial hospitalization programs and residential facilities.

Inpatient care is the most intensive care for acutely ill people (ANA, APNA, & ISPN, 2014). These facilities provide 24-hour nursing care in a safe and structured setting. Such a setting is essential to caring for those who are in need of protection from suicidal ideation, aggressive impulses, medication adjustment and monitoring, crisis stabilization, substance abuse detoxification, and behavior modification. Referrals for inpatient treatment may come from a PCP or mental health provider, agencies, another hospital unit, emergency facilities, or nursing homes. Hospital admissions are made under the services of a psychiatrist, although a PCP also may have admitting privileges.

Patients may be admitted voluntarily or involuntarily (see Chapter 6). Units may be unlocked or locked. Locked units provide privacy and prevent elopement—leaving before being discharged (also referred to as being "away without leave" or AWOL). There may also be psychiatric intensive care units (PICUs) within the general psychiatric units to provide better monitoring of those who display an increased risk for danger to self or others.

The therapeutic milieu is essential to successful inpatient treatment. Milieu refers to the environment in which holistic treatment occurs and includes all members of the treatment team in a positive physical setting, with interactions among those who are hospitalized and activities that promote recovery.

Teamwork and **collaboration** are essential elements of interprofessional teams in acute care inpatient settings. Teamwork refers to a group of people working together to improve patient health with each member of the team performing specialized functions (Box 5-1). There may be a leader of the team—often this is the registered nurse. Collaboration is a type of teamwork that requires team members (including the patient) to work directly together to make decisions and develop strategies to optimize care and achieve successful outcomes. Communication is central to this process. A formal structure for collaboration is a multidisciplinary team meeting where patients are discussed and

TABLE 5-1   Number and Rate of 24-Hour Hospital and Residential Treatment Beds by Type of Mental Health Organization

Type of Organization	1980	1990	2000	2004	2008
Number of 24-Hour Hospital and Residential Treatment Beds					
All organizations	274,713	325,529	214,186	212,231	239,014
State and county mental hospitals	156,482	102,307	61,833	57,034	37,450
Private psychiatric hospitals	17,157	45,952	26,402	28,422	25,406
Nonfederal general hospitals with separate psychiatric services	29,384	53,576	40,410	41,403	54,390
Veterans Administration (VA) medical centers*	33,796	24,799	8,989	—	11,991
Residential treatment centers for emotionally disturbed children	20,197	35,170	33,508	33,835	50,063
All other organizations†	1,433	63,745	43,044	53,536	59,715
24-Hour Hospital and Residential Treatment Beds per 100,000 Civilian Population					
All organizations	124.3	128.5	74.8	71.2	78.6
State and county mental hospitals	70.2	40.4	21.6	19.1	12.3
Private psychiatric hospitals	7.7	18.1	9.2	9.5	8.4
Nonfederal general hospitals with separate psychiatric services	13.7	21.2	14.1	13.9	17.9
VA medical centers	15.7	9.9	3.1	—	3.9
Residential treatment centers for emotionally disturbed children	9.1	13.9	11.7	11.4	16.5
All other organizations†	0.6	25.2	15.0	17.3	19.6

*Department of Veterans Affairs medical centers (VA general hospital psychiatric services and VA psychiatric outpatient clinics) were dropped from the survey in 2004.
†Includes free-standing psychiatric outpatient clinics, partial care organizations, and multiservice mental health organizations.
Data from Substance Abuse and Mental Health Services Administration. (2012). *Mental Health, United States, 2010.* HHS Publication No. (SMA) 12-4681. Rockville, Md.

BOX 5-1   Members of the Treatment Team

- **Psychiatric mental health registered nurses (PMH-RNs)** are registered nurses with specialized skills gained through education and experience in caring for individuals with mental health problems, psychiatric disorders, and substance use disorders. They may or may not have certification in psychiatric mental health nursing.
- **Psychiatric mental health advanced practice registered nurses (PMH-APRNs)** are registered nurses who have completed a master's or doctoral degree. They can assess, diagnose, and treat patients. The two nationally credentialed titles are clinical nurse specialist (PMH-CNS) and nurse practitioner (PMH-NP). Both assess health and psychiatric disorders, provide psychotherapy, and prescribe medications.
- **Psychiatrists** are state-licensed medical doctors who have at least 4 years of additional training in diagnosing and treating psychiatric disorders. Medication prescribing and monitoring is a dominant treatment method used by psychiatrists.
- **Psychologists** are licensed by individual states. They hold a doctoral degree in clinical, educational, counseling, or research. Their expertise lies in evaluation, psychological testing, psychotherapy, and counseling. Some states may allow prescriptive authority for psychologists.
- **Social workers** are licensed by the state and may enter general practice with a bachelor's degree in social work. They may provide counseling and plan for supportive services such as housing, health care, and treatment after the patient is returned to the community. Social workers who hold master's and doctoral degrees are also able to provide assessment and treatment (usually psychotherapy) of psychiatric illness.
- **Licensed professional counselors** possess a master's degree in psychology, counseling, or a related field and are licensed by the state. They are trained to assess and diagnose psychiatric conditions and to provide individual, family, and group counseling.
- **Occupational therapists** are usually state regulated and are prepared at the bachelor's, master's, or doctoral level. They assist individuals to develop or regain independent living skills, activities of daily living, and role performance that have been affected by mental disorders.
- **Physical therapists** possess master's or doctoral degrees and are accredited by the state. Their role is to rehabilitate individuals with physical disabilities that may be present concurrent with psychiatric disabilities.
- **Art therapists** are prepared at the master's level in art therapy and registered through a professional association. They use art to help people understand their problems, enhance healthy development, and reduce the effects of their illnesses.
- **Recreation therapists** are typically bachelor's prepared and may be licensed by the state or be nationally certified. Recreational activities are used to improve emotional, physical, cognitive, and social well-being.
- **Pharmacists** are state licensed and prepared through 6 years of secondary education for a doctor of pharmacy (PharmD) degree. They provide distribution and centralized monitoring of drug regimens. Board Certified Psychiatric Pharmacists possess advanced training and skills in working with psychotropic medications.
- **Medical personnel** are physicians whose focus is the provision of nonpsychiatric care for comorbid conditions.
- **Mental health workers** or psychiatric aides are nonprofessional staff who may be state certified. They have extensive contact with patients while assisting with hygiene and meals and participating in unit activities. Mental health workers communicate important information concerning the patient's condition to professional staff.
- **Pastoral counselors** are clergy who have clinical pastoral education and are certified through the American Association of Pastoral Counselors. They provide individual and group counseling.
- **Peer specialists** are paid or volunteer individuals with serious mental illness who are trained and certified to use their experiences to provide recovery-oriented services and to support others with mental illness. As of 2014, 38 states provide certification programs for peer specialists.

care is planned. As a student you may have a chance to attend team meetings and witness the level of interprofessional collaboration that, ideally, occurs in psychiatric care settings.

Inpatient care provides structure in which patients eat meals, receive medication (if necessary), attend activities, and participate in individual and group therapies on a schedule. For those younger than the age of 18, school attendance is required. Patients are active participants in their plans of care and have the right to refuse treatments as long as they have not been declared incompetent. Advocates are usually available to provide advice and counsel for people who have doubts, and most facilities distribute a patient's bill of rights on admission or have it clearly posted. Box 5-2 provides a sample list of patient's rights.

Inpatient rooms are usually less institutional looking than other hospital rooms and tend to resemble hotel rooms. Showers may be in the individual rooms or dorm-style, with one or two per hallway. Rooms are private, semiprivate, or, occasionally, wards. Units may be made up solely of males or of females, or may be co-ed.

Rooms are designed with safety in mind. Hanging is the most common method of inpatient suicide and strict measures are taken to prevent it. Closet rods and hooks, towel bars, and shower rods are constructed to break if subjected to more than a minimal amount of weight. Sprinkler and shower heads tend to be flush-mounted, and utility pipes are enclosed. Other safety measures include locked windows, platform beds rather than mechanical hospital beds to prevent possible crushing, and furniture with rounded corners to reduce intentional injury. Furniture for inpatient rooms tends to be heavy and durable so that it cannot be thrown or dismantled and used as a weapon.

Inpatient care begins with a medical assessment to rule out or consider co-occurring/comorbid conditions. Comprehensive assessments are conducted by a multidisciplinary team, and a plan of care is developed, monitored, evaluated, and refined (refer to Box 5-1). Crisis intervention and stabilization and patient safety are goals of inpatient care. Psychotropic medication evaluation, prescription, and management are usually part of the plan of care, as is individual therapy. Electroconvulsive therapy (ECT) may be ordered for certain conditions, particularly for patients with depression who have been unresponsive to antidepressants.

Group therapy is an important facet of inpatient care. Coping skills are taught and enhanced through cognitive behavioral groups that focus on symptom management. Occupational therapy provides an opportunity to practice life skills that have been delayed, hampered, or eroded. Psychoeducational groups focus on specific psychiatric disorders, medication, goal setting, life planning, and recovery.

Length of stay varies depending on the severity of the illness and symptoms. Nationwide, the mental health average length of stay is 8 days, and for substance abuse the average length of stay is 4.8 days (Piper Report, 2011). At the state level these averages may vary significantly. Therapeutic passes may be helpful so that the patient may go home for limited periods. In some cases, especially with children and people with severe mental illness, privileges and rewards, such as recreational outings, walks on the hospital grounds, and tokens to buy items from a unit "store," may be earned in order to reinforce adaptive behaviors.

Discharge planning begins on the first day of admission based on the patient's unique needs. Case management and collaboration with the patient's outpatient clinician, PCP, family, and community agencies such as the visiting nurse agency facilitate an integrated approach and establish comprehensive transition plans from inpatient to the community setting. This allows the patient to live effectively and safely in the community. Effective case management and collaboration also reduce recidivism.

At discharge, patients should be stabilized. Discharge instructions include follow-up appointments, medication directions, education and prescriptions, and, if necessary, assistance with living arrangements that may include a private residence, shelter, halfway house, or group home.

Crisis intervention is provided in emergency departments of general hospitals or in community-based *crisis intervention centers* (ANA et al., 2014). Crisis care may be initiated by the individual, friends, family, health care provider, or law enforcement personnel. Some patients are involuntarily committed. Psychiatric emergencies may include suicidal (or homicidal) ideation, acute psychosis, or behavioral responses to drugs. The stay in such facilities tends to be short, usually less than 24 hours. At that point the patient may be discharged to home, referred for inpatient care, or transferred to another community facility such as a shelter.

Residential treatment programs are structured short- or long-term 24-hour living environments in which individuals are provided with varying levels of supervision and support (ANA et al., 2014). Psychoeducation is provided for symptom management and medications. Vocational training and even training for daily activities of living may also be part of the program. The residents learn to access community support as an alternative to hospitalization and are encouraged to achieve maximal independence.

State Acute Care System

Today's state-operated psychiatric hospitals are an extension of what remains of the old system, although the quality of care in state hospitals has improved dramatically. The clinical role of state hospitals is to serve the most seriously ill patients, but this role varies widely, depending on available levels of community care and on payments by state Medicaid programs. In some states, state hospitals primarily provide intermediate treatment for patients unable to be stabilized in short-term general hospital units, and long-term care for individuals judged too ill for community care. In other states the emphasis is on acute care that is reflective of gaps in the private sector, especially for the uninsured or for those who have exhausted limited insurance benefits.

BOX 5-2 Typical Items Included in Hospital Statements of a Patient's Rights

- Right to be treated with dignity
- Right to be involved in treatment planning and decisions
- Right to refuse treatment, including medications
- Right to request to leave the hospital, even against medical advice
- Right to be protected against the possible impulse to harm oneself or others that might occur as a result of a mental disorder
- Right to the benefit of the legally prescribed process of an evaluation occurring within a limited period (in most states, 72 hours) in the event of a request for discharge against medical advice that may lead to harm to self or others
- Right to legal counsel
- Right to vote
- Right to communicate privately by telephone and in person
- Right to informed consent
- Right to confidentiality regarding one's disorder and treatment
- Right to choose or refuse visitors
- Right to be informed of research and to refuse to participate
- Right to the least restrictive means of treatment
- Right to send and receive mail and to be present during any inspection of packages received
- Right to keep personal belongings unless they are dangerous
- Right to lodge a complaint through a plainly publicized procedure
- Right to participate in religious worship

In most states the state hospitals provide forensic (court-related) care and monitoring as part of their function for those found *not guilty by reason of insanity* (NGRI). The state or county system also advises the courts as to defendants' sanity who may be judged to have been so ill when they committed the criminal act that they cannot be held responsible, but require treatment instead. One tragic example is that of Andrea Yates, the Texas woman who in 2001 drowned her five young children under the delusional belief she was saving them from their sinfulness. She was found NGRI and was committed to a Texas state psychiatric facility.

General Hospital Psychiatric Units and Private Psychiatric Hospital Acute Care

Acute care general hospital psychiatric units tend to be housed on a floor or floors of a general hospital. Private psychiatric hospitals are free-standing facilities. As noted, the dramatic growth of acute care psychiatric hospitals and hospital units is the result of a shift away from institutionalization in state-managed hospitals. Since that time, reduced reimbursement, increased managed care, enhanced outpatient options, and expanded availability of outpatient and partial hospitalization programs have resulted in the steady decline of these facilities. Average length of stay was declining, but has stabilized at about 9 days among the general population, 12 days for children's programs, and approximately 15 days for older adults (National Association of Psychiatric Health Systems, 2009).

Role of Psychiatric Nurses in Inpatient Care Settings

As professional care providers available around the clock every day of the week, nurses are at the center of any acute care inpatient facility. Management of these units, ideally, is by nurses with backgrounds in psychiatric mental health nursing, preferably with advanced practice degrees. Staff nurses tend to be nurse generalists, that is, nurses who have basic training as registered nurses. Some registered nurses obtain national certification in psychiatric mental health nursing through the American Nurses Credentialing Center. The psychiatric mental health registered nurse carries out the following nursing responsibilities:

- Completing comprehensive data collection that includes the patient, family, and other health care workers
- Developing, implementing, and evaluating plans of care
- Assisting or supervising mental health care workers (e.g., nursing assistants with or without additional training in working with people who have mental illnesses)
- Maintaining a safe and therapeutic environment
- Facilitating health promotion through teaching
- Monitoring behavior, affect, and mood
- Maintaining oversight of restraint and seclusion
- Coordinating care by the treatment team

Medication management is an essential skill for psychiatric nurses. In this specialty area nurses often exert a strong influence on medication decisions because continual observation of the expected, interactive effects and adverse effects of medications provides the data necessary for medication adjustment. For example, feedback about a patient's excessive sedation or increased agitation will lead to a decision to decrease or increase the dosage of an antipsychotic medication.

A common misperception regarding psychiatric nurses in acute care settings is that because they "just talk" they lose their skills, including physical tasks such as starting and maintaining intravenous (IV) lines and changing dressings. First, therapeutic communication itself is a skill that people are not born with and must learn. Second, patients on the psychiatric unit are not limited to *DSM-5* diagnoses and often have complex health care needs. For example, an older adult male with brittle diabetes and a recent foot amputation may become actively suicidal. In this case,

it is likely he will be transferred to the psychiatric unit, where his blood glucose level will be monitored and wound care completed.

Psychiatric mental health advanced practice registered nurses are also represented in inpatient care settings. These master's or doctoral prepared nurse practitioners and clinical nurse specialists are trained to provide much of the same care as psychiatrists. Assessment of mental health, diagnosis of mental health disorders, and prescription of psychiatric medication fall under the job description with varying levels of state-mandated supervision by a physician. Advanced practice psychiatric nurses are qualified to engage in talk therapy (psychotherapy), group therapy, and managing patient care across the life span.

SPECIALTY TREATMENT SETTINGS

Treatment options are available that provide specialized care for specific groups of people. These options include inpatient, outpatient, and residential care.

Pediatric Psychiatric Care

Children with mental illnesses have the same range of treatment options as do adults but receive them apart from adults in pediatric settings. Inpatient care may be necessary if the child's symptoms become severe. Parental or guardian—including Department of Children and Families—involvement in the plan of care is integral so that they understand the illness, treatment, and the family's role in supporting the child. Additionally, hospitalized children, if able, attend school several hours a day.

Geriatric Psychiatric Care

The older adult population may be treated in specialized mental health settings that take into account the effects of aging on psychiatric symptoms. Physical illness and loss of independence can be strong precipitants in the development of depression and anxiety. Dementia is a particularly common problem encountered in geriatric psychiatry. Treatment is aimed at careful evaluation of the interaction of mind and body and provision of care that optimizes strengths, promotes independence, and focuses on safety.

Veterans Administration Centers

Active military personnel and veterans who were not dishonorably discharged may receive federally funded inpatient or outpatient care and medication for psychiatric and alcohol or substance abuse. One of the greatest challenges veterans face is dealing with the aftereffects of the traumas of active combat. During Civil War times these late effects were termed "soldier's heart." After World War I, soldiers had "shell shock" and after World War II it was termed "battle fatigue." Currently mental health services are inundated by people suffering from posttraumatic stress disorder (PTSD). There is a prevalence of PTSD in the general population of about 7%. Among male and female soldiers aged 18 years or older returning from Iraq and Afghanistan, rates range from 9% shortly after returning from deployment to 31% a year after deployment (Veterans Statistics, 2015). This creates a tremendous need for strong psychiatric services for this population.

Forensic Psychiatric Care

Incarcerated populations, both adult and juvenile, have higher than average incidences of mental disorders or substance abuse. Researchers estimate that there are more people with mental illness in prisons than in hospitals (Torrey et al., 2010). Treatment may be provided within the prison system, where inmates are often separated from the general prison population. State hospitals also treat forensic patients. Most facilities provide psychotherapy, group counseling, medication management, and assistance with transition to the community.

Alcohol and Drug Abuse Treatment

All the mental health settings that were previously described may provide treatment for alcohol and substance abuse, although specialized treatment centers exist apart from the mental health care system. While an estimated 22.7 million people older than age 12 needed treatment for an illicit drug or alcohol use problem in 2013, only 2.5 million received treatment at a specialty facility (Substance Abuse and Mental Health Services Administration [SAMHSA], 2014). This treatment is typically outpatient and includes counseling, education, medication management, and 12-step programs. Because alcohol detoxification can be life-threatening, inpatient care may be required for medical management. Drug rehabilitation facilities provide inpatient care for detoxification of drugs, including opiates and chemicals, and offer all levels of outpatient care.

Self-Help Options

Obtaining sufficient sleep, meditating, eating right, exercising, abstaining from smoking, and limiting the use of alcohol are healthy responses to a variety of illnesses such as diabetes and hypertension. As with other medical conditions, lifestyle choices and self-help responses can have a profound influence on the quality of life and the course, progression, and outcome of psychiatric disorders. If we accept the notion that psychiatric disorders are usually a combination of biochemical interactions, genetics, and environment, then it stands to reason that by providing a healthy living situation, we are likely to fare better. If, for example, a person has a family history of anxiety and has demonstrated symptoms of anxiety, then a good first step (or an adjunct to psychiatric treatment) could be to learn yoga and balance the amounts of life's obligations with relaxation.

A voluntary network of self-help groups operates outside the formal mental health care system to provide education, contacts, and support. Since the introduction of Alcoholics Anonymous in the early twentieth century, self-help groups have multiplied and have proven to be effective in the treatment and support of psychiatric problems. Groups specific to anxiety, depression, loss, caretakers' issues, bipolar disorder, posttraumatic stress disorder, and almost every other psychiatric issue are widely available in most communities.

Consumers, people who use mental health services, and their family members have successfully united to shape the delivery of mental health care. Nonprofit organizations such as the National Alliance on Mental Illness (NAMI) encourage self-help and promote the concept of **recovery,** or the self-management of mental illness. Introduced in Chapter 1 and discussed further in Chapters 3 and 19, these grassroots groups also confront social stigma, influence and policies, and support the rights of people experiencing mental illness.

PAYING FOR MENTAL HEALTH CARE

On March 23, 2010, President Obama, signed into law the **Affordable Care Act.** This groundbreaking piece of legislation will help insure millions of people who could not previously afford health care insurance. This will include millions of children and adults with mental health conditions who will no longer be denied health care because of pre-existing conditions. Some other provisions under this law include:

- Insurance companies can no longer deny a person because of pre-existing conditions or for rescinding or taking away insurance for health/mental health related reasons
- Expansion of coverage for young adults up to the age of 26 under the parents' family policy

- A provision for people over 65 on Medicare—a 50% discount for name-brand drugs that reach the Medicare "doughnut-hole"
- Provides tax credits for small businesses that offer insurance
- Provides affordable coverage to millions of Americans who are not able to afford care
- Insurance to cover preventive services such as depression screening and behavioral assessment for children
- Expands integration between primary care and behavioral health care

Before the Affordable Care Act (ACA) there were 48.6 million people without health care insurance (15.7%). According to a 2015 CDC study the uninsured rate is 9.2%, the lowest rate in 50 years. Although there is present controversy and imperfections in the ACA, it is estimated that over 15 million Americans have health insurance due to the Affordable Care Act. "This is aside from the current 10 million Medicaid sign ups and 3 million on their parents' plan by the start of February 2015" (Obama Care Facts, 2016).

In addition to the Affordable Care Act and state and private insurance coverage, public assistance is available for mental health care and costs of living. Four assistance programs are Medicare, Medicaid, Social Security, and the Veterans Administration (VA). Medicare is a national program that provides benefits to those who are 65 years of age or older and to those who have become totally disabled. In the case of mental illness, benefits are limited and coverage may be 50% for outpatient care compared with 80% for non–mental health outpatient care. Medicaid operates under federal guidelines and state regulations and pays mental health care costs for people who have extreme financial need.

States vary widely in how they fund mental health care, but all states must provide benefits for inpatient care, PCP services, and treatment for those younger than age 21. Social Security has two federal programs designed to help people with disabilities. Social Security Disability Insurance (SSDI) may be awarded to individuals who have worked a required length of time, have paid into Social Security, and are disabled for 12 months or more. About 38% of all SSDI beneficiaries have mental disorders. Supplemental Security Income (SSI) provides benefits based on economic need (Social Security Administration, 2015).

A VISION FOR MENTAL HEALTH CARE IN AMERICA

Despite the availability and variety of community psychiatric treatments in the United States, many patients in this country in need of services are not receiving them. In addition to stigma, there are geographic, financial, and systems factors that limit access to psychiatric care. For example, mental health services are scarce in some rural areas, and many American families cannot afford health insurance even if they are working.

A vision for mental health care in the future includes:

- Americans understand that mental health is essential to overall health.
- Mental health care is consumer and family driven.
- Disparities in mental health services are eliminated.
- Early mental health screening, assessment, and referral to services are common practice.
- Excellent mental health care is delivered and research is accelerated.
- Technology is used to access mental health care and information.

Psychiatric registered nurses are uniquely qualified to address each of the goals mentioned above due to an integrated educational background that includes biology, psychology, and the social sciences.

Nurses specializing in this area will increasingly be in demand. As the population ages, more geropsychiatric nurses will be needed to work with older adult psychiatric patients with complex health problems. Advanced practice psychiatric nurses may collaborate more with primary health care practitioners or in independent practice to fill the gap in existing community services.

The ACA is still evolving and has its critics. The 2016 election may see many changes to the ACA or even a repeal. This could greatly change access to medical care for the mentally ill, those with pre-existing conditions (especially children), and young adults.

We envision a future when everyone with a mental illness will improve, a future when mental illnesses can be mitigated or even prevented or cured, a future when mental illnesses are detected early, and a future when everyone with a mental illness at any stage of life has access to effective treatment supports—essentials for living, working, learning, and participating fully in the community.

KEY POINTS TO REMEMBER

- Compared to seeking care for physical disorders, finding care for psychiatric disorders can be complicated by a two-tiered system of care provided in the private and public sectors.
- Nonspecialist primary care providers treat a significant portion of psychiatric disorders.
- Psychiatric care providers are specialists who are licensed to prescribe medication and conduct therapy. They include psychiatrists, advanced practice psychiatric nurses, physicians' assistants, and, in some states, psychologists.
- Community mental health centers are state-regulated and state-funded facilities that are staffed by a variety of mental health care professionals.
- Other outpatient settings include psychiatric home care, intensive outpatient programs, and partial hospitalization programs.
- Inpatient care is used when less restrictive outpatient options are insufficient in dealing with symptoms. It can be provided in general medical centers, private psychiatric centers, crisis units, and state hospitals.
- Nurses provide the basis for inpatient care and are part of the overall unit milieu that emphasizes the role of the total environment in providing support and treatment.
- Specific populations such as children, veterans, geriatrics, and forensics benefit from treatment geared to their unique needs.
- Financing psychiatric care has been complicated by lack of parity, or equal payment for physical as compared to psychiatric disorders. Legislation has been proposed and passed to improve mental health parity.

APPLYING CRITICAL JUDGMENT

1. You are a community psychiatric mental health nurse working at a local mental health center. A single, 45-year-old patient reports that his thoughts seem to be "all tangled up." He states that he does not know how much longer he can go on, but makes no direct reference to suicidal intent. He is disheveled and has been sleeping poorly at shelters. He becomes agitated when you suggest that it might be helpful for you to contact his family. He refuses to sign any release of information forms. He admits to recent hospitalization at the local veterans' hospital and reports previous treatment at a dual-diagnosis facility even though he denies substance abuse. In addition to his mental health problems,

he says that he has tested positive for human immunodeficiency virus and should be taking multiple medications that he cannot name.

A. What are your biopsychosocial and spiritual concerns about this patient?

B. What is the highest priority problem to address before he leaves the clinic today?

C. Do you feel that you need to consult with any other members of the multidisciplinary team today about this patient?

D. In your role as case manager, what systems of care will you need to coordinate to provide quality care for this patient?

E. How will you start to develop trust with the patient to gain his cooperation with the treatment plan?

CHAPTER REVIEW QUESTIONS

1. A patient diagnosed with major depressive disorder tells the community mental health nurse, "I usually spend all day watching television. If there's nothing good to watch, I just sleep or think about my problems." What is the nurse's best action?
   a. Refer the patient for counseling with a recreational therapist.
   b. Ask the patient, "What kinds of program do you like to watch?"
   c. Suggest to the patient, "Are there some friends you could call instead?"
   d. Advise the patient, "Watching television and thinking about problems makes depression worse."

2. The nurse admits a patient experiencing hallucinations and delusional thinking to an inpatient mental health unit. The plan of care will require which service occurs first?
   a. Social history
   b. Psychiatric history
   c. Medical assessment
   d. Psychological evaluation

3. A nurse working in an acute care unit for adolescents diagnosed with mental illness says, "Our patients have so much energy. We need some physical activities for them." In recognition of needs for safety and exercise, which activity could the treatment team approve?
   a. Badminton tournament
   b. Competitive soccer matches
   c. Intramural basketball games
   d. Line dancing to popular music

4. As Election Day nears, a mental health nurse studies the position statements of various candidates for federal offices. Which candidate's commentary would the nurse interpret as supportive of services for persons diagnosed with mental illness?
   a. "Full parity insurance coverage for mental illness"
   b. "Coverage for biologically based mental illnesses"
   c. "Reimbursement for initial treatment of addictions"
   d. "Managed care oversight for mental illness services"

5. An experienced nurse in a major medical center requests a transfer from a general medical unit to an acute care psychiatric unit. Which organizational feature would best support this nurse's successful transition?
   a. Assignment to medication administration for the first 6 months
   b. Working with a seasoned mental health technician for the first month
   c. Co-assignment with a knowledgeable psychiatric nurse for an extended orientation
   d. Staff development activities focused on developing therapeutic communication skills

REFERENCES

Agency for Healthcare Research and Quality. (2015). *Defining the PCMH*. Retrieved December 29, 2011 from www.pcmh.ahrq.gov-/page/defining-pcmh.

American Psychiatric Nurses Association, International Society of Psychiatric-Mental Health Nurses, & American Nurses Association. (2014). *Psychiatric-mental health nursing: scope and standards of practice* (3rd ed.). Silver Spring, Md: American Nurses Association.

Gradus, J. L. (2010). *Epidemiology of PTSD. In United States Department of Veterans Affairs*. Retrieved April 16, 2011, from www.ptsd.va.gov/professional/pages/epidemiological-facts-ptsd.asp.

National Association of Psychiatric Health Systems. (2009). *2008 NAPHS Annual Survey*. Washington, DC.

National Association of State Mental Health Program Directors. (2014). *The vital role of state psychiatric hospitals*. Retrieved from www.nasmhpd.org/Publications/The%20Vital%20Role%20of%20State%20Psychiatric%20HospitalsTechnical%20Report_July_2014.pdf.

National Conference of State Legislatures. (2010). *State laws mandating or regulating mental health benefits*. Retrieved from www.ncsl.org/default.aspx?tabid=14352.

Piper Report. (2011). *Hospitalizations for mental health and substance abuse disorders: costs, length of stay, patient mix, and payor mix*. Retrieved from www.piperreport.com/blog/2011/06/25/hospitalizations-for-mental-health-and-substance-abuse-disorders.

President's New Freedom Commission on Mental Health. (2003). *Achieving the promise: transforming mental health care in America*. Retrieved from http://govinfo.library.unt.edu/mentalhealthcommission/reports/FinalReport/toc.html.

Social Security Administration. (2015). *Understanding supplemental security income*. Retrieved from www.ssa.gov/ssi/text-eligibility-ussi.htm.

Substance Abuse and Mental Health Services Administration. (2014). *Substance use and mental health estimates from the 2013 national survey on drug use and health*. Retrieved from www.samhsa.gov/data/sites/default/files/NSDUH-SR200-RecoveryMonth-2014/NSDUH-SR200-RecoveryMonth-2014.htm.

Torrey, E. F., Kennard, A. D., Eslinger, D., et al. (2010). *More mentally ill persons are in jails and prisons than hospitals: a survey of the states*. Retrieved from http://74.125.155.132/scholar?q=-cache:_ulTyMxYGAsJ:scholar.google.com/+percent+of+prison+population+with+a+mental+disorder&hl=en&as_sdt=0,36&as_ylo=2009.

United States Census Bureau. (2013). *Health insurance coverage rates by types of insurance: 2013*. Retrieved from www.census.gov/h-hes/www/hlthins/data/incpovhlth/2013/Table1.pdf.

Veterans Statistics. PTSD, Depression, TBI, Suicide. Veterans and PTSD. Retrieved September 20, 2015 from www.veteransandptsd.com/PTSD-statistics.html.

Legal and Ethical Basis for Practice

Penny Simpson Brooke

ⓔ http://evolve.elsevier.com/Varcarolis/essentials

KEY TERMS AND CONCEPTS

abandonment, p. 70
assault, p. 68
autonomy, p. 62
battery, p. 68
beneficence, p. 62
bioethics, p. 62
child abuse reporting statutes, p. 67
civil rights, p. 62
commitment, p. 63
conditional release, p. 64
confidentiality, p. 66
defamation of character, p. 69
discharge, p. 64

duty to warn, p. 67
elder abuse reporting statutes, p. 67
ethical dilemma, p. 61
ethics, p. 62
false imprisonment, p. 68
fidelity, p. 62
foreseeability of harm, p. 69
Health Insurance Portability and Account-
    ability Act (HIPAA), p. 65
implied consent, p. 65
informed consent, p. 65
intentional torts, p. 68
involuntary admission, p. 63

involuntary outpatient commitment, p. 63
justice, p. 62
least restrictive alternative doctrine, p. 63
legal guardian, p. 65
negligence, p. 69
punitive damages, p. 69
right to privacy, p. 66
right to refuse treatment, p. 64
right to treatment, p. 64
tort, p. 68
veracity, p. 62
voluntary admission, p. 63
writ of habeas corpus, p. 63

SELECTED CONCEPT: RIGHT TO TREATMENT

With the enactment of the Hospitalization of the Mentally Ill Act in 1964, the federal statutory right to psychiatric treatment in public hospitals was created. The statute requires that medical and psychiatric care and treatment be provided to everyone admitted to a public hospital.
  Based on the decisions of a number of early court cases, treatment must meet the following criteria:
* The environment must be humane.
* The staff must be qualified and sufficient to provide adequate treatment.
* The plan of care must be individualized.

OBJECTIVES

1. Compare and contrast the different admission procedures including admission criteria.
2. Summarize patients' rights as they pertain to the patient's (a) right to treatment, (b) right to refuse treatment, and (c) right to informed consent.
3. **QSEN** Delineate the steps nurses are advised to take to ensure patient **safety** if they suspect negligence or illegal activity on the part of a professional colleague or peer.
4. **QSEN** Discuss the legal considerations of patient privilege (a) after a patient has died, (b) if the patient tests positive for human

immunodeficiency virus, or (c) if the patient's employer states a "need to know." **(Patient-centered care)**
5. **QSEN** Summarize situations in which health care professionals have a duty to break patient confidentiality. **(Safety)**
6. Discuss a patient's civil rights and describe how they pertain to restraint and seclusion.
7. Discuss in detail the balance between the patient's rights and the rights of society with respect to the following legal concepts relevant in nursing and psychiatric nursing: (a) duty to intervene, (b) documentation and charting, and (c) confidentiality.

INTRODUCTION

This chapter introduces you to current legal and ethical issues that may be encountered in the practice of psychiatric nursing. A fundamental goal of psychiatric care is to strike a balance between the rights of the individual patient and the rights of society at large. This chapter is designed to assist you in understanding the implications of ethical or legal issues on the provision of care in a psychiatric setting.

An ethical dilemma results when there is a conflict between two or more courses of action, each carrying with them favorable and unfavorable consequences. How we respond to these dilemmas is based partly on our own morals (beliefs of right or wrong) and values. Suppose you are caring for a pregnant woman with schizophrenia who wants to carry the baby to term, but whose family insists she get an abortion. In order to promote fetal safety, her antipsychotic medication will need to be reduced, putting her at risk of exacerbation of the illness. Furthermore, there is a question as to whether she can safely care for the child. If you relied on the ethical principle of autonomy, you may conclude that she has the right to decide. Would other ethical principles be in conflict with autonomy in this case?

At times your values may be in conflict with the value system of the institution. This situation further complicates the decision-making process and necessitates careful consideration of the patient's desires. For example, you may experience a conflict in a setting where older adult patients are routinely tranquilized to a degree that you find excessive. Whenever one's value system is challenged, increased stress results.

LEGAL AND ETHICAL CONCEPTS

Ethics is the study of philosophical beliefs about what is considered right or wrong in a society. Bioethics is a more specific term that refers to the ethical questions that arise in health care. The five basic principles of bioethics are as follows:

1. Beneficence: The duty to act so as to benefit or promote the good of others. Spending extra time to help calm an extremely anxious patient is a beneficent act.
2. Autonomy: Respecting the rights of others to make their own decisions. Acknowledging the patient's right to refuse medication is an example of promoting autonomy.
3. Justice: The duty to distribute resources or care equally, regardless of personal attributes. An example of justice is when an intensive care unit (ICU) nurse devotes equal attention both to a patient who has attempted suicide and to another patient who suffered a brain aneurysm.
4. Fidelity (nonmaleficence): Maintaining loyalty and commitment to the patient and doing no wrong to the patient. Maintaining expertise in nursing skill through nursing education demonstrates fidelity to patient care.
5. Veracity: One's duty to communicate truthfully. Describing the purpose and side effects of psychotropic medications in a truthful and nonmisleading way is an example of veracity.

Law and ethics are closely related because law tends to reflect the ethical values of society. It should be noted that although you may feel obligated to follow ethical guidelines, these guidelines should not override laws. For example, if you are aware of a statute or a specific rule or regulation created by the state board of nursing that prohibits a certain action (e.g., restraining patients against their will) and you feel you have an ethical obligation to protect the patient by engaging in such an action (e.g., using restraints), you would be wise to follow the law.

MENTAL HEALTH LAWS

Laws have been enacted to regulate the care and treatment of the mentally ill. Mental health laws, or statutes, vary from state to state; in order to understand the legal climate of your specific state, you are encouraged to review its code. This can be accomplished by visiting the webpage of your state mental health department or by doing an *Internet search using the following key words: 'mental+health+statutes+(your state)'*.

Many of these laws have undergone major revision since 1963, which reflects a shift in emphasis from state or institutional care of the mentally ill to community-based care. This was heralded by the enactment of the Community Mental Health Center Act of 1963 under President John F. Kennedy. Along with this shift in emphasis has come the more widespread use of psychotropic drugs in the treatment of mental illness—which has enabled many people to integrate more readily into the larger community—and an increasing awareness of the need to provide the mentally ill with humane care that respects their civil rights. Parity in health insurance coverage for mental health treatment was addressed in 2010 by two separate laws. The Paul Wellstone and Pete Domenici Mental Health Parity and Addiction Equity Act states that if mental health or substance abuse care is covered by a private insurance plan, then these conditions must receive coverage equitable to other physical medical conditions. The 2010 Health Insurance Exchanges program requires that each state offers mental health care and substance use services equal to other medical services (Bazelon, 2010).

In providing protective coverage for mental health and substance abuse, the Affordable Care Act (ACA) built upon the Mental Health Parity and Addition Equity Act of 2008 (CMHPAE), which provided rehabilitative support services for behavior health needs. The CMHPAE was signed into law on October 3, 2008, and became effective on January 1, 2010 (Beronio et al., 2013). Mental health coverage and substance abuse coverage are included in the essential health benefits provision of the Affordable Care Act (ACA). Mental health coverage must be at parity with medical and surgical benefits, meaning coverage cannot be more restrictive than coverage for general medical benefits. It is projected that the ACA has expanded mental health and substance abuse benefits, with parity protections to between 60 and 62 million Americans. Most health plans must now cover preventive mental services at no cost. Screening for depression and other adult mental health conditions as well as behavioral assessments for children are covered by the ACA. Additionally, as of 2014, insurance plans cannot charge more nor deny coverage for preexisting mental health conditions (Beronio et al., 2013).

However, disparities in state-by-state coverage impact the benefits afforded to mental health patients by the ACA. More than 21 states initially refused the ACA provisions to expand Medicaid coverage following the 2012 United States Supreme Court decision to allow states to opt out. Homeless and low-income persons are impacted by Medicaid coverage. Sixteen states and the District of Columbia set up their own insurance exchanges and thus determine their own essential benefits to be covered (Brink, 2014). Nurses working with mental health and substance abuse patients must inform them of the benefits of coverage in their own jurisdiction.

Civil Rights

People with mental illness are guaranteed the same rights under federal and state laws as any other citizen. Most states specifically prohibit any person from depriving an individual receiving mental health services of his or her civil rights, including the right to vote; the right to civil service ranking; the rights related to granting, forfeit, or denial of a driver's license; the right to make purchases and to enter contractual relationships (unless the patient has lost legal capacity by being incompetent); and the right to press charges against another person. The psychiatric patient's rights include the right to humane care and treatment. The medical, dental, and psychiatric needs of the patient must be met in accordance with the prevailing standards accepted in these professions. The mentally ill in prisons and jails are afforded the same protections. The right to religious freedom and practice, the right to social interaction, and the right to exercise and recreational opportunities are also protected.

In recent years many states have established Mental Health Courts to process criminal cases involving defendants with mental illnesses. These courts attempt to direct the offender to treatment and services in the community (Bazelon, 2011).

ADMISSION AND DISCHARGE PROCEDURES

Due Process in Civil Commitment

The courts have recognized that involuntary civil commitment to a mental hospital is a "massive curtailment of liberty" (*Humphrey v. Cady*, 1972) requiring due process protections in the civil commitment procedure. This right derives from the Fifth Amendment of the U.S. Constitution, which states that "no person shall ... be deprived of life, liberty, or property without due process of law." The Fourteenth Amendment explicitly prohibits states from depriving citizens of life, liberty, and property without due process of law. State civil commitment statutes, if challenged in the courts on constitutional grounds, must afford minimal due process protections to pass the court's scrutiny (*Zinermon v. Burch*, 1990). In most states, a patient can challenge commitments through a writ of habeas corpus, which means a "formal written order" to "free the person." The writ of habeas corpus is the procedural mechanism used to challenge unlawful detention by the government.

The writ of habeas corpus and the least restrictive alternative doctrine are two of the most important concepts applicable to civic commitment cases. The least restrictive alternative doctrine mandates that the least drastic means be taken to achieve a specific purpose. For example, if someone can safely be treated for depression on an outpatient basis, hospitalization would be too restrictive and unnecessarily disruptive.

Admission to the Hospital

All students are encouraged to become familiar with the important provisions of the laws in their own states regarding admissions, discharges, patients' rights, and informed consent.

A medical standard or justification for admission should exist. A well-defined psychiatric problem must be established, based on current illness classifications in the current *Diagnostic and Statistical Manual of Mental Disorders (DSM-5)* authored by the American Psychiatric Association in 2013. The presenting illness should also be of such a nature that it causes an immediate crisis situation or that other less restrictive alternatives are inadequate or unavailable. There should also be a reasonable expectation that the hospitalization and treatment will improve the presenting problems.

In the case of *Olmstead v. L.C.* (1999) the Supreme Court of the United States ruled that states are required to place patients with mental health illness in less restrictive community settings, rather than institutions, when the treatment profession has determined that a community setting is appropriate and the patient is not opposed to the decision to transfer from an institution to a community facility.

Voluntary Admission

Generally, voluntary admission is sought by the patient or the patient's guardian through a written application to the facility. Voluntarily admitted patients have the right to demand and obtain release. However, few states require voluntarily admitted patients to be notified of the rights associated with their status. In addition, many states require that a patient submit a written release notice to the facility staff, who reevaluate the patient's condition for possible conversion to involuntary status according to criteria established by state law.

Involuntary Admission (Commitment)

Involuntary admission is made without the patient's consent. Generally, involuntary admission is necessary when a person is in need of psychiatric treatment, presents a danger to self or others, or is unable to meet his or her own basic needs. Involuntary commitment requires that the patient retain freedom from unreasonable bodily restraints as well as the right to informed consent and the right to refuse medications, including psychotropic or antipsychotic medications.

Three different commitment procedures are commonly available: **judicial determination, administrative determination,** and **agency determination.** In addition, a specified number of physicians must certify that a person's mental health status justifies detention and treatment. Involuntary hospitalization can be further categorized by the nature and purpose of the involuntary admission: emergency hospitalization; observational or temporary hospitalization; long-term or formal commitment; or outpatient commitment.

Emergency involuntary hospitalization. Most states provide for emergency involuntary hospitalization or civil commitment for a specified period (1 to 10 days on average) to prevent dangerous behavior that is likely to cause harm to self or others. Police officers, physicians, and mental health professionals may be designated by law to authorize the detention of mentally ill individuals who are a danger to themselves or others.

Observational or temporary involuntary hospitalization. Civil commitment for observational or temporary involuntary hospitalization is of longer duration than emergency hospitalization. The primary purpose of this type of hospitalization is observation, diagnosis, and treatment for those who have mental illness or pose a danger to themselves or others. The length of time and procedures vary markedly from state to state. A guardian, family member, physician, or other public health officer may apply for this type of admission. Certification by two or more physicians, a judicial review, or administrative review and order is often required for involuntary admission.

Long-term or formal commitment. Long-term commitment for involuntary hospitalization has as its primary purpose extended care and treatment of the mentally ill. Those who undergo extended involuntary hospitalization are committed through medical certification, judicial, or administrative action. Some states do not require a judicial hearing before commitment, but often provide the patient with an opportunity for a judicial review after commitment procedures. This type of involuntary hospitalization generally lasts 60 to 180 days, but may be for an indeterminate period.

Involuntary outpatient commitment. Beginning in the 1990s, states began to pass legislation that permitted outpatient commitment as an alternative to forced inpatient treatment. Recently states have begun using involuntary outpatient commitment as a preventive measure, allowing a court order before the onset of a psychiatric crisis that would result in an inpatient commitment. The order for involuntary outpatient commitment is usually tied to receipt of goods and services provided by social welfare agencies, including disability benefits and housing. To access these goods and services the patient is mandated to participate in treatment and may face inpatient admission if he or she fails to participate in treatment (Chan, 2003; Monahan et al., 2003; Rainey, 2001). Forced treatment raises ethical dilemmas regarding autonomy versus paternalism, privacy rights, duty to protect, and right to treatment; and has been challenged on constitutional grounds.

Discharge from the Hospital

Release from hospitalization depends on the patient's admission status. Patients who sought informal or voluntary admission, as previously discussed, have the right to request and receive release. Some states, however, do provide for conditional release of voluntary patients, which enables the treating physician or administrator to order continued treatment on an outpatient basis if the clinical needs of the patient warrant further care.

Conditional Release

Conditional release usually requires outpatient treatment for a specified period to determine the patient's adherence with medication protocols, ability to meet basic needs, and ability to reintegrate into the community. Generally a voluntarily hospitalized patient who is conditionally released can only be committed through the usual methods for involuntary hospitalization. However, an involuntarily hospitalized patient who is conditionally released may be reinstitutionalized while the commitment is still in effect without recommencement of formal admission procedures.

Unconditional Release

Unconditional release, or discharge, is the termination of a patient-institution relationship. This release may be court ordered or administratively ordered by the institution's officials. Generally, the administrative officer of an institution has the discretion to discharge patients.

Release Against Medical Advice (AMA)

In some cases there is a disagreement between mental health care providers and patients as to whether continued hospitalization is necessary. When treatment seems beneficial, but there is no compelling reason (e.g., danger to self or others) to seek an involuntary continuance of stay, patients may be released against medical advice.

PATIENTS' RIGHTS UNDER THE LAW

Psychiatric facilities usually provide patients with a written list of basic patient rights. These rights are derived from a variety of sources, especially legislation that was developed during the 1960s. Since then, they have been modified to some degree, but most lists share commonalities as stated in the following sections.

Right to Treatment

With the enactment of the Hospitalization of the Mentally Ill Act in 1964, the federal statutory right to psychiatric treatment in public hospitals was created. The statute requires that medical and psychiatric care and treatment be provided to everyone admitted to a public hospital.

Although state courts and lower federal courts have decided that there may be a federal constitutional right to treatment, the U.S. Supreme Court has never firmly defined the right to treatment in a constitutional principle. The evolution of these cases in the courts provides an interesting history of the development and shortcomings of our mental health delivery system. Based on the decisions of a number of early court cases, treatment must meet the following criteria:

- The environment must be humane.
- Staff must be qualified and sufficient to provide adequate treatment.
- The plan of care must be individualized.

The initial cases presenting the psychiatric patient's right to treatment arose in the criminal justice system. An interesting case regarding a person's right to treatment is *O'Connor v. Donaldson* (1975). The Court held that a "state cannot constitutionally confine a nondangerous individual who is capable of surviving safely in freedom by himself or with the help of willing and responsible family members or friends."

Right to Refuse Treatment

A companion to the right to consent to treatment is the right to withhold consent. A patient may also withdraw consent at any time. Retraction of consent previously given must be honored, whether it is verbal or written. However, the mentally ill patient's right to refuse treatment with psychotropic drugs has been debated in the courts, based partly on the issue of mental patients' competency to give or withhold consent to treatment and their status under the civil commitment statutes. These early cases, initiated by state hospital patients, considered medical, legal, and ethical considerations, such as basic treatment problems, the doctrine of informed consent, and the bioethical principle of autonomy. For a summary of the evolution of one landmark set of cases regarding the patient's right to refuse treatment, see Table 6-1.

The notion of refusing treatment becomes especially important if we consider medication to be a "chemical restraint." If it is, then the infringement on a person's liberty is at least equal to that with involuntary commitment. In this circumstance, the noninstitutionalized, competent, mentally ill patient has the right, through substituted judgment, to determine whether to be involuntarily committed or to be medicated.

TABLE 6-1	Right to Refuse Treatment: Evolution of Massachusetts Case Law to Present Law	
Case	**Court**	**Decision**
Rogers v. Okin, 478 F. Supp. 1342 (D. Mass. 1979)	Federal district court	Ruled that involuntarily hospitalized patients with mental illness are competent and have the right to make treatment decisions.
		Forcible administration of medication is justified in an emergency if needed to prevent violence and if other alternatives have been ruled out.
		A guardian may make treatment decisions for an incompetent patient.
Rogers v. Okin, 634 F. 2nd 650 (1st Cir. 1980)	Federal court of appeals	Affirmed that involuntarily hospitalized patients with mental illness are competent and have the right to make treatment decisions.
		The staff has substantial discretion in an emergency.
		Forcible medication is also justified to prevent the patient's deterioration.
		A patient's rights must be protected by judicial determination of competency or incompetency.
Mills v. Rogers, 457 U.S. 291 (1982)	U.S. Supreme Court	Set aside the judgment of the court of appeals with instructions to consider the effect of an intervening state court case.
Rogers v. Commissioner of the Department of Mental Health, 458 N.E.2d 308 (Mass. 1983)	Massachusetts Supreme Judicial Court answering questions certified by federal court of appeals	Ruled that involuntarily hospitalized patients are competent and have the right to make treatment decisions unless they are judicially determined to be incompetent.

Cases involving the right to refuse psychotropic drug treatment are still evolving. Without clear direction from the Supreme Court, there will be different case outcomes in different jurisdictions.

The numerous cases involving the right to refuse medication have illustrated the complex and difficult task of translating social policy concerns into a clearly articulated legal standard.

Right to Informed Consent

The principle of informed consent is based on a person's right to self-determination, as enunciated in the landmark case of *Canterbury v. Spence* (1972):

The root premise is the concept, fundamental in American jurisprudence, that every human being of adult years and sound mind has a right to determine what shall be done with his own body.... True consent to what happens to one's self is the informed exercise of choice, and that entails an opportunity to evaluate knowledgeably the options available and the risks attendant on each.

Proper orders for specific therapies and treatments are required and must be documented in the patient's chart. Consent for surgery, electroconvulsive treatment, or the use of experimental drugs or procedures must be obtained. In some state institutions, consent is required for every medication addition or change. Patients have the right to refuse participation in experimental treatments or research and the right to voice grievances and recommend changes in policies or services offered by the facility, without fear of punishment or reprisal.

For consent to be effective legally, it must be informed. Generally, the informed consent of the patient must be obtained by the physician or other health professional who will perform the treatment or procedure. Patients must be informed of the nature of their problem or condition, the nature and purpose of a proposed treatment, the risks and benefits of that treatment, the alternative treatment options available, the probability that the proposed treatment will be successful, and the risks of not consenting to treatment. It is important for psychiatric nurses to know that the presence of psychotic thinking does not mean that the patient is incompetent or incapable of understanding.

Neither voluntary nor involuntary admission to a mental facility determines whether patients are capable of making informed decisions about the health care they may need. Patients must be considered legally competent until they have been declared incompetent through a legal proceeding. Competency is related to the capacity to understand the consequences of one's decisions. The determination of legal competency is made by the courts. If found incompetent, the court may appoint a legal guardian or representative who is legally responsible for giving or refusing consent for a person the court has found to be incompetent.

Guardians have a duty to act in their wards' best interests. "Courts appoint guardians to care for people who cannot take care of themselves. The person a guardian protects is called that guardian's ward. Wards may be either minor children or incapacitated adults. In some other jurisdictions, "custodial" or "conservator" is used instead of "guardian," and some jurisdictions use different terms to refer to different types of guardianships, for example, calling the protector of elderly wards a "conservator" while calling the protector of minor children wards a "guardian." Where appropriate, courts may appoint guardians with limited authority. "Guardians are fiduciaries of their wards" (*Francine M. Neilson v. Colgate-Palmolive Co.*, 199 f.3d 642 [2d Cir. 1999]; www.law.cornell.edu/wex/guardian).

Guardians are usually selected from among family members. The order of selection is usually (1) spouse, (2) adult children or grandchildren, (3) parents, (4) adult brothers and sisters, and (5) nieces and nephews. In the event that a family member is either unavailable or unwilling to serve as guardian, the court may also appoint a court-trained and court-approved social worker representing the county or state or a member of the community.

Many procedures that nurses perform have an element of implied consent attached. For example, if you approach the patient with a medication in hand and the patient indicates a willingness to receive the medication, implied consent has occurred. It should be noted that many institutions, particularly state psychiatric hospitals, have a requirement to obtain informed consent for every medication given. A general rule for you to follow is that the more intrusive or risky the procedure, the higher the likelihood that informed consent must be obtained. The fact that you may not have a legal duty to be the person to inform patients of the associated risks and benefits of a particular medical procedure does not excuse you from clarifying the procedure to patients and ensuring their expressed or implied consent.

Rights Surrounding Involuntary Commitment and Psychiatric Advance Directives

Patients concerned that they may be subject to involuntary psychiatric commitment can prepare an advance psychiatric directive document that will express their treatment choices. The advance directive for mental health decision making should be followed by health care providers when patients are not competent to make informed decisions for themselves. This document can clarify the patient's choice of a surrogate decision maker and instructions about hospital choices, medications, treatment options, and emergency interventions. Identification of individuals who are to be notified of the patient's hospitalization and who may have visitation rights is especially helpful given the privacy demands of the Health Insurance Portability and Accountability Act (HIPAA) (Bazelon, 2003).

Rights Regarding Restraint and Seclusion

The use of the least restrictive means of restraint for the shortest duration is always the general rule and even the law. Verbal interventions or enlisting the cooperation of patients are examples of first-line interventions. Recent changes in the law regarding the use of restraints and seclusion have prompted agencies to revise their policies and procedures, further limiting these practices. The current trend is toward "restraint free" environments and alternative methods of therapy and cooperation with the patient, which is proving successful.

Typically, medication is considered if verbal interventions fail. Chemical interventions are usually considered less restrictive than mechanical, but can have a greater effect on the patient's ability to relate to the environment. When used judiciously, psychopharmacology is extremely effective and helpful as an alternative to other physical methods of restraint.

The history of mechanical restraint and seclusion is one that is marked by abuses and overuse, and even a tendency to use restraint as punishment. This was especially true before the 1950s, when there were no effective chemical treatments. Legislation has dramatically reduced this problem by mandating strict guidelines. The newest guidelines of the Centers for Medicare & Medicaid Services (CMS) and The Joint Commission guidelines read (2008):

A-0154 (Rev. 37, Issued: 10-17-08; Effective/Implementation Date: 10-17-08) §482.13(e) Standard: **Restraint or seclusion.** All patients have the right to be free from physical or mental abuse, and corporal punishment. All patients have the right to be free from restraint or seclusion, of any form, imposed as a means of coercion, discipline, convenience, or retaliation by staff. Restraint or seclusion may only be imposed to ensure the immediate physical safety of the patient, a staff member, or others and must be discontinued at the earliest possible time.

Information on 42 CFR 482: Medicare and Medicaid Programs; Hospital Conditions of Participation: Patients' Rights. "The Federal Department of Health and Human Services Centers for Medicare & Medicaid Services has rules in place regarding the use of restraint and seclusion in all Medicare and Medicaid participating hospitals. These rules specify that training requirements include:

- Demonstrated competency in the application of restraints.
- Periodic refresher training.
- Training in the use of nonphysical intervention skills.
- Information about and recognition of symptoms of patient distress, such as positional asphyxia.
- Certified in cardio pulmonary resuscitation (CPR)."

(Rev. 37, Issued: 10-17-08; Effective/Implementation Date: 10-17-08) §482.13(e)(8) — Unless superseded by State law that is more restrictive — (i) Each order for restraint or seclusion used for the management of violent or self-destructive behavior that jeopardizes the immediate physical safety of the patient, a staff member, or others may only be renewed in accordance with the following limits for up to a total of 24 hours:

(A) 4 hours for adults 18 years of age or older;

(B) 2 hours for children and adolescents 9 to 17 years of age; or

(C) 1 hour for children under 9 years of age.

In an emergency, *an appropriately trained staff for the proper and safe use of seclusion and restraint interventions* may place a patient in seclusion or restraint and obtain a written order within an hour. With the exception of a patient-initiated request to be placed in seclusion, federal laws require an emergency situation to exist in which an immediate risk of harm to the patient or others can be documented. While in restraints the patient must be protected from all sources of harm. The behavior leading to restraint or seclusion and the time the patient is placed in and released from the restraint must be documented; the patient in restraint must be assessed at regular and frequent intervals (e.g., every 15 to 30 minutes) for physical needs (e.g., food, hydration, toileting), safety, and comfort, and these observations also must be documented (every 15 to 30 minutes). The patient must be removed from restraints when safer and quieter behavior is observed.

MAINTENANCE OF PATIENT CONFIDENTIALITY

Ethical Considerations

Confidentiality of care and treatment is also an important right for all patients, particularly psychiatric patients. Any discussion or consultation involving a patient should be conducted discreetly and only with individuals who have a need and a right to know this privileged information. The American Nurses Association (ANA) *Code of Ethics for Nurses with Interpretive Statements* (2015) asserts the duty of the nurse to protect confidential patient information (Box 6-1). Failure to provide this protection may harm the nurse-patient relationship, as well as the patient's well-being. However, the code clarifies that this duty is not absolute. In some situations disclosure may be mandated to protect the patient, other people, or the public health.

Legal Considerations
Health Insurance Portability and Accountability Act

The psychiatric patient's right to receive treatment and to have confidential medical records is legally protected. The fundamental principle underlying the ANA *Code of Ethics for Nurses* on confidentiality is

---

BOX 6-1   Code of Ethics for Nurses

The House of Delegates of the American Nurses Association approved these nine provisions at its June 30, 2001, meeting in Washington, DC. In July 2001, the Congress of Nursing Practice and Economics voted to accept the new language of the interpretive statements, resulting in a fully approved revised *Code of Ethics for Nurses with Interpretive Statements.*

1. The nurse, in all professional relationships, practices with compassion and respect for the inherent dignity, worth, and uniqueness of every individual, unrestricted by considerations of social or economic status, personal attributes, or the nature of health problems.
2. The nurse's primary commitment is to the patient, whether an individual, family, group, or community.
3. The nurse promotes, advocates for, and strives to protect the health, safety, and rights of the patient.
4. The nurse is responsible and accountable for individual nursing practice and determines the appropriate delegation of tasks consistent with the nurse's obligation to provide optimum patient care.
5. The nurse owes the same duties to self as to others, including the responsibility to preserve integrity and safety, to maintain competence, and to continue personal and professional growth.
6. The nurse participates in establishing, maintaining, and improving health care environments and conditions of employment conducive to the provision of quality health care and consistent with the values of the profession through individual and collective action.
7. The nurse participates in the advancement of the profession through contributions to practice, education, administration, and knowledge development.
8. The nurse collaborates with other health professionals and the public in promoting community, national, and international efforts to meet health needs.
9. The profession of nursing, as represented by associations and their members, is responsible for articulating nursing values, for maintaining the integrity of the profession and its practice, and for shaping social policy.

From American Nurses Association. (2015). *Code of ethics for nurses with interpretive statements.* Washington, DC. ©2014 By American Nurses Association and International Society of Psychiatric-Mental Health Nurses. Reprinted with permission. All rights reserved.

---

a person's constitutional right to privacy. Generally, your legal duty to maintain confidentiality is to protect the patient's right to privacy. The Health Insurance Portability and Accountability Act (HIPAA) became effective on April 14, 2003. Therefore, you may not, without the patient's consent, disclose information obtained from the patient or information in the medical record to anyone except those individuals for whom it is necessary for implementation of the patient's treatment plan. Special protection of notes used in psychotherapy that are kept separate from the patient's health information was created by this HIPAA rule (2003). Discussions about a patient in public places such as elevators and the cafeteria, even when the patient's name is not mentioned, can lead to disclosures of confidential information and liabilities for you and the hospital.

Patients' Employers

Your release of information to the patient's employer about the patient's condition, without the patient's consent, is a breach of confidentiality that subjects you to liability for the tort of invasion of privacy as well as a HIPAA violation. On the other hand, discussion of a patient's history with other staff members to determine a consistent treatment approach is not a breach of confidentiality.

Generally, for a situation to be created in which information is privileged, a patient–health professional relationship must exist and the information must concern the care and treatment of the patient. The health professional may refuse to disclose information to protect the patient's privacy. However, the right to privacy is the patient's right, and health professionals cannot invoke confidentiality for their own defense or benefit.

Rights After Death

A person's reputation can be damaged even after death. It is therefore important not to divulge information after a person's death that could not have been legally shared before the death. The Dead Man's Statute protects confidential information about people when they are not alive to speak for themselves.

A legal privilege of confidentiality is enacted legislatively and in some states exists to protect the confidentiality of professional communications (e.g., nurse-patient, physician-patient, attorney-patient). The theory behind such privileged communications is that patients will not be comfortable or willing to disclose personal information about themselves if they fear that nurses will repeat their confidential conversations.

In some states in which the legal privilege of confidentiality has not been legislated for nurses, you must respond to a court's inquiries regarding the patient's disclosures even if this information implicates the patient in a crime. In these states the confidentiality of communications cannot be guaranteed. If a duty to report exists, you may be required to divulge private information shared by the patient.

Patient Privilege and Human Immunodeficiency Virus Status

Some states have enacted mandatory or permissive statutes that direct health care providers to warn a spouse if a partner tests positive for human immunodeficiency virus (HIV). Nurses must understand the laws in their jurisdiction of practice regarding privileged communications and warnings of infectious disease exposure.

Exceptions to the Rule

Duty to warn and protect third parties. The California Supreme Court, in its 1974 landmark decision *Tarasoff v. Regents of University of California,* ruled that a psychotherapist has a duty to warn a patient's potential victim of potential harm. A university student who was in counseling at a California university was despondent over being rejected by Tatiana Tarasoff. The psychologist notified police verbally and in writing that the young man may be dangerous to Tarasoff. The police questioned the student, found him to be rational, and secured his promise to stay away from his love interest. The student killed Tarasoff 2 months later. This case created much controversy and confusion in the psychiatric and medical communities over breach of patient confidentiality and its effect on the therapeutic relationship in psychiatric care and over the ability of the psychotherapist to predict when a patient is truly dangerous. This trend continues as other jurisdictions have adopted or modified the California rule despite the objections of the psychiatric community. These jurisdictions view public safety to be more important than privacy in narrowly defined circumstances.

The *Tarasoff* case acknowledged that generally there is no common law duty to aid third parties. An exception is when special relationships exist, and the court found the patient-therapist relationship sufficient to create a duty of the therapist to aid Ms. Tarasoff, the victim. The duty to protect the intended victim from danger arises when the therapist determines—or, pursuant to professional standards, should have determined—that the patient presents a serious danger to another. Any action reasonably necessary under the circumstances, including notification of the potential victim, the victim's family, and the police, discharges the therapist's duty to the potential victim.

In 1976, the California Supreme Court issued a second ruling in the case of *Tarasoff v. Regents of University of California* (now known as *Tarasoff II*). This ruling broadened the earlier ruling, the duty to warn, to include the **duty to protect.**

Most states have similar laws regarding the duty to warn third parties of potential life threats. The duty to warn usually includes the following:

- Assessing and predicting the patient's danger of violence toward another
- Identifying the specific individual(s) being threatened
- Taking appropriate action to protect the identified victims

Nursing implications. As this trend toward making it the therapist's duty to warn third parties of potential harm continues to gain wider acceptance, it is important for students and nurses to understand its implications for nursing practice. Although none of these cases has dealt with nurses, it is fair to assume that in jurisdictions that have adopted the Tarasoff doctrine, the duty to warn third parties will be applied to *advanced practice psychiatric mental health nurses* (PMH-APRN) in private practice who engage in individual therapy.

If, however, a staff nurse who is a member of a team of psychiatrists, psychologists, psychiatric social workers, and other psychiatric nurses does not report patient threats of harm against specified victims or classes of victims to the team of the patient's management psychotherapist for assessment and evaluation, this failure is likely to be considered substandard nursing care.

So, too, the failure to communicate and record relevant information from police, relatives, or the patient's old records might also be deemed negligent. Breach of patient-nurse confidentiality should not pose ethical or legal dilemmas for nurses in these situations, because a team approach to the delivery of psychiatric care presumes communication of pertinent information to other staff members to develop a treatment plan in the patient's best interest.

Child and Elder Abuse Reporting Statutes

Because of their interest in protecting children, all 50 states and the District of Columbia have enacted child abuse reporting statutes. Although these statutes differ from state to state, they generally include a definition of child abuse, a list of individuals required or encouraged to report abuse, and the governmental agency designated to receive and investigate the reports. Most statutes include civil penalties for failure to report. Many states specifically require nurses to report cases of suspected abuse.

There is a conflict between federal and state laws with respect to child abuse reporting when the health care professional discovers child abuse or neglect during the suspected abuser's alcohol or drug treatment. Federal laws and regulations governing confidentiality of patient records, which apply to almost all substance use and alcohol treatment providers, prohibit any disclosure without a court order. In this case, federal law supersedes state reporting laws, although compliance with the state law may be maintained under the following circumstances:

- If a court order is obtained, pursuant to the regulations
- If a report can be made without identifying the abuser as a patient in an alcohol or drug treatment program
- If the report is made anonymously (some states, to protect the rights of the accused, do not allow anonymous reporting)

As reported incidents of abuse to other persons in society surface, states may require health professionals to report other kinds of abuse. A growing number of states are enacting elder abuse reporting statutes, which require registered nurses (RNs) and others to report cases of abuse of older adults. Agencies who receive federal funding (i.e., Medicare or Medicaid) must follow strict guidelines for reporting and

BOX 6-2 Contraindications to Seclusion and Restraint

- Extremely unstable medical and psychiatric conditions*
- Delirium or dementia leading to inability to tolerate decreased stimulation*
- Severe suicidal tendencies*
- Severe drug reactions or overdoses or need for close monitoring of drug dosages*
- Desire for punishment of patient or convenience of staff

*Unless close supervision and direct observation are provided.
From Simon, R. I. (2001). *Concise guide to psychiatry and law for clinicians* (3rd ed., p. 117). Washington, DC: American Psychiatric Press.

preventing elder abuse. Older adults are defined as adults 65 years of age and older. These laws also apply to dependent adults—that is, adults between 18 and 64 years of age whose physical or mental limitations restrict their ability to carry out normal activities or to protect themselves—when the RN has actual knowledge that the person has been the victim of physical abuse.

Under most state laws, a person who is required to report suspected abuse, neglect, or exploitation of a disabled adult and who willfully does not do so is guilty of a misdemeanor crime. Most state statutes declare that anyone who makes a report in good faith is immune from civil liability in connection with the report.

You may also report knowledge of, or reasonable suspicion of, mental abuse or suffering. Dependent adults as well as older adults are protected by the law from purposeful physical or fiduciary neglect or abandonment. **Because state laws vary, students are encouraged to become familiar with the requirements of their states.**

TORT LAW APPLIED TO PSYCHIATRIC SETTINGS

Torts are a category of civil law that commonly applies to health care practice. A **tort** is a civil wrong for which money damages may be collected by the injured party (the plaintiff) from the wrongdoer (the defendant). The injury can be to person, property, or reputation. Because tort law has general applicability to nursing practice, this section may contain a review of material previously covered elsewhere in your nursing curriculum.

Bullying has become a recognized form of violence in our society. Nurses may encounter bullying behaviors from nursing supervisors, peers, patients, and even family members of patients. The root of this controlling type of behavior can be anxiety, stress, fear, or possibly even guilt felt by the bully (Boudreaux, 2010).

When nurses in psychiatric settings encounter provocative, threatening, or violent behavior from patients, the use of restraint or seclusion might be required until a patient demonstrates quieter and safer behavior. Accordingly, the nurse in the psychiatric setting should understand the intentional torts of battery, assault, and false imprisonment (described in Boxes 6-2 and 6-3). More on the use of restraints and seclusion is found in Chapters 16 and 24.

Common Liability Issues
Protection of Patients

Legal issues common in psychiatric nursing relate to the failure to protect the safety of patients. If a suicidal patient is left alone with the means to harm himself or herself, the nurse who has a duty to protect the patient will be held responsible for the resultant injuries. Leaving a suicidal patient alone in a room on the sixth floor with an open window is an example of unreasonable judgment on the part of the nurse. Precautions to prevent harm must be taken whenever a patient is restrained.

BOX 6-3 **False Imprisonment and Negligence: Plumadore v. State of New York (1980)**

Mrs. Plumadore was admitted to Saranac Lake General Hospital for a gallbladder condition. Her medical workup revealed emotional problems stemming from marital difficulties, which had resulted in suicide attempts several years before her admission. After a series of consultations and tests, she was advised by the attending surgeon that she was scheduled to have gallbladder surgery later that day. After the surgeon's visit, a consulting psychiatrist who examined Mrs. Plumadore directed her to dress and pack her belongings because he had arranged to have her admitted to a state hospital at Ogdensburg.

Subsequently, two uniformed state troopers handcuffed Mrs. Plumadore and strapped her into the backseat of a patrol car. She was also accompanied by a female hospital employee and was transported to the state hospital. On arrival, the admitting psychiatrist recognized that the referring psychiatrist lacked the requisite authority to order her involuntary commitment. He therefore requested that she sign a voluntary admission form, which she refused. Despite Mrs. Plumadore's protests regarding her admission to the state hospital, the psychiatrist assigned her to a ward without physical or psychiatric examination and without the opportunity to contact her family or her medical physician. The record of her admission to the state hospital noted an "informed admission," which is patient-initiated voluntary admission in New York.

The court awarded $40,000 to Mrs. Plumadore for false imprisonment, negligence, and malpractice.

Miscommunications and medication errors are common in all areas of nursing, including psychiatric care. A common area of liability in psychiatry is abuse of the therapist-patient relationship. Issues of sexual misconduct during the therapeutic relationship have become a source of concern in the psychiatric community. Misdiagnosis is also frequently charged in legal suits. See Table 6-2 for common liability issues.

Violence

Violent behavior is not acceptable in our society. The incidence of violence and violent acts appears to be escalating in our society. Therefore we see nurses confronting increasing amounts of violence in the workplace. Nurses must protect themselves in both institutional and community settings. Employers are not typically held responsible for employee injuries caused by violent patient behavior. Nurses have placed themselves knowingly in the range of danger by agreeing to care for unpredictable patients. It is therefore important for nurses to protect themselves by participating in setting policies that create a safe environment. Good judgment means not placing oneself in a potentially violent situation. Nurses, as citizens, have the same rights as patients—that is, to be free from being threatened or harmed. Appropriate security support should be readily available to the nurse practicing in an institution. When you work in community settings, you must avoid placing yourself unnecessarily in dangerous environments, especially when alone at night. You should use common sense and enlist the support of local law enforcement officers when needed. A violent patient is not being abandoned if placed safely in the hands of the authorities.

The psychiatric mental health nurse must also be aware of the potential for violence in the community when a patient is discharged following a short-term stay. The duty of the nurse to protect the patient as well as others who may be threatened by the violent patient is discussed in the preceding section in this chapter titled Duty to Warn and Protect Third Parties. The nurse's assessment of the patient's potential for violence must be documented and monitored if there is legitimate concern regarding discharge of a patient who is discussing

TABLE 6-2 Common Liability Issues

Issue	Examples
Patient safety	Suicide risks
	Restraints
	Miscommunication
	Medication errors
	Boundary violations (e.g., sexual misconduct)
	Misdiagnosis
Defamation of character	Harms patient's reputation
• Slander (spoken)	Confidential information divulged
• Libel (written)	Truth is a defense
Supervisory liability (vicarious liability)	Inappropriate delegation of duties
	Lack of supervision of those supervising
Intentional torts	Voluntary acts intended to bring a physical or mental consequence
• May carry criminal penalties	
• Punitive damages may be awarded	Purposeful acts
	Carelessness or recklessness
• Not covered by malpractice insurance	No patient consent
	Self-defense or protection of others may serve as a defense to charges of an intentional tort
Negligence or malpractice	Carelessness
	Foreseeability of harm
Assault and battery	Person apprehensive (assault) of harmful or offensive touching (battery)
	Threat to use force (words not enough) with opportunity and ability
	Treatment without patient's consent
False imprisonment	Intent to confine to a specific area
	Indefensible use of seclusion or restraints
	Detain voluntarily admitted patient with no agency or legal policies to support detaining

or exhibiting potentially violent behavior. The psychiatric mental health nurse must communicate his or her observations to the medical staff when discharge decisions are being considered.

Negligence/Malpractice

Negligence or **malpractice** is an act or an omission to act that breaches the duty of due care and results in or is responsible for a person's injuries. The five elements required to prove negligence are (1) duty, (2) breach of duty, (3) cause in fact, (4) proximate cause, and (5) damages. Foreseeability or likelihood of harm is also evaluated.

Duty is measured by a standard of care. When nurses represent themselves as being capable of caring for psychiatric patients and accept employment, a duty of care has been assumed. The duty is owed to psychiatric patients to understand the theory and medications used in the specialty care of these patients. People who represent themselves as possessing superior knowledge and skill, such as psychiatric nurse specialists, are held to a higher standard of care in the practice of their profession. The staff nurse who is assigned to a psychiatric unit must be knowledgeable enough to assume a reasonable or safe duty of care for the patients.

If you are not capable of providing the standard of care that other nurses would be expected to provide under similar circumstances, you have breached the duty of care. **Breach of duty** is the conduct that exposes the patient to an unreasonable risk of harm, through either commission or omission of acts by the nurse. If you do not have the required education and experience to provide certain interventions,

you have breached the duty by neglecting or omitting to provide necessary care. You can also act in such a way that the patient is harmed and can thus be guilty of negligence through acts of commission.

Cause in fact may be evaluated by asking the question, "Except for what the nurse did, would this injury have occurred?" **Proximate cause,** or legal cause, may be evaluated by determining whether there were any intervening actions or individuals that were, in fact, the causes of harm to the patient. **Damages** include actual damages (e.g., loss of earnings, medical expenses, and property damage) as well as pain and suffering. Foreseeability of harm evaluates the likelihood of the outcome under the circumstances.

DETERMINATION OF A STANDARD OF CARE

Professional standards of practice determined by professional associations differ from the standards embodied in the minimal qualifications established by state licensure for entry into the profession of nursing. The ANA has established standards for psychiatric mental health nursing practice and credentialing for the Psychiatric Mental Health Registered Nurse (PMH-RN) and the Psychiatric Mental Health Advanced Practice Nurse (PMH-APRN) in psychiatric mental health nursing (ANA, 2014).

Standards for psychiatric mental health nursing practice differ markedly from minimal state requirements because the primary purposes for setting these two types of standards are different. The state's qualifications for practice provide consumer protection by ensuring that all practicing nurses have successfully completed an approved nursing program and passed the national licensing examination. The professional association's primary focus is to elevate the practice of its members by setting standards of excellence.

Nurses are held to the standard of care provided by other nurses possessing the same degree of skill or knowledge in the same or similar circumstances. In the past, community standards existed for urban and rural agencies. However, with greater mobility and expanded means of communication, national standards have evolved. Psychiatric patients have the right to the standard of care recognized by professional bodies governing nursing, whether they are in a rural or an urban facility. Nurses must participate in continuing education courses to stay current with existing standards of care.

Hospital policies and procedures establish institutional criteria for care, and these criteria, such as the frequency of rounds for patients in seclusion, may be introduced to prove a standard that the nurse met or failed to meet. The shortcoming of this method is that the hospital's policy may be substandard. For example, the state licensing laws for institutions might set a minimal requirement for staffing or frequency of rounds for certain patients, and the hospital policy might fall below that minimum. **Substandard institutional policies do not absolve the individual nurse of responsibility to practice on the basis of professional standards of nursing care.**

Like hospital policy and procedures, customs can be used as evidence of a standard of care. For example, in the absence of a written policy on the use of restraint, testimony might be offered regarding the customary use of restraint in emergency situations in which the combative, violent, or confused patient poses a threat of harm to self or others. Using traditions to establish a standard of care may result in the same defect as in using hospital policies and procedures: customs may not comply with the laws, recommendations of the accrediting body, or other recognized standards of care. Customs must be carefully and regularly evaluated to ensure that substandard routines have not developed. Substandard customs do not protect you when a psychiatric patient charges that a right has been violated or that harm has been caused by the staff's common practices.

Guidelines for Nurses Who Suspect Negligence

It is not unusual for a student or practicing nurse to suspect negligence on the part of a peer. In most states, as a nurse you have a legal duty to report such risks of harm to the patient. It is also important that you document the evidence clearly and accurately before making serious accusations against a peer. If you question a physician's orders or actions, or those of a fellow nurse, it is wise to communicate these concerns directly to the person involved. If the risky behavior continues, you have an obligation to communicate these concerns to a supervisor, who should then intervene to ensure that the patient's rights and well-being are protected.

If you suspect a peer of being chemically impaired or of practicing irresponsibly, you have an obligation to protect not only the rights of the peer but also the rights of all patients who could be harmed. Reporting also allows the impaired health care worker to receive treatment and in many states can retain their license to work. However, if, after you have reported suspected behavior of concern to a supervisor and the danger persists, you have a duty to report the concern to someone at the next level of authority. It is important to follow the channels of communication in an organization, but it is also important to protect the safety of the patients. If the supervisor's actions or inactions do not rectify the dangerous situation, you have a continuing duty to report the behavior of concern to the appropriate authority, such as the state board of nursing.

A useful reference for nurses is the ANA's *Code of Ethics for Nurses with Interpretive Statements*:

> Nurses must be alert to and must take appropriate action regarding all instances of **incompetent, unethical, illegal, or impaired practices(s) or actions that place the rights** or best interests of the patient in jeopardy (ANA, 2015, 3.5 p. 12).

> Nurses must protect the patient, the public, and the profession from potential harm when practice appears to be **impaired.** The nurse's duty is to take action to protect patients and to ensure the impaired individual receives assistance (ANA, 2015, 3.6 p. 13).

Duty to Intervene and Duty to Report

The psychiatric mental health nurse has a duty to intervene when the safety or well-being of the patient or another person is obviously at risk. A nurse who follows an order that is known to be incorrect or that the nurse believes will harm the patient is responsible for the harm that results to the patient. **If you have information that leads you to believe that the physician's orders need to be clarified or changed, it is your duty to intervene and protect the patient.** It is important that you communicate with the physician who has ordered the treatment to explain the concern. If the treating physician does not appear willing to consider your concerns, you should carry out the duty to intervene through other appropriate channels.

It is important for you to express your concerns to the supervisor to allow the supervisor to communicate with the appropriate medical staff for intervention in the physician's treatment plan. *As the patient's advocate,* you have a duty to intervene to protect the patient; at the same time, you do not have the right to interfere with the physician-patient relationship.

It is also important to follow agency policies and procedures for communicating differences of opinion. If you fail to intervene and the patient is injured, you may be partly liable for the injuries that result because of failure to use safe nursing practice and good professional judgment.

The legal concept of abandonment may also arise when a nurse does not leave a patient safely reassigned to another health professional before discontinuing treatment. When the nurse is given an assignment to care for a patient, the nurse must provide the care or ensure that the patient is safely reassigned to another nurse. Abandonment issues arise when accurate, timely, and thorough reporting has not occurred or when follow-through of patient care, on which the patient is relying, has not occurred. The same principles apply for the psychiatric mental health nurse who is working in a community setting. For example, if a suicidal patient refuses to come to the hospital for treatment, you cannot abandon the patient but must take the necessary steps to ensure the patient's safety. These actions may include enlisting the assistance of the legal system in temporarily involuntarily committing the patient.

The duty to intervene on the patient's behalf poses many legal and ethical dilemmas for nurses in the workplace. Institutions that have a chain-of-command policy or other reporting mechanisms offer some assurance that the proper authorities in the administration are notified. Most patient care issues regarding physicians' orders or treatments can be settled fairly early in the process by the nurse's discussion of the concerns with the physician. If further intervention by the nurse is required to protect the patient, the next step in the chain of command can be followed. Generally, the nurse then notifies the immediate nursing supervisor; the supervisor thereupon discusses the problem with the physician, and then with the chief of staff of a particular service, until a resolution is reached. If there is no time to resolve the issue through the normal process because of the life-threatening nature of the situation, the nurse must act to protect the patient's life.

Unethical or Illegal Practices

The issues become more complex when a professional colleague's conduct, including that of a student nurse, is criminally unlawful. Specific examples include the diversion of drugs from the hospital and sexual misconduct with patients. Increasing media attention and the recognition of substance abuse as an occupational hazard for health professionals have led to the establishment of substance abuse programs for health care workers in many states. These programs provide appropriate treatment for impaired professionals to protect the public from harm and to rehabilitate the professional.

The problem previously discussed—of reporting impaired colleagues—becomes a difficult one, particularly when no direct harm has occurred to the patient. Concern for professional reputations, damaged careers, and personal privacy rather than public protection has generated a code of silence regarding substance abuse among health professionals.

Several states now require reporting of impaired or incompetent colleagues to the professional licensing boards. In the absence of such a legal mandate, the questions of whether to report and to whom to report become ethical ones. Chapter 19 deals more fully with issues related to the chemically impaired nurse.

The duty to intervene includes the duty to report known abusive behavior. Most states have enacted statutes to protect children and older adults from abuse and neglect. Psychiatric mental health nurses working in the community may be required by law to report unsafe relationships they discover.

DOCUMENTATION OF CARE

Purpose of Medical Records

The purpose of the medical record is to provide accurate and complete information about the care and treatment of patients and to give health care personnel responsible for that care a means of communicating with one another. The medical record allows for continuity of care.

A record's usefulness is determined by evaluating, when the record is read later, how accurately and completely it portrays the patient's behavioral status at the time it was written. The patient has the right to see the chart, but the chart belongs to the institution. The patient must follow appropriate protocol to view his or her records.

For example, if a psychiatric patient describes to a nurse a plan to harm himself or herself or another person and that nurse fails to document the information, including the need to protect the patient or the identified victim, the information will be lost when the nurse leaves work, and the patient's plan may be executed. The harm caused could be linked directly to the nurse's failure to communicate this important information. Even though documentation takes time away from the patient, the importance of communicating and preserving the nurse's memory through the medical record cannot be overemphasized.

Facility Use of Medical Records

The medical record has many other uses aside from providing information on the course of the patient's care and treatment to health care professionals. A retrospective chart review can provide valuable information to the facility on the quality of care provided and on ways to improve that care. A facility may conduct reviews for risk management purposes to determine areas of potential liability for the facility and to evaluate methods used to reduce the facility's exposure to liability. For example, documentation of the use of restraints and seclusion for psychiatric patients may be reviewed by risk managers. Accordingly, the chart may be used to evaluate care for quality assurance or peer review. Utilization review analysts review the chart to determine appropriate use of hospital and staff resources consistent with reimbursement schedules. Insurance companies and other reimbursement agencies rely on the medical record in determining what payments they will make on the patient's behalf.

Medical Records as Evidence

From a legal perspective, the chart is a recording of data and opinions made in the normal course of the patient's hospital care. It is deemed to be good evidence because it is presumed to be true, honest, and untainted by memory lapses. Accordingly, the medical record finds its way into legal cases for a variety of reasons. Some examples of its use include determining (1) the extent of the patient's damages and pain and suffering in personal injury cases, such as when a psychiatric patient attempts suicide while under the protective care of a hospital; (2) the nature and extent of injuries in child abuse or elder abuse cases; (3) the nature and extent of physical or mental disability in disability cases; and (4) the nature and extent of injury and rehabilitative potential in workers' compensation cases.

Medical records may also be used in police investigations, civil conservatorship proceedings, competency hearings, and commitment procedures. In states that mandate mental health legal services or a patients' rights advocacy program, audits may be performed to determine the facility's compliance with state laws or violation of patients' rights. Finally, medical records may be used in professional and hospital negligence cases.

During the discovery phase of litigation, the medical record is a pivotal source of information for attorneys in determining whether a cause of action exists in a professional negligence or hospital negligence case. Evidence of the nursing care rendered will be found in the notes charted by the nurse.

Nursing Guidelines for Computerized Charting

Accurate, descriptive, and legible nursing notes serve the best interests of the patient, the nurse, and the institution. As computerized charting becomes more widely available, it will also be important for psychiatric mental health nurses to understand how to protect the confidentiality of these records. Institutions must also protect against intrusions into the privacy of the patient record systems.

Concerns for the privacy of the legitimate patient's records have been addressed legally by federal laws that provide guidelines for agencies that use computerized charting. These guidelines include the recommendation that staff be assigned a password for entering patients' records in order to identify staff who have accessed patients' confidential information. There are penalties, including grounds for firing the staff, if staff enter a record for which they are not authorized to have access. Only those staff who have a legitimate need to know about the patient are authorized to access a patient's computerized chart.

It is important for you to keep your password private and never to allow someone else to access a record under your password. You are responsible for all entries into records using your password. The various systems used allow specific time frames within which the nurse must make any necessary corrections if a charting error is made.

Any charting method that improves communication between care providers should be encouraged. Courts assume that nurses and physicians read one another's notes on patient progress. Many courts take the attitude that if care is not documented, it did not occur. Your charting also serves as a valuable memory refresher if the patient sues years after the care is rendered. In providing complete and timely information on the care and treatment of patients, the medical record enhances communication among health professionals. Internal institutional audits of the record can improve the quality of care rendered. Chapter 7 describes common charting forms and gives examples as well as the pros and cons of each.

FORENSIC NURSING

Forensic nursing is the application of psychiatric nursing or any medical specialty principles of practice when used in a court of law to assist the court to utilize this knowledge to reach a decision on a contested issue. The nurse acts as an advocate, educating the court about the science of nursing in this courtroom-based practice of forensic nursing. Examples of psychiatric forensic nursing may include cases related to patient competency, fitness to stand trial, and commitment or responsibility for a crime. The relevance of nursing facts is presented and applied to the legal facts. Forensic cases also pertain to personal injury and murder proceedings. A dentist may serve as a forensic dentist in identifying a tooth as it relates to a corpse.

KEY POINTS TO REMEMBER

- States' power to enact laws for public health and safety and for the care of those unable to care for themselves often pits the rights of society against the rights of the individual.
- Psychiatric nurses frequently encounter problems requiring ethical choices.
- The nurse's privilege to practice nursing carries with it the responsibility to practice safely, competently, and in a manner consistent with state and federal laws.
- Knowledge of the law, the ANA's *Code of Ethics for Nurses with Interpretive Statements,* and the ANA's standards of care from *Psychiatric–Mental Health Nursing: Scope and Standards of Practice* is essential to provide safe, effective psychiatric nursing care and will serve as a framework for decision making when the nurse is presented with complex problems involving competing interests.

APPLYING CRITICAL JUDGMENT

1. Two nurses, Joe and Beth, have worked on the psychiatric unit for 2 years. During the past 6 months, Beth has confided to Joe that she has been experiencing a particularly difficult marital situation. Joe has observed that over the 6 months Beth has become increasingly irritable and difficult to work with. He notices that minor tranquilizers are frequently missing from the unit dose cart on the evening shift. He complains to the pharmacy and is informed that the drugs were stocked as ordered. Several patients state that they have not been receiving their usual drugs. Joe finds that Beth has recorded that the drugs have been given as ordered. He also notices that Beth is diverting the drugs.
   A. What action, if any, should Joe take?
   B. Should Joe confront Beth with his suspicions?
   C. If Beth admits that she has been diverting the drugs, should Joe's next step be to report Beth to the supervisor or to the board of nursing?
   D. Should Joe make his concern known to the nursing supervisor directly by identifying Beth, or should he state his concerns in general terms?
   E. Legally, must Joe report his suspicions to the board of nursing?
   F. Does the fact that harm to the patients is limited to increased agitation affect your responses?

2. A 40-year-old man who is admitted to the emergency department for a severe nosebleed has both nares packed. Because of his history of alcoholism and the probability of ensuing delirium tremens, the patient is transferred to the psychiatric unit. He is admitted to a private room, placed in restraints, and checked by a nurse every hour per physician's orders. While unattended, the patient suffocates, apparently by inhaling the nasal packing, which had become dislodged from the nares. On the next 1-hour check, the nurse finds the patient without pulse or respiration. A state statute requires that a restrained patient on a psychiatric unit be assessed by a nurse every hour for safety, comfort, and physical needs.
   A. If standards are not otherwise specified, do statutory requirements set forth minimal or maximal standards?
   B. Does the nurse's compliance with the state statute relieve him or her of liability in the patient's death?
   C. Does the nurse's compliance with the physician's orders relieve him or her of liability in the patient's death?
   D. Was the order for the restraint appropriate for this type of patient?
   E. What factors did you consider in making your determination?
   F. Was the frequency of rounds for assessment of patient needs appropriate in this situation?
   G. Did the nurse's conduct meet the standard of care for psychiatric nurses? Why or why not?
   H. What nursing action should the nurse have taken to protect the patient from harm?

3. Assume that there are no mandatory reporting laws for impaired or incompetent colleagues in the following clinical situation. In a private psychiatric unit in California, a 15-year-old boy is admitted voluntarily at the request of his parents because of violent, explosive behavior that seems to stem from his father's recent remarriage after his parents' divorce. A few days after admission, while in group therapy, he has an explosive reaction to a discussion about weekend passes for Mother's Day. He screams that he has been abandoned and that nobody cares about him. Several weeks later, on the day before his discharge, he elicits from the nurse a promise to keep his plan to kill his mother confidential. Consider the ANA's *Code of Ethics for Nurses* on patient confidentiality, the

principles of psychiatric nursing, the statutes on privileged communications, and the duty to warn third parties in answering the following questions:
   A. Did the nurse use appropriate judgment in promising confidentiality?
   B. Does the nurse have a legal duty to warn the patient's mother of her son's threat?
   C. Is the duty owed to the patient's father and stepmother?
   D. Would a change in the admission status from voluntary to involuntary protect the patient's mother without violating the patient's confidentiality?
   E. Would your response be different depending on the state in which the incident occurred? Why or why not?
   F. What nursing action, if any, should the nurse take after the disclosure by the patient?

CHAPTER REVIEW QUESTIONS

1. A nurse's sibling happily says, "I want to introduce you to my fiancé. We're getting married in six months." The nurse has encountered the fiancé in a clinical setting and is aware of the fiancé's diagnosis of schizophrenia. What is the nurse's best response?
   a. In private, tell the sibling about the fiancé's diagnosis.
   b. Encourage the sibling to postpone the wedding for at least a year.
   c. Ask the fiancé, "Have you told my sibling about your mental illness?"
   d. Say to the sibling and fiancé, "I hope you will be very happy together."

2. A patient has been disruptive to the therapeutic milieu for two days. A certified nursing assistant says to the nurse, "We need to seclude this patient because this behavior is upsetting everyone on the unit." Considering patients' rights, the nurse should respond,
   a. "Seclusion is not part of this patient's plan of care."
   b. "Let's think of some new ways to help this patient be less disruptive."
   c. "Thank you for that suggestion. I will discuss it with the health care provider."
   d. "Disruptive behavior is expected with mental illness. We must respond therapeutically."

3. A day shift nurse contacts a nurse scheduled for night shift at home and says, "Our unit is full and there are eight patients in the emergency department waiting for a bed." The night shift nurse replies, "Thanks for telling me. I am calling in sick." Which type of problem is evident by the night shift nurse's reply?
   a. Ethical problem of fidelity
   b. Legal problem of negligence
   c. Legal problem of an intentional tort
   d. Violation of the patients' right to treatment

4. In a staff meeting at an inpatient mental health facility for persons, the administrator announces that psychiatric technicians will now be supervised by the milieu director rather than by nurses. What is the nurse's best action?
   a. Confer with colleagues about their opinions regarding the proposed change.
   b. Volunteer to participate on a committee charged with defining job responsibilities of unlicensed assistive personnel.
   c. Ask the administrator to delay implementation of this change until the decision can be reviewed by an interdisciplinary team.
   d. Advise the administrator of regulations in the state nurse practice act regarding supervision of unlicensed assistive personnel.

5. A colleague tells the nurse, "I have not been able to sleep for the past three days. I feel like a robot." What is the nurse's best action?
   a. Direct the colleague to leave the facility immediately.
   b. Observe the colleague closely for evidence of impaired practice.
   c. Offer to administer medications to patients assigned to the colleague.
   d. Confer with the supervisor about the nurse's ability to safely deliver care.

REFERENCES

American Nurses Association (ANA). (2015). *Code of ethics for nurses with interpretive statements.* Washington, DC: APA.

American Psychiatric Association (APA). (2013). *Diagnostic and statistical manual of mental disorders (DSM-5)* (5th ed.). Washington, DC: APA.

Bazelon, D. L. (2003). *Advance psychiatric directives.* Washington, DC: Bazelon Center for Mental Health Law.

Bazelon, D. L. (2010). *Mental health parity.* Washington, DC: Bazelon Center for Mental Health Law. Retrieved March 4, 2011, from http://www.bazelon.org/Where-We-Stand/Access-to-Services/Mental-Health-Parity.aspx.

Bazelon, D. L. (2011). *Diversion from incarceration.* Retrieved March 4, 2011, from http://bazelon.org/where-we-stand/access-toservices/-diversion-from incarceration.

Beronio, K., Po, R., Skopec, L., & Glied, S. (2013, February 20). Office of The Assistant Secretary for Planning and Evaluation. Affordable Care Act expands mental health and substance use disorder benefits and federal parity protections for 62 million Americans. Retrieved from https://aspe.hhs.gov/report/affordable-care-act-expands-mental-health-and-substance-use-disorder-benefits-and-federal-parity-protections-62-million-americans.

Brink, S. (2014, April 29). Mental health now covered under ACA, but not for everyone. U.S.News and World Reports. Retrieved from http://www.usnews.com/news/articles/2014/04/29/mental-health-now-covered-under-aca-but-not-for-everyone.

Boudreaux, A. (2010). Keeping your cool with difficult family members. *Nursing, 40*(12), 50.

Canterbury v. Spence, 464 F.2d 772 (D.C. Cir. 1972), quoting *Schloendorff v. Society of N.Y. Hosp.,* 211 N.Y. 125, 105 N.E. 92, 93 (1914).

Chan, C. (2003). *Mandatory outpatient treatment: issues to consider.* Paper presented at the 153rd Annual Meeting of the American Psychiatric Association. Chicago: American Psychiatric Association.

CMS Manual System Department of Health & Human Services (DHHS) Pub. (2008). *100–07 State Operations Provider Certification Centers for Medicare & Medicaid Services (CMS) Transmittal 37 Date: October 17, 2008.*

Health Insurance Portability and Accountability Act (HIPAA). *U.S.C, 45,* (2003) C.F.R § 164.501.

Monahan, J., Swartz, M., & Bonnie, R. J. (2003). Mandated treatment in the community for people with mental disorders. *Health Affairs, 22*(5), 28–38.

O'Connor v. Donaldson. (1975) . 422 U.S. 563.

Olmstead v. L.C. (98–536). (1999). 527 U.S. 581.

Plumadore v. State of New York. (1980). 427 N.Y.S.2d 90.

Rainey, C. J. (2001). *Mandated outpatient treatment resources and data.* Presented at the American Psychiatric Association 53rd Institute on Psychiatric Services. Orlando, Fla: American Psychological Association.

Tarasoff v. Regents of University of California. (1974). 529 P.2d 553, 118 Cal Rptr 129.

Tarasoff v. Regents of University of California. (1976). 551 P.2d 334, 131 Cal Rptr 14.

Zinermon v. Burch. (1990). 494 U.S. 113, 108 L.Ed.2d 100, 110 S. Ct. 975.

Tools for Practice of the Art

Madeleine Leininger, PhD, RN, LhD, FAAN (1925–2012)
Founder of Transcultural Nursing

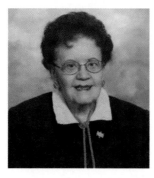

Even during the 1950s, long before "transcultural nursing" became a buzzword in nursing practice, Madeleine Leininger was an adamant supporter of health care workers understanding cultural nuances for the purpose of providing authentic, holistic, patient-centered care.

Leininger was a nurse pioneer in transcultural nursing as well as a scientist, anthropologist, researcher, theorist, leader, certified transcultural nurse specialist, and author and editor of more than 27 books. Leininger developed her Theory of Cultural Care and Universality based on her observations in the 1950s and 1960s of the people of New Guinea, where she lived for 2 years. She recognized the need for nurses to deliver care that combined both humanism and scientific knowledge and that would be meaningful to people from culturally diverse backgrounds.

She was the first graduate-prepared nurse to earn a PhD in cultural and social anthropology. In 1954, Leininger obtained a master's degree in psychiatric nursing from the Catholic University of America in Washington, D.C. Soon afterward, she developed the first master's level clinical specialist program in child psychiatric nursing at the University of Cincinnati. She subsequently developed the first graduate transcultural nursing program in psychiatric nursing, also at the University of Cincinnati.

Simply stated, transcultural nursing is the practice of nursing that provides culturally congruent, competent, and equitable care practices in a world that has become increasingly multicultural in nature.

Leininger (1998) states that when nurses do not take into account a patient's spiritual and religious beliefs, family ties, and economic and educational factors, they are at risk for demonstrating a noncaring attitude that may result in nonbeneficial outcomes. Human care and caring are defined within the context of culture. Leininger's transcultural nursing theory has as its focus "caring." She stated that *"a caring focus must become the dominant focus of all areas of nursing. It is the holistic and most complete and creative way to help people"* (Leininger, 1981).

The twenty-first century has ushered in cultural neuroscience, which studies the differences in brain functions among people of different cultures (e.g., Western and East Asian cultures) and how these differences affect emotions, psychopathology, and cognition. Evidence exists that neurobiological processes underlie social behaviors. Shared cultural meaning and cultural experiences trigger a neurobiological, psychological, and behavioral chain of events (Kim & Sasaki, 2014). Understanding neuroscience and ethnopharmacology can enhance cultural competence in psychiatric nursing.

Kim, H.S. and Sasaki, J.Y. (2014). Cultural neuroscience: biology of the mind in cultural contexts. *Annu Rev Psychol.* 65:487-514.
Leininger, M. M. (1998). *What is transcultural nursing?* Livonia, Mich: Transcultural Nursing Society.
Leininger, M. M. (1981). *Caring: An essential human need.* Thorofare, NJ: Charles B. Slack.

Nursing Process and QSEN: The Foundation for Safe and Effective Care

Elizabeth M. Varcarolis

ⓔ http://evolve.elsevier.com/Varcarolis/essentials

KEY TERMS AND CONCEPTS

evidence-based practice (EBP), p. 76
Health Insurance Portability and Accountability Act (HIPAA), p. 77
health teaching, p. 86
holistic approach to care, p. 77
mental status examination (MSE), p. 80
milieu therapy, p. 86

Nursing Interventions Classification (NIC), p. 85
Nursing Outcomes Classification (NOC), p. 83
outcomes criteria, p. 83
Psychiatric Mental Health Advanced Practice Registered Nurse (PMH–APRN), p. 85

Psychiatric Mental Health Registered Nurse (PMH–RN), p. 85
Quality and Safety Education for Nurses (QSEN), p. 76
self-care activities, p. 86

SELECTED CONCEPT: QUALITY AND SAFETY EDUCATION FOR NURSES (QSEN) PRE-LICENSURE COMPETENCIES

The primary goal of QSEN is to prepare future nurses with the knowledge, skills, and attitudes (KSAs) to increase the quality, care, and safety in the health care setting.

1. Patient-centered care
2. Teamwork and collaboration
3. Quality improvement (QI)
4. Evidence-based practice
5. Safety
6. Informatics

OBJECTIVES

1. Conduct a mental status examination (MSE).
2. Perform a psychosocial assessment including cultural and spiritual components.
3. Explain three principles a nurse follows in planning actions to reach approved outcome criteria.
4. Construct a plan of care for a patient with a mental or emotional health problem.
5. Identify three advanced practice psychiatric nursing interventions.
6. Demonstrate basic nursing interventions and evaluation of care using the *Standards of Practice* (ANA, APNA, ISPN, 2014).
7. Compare and contrast the Nursing Interventions Classification, Nursing Outcomes Classification, and evidence-based nursing practice.
8. **QSEN** Using informatics, access www.qsen.org and read the prelicensure quality and safety competencies for knowledge, skills, and attitudes (KSAs) needed to prepare nurses for employment in the health care system.

INTRODUCTION

The nursing process is a six-step problem-solving approach intended to facilitate and identify appropriate, safe, culturally competent, developmentally relevant, and quality care for individuals, families, groups, or communities. Psychiatric mental health nursing practice bases nursing judgments and behaviors on this accepted theoretical framework (Figure 7-1). Theoretical paradigms such as developmental theory, psychodynamic theory, systems theory, holistic theory, cognitive theory, and biological theory are some examples. Whenever possible, interventions are also supported by scientific theories when we apply evidence-based research to our nursing plans and actions of care (see Chapter 1).

The nursing process is also the foundation of the *Standards of Practice* as presented in *Psychiatric-Mental Health Nursing: Scope and Standards of Practice* (ANA, APNA, ISPN, 2014) which in turn provide the basis for the following:
- Criteria for certification
- Legal definition of nursing, as reflected in many states' nurse practice acts
- National Council of State Boards of Nursing Licensure Examination (NCLEX-RN®)
- The Six Standards of Practice defining the critical thinking model known as the nursing process

Safety and quality care for patients has become the newest standard for nursing education. As of the late 1990s, the Institute of Medicine

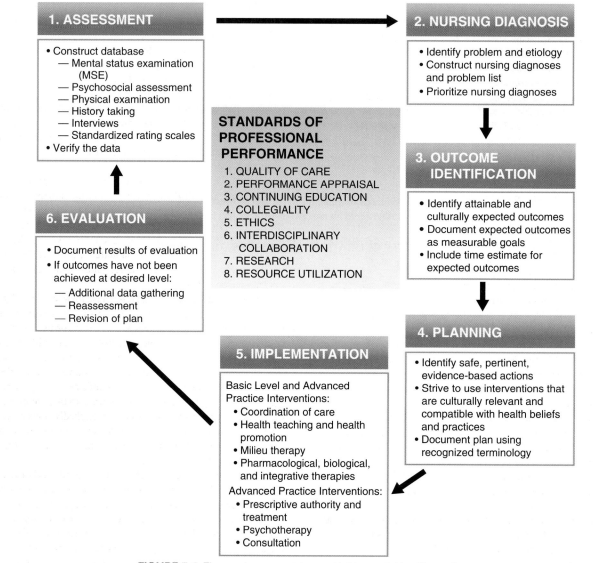

NURSING ASSESSMENT

The assessment interview requires culturally effective communication skills and encompasses a large database (e.g., significant support system; family; cultural and community system; spiritual and philosophical values, strengths, and health beliefs and practices; as well as many other factors).

1. ASSESSMENT

- Construct database
  — Mental status examination (MSE)
  — Psychosocial assessment
  — Physical examination
  — History taking
  — Interviews
  — Standardized rating scales
- Verify the data

2. NURSING DIAGNOSIS

- Identify problem and etiology
- Construct nursing diagnoses and problem list
- Prioritize nursing diagnoses

STANDARDS OF PROFESSIONAL PERFORMANCE

1. QUALITY OF CARE
2. PERFORMANCE APPRAISAL
3. CONTINUING EDUCATION
4. COLLEGIALITY
5. ETHICS
6. INTERDISCIPLINARY COLLABORATION
7. RESEARCH
8. RESOURCE UTILIZATION

3. OUTCOME IDENTIFICATION

- Identify attainable and culturally expected outcomes
- Document expected outcomes as measurable goals
- Include time estimate for expected outcomes

6. EVALUATION

- Document results of evaluation
- If outcomes have not been achieved at desired level:
  — Additional data gathering
  — Reassessment
  — Revision of plan

5. IMPLEMENTATION

Basic Level and Advanced Practice Interventions:
- Coordination of care
- Health teaching and health promotion
- Milieu therapy
- Pharmacological, biological, and integrative therapies

Advanced Practice Interventions:
- Prescriptive authority and treatment
- Psychotherapy
- Consultation

4. PLANNING

- Identify safe, pertinent, evidence-based actions
- Strive to use interventions that are culturally relevant and compatible with health beliefs and practices
- Document plan using recognized terminology

FIGURE 7-1 The nursing process in psychiatric mental health nursing.

(IOM; based on their *Quality Chasm* reports) and other organizations found a need to improve the quality and safety outcomes of health care delivery. The change is evident when one considers that the United States provides lower quality care to its citizens as compared with similar countries. These reports found that the American health care delivery system is lacking in **safety** to patients, lacking in services based on evidence-based practices, lacking in care that was respectful and responsive to patient needs (**patient centered**) and needs to reduce **harmful waits**, **reduce waste,** and provide quality care that is not based on geographic location or **socioeconomic status** (Cronenwett et al., 2007). There was a need for bodies to revise their standards so that students are educated with a core set of competencies. The competencies

mandated by the IOM require changes throughout health professionals' education to better prepare students with the responsibilities and realities in the health care setting. A "national initiative centered on patient safety and quality of care" is known as the Quality and Safety Education for Nurses (QSEN). The primary goal of QSEN is to prepare future nurses with the *knowledge, skills, and attitudes* (KSAs) required to enhance quality, care, and safety in the health care settings in which they are employed (Cronenwett et al., 2007). QSEN bases their work on six competencies (Box 7-1).

As nursing practice focuses more on quality and safety issues, it became evident that graduating nursing students were missing critical competencies for safety and quality of care. As the focus changed to safety and quality, new models of education were needed. These new models offer students more experience in interactive learning that incorporate both knowledge and skills in reality-based situations within a safe environment through simulations. Simulations are defined as activities that mimic the reality of a clinical environment and are designed to demonstrate procedures, decision making, and critical thinking through techniques such as role playing and the use of devices such as interactive videos or mannequins (Jeffries, 2005). Devices used in virtual clinical settings such as avatars, playacting, role playing, or video and audio portrayals of impaired patients give students the chance to implement their knowledge, skills, and attitudes without the potential for patient harm. Nurse educators increasingly incorporate QSEN's six competencies into curricula and teaching modalities. This use of clinical simulations in nursing and medical education is often referred to as *performance-based learning*.

Performance-based learning is a trend that is fundamentally changing medical and nursing education. Performance skills are learned more effectively through interactive strategies, which require changes in the traditional roles of teachers and students. More and more there is less emphasis on lecturing and more on participation with the student in collaborative and simulated hands-on strategies to achieve actual practice competencies.

Suggestions for the use of QSEN competencies in the discussion of *Standards of Practice* can be found in Competency Knowledge, Skills, Attitudes (Pre-Licensure) at the website www.qsen/ksas_pre-licensure.php.

STANDARDS OF PRACTICE FOR PSYCHIATRIC MENTAL HEALTH NURSING

STANDARD 1: ASSESSMENT

The psychiatric mental health registered nurse collects and synthesizes comprehensive health data that are pertinent to the health care consumer's health and/or situation (ANA, APNA, ISPN, 2014, p. 44).

A view of the individual as a complex blend of many parts is consistent with nurses' holistic approach to care. Nurses who care for people with physical illnesses ideally maintain a holistic view that involves an awareness of psychological, social, cultural, environmental, functional, and spiritual issues as well as ethnicity, sexual orientation, and age (e.g.,

child, teenager, older adults). Likewise, nurses who work in the mental health field need to assess, or have access to, past and present medical history, a recent physical examination, and any physical complaints the patient is experiencing, as well as document any observable physical conditions or behaviors (e.g., unsteady gait, abnormal breathing pattern, facial grimacing, or changing position to relieve discomfort).

The nurse collects comprehensive data using therapeutic techniques employing evidence-based assessment skills. Assessments are conducted by a variety of professionals including nurses, psychiatrists, social workers, dietitians, and other therapists. Every patient should have a thorough and formal nursing assessment on entering treatment to develop a basis for the plan of care in preparation for discharge. Subsequent to the formal assessment, data are collected continually and systematically as the patient's condition changes and hopefully improves. Perhaps the patient entered treatment actively suicidal, and the initial focus of care was on protection from injury. In emergency situations, immediate intervention is often based on a minimal amount of data. In all situations, however, legal consent must be given by the patient, who must also receive a copy of the Health Insurance Portability and Accountability Act (HIPAA) guidelines. Essentially, the purpose of the HIPAA privacy rule is to ensure that an individual's health information is properly protected, while at the same time allowing health care providers to obtain personal health information for the purpose of providing and promoting high-quality health care (USDHHS, 2003). HIPAA was first enacted in 1996, but compliance was not mandated until April 14, 2003. Visit www.hhs.gov/ocr/privacy/hipaa/understanding/index.html for a full overview (see chapter 6).

Document relevant data in a retrievable format. Virtually all facilities have standardized nursing assessment forms to aid in organization and consistency among reviewers. These forms will most likely be computerized, although some institutions may still use hardcopy assessments according to the resources and preferences of the institution. The time required for the nursing interview varies, depending on the assessment form and on the patient's response pattern (e.g., a lengthy or rambling historian, a patient prone to tangential thought, or a patient having memory disturbances or markedly slowed responses). In emergency situations, immediate intervention is of essence and may be based on a minimal amount of data. Refer to Chapter 9 for guidelines for setting up and conducting a clinical interview.

Whenever possible involve the patient, family, other health care providers and other support systems in holistic data collection. The nurse's *primary source* for data collection is the patient; however, there may be times when it is necessary to supplement or rely completely on another source for the assessment information. These *secondary sources* can be invaluable when caring for a patient experiencing psychosis, muteness, agitation, or catatonia. Such secondary sources include family, friends, neighbors, police, health care workers, and previous medical records.

Age Considerations
Assessment of Children

It is estimated that 1 in 10 children in our society suffer from a mental illness (Arnold & Boggs, 2016).

An effective interviewer working with children should have familiarity with basic cognitive and social/emotional developmental theory and have some exposure to applied child development (Sommers-Flanagan & Sommers-Flanagan, 2012–2013). The role of the caregiver is central in the interview.

When assessing children it is important to gather data from a variety of sources. Although the child is the best source in determining inner feelings and emotions, the caregivers (parents or guardians) can often best describe the behavior, performance, and conduct of the child. Caregivers also are often helpful in interpreting the child's words and responses. However, a separate interview is advisable when an older child is reluctant to share information, especially in cases of suspected abuse (Arnold & Boggs, 2016).

As mentioned, developmental levels should be considered in the evaluation of children. One of the hallmarks of psychiatric disorders in children is the tendency to regress—that is, to return to a previous level of development. Although it is developmentally appropriate for toddlers to suck their thumbs, such a gesture is unusual in an older child.

Assessment of children should be accomplished by a combination of interview and observation. Watching children at play provides important clues to their functioning. Using age-appropriate storytelling, playing with dolls, drawing, or playing games can be useful as assessment tools when determining critical concerns and painful issues a child may have difficulty expressing. When assessing the child, be sure to position yourself at the child's level and avoid towering over him/her. Always use familiar words and age-based vocabulary. Usually, a clinician/nurse clinician with special training in child and adolescent psychiatry works with young children. Refer to Chapter 26 for further discussion on the assessment of children.

Assessment of Adolescents

All patients are concerned with confidentiality. This is especially true for adolescents. Adolescents may fear that anything they say to the nurse will be repeated to their parents. At least part of the interview should be conducted without the parent/caregiver is present. Adolescents need to be told right from the very beginning that their records are private and should receive an explanation as to how information will be shared among the treatment team. Questions related to sensitive issues such as substance abuse or sexual abuse demand confidentiality (Arnold & Boggs, 2016). However, threats of suicide or homicide, use of illegal drugs, or issues of abuse must be shared with other professionals as well as with the parent(s). Because identifying risk factors is one of the key objectives when assessing adolescents, it is helpful to use a brief structured interview technique called the HEADSSS interview (Box 7-2). Refer to Chapter 26 for more information on the assessment of adolescents.

Assessment of the Older Adult

Older adults often need special attention. The nurse needs to be aware of any physical limitations—any sensory condition (vision or hearing deficits), motor condition (difficulty walking or maintaining balance), or medical condition (cardiac condition)—that could cause increased anxiety, stress, or physical discomfort for the patient while attempting to assess mental and emotional needs.

It is wise to identify any physical deficits the patient may have at the onset of the assessment and make accommodations for them. For example, if the patient is hard of hearing, speak a little more slowly and in clear, louder tones (but not too loud) and seat the patient close to you without invading his or her personal space. Refer to Chapter 28 for more on communicating with the older adult.

Language Barriers

It is becoming more and more apparent that psychiatric mental health nurses can best serve their patients if they have a thorough understanding of the complex cultural and social factors that influence health and illness. Awareness of individual cultural beliefs and health care practices can help nurses to minimize stereotyped assumptions that can lead to ineffective care and interfere with the ability to evaluate care. In fact, it seems that patients from culturally diverse backgrounds respond better when nurses incorporate the clients values and social circumstances into their plan of care (Arnold & Boggs 2016; Knoerl et al., 2011). Unfortunately, there are many opportunities for misunderstandings when assessing a patient from a different cultural or social background from your own, particularly if the interview is conducted in English and the patient speaks a different language or a different form of English.

Often health care professionals require an interpreter to understand the patient's history and health care needs. Federal law mandates the use of a trained professional interpreter in health care settings when language is a barrier to communication. A professionally trained translator needs to be proficient in both English and the patient's spoken language, as well as the patient's culture, dialect, and mores of the patient's background, and is expected to maintain confidentiality and follow specific guidelines (Arnold & Boggs, 2016). Therefore, it is strongly recommended to not use untrained interpreters (e.g., family members, friends, neighbors) who may easily misinterpret or try to "translate" the patient's intent. Unfortunately, professional interpreters are not always readily available in many health care facilities.

Psychiatric Nursing Assessment

The psychiatric nursing assessment has many goals, including the following:

- Establish rapport.
- Obtain an understanding of the current problem or chief complaint.
- Review physical status and obtain baseline vital signs.
- Assess for risk factors affecting the safety of the patient or others. (Suicide/homicide)
- Perform a mental status examination (MSE). (See inside back cover)
- Assess psychosocial status.
- Identify mutual goals for treatment.
- Formulate a plan of care that prioritizes the patient's immediate condition and needs.
- Document data in a retrievable format.

Gathering Data

Review of systems. The mind-body connection is significant in the understanding and treatment of psychiatric disorders. Many patients who are admitted for treatment of psychiatric conditions also are given a thorough physical examination by a primary care provider. Likewise, most nursing assessments include a physical component, such as obtaining a baseline set of vital statistics, a historical and current review of body systems, and a documentation of allergic responses.

BOX 7-2 The HEADSSS Psychosocial Interview Technique

Home environment (e.g., relations with parents and siblings)

Education and employment (e.g., school performance)

Activities (e.g., sports participation, after-school activities, peer relations)

Drug, alcohol, or tobacco use

Sexuality (e.g., whether the patient is sexually active, practices safe sex, uses contraception, or practices alternative sexual lifestyles)

Suicide risk or symptoms of depression or other mental disorder

"**S**avagery" (e.g., violence or abuse in home environment or in neighborhood)

People with certain physical conditions may be more prone to psychiatric disorders such as depression. It is generally believed that the disease process of multiple sclerosis itself may actually cause depression. Other medical diseases that are typically associated with depression are coronary artery disease, diabetes, and stroke. In fact, a 2011 study demonstrated that women with both depression and diabetes have a significantly higher risk for mortality and cardiovascular disease than do women with either depression or diabetes alone (Brauser & Barclay, 2011). Individuals need to be evaluated for any medical origins of their depression or anxiety.

There are many medical conditions that can mimic psychiatric illnesses (Box 7-3). By the same token, when depression is secondary to a

---

BOX 7-3   Some Medical Conditions that May Mimic Psychiatric Illness

Depression
Neurological Disorders
- Cerebrovascular accident (stroke)
- Alzheimer's disease
- Brain tumor
- Huntington's disease
- Epilepsy (seizure disorder)
- Multiple sclerosis
- Parkinson's disease
- Cancer

Infections
- Mononucleosis
- Encephalitis
- Hepatitis
- Tertiary syphilis
- Human immunodeficiency virus (HIV) infection

Endocrine Disorders
- Hypothyroidism and hyperthyroidism
- Cushing's syndrome
- Addison's disease
- Parathyroid disease

Gastrointestinal Disorders
- Liver cirrhosis
- Pancreatitis

Cardiovascular Disorders
- Hypoxia
- Congestive heart failure

Respiratory Disorders
- Sleep apnea

Nutritional Disorders
- Thiamine deficiency
- Protein deficiency
- B_{12} deficiency
- B_6 deficiency
- Folate deficiency

Collagen Vascular Diseases
- Lupus erythematosus
- Rheumatoid arthritis

Anxiety
Neurological Disorders
- Alzheimer's disease
- Brain tumor
- Stroke
- Huntington's disease

Infections
- Encephalitis
- Meningitis
- Neurosyphilis
- Septicemia

Endocrine Disorders
- Hypothyroidism and hyperthyroidism
- Hypoparathyroidism
- Hypoglycemia
- Pheochromocytoma
- Carcinoid

Metabolic Disorders
- Low calcium level
- Low potassium level
- Acute intermittent porphyria
- Liver failure

Cardiovascular Disorders
- Angina
- Congestive heart failure
- Pulmonary embolus

Respiratory Disorders
- Pneumothorax
- Acute asthma
- Emphysema

Drug Effects
- Stimulants
- Sedatives (withdrawal)
- Lead, mercury poisoning

Psychosis
Medical Conditions
- Temporal lobe epilepsy
- Migraine headaches
- Temporal arteritis
- Occipital tumors
- Narcolepsy
- Encephalitis
- Hypothyroidism
- Addison's disease
- HIV infection

Drug Effects
- Hallucinogens (e.g., LSD)
- Phencyclidine
- Alcohol withdrawal
- Stimulants
- Cocaine
- Corticosteroids

known medical condition, it may go unrecognized and thus untreated. *Conversely, psychiatric disorders can result in physical or somatic symptoms such as abdominal pain, headaches, lethargy, insomnia, and intense fatigue.* Therefore all patients presenting to the health care system need to have both a medical and a psychological health evaluation to ensure a correct diagnosis and appropriate care.

Laboratory data. Disorders such as hypothyroidism may have the clinical appearance of depression, and hyperthyroidism may appear to be a manic phase of bipolar disorder; a simple blood test can usually differentiate between a mood disorder and thyroid disorders. Abnormal liver enzyme levels can explain irritability, depression, and lethargy. People who have chronic renal disease often suffer from the same symptoms when their blood urea nitrogen and electrolyte levels are abnormal. Results of a toxicology screen for the presence of either legal (e.g., prescription pain medication, Adderall) or illegal drugs (e.g., designer drugs, hallucinogenic, heroin) also may provide useful information.

Mental status examination. Fundamental to the assessment is a mental status examination (MSE). In fact, an MSE is part of the assessment in all areas of medicine. The MSE in psychiatry is analogous to the physical examination in general medicine. The purpose of the MSE is to evaluate an individual's current cognitive processes. For acutely disturbed patients it is typical for the mental health clinician to administer the MSE every day. Sommers-Flanagan and Sommers-Flanagan (2012 – 2013) advise anyone seeking employment in the medical–mental health field to be competent in communicating with other professionals via MSE reports. Box 7-4 lists the elements of a basic MSE. An example of a **mental status examination is printed on the inside back cover of this text.**

Generally the MSE aids in collecting and organizing *objective data.* The nurse observes the patient's physical behavior, nonverbal communication, appearance, speech patterns, mood and affect, thought content, perceptions, cognitive ability, and insight and judgment.

Psychosocial assessment. A **psychosocial assessment** provides additional information from which to develop a plan of care beyond the MSE. It includes obtaining the following information about the patient:

- Central or chief complaint (in the patient's own words)
- History of violent, suicidal, or self-mutilating behaviors
- Alcohol and/or substance abuse
- Family psychiatric history
- Personal psychiatric treatment including medications and complementary therapies
- Stressors and coping methods
- Quality of activities of daily living
- Personal background
- Social background including support system
- Weaknesses, strengths, and goals for treatment
- Racial, ethnic, and cultural beliefs and practices
- Spiritual beliefs or religious practices

The patient's psychosocial history is most often the *subjective* part of the assessment. The focus of the history is the patient's perceptions and recollections of current lifestyle, and life in general (e.g., family, friends, education, work experience, coping styles, and spiritual and cultural beliefs) (Box 7-5).

BOX 7-4   Content of a Mental Status Examination

Personal Information
- Age
- Gender
- Marital status
- Religious preference
- Race
- Ethnic background
- Employment
- Living arrangements

Appearance
- Grooming and dress
- Level of hygiene
- Pupil dilation or constriction
- Facial expression
- Height, weight, nutritional status
- Presence of body piercing or tattoos, scars, other
- Relationship between appearance and age

Behavior
- Excessive or reduced body movements
- Peculiar body movements (e.g., scanning of the environment, odd or repetitive gestures, level of consciousness, balance and gait)
- Abnormal movements (e.g., tardive dyskinesia, tremors)
- Level of eye contact (keep cultural differences in mind)

Speech
- Rate: slow, rapid, normal
- Volume: loud, soft, normal

- Disturbances (e.g., articulation problems, slurring, stuttering, mumbling)
- Cluttering (e.g., rapid, disorganized, tongue-tied speech)

Affect and Mood
- Affect: flat, bland, animated, angry, withdrawn, appropriate to context
- Mood: sad, labile, euphoric

Thought
- Thought process (e.g., disorganized, coherent, flight of ideas, neologisms, thought blocking, circumstantiality)
- Thought content (e.g., delusions, obsessions, suicidal thought)

Perceptual Disturbances
- Hallucinations (e.g., auditory, visual)
- Illusions

Cognition*
- Orientation: time, place, person
- Level of consciousness (e.g., alert, confused, clouded, stuporous, unconscious, comatose)
- Memory: remote, recent, immediate
- Fund of knowledge
- Attention: performance on serial sevens, digit span tests
- Abstraction: performance on tests involving similarities, proverbs
- Insight
- Judgment

*Refer to the inside back cover for the Saint Louis University Mental Status (SLUMS) exam.

Spiritual and/or religious assessment. The importance of spirituality and religious beliefs is an often overlooked element of patient care, although numerous empirical studies have suggested that being part of a spiritual community is helpful to people coping with illness and recovering from surgery. Spirituality and religious beliefs have the potential to exert an influence on how people understand meaning and purpose in their lives and how they use critical judgment to solve problems (e.g., crises of illness).

The terms spirituality and religion are different although not mutually exclusive. Spirituality refers to how we find meaning, hope, purpose, and a sense of peace in our lives. Spirituality is more of an internal phenomenon centering on universal personal questions and needs. It is the part of us that seeks to understand life. The term spirituality is more about the believer's faith being more personal, less dogmatic, and more inclusive considering that there are many spiritual paths and no one "real path." A person's spiritual beliefs may or may not be connected with the community or with religious rituals.

Religion is an external system that includes beliefs, patterns of worship, and symbols. Religious affiliation is a choice to connect personal spiritual beliefs with a larger organized group or institution and typically involves rituals. Belonging to a religious community can provide support during difficult times. For many individuals, prayer is a source of hope, comfort, and support in healing.

Spiritual and religious practices have been determined to enhance healthy behaviors, social support, and a sense of meaning in people's lives, all of which are linked to decreased overall mental and physical stress, which in turn relate to a decreased incidence of illness in many people. (Refer to Chapter 10 for the effect of stress on health and illness.)

O'Riordan (2010) in an interview with Dr. Donald Lloyd-Jones (Northwestern University Fienberg School of Medicine, Chicago) quoted him as saying:

In general, from the perspective of overall health, healthcare utilization, and outcomes, the suggestion has been from some of the studies that greater religiosity, in terms of participation or spirituality, is typically associated with better health outcomes.

Cultural and social assessment. Because nurses are increasingly faced with caring for culturally diverse populations, there is a growing need for nursing assessment, nursing diagnoses, and subsequent care to be planned around unique cultural health care beliefs, values, and practices. It is becoming more evident that all mental health professionals, and perhaps especially nurses, must have an increased understanding of the complexity of the cultural and social factors that influence health and illness. Knowledge of individual cultural beliefs and health care practices can mitigate against stereotyping, stigmatizing, and labeling of patients.

After the assessment, it is useful to summarize pertinent data with the patient. This summary provides the patient with reassurance that the health care provider understands his or her message, and it gives the patient an opportunity to clarify any misinformation. The patient should be told what will happen next. For example, if the initial assessment takes place in the hospital, you should tell the patient who he or she will be seeing next.

BOX 7-5   Psychosocial Assessment

A. Previous hospitalizations
B. Educational background
C. Occupational background
   1. Employed? Where? What length of time?
   2. Special skills
D. Social patterns
   1. Describe family.
   2. Describe friends.
   3. With whom does the patient live?
   4. To whom does the patient go in time of crisis?
   5. Who makes the decisions in your family?
   6. Describe a typical day.
E. Sexual patterns
   1. Sexually active? Practices safe sex? Practices birth control?
   2. Sexual orientation
   3. Sexual difficulties
F. Interests and abilities
   1. What does the patient do in his or her spare time?
   2. In which sport, hobby, or leisure activity does the patient participate?
   3. Does the patient excel in any particular activity or hobby?
   4. What gives the patient pleasure?
G. Substance use and abuse
   1. What medications does the patient take? How often? How much?
   2. What herbal or over-the-counter drugs does the patient take? How often? How much?
   3. What psychotropic drugs does the patient take? How often? How much?
   4. How many drinks of alcohol does the patient take per day? Per week?
   5. What recreational drugs does the patient take? How often? How much?
   6. Does the patient identify the use of drugs as a problem?

H. Coping abilities
   1. What does the patient do when he or she gets upset?
   2. To whom can the patient talk?
   3. What usually helps to relieve stress?
   4. What did the patient try this time?
I. Spiritual assessment
   1. Does the patient have a spiritual or religious affiliation?
   2. What gives the patient strength and hope?
   3. Does the patient participate in any spiritual/religious activities?
   4. What role does religion/spiritual practice play in the patient's life?
   5. Do the patient's spiritual or religious beliefs help him or her in stressful situations?
   6. Are there any restrictions on diet or medical interventions within the patient's religious, spiritual, or cultural beliefs?
J. Cultural assessment
   1. Does the patient need an interpreter?
   2. What is the first thing the patient does when he or she becomes ill to address the illness?
   3. How has the patient been treating this illness?
   4. How is this condition (medical or mental) viewed in the patient's culture?
   5. Are there special health care practices within the patient's culture that address his or her medical/mental problem?
   6. What are the attitudes toward mental illness in the patient's culture?
   7. Does the patient have culture-specific beliefs that help him or her cope (with racism, prejudice, or discrimination)?
   8. Does the patient's diet consist of culture-specific foods? If so, what foods should not be part of the patient's diet?

If the initial assessment was conducted by a psychiatric nurse in a mental health clinic, the individual will be informed of the future schedule for therapy with a clinician/psychiatric advanced practice nurse. If a referral is necessary, this should be discussed with the patient. For individuals with severe mental health requiring long-term care, some specific assessment guidelines can be helpful. Refer to Chapter 27.

Self-awareness assessment. Self-awareness is a positive trait and a competent and effective interviewer needs to possess a high degree of psychological, emotional, and social/cultural self-awareness to perform optimally (Sommers-Flanagan & Sommers-Flanagan, 2012 – 2013).

We all have personal biases and "off days" (i.e., days we feel sad or upset), and we all hold our own expectations of the outcome of the interview. In addition, we all come from a specific culture/subculture with inherent expectations, traditions, and well-ingrained social beliefs. Being consciously aware of our personal biases and emotional states can help us become cognizant of how these traits can influence and distort our understanding of the individual before us (Sommers-Flanagan & Sommers-Flanagan, 2012 – 2013).

It is a good idea to be aware of your personal cultural and social beliefs that may influence your interactions with a person from another background with inherently different cultural, social, and spiritual/religious beliefs. Also examine how you are feeling at the moment before an interview. We are not always aware of personal feelings or how they are affecting us when we first begin an interview, with the exceptions of students who will always feel anxious in the beginning, a very healthy sign. How do we obtain a good picture of ourselves in relationship to our interviewing skills? One way is clinical supervision from a seasoned and effective psychiatric nurse or clinician. Another effective way is through the use of videotapes of ourselves during an interview (usually a very painful experience, initially). Even seasoned interviewers can be shocked and surprised by their videotapes. Although these insights may be painful they are enormously helpful in becoming more self-aware and they increase our awareness of our patient as well. Taking notes shortly after an interview of what the patient said and what you said (process recordings) is a useful exercise because these "verbatim" notes provide an overall evaluation of your interaction, which may help you reevaluate and review not only what you missed but also what you could have done differently to be more effective. Although these assessment methods are not as popular as they were in the past in nursing education, they offer the opportunity for important learning experiences in improving communication skills (refer to Applying the Art features throughout the clinical chapters).

Validating the Assessment

To gain an even clearer picture of your patient, it is helpful to look to outside sources. Emergency department records can be a valuable resource in understanding an individual's presenting behavior and problems. Police reports may be available in cases in which hostility and legal altercations occurred. Using informatics is a way of checking previous admissions, validating current information, or adding new information to your database. If the patient was admitted to a psychiatric unit in the past, information about the patient's previous level of functioning and behavior gives you a baseline for making clinical judgments. Occasionally consent forms may need to be signed by the patient or other appropriate relative in order to obtain access to records.

Using Rating Scales

A number of standardized rating scales are useful for psychiatric evaluation and monitoring. Rating scales are often administered by a clinician, but many are self-administered. Table 7-1 lists some of the

TABLE 7-1 Standardized Rating Scales*

Use	Scale
Depression	Beck Inventory
	Geriatric Depression Scale (GDS)
	Hamilton Depression Scale
	Zung Self-Report Inventory
	Patient Health Questionnaire (PHQ-9)
Anxiety	Modified Spielberger State Anxiety Scale
	Hamilton Anxiety Scale
Substance use disorders	Addiction Severity Index (ASI)
	Recovery Attitude and Treatment Evaluator (RAATE)
	Brief Drug Abuse Screen Test (B-DAST)
Obsessive-compulsive behavior	Yale-Brown Obsessive-Compulsive Scale (Y-BOCS)
Mania	Mania Rating Scale
Schizophrenia	Scale for Assessment of Negative Symptoms (SANS)
	Brief Psychiatric Rating Scale (BPRS)
Abnormal movements	Abnormal Involuntary Movement Scale (AIMS)
	Simpson Neurological Rating Scale
General psychiatric assessment	Brief Psychiatric Rating Scale (BPRS)
Cognitive function	Mini-Mental State Examination (MMSE)
	Cognitive Capacity Screening Examination (CCSE)
	Alzheimer's Disease Rating Scale (ADRS)
	Memory and Behavior Problem Checklist
	Functional Assessment Screening Tool (FAST)
	Global Deterioration Scale (GDS)
Family assessment	McMaster Family Assessment Device
Eating disorders	Eating Disorders Inventory (EDI)
	Body Attitude Test
	Diagnostic Survey for Eating Disorders

*These rating scales highlight important areas in psychiatric assessment. Because many of the answers are subjective, experienced clinicians use these tools as a guide when planning care and also rely on their knowledge of their patients.

common scales in use today. Many of the clinical chapters in this book include a rating scale.

(QSEN) QUALITY AND SAFETY ALERT

Assessment

Some possible QSEN competencies inherent when assessing patients include the following:
- **Patient-centered care:** Elicit patient values, preferences, and expressed needs as part of the clinical interview.
- **Informatics:** Navigate the electronic health record, research literature, identify appropriate apps for the patient and health care provider alike.
- **Teamwork and collaboration:** Identify the need for an interpreter; recognize contributions of other individuals or groups to help patient/family achieve health goals (not directly from QSEN).

STANDARD 2: DIAGNOSIS

The psychiatric mental health registered nurse analyzes the assessment data to determine diagnoses, problems, and areas of focus for care and treatment, including level of risk. (ANA, APNA, ISPN, 2014, p. 46).

Formulating a Nursing Diagnosis

A nursing diagnosis is a clinical judgment about a patient's response, needs, actual and potential psychiatric disorders, mental health problems, level of risk, and potential comorbid (co-occurring) physical illnesses. An actual or potential problem can be related to a psychiatric disorder (e.g., self-mutilation, hopelessness), a medical disorder (e.g., ineffective breathing pattern), or a potential co-occurring physical illness (e.g., impaired physical mobility). Nursing diagnoses "provide the basis for the selection of nursing interventions to achieve outcomes for which the nurse has accountability." A well-chosen and well-stated nursing diagnosis is the basis for selecting therapeutic outcomes and interventions (NANDA-I, 2015 – 2017). Refer to Appendix B for a list of NANDA-I–approved nursing diagnoses.

Standard Nursing Diagnosis

A standard nursing diagnosis has three structural components: the **problem** (the unmet need), the **etiology** (the probable cause), and the **supporting data** (the signs and symptoms supporting the stated problem).

The problem. The problem or unmet need describes the state of the patient at present. Problems that are within the nurse's domain to treat are termed nursing diagnoses. An example is **self-mutilation.**

The etiology. The etiology includes factors that contribute to or are related to the development or maintenance of a nursing diagnosis title. The related factors tell us what needs to be done to effect change and identifies what needs to be targeted through nursing interventions. An example is **self-mutilation** *related to disturb body image.*

Note that the difference in identifying a plan of care for someone with the same nursing diagnoses is related to a patient's individual and unique "cause and supporting data."

Defining characteristics (supporting data). Supporting signs and symptoms are the "defining characteristics" that make up the patient's objective and measurable signs, plus the more subjective symptoms that reflect the patient's present situation. The defining characteristics may be linked to the diagnosis and probable cause with the words *as evidenced by.*

Supporting data that would validate the diagnosis *self-mutilation related to disturbed body image* might include the following:

- Poor impulse control
- Self-inflicted cutting
- Ineffective coping skills
- Statements like "I'm so ugly, and when I cut myself, I feel better about myself."

Therefore, a completed nursing diagnosis includes (1) **the problem,** which is the area that needs intervention; (2) **the etiology,** which is what is responsible for aggravating the problem; and (3) **the defining characteristics,** which are the objective and subjective data that support the validity of the diagnosis (the problem):

Self-mutilation + related to disturbed body image + as evidenced by self-cutting, impulsivity, and statements that cutting helps relieve painful feelings of inadequacy.

Risk Diagnoses

Risk diagnoses are employed when there is a high probability that a future event may occur in a vulnerable individual. "Risk for" diagnoses are made to help prevent a potential unwanted or dangerous future event in an effort to ensure patient safety (QSEN). For example, assessment in an elderly patient with a recent hip replacement might warrant a nursing diagnosis of "risk for falls + related to (risk factors) postoperative condition and unsteady gait." For a suicidal individual a diagnosis "risk for suicide" would be appropriate for someone who is depressed, has attempted suicide in the past, has poor impulse control, and states that he wants to die.

NANDA-I suggests that when making a "risk for" diagnosis, the diagnosis should include the risk diagnoses + risk factors (risk-related behaviors) that predispose the individual to a potential problem. Since the problem hasn't yet arisen, NANDA-I states that there can be no "related etiological factors." Therefore, an appropriate nursing diagnosis for the suicidal client mentioned above would be *risk for suicide + related to (risk factors, risk behaviors) states he wants to die, diagnosis of depression, and has made previous suicide attempt.*

Health Promotion Diagnoses

Health promotion diagnoses are used when clinical observations and/or patient (family, group, etc.) statements indicate willingness and a wish to enhance specific health behaviors. Health promotion diagnoses are always stated in the form of "readiness for enhanced" and supported by the data/defining characteristics. In cases of health promotion diagnoses, the "related to" factors are already known (motivation to improve health status), so they are not listed in the problem statement. An example is *readiness for enhanced self-concept + (defining characteristics) as evidenced by willingness to enhance self-concept and accept limitations and strengths.*

QSEN QUALITY AND SAFETY ALERT

Diagnosis

Suggested QSEN competencies inherent when planning nursing diagnoses include the following:

- **Patient-centered care:** Integrate understanding of multiple dimensions of patient-centered care, including patient's needs, preferences, and values within their cultural parameters.

STANDARD 3: OUTCOMES IDENTIFICATION

The psychiatric mental health registered nurse identifies expected outcomes and the health care consumer's goals were planned individualized to the health care consumer or to the situation (ANA, APNA, ISPN, 2014, p. 48).

Determining Outcomes

Outcomes criteria are the optimal goal outcomes that reflect the maximal level of patient health that can realistically be achieved through evidence-based nursing interventions. Whereas nursing diagnoses identify nursing problems, outcomes reflect the desired change. **The expected outcomes provide direction for continuity of care and are culturally appropriate. Outcomes are stated in measurable terms and are achievable through evidence-based interventions and include a time estimate for attainment. Therefore outcomes criteria are patient centered, geared to each individual, and documented as obtainable goals** (ANA, 2014).

Moorhead and colleagues (2013) have compiled a standardized list of nursing outcomes in the Nursing Outcomes Classification (NOC). NOC includes a total of 490 standardized outcomes that provide a mechanism for communicating the effect of nursing interventions on the well-being of patients, families, and communities. Each outcome has an associated group of indicators that is used to determine patient status in relation to the outcome. Table 7-2 provides suggested NOC indicators for the outcome of Suicide Self-Restraint along with the Likert scale that quantifies the achievement on each indicator from 1 (never demonstrated) to 5 (consistently demonstrated).

However, NOC does not distinguish between short- and long-term outcomes. It is helpful when assessing the effectiveness of nursing interventions to use long- and short-term outcomes, often stated as

TABLE 7-2 Suicide Self-Restraint (NOC)

Definition:
Personal actions to refrain from gestures and attempts at killing self
Outcome Target Rating:
Maintain at _____. Increase to _____.

Suicide Self-Restraint	Never Demonstrated	Rarely Demonstrated	Sometimes Demonstrated	Often Demonstrated	Consistently Demonstrated	
Overall Rating	1	2	3	4	5	
Indicators						
Expresses feelings	1	2	3	4	5	NA
Expresses sense of hope	1	2	3	4	5	NA
Maintains connectedness in relationship	1	2	3	4	5	NA
Obtains assistance as needed	1	2	3	4	5	NA
Verbalizes suicidal ideas	1	2	3	4	5	NA
Controls impulses	1	2	3	4	5	NA
Refrains from gathering means for suicide	1	2	3	4	5	NA
Refrains from giving away possessions	1	2	3	4	5	NA
Refrains from inflicting serious injury	1	2	3	4	5	NA
Refrains from using nonprescribed mood-altering substance(s)	1	2	3	4	5	NA
Discloses plan for suicide if present	1	2	3	4	5	NA
Upholds suicide contract*	1	2	3	4	5	NA
Maintains self-control without supervision	1	2	3	4	5	NA
Refrains from attempting suicide	1	2	3	4	5	NA
Obtains treatment for depression	1	2	3	4	5	NA
Obtains treatment for substance abuse	1	2	3	4	5	NA
Reports adequate pain control for chronic pain	1	2	3	4	5	NA
Uses suicide prevention resources	1	2	3	4	5	NA
Uses social support group	1	2	3	4	5	NA
Uses available mental health services	1	2	3	4	5	NA
Plans for future	1	2	3	4	5	NA

*Some clinicians question the effectiveness of making a suicide plan.
From Moorhead, S., Johnson, M., Maas, M. L., & Swanson, E. (2013). *Nursing outcomes classification (NOC)* (5th ed.). St. Louis: Elsevier.

goals. The use of long- and short-term outcomes or goals is particularly helpful for teaching and learning purposes. In addition it provides guidelines when planning appropriate interventions. The use of goals guides nurses in building incremental steps toward meeting the desired outcome. What might be a long-term goal for one patient could be a short-term goal or a middle-term goal for another patient. All outcomes (goals) are written in positive terms following the criteria established by the *Standards of Practice*. Table 7-3 shows how a specific outcome criterion might be stated for a suicidal individual with a nursing diagnosis of *Risk for Suicide related to depression and suicide attempt.*

(QSEN) QUALITY AND SAFETY ALERT

QSEN Outcomes

Patient-Centered Care
- Integrate understanding of multiple dimensions of patient-centered care.
- Engage patients or designated surrogates (e.g., family members) and active partnerships that promote health, safety, well-being, and self-management.
- Plan goals that are congruent with the patient/family and are realistic and meet patient's needs (this one not directly from QSEN).

TABLE 7-3 Examples of Long- and Short-Term Goals for a Suicidal Patient

Long-Term Goals or Outcome	Short-Term Goals or Outcomes
1. Patient will remain free from injury throughout the hospital stay.	a. Patient will state he or she understands the rationale and procedure of unit's protocol for suicide precautions.
	b. Patient will find staff and/or friend or family member when feeling overwhelmed or self-destructive during hospitalization.
2. By discharge, patient will state he or she no longer wishes to die and has at least two people to contact if suicidal thoughts arise.	a. Patient will meet with the nurse twice a day for 15 minutes to problem solve alternatives to the situation throughout the hospital stay.
	b. Patient will meet with social worker to find supportive resources in his or her community on discharge.
	c. By discharge, patient will state the purpose of medication, time and dose, adverse effects, and who to call for questions or concerns.

STANDARD 4: PLANNING

The psychiatric mental health registered nurse develops a plan that prescribes strategies and alternatives to assist the health care consumer in attainment of expected outcomes (ANA, APNA, ISPN, 2014, p. 50).

Inpatient and community-based facilities may use standardized tools (e.g., care plans, flowcharts, clinical pathways) for patients with specific diagnoses. Standard tools allow for inclusion of evidence-based practice and newly tested interventions as they become available. Although these tools may be more time efficient, they may not be appropriately focused on the individual's needs. Whatever the care planning procedures in a specific institution, the nurse considers the following specific principles when planning care:

- *Safety.* They must be safe for the patient as well as for other patients, staff, and family.
- *Appropriate.* They must be compatible with other therapies and with the patient's personal goals, spiritual and cultural values, as well as with institutional rules.
- *Individualized to the patient* (patient centered). They should be realistic (1) within the patient's capabilities given the patient's age, physical strength, condition, and willingness to change; (2) consider the patient's preferences, health practices, coping styles, developmental level and the individual's recovery goals (to name but a few); (3) reflective of the actual available community resources and technology.
- *Evidence based.* The plan should integrate current scientific evidence, trends, and research. Using best-evidence interventions and treatments as they become available is being stressed in all areas of medical and mental health care. Evidence-based practice essentially means "a conscientious, explicit, and judicious use of current best evidence in making decisions about the care of individual patients" (Sackett et al., 2000) (refer to Chapter 1). Evidence-based practice (EBP) for nurses is a combination of clinical skills and the use of clinically relevant research in the delivery of effective patient-centered care. Therefore, the use of best available research coupled with patient preferences and sound clinical judgment and skills makes an optimal patient-centered nurse-patient partnership (Sackett et al., 2000). Keep in mind that any interventions that are chosen to be used need to be acceptable and appropriate to the individual patient.

The Nursing Interventions Classification (NIC)(Bulechek et al., 2013) is a research-based standardized listing of 554 interventions that the nurse can use to plan care and reflect current clinical practice. Nurses in all settings can use NIC to support quality patient care and incorporate evidence-based nursing actions. **The nurse partners with the patient, family, and significant others in a realistic and timely manner.** Although many safe and appropriate interventions may not be included in NIC, it is a useful guide for standardized care, **but individualizing interventions to meet an individual's special needs should always be part of the planning.**

When choosing nursing interventions from NIC or other sources, the nurse chooses not only those that fit the nursing diagnosis (e.g., *Risk for Suicide*) but also those that match the defining data. Although the outcome criteria (NOC) might be similar or the same (e.g., Suicide Self-Restraint), the safe and appropriate interventions may be totally different because of the defining data. For example, consider the nursing diagnosis *Risk for Suicide as evidenced by (risk factors/risk behaviors) two recent suicide attempts and repeated statements that "I want to die."*

The planning of appropriate nursing interventions from Nursing Interventions Classifications (2013) might include the following:

- Consider hospitalization of a patient who is at serious risk for suicidal behavior.
- Explain suicide precautions and relevant safety issues to the patient/family/significant others (e.g., purpose, duration, behavioral expectations, and behavioral consequences).

- Initiate suicide precautions (e.g., ongoing observations and monitoring of the patient, provision of a protective environment) for the person who is at serious risk for suicide.
- Search the newly hospitalized patient and personal belongings for weapons or potential weapons during the inpatient admission procedure, as appropriate.
- Use protective interventions (e.g., area restriction seclusion, physical restraints) if the patient lacks the restraint to refrain from harming self, as needed.
- Assign hospitalized patient to a room located near the nursing station for ease in observations, as appropriate.

However, if the defining data are different, so too will be the appropriate interventions, for example, *risk for suicide related (risk factors behaviors) to recent loss of spouse, lack of self-care, and statements evidencing loneliness and hopelessness.*

The nurse might choose the following interventions from NIC (2013) for this patient's plan of care:

- Determine presence and degree of suicidal risk.
- Use direct, nonjudgmental approach in discussing suicide.
- Assist patient to identify network of supportive persons and resources (e.g., clergy, family, providers).
- Facilitate support of the patient by family and friends.
- Consider strategies to decrease isolation and opportunities to act on harmful thoughts.
- Provide information about available community resources and outreach programs.

Chapter 23 addresses assessment of and intervention for the suicidal patient in more depth.

(QSEN) QUALITY AND SAFETY ALERT

Planning

Some possible QSEN competencies inherent in planning care include the following:

- **Patient-centered care:** Respect patient preferences for degree of active engagement in care process toward helping the patient meet his or her needs and goals.
- **Evidence-based practice:** Base individualized care plan on patient's values, clinical expertise, and evidence.
- **Informatics:** Document and plan patient care in an electronic health record.

STANDARD 5: IMPLEMENTATION

The psychiatric mental health registered nurse implements the identified plan (ANA, APNA, ISPN, 2014, p. 52).

Recent graduates and practitioners new to the psychiatric setting will participate in many of these activities with the guidance and support of more experienced health care professionals. The Psychiatric Mental Health Registered Nurse (PMH–RN), who have earned a baccalaureate degree, practices on the basic level of intervention, while the Psychiatric Mental Health Advanced Practice Registered Nurse (PMH–APRN), prepared at the master's level or above, is prepared to function at an advanced level.

The basic level for the psychiatric mental health registered nurses practice is accomplished through the nurse-patient partnership and the use of therapeutic intervention skills. The nurse implements the plan using evidence-based interventions whenever possible, utilizing community resources and collaborating with nursing colleagues. Provision of care implies that interventions are age appropriate and culturally and ethnically sensitive. The following categories of interventions are divided by levels and groups but are not necessarily presented in the order recorded in the Standards in order to more clearly identify those interventions that only apply to the PMH–APRN.

Basic Level and Advanced Practice Interventions
Basic Level: Psychiatric Mental Health Registered Nurse (PMH–RN)

Standard 5A: Coordination of care. **The psychiatric mental health registered nurse (PMH-RN) coordinates care delivery (ANA, APNA, ISPN, 2014, p. 54).**

Coordinates and implements the plan maximizing quality-of-life, independence and optimal recovery. Communicates among family, other health care workers and advocates respectable care for the individual by the interprofessional team. Assists the patient and family to find alternatives to care and documents the coordination of care.

Standard 5B: Health teaching and health promotion. **The psychiatric mental health registered nurse employs strategies to promote health and safe environment (ANA, APNA, ISPN, 2014, p. 55).**

Psychiatric mental health nurses use a variety of health teaching methods adaptive to the patient's special needs (age, culture, ability to learn, readiness), and recovery goals integrating current knowledge and evidence-based psychoeducational strategies in their interventions.

Health teaching includes identifying the health education needs of the patient and provides health care teaching, such as coping skills, self-care activities, stress management, problem-solving skills, relapse prevention, conflict management, and giving information about coping with interpersonal relationships. Among the most vital parts of health promotion is identifying resources for prevention and recovery mental health care services in the community.

Standard 5E: Pharmacological, biological, and integrative therapies. **The psychiatric mental health registered nurse incorporates knowledge of pharmacological, biological, and complementary interventions with applied clinical skills to restore the consumer's health and prevent further disability (ANA, APNA, ISPN, 2014).**

The nurse is knowledgeable regarding the current research findings, intended action, therapeutic dosage, adverse reactions, and safe blood levels of medications being administered and monitors the patient for any untoward effects. The nurse is expected to discuss and provide health care teaching regarding medication to the patient and family for any drug action, adverse side effects, dietary restrictions, and drug interactions, and to provide time for questions. The nurse's assessment of the patient's response to psychobiological interventions is communicated to other members of the mental health team.

Standard 5F: Milieu therapy. **The psychiatric mental health registered nurse provides, structures, and maintains safe, therapeutic, recovery oriented environment collaboration with health care consumers, families, and other health care clinicians (ANA, APNA, ISPN, 2014, p. 60).**

Among other things milieu management includes orienting patients to their rights and responsibilities. Milieu management also includes informing patients in a culturally competent manner about the need for structure, maintenance of a safe environment, and limits set on the unit. The nurse selects activities (both individual and group) that meets the patient's physical and mental health needs. The patient should always be maintained in the least restrictive environment.

Standard 5G: Therapeutic relationship and counseling. **The psychiatric mental health registered nurse (PHM-RN) uses the therapeutic relationship and counseling interventions to assist health care** consumers in their individual recovery journeys by improving and regaining their previous coping abilities, fostering mental health and preventing mental disorder and disability (ANA, APNA, ISPN, 2014, p. 62).

Advanced Practice Interventions: Psychiatric Mental Health Advanced Practice Registered Nurse (PMH–APRN)
Prescriptive Authority and Treatment

Psychiatric mental health advance practice registered nurse (PMH-APRN) uses prescriptive authority, procedures, referrals, treatments, and therapies in accordance with state and federal law and regulation (ANA, APNA, ISPN, 2014).

Psychotherapy

The psychiatric nurse advanced practice registered nurse (PMH-APRN) conducts individual, couples, group, and family psychotherapy using evidence-based psychotherapeutic frameworks and nurse-patient therapeutic relationships (ANA, APNA, ISPN, 2014, p. 63)

Consultation

The psychiatric mental health advanced practice registered nurse (PMH-APRN) provides consultation to influence the identified plan, enhance the abilities of other clinicians to promote services for health care consumers, and effect change (ANA, APNA, ISPN, 2014, p. 57).

QSEN **QUALITY AND SAFETY ALERT**

Implementation

Some possible QSEN competencies for implementing patient-centered care include the following:

Patient-Centered Care
- Provide patient-centered care with sensitivity and respect for the diversity of human experience.
- Recognize the boundaries of therapeutic relationships.
- Participate in building consensus or resolving conflict in the context of patient care.

Safety
- Do the interventions based on your care plan minimize the risk of harm to patients and providers through both system effectiveness and individual performance?

Teamwork and Collaboration
- Initiate request for help when appropriate to the situation.
- Integrate the contributions of others who play a role in helping patient/family achieve health goals in order to achieve quality patient care.

STANDARD 6: EVALUATION

The psychiatric mental registered nurse enhances progress toward attainment expected outcomes (ANA, APNA, ISPN, 2014, p. 65).

Unfortunately, evaluation of patient outcomes is often the most neglected part of the nursing process. Evaluation of the individual's response to treatment should be systematic, ongoing, and criterion-based. Supporting data are included to clarify the evaluation. Ongoing assessment of data allows for revisions of nursing diagnoses, changes to more realistic outcomes, or identification of more appropriate interventions when outcomes are not met.

Evaluation

Suggested QSEN competencies inherent when evaluating care include the following:

Quality Improvement (QI)
- Seek information about outcomes of care populations served in care setting.
- Evaluate and monitor the patient's outcomes (long- and short-term goals) and make changes to improve and increase the quality and safety of patient care (not directly from QSEN).

DOCUMENTATION

Documentation could be considered the seventh step in the nursing process. Keep in mind that patient records are legal documents and may be used in a court of law (refer to Chapter 6 on the legalities of charting). Besides the evaluation of stated outcomes, the notes of all health care workers should record changes in patient condition, record of informed consents (for medications and treatments), reaction to medication, documentation of symptoms (verbatim when appropriate), concerns of the patient, and any untoward incidents in the health care setting. Documentation of patient progress is the responsibility of the entire mental health team.

Suggested QSEN competencies inherent in the documentation of care include the following:
- **Informatics:** Communicates information to the rest of the team on the patient's progress and employs communication technologies to coordinate care for patients.

Documentation of "Nonadherence"

When patients do not follow medication and treatment plans, they are often labeled as "noncompliant." Applied to patients, the term *noncompliant* often has negative connotations because *compliance* traditionally referred to the extent that a patient obediently and faithfully followed the health care providers' instructions. "That patient is noncompliant" often translates into he or she is "bad" or "lazy," subjecting the patient to blame and criticism. Crane (2012) cautions nurses and physicians not to blame noncompliance on a patient's stubbornness or bad mood; this can leave both the nurse and the patient frustrated and angry. The term *noncompliant* is invariably judgmental. A much more useful term would be **nonadherent.** It now invites us to find out what is going on in the patient's life that he is unable to take medication.

Crane (2012) also emphasizes that under the Affordable Care Act, documenting "noncompliance" no longer protects the physician, nurse, manager, or hospital for bad outcomes, which have led to further illness or injury. A finding of noncompliance may void Medicaid or Medicare reimbursements, which can lead to financial losses to the institution and damage to the facility's reputation (Scudder, 2013).

Furthermore, "patient did not comply" does not protect nurses, physicians, or health care workers from malpractice lawsuits. Crane (2012) advises that meticulous records that document the doctor's or nurse's "rationale for treatment, clear explanations of what he or she wants the patient to do, and whether the patient actually complied with that advice" will help prevent health care workers in the event of lawsuits. The lesson is to treat noncompliance/nonadherence seriously. "Each compliance issue, large and small, must be recognized as an indicator of potential trouble and must be addressed early and appropriately" (Scudder, 2013). Probably the biggest issue involved in a malpractice verdict is if the patient was given instructions or printed information sheets, it is possible that the patient did not understand the instructions or didn't realize how important the treatment (medication, a follow-up, etc.) was to their health.

Systems of Charting

Although communication among team members and coordination of services are the primary goals when choosing a system for charting, practitioners in all settings must also consider professional standards, legal issues, requirements for reimbursement by insurers, and accreditation by regulatory agencies.

Information also must be in a format that is retrievable for quality assurance monitoring, utilization management, peer review, and research. Documentation, using the nursing process as a guide, is reflected in many of the different formats that are commonly used in health care settings (Table 7-4). Computerized clinical documentation is preferred in today's medical settings. Nurses need to be trained to use these technologies and the medical setting should be prepared to provide further training for nurses in the use of terminology, progress notes relating to needs assessment, nursing interventions, and nursing diagnoses (Hayrinen, 2010). Any documentation format used by a health care facility must be focused, organized, and pertinent and must conform to certain legal and other generally accepted principles (Box 7-6).

TABLE 7-4 **Narrative versus Problem-Oriented Charting***	
Narrative Charting	**Problem-Oriented Charting: SOAPIE**
Characteristics	
A descriptive statement of patient status written in chronological order throughout a shift. Used to support assessment finding from a flow sheet. In charting by exception, narrative notes are used to indicate significant symptoms, behaviors, or events that are exceptions to norms identified on assessment flow sheet.	Developed in the 1960s for physicians to reduce inefficient documentation. Intended to be accompanied by a problem list. Originally SOAP, with IE added later. Emphasis is on problem identification, process, and outcome.
	S: Subjective data (patient statement)
	O: Objective data (nurse observations)
	A: Assessment (nurse interprets S and O and describes either a problem or a nursing diagnosis)
	P: Plan (proposed intervention)
	I: Interventions (nurse's response to problem)
	E: Evaluation (patient outcome)

Continued

TABLE 7-4 Narrative versus Problem-Oriented Charting—cont'd

Narrative Charting	Problem-Oriented Charting: SOAPIE
Example Date/time/discipline Patient was agitated in the morning and pacing in the hallway. Blinked eyes, muttered to self, and looked off to the side. Stated heard voices. Verbally hostile to another patient. Offered 2 mg of haloperidol (Haldol) prn and sat with staff in quiet area for 20 minutes. Patient returned to community lounge and was able to sit and watch television.	Date/time/discipline S: "I'm so stupid. Get away, get away." "I hear the devil telling me bad things." O: Patient paced the hall, mumbling to self and looking off to the side. Shouted derogatory comments when approached by another patient. Watched walls and ceiling closely. A: Patient was having auditory hallucinations and increased agitation. P: Offered patient haloperidol prn. Redirected patient to less stimulating environment. I: Patient received 2 mg of haloperidol PO prn. Sat with patient in quiet room for 20 minutes. E: Patient calmer. Returned to community lounge, sat, and watched television.
Advantages Uses a common form of expression (narrative writing). Can address any event or behavior. Explains flow sheet findings. Provides multidisciplinary ease of use.	Structured. Provides consistent organization of data. Facilitates retrieval of data for quality assurance and utilization management. Contains all elements of the nursing process. Minimizes inclusion of unnecessary data. Provides multidisciplinary ease of use.
Disadvantages Unstructured. May result in different organization of information from note to note. Makes it difficult to retrieve quality assurance and utilization management data. Frequently leads to omission of elements of the nursing process. Commonly results in inclusion of unnecessary and subjective information.	Requires time and effort to structure the information. Limits entries to problems. May result in loss of data about progress. Not chronological. Carries negative connotation.

*Today most charting is computerized, and each institution has its own system of updating patients' records.

BOX 7-6 Legal Considerations for Documentation of Care

Do's

- Chart in a timely manner all pertinent and factual information.
- Be familiar with the nursing documentation policy in your facility and make your charting conform to this standard. The policy generally states the method, frequency, and pertinent assessments, interventions, and outcomes to be recorded. If your agency's policies and procedures do not encourage or allow for quality documentation, bring the need for change to the administration's attention.
- Chart legibly in ink.
- Chart facts fully, descriptively, and accurately.
- Chart what you see, hear, feel, and smell.
- Chart pertinent observations: psychosocial observations, physical symptoms pertinent to the medical diagnosis, and behaviors pertinent to the nursing diagnosis.
- Chart follow-up care provided when a problem has been identified in earlier documentation. For example, if a patient has fallen and injured a leg, describe how the wound is healing.
- Chart fully the facts surrounding unusual occurrences and incidents.
- Chart all nursing interventions, treatments, and outcomes (including teaching efforts and patient responses), and safety and patient protection interventions.
- Chart the patient's expressed subjective feelings.
- Chart each time you notify a physician and record the reason for notification, the information that was communicated, the accurate time, the physician's instructions or orders, and the follow-up activity.

- Chart physicians' visits and treatments.
- Chart discharge medications and instructions given for use, as well as all discharge teaching performed, and note which family members were included in the process.

Don'ts

- Do *not* chart opinions that are not supported by the facts.
- Do *not* defame patients by calling them names or by making derogatory statements about them (e.g., "an unlikable patient who is demanding unnecessary attention").
- Do *not* chart before an event occurs.
- Do *not* chart generalizations, suppositions, or pat phrases (e.g., "patient in good spirits").
- Do *not* obliterate, erase, alter, or destroy a record. If an error is made, draw one line through the error, write "mistaken entry" or "error," and initial. Follow your agency's guidelines closely.
- Do *not* leave blank spaces for chronological notes. If you must chart out of sequence, chart "late entry." Identify the time and date of the entry and the time and date of the occurrence.
- If an incident report/occurrence is filed, *do not note in the chart that one was filed.* This form is generally a privileged communication between the hospital and the hospital's attorney. Describing it in the chart may destroy the privileged nature of the communication. The incident as it occurred should be documented in the patient's records.

KEY POINTS TO REMEMBER

- The nursing process is a six-step problem-solving approach to patient care to help secure safety and quality care for patients.
- The Institute of Medicine (IOM) and QSEN faculty have established mandates to prepare future nurses with the knowledge, skills, and attitudes (KSAs) necessary for achieving quality and safety as they engage in the six competencies of nursing: patient-centered care, teamwork and collaboration, evidence-based practice (EBP), quality improvement (QI), safety, and informatics.
- The *primary source* of assessment is the patient. *Secondary sources* of information include the family, neighbors, friends, police, and other members of the health team.
- The assessment interview includes gathering objective data (mental or emotional status) and subjective data (psychosocial assessment). A number of tools are provided in this textbook for the evaluation of cultural, spiritual/religious, and mental status.
- Medical examination, history, and systems review complete a comprehensive assessment.
- An important part of planning patient-centered care is to understand how spiritual/religious beliefs play a part in a person's life and how they deal with stress.
- Caregivers should also have an awareness of the person's cultural background and social attachments, and how these issues affect the way a person experiences healing in his or her culture.
- Assessment tools and standardized rating scales may be used to evaluate and monitor a patient's progress. Emphasis needs to be placed on further evaluation of progress and sharing of this information with other members of the health care team.
- Self-assessment is an important part of the assessment process. There are a number of ways that novice interviewers can gain valuable feedback, support, and supervision.
- Determination of the nursing diagnosis (NANDA-I) defines the practice of nursing, improves communication between staff members, and assists in accountability for care.
- A nursing diagnosis consists of (1) an unmet need or problem, (2) an etiology or probable cause, and (3) supporting data.
- Outcomes are variable, measurable, and stated in terms that reflect a patient's actual state. NOC provides 330 standardized outcomes. Planning involves determining desired outcomes.
- Behavioral goals support outcomes. Short- and long-term outcomes are measurable, indicate the desired patient behavior(s), include a set time for achievement, and are short and specific.
- Planning nursing actions (NIC or other sources) to achieve the stated outcomes include the use of the following specific principles: the plan should be (1) safe, (2) evidence based whenever possible, (3) realistic, and (4) compatible with other therapies. NIC provides nurses with standardized nursing interventions that are applicable for use in all settings.
- Practice in psychiatric nursing encompasses basic-level interventions: coordination of care; health teaching and health promotion; milieu therapy; and pharmacological, biological, and integrative therapies.
- Advanced practice interventions are carried out by a nurse who is educated at the master's level or higher. Nurses certified for advanced practice psychiatric mental health nursing may be additionally prepared to practice psychotherapy, prescribe certain medications, and perform consulting work.
- The evaluation of care is a continual process of determining to what extent the outcome criteria have been achieved. The plan of care may be revised on the basis of the evaluation.
- Documentation of patient progress through evaluation of outcome criteria is crucial. The patient's record is a legal document and should accurately reflect the patient's condition, medications, treatment, tests, responses, and any untoward incidents.
- Simply documenting a patient's noncompliance/nonadherence to medical treatment no longer protects nurses, doctors, other health care professionals, and/or institutions from lawsuits when further harm to the patient presents itself. Careful documentation of what has been done to help the individual understand the instructions, understand the reasons behind the medical advice, and follow-up on compliance issues should be included.

APPLYING CLINICAL JUDGMENT

1. Pedro Gonzales, a 37-year-old Hispanic man, arrived by ambulance from a supermarket, where he had fallen. He remains lethargic. On his arrival to the emergency department (ED), his breath smelled "fruity." He appears confused and anxious, saying that "they put the 'evil eye' on me, they want me to die, they are drying out my body … it's draining me dry … they are yelling, they are yelling … no, no I'm not bad … oh God don't let them get me." When his mother arrives in the ED, she tells the staff, through the use of an interpreter, that Pedro is a severe diabetic and has a diagnosis of paranoid schizophrenia, and this happens when he does not take his medications. In a group or in collaboration with a classmate respond to the following:
   A. A number of nursing diagnoses are possible in this scenario. Formulate in writing at least two nursing diagnoses (problems) given the preceding information, and include "related to" and "as evidenced by."
   B. For each of your nursing diagnoses, list one long-term outcome (e.g., the problem, what should change). Include a time frame, desired change, and three criteria that will help you evaluate if the outcome has been met, not met, or partially met.
   C. For each long-term outcome, list two short-term outcomes (goals) (the steps that need to be taken in order for the goal to be accomplished), including time frame, desired outcomes, and evaluation criteria.
   D. What are the four basic principles for planning nursing interventions?
   E. What specific needs might you take into account when planning nursing care for Mr. Gonzales?
   F. Using informatics, evaluate optimal outcomes for Mr. Gonzalez at your current health care setting, or use the charting method employed by the institution.
   G. Give an example of the QSEN competencies you might stress when planning care for Mr. Gonzalez.

CHAPTER REVIEW QUESTIONS

1. A nurse assesses a new patient whose chief concern is "daily crying spells." Which comment from the patient would prompt the nurse to suspect a medical reason is causing the problem rather than depression?
   a. "I usually drink two or three cups of coffee in the morning."
   b. "I often have headaches, especially when the pollen count is high."
   c. "Years ago I had thyroid problems but they cleared up and I stopped the medicine."
   d. "I recently had three moles removed because my doctor thought they were suspicious."

2. A 55-year-old lives 100 miles from her parents and mother-in-law. In the past year, her father had back surgery, her mother broke her hip, and her mother-in-law had a cardiac event. Which nursing diagnosis is most applicable to the 55-year-old?

    a. *Risk for complicated grieving related to impending deaths of parents*

    b. *Risk for injury related to frequent long drives to care for aging parents*

    c. *Risk for chronic low self-esteem related to overwhelming responsibilities*

    d. *Risk for caregiver role strain related to responsibilities for care of aging parents*

3. A patient asks the psychiatric mental health registered nurse, "I'm having so much anxiety. I think hypnosis would help me. Will you do that for me?" When determining a response, which factor should the nurse consider?

    a. The patient's current medication regime

    b. State regulations regarding scope of practice

    c. The patient's level of participation within the therapeutic milieu

    d. The plan of care the multidisciplinary team has developed for the patient

4. The nurse plans care for a newly hospitalized patient experiencing panic level anxiety after an automobile accident. The patient has no physical injuries. When selecting goals from the Nursing Outcomes Classification (NOC), the nurse will

    a. Select outcomes related to patient learning.

    b. Focus first on the long-term goals for the patient.

    c. Individualize outcomes based on the patient's needs.

    d. Confer with the patient about which outcomes the patient wants to achieve.

5. On an inpatient unit, one patient assaults another patient resulting in a small laceration. Considering the patients' right to confidentiality, how will the nurse effectively document this event?

    a. Ensure unit safety by documenting the hostile and combative characteristics of the assaulting patient.

    b. Document in each patient's medical record the events and actions taken, using initials of other patients involved.

    c. Document in both patients' medical records that an occurrence (incident) report was prepared according to agency policy.

    d. Verbally report the events to other team members and minimize written documentation in order to reduce potential legal consequences.

REFERENCES

American Nurses Association (ANA), American Psychiatric Nurses Association, & International Society of Psychiatric–Mental Health Nurses. (2014). *Psychiatric–mental health nursing: scope and standards of practice.* Washington, DC: Nursebooks.org. © 2014 By American Nurses Association, American Psychiatric Nurses Association and International Society of Psychiatric-Mental Health Nurses. Reprinted with permission by ANA. All rights reserved.

Arnold, E. C., & Boggs, K. U. (2016). *Interpersonal relationships: professional communication skills for nurses* (6th ed.). St. Louis: Saunders.

Brauser, D. (2011). *Deadly combination of depression and diabetes doubles mortality risk.* Retrieved from www.Medscape.org/viewarticle/735714?SRE=cmemp.

Bulechek, G. M., Butcher, H. K., Dochterman, J. M., & Wagner, C. M. (2013). *Nursing interventions classification (NIC)* (6th ed.). St. Louis: Elsevier.

Crane, M. (2012). *Documenting noncompliance won't protect you anymore.* Retrieved February 18, 2013, from www.Medscape.com/viewarticle/773918.

Cronenwett, L., Sherwood, G., Bronsteiner, J., Disch, J., Johnson, J., Mitchell, P., Sullivan, D., & Water, J. (2007). Quality and safety education for nurses. *Nursing Outlook, 55*(3), 122–131.

Hayrinen, K. (2010). Evaluation of electronic nursing documentation—nursing process model and standardized terminologies as key to visible and transparent nursing. *International Journal of Medical Informatics, 79*(8), 554–564.

Institute of Medicine (IOM). (2001). Crossing the quality chasm: A new healthcare system for the 21st century. Retrieved December 30, 2015, from http://www.nap.edu/books/0309072808/html/.

Jeffries, P. (2005). A framework for designing, implementing, and evaluate simulations used as teaching strategies in nursing. *Nursing Education Perspectives,* 96–103.

Knoerl, A. M., Esper, K., Hasenau, S. (2011). Cultural sensitivity in patient health education. *Nursing clinics of America, 46*(3), 335–340.

Moorhead, S., Johnson, M., Maas, M. L., & Swanson, E. (2013). *Nursing outcomes classification (NOC)* (5th ed.). St. Louis: Elsevier.

North American Nursing Diagnosis Association International (NANDA-I). (2015 – 2017). Nursing diagnoses—definitions and classification 2015 – 2017. *Copyright 2014,* 1994–2012 by NANDA International, Philadelphia. Used by arrangement with Blackwell Publishing Limited, a company of John Wiley and Sons, Inc.

O'Riordan, M. (2000). *Religion, spirituality not associated with better cardiovascular health.* Retrieved March 16, 2012, from http://www.theheart.org/article/104-5327.do.

Sackett, D. L., Straus, S., Richardson, W., et al. (2000). *Evidence-based medicine: how to practice and teach EBM.* London: Churchill Livingstone.

Scudder, L. (2013). *Nurses and noncompliance: a primer.* Retrieved March 18, 2013, from www.medscape.com/viewarticle/779149_print.

Sommers-Flanagan, J., & Sommers-Flanagan, R. (2012 – 2013). *Clinical interviewing* (5th ed.). Hoboken, NJ: John Wiley & Sons.

Communication Skills: Medium for All Nursing Practice

Elizabeth M. Varcarolis

KEY TERMS AND CONCEPTS

cultural filters, p. 101
double-bind messages, p. 94
double messages, p. 94
feedback, p. 92

information communication
    technologies (ICT), p. 101
mobile medical apps, p. 91
nontherapeutic techniques, p. 95
nonverbal communication, p. 93

telehealth technologies, p. 91
therapeutic communication, p. 92
therapeutic techniques, p. 95
verbal communication, p. 93

SELECTED CONCEPT: NEW AND EVOLVING INFORMATION COMMUNICATION TECHNOLOGIES (ICT)

Telehealth Technologies

"Telehealth is the use of electronic information and telecommunication technologies to support long-distance clinical healthcare in order to eliminate barriers from the delivery of healthcare seer services. Telehealth technologies include such electronic means of communication as videoconferencing, the Internet, telephone/cell phone consultation and counseling, image transmission, and interactive video sessions. These techniques allow for establishing and maintaining therapeutic relationships. However, "particular attention must be directed to confidentiality, informed consent, documentation, maintenance of records, and the integrity of the transmitted information" (ANA, 2014, p. 37).

"Mobile medical apps can monitor, communicate, triage, and even assist in the diagnosis and treatment of psychiatric disorders. Mobile apps can collect real-time patient data, including self-report, behavioral changes, passive data, and physiological parameters" (Peek, 2015). However, privacy and confidential issues are unresolved at present, as well as a lack of current clinical data for efficacy and safety of specific mobile apps (Peek, 2015).

OBJECTIVES

1. Identify three personal and two environmental factors that can impede accurate communication.
2. Discuss the differences between verbal and nonverbal communication and demonstrate at least five areas of nonverbal communication.
3. Identify two attending behaviors that you will work on to increase your communication skills.
4. Relate problems that can arise when nurses are insensitive to cultural differences in patients' communication styles.
5. Compare and contrast the range of verbal and nonverbal communication of your cultural groups with two other cultural groups in the areas of (a) communication style, (b) eye contact, and (c) touch. Give examples.
6. Demonstrate with a classmate the use of four techniques that can enhance communication, highlighting what makes them effective.
7. Demonstrate with a classmate the use of four techniques that can obstruct communication, highlighting what makes them ineffective.
8. Role-play with a classmate the techniques of "What if" and the "Miracle Question" and then switch roles. Identify what new information you might have learned about your classmate, and what new insight you might have about yourself.
9. Identify the advantages of telehealth technologies in the community in which you live.

INTRODUCTION

Humans have a fundamental need to relate to others, and our advanced ability to communicate gives our life sustenance and meaning. We also share a need to be understood and form satisfying relationships with others. This is usually accomplished through the use of effective communication skills. On the other hand, when stress or negative feelings occur within the relationship, effective communication has a higher potential to falter, and there is a greater chance for miscommunication. Our ability to communicate is a fundamental aspect of being human; in fact, all of our actions, words, and expressions convey meaning to others. It is even said that we cannot *not* communicate. Silence, for example, can communicate acceptance, anger, or thoughtfulness. In the provision of nursing care, however, communication has a new emphasis. Just as social relationships are different from therapeutic relationships, basic communication is different from the professional, goal-directed, and scientifically based communication we call therapeutic communication.

The findings of a study using a large body of nursing literature evaluating communication pointed to "increased recovery rates, a sense of safety and protection, improved levels of patient satisfaction, and greater adherence to treatment options" as well-documented results of effective communication (Neese, 2015). Conversely, as many as 440,000 people die each year from preventable medical errors, representing the third leading cause of death in the United States. The Joint Commission estimates that 80% of these deaths involve miscommunication/poor communication techniques (Neese, 2015).

COMMUNICATION

The ability to form patient-centered therapeutic relationships/partnerships is fundamental and essential to effective nursing care, and therapeutic communication is crucial to the formation of a therapeutic relationship. Determining levels of pain in the postoperative patient, listening as parents express feelings of fear concerning their child's diagnosis, or understanding, without words, the needs of the intubated patient in the intensive care unit are essential skills in providing quality nursing.

Ideally, therapeutic communication is a professional skill you learn and practice early in your nursing curriculum. But in psychiatric nursing, communication skills assume a different and new emphasis because psychiatric disorders cause not only physical symptoms (e.g., fatigue, loss of appetite, and insomnia) but also emotional symptoms (e.g., sadness, anger, hopelessness, euphoria, as well as sensory distortions) that affect a person's very ability to relate to others.

It is often in the psychiatric rotation that students discover the importance of communication and increase their ability to utilize "therapeutic communication" and begin to rely on techniques they once considered artificial. NOTE: There is a fundamental difference between performing an *assessment* and the use of *therapeutic communication*. Assessment is an information-gathering approach designed to meet the nurse's needs, whereas therapeutic communication meets the patient's needs (T. Burckhalter, 2015, personal communication).

With continued practice, you will develop your own style and rhythm, and eventually these techniques will become a part of the way you communicate with others.

Novice psychiatric practitioners are often concerned that they may say the wrong thing, especially when learning to apply therapeutic techniques. Will you say the "wrong" thing? The answer is, yes, you probably will. That is how we all learn to find more useful and effective ways of helping individuals reach their goals. The challenge is to recover from your mistakes and use them for learning and growth (Sommers-Flanagan & Sommers-Flanagan, 2012–2013).

Will saying the "wrong" thing be harmful to the patient? Hardly, especially if your intent is honest, your approach is respectful, and you have a genuine concern for the patient. Communication is up to 90% nonverbal, and individuals pay attention to the intent, as discussed in greater detail later in this chapter. Scientific investigations have identified special skills and methods that can aid people in becoming more effective helpers. However, knowledge of skills and techniques is not enough. Being an effective communicator, whether in nursing or in any other area of life, is not just a matter of knowing what techniques to use. Genuine respect for the individual and the ability to listen compassionately and empathetically are the essence of psychological healing.

The Communication Process

A standard communication model is Berlo's classic communication model developed in 1960 and it remains relevant today (Berlo, 1960).

1. One person has a need to communicate with another (**stimulus**). For example, the stimulus for communication can be a need for information, comfort, or advice.
2. The person sending the message (**sender**) initiates interpersonal contact.
3. The **message** is the information sent or expressed to another. The clearest messages are those that are well organized and expressed in a manner familiar to the receiver.
4. The message can be sent through a variety of **media,** including auditory (hearing), visual (seeing), tactile (touch), olfactory (smell), or any combination of these.
5. The person receiving the message (**receiver**) then interprets the message and responds to the sender by providing feedback. The nature of the feedback often indicates whether the meaning of the message sent has been correctly interpreted by the receiver. Validating the accuracy of the sender's message is extremely important. An accuracy check may be obtained by simply asking the sender, "Is this what you mean?" or "I notice you turn away when we talk about your going back to college. Is there a conflict there?"

Figure 8-1 shows this simple model of communication along with some of the many factors that affect communication.

Effective communication within a nurse-patient partnership depends on the nurse understanding what he or she is trying to convey (the purpose of the message), communicating what is really meant to the patient, and comprehending the meaning of what the patient is intentionally or unintentionally conveying (Arnold & Boggs, 2016). Communication is complex and involves a variety of personal and environmental factors that can distort both the sending and the receiving of messages.

Factors that Affect Communication
Personal Factors

Personal factors that can impede accurate transmission or interpretation of messages include *emotional factors* (e.g., mood, responses to stress, personal bias, relationship misunderstandings), *social factors* (e.g., previous experience, cultural differences, language differences, lifestyle differences), and *cognitive factors* (e.g., problem-solving ability, knowledge level, language use).

Environmental Factors

Environmental factors that may affect communication include *physical factors* (e.g., background noise, lack of privacy, uncomfortable accommodations) and *societal determinants* (e.g., sociopolitical, historical, or economic factors; the presence of others; the expectations of others).

Relationship Factors

Relationship factors refer to whether the participants are equal or unequal. When the two participants are equal, such as friends or colleagues, the relationship is said to be **symmetrical.** However, when there is a difference in status or power, such as between nurse and patient or teacher and student, the relationship is characterized by inequality (one participant is "superior" to the other) and is called a **complementary** relationship.

Complementary relationships exist when there is a difference in status between the participants. For example, in all cultures social status, age or developmental differences, gender differences, and educational differences can be influential in the communication process.

In the United States, capitalism intimately ties systems of privilege (high-power groups) with systems of oppression (low-power groups) through economic control. Because high-status groups hold more power, they have more control over lower status groups. One way that

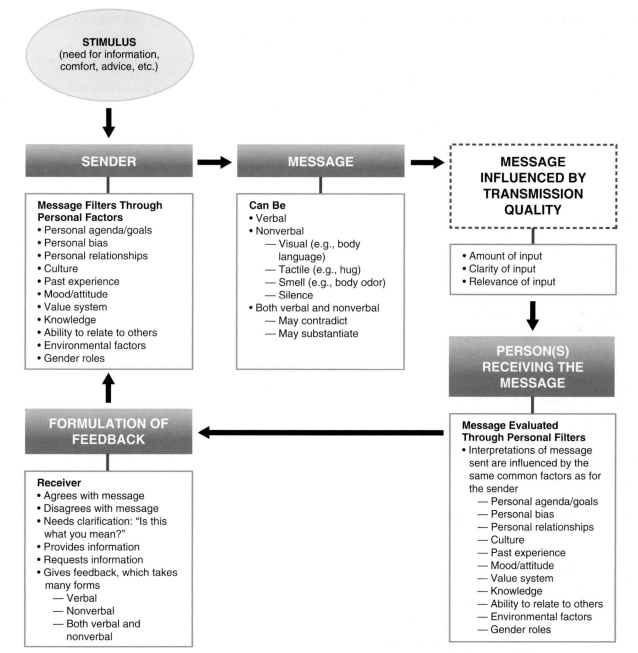

FIGURE 8-1 Operational definition of communication. (Adapted from Ellis, R. B., Gates, B., & Kenworthy, N. [2003]. *Interpersonal communication in nursing: theory and practice.* London: Churchill Livingstone Elsevier.)

power groups retain control (unequal) is through stereotypes, prejudice, and bias. In other words, stigma plays a big part in keeping relationship factors unbalanced (Hays, 2008).

Verbal Communication

Verbal communication consists of all words a person speaks. We live in a society of symbols, and our supreme social symbols are words. Talking is our most common activity—our public link with one another, the primary instrument of instruction, a need, an art, and one of the most personal aspects of our private lives. When we speak, we:

- Communicate our beliefs and values.
- Communicate perceptions and meanings.
- Convey interest and understanding *or* insult and judgment.
- Convey messages clearly *or* convey conflicting or implied messages.
- Convey clear, honest feelings *or* disguised, distorted feelings.

Culture pervades everything and words are often culturally perceived. Clarifying what is meant by certain words is very important. Even if the nurse and patient have the same cultural background, the mental image they have of a given word may not be exactly the same. Although they believe they are talking about the same thing, the nurse and patient may actually be talking about two quite different things. Words are the symbols for emotions as well as mental images.

Nonverbal Communication

The tone and pitch of a person's voice and the manner in which a person paces speech are examples of nonverbal communication. It is important to keep in mind however, that culture influences the pitch and the tone a person uses. For example, the tone and pitch of a voice used to express anger can vary widely within cultures and families (Arnold & Boggs, 2016). Other common examples of nonverbal communication

TABLE 8-1   Nonverbal Behaviors

Behavior	Possible Nonverbal Cues	Example
Body behaviors	Posture, body movements, gestures, gait	The patient is slumped in a chair, puts her face in her hands, and occasionally taps her right foot.
Facial expressions	Frowns, smiles, grimaces, raised eyebrows, pursed lips, licking of lips, tongue movements	The patient grimaces when speaking to the nurse; when alone, he smiles and giggles to himself.
Eye cast	Angry, suspicious, and accusatory looks	The patient's eyes harden with suspicion.
Voice-related behaviors	Tone, pitch, level, intensity, inflection, stuttering, pauses, silences, fluency	The patient talks in a loud sing-song voice.
Observable autonomic physiological responses	Increase in respirations, diaphoresis, pupil dilation, blushing, paleness	When the patient mentions discharge, she becomes pale, her respirations increase, and her face becomes diaphoretic.
Personal appearance	Grooming, dress, hygiene	The patient is dressed in a wrinkled shirt and his pants are stained; his socks are dirty and he is unshaven.
Physical characteristics	Height, weight, physique, complexion	The patient appears grossly overweight and his muscles appear flabby.

(often called **cues**) are physical appearance, facial expressions, body posture, amount of eye contact, eye cast (i.e., emotion expressed in the eyes), hand gestures, sighs, fidgeting, and yawning. Table 8-1 identifies key components of nonverbal behaviors. Nonverbal behaviors need to be observed and interpreted in light of a person's culture, class, gender, age, sexual orientation, and spiritual norms. Cultural influences on communication will be discussed later in this chapter.

Interaction of Verbal and Nonverbal Communication

Many of us may think of communication primarily in terms of what is said; however, it is believed that only 5% to 10% is conveyed by verbal means and nonverbal behaviors comprise from 65% to 95% of a sent message. Therefore it comes as no surprise that nonverbal behaviors and cues drastically influence communication. Effective communicators pay attention to verbal as well as nonverbal cues.

Communication thus involves two radically different but interdependent kinds of symbols. The first type is the **spoken word,** which represents our public selves. Verbal assertions can be straightforward comments or skillfully used to distort, conceal, deny, and generally disguise true feelings. The second type, **nonverbal behaviors,** covers a wide range of human activities, from body movements to responses to the messages of others. How a person listens and uses silence and sense of touch may also convey important information about the private self that is not available from conversation alone, especially when viewed from a cultural perspective.

Some elements of nonverbal communication, such as facial expressions, seem to be inborn and are similar across cultures. Matsumoto (1992) and Matsumoto and Sung Hwang (2011) cited studies that found a high degree of agreement in spontaneous facial expressions or emotions across 10 different cultures. In public, however, some cultural groups (e.g., Japanese) may control their facial expressions when observers are present. Other types of nonverbal behaviors, such as how close people stand to each other when speaking, depend on cultural conventions. Some nonverbal communication is formalized and has specific meanings (e.g., the military salute, the Japanese bow).

Messages are not always simple and can appear to be one thing when in fact they are another. Often, people have more conscious awareness of their verbal messages and less awareness of their nonverbal behaviors. The verbal message is sometimes referred to as the **content** of the message, and the nonverbal behavior is called the **process** of the message.

When the content is congruent with the process, the communication is more clearly understood and is considered healthy. For example, if a student says, "It's important that I get good grades in this class," that is *content.* If the student has purchased the books for the class, takes good notes, and has a study buddy, that is *process.* Therefore the content and process are congruent and straightforward, and there is a "healthy" message. If, however, the verbal message is not reinforced or is in fact contradicted by the nonverbal behavior, the message is confusing. For example, if the student does not have the books, skips several classes, and does not study, that is *process.* Here the student is conveying two different messages.

Conflicting messages are known as double messages or *mixed messages.* One way a nurse can respond to verbal and nonverbal incongruity is to reflect and validate the patient's feelings. "You say you are upset that you did not pass this semester, but I notice that you look more relaxed and less conflicted than you have all term. What do you see as some of the pros and cons of not passing the course this semester?"

Pioneers in the field of family therapy, Bateson and colleagues (1956) coined the term double-bind messages. Messages are sent to create meaning but also can be used defensively to hide what is actually occurring, create confusion, and attack relatedness. A double-bind message is a mix of content (what is said) and process (what is transmitted nonverbally) that has both a neutral/nurturing aspect, as in what is said, and a hurtful/negative aspect, which is often implied. For example:

> **VIGNETTE**
>
> A 17-year-old female who lives at home with her mother wants to go out for an evening with her friends. She is told by her chronically ill but not helpless mother: "Oh, that's okay, go ahead, have fun. I'll just sit here by myself, and I can always call 911 if I don't feel well, but you go ahead and have fun." The mother says this while looking sad, eyes cast down, slumped in her chair, and letting her cane drop to the floor.

The recipient of this double-bind message is caught between contradictory statements that she cannot do the right thing. If she goes out for the evening, the implication is that she is being selfish by leaving her sick mother alone, but if she stays, the mother could say, "I told you to go have fun." If she does go out, the chances are she will not have much fun. No matter what the daughter does, she just cannot win.

With experience in making observations, nurses become increasingly aware of the verbal and nonverbal communication of the patient/person. Nurses can compare patients' dialogue with their nonverbal communication to gain important clues about the real message. What individuals do either expresses and reinforces or contradicts what they say. As in the saying "Actions speak louder than words," actions often reveal the true meaning of a person's intent, whether it is conscious or unconscious.

EFFECTIVE COMMUNICATION SKILLS FOR NURSES

The art of communication was emphasized by Peplau (1952) to highlight the importance of nursing interventions in facilitating achievement of quality patient care and quality of life. Therefore, as stated, the goal of the nurse in the mental health setting is to provide a place of safety and hope where the patient can feel comfortable and understood. Eventually, the long-term goals are to help the patient:

- Identify and explore problems relating to others.
- Discover healthy ways of meeting emotional needs.
- Experience satisfying interpersonal relationships.

Once specific needs and problems have been identified, the nurse can work with the patient on increasing critical thinking skills, learning new coping behaviors, and experiencing more appropriate and satisfying ways of relating to others. To do this the nurse needs to have a sound knowledge of communication skills. Therefore nurses must become more aware of their own interpersonal methods, eliminating obstructive nontherapeutic techniques and developing additional responses that maximize nurse-patient interactions and increase the use of helpful therapeutic techniques.

Useful tools for nurses when communicating with their patients are (1) silence, (2) active listening, and (3) clarifying techniques.

Use of Silence

When used properly, the use of silence can be an effective tool in encouraging individuals to open up. Silence can frighten interviewers as well as patients (Sommers-Flanagan & Sommers-Flanagan, 2012–2013). In our society, and in nursing, there is an emphasis on action. In communication we tend to expect a high level of verbal activity. Many students and practicing nurses find that when the flow of words stops, they become uncomfortable. **Silence** is not the absence of communication; it is a specific channel for transmitting and receiving messages. The practitioner needs to understand that silence is a significant means of influencing and being influenced by others, and if used judiciously, it can be a powerful listening response.

In the initial interview the patient may be reluctant to speak because the newness of the situation may be overwhelming, the fact that the nurse is a stranger may cause unease, or the patient may feel self-conscious, embarrassed, or shy. Talking is highly individualized; some find the telephone a nuisance, but others talk/text on their cell phones almost constantly (e.g., while driving, shopping, in a restaurant with friends, and, yes, sitting in a classroom or meeting). The nurse must recognize and respect individual differences in styles and tempos of responding. People who are quiet, those who have a language barrier or speech impediment, older adults, and those who lack confidence in their ability to express themselves may communicate a need for support and encouragement through their silence.

Although there is no universal rule concerning how much silence is too much, silence has been said to be worthwhile only as long as it is serving some function and not frightening the person. Knowing when to speak during the interview largely depends on the nurse's perception about what is being conveyed through the silence. Icy silence may be an expression of anger and hostility. Being ignored or given the silent treatment is recognized as an insult and is a particularly hurtful form of communication. Silence among some African American patients may relate to anger, insulted feelings, lack of trust, or acknowledgment of a nurse's lack of cultural sensitivity, for example (Smedley et al., 2002).

Furthermore, when appropriately used, silence may provide meaningful moments of reflection for both participants. It gives each individual an opportunity to contemplate thoughtfully what has been said and felt, weigh alternatives, formulate new ideas, and gain a new perspective on the matter under discussion. If the nurse waits to speak and allows the patient to break the silence, the patient may share thoughts and feelings that would otherwise have been withheld.

Nurses who feel compelled to fill every void with words often do so because of their own anxiety, self-consciousness, and embarrassment. When this occurs, the nurse's need for comfort tends to take priority over the needs of the patient. Or conversely, prolonged and frequent silences by the nurse may hinder an interview that requires verbal articulation. Although the untalkative nurse may be comfortable with silence, this mode of communication may make the patient feel uncomfortable and withhold information. Therefore, the nurse needs to check with the patient from time to time since without feedback patients have no way of knowing whether what they said was understood.

Active Listening

People want more than just physical presence in human communication. Most people want the other person to be there for them psychologically, socially, and emotionally. **Active listening** includes the following:

- Observing the patient's nonverbal behaviors
- Listening to and understanding the patient's verbal message
- Listening to and understanding the person in the context of the social setting of his or her life
- Listening for "false notes" (i.e., inconsistencies or things the patient says that need more clarification)
- Providing the patient with feedback about himself or herself of which the patient might be unaware

Sommers-Flanagan and Sommers-Flanagan (2012–2013) advise students, as well as experienced clinicians, to learn to quiet themselves: "They need to rein in any natural urges to help, meet personal needs, and anxieties" (p. 6). Relaxation techniques may help before an interview with the patient (e.g., closing one's eyes and breathing slowly for a few minutes or using mindfulness training/meditation). This usually results in more concentration on the patient and less distraction by personal worries or personal thoughts of what to say next.

Effective interviewers must become accustomed to silence, but it is just as important for effective interviewers to learn to become active listeners when the patient is talking, as well as when the patient becomes silent. During active listening, nurses carefully note what the patient is saying verbally and nonverbally, as well as monitor their own nonverbal responses. Using silence effectively and learning to listen on a deeper, more significant level—to the patient as well as to your own thoughts and reaction—are both key ingredients in effective communication. Both skills take time to develop but can be learned; you will become more proficient with guidance and practice.

Some principles important to active listening are always relevant, such as the following:

- Everything you hear is modified by the patient's filters.
- Everything you hear is modified by your own filters.
- Therefore, every piece of communication must pass through two filters.
- It is okay to feel confused and uncertain.
- Listen to yourself, too.

Active listening helps strengthen the patient's ability to use critical thinking in order to solve problems. By giving the patient undivided attention, the nurse communicates that the patient is not alone. This kind of intervention enhances self-esteem and encourages the patient to direct energy toward finding ways to deal with problems. Serving as a sounding board, the nurse listens as the patient tests thoughts by voicing them aloud. This form of interpersonal interaction often enables the patient to clarify thinking, link ideas, and tentatively decide what should be done and how best to do it. Active listening is an art that develops with practice over time.

Clarifying Techniques

Understanding depends on clear communication, which is aided by verifying with the patient the nurse's interpretation of the patient's messages. The nurse must request feedback on the accuracy of the message received from verbal as well as nonverbal cues. For example, "I'm not quite sure what you were saying. Did you say you are not going to group tonight?" The use of **clarifying techniques** helps both participants identify major differences in their frame of reference, giving them the opportunity to correct misperceptions before these cause any serious misunderstandings. The patient who is asked to elaborate on or to clarify vague or ambiguous messages needs to know that the purpose is to promote mutual understanding.

Paraphrasing (Reflection of Content)

For clarity, the nurse might use **paraphrasing,** which means restating in different (often fewer) words the basic content of a patient's message. Using simple, precise, and culturally relevant terms, the nurse may readily confirm interpretation of the patient's previous message before the interview proceeds. By prefacing statements with a phrase such as, "I'm not sure I understand" or "In other words, you seem to be saying ...," the nurse helps the patient form a clearer perception of what may be a bewildering mass of details. After paraphrasing, the nurse must validate the accuracy of the restatement and its helpfulness to the discussion. The patient may confirm or deny the perceptions through nonverbal cues or by direct response to a question such as, "Was I correct in saying ...?" As a result, the patient is made aware that the interviewer is actively involved in the search for understanding.

Restating

In **restating,** the nurse mirrors the patient's overt and covert messages; thus this technique may be used to echo feeling as well as content. Restating differs from paraphrasing in that it involves repeating the same key words the patient has just spoken. If a patient remarks, "My life is empty ... it has no meaning," additional information may be gained by restating, "Your life has no meaning?" The purpose of this technique is to explore more thoroughly subjects that may be significant. However, too frequent and indiscriminate use of restating might be interpreted by patients as inattention, disinterest, or worse.

It is easy to overuse this tool so that its application becomes mechanical. Parroting or mimicking what another has said may be perceived as poking fun at the person, so that use of this nondirective approach can become a definite barrier to communication. To avoid overuse of restating, the nurse can combine restatements with direct questions that encourage descriptions: "What does your life lack?" "What kind of meaning is missing?" "Describe one day in your life that appears empty to you."

Reflecting of Feelings

Reflection is a means of assisting people to better understand their own thoughts and feelings. **Reflecting** may take the form of a question or a simple statement that conveys the nurse's observations of the patient when sensitive issues are being discussed. The nurse might then describe briefly to the patient the apparent meaning of the emotional tone of the patient's verbal and nonverbal behavior. For example, to reflect a patient's feelings about his or her life, a good beginning might be, "You sound as if you have had many disappointments."

Sharing observations with a patient shows acceptance. The nurse helps make the patient aware of inner feelings and encourages the patient to own them. For example, the nurse may tell a patient, "You look sad." Perceiving the nurse's concern may allow a patient spontaneously to share feelings. The use of a question in response to the patient's question is another reflective technique (Arnold & Boggs, 2016). For example:

Patient: "Nurse, do you think I really need to be hospitalized?"
Nurse: "What do you think, Jane?"
Patient: "I don't know; that's why I'm asking you."
Nurse: "I'll be willing to share my impression with you at the end of this first session. However, you've probably thought about hospitalization and have some feelings about it. I wonder what they are."

Exploring

A technique that enables the nurse to examine important ideas, experiences, or relationships more fully is **exploring.** For example, if a patient tells the nurse that he does not get along well with his wife, the nurse will want to further explore this area. Possible openers include the following:

- *"Tell me* more about your relationship with your wife."
- *"Describe* your relationship with your wife."
- *"Give me an example* of how you and your wife don't get along."

Asking for an example can greatly clarify a vague or generic statement made by a patient.

Patient: "No one likes me."
Nurse: "Give me an example of one person who doesn't like you."
or
Patient: "Everything I do is wrong."
Nurse: "Give me an example of one thing you do that you think is wrong."

Table 8-2 lists more examples of techniques that enhance communication.

Projective Questions: The *"What if"* Question

Projective questions usually start with a *"what if"* to help people articulate, explore, and identify thoughts and feelings. Projective questions can also help people imagine thoughts, feelings, and behaviors they might have in certain situations (Sommers-Flanagan & Sommers-Flanagan, 2012–2013, p. 5):

- If you had three wishes what would you wish for?
- What if you could go back and change how you acted in (X situation/significant life event); what would you do differently now?
- What would you do if you were given $1 million, no strings attached?

Presupposition Questions: The *"Miracle Question"*

- Suppose you woke up in the morning and a miracle happened and this problem had gone away. What would be different? How would it change your life?

These two questions can reveal a lot about a person and can be used to identify goals that the patient may be motivated to pursue, and often get to the crux of what might be the most important issues in a person's thinking/life.

TABLE 8-2 Techniques that Enhance Communication

Technique	Discussion	Examples
Using silence	Gives the person time to collect thoughts or think through a point.	Encourage a person to talk by waiting for the answers.
Accepting	Indicates that the person has been understood. The statement does not necessarily indicate agreement but is nonjudgmental. However, nurses should not imply that they understand when they do not understand.	"Yes." "Uh-huh." "I follow what you say."
Giving recognition	Indicates awareness of change and personal efforts. Does not imply good or bad, or right or wrong.	"Good morning, Mr. James." "You've combed your hair today." "I notice that you shaved today."
Offering self	Offers presence, interest, and a desire to understand. Is not offered to get the person to talk or behave in a specific way.	"I would like to spend time with you." "I'll stay here and sit with you a while."
Offering general leads	Allows the other person to take direction in the discussion. Indicates that the nurse is interested in what comes next.	"Go on." "And then?" "Tell me about it."
Giving broad openings	Clarifies that the lead is to be taken by the patient. However, the nurse discourages pleasantries and small talk.	"Where would you like to begin?" "What are you thinking about?" "What would you like to discuss?"
Placing the events in time or sequence	Puts events and actions in better perspective. Notes cause-and-effect relationships and identifies patterns of interpersonal difficulties.	"What happened before?" "When did this happen?"
Making observations	Calls attention to the person's behavior (e.g., trembling, nail biting, restless mannerisms). Encourages the person to notice the behavior to describe thoughts and feelings for mutual understanding. Helpful with mute and withdrawn people.	"You appear tense." "I notice you're biting your lips." "You appear nervous whenever John enters the room."
Encouraging description of perception	Increases the nurse's understanding of the patient's perceptions. Talking about feelings and difficulties can lessen the need to act them out inappropriately.	"What do these voices seem to be saying?" "What is happening now?" "Tell me when you feel anxious."
Encouraging comparison	Reveals recurring themes in experiences or interpersonal relationships. Helps the person clarify similarities and differences.	"Has this ever happened before?" "Is this how you felt when...?" "Was it something like...?"
Restating	Repeats the main idea expressed. Gives the patient an idea of what has been communicated. If the message has been misunderstood, the patient can clarify it.	Patient: "I can't sleep. I stay awake all night." Nurse: "You have difficulty sleeping?" Patient: "I don't know ... he always has some excuse for not coming over or keeping our appointments." Nurse: "You think he no longer wants to see you?"
Reflecting	Directs questions, feelings, and ideas back to the patient. Encourages the patient to accept his or her own ideas and feelings. Acknowledges the patient's right to have opinions and make decisions and encourages the patient to think of self as a capable person.	Patient: "What should I do about my husband's affair?" Nurse: "What do you think you should do?" Patient: "My brother spends all of my money and then has the nerve to ask for more." Nurse: "You feel angry when this happens?"
Focusing	Concentrates attention on a single point. It is especially useful when the patient jumps from topic to topic. If a person is experiencing a severe or panic level of anxiety, the nurse should not persist until the anxiety lessens.	"This point you are making about leaving school seems worth looking at more closely." "You've mentioned many things. Let's go back to your thinking of 'ending it all'."
Exploring	Examines certain ideas, experiences, or relationships more fully. If the patient chooses not to elaborate by answering no, the nurse does not probe or pry. In such a case, the nurse respects the patient's wishes.	"Tell me more about that." "Would you describe it more fully?" "Could you talk about how it was that you learned your mom was dying of cancer?"
Giving information	Makes available facts the person needs. Supplies knowledge from which decisions can be made or conclusions drawn. For example, the patient needs to know the role of the nurse; the purpose of the nurse-patient relationship; and the time, place, and duration of the meetings.	"My purpose for being here is..." "This medication is for..." "The test will determine..."
Seeking clarification	Helps patients clarify their own thoughts and maximize mutual understanding between nurse and patient.	"I am not sure I follow you." "What would you say is the main point of what you just said?" "Give an example of a time you thought everyone hated you."
Presenting reality	Indicates what is real. The nurse does not argue or try to convince the patient, just describes personal perceptions or facts in the situation.	"That was Dr. Todd, not a terrorist stalking and trying to harm you." "That was the sound of a car backfiring." "Your mother is not here; I am a nurse."
Voicing doubt	Undermines the patient's beliefs by not reinforcing the exaggerated or false perceptions.	"Isn't that unusual?" "Really?" "That's hard to believe."

Continued

TABLE 8-2	Techniques that Enhance Communication—cont'd	
Technique	**Discussion**	**Examples**
Seeking consensual validation	Clarifies that both the nurse and the patient share mutual understanding of communications. Helps the patient become clearer about what he or she is thinking.	"Tell me whether my understanding agrees with yours."
Verbalizing the implied	Puts into concrete terms what the patient implies, making the patient's communication more explicit.	*Patient:* "I can't talk to you or anyone else. It's a waste of time." *Nurse:* "Do you feel that no one understands?"
Encouraging evaluation	Aids the patient in considering people and events from the perspective of the patient's own set of values.	"How do you feel about…?" "What did it mean to you when he said he couldn't stay?"
Attempting to translate into feelings	Responds to the feelings expressed, not just the content. Often termed *decoding*.	*Patient:* "I am dead inside." *Nurse:* "Are you saying that you feel lifeless? Does life seem meaningless to you?"
Suggesting collaboration	Emphasizes working with the patient, not doing things for the patient. Encourages the view that change is possible through collaboration.	"Perhaps you and I can discover what produces your anxiety." "Perhaps by working together we can come up with some ideas that might improve your communications with your spouse."
Summarizing	Combines the important points of the discussion to enhance understanding. Also allows the opportunity to clarify communications so that both nurse and patient leave the interview with the same ideas in mind.	"Have I got this straight?" "You said that…" "During the past hour, you and I have discussed…"
Encouraging formulation of a plan of action	Allows the patient to identify alternative actions for interpersonal situations the patient finds disturbing (e.g., when anger or anxiety is provoked).	"What could you do to let anger out harmlessly?" "The next time this comes up, what might you do to handle it?" "What are some other ways you can approach your boss?"

Adapted from Hays, J. S., & Larson, K. (1963). *Interacting with patients*. New York: Macmillan. Copyright ©1963 Macmillan Publishing.

NONTHERAPEUTIC TECHNIQUES

Although people may use nontherapeutic techniques in their daily lives, they can become problematic when one is working with patients. Table 8-3 offers samples of nontherapeutic techniques and suggestions for more helpful responses.

Asking Excessive Questions

Excessive questioning, or asking multiple questions at the same time, especially closed-ended questions, casts the nurse in the role of interrogator, raising a demand for information without respect for the patient's willingness or readiness to respond. This approach conveys lack of respect for and sensitivity to the patient's needs. Excessive questioning or asking multiple questions at the same time controls the range and nature of the response and can easily result in a therapeutic stall or terminate an interview. It is a controlling tactic and may reflect the interviewer's lack of security in letting the patient tell his or her own story. It is better to ask more open-ended questions and follow the patient's lead. For example:

> *Excessive questioning:* "Why did you leave your wife? Did you feel angry at her? What did she do to you? Are you going back to her?"
>
> *More therapeutic approach:* "Tell me about the situation between you and your wife."

Although you may end up with a lot of facts about a person, it does not mean you understand an individual or the individual's concerns.

Giving Approval or Disapproval

"You look great in that dress." "I'm proud of the way you controlled your temper at lunch." "That's a great quilt you made." What could be bad about giving someone a pat on the back once in a while? Nothing, if it is done without carrying a judgment (positive or negative) by the nurse. We often give our friends and family approval when they do something well. However, in a nurse-patient situation, **giving approval** often becomes much more complex. A patient may be feeling overwhelmed, experiencing low self-esteem, or feeling unsure of where his or her life is going and consequently feel very needy for recognition, approval, and attention. Yet, when people are feeling vulnerable, a value comment might be misinterpreted. For example:

> *Giving approval:* "You did a great job in group telling John just what you thought about how rudely he treated you."

Implied in this message is that the nurse was pleased by the manner in which the patient talked to John. The patient then sees such a response as a way to please the nurse by doing the right thing. To continue to please the nurse (and get approval), the patient may continue the behavior. The behavior might be useful for the patient; but when a behavior is being done to please another person, it is not coming from the individual's own volition or conviction.

Also when the other person whom the patient needs to please is not present, the motivation for the new behavior might not be there either. Thus the new response really is not a change in behavior as much as a ploy to win approval and acceptance from another person. Giving approval also stops further communication. It is a statement of the observer's (nurse's) judgment about another person's (patient's) behavior. A more useful comment would be the following:

> *More therapeutic approach:* "I noticed that you spoke up to John in group yesterday about his rude behavior. How did it feel to be more assertive?"

This opens the way for finding out if the patient was scared or comfortable, wants to work more on assertiveness, or has other issues to discuss. It also suggests that this was a self-choice the patient made. The patient is given recognition for the change in behavior, and the topic is also opened for further discussion.

Disapproving is moralizing and implies that the nurse has the right to judge the patient's thoughts or feelings. Again, an observation should be made instead.

> *Disapproving:* "You really should not cheat, even if you think everyone else is doing it."
>
> *More therapeutic approach:* "Can you give me two examples of how cheating could negatively affect your goal of graduating?"

TABLE 8-3	Nontherapeutic Communication		
Nontherapeutic Technique	**Examples**	**Discussion**	**More Helpful Response**
Giving premature advice	"Get out of this situation immediately."	Assumes the nurse knows best and the patient cannot think for self. Inhibits problem solving and fosters dependency.	*Encouraging problem solving:* "What are the pros and cons of your situation?" "What were some of the actions you thought you might take?" "What are some of the ways you have thought of to meet your goals?"
Minimizing feelings	*Patient:* "I wish I were dead." *Nurse:* "Everyone gets down in the dumps." "I know what you mean." "You should feel happy you're getting better." "Things get worse before they get better."	Indicates that the nurse is unable to understand or empathize with the patient. The patient's feelings or experiences are being belittled, which can cause the patient to feel small or insignificant.	*Empathizing and exploring:* "You must be feeling very upset. Are you thinking of hurting yourself?"
Falsely reassuring	"I wouldn't worry about that." "Everything will be all right." "You will do just fine; you'll see."	Underrates the patient's feelings and belittles the patient's concerns. May cause the patient to stop sharing feelings if the patient thinks he or she will be ridiculed or not taken seriously.	*Clarifying the patient's message:* "What specifically are you worried about?" "What do you think could go wrong?" "What are you concerned might happen?"
Making value judgments	"How come you still smoke when your wife has lung cancer?"	Prevents problem solving. Can make the patient feel guilty, angry, misunderstood, not supported, or anxious to leave.	*Making observations:* "I notice you are still smoking even though your wife has lung cancer. Is this a problem?"
Asking "why" questions	"Why did you stop taking your medication?"	Implies criticism; often has the effect of making the patient feel defensive.	*Asking open-ended questions; giving a broad opening:* "Tell me some of the reasons that led up to you not taking your medications."
Asking excessive questions	*Nurse:* "How's your appetite? Are you losing weight? Are you eating enough?" *Patient:* "No."	Results in the patient's not knowing which question to answer and possibly being confused about what is being asked.	*Clarifying:* "Tell me about your eating habits since you've been depressed."
Giving approval; agreeing	"I'm proud of you for applying for that job." "I agree with your decision."	Implies that the patient is doing the *right* thing—and that not doing it is wrong. May lead the patient to focus on pleasing the nurse or clinician; denies the patient the opportunity to change his or her mind or decision.	*Making observations:* "I noticed that you applied for that job." "What factors led you to change your mind about applying for that job?" *Asking open-ended questions; giving a broad opening:* "What led to that decision?"
Disapproving; disagreeing	"You really should have shown up for the medication group." "I disagree with that."	Can make a person defensive.	*Exploring:* "What was going through your mind when you decided not to come to your medication group?" "That's one point of view. How did you arrive at that conclusion?"
Changing the subject	*Patient:* "I'd like to die." *Nurse:* "Did you go to Alcoholics Anonymous like we discussed?"	May invalidate the patient's feelings and needs. Can leave the patient feeling alienated and isolated and increase feelings of hopelessness.	*Validating and exploring:* *Patient:* "I'd like to die." *Nurse:* "This sounds serious. Have you thought of harming yourself?"

Adapted from Hays, J. S., & Larson, K. (1963). *Interacting with patients.* New York: Macmillan. Copyright ©1963 Macmillan Publishing.

Advising

Although we ask for and give advice all the time in daily life, **giving advice** to a patient is rarely helpful. Often when we ask for advice, our real motive is to discover if we are thinking along the same lines as someone else or if they would agree with us. When the nurse gives advice to a patient who is having trouble assessing and finding solutions to conflicted areas in his or her life, the nurse is interfering with the patient's ability to make personal decisions. Giving a person a solution robs the patient of self-responsibility. When the nurse offers the patient solutions, the patient eventually begins to think that the nurse does not view the patient as capable of making effective decisions.

People often feel inadequate when they are given no choices over decisions in their lives. Giving advice to patients can foster dependency ("I'll have to ask the nurse what to do about …") and can undermine their sense of competence and adequacy. However, people do need information to make informed decisions. Often the nurse can help the patient define a problem and identify what information might be needed to attain an informed decision. A more useful approach would be, "What do you see as some possible actions you can take?" It is much more constructive to encourage critical thinking by the patient. At times the nurse can suggest several alternatives that a patient might consider (e.g., "Have you ever thought of telling your friend about the incident?"). The patient is then free to say yes or no and make a decision from among the suggestions.

Asking "Why" Questions

"Why did you come late?" "Why didn't you go to the funeral?" "Why didn't you study for the exam?" Very often **"why" questions** imply criticism. We may ask our friends or family such questions, and in the context of a solid relationship the "why?" may be understood more as "what happened?" With people we do not know—especially an anxious person who may be feeling overwhelmed—a "why" question from a person in authority (nurse, physician, teacher) can be experienced as intrusive and judgmental, which serves only to make the person defensive.

It is much more useful to ask *what* is happening rather than *why* it is happening. Questions that focus on who, what, where, and when often elicit important information that can facilitate problem solving and further the communication process.

COMMUNICATING ACROSS CULTURES

Communicating across culture poses many challenges for health care workers. We all need a frame of reference to help us function in our world. The trick is to understand that other people use many other frames of reference to help them function in their worlds. Acknowledging that others view the world quite differently and trying to understand other people's ways of experiencing and living in the world can go a long way toward minimizing our personal distortions in listening. Building acceptance and understanding of those culturally different from ourselves is a skill, too.

Awareness of the cultural meaning of certain verbal and nonverbal communications in initial face-to-face encounters with individuals from cultures different from our own can lead to the formation of a positive therapeutic alliance (or lead to frustration and misunderstanding).

Unrecognized differences between aspects of the cultural identities of patient and nurse can result in assessment and interventions that not only are ineffective, but also can appear disrespectful and/or prejudiced. By the same token, nurses/health care workers should also have a strong understanding and awareness of their own cultural identities and biases. Especially important are nurses' attitudes and beliefs from their own cultural background toward those from ethnically diverse populations and subcultures (e.g., alternate lifestyles, different socioeconomic groups, those with disabilities, different ethnic backgrounds, lifestyle differences, the elderly). Unawareness of personal bias invariably affects communication and relationships. Four areas that may prove problematic for the nurse interpreting specific verbal and nonverbal messages of the patient include the following:

1. Communication styles
2. Use of eye contact
3. Perception of touch
4. Cultural filters

One caveat: It is important to recognize that there are varying degrees of diversity among and within cultural groups.

Communication Styles

People from some ethnic backgrounds may communicate in an intense and highly emotional manner. For example, from the perspective of a non-Hispanic person, Hispanic Americans may appear to use dramatic body language when describing their emotional problems. Such behavior may be perceived as out of control and thus viewed as having a degree of pathology that is not actually present. Within the Hispanic culture, however, intensely emotional styles of communication often are culturally appropriate and are to be expected (Kavanaugh, 2008). French and Italian Americans also show animated facial expressions and expressive hand gestures during communication that can be mistakenly interpreted by others.

Conversely, in other cultures, a calm facade may mask severe distress. For example, in Asian cultures, expression of either positive or negative emotions is a private affair, and open expression of emotions is considered to be in bad taste and possibly to be a weakness. A quiet smile by an Asian American may express joy, an apology, stoicism in the face of difficulty, or even anger (USDHHS, 2001). In general, Asian individuals exercise emotional restraint in communication and interpersonal conflicts are not directly addressed or even allowed (Arnold & Boggs, 2016). German and British Americans also value highly the concept of self-control and may show little facial emotion in the presence of great distress or emotional turmoil.

It is important to understand an ethnic minority in light of the historical context in which it evolved and its relationship to the dominant culture. For example, African Americans, whose historical background in the United States is one of slavery and oppression, are likely to be **aware** of a basic need for survival. As a result of their experiences, many African Americans have become highly selective and guarded in their communication with those outside their cultural group, which may explain the distrust that many African Americans have about the American health care system (Eiser & Ellis, 2007). Therefore, a tendency toward guarded and selective communication among African American patients may represent a healthy cultural adaptation (Smedley et al., 2002; USDHHS, 2001).

Eye Contact

The presence or absence of eye contact should not be used to assess attentiveness, to judge truthfulness, or to make assumptions on the degree of engagement one has with the patient. Culture dictates a person's comfort or lack of comfort with direct eye contact. Some cultures consider direct eye contact disrespectful and improper. For example, Hispanic individuals have traditionally been taught to avoid eye contact with authority figures such as nurses, physicians, and other health care professionals. Avoidance of direct eye contact is seen as a sign of respect to those in authority. To nurses or other health care workers, lack of eye contact may be wrongly interpreted by the interviewer as disinterest in the interview or even as a lack of respect.

Similarly, in Asian cultures respect is shown by avoiding eye contact. For example, in Japan direct eye contact is considered to show lack of respect and to be a personal affront; preference is for shifting or downcast eyes or focus on the speaker's neck. Among many Chinese, gazing around and looking to one side when listening to another is considered polite. However, when speaking to an older adult, direct eye contact is used (Kavanaugh, 2008). Philippine Americans may try to avoid eye contact; however, once it is established, it is important to return and maintain eye contact.

Many Native Americans also believe it is disrespectful or even a sign of aggression to engage in direct eye contact, especially if the speaker is younger. Direct eye contact by members of the dominant culture in the health care system can and does cause discomfort for some patients and is considered a sign of disrespect, while listening is considered a sign of respect and essential to learning about the other individual (Kalbfleisch, 2009; Kavanaugh, 2008).

On the other hand, among German Americans, direct and sustained eye contact indicates that the person listens or trusts, is somewhat aggressive, or, in some situations, is sexually interested. Russians also find direct, sustained eye contact the norm for social interactions (Giger & Davidhizar, 2007). In Haiti, it is customary to hold eye contact with everyone but the poor (Kavanaugh, 2008; USDHHS, 2001). French, British, and many African Americans maintain eye contact during conversation; avoidance of eye contact by another person may be interpreted as being disinterested, not telling the truth, or avoiding the sharing of important information. In some Arab cultures, for a woman to make direct eye contact with a man may imply a sexual interest or even promiscuity. In Greece, staring in public is acceptable (Kavanaugh, 2008).

Touch

The therapeutic use of touch is a basic aspect of the nurse-patient relationship, and touch is normally perceived as a gesture of warmth and friendship. However, in some cultures touch can be perceived as an invasion of privacy or an invitation to intimacy by some patients. The response to touch is often culturally defined. For example, many Hispanic Americans are accustomed to frequent physical contact. Holding the patient's hand in response to a distressing situation or giving the patient a reassuring pat on the shoulder may be experienced as supportive and thus help facilitate openness early in the therapeutic relationship (Kavanaugh, 2008).

When the nurse is working with a Mexican American, for example, often the touch of the nurse is welcome because in the minds of some Mexican Americans, this action can both prevent and treat illness (Giger & Davidhizar, 2007). People of Italian and French backgrounds may also be accustomed to frequent touching during conversation (USDHHS, 2001). In the Soviet Union, touch is often an important part of nonverbal communication used freely with intimate and close friends (Giger & Davidhizar, 2007). However, the degree of comfort conveyed by touch in the nurse-patient relationship depends on the country of origin.

Within the context of an interview, touch might easily be experienced as patronizing, intrusive, aggressive, or sexually inviting. For example, among German, Swedish, and British Americans, touch practices are infrequent, although a handshake may be common at the beginning and end of an interaction. In India, men may shake hands with other men but not with women; an Asian Indian man may greet a woman by nodding and holding the palms of his hands together but not touching the woman. In Japan, handshakes are acceptable; however, a pat on the back is not. Chinese Americans may not like to be touched by strangers. Some Native Americans extend their hand and lightly touch the hand of the person they are greeting rather than shake hands (Kavanaugh, 2008).

Even among people of the same culture, the use of touch has different interpretations and rules when the touch is between individuals of different genders and classes. Students are urged to check the policy manual of their facility because some facilities have a *"no touch"* policy, particularly with adolescents and children who may have experienced inappropriate touch and would not know how to interpret the touch of the health care worker.

Cultural Filters

It is important to recognize that it is impossible to listen to people in an unbiased way. In the process of socialization we develop cultural filters through which we listen to ourselves, others, and the world around us. Cultural filters are a form of cultural bias or cultural prejudice that determines what we notice and what we ignore.

We need these cultural filters to provide structure for ourselves and to help us interpret and interact with the world. However, unavoidably, these cultural filters also introduce various forms of bias into our listening because they are bound to influence our personal,

professional, familial, and sociological values and interpretations. If the cultural filters are strong, the likelihood for bias is increased (Egan, 2013). Bias builds a distorted understanding and a tendency to pigeonhole a person because of such factors as race, sexual orientation, nationality, social status, religious persuasion, or lifestyle (Egan, 2013).

COMMUNICATION THROUGH TECHNOLOGIES

Informatics and information technology are increasingly being adopted for medicine, for behavioral health, and mental health care in the United States. Information communication technologies (ICT) are used as live interactive mechanisms, as a way to track clinical progress and provide access to people who otherwise might not receive good medical or psychosocial help (e.g., those in rural areas and chronically ill, home-bound, and underserved individuals).

It is estimated that about one in four adults could be diagnosed with a mental health issue. Mental health issues range from anxiety, stress, marital issues, and depression to substance abuse, for example. Most of these mental health issues are not addressed because of the fear of stigma, the scarcity of health care providers in remote areas, or problems with transportation (e.g., because of anxiety, physical limitations, or lack of transportation). The consequences of not seeking help can be significant. For example, consequences can range from problems at work to domestic violence, increased depression, and suicide—consequences that can result in a host of other ramifications

The U.S. Department of Defense is particularly interested in implementing and expanding the use of these technologies because a large number of service members screened positive for mental health concerns. These technologies can be used for telepsychiatric appointments ranging from treating posttraumatic stress disorder and depression to providing wellness and resiliency interventions, especially in rural areas (Weckerlein, 2011).

As ICTs advance, it is possible that electronic house calls, Internet support groups, and virtual health examination may well be the wave of the future, eliminating office visits altogether (Arnold & Boggs, 2016). It is a valuable tool for patients as well as practitioners to access current psychiatric and medical breakthroughs, diagnoses, and treatment options (Arnold & Boggs, 2016).

Besides providing better health care for those in rural areas or for those who cannot travel, telehealth may help to relieve the impending nursing shortage. Nursing schools are having a difficult time meeting the nursing shortage because of a decrease in financial resources and retiring faculty. The use of telehealth/tele–home care technologies allows nurses to monitor patients' vital signs, including lung sounds, and identify changes in patients' physiological states. Clinicians can conduct remote physical assessment and consults, which are especially helpful in facilities that have limited nursing resources, including schools, prisons, health clinics, or rural hospitals (Castelli, 2010). Social networking tools are becoming increasingly important ways individuals use to gain information and manage their health care. Health care workers use a variety of technologies to maintain contact with patients (e.g., videoconferencing, email and Skype, etc.).

Mobile Apps

According to Peek (2015):

1. Mobile phones are the most quickly adopted consumer technology in human history. (In the United States, 35% owned a smartphone in 2011, 58% in 2014.)

FACILITATIVE SKILLS CHECKLIST

Instructions: Periodically during your clinical experience, use this checklist to identify areas where growth is needed and progress has been made. Think of your clinical client experiences. Indicate the extent of your agreement with each of the following statements by marking the scale: *SA*, strongly agree; *A*, agree; *NS*, not sure; *D*, disagree; *SD*, strongly disagree.

1. I maintain good eye contact.	SA	A	NS	D	SD
2. Most of my verbal comments follow the lead of the other person.	SA	A	NS	D	SD
3. I encourage others to talk about feelings.	SA	A	NS	D	SD
4. I am able to ask open-ended questions.	SA	A	NS	D	SD
5. I can restate and clarify a person's ideas.	SA	A	NS	D	SD
6. I can summarize in a few words the basic ideas of a long statement made by a person.	SA	A	NS	D	SD
7. I can make statements that reflect the person's feelings.	SA	A	NS	D	SD
8. I can share my feelings relevant to the discussion when appropriate to do so.	SA	A	NS	D	SD
9. I am able to give feedback.	SA	A	NS	D	SD
10. At least 75% or more of my responses help enhance and facilitate communication.	SA	A	NS	D	SD
11. I can assist the person to list some alternatives available.	SA	A	NS	D	SD
12. I can assist the person to identify some goals that are specific and observable.	SA	A	NS	D	SD
13. I can assist the person to specify at least one next step that might be taken toward the goal.	SA	A	NS	D	SD

FIGURE 8-2 Facilitative skills checklist. (Adapted from Myrick, D., & Erney, T. [2000]. *Caring and sharing* [2nd ed., p. 168]. Copyright ©2000 by Educational Media Corp., Minneapolis, Minn.)

2. Psychiatric patients own smartphones at high rates and are interested in using them to monitor their mental health, based on published surveys.
3. There are thousands of apps that target psychiatric conditions, however, there is less clinical research on these apps. For depression and bipolar disorder, one review found less than 15 published studies. There are also concerns for unintended adverse effects in app usage.
4. There is growing interest in using "passive data" information.

SAMHSA (Substance Abuse & Mental Health Services Administration) has resources that can help address some of the toughest mental health and substance use challenges, including suicide prevention, bullying prevention, behavioral health following a disaster, and underage drinking prevention.

- **Suicide Safe** helps health care providers integrate suicide prevention strategies into their practice and address suicide risk among their patients.
- **KnowBullying** provides information and guidance on ways to prevent bullying and build resilience in children. A great tool for parents and educators, KnowBullying is meant for kids ages 3 to 18.
- **SAMHSA Disaster App** provides responders with access to critical resources—like psychological first aid and responder self-care—and SAMHSA's behavioral health treatment services locator to help responders provide support to survivors after a disaster.
- **Talk. They Hear You** is an interactive game that can help parents and caregivers prepare for one of the more important conversations they may ever have with children—underage drinking.

Look up SAMHSA's mobile apps at SAMHSA.gov. Ten more approved mental health apps can be found at www.psychiatryadvisor.com/top-10-mental-health-apps/slideshow/2608/.

As previously mentioned, significant concerns remain unresolved (e.g., potential privacy and confidentiality issues, lack of current clinical data for efficacy, safety of specific mobile apps, and liability issues). Future quality clinical trials and evaluation of risks versus benefits still remain to be undertaken. Other issues include ensuring privacy and safety, reviewing legal policies, and creating professional and ethical guidelines (Peek, 2015).

EVALUATION OF CLINICAL SKILLS

After you have had some introductory clinical experience, you may find the facilitative skills checklist in Figure 8-2 useful for evaluating your progress in developing interviewing skills. Note that some of the items might not be relevant for some of your patients (e.g., numbers 11 through 13 may not be possible when a patient is highly psychotic). Self-evaluation of clinical skills is a way to focus on therapeutic improvement. Role-playing can be a useful tool for preparation for the clinical experience as well as a practice in acquiring more effective and professional communication skills.

KEY POINTS TO REMEMBER

- Knowledge of communication and interviewing techniques is the foundation for development of any patient-centered partnership. Goal-directed professional communication is referred to as therapeutic communication.
- Communication is a complex process. Berlo's communication model has five parts: stimulus, sender, message, medium, and receiver. Feedback is a vital component of the communication process for validating the accuracy of the sender's message.
- Effective/therapeutic communication in nursing points to "increased recovery rates, a sense of safety and protection, improved levels of patient satisfaction, and greater adherence to treatment options" (Neese, 2015). Poor communication skills (non-therapeutic) were responsible for 80% of 440,000 medical deaths in the United States in 2013.
- A number of factors can minimize or enhance the communication process. For example, differences in culture, language, and knowledge levels; noise; lack of privacy; the presence of others; and expectations can all influence communication.
- There are verbal and nonverbal elements in communication; the nonverbal elements often play the larger role in conveying a person's message. Verbal communication consists of all words a person speaks. Nonverbal communication consists of the

behaviors displayed by an individual, in addition to the actual content of speech.

- Communication has two levels: the content level (verbal) and the process level (nonverbal behavior). When content is congruent with process, the communication is said to be healthy. When the verbal message is not reinforced by the communicator's actions, the message is ambiguous; we call this a double-bind (or mixed) message.
- Cultural background (as well as individual differences) has a great deal to do with what nonverbal behavior means to different individuals. The degree of eye contact and the use of touch are two nonverbal aspects that can be misunderstood by individuals of different cultures.
- There are a number of communication techniques that nurses can use to enhance their nursing practices. Many widely used communication enhancers are cited in Table 8-2.
- There are also a number of nontherapeutic techniques that nurses can learn to avoid to enhance their effectiveness with people. Some are cited in Table 8-3 along with suggestions for more helpful responses.
- Most nurses are most effective when they use nonthreatening and open-ended communication techniques.
- Effective communication is a skill that develops over time and is integral to the establishment and maintenance of a therapeutic alliance.
- The application of information communication technologies in the psychosocial sciences is relatively new, but it is viewed as an invaluable tool for helping people with mental health and issues in behavioral health and medicine. It is particularly well suited for individuals in rural areas and for those to whom assessing health care/mental health clinics is not possible either physically or financially. The emergence of apps for those with anxiety, depression, and other mental health issues (e.g., posttraumatic stress disorder, bipolar, etc.) can provide greater accessibility to psychiatric care. The one caveat is that an app should be approved and well accepted within the mental health community

APPLYING CRITICAL JUDGMENT

1. Keep a log for 30 minutes a day of your communication pattern (a tape recorder is ideal). Name four effective techniques that you notice you use frequently. Identify two techniques that are obstructive. In your log, rewrite these nontherapeutic communications and replace them with statements that would better facilitate discussion of thoughts and feelings. Share your log and discuss the changes you are working on with one classmate.
2. Role-play with a classmate at least five nonverbal communications and have your partner identify the message he or she was receiving.
3. Using touch and eye contact, act out how the nurse would use the nonverbal messages in three different cultural groups.
4. When interviewing Tom shortly after his return from Afghanistan, he makes the following statement to you. For each of the following techniques, reply using the technique indicated.

I am so afraid to go to sleep at night since I came back from Afghanistan. The nightmares are so real, I can hear the screams of the wounded, and the visions in my mind are terrifying.	Restating Rephrasing Giving information Reflecting feelings	Your responses using each one of these techniques

5. Answer the following questions as honestly as you can to a good friend/partner (Sommers-Flanagan & Sommers-Flanagan, 2012–2013):
    A. Has there ever been a time in your life when you experienced racism or discrimination? What were your thoughts and feelings related to this experience?
    B. Can you relate a time when your own thoughts about people who are different from you affected how you treated them? Would you do anything differently now?
    C. How would you describe the "American culture"? What part of this culture do you embrace? What parts do you reject? How does your internalization of the "American culture" impact what you think constitutes a "mentally healthy individual"?
6. How would information communication technologies (ICTs) be best used in your community? Specifically, which ICTs would you choose if you were opening a telehealth communication center in your community?

CHAPTER REVIEW QUESTIONS

1. An adult experiencing a recent exacerbation of ulcerative colitis tells the nurse, "I had an accident while I was at the grocery store. It was so embarrassing." Select the nurse's therapeutic response.
    a. "Most grocery stores have public restrooms available."
    b. "Tell me more about how you felt when that happened."
    c. "People usually have compassion about those types of events."
    d. "Your disease is now in remission so that is not likely to happen again."
2. A nurse counsels a widow whose husband died 5 years ago. The widow says, "If I'd done more, he would still be alive." Select the nurse's therapeutic response.
    a. "I understand how you feel after such a terrible loss."
    b. "That was a long time ago. Now it's time to move on with your life."
    c. "You did a very good job of caring for him, especially since he was sick so long."
    d. "Your husband was 82 years old with severe chronic obstructive pulmonary disease."
3. A patient has been out of work 3 weeks with a major illness and anticipates another month of recovery. The patient tells the nurse, "I'm trying to keep up with my work email from home. They hired a new person in my department but the person has no experience." Select the nurse's therapeutic response.
    a. "It sounds like you're saying you are worried about your job security."
    b. "No one expects you to keep pace with your job while you're recovering."
    c. "Your employer is required to hold your job for you while you're on sick leave."
    d. "Don't worry about your job right now. It's more important for you to recover."
4. In which nurse-patient interaction would it be appropriate for the nurse to consider using touch?
    a. Comforting a tearful patient of Japanese heritage
    b. Counseling a child who was physically abused by a parent
    c. Welcoming a person of Hispanic heritage to a new group session
    d. Interacting with a Native American who has a hearing impairment
5. A nurse prepares a patient in a rural community for an initial telehealth visit with the health care provider. Select the nurse's priority action.
    a. Ensure that the patient's rights to privacy are respected.
    b. Ask the patient, "How much do you know about the Internet?"
    c. Inform the patient, "This experience will be like appearing on television."
    d. Advise the patient, "You will be able to hear, but not see, your health care provider."

REFERENCES

American Nurses Association (ANA), American Psychiatric Nurses Association, & International Society of Psychiatric–Mental Health Nurses. (2014). *Psychiatric–mental health nursing: scope and standards of practice.* Washington, DC: Nursebooks.org.

Arnold, E. C., & Boggs, K. U. (2016). *Interpersonal relationships: professional communication skills for nurses* (7th ed.). St. Louis: Elsevier Saunders.

Bateson, G., Jackson, D., & Haley, J. (1956). Toward a theory of schizophrenia. *Behavioral Sciences, 1*(4), 251–264.

Berlo, D. K. (1960). *The process of communication.* San Francisco: Reinhart Press.

Castelli, D. (2010). *Telehealth technologies addressing the global impending nursing shortage.* Retrieved August 31, 2011, from www.nursingcenter.com/CareerCenter/static.asp?pageid=800469.

Egan, G. (2013). *The skilled helper: a problem-management approach and opportunity-development approach to helping* (10th ed.). Belmont, Calif: Brooks/Cole, Cengage Learning.

Eiser, A., & Ellis, G. (2007). Cultural competence and the African-American experience with healthcare: the case for specific content and cross-cultural education. *Academic Medicine, 82,* 176–183.

Giger, J. N., & Davidhizar, R. E. (2007). *Transcultural nursing: assessment and intervention* (5th ed.). St. Louis: Mosby Elsevier.

Hays, P. A. (2008). *Addressing cultural complexities in practice.* Washington, DC: American Psychological Association.

Kalbfleisch, P. (2009). Effective health communication in native populations in North America. *Journal of Language and Social Psychology, 28*(2), 158–173.

Kavanaugh, K. H. (2008). Transcultural perspectives in mental health nursing. In M. Andrews & J. Boyle (Eds.), *Transcultural concepts in nursing care* (5th ed.). Philadelphia: Lippincott Williams & Wilkins.

Matsumoto, D. (1992). American-Japanese cultural differences in name recognition of universal facial expressions. *Journal of Cross Cultural Psychology, 23*(1), 72–84.

Matsumoto, D., & Sung Hwang, H. (2011). *Reading facial expressions of emotion.* Retrieved January 2, 2012, from www.apa.org/science/about/psa/2011/05/facial-expressions.aspx.

Neese, B. (2015). *Effective communication in nursing: theory and best practices.* Retrieved January 2, 2016 from http://online.seu.edu/effective-communication-in-nursing/#sthash.hNHpFiV3.dpuf.

Peek, H. (2015). *Evolving potential of mobile psychiatry: current barriers and future solutions.* Retrieved December 30, 2015, from http://www.psychiatrictimes.com/telepsychiatry/technology-psychiatry-year-review?GUID=67CBCF91-8666-442D-9DDD-0FED4DF8E580&rememberme=1&ts=26122015#sthash.0Yr4YTpt.dpuf.

Peplau, H. E. (1952). *Interpersonal relations in nursing: a conceptual frame of reference for psychodynamic nursing.* New York: Putnam.

Smedley, B., Stith, A., & Nelson, A. (2002). *Unequal treatment: confronting racial and ethnic disparities in healthcare* (Institute of Medicine Report). Washington, DC: National Academies Press.

Sommers-Flanagan, J., & Sommers-Flanagan, R. (2012–2013). *Clinical interviewing* (5th ed.). Hoboken, NJ: Wiley.

U.S. Department of Health and Human Services. (2001). *Mental health: culture, race, and ethnicity: supplement to mental health: a report of the Surgeon General.* Rockville, Md: USDHHS, Substance Abuse and Mental Health Services Administration, Center for Mental Health Services.

Weckerlein, J. (2011). *Technology to aid DoD mental health services.* Retrieved August 28, 2011, from http://science.dodlive.mil/2011/08/05/8089/.

Therapeutic Relationships and the Clinical Interview

Elizabeth M. Varcarolis

ⓔ http://evolve.elsevier.com/Varcarolis/essentials

KEY TERMS AND CONCEPTS

SELECTED CONCEPT: CULTURAL SELF-AWARENESS

"Whether two people can understand each other depends not so much on racial or cultural backgrounds, but how strongly each of them believed in their correctness and/or even the superiority of what is personally familiar."

"To the extent that individuals are aware of their culture, they tend to believe in the innate superiority or rightness of their racial–ethnic–culture perspective".

"Truly understanding someone from another culture begins with acceptance of differences as normal, interesting, and even desirable aspects of being human."

(Sommers-Flanagan & Sommers-Flanagan, 2012–2013, p. 35)

OBJECTIVES

1. Compare and contrast the three phases of the nurse-patient relationship.
2. Compare and contrast a social relationship and a therapeutic relationship regarding purpose, focus, communication styles, and goals.
3. Identify at least four patient behaviors a nurse may encounter in the clinical setting.
4. Explore aspects that foster a therapeutic nurse-patient relationship and those that are inherent in a nontherapeutic nursing interactive process.
5. Define and discuss the role of empathy, genuineness, and positive regard on the part of the nurse in a nurse-patient relationship.
6. Role-play with a classmate or group two attitudes and four actions that may reflect the nurse's positive regard for a patient.
7. Analyze what is meant by boundaries and the influence of transference and countertransference on boundary blurring.
8. Act out the use of attending behaviors (eye contact, body language, vocal qualities, and verbal tracking) with a classmate or friend.
9. Discuss the influences of different values and cultural beliefs on the therapeutic relationship.

INTRODUCTION

Psychiatric mental health nursing is based on principles of *science*. A background in anatomy, physiology, and chemistry is the basis for the safe and effective provision of biological treatments. For example, it is assumed the nurse has knowledge of the effects of medications, the indications for use, and the adverse effects based on best-evidence studies and trials. However, it is the caring relationship and the development of the skills needed to enhance and maintain these relationships that include aspects of the *art* of psychiatric nursing. Quinlan (1996) states that "the development of that very human relationship allows a place for caring and healing to occur. This use of the essential humanness of the nurse as a person (use of self) is the most critical part of the way nurses make themselves available to both patients and colleagues" (p. 7). Quinlan goes on to say that how this is achieved remains within the domain of the individual nurse.

NURSE-PATIENT PARTNERSHIP/RELATIONSHIP

The term and concept of the physician-patient relationship/patient-centered care has somewhat more recently been adopted by the medical community and one often sees the phrase "doctor-patient" partnership. Nurses have been using the concept of *nurse-patient relationship* and *patient-centered care* since Hildegard Peplau introduced this concept into nursing. A newer way to look at the relationship between health care provider and patient in light of the recovery model might be *patient-centered partnership*.

The core concepts of patient- and family-centered care consist of (1) dignity and respect, (2) information sharing, (3) patient and family participation, and (4) and the feeling of being heard and understood by patients. These tenants have long been subsumed in the nursing profession as what is known as the nurse-patient relationship, or more recently referred to as the "nurse-patient partnership." A patient-centered partnership implies a patient's allowance for control over his or her health care decisions, hence the term "collaborative patient-centered treatment planning." For our purposes here, the term nurse-patient relationship/partnership implies collaboration with the patient and family regarding health care goals, plans to meet those goals, and appropriate interventions within the framework of the patient's/family's cultural, ethnic, and comfort levels.

The therapeutic nurse-patient relationship/partnership is the basis of all psychiatric nursing treatment approaches regardless of the specific aim. The very first connections between nurse and patient are to establish an understanding that the nurse is safe, reliable, and consistent, and will keep the individuals information private. The relationship/partnership is conducted within appropriate and clear boundaries.

It is true that many disorders, such as schizophrenia and major affective disorders, have strong biochemical and genetic components. However, many accompanying emotional problems such as poor self-image, low self-esteem, and difficulties with adherence to treatment regimen can be significantly improved through a therapeutic patient-centered alliance. All too often individuals who enter treatment have taxed or exhausted their familial and social resources and have found themselves in a position of isolation from people who will listen for more than a few minutes.

The nurse-patient relationship is a creative process and unique to each nurse. Each person brings his or her own uniqueness to this relationship. Each of us has unique gifts that we can learn to use creatively to form positive bonds with others. Historically this has been referred to as the "therapeutic use of self." Therapeutic use of self is an example of the practice of the "art of nursing." *Important to remember,* the efficacy of this therapeutic use of self has been scientifically substantiated as an evidence-based intervention. A positive therapeutic alliance that is collaborative and respectful is one of the best predictors of positive outcomes in therapy (Gordon & Beresin, 2016). On the other hand, nonadherence with treatment and poor outcomes in therapy are related to a patient feeling unheard, disrespected, or otherwise unconnected with the clinician/health care worker (Gordon & Beresin, 2016). Research suggests that therapeutic success is a result of the personal characteristics of the clinician and the patient, not necessarily a result of the particular process employed. Furthermore, there is evidence that psychotherapy (talk therapy) and a therapeutic alliance actually change brain chemistry in much the same way as medication, thus resulting in the adage that the best treatment for most psychiatric problems (less so with psychotic disorders) is a combination of medication and psychotherapy. Cognitive behavioral therapy, in particular, has met with great success in the treatment of depression, phobias, obsessive-compulsive disorders, posttraumatic stress disorder (PTSD), and others.

Establishing a therapeutic alliance or partnership with an individual takes time. Skills in this area gradually improve with guidance from those with more skill and experience. When patients do not engage in a therapeutic alliance, chances are that no matter what plans of care or planned interventions are made, nothing significant will happen except mutual frustration and mutual withdrawal.

Therapeutic versus Other Types of Relationships

The nurse-patient relationship is often loosely defined, but a therapeutic relationship incorporating principles of mental health nursing is more clearly defined and differs from other relationships. A therapeutic nurse-patient relationship has specific goals and functions. Goals in a therapeutic relationship include the following:

- **Facilitating** communication of distressing thoughts and feelings
- **Assisting** patients with problem solving to help facilitate activities of daily living
- **Helping** patients examine self-defeating behaviors and test alternatives
- **Promoting** self-care and independence

A relationship is an interpersonal process that involves two or more people. Throughout life we meet people in a variety of settings and share a variety of experiences. With some individuals we develop long-term relationships; with others the relationship lasts only a short time. Naturally the kinds of relationships we enter vary from person to person and from situation to situation. Generally, relationships can be defined as (1) social or (2) therapeutic.

Social Relationships versus Therapeutic Relationships

A social relationship can be defined as a relationship that is primarily initiated for the purpose of friendship, socialization, enjoyment, or accomplishment of a task. Mutual needs are met during social interaction (e.g., participants share ideas, feelings, and experiences). Communication skills used in social relationships may include giving advice and (sometimes) meeting basic dependency needs, such as lending money and helping with jobs. Often the content of the communication remains superficial. During social interactions, roles may shift. Within a social relationship there is little emphasis on the evaluation of the interaction:

Patient: "Oh, gosh, I just hate to be alone. It is getting me down and sometimes it hurts so much."

Nurse: "I know just how you feel. I don't like it either. What I do is get a friend and go to a movie or something. Do you have someone to hang with?" *(In this response the nurse is minimizing the patient's feelings and giving advice prematurely.)*

Patient: "No, not really, but often I don't even feel like going out. I just sit at home feeling scared and lonely."

Nurse: "Most of us feel like that at one time or another. Maybe if you took a class or joined a group you could meet more people. I know of some great groups you could join. It's not good to be stuck in by yourself all of the time." *(Again, the nurse is not "hearing" the patient's distress, and in so doing, is minimizing again her pain and isolation. The nurse goes on to give the patient banal advice, thus closing off the patient's feelings and experience.)*

Therapeutic Relationships

The therapeutic relationship (patient-centered partnership) between nurse and patient differs from both a social and an intimate relationship in that the nurse maximizes his or her communication skills, understanding of human behavior, and personal strengths to enhance the patient's growth. Patients more easily engage in the relationship when the clinician's interactions address their concerns, respect the patient as a partner in decision making, and use language that is straightforward (Gordon & Beresin, 2016). That suggests the focus of the relationship needs to be on the patient's ideas, experiences, and feelings. Inherent in a therapeutic relationship is the nurse's focus on significant personal issues introduced by the patient during the clinical interview. The nurse and the patient identify areas that need exploration and periodically evaluate the degree of change in the patient.

Although the nurse may assume a variety of roles (e.g., teacher, counselor, socializing agent, liaison), **the relationship is consistently focused on the patient's problem and needs.** Nurses must meet their own needs outside of the therapeutic relationship. When nurses begin to want the patient to "like them," "do as they suggest," "be nice to them," or "give them recognition," the needs of the patient cannot be adequately met, and the interaction could be detrimental (nontherapeutic) to the patient.

Working under supervision is an excellent way to keep the focus and boundaries clear. Communication skills and knowledge of the stages of and phenomena occurring in a therapeutic relationship are crucial tools in the formation and maintenance of that relationship. Within the context of a helping relationship, the following occur:

- The needs of the patient are identified and explored.
- Alternate problem-solving approaches are taken.
- New coping skills may develop.
- Behavioral change is encouraged.

Staff nurses as well as students may struggle with the boundaries between social and therapeutic relationships. There is a fine line. In fact, students often feel more comfortable "being a friend" because it is a more familiar role, especially with people close to their own age. However, when this occurs, the nurse or student needs to make it clear (to themselves and the patient) that the relationship is a therapeutic one. This does *not* mean that the nurse is not friendly toward the patient, and it does *not* mean that talking about innocuous topics (e.g., television, weather, children's pictures) is forbidden. It does mean, however, that the nurse follows the prior stated guidelines regarding a therapeutic relationship; essentially, the focus is on the patient, and the relationship is not designed to meet the nurse's needs. The patient's problems and concerns are explored, potential solutions are discussed by both patient and nurse, and solutions are implemented by the patient:

Patient: "Oh, gosh, I just hate to be alone. It is getting me down and sometimes it hurts so much."

Nurse: "Loneliness can be painful. What is going on now that you are feeling so alone?"

Patient: "Well, my mom died 2 years ago, and last month, my—oh, I am so scared." *(Patient takes a deep breath, looks down, and looks like she might cry.)*

Nurse: (Sits in silence while the patient recovers.) "Go on …"

Patient: "My boyfriend left for an overseas assignment. I haven't heard from him, and I can't get any answers from his boss. He was my best friend and we were going to get married, and if something happens to him I don't want to live."

Nurse: "Have you thought of killing yourself?"

Patient: "Well, if he dies I will. I can't live without him."

Nurse: "Have you ever felt like this before?"

Patient: Yes, when my mom died. I was depressed for about a year until I met my boyfriend."

Nurse: "It sounds like you are going through a very painful and scary time. Perhaps you and I can talk some more and come up with some ways for you to feel less anxious, scared, and overwhelmed. Would you be willing to work on this together?"

The ability of the nurse to engage in interpersonal interactions in a goal-directed manner for the purpose of assisting this young woman with her emotional and, if needed, physical health needs is the foundation of patient-centered care. The nurse-patient relationship is synonymous with a professional helping relationship. Behaviors that have relevance to health care workers, including nurses, are as follows:

- **Accountability:** Nurses assume responsibility for their conduct and the consequences of their actions.
- **Focus on patient needs:** The interest of the patient rather than the nurse, other health care workers, or the institution is given first consideration. The nurse's role is that of patient advocate.
- **Clinical competence:** The criteria on which the nurse bases his or her conduct are principles of knowledge and those that are

appropriate to the specific situation. This involves awareness and incorporation of the latest knowledge made available from research (evidence-based practice).

- **Delaying judgment:** Ideally, nurses refrain from judging patients and avoid transferring their own values and beliefs to others.
- **Supervision** by a more experienced clinician or team is essential to developing one's competence in this area.

Nurses interact with patients in a variety of settings, such as emergency departments, medical-surgical units, obstetric and pediatric units, clinics, community settings, schools, and patients' homes. Nurses who are sensitive to patients' needs and have effective assessment and communication skills can significantly help patients confront current problems and anticipate future choices.

The type of relationship that occurs may be informal and not extensive, such as when the nurse and patient meet for only a few sessions. However, even though it is brief, the relationship may be substantial, useful, and important for the patient. This limited relationship is often referred to as a therapeutic encounter. When the nurse shows true concern for another's circumstances (has positive regard, empathy), even a short encounter with the individual can have a powerful effect on that individual's life.

At other times, the encounters may be longer and more formal, such as in inpatient settings, mental health units, crisis centers, and mental health outpatient facilities, as well as in private practice. This longer time span allows greater development of an effective therapeutic nurse-patient relationship.

Establishing Relationship Boundaries

A well-defined therapeutic relationship allows for the establishment of clear patient boundaries that provide a safe space through which the patient can explore feelings and treatment issues. The nurse's role in the therapeutic relationship is theoretically rather well defined. The patient's needs are separated from the nurse's needs, and the patient's role is different from that of the nurse. Therefore the boundaries of the relationship seem to be well stated. In reality, boundaries are at risk of blurring, and a shift in the nurse-patient partnership may lead to nontherapeutic dynamics. Examples of circumstances that can produce blurring of boundaries include the following:

- When the relationship slips into a social context
- When the nurse's needs are met at the expense of the patient's needs

The following are some warning signals that indicate a nurse may be blurring boundaries.

- **Overhelping:** Doing for patients what they are able to do themselves or going beyond the wishes or needs of patients
- **Controlling:** Asserting authority and assuming control of patients "for their own good"
- Narcissism: Having to find weakness, helplessness, and/or disease in patients to feel helpful, at the expense of recognizing and supporting patients' healthier, stronger, and more competent features

When situations such as these arise, the relationship has ceased to be a helpful one and the phenomenon of control becomes an issue. Role blurring is often a result of unrecognized transference or countertransference.

Transference

Transference is a phenomenon originally identified by Sigmund Freud when he used psychoanalysis to treat patients. **Transference is the process whereby a person unconsciously and inappropriately displaces (transfers) onto individuals in his or her current life those patterns**

of behavior and emotional reactions that originated in relation to significant figures in childhood. The patient may even say, "You remind me of my _____" (e.g., mother, sister, father, brother). See the following example:

> *Patient:* "Oh, you are so high and mighty. Did anyone ever tell you that you are a cold, unfeeling machine, just like others I know?"
>
> *Nurse:* "Tell me about one person who is cold and unfeeling toward you." (*In this example, the patient is experiencing the nurse in the same way she did with significant other[s] during her formative years. It turns out that the patient's mother was very aloof, leaving her with feelings of isolation, worthlessness, and anger.*)

Although the transference phenomenon occurs in all relationships, transference seems to be intensified in relationships of authority. Because the process of transference is accelerated toward a person in authority, physicians, nurses, and social workers are all potential objects of transference. It is important to realize that the patient may experience thoughts, feelings, and reactions toward a health care worker that are realistic and appropriate; these are *not* transference phenomena.

Common forms of transference include the desire for affection or respect and the gratification of dependency needs. The transferential feelings the patient might experience are hostility, jealousy, competitiveness, and love. Requests for special favors (e.g., cigarettes, water, extra time in the session) are concrete examples of transference phenomena.

Countertransference

Countertransference **refers to the tendency of the nurse to displace onto the patient feelings related to people in his or her past.** Frequently, the patient's transference to the nurse evokes countertransference feelings in the nurse. For example, it is normal to feel angry when persistently attacked, annoyed when unreasonably frustrated, or flattered when idealized. A nurse might feel extremely important when depended on exclusively by a patient. If the nurse does not recognize his or her own omnipotent feelings as countertransference, encouragement of independent growth in the patient can be minimized at best. Recognizing our countertransference reactions maximizes our ability to *empower* our patients. When we fail to recognize our countertransferences toward our patients, the therapeutic relationship stalls, and essentially we *disempower* our patients by experiencing them not as individuals but rather as inner projections. See the following examples:

> *Patient:* "Yeah, well I decided not to go to that dumb group. 'Hi, I'm so and so, and I'm an alcoholic.' Who cares?" (*Patient sits slumped in a chair chewing gum, nonchalantly looking around.*)
>
> *Nurse:* (*in a very impassioned tone*) "You always sabotage your chances. You need AA to get in control of your life. Last week you were going to go and now you have disappointed everyone." (*Here the nurse is reminded of her mother who was an alcoholic. The nurse had tried everything to get her mother into treatment and took it as a personal failure and deep disappointment that her mother never sought recovery. After the nurse sorts out her thoughts and feelings, she realizes the frustration and feelings of disappointment and failure come from feelings toward her mother and not the patient. The nurse starts out the next session with the following approach.*)
>
> *Nurse:* "Look, I was thinking about last week and I realize the decision to go to AA or find other help is solely up to you. It is true that I would like you to live a fuller and more satisfying life, but it is your decision. I am wondering, however, what happened to change your mind to not go to AA."

If the nurse feels either a strongly positive or a strongly negative reaction to a patient, the feeling most often signals countertransference

in the nurse. One common sign of countertransference in the nurse is overidentification with the patient. In this situation the nurse may have difficulty recognizing or understanding problems the patient has that are similar to the nurse's own. For example, a nurse who is struggling with an alcoholic family member may feel disinterested, cold, or disgusted toward an alcoholic patient. Other indications of countertransference occur when the nurse becomes involved in power struggles, competition, or arguments with the patient.

Identifying and working through various transference and countertransference issues is crucial if the nurse is to achieve professional and clinical growth and allow for positive change in the patient. These issues are best handled through the use of supervision by either the peer group or the therapeutic team. Regularly scheduled supervision sessions provide the nurse with the opportunity to increase self-awareness, clinical skills, and growth, as well as allow for continued growth of the patient.

Values, Beliefs, and Self-Awareness

Relationships are complex. We bring into our relationships a multitude of thoughts, feelings, beliefs, and attitudes (cultural filters)—some rational and some irrational. We form these from families or cultures, our spiritual beliefs and experiences, and our "heroes." From those we form our values. Values are abstract standards and represent an ideal, either positive or negative. Our values are usually culturally oriented and influenced in a variety of ways through our parents, teachers, religious institutions, workplaces, peers, and political leaders, as well as through films and the media. All these influences attempt to instill their values and to form and influence our values.

Modeling is perhaps one of the most potent means of value education because it presents a vivid example of values in action. We all need role models to guide us in negotiating life's many choices. Young people in particular are hungry for role models and will find them among peers as well as adults. As nurses, parents, bosses, coworkers, friends, lovers, teachers, spouses, and singles, we are constantly (in either a positive or a negative manner) being a role model to others.

Our culture—and more precisely our subculture—defines the guidelines that provide structure to our lives. It is through this that our beliefs, thoughts, behaviors, and feelings are interpreted (Sommers-Flanagan & Sommers-Flanagan, 2012–2013). Our cultural values and beliefs provide meaning to our lives and our environment in the form of an operating system or interpretive system. How we view the world and how we are supposed to behave, think, believe, and live are influenced by this interpretive system.

Most often problems arise when the interpretive system of the clinician and that of the individual seeking guidance are glaringly different. When the nurse is working with an individual from a culturally distinct environment, the interpretive system between them might be so different at times that it is difficult for the patient and the clinician to connect in a clinically meaningful way (Hays, 2008). According to Sommers-Flanagan and Sommers-Flanagan (2012–2013), "Developing cultural self-awareness begins with acceptance of differences as normal, interesting, and even desirable aspects of being human."

It is helpful, even crucial, for us to have an understanding of our *own* values and attitudes so that we may become aware of personal beliefs or attitudes that may interfere with the establishment of a working relationship.

When working with patients, it is important for nurses to understand that our values and beliefs are not necessarily the right ones—and certainly are not right for everyone. It is helpful to realize that our values and beliefs (1) reflect our own culture/subculture, (2) are derived from a range of choices, and (3) are those we have chosen for ourselves from a variety of influences and role models. These chosen values (religious, cultural, societal) guide us in making decisions and taking actions that we hope will make our lives meaningful, rewarding, and fulfilled.

Interviewing and even working with others whose values, beliefs, cultures, or lifestyles are radically different from our own can be a challenge. Several topics that cause controversy in society in general—including religion, gender roles, abortion, war, politics, money, drugs, alcohol, sex/sexual orientation, and corporal punishment—also can cause conflict between clinicians/nurses and their patients (Fontes, 2008). Although we emphasize that the patient and the nurse should identify outcomes together, what happens when the nurse's values, beliefs, and interpretive system are very different from the patient's? Consider the following possible conflicts:

- The patient wants an abortion, which is against the nurse's values.
- The nurse believes the patient who was raped and became pregnant should get an abortion, but the patient refuses.
- The patient engages in unsafe sex with multiple partners, which is against the nurse's concern for safety and values.
- The nurse cannot understand a patient who refuses medications on religious grounds.
- The patient puts material gain and objects far ahead of loyalty to friends and family, in direct contrast to the nurse's values.
- The patient is deeply religious, whereas the nurse has difficulty with organized religion related to an experience with a religious cult.
- The patient's lifestyle includes taking illicit drugs, which is against the nurse's values.

How can nurses develop working relationships and help patients solve problems when patients' values, goals, and interpretive systems are so different from their own? Self-awareness requires that we understand what we value and those beliefs that guide our behaviors. It is critical that as nurses we not only understand and accept our own values and beliefs but also are sensitive to and accepting of the unique and different values and beliefs of others. This is another area in which supervision by an experienced colleague can prove invaluable.

Personal values may change over time; indeed, they may change many times over the course of a lifetime. The values you held as a child are different from those you held as an adolescent and so forth.

Self-Check on Boundary Issues

It is helpful for all of us to take time out to be reflective and to try to be aware of our thoughts and actions with patients, as well as with colleagues, friends, and family. Figure 9-1 is a helpful self-test you can use throughout your career, no matter what area of nursing you choose.

Phases of the Nurse-Patient Relationship

Hildegard Peplau introduced the concept of the nurse-patient relationship in 1952 in her ground-breaking book *Interpersonal Relations in Nursing*. This model of the nurse-patient relationship

---

NURSING BOUNDARY INDEX SELF-CHECK

Please rate yourself according to the frequency with which the following statements reflect your behavior, thoughts, or feelings within the past 2 years while providing patient care.*

1. Have you ever received any feedback about your behavior being overly intrusive with patients and their families?	Never ___	Rarely ___	Sometimes ___	Often ___
2. Do you ever have difficulty setting limits with patients?	Never ___	Rarely ___	Sometimes ___	Often ___
3. Do you ever arrive early or stay late to be with your patient for a longer period?	Never ___	Rarely ___	Sometimes ___	Often ___
4. Do you ever find yourself relating to patients or peers as you might to a family member?	Never ___	Rarely ___	Sometimes ___	Often ___
5. Have you ever acted on sexual feelings you have for a patient?	Never ___	Rarely ___	Sometimes ___	Often ___
6. Do you feel that you are the only one who understands the patient?	Never ___	Rarely ___	Sometimes ___	Often ___
7. Have you ever received feedback that you get "too involved" with patients or families?	Never ___	Rarely ___	Sometimes ___	Often ___
8. Do you derive conscious satisfaction from patients' praise, appreciation, or affection?	Never ___	Rarely ___	Sometimes ___	Often ___
9. Do you ever feel that other staff members are too critical of "your" patient?	Never ___	Rarely ___	Sometimes ___	Often ___
10. Do you ever feel that other staff members are jealous of your relationship with your patient?	Never ___	Rarely ___	Sometimes ___	Often ___
11. Have you ever tried to "match-make" a patient with one of your friends?	Never ___	Rarely ___	Sometimes ___	Often ___
12. Do you find it difficult to handle patients' unreasonable requests for assistance, verbal abuse, or sexual language?	Never ___	Rarely ___	Sometimes ___	Often ___

* Any item that is responded to with "Sometimes" or "Often" should alert the nurse to a possible area of vulnerability. If the item is responded to with "Rarely," the nurse should determine whether it is an isolated event or a possible pattern of behavior.

FIGURE 9-1 Nursing boundary index self-check. (From Pilette, P. C., Berck, C. B., & Achber, L. C. [1995]. Therapeutic management of helping boundaries. *Journal of Psychosocial Nursing and Mental Health Services, 33*[1], 45.)

(patient-centered relationship) is well accepted in the United States and Canada and has become an important tool for all nursing practice. Peplau (1952) proposed that the nurse-patient relationship "facilitates forward movement" for both the nurse and the patient (p. 12). Peplau's interactive nurse-patient process is designed to facilitate the patient's boundary management, independent problem solving, and decision making that promotes autonomy (Haber, 2000).

It is most likely that in the brief period you have for your psychiatric nursing rotation, the phases of the nurse-patient relationship will not have time to develop. However, it is important for you to be aware of these phases because you must be able to recognize and use them later if you will be spending long periods with a specific patient/individual. It is also important to remember that any contact that is caring and respectful and demonstrates concern for the situation of another person can have an enormous positive impact.

Peplau (1952, 1999) described the nurse-patient relationship as evolving through interlocking, overlapping phases. The distinctive phases of the nurse-patient relationship are generally recognized as follows:

- Orientation phase
- Working phase
- Termination phase

Although various phenomena and goals are identified for each phase, they often overlap. Even before the first meeting, the nurse may have many thoughts and feelings related to the first clinical session. This is sometimes referred to as the *preorientation phase*.

Preorientation Phase

Novice health care professionals usually have many concerns and experience a mild to moderate degree of anxiety on their first clinical day. Commonly, nursing instructors will encourage students to identify concerns about working with psychiatric patients in preconference on the first clinical day. These concerns focus on being afraid of people with psychiatric problems, saying "the wrong thing," and being unaware of the proper responses to certain patient behaviors. There really are no magic words. Talking with the instructor and supervised peer group discussion will add confidence, feedback, and suggestions. Chapter 8 discusses the use of communication strategies in clinical practice.

Often, students new to the mental health setting are concerned about being in situations that they may not know how to handle. These concerns are universal and often arise in the clinical setting. Table 9-1 identifies common patient behaviors (e.g., crying, asking the nurse to keep a secret, threatening to commit suicide, giving a gift) and gives examples of an appropriate response, the rationale for the response, and a possible verbal statement. The exact words depend on the situation, but understanding the rationale will aid you in applying the information in future interactions.

Most experienced psychiatric nursing faculty and staff monitor the unit atmosphere and have a sixth sense as it pertains to behaviors that

TABLE 9-1   Common Patient Behaviors and Nurse Responses

Possible Reactions by Nurse	Useful Responses by Nurse
What to Do if the Patient Says He or She Wants to Kill Himself or Herself	
The nurse may feel overwhelmed or responsible for "talking the patient out of it." The nurse may pick up some of the patient's feelings of hopelessness.	The nurse assesses whether the patient has a plan and the lethality of the plan. The nurse tells the patient that this is serious, that the nurse does not want harm to come to the patient, and that this information needs to be shared with other staff. "This is very serious, Mr. Lamb. I do not want any harm to come to you. I will have to share this with the other staff." The nurse can then discuss with the patient the feelings and circumstances that led up to this decision. (Refer to Chapter 23 for strategies in suicide intervention.)
What to Do if the Patient Asks the Nurse to Keep a Secret	
The nurse may feel conflict because the nurse wants the patient to share important information but is unsure about making such a promise.	The nurse *cannot* make such a promise. The information may be important to the health or safety of the patient or others. "I cannot make that promise. It might be important for me to share it with other staff." The patient then decides whether to share the information.
What to Do if the Patient Asks the Nurse a Personal Question	
The nurse may think that it is rude not to answer the patient's question. A new nurse might feel relieved to delay the start of the interview. The nurse may feel uneasy and want to leave the situation. New nurses are often manipulated by a patient into changing roles. This keeps the focus off the patient and prevents the creation of a relationship.	The nurse may or may not answer the patient's query. If the nurse decides to answer a natural question, he or she answers in a word or two, then refocuses back on the patient. *Patient:* Are you married? *Nurse:* Yes. Do you have a spouse? *Patient:* Do you have any children? *Nurse:* This time is for you—tell me about yourself. *Patient:* You can just tell me if you have any children. *Nurse:* This is your time to focus on your concerns. Tell me something about your family.
What to Do if the Patient Makes Sexual Advances	
The nurse feels uncomfortable but may feel conflicted about "rejecting" the patient or making him or her feel "unattractive" or "not good enough."	The nurse needs to set clear limits on expected behavior. "I am not comfortable having you touch (kiss) me. This time is for you to focus on your problems and concerns." Frequently restating the nurse's role throughout the relationship can help maintain boundaries. If the patient does not stop the inappropriate behavior, the nurse might say, "If you can't stop this behavior, I'll have to leave. I'll be back at [time] to spend time with you then." Leaving gives the patient time to gain control. The nurse returns at the stated time.

TABLE 9-1   Common Patient Behaviors and Nurse Responses—cont'd

Possible Reactions by Nurse	Useful Responses by Nurse
What to Do if the Patient Cries	
The nurse may feel uncomfortable and experience increased anxiety or feel somehow responsible for making the person cry.	The nurse should stay with the patient and reinforce that it is all right to cry. Often it is at that time that feelings are closest to the surface and can be best identified. "You seem ready to cry." "You are still upset about your brother's death." "What are you thinking right now?" The nurse offers tissues when appropriate.
What to Do if the Patient Leaves Before the Session Is Over	
The nurse may feel rejected, thinking it was something that he or she did. The nurse may experience increased anxiety or feel abandoned by the patient.	Some patients are not able to relate for long periods without experiencing an increase in anxiety. On the other hand, the patient may be testing the nurse. "I will wait for you here for 15 minutes, until our time is up." During this time, the nurse does not engage in conversation with any other patient or even with the staff. When the time is up, the nurse approaches the patient, says the time is up, and restates the day and time the nurse will see the patient again.
What to Do if the Patient Says He or She Does Not Want to Talk	
The nurse new to this situation may feel rejected or ineffectual.	At first, the nurse might say something to this effect: "It's all right. I would like to spend time with you. We don't have to talk." The nurse might spend short, frequent periods (e.g., 5 minutes) with the patient throughout the day. "Our 5 minutes is up. I'll be back at 10 AM and stay with you 5 more minutes." This gives the patient the opportunity to understand that the nurse means what he or she says and is back on time consistently. It also gives the patient time between visits to assess how he or she feels and what he or she thinks about the nurse, and perhaps to feel less threatened.
What to Do if the Patient Gives the Nurse a Present	
The nurse may feel uncomfortable when offered a gift. The meaning needs to be examined. Is the gift (1) a way of getting better care, (2) a way to maintain self-esteem, (3) a way of making the nurse feel guilty, (4) a sincere expression of thanks, or (5) a cultural expectation?	Possible guidelines: If the gift is expensive, the only policy is to graciously refuse. If it is inexpensive, then (1) if it is given at the end of hospitalization when a relationship has developed, graciously accept; (2) if it is given at the beginning of the relationship, graciously refuse and explore the meaning behind the present. "Thank you, but it is our job to care for our patients. Are you concerned that some aspect of your care will be overlooked?" If the gift is money, it is always graciously refused.
What to Do if Another Patient Interrupts During Time with Your Selected Patient	
The nurse may feel a conflict. The nurse does not want to appear rude. Sometimes the nurse tries to engage both patients in conversation.	The time the nurse had contracted with a selected patient is that patient's time. By keeping his or her part of the contract, the nurse demonstrates that he or she means what is said and views the sessions as important. "I am with Mr. Rob for the next 20 minutes. At 10 AM, after our time is up, I can talk to you for 5 minutes."

indicate escalating tension. They are trained in crisis interventions, and formal security is often available onsite to give the staff support. Your instructor will set the ground rules for safety during the first clinical day. For example, do not enter a patient's room alone, know if there are any patients who should not be engaged, stay in open areas that have other health care personnel, and recognize the signs and symptoms of escalating anxiety. There are certain rules of thumb regarding actions a nurse can take if a patient's anger begins to escalate (see Chapter 24). **You should always trust your own instincts.** If you feel uncomfortable for any reason, excuse yourself for a moment and discuss your feelings with your instructor or a staff member. In addition to obtaining reassurance and support, students can often provide valuable information about the patient's condition by sharing these perceptions.

Orientation Phase

The orientation phase can last for a few meetings or can extend over a longer period. It is the first time the nurse and the patient meet, and they are strangers to each other. When strangers meet, they interact according to their own backgrounds, standards, values, and experiences. This fact—that each person has a unique frame of reference—underlies the need for self-awareness on the part of the nurse. The initial interview includes the following:

- An atmosphere is established in which rapport can grow.
- The nurse's role is clarified, and the responsibilities of both the patient and the nurse are defined.
- The contract containing the time, place, date, and duration of the meetings is discussed.

- Confidentiality is discussed and assumed.
- The terms of termination are introduced (these are also discussed throughout the orientation phase and beyond).
- The nurse becomes aware of transference and countertransference issues.
- Patient problems are articulated, and mutually agreed goals are established.

Establishing rapport. Major emphasis during the first few encounters with the patient is on providing an atmosphere in which trust and understanding can grow and facilitating the establishment of rapport. As in any relationship, rapport can be nurtured by demonstrating genuineness and empathy, developing positive regard, showing consistency, and offering assistance in problem solving and in providing support. It is important for the nurse to first identify how the patient wants to be addressed. In some countries, it is very important that people are addressed by their professional title if they have one. To some people, calling them by their first name, such as a young person addressing an older person by "John" or "Phoebe," would be insulting and likely stall the process. The health care worker simply asks, "What do people call you?" or "How should I address you?"

Parameters of the relationship. The patient needs to know about the nurse (who the nurse is and the nurse's background) and the purpose of the meetings. For example, a student might furnish the following information:

> *Student:* "Hello, Mrs. Rodriquez. I am Jim Thompson from Scottsdale Community College. I am in my psychiatric rotation and will be coming here for the next six Thursdays. I would like to spend time with you each Thursday if you are still here. I'm here to be a support person for you as you work on your treatment goals."

Formal or informal contract. A contract emphasizes the patient's participation and responsibility because it shows that the nurse does something *with* the patient rather than *for* the patient. The contract, either verbal or written, contains the place, time, date, and duration of the meetings. During the orientation phase, the patient may begin to express thoughts and feelings, identify problems, and discuss realistic goals. Therefore the mutual agreement on goals is also part of the contract.

> *Student:* "Mrs. Rodriquez, we will meet at 10 AM each Thursday in the consultation room at the clinic for 45 minutes from September 15 to October 27. We can use that time for further discussion of your feelings of loneliness and anger and explore some things you could do to make the situation better for yourself."

Confidentiality. The patient has a right to know who else will be given the information shared with the nurse and that the information may be shared with specific people, such as a clinical supervisor, the physician, the staff, or other students in conference. The patient also needs to know that the information will *not* be shared with relatives, friends, or others outside the treatment team, except in extreme situations. Safeguarding the privacy and confidentiality of individuals not only is the nurse's ethical obligation but also is a legal responsibility as well.

Extreme situations include (1) child or elder abuse, (2) threats of self-harm or harm to others, or (3) intention not to follow through with the treatment plan. If information must be given to others, this is usually done by the physician, according to legal guidelines (refer to Chapter 6). The nurse must be aware of the patient's right to confidentiality and must not violate that right.

> *Student:* "Mrs. Rodriquez, I will be sharing some of what we discuss with my nursing instructor, and at times I may discuss certain concerns with my peers in conference or with the staff.

However, I will *not* be sharing this information with your husband or any other members of your family or anyone outside the hospital without your permission."

Termination. Termination begins in the orientation phase. It also may be mentioned when appropriate during the working phase if the nature of the relationship is time limited (e.g., six or nine sessions). The date of the termination phase should be clear from the beginning. In some situations the nurse-patient contract may be renegotiated when the termination date has been reached. In other situations, when the therapeutic nurse-patient relationship is an open-ended one, the termination date is not known.

> *Student:* "Mrs. Rodriquez, as I mentioned earlier, our last meeting will be on October 27. We will have three more meetings after today."

Working Phase

The promotion of a strong working relationship develops over a period of time and allows for the patient to experience increased levels of anxiety and demonstrate dysfunctional behaviors in a safe setting while experimenting with new and more adaptive coping behaviors. Moore and Hartman (1988) identified specific tasks of the working phase of the nurse-patient relationship that remain relevant today in current clinical practice:

- Maintain the relationship
- Gather further data
- Promote the patient's problem-solving skills, self-esteem, and use of language
- Facilitate behavioral change
- Overcome resistance behaviors
- Evaluate problems and goals, and redefine them as necessary
- Promote practice and expression of alternative adaptive behaviors

During the working phase, the nurse and patient together identify and explore areas in the patient's life that are causing problems. Often, the patient's present ways of handling situations stem from earlier means of coping devised to survive in a chaotic and dysfunctional family environment. Although certain coping methods may have worked for the patient at an earlier age, they now interfere with the patient's interpersonal relationships and prevent him or her from attaining current goals. The patient's dysfunctional behaviors and basic assumptions about the world are often defensive, and the patient is usually unable to change the dysfunctional behavior at will. Therefore, most of the problem behaviors or thoughts continue because of unconscious motivations and needs that are beyond the patient's awareness.

The nurse can work with the patient to identify these unconscious motivations and assumptions that keep the patient from finding satisfaction and reaching his or her potential. Describing, and often reexperiencing, old conflicts generally awakens high levels of anxiety in the patient. Patients may use various defenses against anxiety and displace their feelings onto the nurse. Therefore during the working phase, intense emotions such as anxiety, anger, self-hatred, hopelessness, and helplessness may surface. Defense mechanisms, such as acting out anger inappropriately, withdrawing, intellectualizing, manipulating, and denying, are to be expected.

During the working phase, the patient may unconsciously transfer strong feelings into the present and onto the nurse that belong to significant others from the past (transference). The emotional responses and behaviors in the patient may also awaken strong countertransference feelings in the nurse. **The nurse's awareness of personal feelings and reactions to the patient are vital for effective interaction with the patient.**

Termination Phase

The termination phase is the final, integral phase of the nurse-patient relationship. Termination is discussed during the first interview, and again during the working stage at appropriate times. Termination may occur when the patient is discharged or when the student's clinical rotation ends. Basically, the tasks of termination are as follows:

- Summarizing the goals and objectives achieved in the relationship
- Discussing ways for the patient to incorporate into daily life any new coping strategies learned during the time spent with the nurse
- Reviewing situations that occurred during the time spent together
- Exchanging memories, which can help validate the experience for both nurse and patient and facilitate closure of that relationship

Termination often awakens strong feelings in both the nurse and patient. Termination of the relationship signifies a loss for both, although the intensity and meaning of termination may be different for each. If a patient has unresolved feelings of abandonment, loneliness, or rejection, these feelings may be reawakened during the termination process. This process can be an opportunity for the patient to express these feelings, perhaps for the first time.

Important reasons for the student or nurse to address the termination phase are as follows:

- Feelings are aroused in both the patient and the nurse with regard to the experience they have shared; when these feelings are recognized and shared, patients learn that it is acceptable to feel sadness and loss when they lose someone for whom they care.
- Termination can be a learning experience; patients can learn that they are important to at least one person.
- By sharing the termination experience with the patient, the nurse demonstrates caring for the patient.
- This may be the first successful termination experience for the patient.

When a nurse/advanced practice nurse has been working with a patient for a while, it is important for the nurse to help the patient acknowledge any feelings and reactions he or she may be experiencing related to separations. If a patient denies that the termination is having an effect (assuming the nurse-patient partnership was strong), the nurse may say something like, "Goodbyes are difficult for people. Often they remind us of other goodbyes. Tell me about another separation in the past." If the patient appears to be displacing anger, either by withdrawing or by being overtly angry at the nurse, the nurse may use generalized statements such as, "People may experience anger when saying goodbye. Sometimes they are angry with the person who is leaving. Tell me how you feel about my leaving." New practitioners as well as students in the psychiatric setting need to consider their last clinical experience with their patient and work with their supervisor or instructor to facilitate communication during this time.

A common response of beginning practitioners, especially students, is feeling guilty about terminating the relationship. These feelings may, in rare cases, be manifested by the student giving the patient his or her telephone number, making plans to get together for coffee after the patient is discharged, continuing to see the patient afterward, or exchanging letters. Maintaining contact after discharge is not acceptable and is in opposition to the goals of a therapeutic relationship. Often this is in response to the student's need to (1) feel less guilty for "using the patient for learning needs," (2) maintain feelings of being "important" to the patient, or (3) sustain the illusion that the student is the only one who "understands" the patient, among other student-centered rationales.

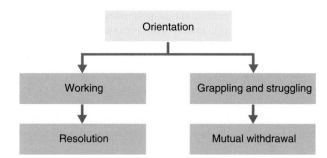

FIGURE 9-2 Phases of therapeutic and nontherapeutic relationships. (From Forchuk, C., Westwell, J., Martin, M., et al. [2000]. The developing nurse-client relationship: nurses' perspectives. *Journal of the American Psychiatric Nurses Association, 6*[1], 3-10.)

Indeed, part of the termination process may be to explore, after discussion with the patient's case manager, the patient's plans for the future: where the patient can go for help, which agencies to contact, and which people may best help the patient find appropriate and helpful resources.

What Hinders and What Helps

Not all nurse-patient relationships follow the classic phases as outlined by Peplau. Some nurse-patient relationships start in the orientation phase but move to a mutually frustrating phase and finally to mutual withdrawal (Figure 9-2).

Forchuk and associates (2000) conducted a qualitative study of the nurse-patient relationship that remains relevant today. They examined the phases of both the therapeutic and the nontherapeutic relationship. From this study they identified certain behaviors that were beneficial to the progression of the nurse-patient relationship as well as those that hampered the development of this relationship. The study emphasized the importance of consistent, regular, and private interactions with patients as essential to the development of a therapeutic alliance. Nurses in this study stressed the importance of listening, pacing, and consistency.

Important evidence-based data so relevant today were found by Forchuk and associates (2000). They identify evidence that the following factors enhance the nurse-patient relationship, allowing it to progress in a mutually satisfying manner:

- **Consistency** includes ensuring that a nurse is always assigned to the same patient and that the patient has a regular routine for activities. Interactions are facilitated when they are frequent and regular in duration, format, and location. Consistency also refers to the nurse being honest and consistent (congruent) in what is said to the patient.
- **Pacing** includes letting the patient set the pace and letting the pace be adjusted to fit the patient's moods. A slow approach helps reduce pressure, and at times it is necessary to step back and realize that developing a strong relationship may take a long time.
- **Listening** includes letting the patient talk when needed. The nurse becomes a sounding board for the patient's concerns and issues. Listening is perhaps the most important skill for nurses to master. Truly listening to another person, attending to what is behind the words, is a learned skill.
- **Initial impressions,** especially positive initial attitudes and preconceptions, are significant considerations in how the relationship will progress. Preconceived negative impressions and feelings toward the patient usually bode poorly for the positive growth of the relationship. In contrast, the nurse's feeling that the patient is "interesting" or "a challenge" and a positive attitude about the relationship are usually favorable signs for the developing therapeutic alliance.

- **Comfort and control,** that is, promoting patient comfort and balancing control, usually reflect caring behaviors. Control refers to keeping a balance in the relationship: not too strict and not too lenient.
- **Patient factors** that seem to enhance the relationship include trust on the part of the patient and the patient's active participation in the nurse-patient relationship.

In relationships that did *not* progress to therapeutic levels, there seemed to be evidence that two major factors hampered the development of positive relationships: **inconsistency** and **unavailability** (e.g., lack of contact, infrequent meetings, meetings in the hallway) on the part of the nurse, patient, or both. When nurse and patient are reluctant to spend time together and meeting times become sporadic and/or superficial, the term **mutual avoidance** is used. This is clearly a lose-lose situation.

The nurse's feelings and lack of self-awareness are major elements that contribute to the lack of progression of positive relationships. Negative preconceived ideas about the patient and negative feelings (e.g., discomfort, dislike, fear, and avoidance) seem to be a constant in relationships that end in frustration and mutual withdrawal. Sometimes these feelings are known, and sometimes the nurse is only vaguely aware of them.

Factors That Enhance Growth

Rogers and Truax (1967) identified three personal characteristics that help promote change and growth in patients, which are classic guidelines that are vital components for establishing a therapeutic alliance or relationship: (1) genuineness, (2) empathy, and (3) positive regard. These are some of the intangibles that are at the heart of the art of nursing.

Genuineness

Genuineness, or self-awareness of one's feelings as they arise within the relationship and the ability to communicate them when appropriate, is a key ingredient in building trust. When a person is genuine, one gets the sense that what is displayed on the outside of the person is congruent with the internal processes. It is conveyed by listening to and communicating with others without distorting their messages, and being clear and concrete in communications with patients. Being genuine in a therapeutic relationship implies the ability to use therapeutic communication tools in an appropriately spontaneous manner, rather than rigidly or in a parrot-like fashion.

Empathy

Empathy is a complex multidimensional concept that has moral, cognitive, emotional, and behavioral components. Perhaps Carl Rogers (1980) explained empathy most clearly:

> It means entering the private perceptual world of the other and becoming thoroughly at home with it. It involves being sensitive, moment by moment, to the changing felt meanings which flow in this other person, to the fear or rage or tenderness or confusion or whatever that he or she is experiencing. It means temporarily living in the other's life, moving about in it delicately without making judgments (p. 142).

Therefore, empathy signifies a central focus and feeling with and in the patient's world. According to Mercer and Reynolds (2002) it involves the following:

- Accurately perceiving the patient's situation, perspective, and feelings
- Communicating one's understanding to the patient and checking with the patient for accuracy
- Acting on this understanding in a helpful (therapeutic) way toward the patient

Empathy versus sympathy. There is much confusion regarding empathy versus sympathy. A simple way to distinguish them is that in empathy we *understand* the feelings of others. In sympathy we *feel* the feelings of others. When a helping person is feeling sympathy for another, objectivity is lost, and the ability to assist the patient in solving a personal problem ceases. Furthermore, sympathy is associated with feelings of pity and commiseration. Although these are considered nurturing human traits, they may not be particularly useful in a therapeutic relationship. When people express sympathy, they express agreement with another, which in some situations may discourage further exploration of a person's thoughts and feelings.

The following examples are given to clarify the distinction between empathy and sympathy. A friend tells you that her mother was just diagnosed with inoperable cancer. Your friend then begins to cry and pounds the table with her fist.

> *Sympathetic response:* "I know exactly how you feel. My mother was hospitalized last year and it was awful. I was so depressed. I still get upset just thinking about it." (*You go on to tell your friend about the incident.*)

Sometimes when nurses try to be sympathetic, they are apt to project their own feelings onto those of the patient, which thus limits the patient's range of responses. A more useful response might be as follows:

> *Empathic response:* "How upsetting this must be for you. Something similar happened to my mother last year and I had so many mixed emotions. What thoughts and feelings are you having?" (*You continue to stay with your friend and listen to his or her thoughts and feelings.*)

In the practice of psychotherapy or counseling, empathy is an essential ingredient in a therapeutic relationship both for the better-functioning patient and for the patient who functions at a more primitive level.

Positive Regard

Positive regard implies respect. It is the ability to view another person as being worthy of caring about and as someone who has strengths and achievement potential. Positive regard is usually communicated indirectly by the following actions rather than directly by words.

Attitudes. One attitude through which a nurse might convey respect is willingness to work with the patient. That is, the nurse takes the patient and the relationship seriously. The experience is viewed not as "a job," "part of a course," or "time spent talking," but as an opportunity to work with patients to help them develop personal resources and actualize more of their potential in living.

Actions. Some actions that manifest an attitude of respect are attending, suspending value judgments, and helping patients develop their own resources.

Attending. Attending behavior is a crucial element in a successful interview. To succeed, nurses must pay attention to their patients in culturally and individually appropriate ways (Sommers-Flanagan & Sommers-Flanagan, 2012–2013). *Attending* is a special kind of listening that refers to an intensity of presence, or being with the patient. At times, simply being with another person during a painful time can make a difference.

Body posture, eye contact, and body language are nonverbal behaviors that reflect the degree of attending and are highly culturally influenced. The cultural components of body posture, eye contact, and body language are covered in more depth in The Clinical Interview section of this chapter.

Suspending value judgments. Although we will always have personal opinions, nurses are more effective when they guard against using their own value systems to judge patients' thoughts, feelings, or behaviors. For example, if a patient is taking drugs or is involved in sexually risky behavior, you might recognize that these behaviors are hindering the patient from living a more satisfying life, posing a potential health threat, or preventing the patient from developing satisfying relationships. However, labeling these activities as bad or good is not useful. Rather, focus on exploring the behavior of the patient and work toward identifying the thoughts and feelings that influence this behavior. Judgmental behavior on the part of the nurse will most likely interfere with further exploration and hinder communication.

The first steps in eliminating judgmental thinking and behaviors are to (1) recognize their presence, (2) identify how or where you learned these responses to the patient's behavior, and (3) construct alternative ways to view the patient's thinking and behavior. Refer to the following example (Sommers-Flanagan & Sommers-Flanagan, 2012–2013).

Denying judgmental thinking will only compound the problem.

Patient: "I am really sexually promiscuous and I love to gamble when I have money. I have sex whenever I can find a partner and spend most of my time in the casino. This has been going on for at least 3 years."

A judgmental response would be the following:

Nurse A: "So your promiscuous sexual and compulsive gambling behaviors really haven't brought you much happiness, have they? You are running away from your problems and could end up with AIDS, broke, or even dead."

A more helpful response would be the following:

Nurse B: "So, your sexual and gambling activities are part of the picture also. You sound as if these activities are not making you happy."

In this example, Nurse B focuses on the patient's behaviors and the possible meaning they might have to the patient. Nurse B does not introduce personal value statements or prejudices regarding promiscuous behavior, as does Nurse A. Empathy and positive regard are essential qualities in a successful nurse-patient relationship.

Helping patients develop resources. The nurse becomes aware of patients' strengths and encourages patients to work at their optimal level of functioning. The nurse does not act for patients unless absolutely necessary, and then only as a step toward helping them act on their own. It is important that patients remain as independent as possible to develop new resources for problem solving.

Patient: "This medication makes my mouth so dry. Could you get me something to drink?"

Nurse: "There is juice in the refrigerator. I'll wait here for you until you get back."

or

Nurse: "I'll walk with you while you get some juice from the refrigerator."

or

Patient: "Could you ask the doctor to let me have a pass for the weekend?"

Nurse: "Your doctor will be on the unit this afternoon. I'll let her know that you want to speak with her."

Consistently encouraging patients to use their own resources helps minimize the patients' feelings of helplessness and dependency and validates their potential for change.

THE CLINICAL INTERVIEW

The content and direction of the clinical interview are decided by the patient. The patient leads. The nurse employs communication skills and active listening to better understand the patient's situation.

During the clinical interview, the nurse provides the opportunity for the patient to reach specific goals, including the following:

- To feel safe
- To feel understood and comfortable
- To identify and explore problems relating to others
- To discuss healthy ways of meeting emotional needs
- To experience a satisfying interpersonal relationship

Preparing for the Interview

Helping a person with an emotional or medical problem is rarely a straightforward task. The goal of assisting a patient to regain psychological or physiological stability can be difficult to achieve. Extremely important to any kind of counseling is permitting the patient to set the pace of the interview, no matter how slow the progress may be (Arnold & Boggs, 2016).

Setting

Effective communication can take place almost anywhere. However, because the quality of the interaction—whether in a clinic, a clinical unit, an office, or the patient's home—depends on the degree to which the nurse and patient feel safe, establishing a setting that enhances feelings of security can be important to the helping relationship. A health care setting, a conference room, or a quiet part in the unit that has relative privacy but is within view of others is ideal. When the interview takes place in the home, it offers the nurse a valuable opportunity to assess the person in the context of everyday life.

Seating

In all settings, chairs need to be arranged so that conversation can take place in normal tones of voice and eye contact can be comfortably maintained or avoided. For example, a nonthreatening physical environment for nurse and patient would involve the following:

- Assuming the same height, either both sitting or both standing.
- Avoiding a face-to-face stance when possible; a 90- to 120-degree angle or side-by-side position may be less intense and the patient and nurse can look away from each other without discomfort.
- Providing safety and psychological comfort in terms of exiting the room. The patient should not be positioned between the nurse and the door, nor should the nurse be positioned in such a way that the patient feels trapped in the room.
- Avoiding a desk barrier between the nurse and the patient.

Introductions

In the orientation phase, students tell the patient who they are, what the purpose of the meeting is, and how long and at what time they will be meeting with the patient. The issue of confidentiality is addressed during the initial interview. Please remember that all health care professionals must respect the private, personal, and confidential nature of the patient's communication except in specific situations as outlined earlier (e.g., harm to self or others, child abuse, elder abuse). What is discussed with staff and your clinical group in conference should not be discussed outside with others, no matter who they are (e.g., patient's relatives, news media, friends). The patient needs to know that whatever is discussed will stay confidential unless permission is given for it to be disclosed.

The nurse can then ask the patient how he or she would like to be addressed. This question accomplishes a number of tasks (Arnold & Boggs, 2016). For example:

- It conveys respect.
- It gives the patient direct control over an important ego issue. (Some patients like to be called by their last names; others prefer being on a first-name basis with the nurse.)

Initiating the Interview

Once introductions have been made, the nurse can turn the interview over to the patient by using one of a number of open-ended statements such as the following:

- "Where should we start?"
- "Tell me a little about what has been going on with you."
- "What are some of the stresses you have been coping with recently?"
- "Tell me a little about what has been happening in the past couple of weeks."
- "Perhaps you can begin by letting me know what some of your concerns have been recently."
- "Tell me about your difficulties."

Communication can be facilitated by appropriately **offering leads** (e.g., "Go on"), making **statements of acceptance** (e.g., "Uh-huh"), or otherwise conveying interest.

Tactics to Avoid

The nurse needs to avoid certain behaviors as outlined by Moscato (1988); they still serve as important guidelines today. For example:

Do Not:	**Try To:**
Argue with, minimize, or challenge the patient.	Keep the focus on facts and the patient's perceptions.
Give false reassurance.	Make observations of the patient's behavior. "Change is always possible."
Interpret to the patient or speculate on the dynamics.	Listen attentively, use silence, and try to clarify the patient's problem.

Do Not:	**Try To:**
Question or probe patients about sensitive areas that they do not wish to discuss.	Pay attention to nonverbal communication. Strive to keep the patient's anxiety decreased.
Try to sell the patient on accepting treatment.	Encourage the patient to look at pros and cons.
Join in attacks patients launch on their mates, parents, friends, or associates.	Focus on facts and the patient's perceptions. Be aware of nonverbal communication.
Participate in criticism of another nurse or any other staff member.	Focus on facts and the patient's perceptions.
	Check out serious accusations with the other nurse or staff member.
	Have the patient meet with the nurse or staff member in question and senior staff or clinician and clarify perceptions.

Helpful Guidelines

Classic guidelines for conducting the initial interviews that are valid today were summed up by Meier and Davis (2001):

- Speak briefly.
- When you do not know what to say, say nothing.
- When in doubt, focus on feelings.
- Avoid advice.
- Avoid relying on questions.
- Pay attention to nonverbal cues.
- Keep the focus on the patient.

Attending Behaviors: The Foundation of Interviewing

Engaging in attending behaviors and listening well are two key principles of counseling on which just about everyone agrees (Sommers-Flanagan & Sommers-Flanagan, 2012–2013). Attending behaviors were addressed earlier but are covered more thoroughly here as they relate to the clinical interview. Ivey and Ivey (1999) define attending behaviors as "culturally and individually appropriate … eye contact, body language, vocal qualities, and verbal tracking" (p. 15). Sommers-Flanagan and Sommers-Flanagan (2012–2013) state that positive attending behaviors can open up communication and encourage free expression. However, negative attending behaviors are more likely to inhibit expression. These behaviors need to be evaluated in terms of cultural patterns and past experiences of both the interviewer and the interviewee. There are no universals; however, there are guidelines that students can follow.

Eye Contact

Even among people from similar cultural backgrounds there may be variation in what an individual is personally comfortable with in terms of eye contact. For some patients and interviewers, sustained eye contact is normal and comfortable, whereas for other patients and interviewers it may be more comfortable and natural to make brief eye contact but look away or down much of the time. Sommers-Flanagan and Sommers-Flanagan (2012–2013) state that it is appropriate for most nurse clinicians to maintain more eye contact when the patient speaks and less constant eye contact when the nurse speaks. However, in general, white patients are more comfortable with more sustained eye contact much of the time; Native Americans, African Americans, and Asian patients often prefer less eye contact.

Body Language

Body language involves two elements: kinesics and proxemics. *Kinesics* is associated with physical characteristics such as body movements and postures. The way someone holds the head, legs, and shoulders; facial expressions; eye contact or lack thereof; and so on convey a multitude of messages. For example, a person who slumps in a chair, rolls the eyes, and sits with arms crossed in front of the chest can be perceived as resistant and unreceptive to what another wants to communicate.

On the other hand, positive body language may include leaning in slightly toward the speaker, maintaining a relaxed and attentive posture, making direct eye contact, making hand gestures that are unobtrusive and smooth while minimizing the number of other movements, and matching one's facial expressions to one's feelings or to the patient's feelings.

Proxemics refers to personal space and what distance between oneself and others is comfortable for an individual. Proxemics takes into account that these distances may be different for different cultural groups. Intimate distance in the United States is 0 to 18 inches and is reserved for those we trust most and with whom we feel most safe. Personal distance (18 to 40 inches) is for personal communications such as those with friends or colleagues. Social distance (4 to 12 feet) is applied to strangers or acquaintances, often in public places or formal social gatherings. Public distance (12 feet or more) relates to public space (e.g., public speaking). In public space one may hail another, and the parties may move about while communicating with one another.

Vocal Qualities

Vocal quality, or **paralinguistics,** encompasses voice loudness, pitch, rate, and fluency. Sommers-Flanagan and Sommers-Flanagan (2012–2013) state that "effective interviewers use vocal qualities to enhance rapport, communicate interest and empathy and to emphasize special issues or conflicts" (p. 56). This supports the old adage, "It's not *what* you say, but *how* you say it." Speaking in soft and gentle tones is apt to encourage a person to share thoughts and feelings, whereas speaking in a rapid, high-pitched tone may convey anxiety and create it in the patient. Consider, for example, how tonal quality can affect communication in a simple sentence like "I will see you tonight."

1. "*I* will see you tonight." (I will be the one who sees you tonight.)
2. "I *will* see you tonight." (No matter what happens, or whether you like it or not, I will see you tonight.)
3. "I will see *you* tonight." (Even though others are present, it is you I want to see.)
4. "I will see you *tonight*." (It is definite, tonight is the night we will meet.)

Verbal Tracking

Verbal tracking is just that: tracking what the patient is saying. Individuals cannot know if you are hearing or understanding what they are saying unless you provide them with cues. Verbal tracking is giving neutral feedback in the form of restating or summarizing what the patient has already said. It does not include personal or professional opinions of what the patient has said (Sommers-Flanagan & Sommers-Flanagan, 2012–2013). For example:

> *Patient:* "I don't know what the fuss is about. I smoke marijuana to relax and everyone makes a fuss."
> *Nurse:* "Do you see this as a problem for you?"
> *Patient:* "No, I don't. It doesn't affect my work … well, most of the time, anyway. I mean, of course, if I have to think things out and make important decisions, then obviously it can get in the way. But most of the time I'm cool."
> *Nurse:* "So when important decisions have to be made, then it interferes; otherwise, you don't see it affecting your functioning."
> *Patient:* "Yeah, well, most of the time I'm cool."

Verbal tracking involves pacing the interview with the patient by sticking closely with the patient's speech content (as well as speech volume and tone as discussed earlier). It can be difficult to know which leads to follow if the patient introduces many topics at once.

Clinical Supervision and Process Recordings

Communication and interviewing techniques are acquired skills. Nurses learn to increase their ability to use communication and interviewing skills through practice and clinical supervision. In **clinical supervision,** the focus is on the nurse's behavior in the nurse-patient relationship. The nurse and the supervisor examine and analyze the nurse's feelings and reactions to the patient and the way they affect the relationship.

> *"And I would emphasize that, no matter how good we become at being our own inner supervisor, professional help and support from experienced (external) supervisor is essential to good practice"* (Fox, 2008, p. 21).

Clinical supervision can be a therapeutic process for the nurse. During the process, feelings and concerns are ventilated as they relate to the developing nurse-patient relationship. The opportunity to examine interactions, obtain insights, and devise alternative strategies for dealing with various clinical issues enhances clinical growth and minimizes frustration and burnout. Clinical supervision is a necessary professional activity that fosters professional growth and helps minimize the development of nontherapeutic nurse-patient relationships.

The best way to increase communication and interviewing skills is to review clinical interactions exactly as they occur. This process offers students the opportunity to identify themes and patterns in their own, as well as their patients', communications. Students also learn to deal with the variety of situations that arise in the clinical interview.

In some clinics, institutes, and other places of learning there is an increased use of taping and videotaping interactions or role-playing for the purpose of learning. However, if taping or videotaping the interaction is not available, the use of process recordings is a good mechanism to identify patterns in the student's and the patient's communication. Process recordings are written records of a segment of the nurse-patient session that reflect as closely as possible the verbal and nonverbal behaviors of both patient and nurse, which were introduced in Chapter 7.

KEY POINTS TO REMEMBER

- The nurse-patient relationship/partnership is well defined, and the roles of the nurse and the patient must be clearly stated.
- It is important that the nurse be aware of the differences between a therapeutic relationship and a social or intimate relationship. In a therapeutic nurse-patient relationship, the focus is on the patient's needs, thoughts, feelings, and goals. The nurse is expected to meet personal needs outside this relationship in other professional, social, or intimate arenas.
- Genuineness, positive regard, and empathy are personal strengths in the helping person that foster growth and change in others.
- Although the boundaries of the nurse-patient relationship generally are clearly defined, they can become blurred; this blurring can be insidious and may occur on an unconscious level. Usually, transference and countertransference phenomena are operating when boundaries are blurred.
- It is important to have a grasp of common countertransferential feelings and behaviors and of the nursing actions to counteract these phenomena.
- Supervision aids in promoting the professional growth of the nurse as well as in the nurse-patient relationship, allowing the patient's goals to be addressed and met.
- The phases of the nurse-patient relationship include the orientation, working, and termination phases, which are in reality very fluid.
- The clinical interview is a key component of psychiatric mental health nursing. Presented are considerations needed for establishing a safe setting and planning for appropriate seating, introduction, and initiation of the interview.
- Attending behaviors (e.g., eye contact, body language, vocal qualities, and verbal tracking) are a key element in effective communication.
- Cultural background (as well as individual values and beliefs) has a great deal to do with what nonverbal behavior means to different individuals. The degree of eye contact and the use of touch are two nonverbal aspects that can be misunderstood by individuals of different cultures.
- A meaningful therapeutic relationship is facilitated when values and cultural influences are considered. It is the nurse's responsibility to seek to understand the patient's perceptions.

APPLYING CRITICAL JUDGMENT

1. On your first clinical day you spend time with an older woman, Mrs. Schneider, who is very depressed. Your first impression is "Oh, my, she looks like my mean Aunt Helen. She even sits like her." Mrs. Schneider asks you, "Who are you and how can you help me?" She tells you that "a student" could never understand what she is going through. She then says, "If you really wanted to help me you could get me a good job after I leave here."
   A. Identify transference and countertransference issues in this situation. What is your most important course of action? What in the classic study of Forchuk and associates indicates that this is a time for you to exercise self-awareness and self-insight to establish the potential for a therapeutic encounter or relationship?

B. How could you best respond to Mrs. Schneider's question about who you are? What other information will you give her during this first clinical encounter? Be specific.

C. What are some useful responses you could give her regarding her legitimate questions about ways you could be of help to her?

D. Analyze Mrs. Schneider's request that you find her a job. How does this request relate to boundary issues, and how can this be an opportunity for you to help Mrs. Schneider develop resources? Keeping in mind the aim of Peplau's interactive nurse-patient process, describe some useful ways you could respond to this request.

2. You are attempting to conduct a clinical interview with a very withdrawn patient. You have tried silence and open-ended statements, but all you get is one-word answers. What other actions could you take at this time?

CHAPTER REVIEW QUESTIONS

1. Which comment by the nurse would be appropriate to begin a new nurse-patient relationship?
   a. "Which of your problems is most serious?"
   b. "I want you to tell me about your problems."
   c. "I'm an experienced nurse. You can trust me."
   d. "What would you like to tell me about yourself?"

2. A neighbor telephones the nurse daily, giving lengthy details about multiple somatic complaints and relationship problems. Which limit-setting strategy should the nurse employ?
   a. Suggest the neighbor call other people in the community.
   b. Say to the neighbor, "I can talk to you for 15 minutes twice a week."
   c. Use the telephone's caller identification to screen calls from the neighbor.
   d. Tell the neighbor, "You should discuss these concerns with your personal physician rather than me."

3. A patient has been oppositional, demanding, and resistant to working on goals. A mental health nurse tells the nursing supervisor, "We finally had a serious talk. I let that patient know it's time to get right with God and stop this behavior." Recognizing the nurse's actions were not acceptable, select the supervisor's responding action.
   a. Review the facility policies regarding patient's rights with the nurse.
   b. Ask the nurse about documentation related to this patient interaction.
   c. Schedule the nurse for a staff development activity on cultural sensitivity.
   d. Work with the nurse to prepare and analyze a process recording of the interaction.

4. A nurse participating in a community health fair interviews an adult who has had no interaction with a health care professional for more than 10 years. The adult says, "I like to keep to myself. Crowds make me nervous." Which action should the nurse employ?
   a. Refer the adult for a full health assessment.
   b. Explore the adult's family and social relationships.
   c. Ask the adult, "How do you feel about the quality of your life?"
   d. Explain to the adult, "We can help you feel better about yourself."

5. A group of nurses privately discuss patients under their care. Which nurse's comment indicates the need for clinical supervision regarding countertransference?
   a. "My patient is always asking my permission to do something, just like a child."

b. "When our unit is understaffed, it seems like we have more incidents of disruptive behavior."
   c. "My patient tries to tell me what to do all the time. I got a divorce because my spouse used to do that."
   d. "Our patients have had so many traumatic life experiences. I find myself feeling sympathetic sometimes."

REFERENCES

Arnold, E. C., & Boggs, K. U. (2016). *Interpersonal relationships: professional communication skills for nurses* (6th ed.). St. Louis: Saunders.

Fontes, L. A. (2008). *Interviewing clients across cultures: a practitioner's guide.* New York: Guilford Press.

Forchuk, C., Westwell, J., Martin, M., et al. (2000). The developing nurse-client relationship: nurse's perspectives. *Journal of the American Psychiatric Nurses Association, 6*(1), 3–10.

Fox, S. (2008). *Relating to clients: the therapeutic relationship for complementary therapists.* London and Philadelphia: Jessica Kingsley Publishers.

Gordon, C., & Beresin, E. V. (2016). The doctor-patient relationship. In T. Stern, M. Fava, T. Wilens, et al. (Eds.), *Massachusetts General Hospital: comprehensive clinical psychiatry* (2nd ed.). Philadelphia: Saunders/Elsevier.

Haber, J. (2000). Hildegard E. Peplau: the psychiatric nursing legacy of a legend. *Journal of the American Psychiatric Nurses Association, 6*(2), 56–62.

Hays, P. (2008). *Addressing cultural complexities in practice* (2nd ed.). Washington, DC: American Psychological Association.

Ivey, A. E., & Ivey, M. (1999). *Intentional interviewing and counseling* (4th ed.). Pacific Grove, Calif: Brooks/Cole.

Meier, S. T., & Davis, S. R. (2001). *The elements of counseling* (4th ed.). Pacific Grove, Calif: Brooks/Cole.

Mercer, S. W., & Reynolds, W. (2002). Empathy and quality of care. *British Journal of General Practice, 52*(Suppl), S9–S12.

Moore, J. C., & Hartman, C. R. (1988). Developing a therapeutic relationship. In C. K. Beck, R. P. Rawlins, & S. R. Williams (Eds.), *Mental health–psychiatric nursing.* St. Louis: Mosby.

Moscato, B. (1988). The one-to-one relationship. In H. S. Wilson & C. S. Kneisel (Eds.), *Psychiatric nursing* (3rd ed.). Menlo Park, Calif: Addison-Wesley.

Peplau, H. E. (1952). *Interpersonal relations in nursing: a conceptual frame of reference for psychodynamic nursing.* New York: Putnam.

Peplau, H. E. (1999). *Interpersonal relations in nursing: a conceptual frame of reference for psychodynamic nursing.* New York: Springer.

Pilette, P. C., Berck, C. B., & Achber, L. C. (1995). Therapeutic management of helping boundaries. *Journal of Psychosocial Nursing and Mental Health Services, 33*(1), 40–47.

Quinlan, J. C. F. (1996). *Co-creating personal and professional knowledge through peer support and peer approval in nursing.* Submitted for degree of PhD of the University of Bath. 1996. Retrieved July 17, 2006, from www.bath.ac.uk/carpp/jquinlan/titlepage.htm.

Rogers, C. R. (1980). *A way of being.* Boston: Houghton Mifflin.

Rogers, C. R., & Truax, C. B. (1967). The therapeutic conditions antecedent to change: a theoretical view. In C. R. Rogers (Ed.), *The therapeutic relationship and its impact.* Madison: University of Wisconsin Press.

Sommers-Flanagan, J., & Sommers-Flanagan, R. (2012-2013). *Clinical interviewing* (4th ed.). Hoboken, NJ: Wiley.

Caring for Patients with Psychobiological Disorders

Sheila Rouslin Welt, MS, APN

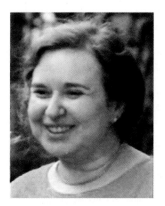

Sheila Rouslin Welt is a Clinical Specialist in Psychiatric Nursing; she established the first position for clinical specialists in community mental health centers in the state of New Jersey and was among the first private practice nurses in psychotherapy. A long-time editor of *Perspectives in Psychiatric Care*, Rouslin Welt was the first nurse to coauthor a book on group psychotherapy (the first of 6 books) and has authored more than 15 articles and book chapters. For 12 years she taught in the graduate psychiatric nursing program at Rutgers University. In addition to being a national and international lecturer, for the past 30 years Rouslin Welt has maintained a private psychotherapy, supervision, and consultation practice in New Jersey.

Rouslin Welt was part of the movement to gain certification for the practice of Clinical Specialists in Psychiatric Nursing. The following is her story.

The credentialing process began in the early 1970s. Marcia Stachyra, a fellow graduate of Peplau's program, spearheaded the process. Although graduate education at the time permitted a nurse to attain the title of Clinical Specialist in Psychiatric Nursing and act as a psychotherapist, the practice of nurse psychotherapy was unprotected by existing Nurse Practice Acts or specialty certification. Therefore, the need for credentialing criteria arose. Indeed, changes or advances in clinical practice typically precede laws that protect and govern the professionals or the public. For example, in the state of New York anyone could practice as a psychotherapist. In New Jersey, however, the Psychology Practice Act specified psychotherapy as within the purview of some disciplines, but not nursing.

With the help of psychologist Allan Williams, the New York State Psychological Association's executive director and a member of their legal team, several of us began the process of certification that would legitimize our practice. We worked with the New York State Nurses Association in a process that included revising the Nurse Practice Act in a way that, through regulations guiding practice, psychotherapy by a properly prepared nurse could be included as a legitimate treatment process. This led to the development of postdegree certification through a designated process of clinical supervision and testing. Not only did the process become a model for New Jersey, the next battleground, but also it became the prototype for national certification, demonstrating growth of the profession.

Trauma and Stress-Related Disorders

Elizabeth M. Varcarolis

http://evolve.elsevier.com/Varcarolis/essentials

KEY TERMS AND CONCEPTS

acute stress disorder, p. 126
compassion fatigue/secondary stress
   trauma, p. 127

distress, p. 120
eustress, p. 120
flashbacks, p. 123

posttraumatic stress disorder (PTSD),
   p. 122
stress response, p. 121

SELECTED CONCEPT: COMPASSION FATIGUE/SECONDARY STRESS TRAUMA

Secondary stress trauma and *compassion fatigue* are synonymous terms. Compassion fatigue/secondary stress trauma is the cumulative physical, emotional, and psychological effect of working closely with those suffering from the consequences of heart-wrenching/traumatic events. "Compassion stress" when not managed properly can lead to compassion fatigue. Nurses and all health care workers who are experiencing compassion stress need to practice self-care to prevent compassion fatigue, posttraumatic stress disorder (PTSD), and potential destructive behaviors that may manifest (e.g., isolation, depression, self-medication, and the long list of symptoms associated with traumatic stress disorder are common in compassion fatigue) (American Bar Organization, 2014; Compassion Fatigue Awareness Project, 2015).

OBJECTIVES

1. Discuss four examples of how *eustress* has helped you in your life and two examples of how *distress* has affected you in your life.
2. Describe some of the common symptoms people experience when they are stressed.
3. Describe the physiological manifestations of the fight-or-flight response of the autonomic nervous system when triggered by a stressor.
4. Describe the physiological manifestations of the hypothalamus-pituitary-adrenal cortex axis in the role of chronic stress in terms of the fight-or-flight response.
5. Teach a classmate about posttraumatic stress disorder (PTSD), including (a) the symptoms, (b) the way it could affect our war veterans and others exposed to trauma, (c) possible sequelae

(results) of untreated PTSD, (d) potential treatments, and (e) the potential for PTSD in first responders.
6. Discuss how health care workers are vulnerable to compassion stress and compassion fatigue and describe the steps to take to mitigate/prevent its occurrence.
7. Explain how assessing for traumatic brain injury (TBI) is best practice when working with returning war veterans, as well as other members of the population who are involved in traumatic injury (e.g., head injuries, sports injuries, physical abuse).
8. Compare and contrast the differences between PTSD and acute stress disorder.
9. Describe what is meant by secondary traumatic stress/compassion fatigue in terms of (a) symptoms and (b) health care workers who might be the most vulnerable.

INTRODUCTION

As of 2014, the American Psychological Association annual study found that average stress levels in America seem to be trending downward (4.9 in 2014 vs. 6.2 in 2007 on a 10-point scale). Those that are not faring so well are parents, younger generations, and those living in lower-income households (making less than $50,000 per year). These groups report higher levels of stress than Americans overall (American Psychological Association, 2015).

We all experience stress. Actually, some stress is "good" stress, or eustress. Eustress is beneficial stress; it motivates people to develop the skills they need to solve problems and meet personal goals. However, it is distress that causes problems both emotionally and physically. Increased stress and anxiety can trigger depression, cause confusion, instill

helplessness/hopelessness, and cause fatigue and more. When individuals feel "stressed-out" they often have trouble sleeping or eating, experience headaches or back pain, lose interest in favorite activities, feel tense and become irritable, and often feel powerless. Long-term chronic stress can cause us physiological harm and more chronic emotional difficulties.

A stressor—that which triggers stress—can be real or perceived. Stress can be psychological (e.g., anxiety, guilt, or joy) or physical (e.g., stressful environment, such as loud noises, extreme heat or cold, or other disturbing physical condition). Stress can be psychosocial (e.g., triggered by threat to self-esteem, lack of acceptance in a group, or low social status, and feeling disrespected or stigmatized). Stress can also be triggered by spiritual distress, for example, or an existential crisis: "What should I be doing with my life?" "Where am I going in life?" "Who am I really?" "Is there a God? What does God want of me?"

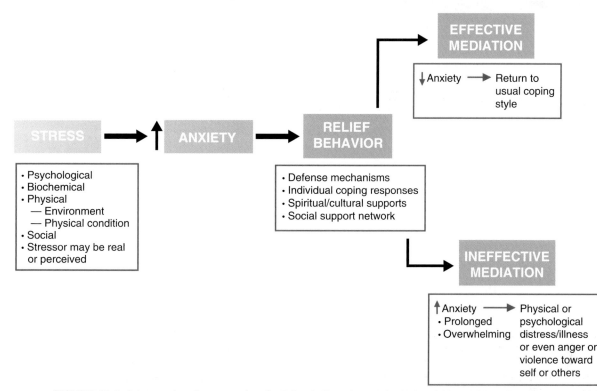

FIGURE 10-1 Stress and anxiety operationally defined. (From Varcarolis, E. M., & Halter, M. J. *Foundations of psychiatric mental health nursing.* [6th ed.]. St Louis: Elsevier.)

Socioeconomic status also plays a role. Wahowiac (2015) contends that poverty is one of the major risk factors in stress and mental health.

We all have individual thresholds for stress, and everyone expresses stress differently (e.g., headaches, digestive problems, anxiety disorder). Also, some people are more resilient than others to stress, but stress is a part of everyday life for everyone. Response to stress can be operationally defined (Figure 10-1).

PHYSIOLOGICAL AND PSYCHOLOGICAL RESPONSES TO STRESS

The Autonomic Nervous System—Fight-or-Flight Response

The stress response is also referred to as the "fight-or-flight response." The fight-or-flight response is a survival mechanism by which our body and mind become immediately ready to meet a threat or stress.

When a threat appears imminent the hypothalamus receives information from almost all parts of the brain including the **limbic system (considered the emotional brain),** particularly the amygdala (the component of the limbic system that contributes to emotional processing). The **hypothalamus functions as the command-and-control center when receiving stressful signals.** The hypothalamus responds to signals of stress by engaging the autonomic nervous system. The autonomic nervous system is comprised of the sympathetic (fight-or-flight response) and parasympathetic nervous systems (relaxation response).

In times of stress the **sympathetic nervous system assumes** control (fight-or-flight response) and sends signals to the adrenal glands, releasing epinephrine (or adrenaline). The circulating adrenaline increases heart rate, elevates blood pressure, increases blood flow to the skeletal muscles, and increases muscle tension. Respirations also increase, bringing more oxygen to the lungs, which is then sent to the brain, increasing alertness.

As the initial rush of epinephrine subsides, the hypothalamus stimulates the HPA axis (hypothalamus, pituitary gland, and adrenal glands). If the stress is prolonged, the hypothalamus releases corticotropin-releasing hormone (CRH), which in turn travels to the pituitary gland and triggers the release of adrenocorticotropic hormone (ACTH) (Harvard Health Publications, 2011). ACTH then travels to the adrenal glands, stimulating release of cortisol. Cortisol is the primary stress hormone. Cortisol helps to supply cells with amino acids and fatty acids for energy, as well as diverts glucose from muscles for use by the brain to maintain vigilance.

As the threat passes, the **parasympathetic branch** of the autonomic nervous system, the part that helps maintain homeostasis and relaxation, takes over. Cortisol levels drop as the body returns to a more normal and healthier state that allows individuals to function as they did before the threat.

However, when stress is prolonged or people are not able to relax, they remain in chronic low levels of stress. The body stays alert for a prolonged period of time. A sustained increase in the chemicals produced by the stress response (cortisol, adrenaline, and other catecholamines) can have damaging effects on the body, causing physical diseases including a substantial negative effect on the immune system, leaving individuals vulnerable to autoimmune diseases. It is believed that as many as 90% of diseases are stress-related. Stress alone does not cause disease, but it does contribute to it.

The stress response is pictorially presented in Figure 10-2.

STRESS REDUCTION TECHNIQUES

Some of the most common techniques that people use to combat stress include the following:

- Trigger the parasympathetic nervous system using techniques to elicit the relaxation response (e.g., meditation, prayer, mindfulness).
- Perform physical activity, which deepens breathing, relieves muscle tension, and can elevate levels of the body's own

THE STRESS RESPONSE

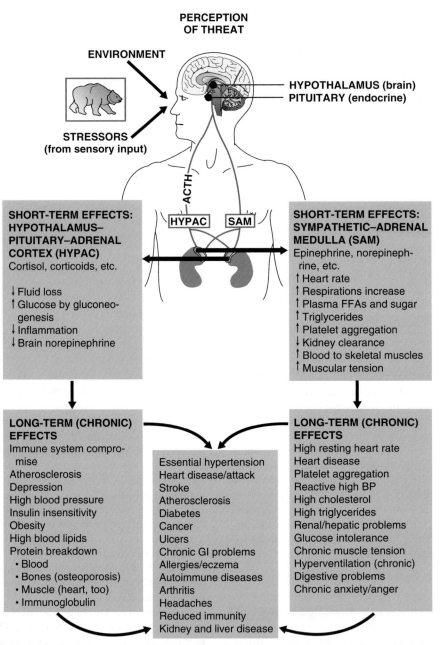

FIGURE 10-2 **The stress response.** (From Brigham, D. D. [1994]. *Imagery for getting well: clinical applications of behavioral medicine.* New York: WW Norton.)

endorphins, which induces a sense of well-being (e.g., yoga, tai chi, running, walking briskly).

- Seek social support (e.g., close family ties, acquaintances, spouses, friends). Studies have shown that social interactions provide great buffers for stress and help people cope better with stress.

For more on selected stress reduction techniques, refer to Box 10-1.

TRAUMA AND STRESS-RELATED DISORDERS

DSM-5 (APA, 2013) added a new diagnostic category called Trauma and Stress-Related Disorders. Included in this category are the Reactive

Attachment Disorder and Disinhibited Social Engagement Disorder. Since these two disorders are essentially disorders of children, they will be addressed in Chapter 26. This chapter will address posttraumatic stress disorder (PTSD) and acute stress disorder (ASD).

Posttraumatic Stress Disorder

The diagnosis of posttraumatic stress disorder (PTSD) and its deleterious effects have received increased awareness over the past decade and more as active-duty military men and women return from war-torn Iraq and Afghanistan. However, **PTSD** is not limited to active-duty military personnel; it can occur in *any individual who has had exposure to a trauma severe enough to be outside the range of normal*

BOX 10-1 Selected Stress Reduction Techniques

Relaxation Techniques

1. These techniques can induce a relaxation state more physiologically refreshing than sleep.

2. They help neutralize stress energy and produce a calming effect.

Reframing

1. Changes the way we look at and feel about things.

2. There are many ways to interpret the same reality (e.g., seeing the glass as half full rather than half empty).

3. Reassess the situation. We can learn from most situations by asking some of the following questions:
   - "What positive thing came out of the situation/experience?"
   - "What did you learn in this situation?"
   - "What would you do differently next time?"

4. Considering life from another person's point of view can help dissipate tension and develop empathy. We might even feel some compassion toward the person.
   - "What might be going on with your (spouse, boss, teacher, friend) that would cause him/her to say/do that?"
   - "Is he/she having problems? Feeling insecure? Under pressure?"

Sleep

1. Chronically stressed people are often fatigued.

2. Go to sleep 30 to 60 minutes earlier each night for a few weeks.

3. If still fatigued, try going to bed another 30 minutes earlier.

4. Sleeping later in the morning is not helpful and can disrupt body rhythms.

Exercise (Aerobic)

1. Exercise can dissipate chronic and acute stress.

2. It is recommended for at least 30 minutes, three times a week.

Lower/Eliminate Caffeine Intake

1. Such a simple measure can lead to more energy, fewer muscle aches, and greater relaxation.

2. Wean yourself off coffee, tea, colas, and chocolate drinks.

Stress-Lowering Tips for Life

1. Engage in meaningful, satisfying work.

2. Live with and/or love whom you choose.

3. Associate yourself with gentle people who affirm your personhood.

4. Guard your personal freedom, especially your freedom to:
   - Choose your friends.
   - Live with and/or love whom you choose.
   - Think and believe as you choose.
   - Structure your time as you desire.
   - Set your own life goals.

---

human experience. Specific examples include childhood physical abuse, torture/kidnap, military combat, sexual assault, natural disasters (e.g., floods, tornados, earthquakes, tsunamis), human disasters (plane and train accidents, crime-related events, terrorist attacks, assault, mugging), and even the diagnosis of a severe illness. Posttraumatic stress disorder not only occurs in people who have experienced a traumatic event but also can *occur in people who have witnessed* an unbearable event (e.g., watching a friend die an atrocious death, first responders answering a call to a graphically violent event, or emergency room personnel and hospice nurses). Even those who have been repeatedly exposed to stories about a traumatic event in graphic terms can become traumatized. The common element in all these experiences is the individual's extraordinary helplessness or powerlessness in the face of overwhelming circumstances.

> *We have not been directly exposed to the trauma scene, but we hear the story told with much intensity, or we hear similar stories so often, or we have the gift and a curse of extreme empathy and we suffer. We feel the feelings of our clients. We experienced their fears. We dream their dreams. Eventually, we lose a certain spark of optimism, humour and hope. We tire. We are not sick, but we are not ourselves. (C. Figley, 1995, p. 7)*

Four cardinal symptoms of posttraumatic stress disorder (PTSD) (APA, 2013; Black and Andreasen, 2014; Lowry, 2015; Scheier et al., 2014).

- **Intrusive reexperiencing of the initial trauma** (flashbacks, nightmares, unwanted distressing memories of the event, feelings of unreality)
- **Avoidance** (avoid all memories and feelings as well as people or places that might recall the event)
- **Persistent negative alterations in cognitions and mood** (distorted cognitions about themselves and others [fear, guilt] and feelings of detachment)
- **Alteration and arousal and activity** (irritability, angry outbursts, self-destructive behavior, exaggerated startle response, hypervigilance, sleep difficulties)

The symptoms of posttraumatic stress disorder are terrifying and often disrupt a person's ability to carry out his or her daily activities. The symptoms have to last longer than a month for a diagnosis to be made (APA, 2013).

DSM-5 DIAGNOSTIC CRITERIA

for Posttraumatic Stress Disorder

NOTE: The following criteria apply to adults, adolescents, and children older than 6 years. For children 6 years and younger, see corresponding criteria below.

A. Exposure to actual or threatened death, serious injury, or sexual violence in one (or more) of the following ways:

1. Directly experiencing the traumatic event(s).

2. Witnessing, in person, the event(s) as it (they) occurred to others.

3. Learning that the traumatic event(s) occurred to a close family member or close friend. In cases of actual or threatened death of a family member or friend, the event(s) must have been violent or accidental.

4. Experiencing repeated or extreme exposure to aversive details of the traumatic event(s) (e.g., first responders collecting human remains; police officers repeatedly exposed to details of child abuse).

NOTE: Criterion A4 does not apply to exposure through electronic media, television, movies, or pictures, unless this exposure is work related.

B. Presence of one (or more) of the following intrusion symptoms associated with the traumatic event(s), beginning after the traumatic event(s) occurred:

1. Recurrent, involuntary, and intrusive distressing memories of the traumatic event(s).

Continued

DSM-5 DIAGNOSTIC CRITERIA—cont'd

for Posttraumatic Stress Disorder

NOTE: In children older than 6 years, repetitive play may occur in which themes or aspects of the traumatic event(s) are expressed.

   2. Recurrent distressing dreams in which the content and/or effect of the dream is/are related to the traumatic event(s).

NOTE: In children, there may be frightening dreams without recognizable content.

   3. Dissociative reactions (e.g., flashbacks) in which the individual feels or acts as if the traumatic event(s) were recurring. (Such reactions may occur on a continuum, with the most extreme expression being a complete loss of awareness of present surroundings.)

NOTE: In children, trauma-specific reenactment may occur in play.

   4. Intense or prolonged psychological distress at exposure to internal or external cues that symbolize or resemble an aspect of the traumatic event(s).

   5. Marked physiological reactions to internal or external cues that symbolize or resemble an aspect of the traumatic event(s).

C. Persistent avoidance of stimuli associated with the traumatic event(s), beginning after the traumatic event(s) occurred, as evidenced by one or both of the following:

   1. Avoidance of or efforts to avoid distressing memories, thoughts, or feelings about or closely associated with the traumatic event(s).

   2. Avoidance of or efforts to avoid external reminders (people, places, conversations, activities, objects, situations) that arouse distressing memories, thoughts, or feelings about or closely associated with the traumatic event(s).

D. Negative alterations in cognitions and mood associated with the traumatic event(s), beginning or worsening after the traumatic event(s) occurred, as evidenced by two (or more) of the following:

   1. Inability to remember an important aspect of the traumatic event(s) (typically due to dissociative amnesia and not to other factors such as head injury, alcohol, or drugs).

   2. Persistent and exaggerated negative beliefs or expectations about oneself, others, or the world (e.g., "I am bad," "No one can be trusted," "The world is completely dangerous," "My whole nervous system is permanently ruined").

   3. Persistent, distorted cognitions about the cause or consequences of the traumatic event(s) that lead the individual to blame himself/herself or others.

   4. Persistent negative emotional state (e.g., fear, horror, anger, guilt, or shame).

   5. Markedly diminished interest or participation in significant activities.

   6. Feelings of detachment or estrangement from others.

   7. Persistent inability to experience positive emotions (e.g., inability to experience happiness, satisfaction, or loving feelings).

E. Marked alterations in arousal and reactivity associated with the traumatic event(s), beginning or worsening after the traumatic event(s) occurred, as evidenced by two (or more) of the following:

   1. Irritable behavior and angry outbursts (with little or no provocation) typically expressed as verbal or physical aggression toward people or objects.

   2. Reckless or self-destructive behavior.

   3. Hypervigilance.

   4. Exaggerated startle response.

   5. Problems with concentration.

   6. Sleep disturbance (e.g., difficulty falling or staying asleep or restless sleep).

F. Duration of the disturbance (Criteria B, C, D, and E) is more than 1 month.

G. The disturbance causes clinically significant distress or impairment in social, occupational, or other important areas of functioning.

H. The disturbance is not attributable to the physiological effects of a substance (e.g., medication, alcohol) or another medical condition.

Specify whether:

With dissociative symptoms: The individual's symptoms meet the criteria for posttraumatic stress disorder, and in addition, in response to the stressor, the individual experiences persistent or recurrent symptoms of either of the following:

   1. Depersonalization: Persistent or recurrent experiences of feeling detached from, and as if one were an outside observer of, one's mental processes or body (e.g., feeling as though one were in a dream; feeling a sense of unreality of self or body or of time moving slowly).

   2. Derealization: Persistent or recurrent experiences of unreality of surroundings (e.g., the world around the individual is experienced as unreal, dreamlike, distant, or distorted).

NOTE: To use this subtype, the dissociative symptoms must not be attributable to the physiological effects of a substance (e.g., blackouts, behavior during alcohol intoxication) or another medical condition (e.g., complex partial seizures).

Specify if:

With delayed expression: If the full diagnostic criteria are not met until at least 6 months after the event (although the onset and expression of some symptoms may be immediate).

Posttraumatic Stress Disorder for Children 6 Years and Younger

A. In children 6 years and younger, exposure to actual or threatened death, serious injury, or sexual violence in one (or more) of the following ways:

   1. Directly experiencing the traumatic event(s).

   2. Witnessing, in person, the event(s) as it (they) occurred to others, especially primary caregivers.

NOTE: Witnessing does not include events that are witnessed only in electronic media, television, movies, or pictures.

   3. Learning that the traumatic event(s) occurred to a parent or caregiving figure.

B. Presence of one (or more) of the following intrusion symptoms associated with the traumatic event(s), beginning after the traumatic event(s) occurred:

   1. Recurrent, involuntary, and intrusive distressing memories of the traumatic event(s).

NOTE: Spontaneous and intrusive memories may not necessarily appear distressing and may be expressed as play reenactment.

   2. Recurrent distressing dreams in which the content and/or effect of the dream are related to the traumatic event(s).

NOTE: It may not be possible to ascertain that the frightening content is related to the traumatic event.

   3. Dissociative reactions (e.g., flashbacks) in which the child feels or acts as if the traumatic event(s) were recurring. (Such reactions may occur on a continuum, with the most extreme expression being a complete loss of awareness of present surroundings.) Such trauma-specific reenactment may occur in play.

   4. Intense or prolonged psychological distress at exposure to internal or external cues that symbolize or resemble an aspect of the traumatic event(s).

   5. Marked physiological reactions to reminders of the traumatic event(s).

C. One (or more) of the following symptoms, representing either persistent avoidance of stimuli associated with the traumatic event(s) or negative alterations in cognitions and mood associated with the traumatic event(s), must be present, beginning after the event(s) or worsening after the event(s).

Persistent Avoidance of Stimuli

   1. Avoidance of or efforts to avoid activities, places, or physical reminders that arouse recollections of the traumatic event(s).

   2. Avoidance of or efforts to avoid people, conversations, or interpersonal situations that arouse recollections of the traumatic event(s).

DSM-5 **DIAGNOSTIC CRITERIA—cont'd**

for Posttraumatic Stress Disorder

Negative Alterations in Cognitions

3. Substantially increased frequency of negative emotional states (e.g., fear, guilt, sadness, shame, confusion).
4. Markedly diminished interest or participation in significant activities, including constriction of play.
5. Socially withdrawn behavior.
6. Persistent reduction in expression of positive emotions.

D. Alterations in arousal and reactivity associated with the traumatic event(s), beginning or worsening after the traumatic event(s) occurred, as evidenced by two (or more) of the following:

1. Irritable behavior and angry outbursts (with little or no provocation) typically expressed as verbal or physical aggression toward people or objects (including extreme temper tantrums).
2. Hypervigilance.
3. Exaggerated startle response.
4. Problems with concentration.
5. Sleep disturbance (e.g., difficulty falling or staying asleep or restless sleep).

E. The duration of the disturbance is more than 1 month.

F. Thedisturbancecausesclinicallysignificantdistressorimpairmentinrelationships with parents, siblings, peers, or other caregivers or with school behavior.

G. The disturbance is not attributable to the physiological effects of a substance (e.g., medication or alcohol) or another medical condition.

Specify whether:

With dissociative symptoms: The individual's symptoms meet the criteria for posttraumatic stress disorder, and the individual experiences persistent or recurrent symptoms of either of the following:

1. Depersonalization: Persistent or recurrent experiences of feeling detached from, and as if one were an outside observer of, one's mental processes or body (e.g., feeling as though one were in a dream; feeling a sense of unreality of self or body or of time moving slowly).
2. Derealization: Persistent or recurrent experiences of unreality of surroundings (e.g., the world around the individual is experienced as unreal, dreamlike, distant, or distorted).

NOTE: To use this subtype, the dissociative symptoms must not be attributable to the physiological effects of a substance (e.g., blackouts) or another medical condition (e.g., complex partial seizures).

Specify if:

With delayed expression: If the full diagnostic criteria are not met until at least 6 months after the event (although the onset and expression of some symptoms may be immediate).

From the American Psychiatric Association. (2013). *Diagnostic and statistical manual of mental disorders.* (5th ed.). Washington, DC: APA.

Although the prevalence of PTSD is about 3% to 7% in the general population (Black & Andreasen, 2014), the incidence of PTSD in Afghanistan and Iraq war veterans has been estimated to be up to 20%. War veterans who have screened positive for PTSD were up to four times more likely to experience suicidal ideation then non-PTSD veterans. In addition, those diagnosed with PTSD are more likely to have co-occurring medical conditions, including osteoarthritis, diabetes, heart disease, obesity, and elevated lipid levels (Weiss & Skelton, 2011) and/or depression; suffer from chronic pain; and self-medicate with alcohol/nonprescribed medications (Hoge, 2011). When PTSD and a major depressive disorder (MDD) are untreated or undertreated, there is a long list of painful repercussions: marital problems, unemployment, heavy substance use, suicide attempts, and all too often completed suicides, to name a few.

Studies of patients with PTSD suggest that the stress response of the hypothalamus-pituitary-adrenal cortex is abnormal in these individuals. Repeated trauma or stress not only alters the release of neurotransmitters but also changes the anatomy of the brain—neuroimaging shows reduced hippocampal volume and increased metabolic activity in the limbic regions.

Besides PTSD, it has been estimated that up to 20% of our combat veterans suffer some degree of traumatic brain injury (TBI). Left untreated, TBI can result in permanent disability and permanent brain damage. Traumatic brain injury is a great concern in our civilian population as well. TBI is being diagnosed in both children and professional athletes who are involved in contact sports, as well as those individuals who have been involved in accidents, falls, or shaken baby syndrome, for example. Therefore returning veterans of war should be closely assessed not just for PTSD, but also for signs and symptoms of TBI as well. A study reported in the *Journal of American Medical Association Psychiatry* found that "Even when accounting for pre-deployment symptoms, prior TBI, and combat intensity, TBI during the most recent deployment is the strongest predictor of post-deployment PTSD symptoms" (*JAMA Psychiatry*, 2014).

PTSD symptoms often begin within a few months after the trauma, but a delay of months or years is not uncommon. Survivors benefit from receiving treatments for PTSD within months after the event. If left for a year or more, and severe symptoms are not treated, they most likely will become chronic and natural recovery is unlikely. It is helpful to keep in mind that most people who go through a traumatic event may have symptoms in the beginning; however, they do not go on to develop PTSD.

Difficulty with interpersonal, social, or occupational relationships nearly always accompanies PTSD, and trust is a common issue of concern. Child and spousal abuse may be associated with hypervigilance and irritability. Chemical abuse (alcohol or other mind-altering substances) may begin as an attempt to decrease anxiety and/or depression

It is important for health care workers to realize that exposure to stimuli reminiscent of those associated with the original trauma may cause an exacerbation of the trauma.

There has been much written about the higher rates of suicide and suicide attempts in military personnel. A recent report of a study comparing deployed veterans with nondeployed veterans identified some unexpected results (U.S. Department of Veterans Affairs, 2015) such as the risk comparison among veterans serving during the Iraq and Afghanistan wars from 2001 to 2007:

- Deployed veterans had a 41% higher suicide risk compared with the general U.S. population.
- Non-deployed veterans had a 61% higher suicide risk compared with the general U.S. population.
- Deployed veterans had a 25% lower overall risk of death from all causes compared with the general U.S. population.
- Non-deployed veterans had a 24% lower risk of death from all causes compared with the general U.S. population.

GOALS OF TREATMENT

According to Scheier and colleagues (2014) factors predictive of positive outcomes for individuals with PTSD include a solid social support system, the possession of premorbid good psychiatric and medical health care, and the rapid onset of symptoms.

The following are the optimal outcomes for the individual with PTSD:
- Patient and others (e.g., family, friends) will remain safe.
- Patient will receive treatment for co-occurring conditions, which is always part of active treatment (e.g., alcohol/drug addiction, depression, anxiety disorders, specifically panic attacks).
- Patient will attend support group meetings.
- Patient will expand social support network.
- Patient will exhibit an increase in restful sleep periods.
- Patient will have fewer nightmares and flashbacks.
- Patient will express decreased irritability.
- Patient will be able to demonstrate effective anxiety reduction techniques (cognitive or behavioral).

(Refer to Chapters 20 and 22 for more information about PTSD.)

PSYCHOTHERAPEUTIC TREATMENT STRATEGIES

The U.S. Department of Defense and Veterans' Affairs has implemented numerous programs in the area of screening, education, stigma reduction, and clinical care for veterans. However, veterans with PTSD are reluctant to seek care, with only 50% of those diagnosed utilizing mental health services. New research among veterans found negative perceptions of mental health care, which included distrust of mental health professionals and consideration of treatment as "unhealthy" or a "last resort." *This may be due to the belief that the roles of military personnel are similar to those of police and other first responders—they are trained to deal with multiple traumatic events.* They do not normally perceive themselves as victims, nor do they see their reactions as pathological. The paradox of war-related PTSD is that reactions labeled "symptoms" upon return home can be highly effective in combat—hypervigilance and the ability to deny emotions (Hoge, 2011).

The first step in treatment is establishing a sense of safety. Medical treatment for people diagnosed with PTSD includes antidepressants, particularly selective serotonin reuptake inhibitors (SSRIs, sertraline and paroxetine are approved for PTSD). An atypical antipsychotic may be added to an antidepressant for patients who do not respond to an SSRI alone.

PSYCHOTHERAPY

Cognitive behavioral therapy (CBT) teaches individuals skills for controlling anxiety and countering dysfunctional thoughts. Therapy guides individuals to focus awareness on current thoughts/feelings and utilize psychoeducation and learning skills to adapt to real-world practices to reduce distress in situations that have been previously avoided. (Refer to Table 10-1 for other useful therapeutic interventions.)

As mentioned above, the antidepressant group, SSRIs, are an integral part of the treatment for most individuals with PTSD. However, when target symptoms arise and become serious (e.g., nightmares), medications can be used and may serve to help the patient achieve emotional control (Black & Andreasen, 2014).

Refer to Table 10-2 for medications used to ease some of the target symptoms of PTSD. The IOM (Institute of Medicine) is actively involved in the study of "innovative" treatments for PTSD such as acupuncture, yoga, and the therapeutic use of animals (IOM, 2011). Other successful strategies are eye movement desensitization reprocessing (EMDR)—focusing on mental images and muscular tension and adopting positive thoughts/images while performing particular eye movements and using creative narration—imagining different scenarios to the reality of trying to be at the actual traumatic event (Lahad et al., 2010).

TABLE 10-1 Therapeutic Approach

Disorder	Therapeutic Modality	Comments
Posttraumatic stress disorder	Psychotherapy (e.g., exposure-based cognitive behavioral therapy [CBT]) Family therapy Vocational rehabilitation Group therapy with others who have shared similar experiences (e.g., veterans, partner abuse, sexual violence) Relaxation techniques Psychoeducation and methods to help obtain control of thoughts and feelings Learning skills	More than one treatment modality should be used: a. Establish support b. Focus on abreaction, survivor guilt or shame, anger, and helplessness

TABLE 10-2 Pharmacology for Target Symptoms for PTSD Patients

Target Symptoms	Potential Treatment
Intrusive experiences; "flashbacks," avoidance, and numbing	SSRI antidepressants, buspirone augmentation of SSRI, second-generation antipsychotics
Hyperarousal	Antidepressants, benzodiazepines, α_2-adrenergic agonists, anticonvulsants
Transient psychosis, marked derealization	Low-dose antipsychotics
Nightmares	Prazosin (Minipress)
Treatment-resistant PTSD	Second-generation antipsychotics, anticonvulsants
Depression	Antidepressants
Panic attacks	Antidepressants, MAO inhibitors, high-potency benzodiazepines

From Preston, J. D., O'Neal, J. H., & Talaga, M. C. (2013). *Handbook of clinical psychopharmacology for therapists* (7th ed., p. 143, Fig. 12-B). Oakland, Calif: New Harbinger Publications.

More recently, researchers are finding that a drug usually associated with attention-deficit/hyperactivity disorder (ADHD)—methylphenidate (multiple brands)—may be helpful. Early studies demonstrate marked improvement in people with PTSD symptoms who are given methylphenidate, as well as improvement in depression and postconcussive symptoms in individuals with PTSD, TBI, or both (Davenport, 2015).

Individuals with mild brain injury as well as posttraumatic stress disorder report with cognitive complaints (e.g., problems with concentration, attention, and memory). In both cases, another small study demonstrated that methylphenidate use was associated with significant improvements in cognitive complaints (Davenport, 2015; Brown University Psychopharmacology Update, 2016).

Acute Stress Disorder

Acute stress disorder can occur after the same kind of triggers that exist in posttraumatic stress disorder, which include experiencing a violent event or repeatedly witnessing a violent or traumatic event (e.g., first responders at the scene of a mass casualty incident, police officers repeatedly exposed to details of child abuse). Possible precipitating traumatic events are the same as those listed under Posttraumatic Stress Disorder. However, in an acute stress disorder, the resolution of the symptoms is within 1 month.

APPLYING EVIDENCE-BASED PRACTICE (EBP)

Problem A 29-year-old female is called in by her director of nursing (DON) to discuss an increase in her recent sick days off as well as patient complaints of the nurse being rude to them. The employee begins crying almost immediately and says "I don't know what's wrong; I just don't feel good lately. I wanted to be a nurse so badly and now I dread coming to work." The DON has recently attended a seminar on compassion fatigue and suspects this might be going on with her employee, a fairly new nurse who graduated just about a year ago. Further discussion reveals that patients the employee has worked with recently have had dismal outcomes, she has not felt support from her coworkers, and the employee's nursing mentor recently left the job due to feeling burned out.

EBP Assessment

A. **What do you already know from experience?** The workload on this general medical unit has been high. New nurses do better with support and ongoing mentoring. Demands on nurses are higher than ever, with the prevailing expectation of doing more with less.

B. **What does the literature say?** The literature defines compassion fatigue (CF) as a loss of job satisfaction, or when the distress outweighs the good parts. Symptoms of CF include impaired job performance, absenteeism and high turnover, and physical or mental exhaustion. Burnout can be caused by unfair or uncivil treatment by coworkers or especially by one's supervisor. There is a higher than average turnover rate within the first 1 to 3 years of a nurse's career.

C. **What does the patient want?** The nurse wants to feel good about work again, that she is making a difference, and is supported in the job. She wants to feel confident in her abilities and not be overwhelmed by the workload.

Plan The DON recognized that the nurse had not really received her full orientation due to low staffing and high acuity on the unit when she was hired. The DON also recognized that the employee did not have a mentor anymore. She acknowledged that the employee wanted to do a good job and had an appropriate skill set for her experience level. They made a plan together to assign a new mentor, complete the orientation program, and meet periodically to make sure the employee was feeling supported and confident. In addition, the DON scheduled training for the entire staff on self-care and recognizing compassion fatigue.

QSEN **QSEN Prelicensure Knowledge, Skills, and Attitudes (KSAs) Addressed:**

Evidence-based practice as the DON recognized compassion fatigue and used findings from the literature to assist the nurse and the entire team.

Team work and collaboration by listening to nursing concerns and fostering, resolving conflict, and encouraging improved professional interactions.

From Robert Wood Johnson Foundation. (2014). *Nearly one in five new nurses leaves first job within a year, according to survey of newly-licensed registered nurses.* Retrieved from www.rwjf.org/en/library/articles-and-news/2014/09/nearly-one-in-five-new-nurses-leave-first-job-within-a-year--acc.html; Sheppard, K. (2015). Compassion fatigue among registered nurses: connecting theory and research. *Applied Nursing Research, 28*(1), 57–59.

CRITICAL INCIDENT DEBRIEFING

Critical incident stress debriefing may be valuable for ameliorating symptoms in people with an acute stress response. Benzodiazepines may be used to treat daytime anxiety, and sedative-hypnotics may be used for sleep. However, these medications are prescribed short term and are used in conjunction with crisis intervention and other psychological treatments because of their abuse potential. Refer to Chapter 24 for more information on critical incident debriefing.

SELF-CARE FOR NURSES

Compassion fatigue is different from **burnout** in that burnout is related to emotional exhaustion and withdrawal associated with increased workload and institutional stress.

Nurses should be alert to compassion fatigue/secondary traumatic stress. These terms are used interchangeably and describe the emotional effect that nurses and other health care workers may experience by being indirectly traumatized when helping or trying to help a person who has experienced primary traumatic stress. The American Bar Organization (2014) summarizes some of the secondary traumatic stress/compassion fatigue symptoms:

- Feeling overwhelmed, physically and mentally exhausted
- Interferes with ability to function
- Intrusive thoughts/images of another's critical experience
- Difficulty separating work from personal life
- Becoming pessimistic, critical, irritable, prone to anger
- Dread of working with certain individuals
- Depression
- Ineffective and/or destructive self-soothing behaviors
- Withdrawing socially and becoming emotionally disconnected from others
- Becoming demoralizing and questioning one's professional competence and effectiveness
- Becoming easily frustrated
- Insomnia
- Lowered self-esteem in nonprofessional situations
- Loss of hope

Nurses who work with patients with posttraumatic stress disorder and hear their stories and nurses who are constantly exposed to patients who describe traumatic events in their lives may be vulnerable to compassion fatigue or secondary traumatic stress or may even develop posttraumatic stress disorder themselves.

Examples of nurses who are at high risk for secondary trauma stress are those who work in hospice care, pediatrics, emergency departments (EDs), oncology, and forensic nursing, and certainly psychiatric nurses and social workers who work closely with traumatized individuals. Also, the emotional character of the nurse can potentiate compassion fatigue; for example, if the nurse has unrealistic self-expectations, is overinvolved with the patient, is inexperienced, or is having a personal crisis or risk. Studies show that psychiatrists, in particular, are prone to high levels of stress as evidenced by high rates of suicide, severe depression, and secondary general compassion fatigue.

Nurses need to practice self-care in any kind of work they do. Some guidelines for finding balance in your life include:

- Make a concerted effort to put activities in your schedule that add an experience of joy, pleasure, and diversion.
- Allow for mini–escapes to relieve the intensity of your work.
- Get medical care to relieve symptoms that interfere with your daily functioning.

- Refrain from the use of alcohol or drugs to self-medicate.
- Reframe the negative aspects of your work by challenging the negativity, finding meaning, and finding aspects in your life for which you are grateful.

KEY POINTS TO REMEMBER

- Some stress is useful in our lives; *eustress* is stress that makes us strive to reach our goals, repair important relationships, improve our work, and stimulate creative problem-solving processes and improve critical thinking.
- Stress is common in our lives, but when stress is prolonged and increased it may be experienced more as *distress,* which is a negative experience. When stress becomes chronic it can cause physiological harm and emotional difficulties.
- When we are confronted with a serious stressor, our autonomic nervous system reacts with the fight-or-flight response. This response involves a complex network of nerve pathways, brain structures, and glands to help our bodies and mind deal with the stressor.
- The second part of the fight-or-flight response is caused by the hypothalamus-pituitary-adrenal (HPA) cortex, which activates the response.
- When the stress response is prolonged and becomes chronic, it can have damaging effects on the body by lowering the resistance of the immune system and contributing to both physical illness and mental trauma (e.g., depression, hopelessness, helplessness, increased sustained anxiety).
- Some suggestions for stress reduction are given in Box 10-1.
- Posttraumatic stress disorder (PTSD) usually occurs after a severe traumatic event (e.g., childhood abuse, torture/kidnap, military combat, sexual assault, incest, natural disasters, and life-threatening illness). It is estimated that up to 20% of our combat veterans returning from combat have PTSD.
- If PTSD is not treated, serious consequences often result, including severe depression, alcohol/substance abuse, suicide, inability to trust, and social and occupational disruptions, as well as a host of mentally damaging symptoms and/or disorders.
- The major symptoms of PTSD and acute stress disorder have been addressed in this chapter.
- Pharmacological and therapeutic interventions that have proven successful with PTSD have been identified.
- Nurses, physicians, and first responders are cautioned to be alert for secondary traumatic stress and practice self-care since they also can be at risk for compassion fatigue/posttraumatic stress disorder if not properly managed.
- Symptoms a health care worker might experience are included in this chapter. Health care workers who might be vulnerable to compassion fatigue stress/compassion fatigue/PTSD have been identified; however, this is not an exclusive list.

APPLYING CRITICAL JUDGMENT

1. A friend of yours, Juan, arrives to class breathing hard and looking pale and shaken. He tells you that he just missed getting run over by a car and that his heart keeps pounding.
   A. Once Juan becomes calm, how would you explain to Juan his body's physiological response to the fight-or-flight response?
2. Another friend of yours, Teresa, tells you that after failing the midterm exam she just cannot stop thinking about her failure. She feels preoccupied and stressed all the time.
   A. If Teresa is experiencing chronic stress, describe what is happening physiologically.
   B. If this response continues for a long time, what might be some of the sequelae (results)?
   C. Depending on the situation, what are some suggestions that you could offer both Juan and Teresa that might help reduce their stress?
3. After witnessing a brutal murder of four bank guards 3 months ago, Laura continues to have nightmares and jumps at any loud noise. At the health clinic where you work, she tells you that she does not sleep well at night and cannot stop thinking about the traumatic event.
   A. If Laura is diagnosed with PTSD, identify and define other signs and symptoms you might notice.
   B. Besides her symptoms, what would you include in your assessment in order to plan effective interventions for Laura?
   C. If Laura tells you she has flashbacks and cannot function at school and work, what medication might alleviate her symptoms?

CHAPTER REVIEW QUESTIONS

1. A mature, professional couple plans a large wedding in a city 100 miles from their home. Which response is most likely to be associated with this experience?
   a. Distress
   b. Eustress
   c. Acute stress
   d. Depersonalization
2. A college student has been experiencing significant stress associated with academic demands. Last month, the student began attending yoga sessions three times a week. Which outcome indicates this activity has been successful?
   a. The student reports improved feelings of well-being.
   b. The student increases use of caffeine to enhance concentration.
   c. The student reports, "Now I am sleeping about 10 hours every day."
   d. The student says, "I withdrew from two courses to reduce my academic load."
3. An adult required a heart transplant 5 years ago. Multiple medical complications followed, resulting in persistent irritability, depression, and insomnia. The adult's spouse says, "I've walked on eggshells for five years, never knowing when something else will go wrong." What is the nurse's priority intervention regarding the spouse?
   a. Explore the spouse's feelings, showing care and compassion.
   b. Encourage the spouse to attend a community support group.
   c. Teach stress reduction and relaxation techniques to the spouse.
   d. Refer the spouse to the primary care provider for health assessment.
4. A veteran of the war in Afghanistan tells the nurse, "Everyday, something happens that makes me feel like I'm still there. My family has grown impatient with me. They say it's time for me to move on from that time in my life but I can't." What is the nurse's first priority?
   a. Assess the veteran for suicide risk.
   b. Refer the veteran for specialized mental health services.
   c. Assess the veteran for evidence of traumatic brain injury.
   d. Refer the veteran's family to a posttraumatic stress disorder group.
5. An individual lives in a community adjacent to a military base. Loud jets fly overhead multiple times daily. The person tells the nurse, "They're so loud I can't hear myself think." What is the nurse's best first action?
   a. Direct the individual to report the jet noise to local authorities.
   b. Teach relaxation and stress reduction techniques to the individual.

c. Assess the individual for sensory impairments, particularly auditory.

d. Encourage the individual to form a community action group to oppose noise pollution.

REFERENCES

American Bar Organization. (2014). *Compassion fatigue: what is compassion fatigue?*. Retrieved May 6, 2014, from www.americanbar.org/groups/lawyers-assistance/resources/compassion-fatigue.HTML.

American Psychiatric Association. (2013). *Diagnostic and statistical manual of mental disorders (DSM-5)* (5th ed.). Washington, DC: APA.

American Psychological Association. (2015). *Stress in America™; paying with our health*. Washington, DC: APA.

Black, D. W., & Andreasen, N. A. (2014). *Introductory textbook of psychology* (6th ed.). Washington, DC: American Psychiatric Publishing.

Brown University Psychopharmacology Update. (2016). *Methylphenidate effective on range of symptoms in PTSD, brain injury, 27*(2), 1–7.

Compassion Fatigue Awareness Project. (2015). *Did you know?*. Retrieved March 4, 2015, from www.compassionfatigue.org.

Davenport, L. (2015). *ADHD drug may improve PTSD, TBI symptoms*. Retrieved January 15, 2016, from http://www.medscape.com/viewarticle/854472#vp_2.

Figley, C. R. (Ed.). (1995). *Compassion fatigue: coping with secondary trauma stress disorder in those who treat the traumatized* (p. 7). London, UK: Brunner-Routledge.

Harvard Health Publications. (2011). *Understanding the stress response*. Retrieved July 27, 2011, from www.health.harvard.edu/newsletters/Harvard_Mental_Health.

Hoge, C. (2011). Interventions for war-related PTSD: meeting veterans where they are. *Journal of the American Medical Association, 306*(5), 549–551.

Institute of Medicine (IOM). (2011). Assessment of ongoing efforts in treatment of PTSD. *IOM do you abuse on Newsletter* July 11, 2011.

Journal of American Medical Association. (2014). Psychiatry. *JAMA Psychiatry, 71*(2), 149–157.

Lahad, M., et al. (2010). Preliminary study of a new integrative approach in treating PTSD. *Arts in Psychotherapy, 37*, 391–399.

Lowry, F. (2015). *Emergency staff not immune to traumatic stress*. Retrieved June 6, 2015, from www.Medscape.com/viewarticle/840980.

Preston, J. D., O'Neal, J. H., & Talaga, M. C. (2013). *Handbook of clinical psychopharmacology for therapists* (7th ed.). Oakland, Calif: New Harbinger Publications.

Scheier, F. R., Vidair, H. B., Vogel, L. R., et al. (2014). Anxiety, obsessive-compulsive, and stress disorders. In Janice L. Cutler (Ed.), *Psychiatry* (3rd ed.). New York: Oxford University Press.

U.S. Department of Veterans Affairs. (2015). *Suicide risk and risk of death among recent veterans*. Retrieved January 5, 2016, from http://www.publichealth.va.gov/epidemiology/studies/suicide-risk-death-risk-recent-veterans.asp#sthash.5b2WGSA5.dpuf.

Wahowiac, L. (2015). *Addressing stigma, disparities in minority mental health: Access to care among barriers*. Retrieved December 15, 2015, from http://thenationshealth.aphapublications.org/content/45/1/1.3.full.

Weiss, T., & Skelton, K. (2011). PTSD is a risk factor for metabolic syndrome in an impoverished urban population. *General Hospital Psychiatry, 33*, 135–142.

Anxiety, Anxiety Disorders, and Obsessive-Compulsive and Related Disorders

Elizabeth M. Varcarolis

e http://evolve.elsevier.com/Varcarolis/essentials

KEY TERMS AND CONCEPTS

acting-out behaviors, p. 135
acute anxiety, p. 131
agoraphobia, p. 139
altruism, p. 133
anxiety, p. 131
anxiolytic drugs, p. 147
burnout, p. 143
chronic anxiety, p. 137
compassion fatigue/secondary traumatic
    stress, p. 143
compulsions, p. 141
denial, p. 136
devaluation, p. 135
displacement, p. 134

dissociation, p. 135
fear, p. 131
generalized anxiety disorder (GAD), p. 139
hoarding, p. 141
idealization, p. 135
mild anxiety, p. 131
moderate anxiety, p. 131
normal anxiety, p. 131
obsessions, p. 141
obsessive-compulsive disorder (OCD), p. 141
panic attack, p. 138
panic disorders (PDs), p. 138
panic level of anxiety, p. 131
passive aggression, p. 135

pathological anxiety, p. 131
phobia, p. 139
projection, p. 136
rationalization, p. 135
reaction formation, p. 134
repression, p. 134
severe anxiety, p. 131
social phobia, p. 139
somatization, p. 135
specific phobias, p. 139
splitting, p. 136
sublimation, p. 134
suppression, p. 134
undoing, p. 135

SELECTED CONCEPT: BURNOUT

Burnout can occur in any work-related situation. Burnout occurs among health care professionals when feelings of disengagement, blunted emotions, frustration, depression, and negative feelings affect motivation and drive, and results in demoralization. Burnout produces a sense of helplessness and hopelessness.

    When working long periods of time in demanding situations, nurses and other health care professionals may no longer be able to function effectively and feel constantly overwhelmed, depressed, and ineffectual.

(Reese, 2011)

OBJECTIVES

1. Differentiate among normal anxiety, acute anxiety, and chronic anxiety.
2. Contrast and compare the four levels of anxiety in relation to perceptual field, ability to learn, and physical and other defining behavioral characteristics.
3. Summarize five properties of the defense mechanisms.
4. Give a definition for at least six defense mechanisms.
5. Rank the defense mechanisms from healthy to highly detrimental.
6. Describe clinical manifestations of each anxiety disorder.
7. Formulate four NANDA International nursing diagnoses that might be appropriate in the care of an individual with an anxiety disorder.
8. Name three defense mechanisms commonly used in excess by patients with anxiety disorders.

9. Propose realistic outcome criteria for patients with (a) generalized anxiety disorder, (b) panic disorder, and (c) obsessive-compulsive disorder.
10. **QSEN** Discuss three classes of medications that have demonstrated **evidence-based** effectiveness in treating anxiety disorders.
11. **QSEN** Identify the patient's experience and needs when planning **patient-centered care** for a person with obsessive-compulsive disorder.
12. Compare and contrast the differences between hoarding behaviors with obsessive-compulsive disorder (OCD) and hoarding behaviors without OCD.

INTRODUCTION

An understanding of anxiety and anxiety defense mechanisms is basic to the practice of psychiatric nursing. One of the greatest contributions to psychiatric nursing by Hildegard Peplau (1909 to 1999) was the operational definition of the four levels of anxiety and the recommendation of appropriate interventions to treat each level of anxiety. Anxiety is the most basic of human emotions to which no one is a stranger. Dysfunctional behaviors are often a defense against anxiety. When the behavior is recognized as dysfunctional, interventions to reduce anxiety can be initiated by the nurse. As anxiety decreases, dysfunctional behavior will frequently decrease.

ANXIETY

Anxiety and fear are indistinguishable except for the cause. Simply put, anxiety can be defined as a feeling of apprehension, uneasiness, uncertainty, or dread resulting from a real or perceived threat whose actual source is unknown or unrecognized. According to the *DSM-5*, the physiological response of anxiety is more often "associated with muscle tension and vigilance in preparation for future danger with cautious or avoidant behaviors" (APA, 2013, p. 189). Fear, on the other hand, is a reaction to a specific danger, and more often the body reacts "with surges of autonomic arousal necessary for fight or flight, thoughts of immediate danger, and escape behaviors" (APA, 2013, p. 189).

Another important distinction between anxiety and fear is that anxiety affects us at a deeper level than does fear. Anxiety invades the central core of the personality. It erodes the individual feelings of self-esteem and personal worth that contribute to a sense of being fully human.

Normal anxiety is a healthy life force that is necessary for survival. It provides the energy needed to carry out the tasks involved in living and striving toward goals. Anxiety motivates people to make and survive change. It prompts constructive behaviors, such as studying for an examination, being on time for a job interview, preparing for a presentation, and working toward a promotion.

Acute anxiety is precipitated by an imminent loss or change that threatens an individual's sense of security. Acute anxiety is a normal and expected response to stress. For example, many entertainers experience acute anxiety before live concerts or theater performances. Students may experience acute anxiety before an examination. Patients preparing for surgery often experience acute anxiety. The death of a loved one can stimulate acute anxiety when there is great disruption in the life of the bereaved person. In general, crisis involves the experience of acute anxiety.

Pathological anxiety differs from normal anxiety in terms of duration, intensity, and disturbance in a person's ability to function (e.g., dysfunctional behaviors or extreme withdrawal). Pathological anxiety "occurs with an intensity that is out of proportion to the threat, persists after the threat is resolved, becomes generalized to benign situations, or occurs in the complete absence of a stressor" (Schneir et al., 2014, p. 169).

These are the kinds of responses that we see in the anxiety disorders. An understanding of the types, levels, and defensive patterns used in response to anxiety is basic to psychiatric nursing care. This understanding is essential for effectively assessing and planning interventions to help both patients and nurses lower their levels of anxiety.

LEVELS OF ANXIETY

Levels of anxiety range from mild, to moderate, to severe, to panic. Peplau's (1968) classic delineation of these four levels of anxiety is based on the work by Harry Stack Sullivan (1953) (American psychiatrist and theorist, 1892 to 1949). Assessment of a patient's level of anxiety is basic to therapeutic intervention in any setting—psychiatric, hospital, general hospital, or community. Identification of a specific level of anxiety can be used as a guideline in selecting interventions. Although four levels of anxiety from mild to panic have been defined, the boundaries between these levels are not distinct, and the behaviors and characteristics shown by individuals experiencing anxiety can and often do overlap these categories. Use Table 11-1 as a guide for making observations.

Mild Anxiety

Mild anxiety occurs in the normal experience of everyday living. A person's ability to perceive reality is brought into sharp focus. A person sees, hears, and grasps more information, and problem solving becomes more effective. A person may display physical symptoms such as slight discomfort, restlessness, irritability, or mild tension-relieving behaviors (e.g., nail biting, foot or finger tapping, fidgeting).

Moderate Anxiety

As anxiety escalates, the patient's perceptual field narrows and some details are excluded from observation. An individual experiencing moderate anxiety sees, hears, and grasps less information than someone who is not in that state. Individuals may demonstrate **selective inattention,** in which only certain things in the environment are seen or heard. The ability to think clearly is hampered, but learning and problem solving can still take place, although not at an optimal level. At the moderate level of anxiety, the person's ability to solve problems is enhanced greatly by the supportive presence of another person. Physical symptoms include tension, pounding heart, increased pulse and respiration rates, perspiration, and mild somatic symptoms (e.g., gastric discomfort, headache, urinary urgency). Voice tremors and shaking may be noticed. Mild or moderate anxiety levels can be constructive, because anxiety can be viewed as a signal that something in the person's life needs attention.

Severe Anxiety

The perceptual field of a person experiencing severe anxiety is greatly reduced. A person with severe anxiety may focus on one particular detail or many scattered details. The person will have difficulty noticing events occurring in the environment, even when they are pointed out by another. Learning and problem solving are not possible at this level, and the person may be dazed and confused. Behavior is automatic and aimed at reducing or relieving anxiety. Often the individual complains of increased severity of somatic symptoms (e.g., headache, nausea, dizziness, insomnia), trembling, and pounding heart. The most classic experiences are hyperventilation and a sense of impending doom or dread.

Panic Level of Anxiety

The panic level of anxiety is the most extreme form and results in markedly disturbed behavior. An individual is not able to process events in the environment and may lose touch with reality. The resulting behavior may be confusion, shouting, screaming, or withdrawal. Hallucinations, or false sensory perceptions such as seeing people or objects that are not present, may be experienced by people at panic levels of anxiety. Physical behavior may be erratic, uncoordinated, and impulsive. Automatic behaviors are used to reduce and relieve anxiety, although such efforts may be ineffective. Acute panic may lead to exhaustion. Review Table 11-1 to identify the levels of anxiety and review how the level affects (1) perceptual field, (2) ability to learn, and (3) physical manifestations and other defining characteristics.

TABLE 11-1   Anxiety Levels and Their Characteristics

Mild	Moderate	Severe	Panic
Perceptual Field			
May have heightened perceptual field	Has narrow perceptual field; grasps less of what is occurring	Has greatly reduced perceptual field	Unable to focus on the environment
Is alert and can see, hear, and grasp what is happening in the environment	Can attend to more *if pointed out by another* (selective inattention)	Focuses on details or one specific detail	Experiences the utmost state of terror and emotional paralysis; feels he or she "ceases to exist"
Can identify issues that are disturbing and are producing anxiety		Attention scattered	In panic, may have hallucinations or delusions that take the place of reality
		Completely absorbed with self	
		May not be able to attend to events in environment *even when pointed out by others*	
		In severe to panic levels of anxiety, the environment is blocked out; it is as if these events are not occurring	
Ability to Learn			
Able to work effectively toward a goal and examine alternatives	Able to solve problems but not at optimal ability	Unable to see connections between events or details	May be mute or have extreme psychomotor agitation leading to exhaustion
	Benefits from guidance of others	Has distorted perceptions	Shows disorganized or irrational reasoning
Mild and moderate levels of anxiety can alert the person that something is wrong and can stimulate appropriate action		*Severe and panic levels prevent problem solving and discovery of effective solutions*	
		Unproductive relief behaviors are implemented, thus perpetuating a vicious cycle	
Physical or Other Characteristics			
Slight discomfort	Voice tremors	Feelings of dread	Experience of terror
Attention-seeking behaviors	Change in voice pitch	Ineffective functioning	Immobility or severe hyperactivity or flight
Restlessness	Difficulty concentrating	Confusion	Dilated pupils
Irritability or impatience	Shakiness	Purposeless activity	Unintelligible communication or inability to speak
Mild tension-relieving behavior: foot or finger tapping, lip chewing, fidgeting	Repetitive questioning	Sense of impending doom	Severe shakiness
	Somatic complaints (e.g., urinary frequency and urgency, headache, backache, insomnia)	More intense somatic complaints (e.g., dizziness, nausea, headache, sleeplessness)	Sleeplessness
	Increased respiration rate	Hyperventilation	Severe withdrawal
	Increased pulse rate	Tachycardia	Hallucinations or delusions; likely out of touch with reality
	Increased muscle tension	Withdrawal	
	More extreme tension-relieving behavior; pacing, banging hands on table	Loud and rapid speech	
		Threats and demands	

INTERVENTIONS

Mild to Moderate Levels of Anxiety

A patient experiencing a mild to moderate level of anxiety is still able to solve problems; however, the ability to concentrate decreases as anxiety increases. The nurse can help the patient focus and solve problems with the use of specific communication techniques, such as employing open-ended questions, giving broad openings, and exploring and seeking clarification. These techniques can be useful to a patient experiencing mild to moderate anxiety. Restricting topics of communication and introducing irrelevant topics can increase a person's anxiety and are tactics that usually make the *nurse,* not the patient, feel better.

Helpful Interventions

Reducing the patient's level of anxiety and preventing escalation of anxiety can be accomplished by being calm, recognizing the anxious patient's distress, and being willing to listen. Evaluation of effective past coping mechanisms is useful. Often the nurse can help the patient consider alternatives to problem situations and offer activities that may temporarily relieve feelings of inner tension. Table 11-2 identifies counseling interventions useful in assisting people experiencing mild to moderate levels of anxiety.

Severe to Panic Levels of Anxiety

A patient experiencing a severe to panic level of anxiety is unable to solve problems and may have a poor grasp of events occurring in the environment. Unproductive relief behaviors may predominate and the person may not be in control of his or her actions. Extreme regression and aimless behaviors are behavioral manifestations of a person's intense psychic pain. The nurse must be concerned with the patient's safety and, at times, with the safety of others. Physical needs (e.g., for fluids and rest) must be met to prevent exhaustion.

Helpful Interventions

Anxiety reduction measures may take the form of moving the person to a quiet environment in which there is minimal stimulation and providing gross motor activities to drain some of the tension. The use of medications may have to be considered, but medications and restraints should be used only after other more personal and less restrictive interventions have failed to decrease anxiety to safer levels. Although communication may be scattered and disjointed, themes can often be heard that the nurse must address. The feeling that one is understood can decrease the sense of isolation and reduce anxiety.

TABLE 11-2 Interventions for Mild to Moderate Levels of Anxiety*

NURSING DIAGNOSIS: *Anxiety* (moderate) related to situational event or psychological stress, as evidenced by increase in vital signs, moderate discomfort, narrowing of perceptual field, and selective inattention

Intervention	Rationale
1. Help the patient identify anxiety. "Are you comfortable right now?"	1. It is important to validate observations with the patient, name the anxiety, and start to work with the patient to lower anxiety.
2. Anticipate anxiety-provoking situations.	2. Escalation of anxiety to a more disorganizing level is prevented.
3. Use nonverbal language to demonstrate interest (e.g., lean forward, maintain eye contact, nod your head).	3. Verbal and nonverbal messages should be consistent. The presence of an interested person provides a stabilizing focus.
4. Encourage the patient to talk about his or her feelings and concerns.	4. When concerns are stated aloud, problems can be discussed and feelings of isolation decreased.
5. Avoid closing off avenues of communication that are important for the patient. Focus on the patient's concerns.	5. When staff anxiety increases, changing the topic or offering advice is common but leaves the person isolated.
6. Ask questions to clarify what is being said. "I'm not sure what you mean. Give me an example."	6. Increased anxiety results in scattering of thoughts. Clarifying helps the patient identify thoughts and feelings.
7. Help the patient identify thoughts or feelings before the onset of anxiety. "What were you thinking right before you started to feel anxious?"	7. The patient is assisted in identifying thoughts and feelings, and problem solving is facilitated.
8. Encourage problem solving with the patient.*	8. Encouraging patients to explore alternatives increases sense of control and self-sufficiency, while decreasing anxiety.
9. Assist in developing alternative solutions to a problem through role play or modeling behaviors.	9. The patient is encouraged to try alternative behaviors and solutions to gain confidence and develop alternate skills in dealing with anxiety.
10. Explore behaviors that have worked to relieve anxiety in the past.	10. The patient is encouraged to mobilize successful coping mechanisms and strengths.
11. Provide outlets for dissipating excess energy (e.g., walking, playing table tennis, dancing, exercising).	11. Physical activity can provide relief of built-up tension, increase muscle tone, and increase endorphin levels.

*Patients experiencing mild to moderate anxiety levels are still able to problem solve.

Because individuals experiencing severe to panic levels of anxiety are unable to solve problems, techniques suggested for communicating with people with mild to moderate levels of anxiety are not always effective. Patients experiencing severe to panic anxiety levels are out of control, so they need to know that they are safe from their own impulses. **Firm, short, and simple statements are useful.**

Reinforcing commonalities in the environment and recognition of reality when there are distortions can also be useful interventions for severely anxious persons. Table 11-3 suggests some basic nursing interventions for patients with severe to panic levels of anxiety.

DEFENSE MECHANISMS

Responses to stress and anxiety are affected by factors such as age, gender, culture, life experiences, and lifestyle. Vaillant and Vaillant (2004) identified the classic three distinct classes of coping mechanisms that people use to overcome stressful and anxiety-provoking situations. It is important to note that social support is one mediating factor that has been heavily researched and has significant implications for nurses and other health care professionals. The fact that strong social supports from significant others can enhance mental and physical health and act as a significant buffer against distress has been well documented in the literature. Numerous studies have found a strong correlation between lower mortality rates and intact support systems.

All defense mechanisms are employed on an unconscious level, with the exception of sublimation. Defense mechanisms protect people from painful awareness of feelings and memories that can provoke overwhelming anxiety. Adaptive use of defense mechanisms helps people lower anxiety levels to achieve goals in acceptable ways.

Defense mechanisms operate all the time. However, when an individual is faced with a situation that triggers high levels of anxiety, that person may become more rigid in the use of defense mechanisms and

may revert to using less mature defenses. The degree of distortion of reality and disruption in interpersonal relationships determines if the use of a defense mechanism is adaptive (healthy) or maladaptive (unhealthy).

Sigmund Freud and his daughter Anna outlined most of the defense mechanisms that we recognize today. Five of the most important properties of defense mechanisms are as follows:
1. Defenses are a major means of managing conflict and affect.
2. Defenses are for the most part unconscious.
3. Defenses are discrete from one another.
4. Although defenses are often the hallmarks of major psychiatric syndromes, they are reversible.
5. Defenses are adaptive as well as pathological.

All defense mechanisms except sublimation and altruism can be used in both healthy and unhealthy ways. (Sublimation and altruism are considered very healthy coping mechanisms.) Specifically, the defense mechanism of **repression** is the foundation of all defense mechanisms that are used on an unconscious level. Most people use a variety of defense mechanisms but not always at the same level. Keep in mind that whether the use of defense mechanisms is adaptive or maladaptive is determined for the most part by their *frequency, intensity,* and *duration* of use.

The defense mechanisms are discussed in the following sections starting with the most mature and healthy, followed by those that are less healthy, and then by those that result in a greater degree of reality distortion and disruption in relationships and personal functioning.

Healthy Defenses
Altruism

In altruism, emotional conflicts and stressors are addressed by meeting the needs of others. Unlike in self-sacrificing behavior, in altruism the person receives gratification either vicariously or from the response of others.

TABLE 11-3 Interventions for Severe to Panic Levels of Anxiety*

NURSING DIAGNOSIS: *Anxiety* (severe, panic) related to severe threat (biochemical, environmental, psychosocial), as evidenced by verbal or physical acting out, extreme immobility, sense of impending doom, inability to differentiate reality (possible hallucinations or delusions), and inability to problem solve

Intervention	Rationale
1. Maintain a calm manner.	1. Anxiety is communicated interpersonally. The quiet calm of the nurse can serve to calm the patient. The presence of anxiety can escalate anxiety in the patient.
2. Always remain with the person experiencing an acute severe to panic level of anxiety.	2. Alone with immense anxiety, a person feels abandoned. A caring face may be the patient's only contact with reality when confusion becomes overwhelming.
3. Minimize environmental stimuli. Move to a quieter setting and stay with the patient.	3. Helps minimize distractions and triggers which can further escalate the individual's anxiety.
4. Use clear and simple statements and repetition.	4. A person experiencing a severe to panic level of anxiety has difficulty concentrating and processing information.
5. Use a low-pitched voice; speak slowly.	5. A high-pitched voice can convey anxiety. Low pitch can decrease anxiety.
6. Reinforce reality if distortions occur (e.g., seeing objects that are not there or hearing voices when no one is present).	6. Anxiety can be reduced by focusing on and validating what is happening in the environment.
7. Listen for themes in communication.	7. In severe to panic levels of anxiety, verbal communication themes may be the only indication of the patient's thoughts or feelings.
8. Attend to physical and safety needs when necessary (e.g., need for warmth, fluids, elimination, pain relief, family contact).	8. High levels of anxiety may obscure the patient's awareness of physical needs.
9. Because safety is an overall goal, physical limits may need to be set. Speak in a firm, authoritative voice: "You may not hit anyone here. If you can't control yourself, we will help you."	9. A person who is out of control is often terrorized. Staff must offer the patient and others protection from destructive and self-destructive impulses.
10. Provide opportunities for exercise (e.g., walk with nurse, use a punching bag, play table tennis).	10. Physical activity helps channel and dissipate tension and may temporarily lower anxiety.
11. When a person is constantly moving or pacing, offer high-calorie fluids.	11. Dehydration and exhaustion must be prevented.
12. Assess need for medication.	12. Exhaustion and physical harm to self and others must be prevented.

*Patients who are experiencing severe to panic levels of anxiety are no longer able to problem solve.

> **VIGNETTE**
>
> Six months after losing her husband in a car accident, Jeanette began to spend 1 day a week doing grief counseling with families who had lost a loved one. She found that she was effective in helping others in their grief, and she obtained a great deal of satisfaction and pleasure from helping others work through their pain.

Sublimation

Sublimation is an unconscious process of substituting constructive and socially acceptable activity for strong impulses that are not acceptable in their original form. Often these impulses are sexual or aggressive. A man with strong hostile feelings may choose to become a butcher, or he may participate in rough contact sports. A person who is unable to experience sexual activity may channel this energy into something creative, such as painting or gardening.

Humor

Humor makes life easier. An individual may deal with emotional conflicts or stressors by emphasizing the amusing or ironic aspects of the conflict or stressor through **humor.**

> **VIGNETTE**
>
> A man goes to an interview that means a great deal to him. He is being interviewed by the top executives of the company. He has recently had foot surgery and, on entering the interview room, he stumbles and loses his balance. There is a stunned silence, and then the man states calmly, "I was hoping I could put my best foot forward." With everyone laughing, the interview continues in a relaxed manner.

Suppression

Suppression is the conscious denial of a disturbing situation or feeling. For example, a student who has been studying for the state board examinations says, "I can't worry about paying my rent until after my exam tomorrow."

Intermediate Defenses
Repression

Repression is the exclusion of unpleasant or unwanted experiences, emotions, or ideas from conscious awareness. Examples include forgetting the name of a former boyfriend or girlfriend or forgetting an appointment to discuss poor grades. *Repression is considered the cornerstone of the defense mechanisms, and it is the first line of psychological defense against anxiety.*

Displacement

Transfer of emotions associated with a particular person, object, or situation to another person, object, or situation that is nonthreatening is called displacement. The frequently cited example in which the boss yells at the man, the man yells at his wife, the wife yells at the child, and the child kicks the cat demonstrates the successive use of displaced hostility. The use of displacement is common but not always adaptive. Spousal, child, and elder abuse are often cases of displaced hostility.

Reaction Formation

In reaction formation (also termed **overcompensation**), unacceptable feelings or behaviors are kept out of awareness by developing the opposite behavior or emotion. For example, a person who harbors hostility toward children becomes a Boy Scout leader.

Somatization

Somatization occurs when anxiety is repressed to an unconscious level but is revealed on a physical level in the form of physical symptoms that have no organic cause. Often the symptom functions as an attention-seeking device or as an excuse.

> **VIGNETTE**
>
> A professor develops laryngitis on the day he is scheduled to defend a research proposal to a group of peers.
>
> A woman who does not want to go out with the brother of her boss calls to say "her back went out," and she cannot make the date (and, in fact, her back is sore).

Undoing

Undoing compensates for an act or communication (e.g., giving a gift to undo an argument). A common behavioral example of undoing is compulsive hand washing. This can be viewed as cleansing oneself of an act or thought perceived as unacceptable.

Rationalization

Rationalization consists of justifying illogical or unreasonable ideas, actions, or feelings by developing acceptable explanations that satisfy the teller as well as the listener. Common examples are, "If I had Lynn's brains, I'd get good grades, too," or "Everybody cheats, so why shouldn't I?" Rationalization is a form of self-deception.

Immature Defenses
Passive Aggression

A passive-aggressive individual deals with emotional conflict or stressors by indirectly and unassertively expressing aggression toward others. On the surface, there is an appearance of compliance that masks covert resistance, resentment, and hostility. In passive aggression, aggression toward others is expressed through procrastination, failure, inefficiency, passivity, and illnesses that affect others more than oneself. Such passive-aggressive behaviors occur especially in response to assigned tasks or demands for independent action, responsibilities, or obligations.

> **VIGNETTE**
>
> Sam promises his boss that he is working on the presentation for important patients, even though he constantly "forgets" to bring in samples of the presentation. The day of the presentation, Sam calls in sick with the flu.
>
> A young woman unconsciously jealous of her roommate promises over and over to bring the special salad over to her roommate's mother's house for Thanksgiving. When putting the food out for dinner, it is noticed that the young woman "forgot" the special salad, forcing her roommate to go back to fetch it, costing her an hour and a half of drive time.

Acting-Out Behaviors

In acting out, an individual addresses emotional conflicts or stressors by actions rather than by reflections or feelings. For example, a person may lash out in anger verbally or physically to distract the self from threatening thoughts or feelings. The verbal or physical expression of anger can make a person feel temporarily less helpless or vulnerable. By lashing out at others, an individual can transfer the focus from personal doubts and insecurities to some other person or object. Acting-out behaviors are a destructive coping style.

> **VIGNETTE**
>
> When Harry was turned down a third time for a promotion, he went to his office and tore apart every patient file in his file cabinet. His initial feelings of worthlessness and lowered self-esteem related to the situation were interpreted by Harry to mean "I am no good." This thinking resulted in Harry quickly transforming these painful feelings into actions of anger and destruction. Temporarily, Harry felt more powerful and less vulnerable.

Dissociation

A disruption in the usually integrated functions of consciousness, memory, identity, or perception of the environment is known as dissociation.

> **VIGNETTE**
>
> A young mother who saw her son struck by a car was taken to a neighbor's house while the police dealt with the accident. Later she told the policeman, "I really don't remember what happened. The last thing I remember is going out the door to check on Johnny." At that moment, to protect herself from an unbearable situation, she separated the threatening event from awareness until she could begin to deal with her feelings of devastation.

Devaluation

Devaluation occurs when emotional conflicts or stressors are handled by attributing negative qualities to self or others. When devaluing another, the individual then appears good by contrast.

> **VIGNETTE**
>
> A woman who is very jealous of a coworker says, "Oh, yes, she won the award. Those awards don't mean anything anyway, and I wonder what she had to do to be chosen." In this way she minimizes the other woman's accomplishments and keeps her own fragile self-esteem intact.

Idealization

In idealization, emotional conflicts or stressors are addressed by attributing exaggerated positive qualities to others. Idealization is an important aspect of the development of the self. Children who grow up with parents they can respect and idealize develop healthy standards of conduct and morality.

When people idealize and overvalue a person in a new relationship, they are sure to be disappointed when the object of the idealization turns out to be human. This leads to a great deal of disappointment and painful lowering of self-esteem. Such individuals may then devalue and reject the object of their affection to protect their own self-esteem. This pattern can be repeated over and over on a job, in friendships, in intimate relationships, and in marriage.

> **VIGNETTE**
>
> Mary met the most "wonderful and perfect" man. No one could tell Mary that Jim was nice but had some quirks, like everyone else. Mary would not listen. When Jim failed to live up to Mary's expectations of giving her constant attention, adoration, and gifts, Mary was devastated. Shortly thereafter, she started saying that Jim was, like all men, a brute, and that she wanted no more to do with such an insensitive person.

Splitting

Splitting is the inability to integrate the positive and negative qualities of oneself or others into a cohesive image. Aspects of the self and of others tend to alternate between opposite poles; for example, either good, loving, worthy, and nurturing; or bad, hateful, destructive, rejecting, and worthless. Use of this defense mechanism is prevalent in personality disorders, especially in people who have borderline components, and will be discussed at greater length in Chapter 13.

VIGNETTE

Alice viewed her therapist as the most wonderful, loving, and insightful therapist she had ever seen. When her therapist refused to write her a prescription for Valium, Alice shouted at her that she was the "stupidest, most uncaring, and thickheaded person," and she demanded another therapist "right away."

Projection

A person unconsciously rejects emotionally unacceptable personal features and attributes them to other people, objects, or situations through **projection**. Projection is the hallmark of blaming, scapegoating, prejudicial thinking, and stigmatization. People who always feel that others are out to deceive or cheat them may be projecting onto others those characteristics in themselves that they find distasteful and cannot consciously accept.

Projection of anxiety can often be seen in systems (family, hospital, school, business, politics). In a family in which there are problems, the child is often scapegoated, and the pain and anxiety within the family are projected onto the child: "The problem is Tommy." In a larger system in which anxiety and conflict are present, the weakest members are scapegoated: "The problem is the nurses' aides … the students … the new salesman … the Democrats/Republicans who are to blame for the mess we're in today." When pain and anxiety exist within a system, projection can be an automatic relief behavior. Once the cause of the anxiety is identified, changes in relief behavior can ensue, and the system can become more functional and productive.

Denial involves escaping unpleasant realities by ignoring their existence. For example, a man believes that physical limitations reflect negatively on one's manhood. Thus he may deny chest pains, even though his family has a history of heart attacks, because of a threat to his self-image as a man. A woman whose health has deteriorated because of alcohol abuse denies she has a problem with alcohol by saying she can stop drinking whenever she wants. Table 11-4 gives examples of adaptive and maladaptive uses of some common defense mechanisms.

TABLE 11-4 Defense Mechanisms

Defense Mechanism	Adaptive/Within Normal Limits	Maladaptive
Repression	Man forgets his wife's birthday after a marital fight.	Woman is unable to enjoy sex after having pushed out of awareness a traumatic sexual incident from childhood.
Sublimation	Woman who is angry with her boss writes a short story about a heroic woman. By definition, use of sublimation is always constructive.	None
Regression	Four-year-old boy with a new baby brother starts sucking his thumb and wanting a bottle.	Man who loses a promotion starts complaining to others, does sloppy work, misses appointments, and arrives late for meetings.
Displacement	Patient criticizes a nurse after his family fails to visit.	Child who is unable to acknowledge fear of his father becomes fearful of animals.
Projection	Man who is unconsciously attracted to other women teases his wife about flirting.	Woman who has repressed an attraction toward other women refuses to socialize. She fears another woman will make homosexual advances toward her.
Compensation	Short man becomes assertively verbal and excels in business.	Individual drinks alcohol when self-esteem is low to diffuse discomfort temporarily.
Reaction formation	Recovering alcoholic constantly preaches about the evils of alcoholic beverages.	Mother who has an unconscious hostility toward her daughter is overprotective to protect daughter from harm, interfering with daughter's normal growth and development.
Denial	Man reacts to news of the death of a loved one by saying, "No, I don't believe you. The doctor said he was fine."	Woman whose husband died 3 years earlier still keeps his clothes in the closet and talks about him in the present tense.
Conversion	Student is unable to take a final examination because of a terrible headache.	Man becomes blind after seeing his wife flirt with other men.
Undoing	After flirting with her male secretary, a woman buys her husband tickets to a show.	Man with rigid and moralistic beliefs and repressed sexuality is driven to wash his hands to gain composure when around attractive women.
Rationalization	Employee says, "I didn't get the raise because the boss doesn't like me."	Father who thinks his son was fathered by another man excuses his malicious treatment of the boy by saying, "He is lazy and disobedient," when that is not the case.
Identification	Five-year-old girl dresses in her mother's shoes and dress and meets her father at the door.	Young boy thinks a neighborhood pimp with money and drugs is someone to emulate.
Introjection	After his wife's death, the husband has transient complaints of chest pains and difficulty breathing—the symptoms his wife had before she died.	Young child whose parents were overcritical and belittling grows up thinking that she is inferior. She has taken on her parents' evaluation of her as part of her self-image.
Suppression	Businessman who is preparing to make an important speech later in the day is told by his wife that morning that she wants a divorce. Although visibly upset, he puts the incident aside until after his speech, when he can give the matter his total concentration.	A woman who feels a lump in her breast shortly before leaving for a 3-week vacation puts the information in the back of her mind until after returning from her vacation.

ANXIETY DISORDERS

Anxiety is a normal response to threatening situations, and everyone experiences occasional distress. Anxiety becomes a problem when it interferes with adaptive behavior, causes physical symptoms, or exceeds a tolerable level. In individuals with anxiety disorders, the experience is often one of considerable functional impairment and distress.

Anxiety is painful. Defenses employed are often rigid, repetitive, and ineffective in an attempt to control anxiety and ward off painful feelings. The common element in anxiety disorders is that individuals experience a degree of anxiety that is so uncomfortably high and often persistent that it causes dysfunction at work and in social situation, and interferes with family functioning.

Anxiety can also be one of the first symptoms of a medical disorder, which is discussed later in this chapter. Conversely, anxiety disorders can mimic medical illnesses as well. Patients may visit a variety of medical practitioners seeking an explanation for their symptoms when in fact the basis of their complaints is an anxiety disorder.

PREVALENCE AND COMORBIDITY

Anxiety disorders are the most prevalent lifetime psychiatric disorders leading to stress and impairment worldwide (Black & Andreasen, 2014). Approximately one in four (25%) individuals in the United States will experience an anxiety disorder in his or her lifetime (Preston et al., 2013). Women have a lifetime prevalence rate of approximately 30% while for men the lifetime rate of anxiety disorders is approximately 19% (Sadock et al., 2015).

As mentioned, people with anxiety disorders frequently seek health care services for relief of physical symptoms. For example, 70% of patients with panic disorder (PD) had seen at least 10 medical practitioners without receiving a diagnosis or adequate treatment (Pollock et al., 2010) and others had developed symptoms of generalized anxiety disorder (GAD) shortly before exhibiting somatic symptoms. Often, many individuals go untreated.

Anxiety disorders are highly **comorbid/co-occurring** with each other, with major depressive disorders, and with alcohol and/or drug abuse. Major depressive disorder (MDD) co-occurs in up to half of people with anxiety disorders and produces greater impairment and poorer response to treatment. Substance abuse is also frequently present and has a similar negative effect on treatment as well. Anxiety disorders frequently co-occur with many other psychiatric disorders (e.g., eating disorders, bipolar disorders, dysthymia); several studies suggest that up to 90% of people with an anxiety disorder develop another psychiatric disorder during their lifetime.

Other co-occurring conditions that are medical in nature and have been well documented in the literature include cancer, heart disease, high blood pressure, irritable bowel syndrome, kidney and liver dysfunction, reduced immunity, and others. Chronic anxiety is thought to be associated with increased risk for cardiovascular morbidity and mortality. Usually anxiety disorders begin in childhood, adolescence, and early adulthood.

THEORY

Anxiety disorders are most likely caused by a complex interaction of biological, psychological, and environmental factors. There is no longer any doubt that biological factors such as genetic vulnerability may interact with stress or trauma to trigger pathological anxiety states in some individuals (e.g., phobias, panic attacks). By the same token, traumatic life events (witnessing spousal abuse, child abuse, muggings, sexual assault), psychosocial factors, and sociocultural factors also are etiologically significant.

Neurobiology

Although the neurobiology of anxiety and anxiety disorders is vastly complex, the following identifies some of the major factors in anxiety that relate directly to evidence-based nursing care. Refer to Chapter 4 for more information on the neurotransmitters and how medications work, and refer to Chapter 10 for more information on the stress response.

Certain anatomical pathways (the limbic system) provide structure for electrical impulses that either receive or send anxiety-related responses. Neurons release neurotransmitter messages.

The limbic system, referred to by some as "the emotional brain," consists of the amygdala, hippocampus, thalamus, hypothalamus, basal ganglia, and cingulate gyrus (Boundless, 2015). All of the components of the lymbic system work together to regulate some of the brain's most important processes. The three functions of the limbic system include:

- Scan the environment for threat-relevant cues and assess magnitude of the threat.
- Initiate the body's readiness to respond by eliciting the fight-or-flight response (see Chapter 10).
- Terminate reactivity after external stressors subside and restore the nervous system to a state of homeostasis.

The part of the limbic system most associated with anxiety disorders as well as the obsessive-compulsive disorders is the cingulate, where the neural pathways connect to the limbic system and prefrontal lobes that result in the regulation of emotions. The limbic system is involved in storing memories and creating emotions and is thought to be a major factor in processing anxiety-related information. Some of the other parts of the brain involved in anxiety and anxiety-related disorders are:

- Frontal cortex: cognitive interpretations (e.g., potential threat)
- Hypothalamus: activation of the stress response (fight-or-flight response; refer to Chapter 10)
- Hippocampus: associated with memory related to fear responses
- Amygdala: fear, especially related to phobic and panic disorders

There is a link between anxiety and specific areas of the brain. When anxiety occurs it causes an imbalance in certain neurotransmitters in the brain that regulate anxiety. Based on animal studies and responses to drug treatment, at present there are three main mediators of anxiety in the central nervous system that regulate anxiety responses; these are serotonin (5-HT), norepinephrine (NE), and γ-aminobutyric acid (GABA) (Sadock et al., 2015).

- Serotonin (5-HT): Serotonin levels are thought to be decreased in anxiety disorders. Therefore, it is hypothesized that serotonin dysfunction contributes to anxiety disorders. The selective serotonin reuptake inhibitors (SSRIs), which increase serotonin levels in the brain, are often first-line medications for the treatment of many anxiety disorders.
- Norepinephrine (NE): Norepinephrine is known to mediate arousal. When a person feels threatened (real or perceived), the level of norepinephrine (adrenaline) increases and can cause hyperarousal and increased anxiety. In some people with anxiety disorders, it is thought that the noradrenergic system is poorly regulated and can cause bursts of activity. Noradrenergic drugs such as propranolol (which blocks adrenergic receptor activity) and clonidine (which stimulates α-adrenergic receptors) are used to help lower anxiety.
- GABA (γ-aminobutyric acid): GABA is an inhibitory neurotransmitter in the brain. The release of GABA slows neural transmission, which has a calming effect. It is believed that people with anxiety disorders (e.g., panic disorder) diminish benzodiazepine receptor sensitivity. When benzodiazepine medications are given the benzodiazepine receptors can more readily facilitate the action of GABA. A number of drugs including antianxiety agents,

sedative-hypnotics, general anesthetics, and anticonvulsant drugs are the targets of the GABA receptor system, thus slowing neural transmission and lowering anxiety. Abnormalities of these benzodiazepine receptors may lead to unregulated anxiety levels.

Genetics

The fact that there are **genetic** components is substantiated by numerous studies that find anxiety disorders tend to cluster in families (Sadock et al., 2015). Twin studies indicate the existence of a genetic component to panic disorders (PDs). For example, there is a high concordance rate in monozygotic twins as compared with dizygotic twins; however, it is still uncertain if the genetic influence is specific to panic disorder or represents general anxiety proneness.

People with obsessive-compulsive disorder (OCD) also show genetic components as referred to in the section later in this chapter on OCD. Twin and family studies report that panic disorder has a hereditability of approximately 40%.

Cognitive Behavioral Theory
Behavioral Theory

Learning theories provide another view. Behavioral psychologists conceptualize anxiety as a learned response that can be unlearned. Some individuals may learn to be anxious from the modeling provided by parents or peers. For example, a mother who is fearful of thunder and lightning and who hides in closets during storms may transmit her anxiety to her children, who continue to adopt her behavior even into adult life. Such individuals can unlearn this behavior by observing others who react normally to a storm. For example, behavioral therapy in the form of gradually exposing a highly anxious person to a feared object or situation (such as that in agoraphobia) over time with support can help the person overcome his or her fear of the object or situation.

Cognitive Theory

Cognitive theorists believe that anxiety disorders are a result of distortions in an individual's thinking and perceiving. Because individuals with such distortions believe that any mistake they make will have catastrophic results, they experience acute anxiety. Brain scans taken before and after cognitive therapy treatment support the hypothesis that learning to reframe one's thinking can literally change the chemistry and function of the brain. Cognitive behavioral therapy seems to have the best evidence not only for effective psychotherapeutic treatment of anxiety disorders but also for more lasting results in other disorders and problematic situations.

CULTURAL CONSIDERATIONS

Reliable data on the incidence of anxiety disorders among cultures are sparse, but sociocultural variation in symptoms of anxiety disorders has been noted. In some cultures, individuals express anxiety through somatic symptoms, whereas in other cultures cognitive symptoms predominate. Panic attacks in Latin Americans and Northern Europeans often involve sensations of choking, smothering, numbness, or tingling, as well as fear of dying. In other cultural groups, panic attacks involve fear of magic or witchcraft. Social phobias in Japanese and Korean cultures may relate to a belief that the individual's blushing, eye contact, or body odor is offensive to others.

One of the barriers for some cultural groups seeking health care for anxiety disorders is the stigma that various cultures are associated with mental disorders. For example, African Americans are much less likely to seek mental health services than those from other cultural backgrounds, and Asian Americans are even more reticent to seek help (Satcher et al., 2005).

Interestingly, the incidence of anxiety disorders seems to vary among cultures and countries. Anxiety disorders also vary among immigrants from generation to generation. One must be aware of the cultural norm before hastily making a diagnosis (e.g., labeling ritualistic behavior as obsessive-compulsive disorder).

CLINICAL PICTURE

The term *anxiety disorder* refers to a number of disorders, including panic disorders, phobias, and general anxiety disorders, among others.

Panic Disorders

Panic disorder (PD) consists of recurrent and unexpected "out of the blue" panic attacks. The panic attack is the key feature of panic disorders (PDs). A panic attack is the sudden onset of extreme apprehension or fear, usually associated with feelings of impending doom: "I am going to die." Typically, panic attacks occur suddenly (not necessarily in response to stress), are extremely intense, and can last for 1 to 30 minutes before they subside. Panic attacks can happen at any time during the day or can occur while sleeping at night, causing a person to wake up terrified. The feelings of terror present during a panic attack are so severe that normal function is suspended, the perceptual field is severely limited, and misinterpretation of reality may occur. Severe personality disorganization is evident.

People experiencing panic attacks may believe that they are losing their minds or are having a heart attack; the attacks are often accompanied by highly uncomfortable physical symptoms. Some of the symptoms a person may experience are palpitations, chest pain, diaphoresis, muscle tension, urinary frequency, hyperventilation, breathing difficulties, nausea, feelings of choking, chills, hot flashes, and gastrointestinal symptoms. During the intervals between panic attacks, the person may experience low-level constant anxiousness and anticipatory anxiety. It is not uncommon for someone rushed to the emergency department (ED) with all the signs and symptoms of a heart attack (chest pain, difficulty breathing, dizziness, and excessive fatigue) to have an extensive medical workup that proves negative for cardiac problems. At that point the person needs to be referred to a counselor for potential diagnosis and treatment of an anxiety disorder. Major depression occurs in the majority of individuals with PD and complicates the course of the disorder considerably.

Panic attacks are usually terrifying and painful for the person who is experiencing them. Some studies have demonstrated that people with panic attacks have an 18% higher rate of suicide attempts as well as a higher suicide rate in the general population (Preston et al., 2013; Sadock et al., 2015).

The incidence of panic attacks over time may lead to complications such as persistent anxiety, phobic avoidance, depression, alcoholism, or other drug overuse. At times, people with panic disorder may also have agoraphobia. If agoraphobia is present, it is noted as a specifier on a *DSM-5* diagnosis.

Preston and Johnson (2015) cite the following pharmacological treatments as efficacious in the treatment of panic disorders:
- High-potency benzodiazepines, such as alprazolam, clonazepam, and lorazepam usually used on a short-term basis.
- Antidepressants such as tricyclics and SSRIs
- Monoamine oxidase inhibitors (MAOIs)
- Use of cognitive and behavioral therapy in conjunction with medications can help people learn skills to combat their panic, and is effective in the treatment among some individuals with panic attacks

Phobias

A phobia is a persistent, intense irrational fear of a specific object, activity, or situation that leads to a desire for avoidance, or actual avoidance, of the object, activity, or situation.

Specific phobias are characterized by the experience of high levels of anxiety or fear in response to specific objects or situations, such as dogs, spiders, heights, storms, water, blood, closed spaces, tunnels, and bridges. Specific phobias are common and usually do not cause much difficulty because people can contrive ways to avoid the feared object, such as cats or spiders, flying, or heights. However, the fear, anxiety, or avoidance in some cases may cause impairment in social, occupational, or other areas of functioning when faced with the feared object or situation. Clinical names for common phobias are provided in Table 11-5.

There is no evidence that these disorders are related to biological dysfunction and need medication to be treated. In fact, behavioral therapy seems to be the only therapy effective with specific phobias. According to the *DSM-5*, the prevalence rate for a specific phobia is approximately 7% to 9% over a 12-month period of time (APA, 2013).

Social anxiety disorders (SADs), or social phobias, are characterized by severe anxiety or fear provoked by exposure to a social situation or a performance situation, resulting in humiliation or embarrassment (e.g., fear of saying something that sounds foolish in public, fear of being unable to answer questions in a classroom, fear of eating in the presence of others, fear of performing on stage). The intense terror in these situations is fear of being evaluated or being rejected by others. Fear of public speaking is the most common social phobia. Many well-known performers suffer from terrific bouts of performance anxiety when appearing in front of an audience.

Social anxiety disorders are believed to be influenced by psychological factors such as the quality of early attachments, the development of appropriate social skills, inadequate experiences interacting with others, and other negative environmental influences (Sadock et al., 2015).

However, first-degree relatives of persons with a social anxiety disorder are three times more likely to develop a social anxiety disorder than those in the general population (Sadock et al., 2015). Twin studies suggest a complex genetic transmission of this disorder. There are currently ongoing biological studies to identify specific neurobiological factors associated with anxiety and fear.

The beta-blocker propranolol reduces the physiological symptoms of anxiety, although not the cognitive (e.g., worry) symptoms. Propranolol is used effectively by many performers or lecturers before appearing on stage to act, conduct, speak, and otherwise make a presentation in front of an audience. More pervasive social anxiety may

respond to monoamine oxidase inhibitors (MAOIs) and selective serotonin reuptake inhibitors (SSRIs). Cognitive therapy interventions along with social skills training are helpful for many.

Agoraphobia

Agoraphobia is an intense, excessive anxiety about or fear of being in places or situations where help might not be available and escape might be either difficult or embarrassing. The feared places or situations are avoided by the individual in an effort to control anxiety. Examples of situations that are commonly avoided by patients with agoraphobia are being alone outside the home; using public transportation (e.g., traveling in a car, bus, or airplane); being in open spaces (e.g., bridges, marketplaces, or parking lots); being in an enclosed place (e.g., elevators, churches, or theaters); or being in a crowd (APA, 2013). A *DSM-5* diagnosis is made when a person experiences fear or anxiety in at least two of the aforementioned situations. Avoidance behaviors can be debilitating and life constricting.

Agoraphobia is perhaps the most limiting and debilitating of all of the phobias. In its most extreme form, patients may simply refuse to leave their homes, putting great strain on family and friends and resulting in problems in their marriages. Characteristically, individuals with agoraphobia experience overwhelming and crippling anxiety when they are faced with the provoking object or situation. Even thinking about or visualizing the object or situation can cause a person to become severely anxious.

Consider the effects on a father whose avoidance renders him unable to leave home and who thus cannot work or participate in his children's school activities, such as attending school sports. Or consider the businesswoman whose avoidance of flying prevents her from attending business conferences or sales promotions.

The life of a person with agoraphobia becomes even more restricted when the symptoms become more severe and activities are discontinued. When the fears and anxieties become too intense, an individual may not be able to leave home and must rely on others to help him or her meet basic needs and provide everyday services such as shopping, walking the dog, and so on. All too frequently, complications ensue when individuals attempt to decrease anxiety or depression through self-medication with alcohol or drugs.

This disorder is thought to be primarily due to psychogenic causes that lead to a conditioned response of fear and anxiety. The disorder is chronic, although it responds well to cognitive behavioral therapy (CBT) and SSRI medications to help reduce the anxiety as well as treat the depression. Panic attacks may precede agoraphobia 30% to 50% of the time, depending on the specific source (APA, 2013).

Generalized Anxiety Disorder

Generalized anxiety disorder (GAD) is a chronic psychiatric disorder associated with severe distress different from other anxiety disorders in that there is pervasive cognitive dysfunction, impaired functioning, and poor health-related outcomes. GAD is highly comorbid with other mental disorders in particular social phobia, specific phobia, panic disorder, and depression. Self-medication may lead to alcohol or substance use disorder (see *DSM-5* box).

GAD also differs from other anxiety disorders in that patients do not fear a specific external object or situation, and there is no distinct symptomatic reaction pattern. Basically, GAD is characterized by excessive, persistent, and uncontrollable anxiety, and by excessive and constant worrying. It is sometimes referred to as the "worry disease" (e.g., What if I'm late? …What if I fail? …What if I am fired?). A diagnosis of GAD is made if at least three of the following symptoms are present: restlessness, fatigue, poor concentration, irritability, muscle tension, and sleep disturbance (APA, 2013).

TABLE 11-5 Clinical Names for Common Phobias

Clinical Name	Feared Object or Situation
Acrophobia	Heights
Agoraphobia	Open spaces
Astraphobia	Electrical storms
Claustrophobia	Closed spaces
Glossophobia	Talking
Hematophobia	Blood
Hydrophobia	Water
Monophobia	Being alone
Mysophobia	Germs or dirt
Nyctophobia	Darkness
Pyrophobia	Fire
Xenophobia	Strangers
Zoophobia	Animals

DSM-5 DIAGNOSTIC CRITERIA
for Generalized Anxiety Disorder

A. Excessive anxiety and worry (apprehensive expectation), occurring more days than not for at least 6 months, about a number of events or activities (such as work or school performance).

B. The individual finds it difficult to control the worry.

C. The anxiety and worry are associated with three (or more) of the following six symptoms (with at least some symptoms having been present for more days than not for the past 6 months):

NOTE: Only one item is required in children.

1. Restlessness or feeling keyed up or on edge
2. Being easily fatigued
3. Difficulty concentrating or mind going blank
4. Irritability
5. Muscle tension
6. Sleep disturbance (difficulty falling or staying asleep, or restless, unsatisfying sleep)

D. The anxiety, worry, or physical symptoms cause clinically significant distress or impairment in social, occupational, or other important areas of functioning.

E. The disturbance is not attributable to the physiological effects of a substance (e.g., a drug of abuse, a medication) or another medical condition (e.g., hyperthyroidism).

F. The disturbance is not better explained by another mental disorder (e.g., anxiety or worry about having panic attacks in panic disorder, negative evaluation in social anxiety disorder [social phobia], contamination or other obsessions in obsessive-compulsive disorder, separation from attachment figures in separation anxiety disorder, reminders of traumatic events in posttraumatic stress disorder, gaining weight in anorexia nervosa, physical complaints in somatic symptom disorder, perceived appearance flaws in body dysmorphic disorder, having a serious illness in illness anxiety disorder, or the content of delusional beliefs in schizophrenia or delusional disorder).

From the American Psychiatric Association. (2013). *Diagnostic and statistical manual of mental disorders*. (5th ed.). Washington, DC: APA.

The individual's worry is out of proportion to the true effect of the event or situation about which the individual is focused for most days during a 6-month period in order to qualify for *DSM-5* diagnosis. Examples of worries typical in GAD are inadequacy in interpersonal relationships, job responsibilities, finances, health of family members, household chores, and lateness for appointments. In fact, these excessive worries are conducive to disturbances in relationships and family life, impaired functioning at work, and disturbances in social roles. Sleep disturbance is common because the individual worries about the day's events and real or imagined mistakes, reviews past problems, and anticipates future difficulties during sleep hours. These constant worries leave the limbic system in a perpetual state of alertness. Decision making is difficult because of poor concentration and dread of making a mistake. Somatic symptoms are not uncommon and include sweating, nausea, and diarrhea.

GAD is thought by many to be a psychogenic disorder. However, there is also speculation that GAD may be biologically mediated. For example, buspirone and 5-HT serotonin antagonists (SSRIs) are effective in reducing the "what if's" and worrying in GAD patients (Preston & Johnson, 2015). An overview of medications and therapies for specific anxiety disorders is found in Table 11-6.

Anxiety Due to Medical Conditions

In anxiety attributable to medical conditions, the individual's symptoms of panic attacks and anxiety are a direct physiological result of a medical condition. Examples include the following:

TABLE 11-6   Potential Nursing Diagnoses for the Anxious Patient

Signs and Symptoms	Nursing Diagnoses
• Concern that a panic attack will occur	*Anxiety (moderate, severe, panic)*
• Exposure to phobic object or situation	*Fear*
• Presence of obsessive thoughts	
• Recurrent memories of traumatic event	
• Fear of panic attacks	
• High levels of anxiety that interfere with the ability to work, disrupt relationships, and change ability to interact with others	*Ineffective coping* *Deficient diversional activity*
• Avoidance behaviors (phobia, agoraphobia)	*Social isolation*
• Hypervigilance after a traumatic event	*Ineffective role performance*
• Inordinate time taken for obsession and compulsions	*Impaired social interaction*
	Ineffective relationship
• Difficulty with concentration	*Post-trauma syndrome*
• Preoccupation with obsessive thoughts	
• Disorganization associated with exposure to phobic object	
• Intrusive thoughts and memories of traumatic event	
• Excessive use of reason and logic associated with overcautiousness and fear of making a mistake	
• Inability to go to sleep related to intrusive thoughts, worrying, replaying of a traumatic event, hypervigilance, fear	*Sleep deprivation* *Disturbed sleep pattern* *Fatigue*
• Feelings of hopelessness, inability to control one's life, low self-esteem related to inability to have some control in one's life	*Hopelessness* *Chronic low self-esteem* *Spiritual distress*
• Inability to perform self-care related to rituals	*Self-care deficit*
• Skin excoriation related to rituals of excessive washing or excessive picking at the skin	*Impaired skin integrity*
• Inability to eat because of constant ritual performance	*Imbalanced nutrition: less than body requirements*
• Feeling of anxiety or excessive worrying that overrides appetite and need to eat	
• Excessive overeating to appease intense worrying or high anxiety levels	*Imbalanced nutrition: more than body requirements*

Herdman, T.H. (Ed.) *Nursing Diagnoses-Definitions and Classification 2015-2017*. Copyright 2014, 1994-2014 NANDA International. Used by arrangement with John Wiley & Sons Limited. In order to make safe and effective judgments using NANDA-I nursing diagnoses it is essential that nurses refer to the definitions and defining characteristics of the diagnoses listed in this work.

- **Respiratory:** asthma, hypoxia, pulmonary edema, chronic obstructive pulmonary disease (COPD), pulmonary embolism
- **Cardiovascular:** cardiac dysrhythmias such as torsades de pointes, angina, congestive heart failure, mitral valve prolapse, hypertension
- **Endocrine:** hyperthyroidism, hypoglycemia, hypercortisolism, pheochromocytoma
- **Neurological:** Parkinson's disease, akathisia, postconcussion syndrome, complex partial seizures
- **Metabolic:** hypercalcemia, hyperkalemia, hyponatremia, porphyria

To determine whether the anxiety symptoms are caused by a medical condition, a careful and comprehensive assessment of multiple factors is necessary. Evidence must be present in the history, physical examination, and/or laboratory findings to diagnose the medical condition. Anxiety also can be caused by medications or substances, and when that occurs a *DSM-5* diagnosis would be made of substance/medication-induced anxiety disorder.

Separation anxiety in children, now under the heading of Anxiety Disorders, will be discussed in Chapter 26. It is important to note, however, that separation anxiety exists in the adult population as well.

OBSESSIVE-COMPULSIVE AND RELATED DISORDERS

Obsessive-compulsive disorder (OCD) usually begins the late teens or early twenties and ranges from mild to severe. There is substantial evidence that OCD has biological origins and is thought by many to be a neurologically based disorder. OCD seems to occur more often in patients with other neurological disorders, such as in Huntington's chorea epilepsy, Sydenham's chorea, and brain trauma (Black & Andreasen, 2014). OCD is related to Tourette's disorder; there is a high frequency of one disorder co-occurring with the other. Other factors that support OCD as a neurological disorder include the following (Black & Andreasen, 2014; Sadock et al., 2015).

1. Brain imaging studies show an increase in metabolic activity in patients with OCD, specifically hyperactivity in the prefrontal cortex and dysfunction in the basal ganglia and cingulum. Some researchers speculate that the basal ganglia dysfunction is responsible for the complex motor programs involved in OCD, whereas the tendency to worry and plan excessively is a result of the prefrontal cortex hyperactivity.

2. There is evidence that OCD has a significant genetic component based on family and twin studies.

3. The hypothesis is that dysregulation of serotonin levels is involved in the etiology of OCD. Clinical studies have shown that OCD patients are responsive to SSRIs whereas other antidepressants are ineffective, with the exception of the tricyclic antidepressant *clomipramine* that has proven especially effective in people with OCD.

Obsessive-compulsive (OC) symptoms are common, but obsessive-compulsive disorders (OCDs) can be extremely disabling and painful. OCD is no longer considered uncommon.

Obsessions are defined as thoughts, impulses, or images that persist and recur so that they cannot be dismissed from the mind. Obsessions often seem senseless to the individual who experiences them, although they still cause the individual to experience severe anxiety. Common obsessions include fear of hurting a loved one or fear of contamination.

Compulsions are ritualistic behaviors that an individual feels driven to perform in an attempt to reduce anxiety. Common compulsions are repetitive hand washing and checking a door multiple times to make sure it is locked. Compulsions can include mental acts as well, such as counting, praying, or performing a compulsive act that temporarily reduces high levels of anxiety. The primary gain is achieved by compulsive rituals, but because the relief is only temporary, the compulsive act must be repeated many times.

Although obsessions and compulsions can exist independently of each other, they almost always occur together as in **obsessive-compulsive disorder (OCD)**. OCD behavior exists along a continuum. "Normal" individuals may experience mildly obsessive-compulsive behavior. Nearly everyone has experienced having a song playing persistently through the mind, despite attempts to push it away. Many people have had nagging doubts as to whether a door is locked or the stove is turned off. These doubts require the person to go back to check the door or stove. Minor compulsions, such as touching a lucky charm, knocking on wood, and making the sign of the cross upon hearing disturbing news, are not harmful to the individual. Mild compulsions

(timeliness, orderliness, and reliability) are valued traits in selective contexts in the U.S. society.

At the more severe end of the continuum are obsessive-compulsive symptoms that typically center on dirtiness, contamination, and germs and occur with corresponding compulsions, such as cleaning and hand washing. A smaller number focus on safety issues and engage in repetitive checking rituals. At the most severe levels are persistent thoughts of sexuality, violence, illness, or death. These obsessions or compulsions cause marked distress to the individual. People often feel humiliation and shame regarding these behaviors. The rituals are time-consuming and interfere with normal routine, social activities, and relationships with others. Severe OCD consumes so much of the individual's mental processes that the performance of cognitive tasks may be impaired. Suicide can be a risk for these individuals, especially in the presence of a co-occurring depression.

Body Dysmorphic Disorder

Body dysmorphic disorder (BDD) is a highly distressing and impairing disorder that ranges along the continuum from distressing to delusional severity. Patients with BDD usually have a normal appearance, although a small number do show minor defects. The average age of onset is younger than 20 years. A *DSM-5* diagnosis includes preoccupation with an imagined "defective body part"; obsessional thinking (e.g., thinking they are ugly or deformed) and compulsive behaviors (e.g., such as mirror checking, skin picking, or excessive grooming); and impairment of normal social activities related to academic or occupational functioning. Individuals with BDD are frequently concerned with the face, skin, genitalia, thighs, hips, and hair.

Usually the person feels great shame and hides or withdraws from others. Many will alter their appearance through plastic surgeries, wrongly perceiving themselves as being ugly or having "hideous physical flaws." (People with BDD may have multiple plastic surgeries.) Unfortunately, cosmetic surgery often does not relieve the symptoms.

Researchers have found that BDD patients who have plastic surgery (e.g., rhinoplasty or breast enlargement) are rarely satisfied with the results. Among the most common co-occurring disorders include major depression, substance use disorder, and social phobia.

Individuals with BDD have higher rates of suicidal ideation, suicide attempts, and completed suicides than individuals who did not meet criteria for BDD. The disorder is often kept secret for many years, and the patient does not respond to reassurance. The pharmacological agents of choice for treating people with BDD are SSRIs, antidepressants, and clomipramine (a tricyclic antidepressant) and cognitive behavioral therapy (CBT). A second-generation antipsychotic added to an SSRI may help in the more severe delusional form of BDD.

Hoarding

Compulsive hoarding is associated with excessive collecting of items that are essentially worthless (although wealthy individuals have been known to hoard paintings, statues, and other valuable items from all over the world). These individuals often feel shame for their failure to discard excessive amounts of these items. People with compulsive hoarding suffer extreme disruption in daily living and severe distress, and hoarding can be disabling and result in self-imposed social isolation. Often these individuals live in unsafe conditions. Their homes may be cluttered to the point where getting from room to room is almost impossible. The items hoarded may include garbage and trash, broken objects, old newspapers, books, and old clothing piled indiscriminately in their home. Kitchens may not be usable, beds cannot be slept in, and chairs, couches, and tables may be buried under piles of hoarded items. It has been noted by clinicians that in people with OCD excessive hoarding is associated with the following:

- Increased co-occurring mood or anxiety disorder
- Impairment in the performance of activities of daily living
- Distractibility
- Reduced insight and indecisiveness
- Poor response to standard psychological and pharmacological treatments
- A distinct genetic and neurobiological profile

Compulsive hoarding does not meet the *DSM-5* criteria for OCD.

APPLICATION OF THE NURSING PROCESS

ASSESSMENT

Symptoms of Anxiety

People with anxiety disorders rarely need hospitalization unless they are suicidal or have compulsions causing injury (e.g., cutting self). Therefore most patients prone to anxiety are encountered in a variety of community settings. A common example of an acute anxiety episode occurs when an individual who is taken to an emergency department to rule out a heart attack is found to be experiencing a panic attack. Therefore one of the first things that may need to be determined is whether the anxiety is from a secondary source (medical condition or substances) or a primary source, as in an anxiety disorder.

Defenses Used in Anxiety Disorders

People use a variety of ego defenses and behaviors to lessen the uncomfortable levels of anxiety. Psychodynamic theorists believe that people who suffer from anxiety disorders employ specific defenses. A comprehensive and sophisticated assessment tool is the Hamilton rating scale. *A word of caution:* The Hamilton scale highlights important areas in the assessment of anxiety. But because many answers are subjective, experienced clinicians use this tool as a guide when planning care and draw on their knowledge of their patients.

≫ Assessment Guidelines
Anxiety Disorders

1. Ensure that a sound physical and neurological examination is performed to help determine whether the anxiety is primary or secondary to another psychiatric disorder, a medical condition, or substance use.
2. Assess potential for self-harm and/or suicide. It is known that people suffering from high levels of intractable anxiety may contemplate, attempt, or complete suicide.
3. Perform a psychosocial assessment. Always ask the person, "What has happened recently that might be increasing your anxiety?" The patient may identify a problem that should be addressed through counseling or therapy (e.g., stressful marriage, recent loss, stressful job or school situation). In some situations, there may be no identifiable recent event.
4. Assess cultural beliefs and background. Differences in culture can affect how anxiety is manifested.

DIAGNOSIS

NANDA International (NANDA-I, 2015–2017) provides many nursing diagnoses that are appropriate for individuals experiencing high or extreme levels of anxiety and anxiety disorders. The "related to" component will vary with the individual. Table 11-6 identifies potential nursing diagnoses for the anxious patient. Included are the signs and symptoms that might be found on assessment that support the diagnoses.

OUTCOMES IDENTIFICATION

The Nursing Outcomes Classification (NOC) identifies a number of desired outcomes for patients with anxiety or anxiety-related disorders (Moorhead et al., 2012). *Psychiatric–Mental Health Nursing: Scope and Standards of Practice* (ANA, 2014) emphasizes that outcomes should, among other considerations:

- Reflect patient values and ethical and environmental situations.
- Be culturally appropriate.
- Be documented as measurable goals.
- Include a time estimate of expected outcomes.

Table 11-7 identifies short- and long-term outcomes using the criteria from *Psychiatric–Mental Health Nursing: Scope and Standards of Practice* (ANA, 2014).

PLANNING

Anxiety disorders are encountered in numerous settings. Nurses care for people with concurrent anxiety disorders in medical-surgical units and in outpatient settings, such as homes, day programs, and clinics. Usually patients with anxiety disorders do not require admission to inpatient psychiatric units. Therefore, planning for care usually involves selecting interventions that can be implemented in a community setting.

Whenever possible, individuals with anxiety disorders should be encouraged to participate actively in planning. By sharing decision making with the patient, the nurse increases the likelihood of positive outcomes. Shared planning is especially appropriate for a patient with mild or moderate anxiety. When the patient is experiencing severe levels of anxiety, he or she may be unable to participate in planning, which requires the nurse to take a more directive role.

TABLE 11-7	Short- and Long-Term Outcomes for Specific Anxiety Disorders
Anxiety Disorder	**Short- or Long-Term Outcomes**
Phobia	Patients will: • Develop skills at reframing anxiety-provoking situation (by date). • Work with nurse/clinician to desensitize self to feared object or situation (by date). • Demonstrate one new relaxation skill that works well for them (by date).
Generalized anxiety disorder	Patients will: • State increased ability to make decisions and problem solve. • Demonstrate ability to perform usual tasks even though still moderately anxious (by date). • Demonstrate one cognitive or behavioral coping skill that helps reduce anxious feelings (by date).
Obsessive-compulsive disorder	Patients will: • Demonstrate techniques that can distract and distance self from thoughts that are anxiety producing (by date). • Decrease time spent in ritualistic behaviors. • Demonstrate increased amount of time spent with family and friends and on pleasurable activities. • State they have more control over intrusive thoughts and rituals (by date).

Self-Care for Nurses

Anxiety is communicated empathetically from person to person. Therefore, it is not surprising that being around an anxiety-disordered person may cause the nurse to experience intense and uncomfortable emotions. When working with highly anxious patients, students and new clinicians will do best to work under supervision of a more experienced health care professional. Supervision can help nurses/health care professionals identify and intervene with their emotions when they become negative and problematic. When nurses in any situation feel anger, frustration, or other negative feelings toward the patient, the nurse and patient will most likely experience a situation of mutual withdrawal.

Common responses when working with anxiety-disordered clients include increased anxiety, frustration, anger, and other negative emotions. For example, in communication techniques used with people with OCD, the nurse provides very clear and structured communication, because a person with OCD tends to correct and clarify repeatedly as though he or she cannot let go of any topic. This can cause frustration and anger in the nurse/clinician. When working with people who are phobic and/or agoraphobic, angry feelings may arise when the person does not make rapid progress. Feelings of frustration, anger, and anxiety and negative feelings can cause tension and fatigue from mental strain. These feelings of frustration and mental strain, especially over a period of time, may lead to burnout. Burnout is defined as "a state of physical, emotional, and mental exhaustion caused by long-term involvement in emotionally demanding situations" (Pines & Aronson, 2008), as opposed to compassion fatigue/secondary traumatic stress, described under PTSD in Chapter 10. Supervision, stress management courses, mindfulness, yoga, exercise, creative activities, and humor are all examples of stress reduction techniques (refer to Box 10-1 for selected stress reduction techniques). As instructors often tell their students, "keep your bucket full," meaning students as well as health care providers need to work at keeping a healthy balance in their personal lives.

IMPLEMENTATION

The nurse follows the *Psychiatric–Mental Health Nursing: Scope and Standards of Practice* (ANA, 2014) when intervening with patients. Whenever possible, interventions should be based on the *best evidence available*. Overall guidelines for basic nursing interventions are as follows:

1. Identify community resources that can offer specialized treatment that is proven to be highly effective for people with a variety of anxiety disorders.
2. Identify community support groups for people with specific anxiety disorders and their families.
3. Use therapeutic communication, milieu therapy, promotion of self-care activities, psychotherapy, and health teaching and health promotion as appropriate.

Communication Guidelines

Psychiatric mental health nurses use therapeutic communication skills to assist patients with anxiety disorders to reduce anxiety, enhance coping and communication skills, and intervene in crises. When patients request or prefer to use integrative therapies, the nurse performs assessment and teaching as appropriate.

Health Teaching and Health Promotion

Health teaching is a significant nursing intervention for patients with anxiety disorders. Patients may conceal symptoms for years before seeking treatment, with problems frequently being disclosed during examination of a comorbid condition. More than 50% of people who experience panic attacks seek medical treatment at one time or another. Teaching about the specific disorder and available effective treatments

is a major step toward improving the quality of life of these patients. Giving patients written information about support groups/telephone support groups, Internet sites, nearby clinics, and medication handouts, for example, is all part of health teaching and health promotion.

In the community or hospital setting, the nurse teaches the patient about signs and symptoms of the disorder, theory regarding causes or risk factors, and risk of co-occurrence with other disorders, especially substance use disorder and/or depression. Medication to target the individual's specific disorder, use of relaxation exercises, and availability of specialized treatments such as cognitive behavioral therapy are part of health teaching and health promotion.

People with anxiety disorders are usually able to meet their own basic physical needs. Sleep, however, can be a real and serious problem. Patients with anxiety disorders often experience sleep disturbance and nightmares. Teaching people ways to promote sleep (e.g., warm bath, warm milk, relaxing music) and monitoring sleep through a journal are useful interventions.

Milieu Therapy

As mentioned, most patients with anxiety disorders can be treated successfully as outpatients. Hospital admission is necessary only if severe anxiety or symptoms that interfere with the individual's health are present, or if the individual is suicidal. If or when hospitalization is necessary, the following features of the therapeutic milieu can be especially helpful to the patient:

- Structuring the daily routine to offer physical safety and predictability, thus reducing anxiety over the unknown
- Providing daily activities to promote sharing and cooperation
- Providing therapeutic interactions, including one-on-one nursing care and behavior contracts
- Including the patient in decisions about his or her own care

Psychotherapy

Among the most useful therapies are cognitive behavioral therapies (CBTs), which provide education, address cognitive distortions, and present behavioral approaches in an attempt to reduce symptoms and increase involvement with others and the environment. The cognitive element of CBT refers to teaching people to restructure their thinking and examine their assumptions, problems, concerns, and/or fears so that problems or concerns seem more amenable to change, and hold less negative emotional impact. Essentially, the therapist helps patients correct their faulty conceptions and helps them change their "self signals" or "self talk." Teaching people to successfully redefine their fears and to look at themselves in a new and more positive way can trigger chemical changes in the brain similar to those caused by medications.

CBT essentially challenges core beliefs that are causing a person distress. The following are examples of such beliefs (Sadock et al., 2015):

- Panic attacks: catastrophic misinterpretations of bodily and mental disturbances
- Phobias: danger in specific avoidable situations
- Obsessive-compulsive disorders: repeated warnings or doubting about safety and repetitive acts to ward off threats
- Anxiety disorders: fear of physical or psychological threats

Mindfulness meditation (MM) is often used as an important tool in the practice of CBT. Mindfulness practice is not a new idea. Religions have advocated mindfulness for centuries and it is central to Buddhism and other contemplative traditions. Over the past 30 years, MM has increasingly found a place in mainstream health care because it has been shown not only to reduce symptoms of depression but also to alleviate anxiety, headaches, psoriasis, high blood pressure, high cholesterol levels, eating disorders, substance abuse, and chronic pain (Holzel & Carmody, 2011). With advances in imaging, scientists have begun to explore the brain mechanisms that may underlie these benefits. MM impacts the synthesis of neurotransmitters, particularly serotonin and norepinephrine, which influences mood, increases activity in telomerase (an enzyme important to the long-term health of cells), and affects the concentration of gray matter in the amygdala (a region of the brain associated with fear, anxiety, and stress). Some studies suggest it can improve immune function (Holzel & Carmody, 2011).

APPLYING THE ART

A Person with Obsessive-Compulsive Disorder

Scenario

Eight-year-old Tommy Jansen came to see the school nurse I worked with during my community nursing leadership rotation. His productive cough and a temperature of 101.2° F prompted a call to his mother. While we waited, Tommy looked worried. "Germs make people sick," he said. I nodded. "But how did I get sick when [holding out his red dry hands] I wash my hands lots of times just like Mommy does?" Tommy took a tissue for a cough. "Maybe I got sick because I forgot to use a tissue to hold the doorknob like Mommy does." When Mrs. Jansen arrived, I introduced myself and we talked privately while Tommy's make-up assignments were being gathered.

Therapeutic Goal

By the end of this interaction, Tommy will acknowledge needing help to manage his anxiety and ritualistic hand washing.

Student-Patient Interaction	Thoughts, Communication Techniques, and Mental Health Nursing Concepts
Mrs. Jansen: "I'm going to get Tommy to his pediatrician this afternoon. He didn't have a fever this morning, though he did act a little grouchy."	Tommy looked relieved to see his mother. I don't observe any signs of abuse or neglect.
Student's feelings: *Poor little guy—I wonder about that.*	
Student: "You're concerned about him." *She nods.* "Mrs. Jansen, Tommy worried that he got sick from germs, despite, as he said, 'washing my hands lots of times like Mommy'."	*He's already a worrier at 8 years old. Sounds like he's afraid that getting sick is his fault.*
Student's feelings: *I just met this person yet here I am jumping in, which means I might make a mistake. I guess I'd rather make a mistake by trying to help than by saying nothing. Guess I'm anxious.*	
Mrs. Jansen: *Looking stricken.* "My poor baby! I didn't want my problem to affect him."	I *give information* about Tommy. From looking at Tommy's hands and from what he is saying, this could be a problem. I am concerned that his mother has some obsessive-compulsive traits.
Student: "Your problem?"	I use *restatement.* Because Mrs. Jansen is able to identify a problem, she may be showing some *insight.* She uses *denial* and *rationalization.*
Mrs. Jansen: "Until now I've been convincing myself that I just wanted my house clean."	
Student's feelings: *How could she not see that her behavior represents more than just keeping her house clean?*	

Student-Patient Interaction	Thoughts, Communication Techniques, and Mental Health Nursing Concepts
Student: "How do you explain all the hand washing and using tissues to not touch doorknobs?"	Although I asked an *open* question, this came out like I was being critical of her, like I'm *challenging* or even accusing her.
Student's feelings: *I didn't mean to sound like I'm blaming her. This isn't about a logical decision. It's about a disorder.*	
Mrs. Jansen: *Looks down. Silent.*	
Student: "I'm sorry I pushed you for an explanation. This must be so difficult."	I work on restoring trust by attempting to translate into feelings. I hope I did the right thing by saying I'm sorry.
Mrs. Jansen: *Nods, then makes brief eye contact.* "Since Tommy's dad was sent back to Afghanistan as part of a special forces, I worry all the time. I know I sound crazy, but when I try to stop washing my house, my hands, the doorknobs, I see Tom, Sr., getting blown up by a suicide bomber."	Worrying "all the time" sounds like generalized anxiety disorder. The obsessive worry that gets relieved by the washing rituals sounds like OCD. Both disorders cause such distress. Her self-esteem sounds low, especially about her mothering role.
Student's feelings: *I would worry too with my loved one in a war zone. She worries about "sounding crazy." The stigma of mental illness interferes with people feeling okay about seeking treatment. I feel concern toward her.*	
Student: "You feel kind of scared so often and so alone."	I attempt to *translate* into feelings.
Student's feelings: *I want to always show nonjudgmental acceptance. I show empathy when I reflect underlying feelings. I feel sad at all she has to carry. She obviously cares about her son.*	
Mrs. Jansen: *Tears in her eyes.* "While I wash things, my mind rests a minute. Then I look at my bloody raw hands! Now, I've worried Tommy. Poor kid deserves better than me."	
Student: "Mrs. Jansen, sounds like you're feeling really down on yourself."	I assess her *self-esteem.* Low self-esteem, *depressed mood,* and *suicide* ideation go hand-in-hand. I *validate* to see if I've understood her meaning.

Applying the Art

A Person with Obsessive-Compulsive Disorder—cont'd

Student-Patient Interaction	Thoughts, Communication Techniques, and Mental Health Nursing Concepts	Student-Patient Interaction	Thoughts, Communication Techniques, and Mental Health Nursing Concepts
Mrs. Jansen: "Sometimes I feel panicky...like giving up." **Student:** "Like giving up...as in suicide?" **Student's feelings:** I feel awkward asking about suicide, but I would rather feel funny asking, than overlook a suicide cue.	*Asking* about suicide does not plant the idea of suicide.	**Student's feelings:** I called the behavior "compulsive." I hope that naming the behavior with the word "compulsive" does not threaten her. **Mrs. Jansen:** "Proud of myself, but also scared for Tom, Sr. You said 'compulsive.' I've heard of that on Dr. Phil."	Mrs. Jansen identified hearing about *OCD* on television. Maybe that helped her readiness to talk about her ritualistic behaviors.
Mrs. Jansen: "No, never. I wouldn't do that to Tommy, Jr. The only time I can resist cleaning for a while is when Tommy needs me to help him with something at home or when I watch him play soccer." **Student's feelings:** I'm so relieved that she answered "no" immediately even if the reason is Tommy rather than self.	She focuses so many of her responses in terms of her son. Mrs. Jansen recognizes that resisting the compulsion is healthy behavior. I *validate* the meaning.	**Student:** *Nods.* "Obsessive-compulsive disorder responds to medication and therapy. You don't have to do this all by yourself." **Student's feelings:** I feel hopeful that Mrs. Jansen really will seek treatment.	I *validate* the meaning and *assess* her feelings. I do a little teaching as I give information that OCD responds to treatment.
Student: "So sometimes you are able to delay the compulsive washing behavior. How do you feel then?"	I *give support* by saying, "you are able to...." I then ask an *open question*.	**Mrs. Jansen:** *Looking down at her red raw hands.* "I'm ready for Tommy's sake." *I watch and wait.* "And for myself." *As Tommy rejoins us, Mrs. Jansen asks the school nurse for the community mental health number.*	

APPLYING EVIDENCE-BASED PRACTICE (EBP)

Problem A 37-year-old male with a history of anxiety presents to urgent care hyperventilating and experiencing chest pain. The symptoms started in response to an unexpected increase in his job responsibilities to begin on Monday. The patient is a single father and is fearful about not being able to perform, losing his job, and being unable to support his children. After an examination and ECG are performed, the symptoms are diagnosed as a panic attack. The NP listens empathetically, and then practices a breathing technique with the patient: breathe in slowly for the count of 4, hold for the count of 4, and breathe out slowly for the count of 8. The NP modeled the breathing along with the patient for several cycles. The patient expressed surprise at how well the technique worked to settle him down and stop the panic attack.

EBP Assessment

A. **What do you already know from experience?** Anxiety can interfere with all areas of life. Panic attacks can feel like respiratory distress or even a heart attack, causing fearfulness in the patient. Patients frequently want benzodiazepines to quickly resolve their symptoms. Relaxation and breathing exercises can be very effective if patients are willing to give them a try.

B. **What does the literature say?** There is extensive research supporting relaxation and guided imagery, mindfulness, breathing exercises, yoga, massage, exercise, pet therapy, and other alternative therapies in decreasing anxiety. Benzodiazepines can be very effective, but need to be used with caution due to addictive potential, rebound anxiety, dangerous combinations

with other medications such as narcotics, the connection between long-term benzodiazepine use and dementia, contribution to depression, and the general recommendation to use these medications for short periods of time in acute situations.

C. **What does the patient want?** The patient initially requested a prescription for benzodiazepines and stated that was the only thing that worked for him. By the end of the appointment, however, he was open to continuing the breathing exercise he had practiced with the NP as well as following the other NP recommendations.

Plan The NP referred the patient to a relaxation class at a nearby community mental health clinic. The NP discussed relaxation and guided imagery with the patient, gave information on obtaining a CD to use at home, and encouraged the patient to continue the breathing exercises they practiced during the appointment. In addition, a 7-day temporary supply of Klonopin was given to help the patient get through his first week of new responsibilities, until he could get started with the other recommendations.

QSEN QSEN Prelicensure Knowledge, Skills, and Attitudes (KSAs) Addressed:

Safety as the NP ruled out a cardiac etiology, and used benzodiazepines in a sparing and appropriate manner.

Patient-centered care by providing access to resources, listening attentively, and developing an individualized plan of care.

From Billioti de Gage, S., Moride, Y., Ducruet, T., et al. (2014). Benzodiazepine use and risk of Alzheimer's disease: case-control study. *British Medical Journal, 349*(g5205); WebMD. (2015). *Mindfulness-based stress reduction - topic overview.* Retrieved from www.webmd.com/balance/tc/mindfulness-based-stress-reduction-topic-overview.

Neurobiology of Anxiety Disorders and the Effects of Anti-Anxiety Medications

An imbalance of certain neurotransmitters are thought to disrupt specific brain regions that contribute to various anxiety disorders.
Frontal cortex: cognitive interpretations (e.g., potential threat)
Hypothalamus: activation of the stress response (fight-or-flight response)
Hippocampus: associated with memory related to fear responses
Amygdala: fear, especially related to phobic and panic disorders

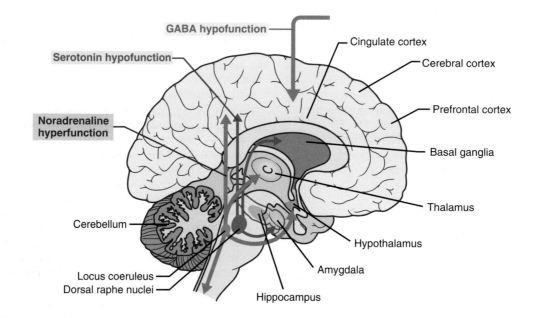

Serotonin: Midbrain, VTA, Cerebral Cortex, and Hypothalamus. Helps regulate mood, sleep, sexual desire, appetite, and inhibits pain. In the anxiety disorders it is believed that there are reduced levels of serotonin transmission and low levels of serotonin are believed to play a role in anxiety disorders as well as depression.

Gamma-aminobutyric acid (GABA): neurotransmitters are widely distributed in the brain. GABA slows neuron activity which plays a role in lowering anxiety and also affects memory. There appears to be strong support that problems with the GABA neurotransmitter system in the brain are related to anxiety disorders.

Norepinephrine (also called Noradrenaline) midbrain, VTA, cerebral cortex, hypothalamus: plays a role in sensitization, fear conditioning, stress response (increases blood pressure and heart rate). Excessive and unregulated norepinephrine is thought to be related to anxiety disorders.

Antianxiety Agent	How it Works	Examples of Use
SSRIs–first-line treatment	Block reuptake of serotonin-increasing levels in the brain	Paroxetine (Paxil)—helpful in GAD
SNRI–first-line treatment	Blocks both serotonin and norepinephrine in the brain	Venlafaxine (Effexor)—mixed anxiety/depression, anxiety and nerve pain
Noradrenergic drugs	Propranolol—blocks adrenergic receptor activity Clonidine—stimulates-adrenergic receptors	Propranolol—short-term relief of social anxiety and performance anxiety Clonidine—anxiety disorders, panic attacks
Benzodiazepines	Binds to benzodiazepine receptors, facilitates action of GABA, slowing neural transmission thus lowering anxiety	Alprazolam—may be used short-term to treat panic disorder and agoraphobia
Buspirone (BuSpar)	Buspirone functions as a serotonin 5-HT$_{1A}$ receptor partial agonist resulting in anxiolytic and antidepressant effects	Can treat the worry associated with GAD rather than the muscle tension

BEHAVIOR MODIFICATION THERAPY

There are currently several forms of behavioral therapy, which involves teaching and physical practice of activities to decrease anxious or avoidant behaviors. As noted earlier, one form of behavioral therapy is relaxation training, examples of which include the following:

- *Modeling*—mimicking appropriate behaviors in situations
- *Systematic desensitization*—gradually exposing a person to the feared object or situation until the person is free of incapacitating anxiety
- *Response prevention*—starts with the therapist preventing the compulsion, such as hand washing, and gradually helping the patient limit the time between rituals until the urge dissipates
- *Thought stopping*—examples include snapping a rubber band on one's wrist to stop an obsession or negative thought

Pharmacological, Biological, and Integrative Therapies

Anxiety disorders are chronic and incurable conditions, although in most cases treatable, and there are many helpful treatments available. Several classes of medications have been found to be effective in the treatment of anxiety disorders. Psychopharmacology is an important adjunct to use with other therapies, especially CBT. Best evidence research points to the fact that when the serotonergic system is modulated (SSRIs, CBT) by itself, or with the noradrenergic system (serotonin-norepinephrine reuptake inhibitors [SNRIs]), anxiety symptoms are alleviated much more often than by using traditional antidepressants (tricyclics) alone. The following medications have been shown to be helpful (Preston et al., 2013):

1. Benzodiazepines: Prescribed for *short-term treatment only;* not recommended for use by patients with substance use problems. Benzodiazepines can be highly addictive and are prescribed for short periods of time, especially when used to self-medicate for anxiety/depression.
2. Buspirone: Management of anxiety disorders; this medication is nonaddictive, an excellent medication for people needing long-term relief of anxiety symptoms (e.g., GAD).
3. SSRIs: First-line treatment for all anxiety disorders, and OCD and BDD.
4. SNRIs: Examples include venlafaxine, milnacipran, and duloxetine; only venlafaxine is currently approved for panic disorder (PD), generalized anxiety disorder (GAD), and social affective disorder (SAD).
5. Tricyclic antidepressants: Second- or third-line use in people with PD, GAD, and SAD; clomipramine is effective in OCD.
6. MAOIs: Recently being used in people with SAD and rejection sensitivity.

Refer to Table 11-8 for trade and generic names of common medications and see Table 11-9 for therapeutic modalities used to treat specific anxiety disorders.

Antidepressants

As stated previously, SSRIs are the first-line treatment for anxiety disorders, OCD, and BDD. They are preferable to the tricyclic antidepressants (TCAs) because they have a more rapid onset of action, have fewer problematic side effects, and are more effective. Monoamine oxidase inhibitors (MAOIs) are reserved for treatment-resistant conditions because of the risk of life-threatening hypertensive crisis if the patient does not follow dietary restrictions. (Patients cannot eat foods containing tyramine and must be given specific dietary instructions.) Venlafaxine (Effexor) and duloxetine (Cymbalta) are SNRIs used to treat anxiety disorders.

Antidepressants have the secondary benefit of treating co-occurring depressive disorders in patients. Because anxiety and depression frequently occur together, these agents may bring welcome benefits. However, there are three notes of caution. First, when treatment is started, low doses of SSRIs must be used because of the activating effect, which temporarily increases anxiety symptoms. Second, in patients with co-occurring bipolar disorder, use of an antidepressant may cause a manic episode, which requires the addition of mood stabilizers or even antipsychotic agents. Third, use of MAOIs is contraindicated in patients with co-occurring substance use disorder; because of the risk of hypertensive crisis with use of stimulant drugs.

Anxiolytics

Anxiolytic drugs (also called *antianxiety drugs*) are often used to treat the somatic and psychological symptoms of anxiety disorders. When moderate or severe anxiety is reduced, patients are better able to participate in treatment directed at their underlying problems. Benzodiazepines are most commonly prescribed because they have a quick onset of action. Because of the potential for dependence, however, these medications should ideally be used for *short periods only* until other medications or treatments reduce symptoms. It is important for the nurse to monitor for side effects of the benzodiazepines, including sedation, ataxia, and decreased cognitive function. As previously mentioned benzodiazepines are not recommended for patients with a known substance use problem and should not be given to women who are pregnant or breast-feeding. Box 11-1 lists important information on patient and family medication teaching.

Buspirone (BuSpar) is an alternative anxiolytic medication that does not cause dependence; however, 2 to 4 weeks are required for it to become fully effective. Its usefulness in anxiety disorders is probably limited to the treatment of GAD.

Other Classes of Medication

Other classes of medication sometimes used to treat anxiety disorders include beta-blockers, antihistamines, and anticonvulsants. These agents are often added if the first course of treatment is ineffective. Beta-blockers have been used to treat panic disorder and social anxiety disorder (SAD). Anticonvulsants have shown some benefit in the management of GAD, SAD, and co-occurring depression with SAD or panic disorder. See Box 11-1 for information on patient and family medication teaching.

Complementary and Alternative Medicine (CAM)

Among the primary "natural" substances purported to relieve anxiety are kava kava and valerian root. Although randomized controlled studies are under way, available scientific evidence regarding the efficacy of any of these agents in the treatment of anxiety disorders is sparse.

Kava Kava

For hundreds of years, kava kava has been used as part of a ceremonial drink in the Pacific Islands. It has been believed that this herb can elevate mood, well-being, contentment, and feelings of relaxation. However, now the medical community believes kava kava may increase psychiatric symptoms and can be dangerous. Even though some countries have removed kava kava from the market, it is still available in the United States. However, in March 2002 the Food and Drug Administration issued a consumer advisory warning of potential risk of liver failure associated with kava kava (UMM, 2009). Kava kava can have multiple drug interactions and potentiate the effects of certain medications, such as anticonvulsants, antianxiety agents, diuretics, and many others.

TABLE 11-8   Medications Commonly Used in the Treatment of Anxiety Disorders

Generic Name	Trade Name	Comments
Benzodiazepines		
Alprazolam*	Xanax	Anxiolytic effects result from depressing neurotransmission in the limbic system and cortical areas. Useful
	Xanax XR	for short-term treatment of anxiety; dependence and tolerance develop. These drugs are NOT indicated
Diazepam	Valium	as a primary treatment for OCD or PTSD.
Lorazepam*	Ativan	
Oxazepam	Serax	
Chlordiazepoxide	Librium	
Clorazepate	Tranxene	
Buspirone		
Buspirone hydrochloride†	BuSpar	Alleviates anxiety, but works best before benzodiazepines have been tried. Less sedating than benzodiaze-pines. Does not appear to produce physical or psychological dependence. Requires 3 or more weeks to be effective.
Selective Serotonin Reuptake Inhibitors (SSRIs)		
First Line		
Citalopram	Celexa	
Escitalopram	Lexapro	Escitalopram not useful with seasonal affective disorder or PD.
Fluoxetine	Prozac	
Fluvoxamine	Luvox	
Paroxetine	Paxil	
Sertraline	Zoloft	
Dual-Action Reuptake Inhibitors (Serotonin and Norepinephrine) (SNRIs)		
First Line		
Duloxetine	Cymbalta	Acts within 1 to 2 weeks.
Venlafaxine	Effexor	
Tricyclic Antidepressants (TCAs)		
Second or Third Line		
Amitriptyline	Elavil	Clomipramine effective with OCD, PD, GAD, seasonal affective disorder; may also respond to Surmontil.
Clomipramine	Anafranil	
Desipramine	Norpramin	
Doxepin	Sinequan	
Imipramine	Tofranil	
Maprotiline	Ludiomil	
Nortriptyline	Pamelor	
Trimipramine	Surmontil	
Amoxapine	Asendin	
Beta-Blockers		
Propranolol	Inderal	Used to relieve physical symptoms of anxiety, as in performance anxiety (stage fright). Act by attaching to
Atenolol	Tenormin	sensors that direct arousal messages.

GAD, Generalized anxiety disorder; *OCD*, obsessive-compulsive disorder; *PD*, panic disorder; *PTSD*, posttraumatic stress disorder.

*Most commonly used benzodiazepines for treating chronic or unpredictable anxiety syndromes.

†Useful as a first-line treatment in GAD.

Adapted from Varcarolis, E. M. (2014). *Manual of psychiatric mental health nursing care plans* (5th ed., p. 151). St Louis: Saunders. Benzodiazepine dosages updated from Lehne, R. A. (2011). *Pharmacology for nursing care* (7th ed.). St Louis: Saunders.

Valerian

Valerian is used for conditions related to anxiety and psychological stress, but it is most commonly used for insomnia (inability to sleep). Although it is not FDA approved, it has proven effective for insomnia. Valerian, unlike kava kava, is considered safe for most people when used in medical amounts on a short-term basis. Some side effects of valerian are headaches, excitability, uneasiness, and even insomnia (MEDLINEplus, 2010). There are, however, many contraindications for its use (Everyday Health Media, 2016). Go to http://www.everydayhealth.com/drugs/valerian-root-valeriana-officinalis for contraindications and a more thorough list of side effects.

Herbs and dietary supplements are not subject to the same rigorous testing as prescription medications. Also, herbs and dietary supplements are not required to be uniform, and there is no guarantee of bioequivalence of the active compound across preparations. Problems that can occur with the use of psychotropic herbs include toxic side effects and herb-drug interactions.

TABLE 11-9 Accepted Treatments for Selected Anxiety Disorders*

Disorder	Pharmacotherapy	Therapeutic Modality	Comments
Panic disorder (PD)	SSRIs are treatment of choice; if patients do not respond to SSRIs, short-term treatment with a benzodiazepine may be used, or patients may switch to another type of antidepressant such as venlafaxine or tricyclics	CBT (cognitive behavioral therapy) • Relaxation techniques • Breathing techniques • Cognitive restructuring • Systematic desensitization • In vivo exposure aimed at eliminating avoidance behaviors	Benzodiazepines (short term) to reduce or eliminate panic attacks in initial phase of treatment Antidepressants may decrease panic episodes and treat underlying depression CBT teaches new coping skills and ways to reframe thinking
Generalized anxiety disorder (GAD)	When medications are indicated: • Buspirone (BuSpar) reduces rumination and worry, not addictive • SSRI and TCA antidepressants are effective with chronic anxiety • Investigational drugs include pregabalin and other anticonvulsants	Cognitive behavioral therapy or anxiety management therapy Anxiety management therapy involves education, relaxation training, and exposure to anxiety-provoking stimuli	Many patients are helped with psychological approaches and may not need medications
Social phobia/social anxiety disorder (SAD)	SSRIs or venlafaxine are first-line drug treatments SSRIs may help lessen rejection sensitivity Beta-blockers target physical symptoms of anxiety (e.g., propranolol) Anticonvulsants such as gabapentin (Neurontin) and pregabalin (Lyrica) are being investigated	Cognitive behavioral therapy can help improve symptoms after 6 to 12 weeks	*Benzodiazepines can be addictive over the long term and are not really a drug of choice for social anxiety disorder*
Obsessive-compulsive disorder (OCD)	SSRIs reduce OCD symptoms directly (e.g., fluvoxamine [Luvox] and fluoxetine [Prozac]) TCAs (e.g., clomipramine [Anafranil])	Exposure and response prevention (ERP) emotionally difficult treatment for patients yet up to 75% to 80% successful SSRIs reduce OCD symptoms directly	Effective and necessary in addition to serotonergic medications Exposure in vivo plus response prevention are the crucial essential factors Complete remission is not common

MAOI, Monoamine oxidase inhibitor; *SSRI,* selective serotonin reuptake inhibitor; *TCA,* tricyclic antidepressant.
*The sooner the treatment is initiated, the greater the chance of successful recovery.
Updated from Varcarolis, E. (2012). *Essentials of psychiatric mental health nursing.* Philadelphia: WB Saunders; reprinted with permission; Preston, J. D., O'Neal, J. H., & Talaga, M. C. (2013). *Handbook of clinical psychopharmacology for therapists* (6th ed.). Oakland, Calif: New Harbinger Publications; Preston, J., & Johnson, J. (2015). *Clinical psychopharmacology made ridiculously simple* (6th ed.). Miami, Fla: MedMaster.

BOX 11-1 Patient and Family Medication Teaching: Anxiolytic Drugs

1. Caution the patient and family:
   - Not to increase dose or frequency of ingestion without prior approval of therapist
   - That these medications reduce the ability to handle mechanical equipment (e.g., cars, saws, and other machinery)
   - Not to drink alcoholic beverages or take other antianxiety drugs because depressant effects of both would be potentiated
   - To avoid drinking beverages containing caffeine because they decrease the desired effects of the drug
2. Recommend that the patient taking benzodiazepines avoid becoming pregnant because these drugs increase the risk of congenital anomalies.
3. Advise the patient not to breast-feed because these drugs are excreted in the milk and would have adverse effects on the infant.
4. Teach a patient who is taking monoamine oxidase inhibitors about the details of a tyramine-restricted diet.
5. Teach the patient that:
   - Abrupt cessation of benzodiazepine use after 3 to 4 months of daily use may cause withdrawal symptoms such as insomnia, irritability, nervousness, dry mouth, tremors, convulsions, confusion, and even psychosis.
   - Medications should be taken with, or shortly after, meals or snacks to reduce gastrointestinal discomfort.
   - Drug interactions can occur: antacids may delay absorption; cimetidine interferes with metabolism of benzodiazepines, causing increased sedation; central nervous system depressants, such as alcohol and barbiturates, cause increased sedation; serum phenytoin concentration may become too high because of decreased metabolism.

EVALUATION

Identified outcomes serve as the basis for evaluation. In general, evaluation of outcomes for patients with anxiety disorders deals with questions such as the following:

- Is the patient experiencing a reduced level of anxiety? Describe the level of anxiety supported by the patient's present symptoms.
- Does the patient recognize symptoms as anxiety related? What symptoms does he or she experience when anxiety levels are rising?

- Does the patient continue to display obsessions, compulsions, phobias, worrying, or other symptoms of anxiety disorders? If so, ask the patient to quantify the number of increased or decreased symptoms during the day/night/situation. How does the patient describe the change in the level of intensity?
- What newly learned behaviors does the patient use to help manage anxiety?
- Can the patient adequately perform self-care activities? Describe changes in ability to manage health care needs.

- Can the patient maintain satisfying interpersonal relations? How does the patient describe close relationships now as compared with before treatment?
- Can the patient assume usual roles? Describe the ways certain role performances have improved, and identify role performances that still require interventions.
- Is the patient compliant with medication?

KEY POINTS TO REMEMBER

- A simple explanation for the difference between anxiety and fear is that anxiety has an unknown or unrecognized source, whereas fear is a reaction to a specific threat.
- Anxiety can be normal, acute, or chronic, as well as adaptive or maladaptive.
- Peplau operationally defined four levels of anxiety. The patient's perceptual field, ability to learn, and physical or other characteristics are different at each level (see Table 11-1).
- Effective psychosocial interventions are different for people experiencing mild to moderate levels of anxiety and for individuals experiencing severe to panic levels of anxiety. Effective psychosocial nursing approaches are suggested in Tables 11-2 and 11-3.
- Defenses against anxiety can be adaptive or maladaptive. Defenses are presented in a hierarchy from healthy to intermediate to immature. Table 11-4 provides examples of adaptive and maladaptive uses of many of the more common defense mechanisms.
- Anxiety disorders are the most common psychiatric disorders in the United States and frequently co-occur with major depression and/or substance use disorders; OCD and BDD also have high rates of co-occurring with major depression.
- Research has identified genetic and biological factors in the etiology of anxiety disorders and OCD.
- Psychological theories, cultural influences, and socioeconomic status also are pertinent to the understanding of anxiety disorders.
- Patients with anxiety disorders suffer from panic attacks, irrational fears, excessive worrying, uncontrollable rituals, or severe reactions to stress.
- People with anxiety disorders and hoarding disorder are often too embarrassed or ashamed to seek psychiatric help. People with anxiety disorders may consult their primary care providers about multiple somatic complaints.
- One form of psychotherapy that is effective for treating anxiety disorders, OCD, and milder forms of BDD is cognitive behavioral therapy (CBT) in conjunction with medication.
- Interventions include counseling, milieu therapy, promotion of self-care activities, psychobiological intervention, and health teaching.

APPLYING CRITICAL JUDGMENT

1. Ms. Smith, a patient with OCD, washes her hands until they are cracked and bleeding. Your nursing goal is to promote healing of her hands. What interventions will you plan?
2. This is Mr. Olivetti's third emergency department visit in a week. He is experiencing severe anxiety accompanied by many physical symptoms. He clings to you, desperately crying, "Help me! Help me! Don't let me die!" Diagnostic tests have ruled out a physical disorder. The patient outcome has been identified as "Patient anxiety level will be reduced to moderate/mild within 1 hour." What are some of the effective interventions you should use?
3. Mrs. Zeamans is a patient with GAD. She has a history of substance use disorder and is a recovering alcoholic. During a clinic visit, she tells you she plans to ask the psychiatrist to prescribe diazepam (Valium) to use when she feels anxious. She asks whether you think this is a good idea. How would you respond? What other kinds of medications might the physician order?

CHAPTER REVIEW QUESTIONS

1. Friends invite an adult diagnosed with type 2 diabetes to go on a mountain hike next week. The adult replies, "I can't go because I don't have any hiking shoes." In actuality, this adult fears difficulty with blood glucose management during strenuous activity. Which defense mechanism is evident?
   a. Displacement
   b. Rationalization
   c. Passive aggression
   d. Reaction formation
2. A nurse analyzes reports from four adult patients of frightening events they encountered. Which patient's report most clearly indicates that the resulting fear was mentally healthy?
   a. "I saw a large spider crawling along my kitchen wall."
   b. "I was at the mall when a gunman began firing an assault weapon."
   c. "I was at home when a storm with heavy thunder and lightning lasted over an hour."
   d. "I was trapped on an elevator that stopped between floors when the power went out."
3. A nursing student arrives late for a clinical experience and is not wearing the correct attire. When the instructor privately criticizes the behavior, the student responds, "I'm always the one who gets caught. You're going to cause me to fail." Select the instructor's best response.
   a. "Other students get caught as well."
   b. "I am not trying to cause you to fail. I am here to help you."
   c. "I am sorry you feel that way. I try to treat all my students equally."
   d. "The requirements for this experience were discussed during our orientation."
4. Select the best example of altruism.
   a. After recovering from a gunshot wound, a police officer attends a local support group.
   b. After recovering from open heart surgery, an individual plays tennis three times a week.
   c. An individual who received a liver transplant volunteers at a local organ procurement agency.
   d. An individual with a long-standing fear of animals volunteers at a community animal shelter.
5. An outpatient psychiatric nurse assesses a patient diagnosed with hoarding disorder. The patient has lost 12 pounds in the past two months, appears disheveled, and is wearing dirty clothing with poor hygiene. What is the nurse's priority action?
   a. Review the patient's medication regimen.
   b. Ask the patient, "What types of foods have you been eating?"
   c. Refer the patient to a psychologist for cognitive behavioral therapy (CBT).
   d. Schedule a home visit to assess the safety of the patient's living conditions.

REFERENCES

American Nurses Association, American Psychiatric Nurses Association, & International Society of Psychiatric-Mental Health Nurses. (2014). *Psychiatric–mental health nursing: scope and standards of practice.* Silver Springs, Md: Nursesbooks.org.

American Psychiatric Association. (2013). *Diagnostic and statistical manual of mental disorders (DSM-5)* (5th ed.). Washington, DC: APA.

Black, D. W., & Andreasen, N. A. (2014). *Introductory textbook of psychology* (6th ed.). Washington, DC: American Psychiatric Publishing.

Boundless. (2015). Retrieved April 5, 2016 from https://www.boundless.com/psychology/textbooks/boundless-psychology-textbook/biological-foundations-of-psychology-3/structure-and-function-of-the-brain-35/the-limbic-system-154-12689/.

Holzel, B., & Carmody, J. (2011). Mindfulness practice leads to increases in regional brain gray matter density. *Psychiatry Research: Neuroimaging, 191,* 36–43.

MEDLINEplus, U.S. National Library of Medicine, & NIH. (2010). *Valerian.* Retrieved February 11, 2011, from www.nlm.nih.gov/MEDLINEplus/druginfo/natural/870.html.

Moorhead, S., Johnson, M., Maas, M. L., et al. (2012). *Nursing outcomes classification (NOC)* (5th ed.). St Louis: Mosby.

North American Nursing Diagnosis Association International (NANDA-I). (2015). *NANDA nursing diagnoses: definitions and classification 2015–2016.* Philadelphia: NANDA-I.

Peplau, H. E. (1968). A working definition of anxiety. In S. F. Burd & M. A. Marshall (Eds.), *Some clinical approaches to psychiatric nursing.* New York: Macmillan.

Pines, A., & Aronson, E. (2008). *Career burnout: causes and cures.* New York: Free Press.

Pollock, M. H., Otto, M. W., Whittmann, et al. (2010). Anxious patients. In T. A. Stern, G. L. Fricchione, N. H. Cassem, et al. (Eds.), *Massachusetts General Hospital: handbook of general hospital psychiatry* (6th ed.). Philadelphia: Saunders.

Preston, J., & Johnson, J. (2015). *Clinical psychopharmacology: made ridiculously simple* (8th ed.). Miami, Fla: MedMaster, Inc.

Preston, J. D., O'Neal, J. H., & Talaga, M. C. (2013). *Handbook of clinical psychopharmacology for therapists* (7th ed.). Oakland, Calif: New Habinger Publications.

Reese, S. M. (2011). *Burned out? How doctors recover their spark.* Retrieved July 28, 2011, from www.medscape.com/viewarticle/746117?src=nl_topic.

Sadock, B. J., Sadock, V. A., & Ruiz (2015). *Kaplan and Sadock's synopsis of psychiatry* (11th ed.). Philadelphia: Wolters/Lippincott Williams & Wilkins.

Satcher, D., Delgado, P. L., & Masand, P. S. (2005). A surgeon general's perspective on the unmet needs of patients with anxiety disorders. *Medscape Psychiatry & Mental Health, 10*(2).

Schneir, F. A., Vidar, H. B., Vogel, L. R., et al. (2014). Anxiety, obsessive-compulsive, and stress disorders. In L. Janis Cutler (Ed.), *Psychiatry* (3rd ed.). New York: Oxford University Press.

Sullivan, H. S. (1953). *The interpersonal theory of psychiatry.* New York: Norton.

University of Maryland Medical Center (UMM). (2009). *Kava kava.* Retrieved February 11, 2011, from www.umm.edu/almed/articles/kava-kava-000259.htm.

Vaillant, G. E., & Vaillant, C. O. (2004). Normality and mental health. In B. J. Sadock & V. A. Sadock (Eds.), *Kaplan and Sadock's comprehensive textbook of psychiatry* (8th ed.) vol. 1. (pp. 583–597). Philadelphia: Lippincott Williams & Wilkins.

Somatic Symptom Disorders and Dissociative Disorders

Susan L. Frost, Chyllia D. Fosbre, Elizabeth M. Varcarolis

ⓔ http://evolve.elsevier.com/Varcarolis/essentials

KEY TERMS AND CONCEPTS

alternate personality (alter), p. 160
assertiveness training, p. 158
depersonalization/derealization disorder,
    p. 159
dissociative amnesia, p. 160
dissociative amnesia with fugue, p. 160
dissociative disorders, p. 152

dissociative identity disorder (DID), p. 160
factitious disorder, p.155
functional neurological disorder (conver-
    sion disorder), p. 153
hypochondriasis, p. 154
la belle indifférence, p. 155
malingering, p. 155

secondary gains, p. 156
somatic symptom disorder, p. 152

SELECTED CONCEPT: SOMATIZATION

To somatize is the process of experiencing and communicating psychological distress through physical symptoms. The symptoms may or may not have a medical basis that can be identified. A key identifying feature is the patient's disproportionate and excessive distressful reaction to the physical symptoms, which causes life impairment. This is an unconscious process in most cases, with the exception of factitious disorder, and will be discussed in more depth in this chapter.

(APA, 2013, p. 309)

SELECTED CONCEPT: DISSOCIATION

Everyone uses dissociation to an extent. Daydreaming, fantasizing, and zoning-out are all examples of healthy dissociation and can be used in creative ways to solve problems or relax.

However, severe dissociation differs from normal daydreaming and is caused by major trauma in which an individual is unable to integrate the trauma into his/her psyche. Depending on the severity and impact of the events, a person may be unable to recall a specific event, feel unreal or detached for short or long periods of time, or, in the most severe cases, develop more than one personality to help carry the load of extremely severe trauma or abuse.

OBJECTIVES

1. Compare and contrast the etiologies and basic symptoms of somatic system disorders and dissociative disorders.
2. Differentiate the significant differences between the bulk of the somatic symptom disorders and factitious disorder. Understand how this would affect your thought process while giving nursing care.
3. Identify factors that can make it difficult to identify somatic symptom disorders.
4. Keeping in mind that dissociative disorders are trauma based, describe how this might change your approach in providing nursing care to this population.

INTRODUCTION

This chapter will cover the two categories of somatic symptom disorders and dissociative disorders.

Somatic symptom disorder and related disorders (formerly called somatoform disorders) are an umbrella group of disorders characterized by the presence of one or more physical symptoms accompanied by abnormal thoughts, feelings, and behavioral reactions in response to these symptoms, often in the absence of known physical findings or medical illnesses that would explain them. These symptoms are associated with extreme distress and/or dysfunction contributing to life impairment (Frances, 2013).The emphasis in the *DSM-5* is not only on the presence of physical symptoms but also on the way an individual presents and interprets the symptoms in a persistent and excessive manner. Often, people with somatic symptom disorders are associated with increased health care use, functional impairment, dissatisfaction with and changing providers, psychiatric comorbidity, and failure to respond to standard treatment. Individuals with somatic symptom disorders are often seen in medical clinics and not psychiatric settings because the distressing symptoms present as primarily physical in nature. Actual diagnosed medical issues and somatic syndrome disorders can be present concurrently, which can make it difficult to diagnose.

Dissociative disorders are an umbrella group of disorders characterized by varying degrees of mental detachment from conscious awareness. Dissociative disorders differ from the normal process of daydreaming in their intensity and in the fact that they derive as a reaction to abuse and, at some level, cause impairment in the patient's ability to function. Dissociative disorders range from feeling unreal through actually creating more than one personality as a coping mechanism to disperse the psychological effects of severe abuse memories and reactions. People with dissociative identity disorder (formerly called multiple personality disorder) are often misdiagnosed as schizophrenic or psychotic due to hearing voices, seeing people in their mind, and the tendency to decompensate and present as unstable.

SOMATIC SYMPTOM DISORDER

People with somatic symptom disorders are extremely and persistently preoccupied with and distressed by their perceived health issues. They may demand unnecessary tests, and may be noncompliant with provider recommendations. Individuals with this disorder experience significant life impairment as a result of their symptoms, preoccupation, and high anxiety. They tend to incur large health care costs, with the person usually failing to respond to standard treatment.

When patients do not obtain an answer from a physician concerning their physical distress, they may become frustrated and visit several medical facilities seeking relief (referred to as "doctor shopping"). Unfortunately, these individuals often undergo unnecessary surgeries, invasive diagnostic procedures, and drug trials, all of which can be life-threatening (Braun et al., 2010). This situation can also be frustrating for the medical professionals involved because of the inability to find causes and the high emotionality of the patients.

It is important to remember that in most somatic symptom disorders, with the exception of factitious disorders, these symptoms are not intentional or under the conscious control of the patient. If, after a thorough medical examination, no physical reasons for the patient's signs and symptoms can be found, a mental health evaluation should be performed to determine if a somatic symptom disorder is the cause or a contributing factor. Yates (2014) advises that anxiety or mood disorders be considered before leaning toward a somatic symptom disorder because depression and anxiety can worsen physical pain or symptoms. Cultural factors need to be assessed because in some cultures, the predominant means of expressing psychological stress presents with physical signs and symptoms (Frances, 2013). For example, in African and Latin cultures, anxiety is expressed initially as stomach or other physical pain, whereas in Western cultures anxiety initially presents as mental distress and if prolonged can then translate into physical discomfort (Frances, 2013).

PREVALENCE AND COMORBIDITY

Prevalence rates of somatic symptom disorders in the general population are about 4% (Creed et al., 2012). It is estimated, however, that 30% of patients seen by their primary care providers present with unexplained symptoms, and 30% of these patients are diagnosed with no serious medical basis for their symptoms (Black & Andreasen, 2014). No differences in the rates of somatic syndrome disorders were found across cultures, although the unique expression of the disorder may vary (Zaroff et al., 2012).

Differentiating somatic symptom disorders from physical disorders and identifying co-occurring/**comorbid medical or psychiatric conditions** are significant issues for the primary care provider. Research shows that half of all frequent users of medical care have psychological problems. Psychiatric disorders are frequently present in people who have unexplained medical complaints, including **depressive disorders** and **anxiety disorders** in approximately 50% of patients (Burton et al., 2011). Although there is no evidence specifically linking somatic syndrome

disorders with suicide, because of the comorbidity with depression, this tendency should be monitored. Because actual diagnosed medical disorders and somatic syndrome disorders can exist concurrently, a comprehensive physical and psychosocial examination is imperative.

THEORY

Genetic Factors

Several factors may contribute to the development of somatic symptom disorders. These include genetic vulnerabilities such as low tolerance to pain, early trauma, learning disorders (such as attention during illness or failure to learn emotional coping methods), and societal recognition of physical problems while devaluing psychological distress (APA, 2013). School stressors are a common environmental factor in the development and continuation of these symptoms (Hart et al., 2011). There is no direct evidence of a genetic etiology for any one *specific* somatic symptom disorder. However, data do support a genetic theory that somatic symptom disorder tends to occur in families, presenting in 10% to 20% of first-degree relatives with somatization disorder (Spratt, 2014). Rates may also be higher in monozygotic twins (Ask et al., 2016) and in women (Kurlansik & Maffei, 2016). Twin studies looking at the construct of "health anxiety" support somatic symptom disorders as being moderately heritable (Ask et al., 2016).

Environmental Factors

Antecedents of somatization may include living around a family member with an illness, receiving attention for an illness, or having an overprotective parenting style, childhood expectation of perfection, or history of divorce, maltreatment, or trauma (Kurlansik & Maffei, 2016). This may reflect a learned process where experiencing illness in the environment or the self can lead to a heightened focus on symptoms (Ibeziako & Bujoreanu, 2011). In addition, children may not have the ability or training to express distress verbally, which can plant the seeds of somatic behavior. This pattern of focus can carry over into adulthood and be reinforced over time. Before pubescence the rates of somatizing are equal between boys and girls with the rate in females being higher after this time (Spratt, 2014).

Psychological Theory

Somatizing behavior may be understood as being driven by a maladaptive and anxious attachment style. The behavior is fostered by real or perceived rejection from significant others and is geared toward attempts to elicit care or nurturing. Difficulty with expressing distress verbally is thought to underlie the expression through physical symptoms (Spratt, 2014). Positive and negative responses from parents or role models can lead to reinforcement and operant conditioning of somatic and illness behaviors (Spratt, 2014). There are both positive and negative rewards associated with somatizing behaviors and assuming the sick role. Positive reinforcers include lessened expectations at work or home, time off from work or school, disability payments, and justification for life conflicts. At the same time there is a loss of career, status, and independence (Lubkin & Larson, 2013).

Interpersonal Model

There is growing evidence that childhood adversity is linked to adult somatic symptom disorder. Many patients report traumatic events and substance abuse in their families compared with controls. Yates (2010) identified some childhood influences that are thought to contribute to somatization:

- Children raised in homes where there is a high degree of parental somatization may model somatization.
- Early physical or sexual abuse may be associated with increased risk of somatization or functional neurological disorder (conversion

disorder) later in life, in addition to other psychiatric disorders (Koelen et al., 2014).

- Exposure to illness in parents or other family members during development can result in learned behaviors (Spratt, 2014).

CULTURAL CONSIDERATIONS

Cultural factors can influence an individual's tendency to develop somatic symptoms, as well as the types of symptoms that may be unconsciously expressed. Every culture allows for different expression of distress and has a unique set of idioms aimed toward impelling help (Lind et al., 2014). In some cultures, somatic symptoms may be the first indicator of an underlying anxiety or depressive disorder.

Interestingly, there is no difference in the rates of somatic symptom disorders across cultures, although the expressions of the disorders are varied and unique (Zaroff et al., 2012). One example in lower class Africans who are members of the Pentecostal church involves a condition of "spiritual heart trouble" with symptoms that include a heavy heart, loss of joy, and saying things not typically said by the person. Mal de ojo, or "evil eye," is seen in Hispanic cultures where gazing upon a child with malicious intent results in a curse of illness or even death. Passing a raw egg over the child or tying a red ribbon on the ankle is believed to absorb negative energy (Carteret, 2011).

CLINICAL PICTURE

When a patient presents with severe preoccupation with and distress surrounding unexplained physical symptoms that cannot be explained by a medical disorder, substance use, or another mental disorder, then a somatic disorder may be diagnosed. In addition, factitious disorder or the behavior of malingering should be considered. Because anxiety disorders and mood disorders often present with physical symptoms, these disorders must be ruled out (Yates, 2010). Therefore, both a medical and a psychological workup are used to diagnose these disorders.

SOMATIC SYMPTOM DISORDER (FORMERLY SOMATIZATION DISORDER)

According to the *DSM-5* (APA, 2013), individuals with somatic symptom disorder present with multiple physical/medical symptoms, considerable distress, and impaired functioning in daily life. In addition to the symptoms, patients present with excessive time, rumination, and focus spent on health concerns. Somatic symptom disorder can present with pain as the predominant symptom; is persistent in nature, lasting longer than 6 months; and is specified as mild, moderate, or severe.

The individual with this disorder typically has a long history of multiple complaints and medical visits to numerous providers. The most common symptoms are pain, gastric or intestinal distress, palpitations, dizziness, shortness of breath, sexual dysfunction, neurological symptoms, and fatigue. Patients may describe their symptoms in an exaggerated or dramatic way or have symptoms that are atypical for the disease. Medical findings are lacking or less than expected for the magnitude of the complaint. Their histories include multiple treatments and surgeries, substance abuse, marital difficulties, suicide attempts, chronic pain, and impaired work and life functioning including disability and high health care costs. It is important to recognize and treat co-occurring depression and anxiety. Antidepressants can sometimes help relieve pain symptoms

---

DSM-5 DIAGNOSTIC CRITERIA
for Somatic Symptom Disorder

A. One or more somatic symptoms that are distressing or result in significant disruption of daily life.

B. Excessive thoughts, feelings, or behaviors related to the somatic symptoms or associated health concerns as manifested by at least one of the following:
1. Disproportionate and persistent thoughts about the seriousness of one's symptoms.
2. Persistently high level of anxiety about health or symptoms.
3. Excessive time and energy devoted to these symptoms or health concerns.

C. Although any one somatic symptom may not be continuously present, the state of being symptomatic is persistent (typically more than 6 months).

Specify if:
With predominant pain (previously pain disorder): This specifier is for individuals whose somatic symptoms predominantly involve pain.

Specify if:
Persistent: A persistent course is characterized by severe symptoms, marked impairment, and long duration (more than 6 months).

Specify current severity:
Mild: Only of the symptoms specified in Criterion B is fulfilled.
Moderate: Two or more of the symptoms specified in Criterion B are fulfilled.
Severe: Two or more of the symptoms specified in Criterion B are fulfilled, plus there are multiple somatic complaints (or one very severe somatic symptom).

From the American Psychiatric Association. (2013). *Diagnostic and statistical manual of mental disorders* (5th ed.). Washington, DC: APA.

---

as well (Yates, 2010). Unfortunately, these individuals frequently refuse psychiatric assistance because they believe their symptoms are medical, even when presented with negative test findings. They tend to not recognize the underlying mental problem and may pressure providers for repeated and unnecessary procedures (Dimsdale, 2015). Secondary gains such as freedom from responsibilities or stressful situations can reinforce the disorder. Pain response is individual and difficult to measure objectively, making the disorder even more difficult to identify and treat. Patients with somatic symptom disorder are at risk for excessive narcotic use in pursuit of relief (Yates, 2010).

Illness Anxiety Disorder (Formerly Hypochondriasis)

According to the *DSM-5* (APA, 2013), individuals with Illness Anxiety Disorder are preoccupied with having or eventually developing a serious illness. Individuals with this disorder may or may not present with somatic symptoms, and if they do, the symptoms are usually mild. What they do exhibit is a high level of anxiety and alarm about their health lasting at least 6 months, and may either excessively check for problems or avoid medical care. It is important to consider other possible diagnoses such as anxietydisorders.

The preoccupation with health leads to an encompassing anxiety that severely impairs functioning. They are more alarmed by the potential implications of any disorder than with the disorder itself, and are alarmed with any new bodily sensations. Patients can misinterpret normal physical sensations such as sweating, abdominal cramping, or awareness of heartbeat as indicative of disease (Dimsdale, 2015).

Conversion Disorder (also Called Functional Neurobiological Symptom Disorder)

According to the *DSM-5* (APA, 2013), this disorder presents with one or more symptoms of impaired motor or sensory function. Findings are incompatible with or an exaggeration of recognized neurological conditions and are not better explained by another mental or medical disorder.

The deficit causes significant distress to the patient and impaired social or occupational functioning. Symptoms are further specified as including weakness or paralysis, abnormal movement, swallowing or speech difficulties, seizures or attacks, sensory loss or anesthesia, or symptoms involving the senses (blindness or loss of smell). Symptoms can also be mixed with elements of more than one specifier.

The symptoms are not voluntarily controlled or created. Patients may be highly distressed or show a lack of emotional concern known as la belle indifférence (Braun et al., 2010). Episodes are typically brief but may become chronic. Some symptoms such as tremor may disappear when the patient is distracted (Dimsdale, 2015).

The long-held view of conversion disorders is based on psychoanalytic theory. Now competing theories dispute a purely psychological origin. Functional brain imaging studies are pointing to the understanding of conversion disorders as symptoms related to the brain as well as encompassing the mind-body perspective of disease. A number of studies in people with stress-related disorders have found there is often smaller hippocampal volume in the brain, lending scientific support to the notion that conversion disorders are not purely psychological in nature (Stone et al., 2010).

Conversion disorders are among the most common of the somatic symptom disorders; they are more prevalent in women, in the elderly, and among lower educated and rural populations. Comorbidities include childhood abuse, depression, anxiety, and personality disorders (Black & Andreasen, 2014). It is estimated that one fourth of patients admitted to neurological units have conversion symptoms. The course of the disorder is related to its acuity. If symptoms have been present for more than 6 months, the remission rate is about 50%.

> **VIGNETTE**
>
> An 18-year-old female was brought to the emergency department during a seizure-like episode. She had been having incidents where she would fall to the ground with jerky muscle movements, and also less severe periods of muscle shaking and anxiety. The episodes began after her fiancé broke off their relationship and began dating someone else. The patient's EEG was completely normal, and the episodes had not decreased with the use of the antiseizure medication Keppra. Although the patient was still being followed by a neurologist, she was also referred for a psychiatric evaluation and treatment. During the initial assessment it was discovered that the patient had similar episodes after her parents' divorce while she was in third grade, but they had resolved since then. The patient had never been able to discuss her feelings about the divorce with either parent, but she was allowed to stay home from school and spend more time with them whenever she was ill.

Psychological Factors Affecting Other Medical Conditions

According to the *DSM-5* (APA, 2013), an actual medical condition must be present, with adverse effects on the condition resulting from psychological or behavioral factors. These factors may exacerbate the medical condition or delay recovery and elevate health risks for the patient. Severity is specified as mild, moderate, severe, or extreme (life-threatening).

Conditions that may be affected in this disorder include endocrine, gastrointestinal, cardiac, and skin conditions (Falvo, 2014). Psychological or behavioral factors such as dysfunctional interpersonal patterns, distress, and denial of symptoms or noncompliance with medical treatment increase suffering, disability, and risk of death. Common examples are asthma, psoriasis, migraine, or irritable bowel syndrome that are exacerbated by anxiety. The association between the medical and psychological factors should be evident to make this diagnosis.

Factitious Disorder Imposed on Self (Formerly Munchausen Syndrome)

According to the *DSM-5* (APA, 2013), factitious disorder **imposed on self** refers to the deliberate fabrication of symptoms or self-injury, without obvious external reward or gain. The patient identifies himself/herself in a deceptive manner to others as sick or impaired. This disorder is further specified as a single episode or recurrent.

Factitious disorders are differentiated from the behavior of malingering by the intent to receive reward or gain through the fabricated or exaggerated symptoms. Malingerers attempt to receive an obvious gain, an example being continued visits to a chiropractor when the neck strain has been resolved in order to inflate an insurance claim. Malingering is not a *DMS-5* diagnosis but is considered a behavior (Spratt, 2014).

The unconscious motivation is thought to be for the purpose of assuming the sick role and receiving nurturance, comfort, and attention although this is not clear. The cause is unknown although stress and often borderline personality disorder are implicated. The patient is often intelligent, resourceful, and sophisticated regarding medical practices (Dimsdale, 2015). A person may exaggerate, fabricate, simulate, or induce a symptom. For example, a person might inject a caustic substance into the skin to form an abscess, injure him- or herself, use medication inappropriately, or falsify lab results or medical reports, or describe suicidal thoughts after the death of a spouse who did not exist. About 1% of hospitalized patients meet the criteria for factitious disorder, although underreporting is likely due to the inherent deception.

> **VIGNETTE**
>
> A 52-year-old man was being treated for complaints of abdominal pain and rectal bleeding by his primary care provider (PCP). As part of the workup, the patient was sent to a surgeon for consultation and further diagnostics. The patient was told that cancer was one of several possibilities, but was unlikely. The patient refused to have a colonoscopy or other testing. He returned to the psychiatrist he had been seeing and also to his PCP for care. The patient told his health care providers and children that he had colon cancer and was dying. Every appointment was spent ruminating about his weakness, wasting muscles, and bleeding during defecation, presenting photographs of the bloody stool in the toilet and complaining about his medical care. The patient was a very angry individual who did not express emotions well. He had a history of being raped by his father in childhood and having never worked through this, he lashed out at the world as a matter of course. He went into hospice status and was receiving assistance at home. During this time, his PCP was obtaining records for collaboration of care and discovered that cancer had never been diagnosed. Both somatic symptom disorder and factitious disorder were considered in this case. The patient was receiving benefits in that he had hospice status, narcotic pain medication, and attention from his providers and children. It was determined with consultation between the PCP and psychiatrist that this was a somatic symptom disorder, without a conscious production of symptoms for gain. In this case, the correlation between the emotional distress (rape) and the symptoms (rectal bleeding) can be clearly made, although this is not always evident.

Factitious disorder imposed on another (formerly Munchausen by proxy) has the same criteria as a factitious disorder, except the deliberate fabrication of symptoms or injury is imposed upon another person, often a child or dependent victim. The perpetrator is often a parent or caregiver, and the motivation is to receive attention or nurturing. The diagnosis is given to the perpetrator, not the victim; the victim may be given a diagnosis of abuse. There is a criminal aspect to this disorder because another person is being harmed.

The diagnosis of *Other specified somatic symptom and related disorders* does not meet the full *DSM-5* criteria for the main somatic symptom and related disorders. They include brief somatic symptom disorder (less than 6 months' duration); brief illness anxiety disorder (less than 6 months' duration); illness anxiety disorder without excessive health-related behaviors (all criterion for illness anxiety disorder not met); and pseudocyesis (false belief of being pregnant with objective signs).

The diagnosis of *Unspecified somatic symptom and related disorder* is used when the symptoms and impairment do not meet the full criteria for any specific disorder.

NURSING PROCESS: SOMATIC SYMPTOMS AND RELATED DISORDERS

Assessment of patients with somatic symptom disorders is a complex process that requires careful and complete medical examination. Between 13% and 30% of people diagnosed with a somatic symptom disorder eventually developed an organic condition that was related to the original symptom (Braun et al., 2010). Somatic symptoms and actual medical conditions may occur in the same patient at some point. Full assessment cannot be ignored because of a diagnosis of a somatic symptom disorder. The following sections outline several areas that are not normally included in a nursing assessment, but are important to assess in a patient with suspected somatic symptom disorders.

APPLICATION OF THE NURSING PROCESS

ASSESSMENT

Symptoms and Needs

Assessment should begin with collection of data about the nature, location, onset, character, and duration of the symptom(s). Often, patients with conversion disorder report having a sudden loss in function of a body part. "I woke up this morning and couldn't move my arm." Patients with any of the somatic symptom disorders may discuss their symptoms in dramatic terms. They may use colorful descriptions such as "the pain was searing, like a hot sword drawn across my forehead" or "my symptoms are so rare that none of the doctors can figure it out."

Information should be sought about patients' ability to meet their own basic needs. As in all patients, they should be met where they are and gradually guided toward independence. This process is different for each individual. Anxiety may cause or exacerbate tachypnea and tachycardia. Nutrition, fluid balance, and elimination needs should be evaluated because patients with somatic symptom disorders often complain of gastrointestinal distress, diarrhea, constipation, and anorexia. Sexual desire or performance may be altered by experiences of painful intercourse or pain in another part of the body.

Rest, comfort, recreational activity, and hygiene needs may be altered as a result of problems such as fatigue, weakness, insomnia, muscle tension, and pain. Safety and security needs may be threatened by patient experiences of blindness, deafness, loss of balance and falling, and anesthesia of various parts of the body.

Voluntary Control of Symptoms

During assessment it is important to determine if the symptoms are under the patient's voluntary control. People with somatic symptom disorder and related disorders do not have voluntary control over their symptoms, with the exception of factitious disorders. The patient does not understand the relationship between symptoms and interpersonal conflicts that may be obvious to others and often suffers extreme physical discomfort and mental anguish.

Secondary Gains

The nurse should consider the benefits a person might be receiving from the symptoms. Secondary gains are those benefits derived from the symptoms alone. For example, in the sick role, the patient is not able to perform normal family, work, and social functions and receives extra attention from loved ones. If a patient derives personal benefit from the symptoms, relinquishing the symptoms is more difficult. The clinician works with the patient to achieve the same benefits through healthier avenues, such as assertiveness training. It should be recognized that it will likely be difficult for the patient to give up the sick role, as this has been his/her primary identity. One approach to identifying the presence of secondary gains is to ask the patient questions such as the following:

- What abilities have you lost since the development of your symptom(s)?
- How has this problem affected your life? Are there things you can no longer do?
- Depending upon the individual patient and your rapport, the nurse might gently approach whether there is anything positive obtained because of the disorder.

Cognitive Style

In general, patients with these disorders misinterpret physical stimuli and distort reality regarding their symptoms. For example, sensations a normal individual might interpret as a headache might suggest a brain tumor to a patient with anxiety illness disorder. Exploring the patient's thought processes is enlightening in identifying these distortions. The patient with a somatic symptom disorder may exhibit an obsessive attention to detail about symptoms or health topics and a preoccupation with the consequences of serious illness. The patient may be vague about details, identify disconnected symptoms, and have a long history of medical appointments with different providers. Some patients will present with a large folder or notebook containing a plethora of letters, documentation, and test results.

Ability to Communicate Feelings and Emotional Needs

Patients with somatic symptom disorders have difficulty communicating their emotional needs. As children, their family communication style may have neglected the appropriate expression of anger, depression, fear, and other emotions, and thus they do not recognize feelings nor understand how to relate to them. For example, the feeling of anxiety may cause tightness in the stomach, nausea, rapid heartbeat, shortness of breath, dizziness, sweating, and tensing of muscles such as the hands or jaw. If a person is taught to consider the relationship of emotions to physical symptoms, the person will likely identify that he or she is anxious. If this emotional coaching has not occurred, the stage is set to believe only a medical problem could be the cause. Somatization may be a predominant method of expressing feelings in the family, or the child may have received attention for normal symptoms during his or her developmental phases and somatization was reinforced. Sometimes there is an obvious connection between symptom and stressor, such as blindness when someone cannot face a situation. More often the connection is not obvious to the patient or provider.

Dependence on Medication

Individuals experiencing many somatic complaints often become dependent on medication to relieve pain, anxiety, or depression or to induce sleep. Taking anxiolytic agents such as benzodiazepines is common in this population because of high anxiety and concern about symptoms. These medications can become addictive and cause "rebound anxiety" when the dosage wears off, exacerbating the anxiety problem over time. It is important that the nurse assess the type and amount of medications being used and be alert for a history of numerous prescribers.

Assessment Guidelines

It is always important to ensure that an underlying medical condition has been eliminated from the differential diagnosis, which could be any medical condition including autoimmune disorders, cardiac disease, and endocrine imbalances. However, as you recall, both a true medical condition and a somatic symptom disorder can co-occur

Somatic Symptoms and Related Disorders

1. Ensure that a thorough physical examination with appropriate medical tests has been completed.
2. Assess for nature, location, onset, characteristics, and duration of the symptom(s).
3. Assess the patient's ability to meet basic needs (level of independence).
4. Assess risks to safety and security needs of the patient as a result of the symptom(s).
5. Determine whether the symptoms are under the patient's voluntary control.
6. Consider any secondary gains that the patient is deriving from the symptom(s).
7. Explore the patient's thought processes and ability to communicate feelings and needs.
8. Determine the type and amount of medication the patient is using.

DIAGNOSIS

Patients with somatic symptoms and related disorders present various nursing problems. *Ineffective coping* is frequently diagnosed. Causal statements might include the following:
- Distorted perceptions of body functions and symptoms
- Chronic pain of psychological origin
- Dependence on pain relievers or anxiolytics

Table 12-1 identifies potential nursing diagnoses for patients with somatic symptom disorders.

OUTCOMES IDENTIFICATION

The overall long-term goal in treating individuals with somatic symptom disorders is that people with these disorders will eventually be able to live as normal a life as possible. This includes symptom or pain reduction, improved level of independence, and a better overall quality of life.

The following are examples of potential long-term outcome criteria:
- Patient will identify and articulate feelings such as anger, shame, guilt, and remorse.
- Patient will resume performance of work role behaviors.
- Patient will identify ineffective coping patterns.
- Patient will make realistic appraisal of strengths and weaknesses.

PLANNING

Because patients are seldom admitted to psychiatric units specifically because of these disorders, long-term interventions usually take place on an outpatient basis. Short-term planning, such as a referral to a psychiatric provider, may be initiated during a medical-surgical admission, which is often of brief duration.

Nursing interventions should focus initially on establishing rapport with the patient. The therapeutic relationship is vital to treatment success given the tendency toward defensiveness in these patients. Broaching a nonmedical or psychiatric etiology to the patient's symptoms is threatening. Therapeutic interventions must address helping the patient learn to meet needs without resorting to somatization. The

TABLE 12-1 Potential Nursing Diagnoses for Somatic Symptom Disorders

Signs and Symptoms	Nursing Diagnoses (NANDA)
Inability to meet occupational, family, or social responsibilities because of symptoms	*Ineffective coping*
	Ineffective role performance
	Impaired social interaction
Inability to participate in usual community activities or friendships because of psychogenic symptoms	*Ineffective relationship*
Dependence on pain relievers; distortion of body functions and symptoms; presence of secondary gains by adoption of sick role	*Powerlessness*
	Disturbed body image
	Pain (acute or chronic)
Inability to meet family role function and need for family to assume role function of the somatic individual	*Interrupted family processes*
	Ineffective sexuality pattern
Assumption of some of the roles of the somatic parent by the children	*Impaired parenting*
Shifting of the sexual partner's role to that of caregiver or parent and of the patient's role to that of recipient of care	*Risk for caregiver role strain*
Feeling of inability to control symptoms or understand why he or she cannot find help	*Chronic low self-esteem*
	Spiritual distress
Development of negative self-evaluation related to losing body function, feeling useless, or not feeling valued by significant others	
Inability to take care of basic self-care needs related to conversion symptom (paralysis, seizures, pain, fatigue)	*Focus on self-care deficit (hygiene, dressing, feeding, toileting)*
Inability to sleep related to psychogenic pain	*Disturbed sleep pattern*

Herdman, T.H. (Ed.) *Nursing Diagnoses-Definitions and Classification 2015-2017*. Copyright 2014, 1994-2014 NANDA International. Used by arrangement with John Wiley & Sons Limited. In order to make safe and effective judgments using NANDA-I nursing diagnoses it is essential that nurses refer to the definitions and defining characteristics of the diagnoses listed in this work.

secondary gains the patient has derived from illness behaviors will hopefully become less important to the patient when underlying needs can be met directly. The optimal goal is not only to relieve but also to increase quality of life and independence. Collaboration with family or significant others can be supportive to patient success; however, each situation must be assessed individually; families can also be sources of stress or dysfunction.

IMPLEMENTATION

Communication Guidelines

Generally for patients with somatic symptom disorders, nursing interventions take place in the outpatient setting. The nurse attempts to help the patient improve overall functioning through the development of effective coping and communication strategies. Through the use of identification and expression of emotions or issues, patients no longer rely only on medical symptoms to unconsciously display their needs. Remember, when patients complain of physical symptoms, take the symptoms seriously. Even if a medical explanation is not found understandable, the symptoms are real and distressing to the patient. Table 12-2 lists possible interventions for patients with somatic symptom disorders.

TABLE 12-2 **Interventions for Somatic Symptom Disorders**	
Intervention	**Rationale**
1. Offer explanations and support during diagnostic testing.	1. Reduces anxiety while ruling out organic illness.
2. After physical complaints have been investigated, avoid further reinforcement of the somatic complaints.	2. Directs focus away from physical symptoms.
3. Spend time with the patient at times other than when he/she is expressing a physical complaint (e.g., when talking about a pet or TV program and give the "reward" of extra attention during those times).	3. Rewards non–illness-related behaviors and encourages repetition of desired behavior.
4. Observe and record frequency and intensity of somatic symptoms.	4. Establishes a baseline and later enables evaluation of effectiveness of interventions.
5. Do not imply that symptoms are not real.	5. Acknowledges that psychogenic symptoms are real to the patient.
6. Shift focus from somatic complaints to feelings or to neutral topics.	6. Conveys interest in patient as a person rather than in patient's symptoms; reduces need to gain attention via symptoms.
7. Assess secondary gains that physical illness provides for patient, such as attention, lack of work responsibility, or guilt of a spouse causing them to stay rather than leave the patient.	7. Allows these needs to be met in healthier ways and thus minimizes secondary gains.
8. Use straightforward approach to patient exhibiting resistance or covert anger.	8. Avoids power struggles, demonstrates acceptance of anger, and permits discussion of angry feelings.
9. Have patient direct all requests to a designated nurse or clinician.	9. Reduces manipulation.
10. Show concern for patient, but avoid fostering dependency needs.	10. Shows respect for patient's feelings while minimizing secondary gains from illness; encourages progress toward independence.
11. Reinforce patient's strengths and problem-solving abilities.	11. Contributes to positive self-esteem; helps patient realize that needs can be met without resorting to somatic symptoms.
12. Teach assertive communication skills and techniques.	12. Provides patient with a positive way of identifying feelings and meeting emotional needs; reduces feelings of helplessness and need for manipulation.
13. Teach patient stress reduction techniques, such as meditation, relaxation, and mild physical exercise.	13. Provides alternate coping strategies; reduces need for medication.

Working with people who have somatic symptom disorders can be frustrating, and you and other staff may find yourself avoiding interaction with them. However, when people feel they are receiving care and attention, the intensity of symptoms tends to diminish. As the symptoms are alleviated and rapport is established, it becomes easier to address emotional issues.

Health Teaching and Health Promotion

When somatization is present, the patient's ability to perform self-care activities may be impaired. In general, nursing interventions involve the use of a straightforward approach to support the highest level of functioning. For example, the patient who demonstrates arm paralysis can be encouraged to eat using the other arm. The patient who is experiencing blindness can be told where foods are located on his or her plate by comparing the plate to a clock face. These strategies are effective in reducing secondary gain.

Assertiveness training is often appropriate to teach a direct means of meeting needs and thereby decreases the need for somatic symptoms. Teaching an exercise regimen, such as doing range-of-motion exercises for 15 to 20 minutes daily, can help the patient feel in control, increase endorphin levels, and help decrease anxiety.

Assertiveness Training

"Assertiveness training is a form of behavior therapy designed to help people stand up for themselves—to empower themselves, in more contemporary terms. Assertiveness is a response that seeks to maintain an appropriate balance between passivity and aggression. Assertive responses promote fairness and equality in human interactions, based on a positive sense of respect for self and others" (Encyclopedia of Mental Disorders, http://www.minddisorders.com/A-Br/Assertiveness-training.html#ixzz3yHMZ9Tle).

Assertiveness training uses "I" statements to help defuse a combative/aggressive response. Instead of saying *"you always say you're going to study and you don't study, you'll never amount to anything,"* a less accusatory approach using "I" statements could decrease an aggressive tone and help the listener feel less defensive ("when you… I feel…"). For example, *"When you don't study, I feel so upset and frustrated because I want you to get the skills that will make you successful in life."*

Case Management

"Doctor shopping" is common among patients with these disorders. The patient constantly changes providers, hoping to establish a physical basis for his or her distress. Repeated diagnostic tests are often documented in the medical record. Case management can help limit health care costs by recommending to the provider that the patient be seen at regular intervals to instill security and avoid frantic and frequent demands. The patient who establishes a relationship with the case manager often feels less anxiety because he or she has an advocate and feels someone is managing and aware of his or her care.

Psychotherapy

Cognitive and behavioral approaches can be effective and may prove to be the therapy of choice for patients with somatic symptom disorders (Braun et al., 2010; Sharma & Manjula, 2012). Behavior modification can provide incentives, motivation, and rewards to help patients control their symptoms. Family and group therapy can increase awareness of communication patterns and help patients gain strategies to improve social skills (Koelen et al., 2014). Nurses may be involved with teaching patients alternative coping skills as well, such as relaxation and breathing techniques, or cognitive restructuring to aid in controlling anxiety and reframing faulty thinking.

Pharmacological Therapies

Currently antidepressants, specifically selective serotonin reuptake inhibitors (SSRIs), show the greatest promise for helping patients suffering from somatic symptom disorders (Black & Andreasen, 2014).

Patients may also benefit from short-term use of antianxiety medication, including benzodiazepines, which must be monitored carefully because of the risk of dependence. Nursing responsibilities include administering these medications and providing patient teaching.

EVALUATION

Evaluation of progress toward therapeutic goals is a straightforward process when measurable behavioral outcomes have been written clearly and realistically in the care plan. Even partially met goals are considered a success because of the considerable resistance to change in this population. Remission of symptoms is a process over time, and patients are likely to report the continuing presence of somatic symptoms, although they report less intensity and focus on the symptoms.

DISSOCIATIVE DISORDERS

The hallmark of the **dissociative disorders** is a disturbance in the normally well-integrated continuum of consciousness, memory, identity, and perception. Dissociation is an unconscious defense mechanism to protect the individual against overwhelming anxiety related to past trauma, and ranges from minor to severe in presentation. Patients with dissociative disorders have intact reality testing, meaning they are not delusional or hallucinating.

We all dissociate. Fantasy, daydreaming, absorption in activities, and night dreaming are considered normal dissociations. For example, we say we are on automatic pilot when we drive home from work but cannot recall the last 15 minutes before reaching home. However, these common experiences are distinctly different from the processes of pathological dissociation where the dissociation becomes prevalent and interferes with the person's functioning (Black & Andreasen, 2014). People with these disorders routinely experience significant emotional pain and struggle with overall functioning and safety.

Prevalence and Comorbidity

The actual **prevalence of dissociative disorders** in the general population is difficult to determine. A study conducted by Sar and colleagues (2011) determined the prevalence of dissociative disorders ranges from 5% to 29%. About 20% to 40% of the general population has had a transient period of depersonalization. Patients with dissociative disorders often present in emergency or outpatient settings with symptoms of self-harming behavior, suicidal ideations, addictions, mood swings, trauma, flashbacks, nightmares, and instability or disruption in work and relationships. Often identification of the dissociative process is overlooked by mental health clinicians who are not trained to recognize these processes. **Dissociative disorders can co-occur** with a wide range of other psychiatric disorders including posttraumatic stress disorder, body dysmorphic disorder, borderline personality disorder, childhood sexual abuse, and attention deficit disorder. Dissociative disorders may be misdiagnosed as psychosis due to hearing voices or presenting as unstable, although the etiologies and treatment of these disorders are very different.

THEORY

The cause of dissociative disorders is thought to be a protective response to past trauma. In the most severe presentation, dissociative identity disorder (formerly multiple personality disorder), the trauma began at an early age and has been severe and repetitive. Physical, sexual, or emotional abuse or other traumatic life experiences have been implicated. In addition to trauma, other etiological factors are discussed in the following sections.

Biological Factors

Current research suggests that the limbic system is involved in the development of dissociative disorders. Traumatic memories are processed in the limbic system, and the hippocampus stores this information. Animal studies show that early prolonged detachment from the caretaker negatively affects the development of the limbic system. Significant early trauma and lack of attachment have also been demonstrated to have effects on neurotransmitters, specifically on serotonin.

Extreme stress can cause alterations in the brain that may manifest as brain scan abnormalities. One study found that the hippocampus, essential for memory and learning, and the amygdala, which regulates emotions, are significantly smaller in people with dissociative identity disorder as compared with control subjects (Vermetten et al., 2006). Other studies have found no differences in brain structures in patients with dissociative disorders (Staniloiu et al., 2012).

Altered perceptions of self and fugue states occur with neurological diseases such as brain tumors and epilepsy, especially complex partial seizure disorder, suggesting a neurological component to the dissociative disorders. Depersonalization is also experienced by individuals under the influence of certain drugs, such as alcohol, barbiturates, and hallucinogens.

Genetic Factors

Several studies suggest that dissociative identity disorder (DID) is more common among first-degree biological relatives of individuals with the disorder than in the population at large. There is also evidence that patient histories recount multiple generations of dissociative symptoms and disorders and occurrence among siblings (Black & Andreasen, 2014).

Psychosocial Factors

Learning theory suggests that dissociative disorders can be explained as learned methods for avoiding stress and anxiety. The pattern of avoidance occurs when an individual deals with an unpleasant event by consciously deciding not to think about it. The more anxiety-provoking the event, the greater the need to emotionally escape. The more this technique is used, the more likely it is to become automatically utilized as a coping mechanism in response to stress. When stress is intolerable—for example, in a severely abused child—the individual may develop dissociation to defend against the overwhelming pain and helplessness of the situation. In about half the cases of depersonalization/derealization disorder, a recent traumatic antecedent cannot be identified (Armour et al., 2014). This may reflect a learned or biological etiology, but may also indicate a lack of recognition on the patient's part of the abuse. Rather than an obvious incident of rape, for example, the trauma may have been a daily pattern of parental conflict. While these coping mechanisms first develop in childhood, they carry on into adulthood where they create difficulties in the patient's life.

CULTURAL CONSIDERATIONS

Certain culturally bound disorders exist in which there is a high level of activity, a trancelike state, and running or fleeing, followed by exhaustion, sleep, and amnesia regarding the episode. These syndromes include *piblokto* among native people of the Arctic, Navajo *frenzy* witchcraft, and *amok* among western Pacific natives. These syndromes must be differentiated from dissociative disorders.

CLINICAL PICTURE

Depersonalization/Derealization Disorder

According to the *DSM-5* (APA, 2013) this disorder is characterized by recurrent periods of feeling unreal, detached, outside of the body, numb, dreamlike, or a distorted sense of time or visual perception. During the episodes, reality testing remains intact. The symptoms cause significant distress and life impairment and are not related to a medical condition or substance use. Other conditions to be ruled out include schizophrenia and posttraumatic stress disorder.

> **VIGNETTE**
>
> A 48-year-old female is admitted to a medical-surgical unit with complaints of a generalized numb feeling in her body. During a thorough assessment, she describes an odd perception when she looks in the mirror of not appearing or feeling like herself. "I don't know how to explain it, it just doesn't seem like me." She also reports the numb feeling and a detached or floating sensation, as well as not being fully alert. These symptoms began after her son sat down with her and confided that he was gay and HIV positive. In addition to considering neurological causes, depersonalization in response to her emotional trauma is probable.

Dissociative Amnesia, Dissociative Amnesia with Fugue

The *DSM-5* describes this disorder as the inability to recall specific information about the self, usually of a traumatic nature. The memory impairment may be selective for the traumatic event(s) or a particular time period, or generalized for the entire life history. The symptoms are not a result of drugs or a medical condition. Head injury, posttraumatic stress disorder, or a neurological disorder should also be considered. Dissociative amnesia is related to a traumatic incident, and may be accompanied by a fugue where the patient flees from their normal life to another location and starts a new life. Gradually over time, memories of the original life may be triggered. Patients can become confused and embarrassed when the amnesia subsides and memory returns. Black and Andreasen (2014)

> **VIGNETTE**
>
> A real-life example of dissociative fugue is the story of Raymond Powers, Jr., a New York attorney who disappeared one day. After his photo was displayed on the television show *America's Most Wanted* he was recognized by a resident at a homeless shelter in Chicago where he had been living for 6 months. Even after speaking with his wife by phone, Mr. Powers was unable to remember his children or life. Mr. Powers had been traumatized during the Vietnam War, and his trauma was brought to the surface after the terrorist attack on the World Trade Center on September 11, 2001. Mr. Powers had left work early that day, or would have been a victim of the tragedy. It is believed that memories of these traumas led to his dissociative fugue episode.
>
> Some cases of dissociative fugue prove to be false, such as the "runaway bride" Jennifer Wilbanks, who was under extreme stress before her wedding and knowingly fled to another state. Once she began to realize the consequences of her actions, she called home but fabricated a false story that she had being abducted. Ms. Wilbanks may have had amnesia for portions of her experience.

report that between 5% and 20% of veterans were amnesic for some parts of their combat experience.

Dissociative Identity Disorder (Formerly Multiple Personality Disorder)

Dissociative identity disorder (DID) is the most severe of the dissociative disorders. The *DSM-5* criteria include disruption of identity by two or more distinct personality states. The disruption in identity involves discontinuity in the sense of self, accompanied by alterations in affect, behavior, memory, and functioning. Patients "lose time," meaning they do not have memory of periods of time ranging from minutes to weeks. During the periods of lost time, an alter personality will be in control of the host person. The patient is often unaware of the other personalities before obtaining psychological treatment. The etiology of DID is severe and involves repetitive childhood abuse or trauma, with a mean duration of 10 years and beginning before the age of 6 years (Boysen & Van Bergen, 2013; Paris, 2012). In more than 600 patients with DID, sexual abuse was reported by 83%, physical abuse by 81%, and other or combined trauma by 94% (Paris, 2012). Although once considered rare, DID is now known to exist in 1% of the population, a rate equal to that of schizophrenia (Sar et al., 2007). Up to 90% of patients with this disorder are women, which is consistent with higher rates of abuse or more severe abuse in females (Black & Andreasen, 2014). Each alternate personality (alter) has its own pattern of personality, perception, and memories. The traumas that are overwhelming or intolerable to one small child are shared among the alters to protect the host individual (APA, 2013). Signs of this disorder in adulthood may include finding clothing or other unfamiliar items, being recognized by unfamiliar persons, differing handwriting on documents, and losing time. The change or switch between personalities may be subtle or more noticeable to an observer. Alter personalities often fall into common categories such as child alters and protector alters, which protect the secrets and may be violent. Borderline personality disorder traits including self-harm often co-occur with DID because of their common etiology of childhood trauma. The constant disruption of the main personality causes significant distress or impairment in social, occupational, or other important areas of functioning.

> **VIGNETTE**
>
> A 28-year-old woman is being seen for medication management by a doctoral level psychiatric nurse practitioner (DNP). The DNP notices a change in presentation during subsequent appointments. In the initial psychiatric evaluation, the patient was conservative, well-dressed, and articulate. In the third appointment, the patient was wearing a sweatshirt and jeans and had an arrogant air about her. A few appointments later, the patient was almost childlike, was wearing a pony tail, and was talking in a higher, lisping tone of voice. The DNP began to suspect dissociative identity disorder (DID) and started assessing more specifically for this disorder. When questioned, the patient recognized lapses in time, clothing that is not her usual style in the closet, and differing handwriting in her documentation at work. It was uncovered through the following months of treatment that the patient had three personalities or "alters": the main personality, who is an electrical engineer; a teenage male, who is a protector; and a young girl, who has memories of abuse. The patient had a history of severe sexual abuse beginning at age 2 and continuing until she graduated high school and moved out of the house. She had never had therapy for the abuse, but had periods during her life where she became very depressed, disorganized, and would attempt suicide. She initially came for treatment during a depressed phase.

ASSESSMENT

Medical Workup

In order for one of the dissociative disorders to be diagnosed, medical and neurological illnesses, substance use, and other coexisting psychiatric disorders must be considered as well. Medical and psychological clinicians may collect objective data from physical examination, electroencephalography, imaging studies, projective tests such as the Rorschach inkblot test, structured personality tests, and specific questionnaires designed to identify dissociative symptoms.

Identity and Memory

Assessing patients' ability to identify themselves requires more than asking patients to state their names. Changes in behavior, voice, dress, and demeanor might signal the presence of an alternate personality. Often the clinician will notice a childlike or angry personality first. Referring to self by another name or in the third person and using the word *we* instead of *I* are indications that the patient may have DID. The nurse should consider the following when assessing for memory and for dissociation:

- Does the patient report feeling unreal, like in a dream, or not feeling like himself/herself?
- Does the patient have a history of childhood abuse or trauma?
- Does the patient have gaps in memory, for specific events, or periods of time?
- Has the patient noticed any unfamiliar clothing or other objects or been recognized by unfamiliar persons?
- Have friends or family members told the patient that he/she acts like a different person sometimes?
- Has the patient ended up someplace and not known how he or she got there?
- Has the patient harmed him- or herself, such as cutting on arms or legs, with no recall of the event?

Patient History

The nurse must gather information about events in the person's life. Has the patient sustained a recent injury, such as a concussion? Does the patient have a history of seizures, especially temporal lobe epilepsy? Does the patient have a history of early trauma, such as physical, mental, or sexual abuse? Also refer to questions under the Identity and Memory section.

Mood

Is the individual depressed, anxious, or unconcerned? Many patients with DID seek help when the primary personality is depressed. Have there been suicidal thoughts, self-harm behavior, or suicide attempts? The nurse also observes for mood shifts. When alter personalities of DID assume control, their predominant moods may be different from that of the principal personality. If the alters shift frequently, marked mood swings and erratic behaviors may be noted.

Use of Alcohol and Other Drugs

Specific questions should be asked to identify drug or alcohol use. Dissociative episodes may be associated with recent use of alcohol or other substances—such as cocaine, opioids, sedatives, or stimulants—rather than related to childhood abuse. In addition, patients with dissociative disorders may have co-occurring substance abuse diagnoses.

Effect on Patient and Family

The effect of dissociation or alter personalities on the person's individual and family life should be assessed. Patients often present for treatment reporting a job loss, relationship strain, or severe depression and suicidality. In fugue states, individuals may function adequately in their new identities by choosing simple histories, undemanding occupations, and a relatively solitary lifestyle. The families of patients in fugue states report being highly distressed over the patient's disappearance. Patients with amnesia may be more dysfunctional. Their perplexity often renders them unable to work, and their memory loss impairs normal family relationships.

Suicide Risk

Whenever a patient's life has been substantially disrupted, he or she may have thoughts of suicide. According to the *DSM-5*, more than 70% of patients with dissociative identity disorder have attempted suicide, and self-mutilation and self-harm behaviors are common (APA, 2013). The nurse gathering data should be alert for expressions of hopelessness, verbalization that indicates the intent to engage in self-destructive behaviors, or visual observation of scarring, bruising, or other bodily damage that could indicate self-harm. Asking about suicidal thoughts or self-harming behaviors should be a routine part of assessment in this population.

▶▶ Assessment Guidelines
Dissociative Disorders

1. Assess for a history of a similar episode in the past.
2. Establish whether the person suffered abuse, trauma, or loss as a child.
3. Identify relevant psychosocial distress issues by performing a basic psychosocial assessment. (See Chapter 7 for information on the basic psychosocial assessment.)

See previous sections for specific questions indicating dissociation.

DIAGNOSIS

Nursing diagnoses for patients with dissociative disorders are suggested in Table 12-3.

OUTCOMES IDENTIFICATION

Outcomes must be established for each nursing diagnosis. General goals are to develop trust, correct faulty perceptions, heal emotional damage resulting from abuse, and encourage the patient to live in the present instead of dissociating (Moorhead et al., 2013). Recovery from DID can take long-term therapy to address the abuse, dissolve the amnesic barriers between alter personalities leading to integration, and develop healthier coping skills.

Specific examples of indicators that the outcomes are being achieved include the following:

- Patient will verbalize a clear sense of personal identity.
- Patient will report a decrease in stress (using a scale of 1 to 10).
- Patient will report comfort with role expectations.
- Patient will plan coping strategies for stressful situations.
- Patient will refrain from injuring self.

PLANNING

The planning of nursing care for the patient with a dissociative disorder is influenced by the setting and presenting problem. Nurses may encounter such a patient in times of crisis either in the emergency department or when the patient is admitted to the hospital for suicidal or homicidal behavior. The care plan will focus on safety and crisis intervention. The patient also may seek treatment of a comorbid depressive or anxiety disorder in the community setting. Planning will

TABLE 12-3 Potential Nursing Diagnoses for Dissociative Disorders

Signs and Symptoms	Nursing Diagnoses (NANDA)
Amnesia or fugue related to a traumatic event	Disturbed personal identity
Symptoms of depersonalization; feelings of unreality or body image distortions	Disturbed body image
Alterations in consciousness, memory, or identity	Ineffective coping
Abuse of substances related to dissociation	Ineffective role performance
Disorganization or dysfunction in usual patterns of behavior (absence from work, withdrawal from relationships, changes in role function)	Ineffective coping Ineffective family coping
Disturbances in memory and identity	Interrupted family processes
Interrupted family processes related to amnesia or erratic and changing behavior	Impaired parenting Ineffective impulse control
Feeling of being out of control of memory, behaviors, and awareness	Anxiety
Inability to explain actions or behaviors when in an altered state	Spiritual distress Risk for other-directed violence Risk for self-directed violence
Obsessive fear of contracting or having a serious or terminal illness	Death anxiety

Herdman, T.H. (Ed.) *Nursing Diagnoses-Definitions and Classification 2015-2017.* Copyright 2014, 1994-2014 NANDA International. Used by arrangement with John Wiley & Sons Limited. In order to make safe and effective judgments using NANDA-I nursing diagnoses it is essential that nurses refer to the definitions and defining characteristics of the diagnoses listed in this work.

TABLE 12-4 Interventions for Dissociative Disorders

Intervention	Rationale
1. Ensure patient safety by providing safe, protected environment and frequent observation.	1. Sense of bewilderment may lead to inattention to safety needs; some alter personalities may be angry or suicidal.
2. Provide nondemanding, simple routine.	2. Reduces anxiety.
3. Confirm identity of patient and orientation to time and place.	3. Supports reality and promotes ego integrity.
4. Encourage patient to do things for self and make decisions about routine tasks.	4. Enhances self-esteem by reducing sense of powerlessness and secondry gain associated with dependence; promotes independence.
5. Assist with other decision making until memory improves.	5. Lowers stress and prevents patient from having to live with the consequences of unwise decisions.
6. Support patient during exploration of feelings surrounding the stressful event.	6. Helps patient use support rather than dissociation to cope.
7. Do not overwhelm patient with data regarding past events.	7. Memory loss serves the purpose of preventing severe anxiety from overwhelming the individual.
8. Allow patient to progress at own pace as memory is recovered.	8. Prevents undue anxiety and resistance, keeps patient safe from acting out to escape emotional pain.
9. Provide support during disclosure of painful experiences.	9. Can be healing while minimizing feelings of isolation.
10. Accept patient's expression of negative feelings.	10. Conveys permission to have negative or unacceptable feelings.
11. Teach stress reduction methods.	11. Provides alternatives for anxiety relief.

address the major complaint with appropriate referrals for treatment of the dissociative disorder.

IMPLEMENTATION

Most of the time the patient with DID or other dissociative disorders is treated in the community, but may be admitted to a psychiatric unit when suicidal or in need of crisis stabilization. Once a complete history has been obtained and a nursing care plan established, the nurse will follow and evaluate progress of the interventions.

Communication Guidelines

Nurses can offer emotional presence during the recall of painful experiences, provide a sense of safety, and encourage an optimal level of functioning. Trust is a central issue in DID because of the etiology of abuse. A gentle and supportive approach will help to build therapeutic rapport. Table 12-4 offers examples of interventions for patients with dissociative disorders.

Health Teaching and Health Promotion

Patients with dissociative disorders need teaching about the illness and instruction in coping skills and stress management. They may need to develop techniques to interrupt a dissociative episode. Staff and significant others are made aware of the plan in order to foster cooperation and support. Patients need to keep a daily journal to increase their awareness of feelings and to identify triggers to dissociation. If a patient has never utilized journaling as a therapeutic tool, the nurse can suggest short writing exercises.

Milieu Therapy

When the patient is in a crisis that requires hospitalization, providing a safe environment is fundamental. Other desirable characteristics include that the environment be quiet, structured, and supportive. Confusion and noise increase the potential for depersonalization, anxiety, switching alter personalities in relation to negative memories being triggered, or other acting-out behavior. Task-oriented therapy or occupational and art therapy can be useful for these patients to calm and express internal feelings.

Psychotherapy

Psychotherapy has been proven to be the primary and most effective treatment modality in dissociative identity disorder patients (Brand et al., 2012). Therapists who treat this population need special training in dissociation and trauma. According to Brand and colleagues (2012), therapy needs to be very flexible. From their years of experience they found applying specific techniques within an overall psychodynamic framework effective. Such techniques include psychoeducation, processing memories and traumas through talking, traumatic reenactment, safety planning, journaling, relaxation techniques, hypnosis, and artwork.

APPLYING THE ART

A Person with Dissociative Disorder

Scenario

A student nurse attended a coping skills group at a local psychiatric inpatient facility during her psychiatric nursing rotation and noticed a patient staring out the window and seemingly not paying attention.

Therapeutic Goal

By the end of this interaction, the patient will report one concept or coping skill he or she has learned during group.

Student-Patient Interaction	Thoughts, Communication Techniques, and Mental Health Nursing Concepts
Student: "Hello. I'm a nursing student. May we sit down and talk for a bit?" **Patient:** "Sure, that's fine." **Student's feelings:** *Relief that patient was willing to talk.*	Giving information, general leads, offering self
Student: "During the group today, I noticed that you were staring out the window and kind of blanking out. Were you able to gain anything from the group session?" **Patient:** "I really wasn't paying attention after the beginning. I wanted to hear what she had to say; I like that group leader, but next thing I know I was out of it. I don't remember what she was teaching." **Student's feelings:** *Not what I was expecting; I thought she was just ignoring the group.*	Making observations, seeking information

Student-Patient Interaction	Thoughts, Communication Techniques, and Mental Health Nursing Concepts
Student: "What was the last thing you remember before feeling out of it?" **Patient:** "I was looking at her outfit, the pink flowered shirt and gray skirt…it looked so much like an outfit my mother had." **Student's feelings:** *I'm really not sure what to say now.*	Seeking information, placing event in time or sequence; student is noticing a probable dissociative event; patient is bringing up a connection with her mother
Student: "Would that be a good or bad memory related to your mother's outfit?" **Patient:** "There weren't too many good memories with my mother." **Student's feelings:** *I don't know if I have the skills to go down this road with her, not sure what all will come up. Will I hurt her by asking questions about sad memories?*	Focusing, exploring; student recognizing there may be some trauma or abuse related to patient's mother
Student: "Would it be alright if I passed this information on to your therapist? You could process some of the feelings about your mother. The therapist might be able to help you with some techniques to use when you feel triggered and want to blank out mentally." **Patient:** "That would be fine, I appreciate you noticing that I wasn't all there, and taking the time to sit and talk with me." **Student's feelings:** *I feel good about this. She appreciated my support, and I can help the treatment team with more information.*	Formulating a plan of action, suggesting collaboration, offering support; student recognizing some trained professional help is needed to explore childhood issues Goal was not met—my patient did not really pay attention in group to report a new skill. But, the interaction was still therapeutic and successful.

Pharmacological, Biological, and Integrative Therapies

There are no specific medications for dissociative disorders, but appropriate antidepressants or anxiolytic medications are given for comorbid symptoms. Substance use disorders and suicidal risk, which are common, must be assessed carefully if medication is prescribed. In the acute inpatient setting, the nurse may witness dramatic memory retrieval in patients with dissociative amnesia or fugue after treatment with intravenous benzodiazepines, although this approach is not common (Lee et al., 2011).

EVALUATION

Treatment is considered successful when outcomes are met. In the final analysis, the evaluation is positive when the following are achieved:
- Patient safety has been maintained.
- Anxiety has been reduced and the patient has returned to a functional state.
- Conflicts have been explored.
- New coping strategies have permitted the patient to function at a better level.
- Stress is handled adaptively, without the use of dissociation.
- Therapeutic alliances have been fostered.

APPLYING EVIDENCE-BASED PRACTICE (EBP)

Problem A 30-year-old woman has been referred for a psychiatric evaluation by her PCP. She brings pillows for joint support and asks that the lights be turned down during appointments. The first two sessions have been spent talking about her numerous medical conditions, and she has shared a three-ring binder of medical records with the psychiatric nurse practitioner. Her complaints include back, neck, and knee pain as well as migraine headaches. Her records indicate mild osteoarthritis that is inconsistent with the level of pain and inability to work that she reports. She has had second and third opinions with similar findings. She has an appointment with a neurologist because she is concerned her headaches may be indicative of a tumor. Her husband and friends avoid her, stating they are tired of hearing about her medical problems all the time.

APPLYING EVIDENCE-BASED PRACTICE (EBP)—cont'd

EBP Assessment

A. **What do you already know from experience?** This patient seems significantly more concerned about her conditions in comparison to the average person. Mild osteoarthritis is unlikely to present with a severe level of pain or result in the inability to work. Similar patients have tended to be defensive when possible psychiatric aspects to their problems have been broached.

B. **What does the literature say?** People with somatic symptom disorder often present with several medical issues. Symptoms are often exaggerated in comparison to the medical findings. Patients with this disorder focus on medical problems to a degree that creates high anxiety and interferes with life functioning. Several providers may have been consulted, and patients are frequently unaware of psychological aspects to their condition. Antidepressants, anxiolytics, cognitive behavioral therapy, and hypnotherapy have been shown to be helpful.

C. **What does the patient want?** This client is seeking help with a disability claim that had been denied. She requests assistance with anxiety related to the denied claim. She is interested in the nurse practitioner's opinion of her medical records and the quality of care she has received.

Plan Although this patient does not see the connection between her psychological stressors and her medical problems, treating her anxiety is a good place to start. She has requested help with this, so she should be cooperative, and the treatment of anxiety will likely improve her physical symptoms as well. As therapeutic rapport is established, the connection between psychological and physical symptoms can be gently discussed. An SSRI antidepressant such as sertraline will be prescribed, and a referral given for counseling to help with anxiety and relationships.

QSEN **QSEN Prelicensure Knowledge, Skills, and Attitudes (KSAs) Addressed:**

Team work and collaboration by referring the patient for therapy, reviewing medical records, and making contact with other providers.

Evidence-based care by utilizing what the literature says about best practice, past experience, and patient desires in the plan of care.

From Dimsdale, J. E. (2015). *Somatic symptom disorder. Merck Manual Professional Version.* Retrieved from www.merckmanuals.com/professional/psychiatric-disorders/somatic-symptom-and-related-disorders/somatic-symptom-disorder.

KEY POINTS TO REMEMBER

- Somatic symptom disorders are characterized by the presence of multiple, real physical symptoms for which there is most often no evidence of medical illness.
- Dissociative disorders involve a disruption in consciousness with a significant impairment in memory, identity, or perceptions of self.
- Emergences of both somatic symptom disorders and dissociative symptoms are believed to be responses to extreme psychological stress, which may result in faulty coping patterns.
- Patients with somatic symptom disorders and dissociative disorders often have a number of comorbid psychiatric illnesses, primarily depression, anxiety, substance abuse, and borderline personality disorder.
- A suicide assessment should be performed with any psychiatric patient. Somatic symptom disorders and related disorders and also dissociative disorder patients may be especially prone to self-harm behaviors.
- Because these patients may not seek psychiatric treatment, the nurse may often see these patients in a medical setting first.
- The nursing assessment is especially important to clarify the history and course of past symptoms, as well as to obtain a complete picture of the current physical and mental status.
- Although these patients do respond to crisis intervention, they usually require referral for long-term psychiatric treatment.

APPLYING CRITICAL JUDGMENT

1. A patient with suspected somatic symptom disorder has been admitted to the medical-surgical unit after an episode of chest pain. While on the unit, she frequently complains of palpitations, asks the nurse to check her vital signs, and begs staff to stay with her. She does not believe that her electrocardiogram was normal, and asks repeatedly for it to be interpreted again. Some nurses retake her pulse and blood pressure measurements when she asks. Others evade her requests. Most staff try to avoid spending time with her. Consider why staff tend to avoid her.
   A. What could you do as a nursing team to improve care and support each other with this difficult patient? Think about both communication and structured interventions.

2. A patient with DID has been admitted to the crisis unit for a short-term stay after a suicide threat. On the unit, the patient has repeated the statement that she will kill herself to get rid of "all the others," meaning her alter personalities.
   A. What safety concerns might you have about this patient?
   B. Knowing that she has DID, what types of information should you gather?

CHAPTER REVIEW QUESTIONS

1. A patient at a general medical clinic tells the nurse, "I have so many ailments that I need to see six different doctors. None of them has discovered what is really wrong with me." Which comment should the nurse offer next?
   a. "Let's review all the medications you currently take."
   b. "Tell me about allergic reactions you've had to medication."
   c. "Selecting one primary care provider would be better for you."
   d. "I'm not sure I understand how you can afford these expenses."

2. A combat veteran from two tours of the war in Afghanistan tells the nurse, "Some guys in my unit have posttraumatic stress disorder, but I never had any problems other than my hearing is not as good as it once was." Which explanation for this comment should the nurse consider?
   a. The veteran wants to demonstrate toughness and strength.
   b. The veteran shows indicators of derealization and depersonalization.
   c. The veteran may be rationalizing this reaction to memories of combat.
   d. The veteran may have amnesia associated with the combat experience.

3. A patient diagnosed with dissociative identity disorder is hospitalized on an acute care psychiatric unit after a suicide attempt. During a team meeting, which staff nurse's comment should prompt the nursing supervisor to intervene?
   a. "I have never taken care of a patient diagnosed with this disorder."
   b. "I think this patient was misdiagnosed and probably has schizophrenia."

c. "I find myself more fascinated and engaged with this patient than others."

d. "I recently read an autobiographical book about someone with this problem."

4. A nurse in an outpatient medical clinic talks to a patient with a long history of malingering and doctor-shopping. The patient continues to express complaints of multiple problems. Select the nurse's best comment to the patient.

a. "The treatment team believes you would benefit more from seeing a mental health professional."

b. "The treatment team discussed your case and wants to begin a special case management program for you."

c. "Because you take a number of medications, it would be safer to have them all filled at the same pharmacy."

d. "Diagnostic testing has shown no medical problems and you are using more than your fair share of health care services."

5. A patient in the emergency department was seen for the third time in a month with complaints of tremors and paresthesia in the lower extremities. Conversion disorder was diagnosed. While preparing for discharge, the patient says, "Now I'm having chest pain but it's probably nothing." How should the nurse respond?

a. Assess the patient's most current laboratory values.

b. Interrupt the discharge and arrange additional medical evaluation of the patient.

c. Remind the patient, "The diagnostic tests showed you did not have a medical problem."

d. Tell the patient, "Being in the emergency department a long time can be very distressing."

REFERENCES

American Psychiatric Association. (2013). *Diagnostic and statistical manual of mental disorders (DSM-5)* (5th ed.). Washington, DC: APA.

Armour, C., Contractor, A. A., Palmieri, P. A., et al. (2014). Assessing latent level associations between PTSD and dissociative factors: is depersonalization and derealization related to PTSD factors more so than alternative dissociative factors? *Psychological Injury and Law, 7*(2), 131–142.

Ask, H., Waaktaar, T., Seglem, K. B., & Torgersen, S. (2016). Common etiological sources of anxiety, depression, and somatic complaints in adolescents: a multiple rater twin study. *Journal of Abnormal Childhood Psychology, 2016*(44), 101–114.

Black, D. W., & Andreasen, N. C. (2014). *Introductory textbook of psychiatry* (6th ed.). Washington, DC: American Psychiatric Publishing.

Boysen, G. A., & Van Bergen, A. (2013). A review of published research on adult dissociative identity disorder: 2000-2012. *Journal of Nervous & Mental Disease, 201*(1), 5–11.

Brand, B. L., Myrick, A. C., Lowenstein, R. J., et al. (2012). A survey of practices and recommended treatment interventions among expert therapists treating patients with dissociative identity disorder and dissociative disorder not otherwise specified. Psychological trauma: theory. *Research, Practice, and Policy, 4*(5), 490–500.

Braun, I. M., Greenberg, D. B., Smith, F. A., et al. (2010). Functional somatic symptoms, deception syndromes, and somatic symptom disorders. In T. A. Stern, G. L. Friccione, N. H. Cassem, et al. (Eds.), *Massachusetts General Hospital handbook of general hospital psychiatry* (6th ed.). Philadelphia: Saunders/Elsevier.

Burton, C., McGorm, K., Weller, D., & Sharpe, M. (2011). Depression and anxiety in patients repeated referred to secondary care with medically unexplained symptoms: a case-control study. *Psychological Medicine, 2011*(41), 555–563.

Carteret, M. (2011). *Folk illnesses and remedies in Latino communities. Dimensions of culture.* Retrieved from http://www.dimensionsofculture.com/2010/10/folk-illnesses-and-remedies-in-latino-communities/.

Creed, F. H., Davies, I., Jackson, J., et al. (2012). The epidemiology of multiple somatic symptoms. *Journal of Psychosomatic Research, 72*(4), 311–317.

Dimsdale, J. E. (2015). Somatic symptom disorder. *Merck manual professional version.* Retrieved from www.merckmanuals.com/professional/psychiatric-disorders/somatic-symptom-and-related-disorders/somatic-symptom-disorder.

Falvo, D. R. (2014). *Medical and psychosocial aspects of chronic illness and disability* (5th ed.). Burlington, Mass: Jones & Bartlett Learning.

Frances, A. (2013). DSM-5 somatic symptom disorder. *Journal of Nervous and Mental Disease, 201*(6), 530–531.

Hart, S. L., Hodgkison, S. C., Belcher, H. M. E., Hyman, C., & Cooley-Strickland, M. (2011). Somatic symptoms, peer and school stress, and family and community violence exposure among urban elementary school children. *Journal of Behavioral Medicine, 2013*(36), 454–465.

Ibeziako, P., & Bujoreanu, S. (2011). Approach to psychosomatic illness in adolescents. *Current Opinion, 23*(4), 483–489.

Koelen, J. A., Houtveen, J. H., Abbass, A., et al. (2014). Effectiveness of psychotherapy for severe somatoform disorder: meta-analysis. *British Journal of Psychiatry, 204*(1), 12–19.

Kurlansik, S. L., & Maffei, M. S. (2016). Somatic symptom disorder. *American Family Physician, 93*(1), 49–54a http://www.aafp.org/.

Lee, S., Park, S., & Park, S. (2011). Use of lorazepam in drug-assisted interviews: two cases of dissociative amnesia. *Psychiatry Investigation, 8*(4), 377–380.

Lind, A. B., Delmar, C., & Nielsen, K. (2014). Struggling in an emotional avoidance culture: a qualitative study of stress as a predisposing factor for somatoform disorders. *Journal of Psychosomatic Research, 76*(2), 94–98.

Lubkin, I. M., & Larson, P. (2013). *Chronic illness: impact and intervention* (8th ed.). Burlington, Mass: Jones & Bartlett Learning.

Moorhead, S., Johnson, M., Maas, M. L., et al. (2013). *Nursing outcomes classification (NOC)* (4th ed.). St Louis: Mosby.

Paris, J. (2012). The rise and fall of dissociative identity disorder. *Journal of Nervous & Mental Disease, 200*(12), 1076–1079.

Sar, V., et al. (2011). *Epidemiology of dissociative disorders: an overview. Epidemiology Research International.*

Sar, V., Akyuz, G., & Dogan, O. (2007). Prevalence of dissociative disorders among women and the general population. *Psychiatry Research, 149*(1–3), 169.

Sharma, M. P., & Manjula, M. (2012). Behavioral and psychological management of somatic symptom disorder: an overview. *International Review of Psychiatry, 25*(1), 116–124.

Spratt, E. G. (2014). Somatoform disorder. *Medscape.* Retrieved from http://emedicine.medscape.com/article/918628-overview.

Staniloiu, A., Vitcu, I., & Markowitsch, H. J. (2012). Neuroimaging and dissociative disorders: advances in brain imaging. In V. Chaudhary (Ed.), *InTech.* Retrieved from www.intechopen.com/books/advances-in-brain-imaging/neuroimaging-and-dissociative-disorders.

Stone, J., LaFrance, C., Levenson, J. L., et al. (2010). Issues for DSM-5: conversion disorder. *American Journal of Psychiatry, 167*, 626–627. Retrieved from http://ajp.psychiatryonline.org/cgi/content/full/167/6/626.

Vermetten, E., Schmahl, C., Lindner, S., et al. (2006). Hippocampal and amygdalar volumes in dissociative identity disorder. *American Journal of Psychiatry, 163*, 630–636.

Yates, W. R. (2014). *Somatic symptom disorders: treatment and medication.* Updated 2010. Retrieved from http://emedicine.Medscape.com/article/294908-treatment.

Zaroff, C. M., Davis, J. M., Chio, P. H., et al. (2012). Somatic presentations of distress in China. *Australia New Zealand Journal of Psychiatry, 46*(11), 1053–1057.

Personality Disorders

Elizabeth M. Varcarolis

http://evolve.elsevier.com/Varcarolis/essentials

KEY TERMS AND CONCEPTS

antisocial personality disorder, p. 169
avoidant personality disorder, p. 171
borderline personality disorder
(BPD), p. 169
dialectical behavior therapy (DBT), p. 176
entitlement, p. 169

manipulation, p. 169
narcissistic personality disorder, p. 170
obsessive-compulsive personality
disorder (OCPD), p. 171
paranoid personality disorder, p. 168
passive-aggressive personality traits, p. 172

personality, p. 166
personality disorders (PDs), p. 166
schizoid personality disorder, p. 168
schizotypal personality disorder, p. 168
splitting, p. 170

SELECTED CONCEPT: PERSONALITY

"**Personality** refers to the habitual patterns of behavior, cognition, motivation, and ways of relating to others that are characteristic of the individual" (Caligor et al., 2014, p. 257).

Mayer (2005) identified three personality traits needed to guide a person toward effective social and interpersonal functioning:

- A stable and realistic sense of self
- A system for the interpretation of social situations and the understanding of the relational motives and actions of others
- The capacity to serve the self as it relates with others

OBJECTIVES

1. Summarize four characteristics shared by people with personality disorders.
2. Describe at least four co-occurring conditions that are often present in people with a personality disorder.
3. Define and differentiate among at least three examples of primitive or immature defenses.
4. Compare and contrast the behaviors seen in borderline personality disorder and narcissistic personality disorder.
5. Identify some disconcerting feelings that health care professionals frequently experience when working with individuals with personality disorders.
6. **QSEN** Discuss how you would use **teamwork and collaboration** when working with a patient who is extremely manipulative.
7. **QSEN** In planning **patient-centered care** for an individual who demonstrates impulsive behaviors, explain how to use at least four effective communication strategies.
8. **QSEN** Identify those individuals with personality disorders who have the highest potential for self-harm (e.g., **safety** risks).

INTRODUCTION

Personality is essentially an enduring pattern of inner experience and behavior that deviates from the individual's culture. These enduring traits are usually first evident in adolescent disorders (Black & Andreasen, 2014). Essentially, personality is a "style" a person adopts to deal with the world. Personality traits are stylistic peculiarities that all people bring to social relationships, including shyness, seductiveness, rigidity, suspiciousness, or passive-aggressive traits. In ordinary/nonpathological states, personality traits are flexible and adaptive and defenses against anxiety tend to be more mature. In people with personality disorders (PDs), personality traits tend to be inflexible and unpredictable, and coping strategies tend to be more primitive and immature (Blaise et al., 2016). Personality pathology exists on a continuum. Personality disorders range from mild to moderate to severe based on disturbances in functionality. Most people with PDs do suffer. Their relationships with others are problematic, and they rarely reach their potential. They are often socially isolated because of their rigidity, maladaptive coping skills, and control issues that complicate their interpersonal as well as interactions with society. These patients can act bizarre, anxious, withdrawn, manipulative, or violent, and their behaviors tend to alienate them from the population. Because people with personality disorders are unaware that traits in their own personality makeup are causing problems, they often blame others for their difficulties or even deny they have a problem.

NOTE: Often nurses and other medical personnel loosely refer to various patients as "difficult" because they themselves have not yet figured out how best to work with patients with certain peculiarities. Having heard a patient is "difficult," staff members may approach that patient ready for trouble. Gordon (2013) suggests reframing the situation as a professional (as in, "I am having difficulties dealing with this particular patient"). Reframing allows us to look for more creative or alternatives solutions and approaches. Having said that, there *are* patients who may deserve that characterization.

People with PDs present the most complex, difficult behavioral challenges for themselves and people around them. In the health care community a truly "difficult patient" is usually an individual with a PD. Personality disorders are among the most frequently treated disorders by psychiatrists and mental health practitioners, although the initial focus of treatment is usually a co-occurring symptom or disorder (e.g., anxiety disorder, depressive disorder, substance use disorder, eating disorder, or a medical condition). Besides having extensive disability in work and personal relationships, people with personality disorders often have difficulty with **accurately perceiving and interpreting** the world and others around them. They also can have **inappropriate emotional responses** (range and intensity) to stress, occurrences in the environment, or interpersonal interactions. People with personality disorders may often have a great deal of difficulty with **impulse control** as well (APA, 2013).

These individuals assume that everyone thinks and functions as they do; therefore, within relationships they do not view their behavior as a problem; they do not see a need to make changes or accommodate others. They believe that they are normal and that others have a problem. This thinking leads to problems with self-concept, relationships, and ability to function in society. Although some individuals with PDs may desire closer relationships with others, the following are some of the reasons personal and work relationships often fail for individuals with PDs:

- Avoidance and fear of rejection
- Blurring of boundaries between the self and others so that closeness seems to lead to fusion, an intense and undesirable effect on both parties
- Insensitivity to the needs of others
- Demanding
- Fault finding (grievance collectors)
- Inability to trust
- Lack individual accountability
- Passive-aggressive traits
- Tendency to evoke intense interpersonal conflict

Since people with PDs fail to see themselves objectively and they lack the desire to alter aspects of their behavior in order to enrich or maintain important relationships, relationships are often marked by intense emotional upheavals and hostility that lead to serious interpersonal conflict, and in some cases violence (self-violence or violence toward others).

PREVALENCE AND COMORBIDITY

Individuals with personality disorders are frequently seen in psychiatric and medical settings. Caligor and colleagues (2014) estimate that 50% or more of patients who come for medical advice may have a personality disorder. In the clinical population of people already diagnosed with a psychiatric disorder, studies find that between 30% and 50% have a co-occurring personality disorder. For example, some studies indicate that up to 51% of people with a major depressive disorder and more than 60% of people with generalized anxiety disorder may have a comorbid personality disorder (Black & Andreasen, 2014).

Co-occurring Disorders/Comorbid

Personality disorders often co-occur with other PDs, with other mental health disorders (e.g., substance use disorder, somatic symptom disorders, eating disorders, posttraumatic stress disorder [PTSD], depression, anxiety disorders, etc.) or with general medical conditions.

In fact, comorbidity seems to be the rule and not the exception. The co-occurrence of personality disorder with other disorders often portends a poor response to treatment.

Because most people with PDs do not believe there is anything wrong with them, they rarely enter treatment for their personality disorder alone. Most often the disorder is not the initial focus of treatment. Many clinicians advocate that PDs should be evaluated in all psychiatric patients because their presence can influence the course and treatment of an existing psychiatric disorder or a medical disorder for which the patient sought help initially.

THEORY

It is unlikely that there is any single cause for a discrete PD. Personality traits and their exaggerations are probably largely caused by a combination of hereditary temperamental traits and environmental and neurodevelopmental events. The contribution of genetic, biological, and environmental factors will vary with each specific disorder and individual. The personality traits are thought to be present from infancy, but in most cases it is not until adolescence that the disorder emerges.

Genetic Factors

Research results support a more dominant role of genetics. In a definitive study of identical and fraternal twins who were raised apart, identical twins were found to have more similar personality traits than fraternal twins (Sadock et al., 2015).

Genetics seem to play a significant role in the development of schizotypal personality disorder, which is more common in families with a history of schizophrenia. Obsessive-compulsive personality disorder seems to have a genetic link as well. A strong genetic link is found in family and adoption studies for the presence of borderline and antisocial personality disorders (Black & Andreasen, 2014). Depression is more common in the background in patients with borderline personality disorders; antisocial disorders have a high rate of concordance with alcohol/substance use disorders (Sadock et al., 2015).

Neurobiological Factors
Impulsive and Aggressive Behaviors

Disturbances in the levels of the neurotransmitter serotonin (5-hydroxytryptamine [5-HT]) have been linked with irritability, impulsivity, and hypersensitivity. Brain imaging studies suggest abnormalities in prefrontal, corticostriatal, and limbic networks that may be related to lower serotonin neurotransmission (5-HT) and behavioral disinhibition in people with borderline and antisocial personality disorders (Black & Andreasen, 2014).

In people with borderline personality disorder, abnormal brain structure and function have been found. Findings include abnormalities in the size of the hippocampus, in the size and functioning of the amygdala, and in the functioning of the frontal lobes. These areas of the brain are associated with regulating emotions and integrating thoughts with emotions (Dryden-Edwards, 2016). Individuals with antisocial personality disorder have shown altered metabolism in the prefrontal regions of the brain. An image study identified reduced prefrontal gray matter within areas of the brain implicated in empathic processing, moral reasoning, and the processing of emotions such as guilt and embarrassment, whereas another study also found specific abnormalities in the processing of emotions in psychopathic criminals (Black & Andreasen, 2014; Gregory, 2012).

Affective Instability

Affective instability, seen in borderline personality disorder, is characterized by brief shifts of mood from depression, to irritability, to anxiety lasting up to a couple of hours in length. Affective instability is thought to be a result of excessive limbic reactivity in GABAergic/glutamatergic/cholinergic circuits. "These shifts are dramatic and trigger impulsive aggression and self-destructive behavior, including drug and alcohol abuse, reckless driving, promiscuity, direct self-injurious actions, as well as suicidal gestures or attempts" (Siever & Weinstein, 2009, p. 370).

Psychological Influences

Children suffering from abuse or trauma or children living in homes in which there is domestic abuse, divorce, separation, or parental absence are at risk for development of personality disorders; neglect seems to be particularly damaging (Black & Andreasen, 2014). Childhood trauma may be a risk factor for any personality disorder in general and for borderline and antisocial personality disorders in particular (Black & Andreasen, 2014). Individuals diagnosed with antisocial personality disorder often have a history that includes excessively harsh or erratic discipline, alcoholic/substance using parent(s), and/or an abusive/chaotic home life.

This is particularly true for people with borderline personality disorder (BPD). There is consistent evidence that sexual abuse is a common risk factor for BPD, which also may entail significant parental conflict or loss. Linehan (1993), an early pioneer in the successful treatment of people with borderline personality disorder, made the observation that those with borderline personality disorder frequently were raised in families in which they were subjected to constant belittling, devaluation, and validation. If the history of sexual abuse was before the age of 13, PTSD may also be present as well as borderline traits or diagnoses.

Cultural Considerations

It is important when making a psychiatric diagnosis to be aware of the cultural implications and what is considered normal so that culturally unsanctioned behaviors can be differentiated. This is especially true when a clinician is making a diagnosis of personality disorder. However, it appears that certain groups of the population are at a greater risk than others for certain PDs. In general, other risk factors include being Native American or African American, being a young adult, having low socioeconomic status, and being divorced, separated, widowed, or never married.

Cross-cultural studies indicate low rates of antisocial personality disorder in Taiwan, China, and Japan, as well as in Jewish families, which might be attributed to their strong family ties (Black & Andreasen, 2014).

CLINICAL PICTURE

The following A, B, C clusters are useful in research and for educational purposes (refer to the box below). However, there are some limitations to using these categorizations too rigidly. One caveat is that many people invariably present with more than one personality disorder, and a second personality disorder may come from a different cluster.

Cluster A	Cluster B	Cluster C
Odd or eccentric behavior	Dramatic, emotional behavior	Anxious, fearful behavior
Suspicious	Attention-seeking	Tense
Cold	Labile	Overcontrolled
Withdrawn	Shallow	Depressed
Irrational	Increased rates of substance use and suicide	

For educational purposes, the personality disorders are presented within these ABC clusters, along with a clinical picture, major pathological personality traits, and clinical vignettes.

CLUSTER A DISORDERS

These individuals, often seen as **"odd" or eccentric,** have been established to have some relationship to schizophrenia. Of the cluster A disorders,

schizotypal is the most strongly related to schizophrenia. Individuals with cluster A disorders avoid interpersonal relationships, have unusual beliefs, and may be indifferent to the reactions of others in their lives. They come into the health care system either because of a co-occurring disorder or because of a brief psychotic episode. These individuals refuse responsibility of their own feelings and assign responsibility to others. Prominent stages for the following disorders are listed and illustrated by vignettes. Cluster A disorders include schizotypal personality disorder, schizoid personality disorder, and paranoid personality disorder.

Schizotypal Personality Disorder
Pathological Personality Traits

Individuals with schizotypal personality disorders are characterized by a pattern of **peculiar behavior and odd speech and by the presence of cognitive perceptual distortions in the absence of psychosis** (APA, 2013; Black & Andreasen, 2014). These individuals avoid interpersonal relationships, and may be indifferent to the reactions of others in their lives.

They most closely resemble people with schizophrenia and are perceived by others as **strikingly odd, strange, or eccentric.** Individuals with schizotypal personality disorders often possess and demonstrate **magical thinking and rituals,** hold beliefs that they can control the actions of others, or have bizarre fantasies or preoccupations that are *not* consistent with cultural norms. Their **speech is peculiar in phrasing and syntax and may have meaning only to them.** Reactions of confusion by others to their apparent illogical speech may cause these individuals to become **suspicious of others and eventually to develop paranoid thinking.** Their eccentric and **unkempt appearances, strange behaviors, and nonadherence to social conventions** make it impossible for them to have give-and-take conversations. Because of these odd styles of behavior and inattention to social conventions, they lack friends. People with this disorder are genuinely unhappy about their lack of relationships and their social anxiety and unhappiness increase over time. Under increased stress, these individuals may exhibit psychotic symptoms (APA, 2013; Sadock et al., 2015).

Up to 10% of people with schizotypal personality disorder commit suicide and some may develop schizophrenia (Sadock et al., 2015). These individuals enter the health care system either because of a co-occurring disorder or because of a psychotic episode.

> **VIGNETTE**
>
> Ms. Sands is 36 years old, lives alone, and is a "writer" and lives on social security benefits. She goes out every night, only at night, to a nearby grocery store (because "their magic does not work at night"). She dresses in several layers of multicolored and mismatched clothes, even in warmer weather. She wears a turban on her head to "keep them from seeing my thoughts." Each night she tells the grocer in a flat and formal manner that she is going to be a famous director and star. She knows this because "it hasn't snowed yet, and that means the coast is clear."

Paranoid Personality Disorder
Pathological Personality Traits

People with paranoid personality disorder (PPD) exhibit traits that are characterized by **pervasive, persistent, and inappropriate suspiciousness and distrust of others** without the slightest justification (APA, 2013). Individuals with PPD are no strangers to the health care system. Nurses encounter people who are **hostile, irritable, angry, injustice collectors, pathologically jealous of their partner, and litigious cranks;** they are constantly suspicious and believe that others are lying, cheating, exploiting, or trying to harm them in some way. These individuals **lack warmth, pay close attention to power and rank, and express disdain to those who are weak, sickly, and impaired.** Although they may appear businesslike and efficient, they often generate fear and conflict in others through their hostile, stubborn, and sarcastic expressions (APA, 2013; Sadock et al., 2015). People with paranoid traits are constantly suspicious of the intentions of others, and find hidden malicious meaning in benign comments and behaviors (**ideas of reference**). Even when people are loyal to them (e.g., spouse, partner) they usually make others uncomfortable; they are **keenly aware of the weaknesses of others and exploit these weaknesses** to keep interpersonal distance. It has been said that individuals with personality traits "lack the milk of human kindness."

VIGNETTE

Mr. Cole, a 58-year-old man, comes into the emergency department (ED) with chest pains. He refuses to give background information "because the information could be used against me," and he is haughty and demeaning to the nurse, saying, in a loud and angry voice, "Get someone in here who knows something. I know when I am being treated unfairly."When the nurse turned her back to Mr. Cole to speak to the physician, Mr. Cole shouted, "What lies is she telling you about me? Do either one of you know what you are doing? Are you both in this together?"

Schizoid Personality

People with schizoid personality traits are characterized by an **inability to establish relationships with others and a restricted range of emotions in interpersonal settings** (APA, 2013). They are seen by others as **eccentric, isolated, or lonely.** They may exist on the periphery of society content to avoid relationships of even the most superficial nature. Their **affect is usually flat, which projects emotional coldness.** They appear indifferent to praise or criticism by others. Although they invest **no interest or energy into human relationships of any kind, they may invest enormous energy into nonhuman interests** such as mathematics and astronomy. Typically loners, they spend much time daydreaming and are often very attached to animals. There is some evidence that people with schizoid personality traits may later develop schizophrenia or a delusional disorder. Although aloof, some individuals with schizoid traits have conceived, developed, and given our world genuinely original and creative ideas.

VIGNETTE

Mr. Ortiz, a 38-year-old unmarried bookkeeper, was assaulted on his way home from work. A bystander called 911 and Mr. Ortiz was taken to the emergency department in an unconscious state. Once awake, he answers questions in a monotonal voice and avoids making eye contact. He often looks away and does not respond at all. He is compliant and remains a passive recipient of his treatment. Mr. Ortiz rejects all nursing interventions aimed at increasing socialization.

CLUSTER B PERSONALITY DISORDERS

Cluster B disorders appear to share **emotional reactivity** (e.g., dramatic, erratic, flamboyant), **poor impulse control,** and an **unclear sense of identity** (Caligor et al., 2014). There seems to be a great deal of overlap among these disorders with other mental health disorders such as substance use, depression, and eating disorders. Manipulation is a common defensive mechanism among people with these disorders, and their behaviors are always challenging no matter what part of the health care system is caring for their needs.

These disorders include antisocial, borderline, histrionic, and narcissistic personality disorders.

Antisocial Personality Disorder
Pathological Personality Traits

Antisocial personality disorder is characterized by **persistent disregard for and violation of the rights of others with an absence of remorse for hurting others** (APA, 2013, p. 659).

People with antisocial PD have a sense of entitlement, which means they believe they have the right to hurt others, take what they want,

treat others unfairly, destroy the property of others, and so on (**callousness**). They do not adhere to traditional values or standards of morality as boundaries for their actions. Therefore, there is no restraint on their behavior, nor do they feel any sense of responsibility for their actions. People who have antisocial personality disorders **lack regard for the law and the rights of others and have a history of persistent lying, use of aliases, conning others for personal profit or pleasure, and stealing (deceitfulness).** However, they do rely on others to conform to the social norms.

Verbally these patients may be charming, engaging, and uncanny in their ability to find just the right angle to lure a person into their intrigue with the intent to exploit them for money, favors, or more sadistic purposes (**manipulation**). Promiscuity, reckless disregard for the safety of others, failure to honor work or financial commitments, and drunk driving are common events in their lives. Their lives are marked by chronic irresponsibility and unreliability. They may have a history of violence, partner abuse, child abuse, anger in response to minor slights, and vindictive behavior toward others that can result in physical or emotional pain. General reckless disregard for the safety of others is a common trait of these individuals. However, this same recklessness applies to themselves as well in their pursuit of thrill-seeking activities. People with antisocial personality disorder often become bored and engage in **impulsive/risky** and dangerous sports or other activities, some claiming they participate in such behaviors just to "feel alive." This diagnosis is made in people 18 years of age or older. Often there is evidence of *conduct disorder* (e.g., fire setting, cruelty to animals, stealing) with onset before the age of 15 years (APA, 2013).

These individuals account for a disproportionate number of crimes including violent offenses (Verona & Patrick, 2015).

VIGNETTE

Mr. Jones has been extorting money from lonely widows by charming them, "helping them with their finances," promising to marry them, and then taking off with their money. When in court, he laughed when he was asked if he felt guilty for taking the life savings of these elderly lonely widows, "Hey, I gave them what they wanted." Fingerprints revealed that his name was really Oliver Torres, with a long list of aliases, as well as a history of family violence and burglary. He had abandoned his wife and three children eight years previously.

Borderline Personality Disorder (BPD)

Central to the character of people with borderline personality disorder (BPD) is their **unstable and intense relationship, and, instability of affect**, marked by unstable and frequent mood changes. Feelings of anxiety, dysphonia, and irritability can be intense though short lived (**emotional lability**). **Poor impulse control** is evidenced by recurrent suicide attempts, self-mutilation, and other self-destructive behaviors. Chronic depression is common. The use of the primitive defense mechanism of **projected identification** is common in patients with BPD. This occurs when the person projects on an undesirable aspect of the self. Individuals with BPD often exhibit patterns of high emotional sensitivity, acute responsiveness, and slow return to normal as **"emotional dysregulation."** This cycle may lead to feelings of deadness, panic, and fury as well as *self-mutilation* and *suicide-prone behaviors*. These are common responses to threats of separation or rejection. People with BPD desperately seek relationships to avoid **feelings of abandonment and chronic feelings of emptiness.** However, their excessive demands, impulsive behavior, and/or uncontrolled anger drives others away. Their relationships are stormy, marked by intense neediness and lack of trust. Their perception of the person in the relationship alternates between idealization and devaluation and between overinvolvement and withdrawal. When relationships end, the person with borderline personality disorder is often left with feelings of deadness, panic, fury, and intense abandonment. A person with BPD can experience dissociative states under stress. Their frequent use of the defense of splitting not only strains personal relationships but also creates turmoil in health care settings. Splitting is the inability to integrate both the positive and the negative qualities of an individual into one person. The individual tends to think in extremes (i.e., an individual's actions and motivations are all good or all bad with no middle ground). Therefore an individual is viewed as either highly valued or extremely bad, either black or white. Often, initially a health care provider (or friend, teacher, boss, or lover) is idealized (e.g., "he/she is wonderful!"). But, at the first sign of disappointment or perceived rejection, the individual is experienced as "intensely bad" and thus goes from idealized to devalued/despised in a matter of minutes. Holding alternating strong and intense positive and negative feelings toward the same person results in unstable and difficult interpersonal relationships. According to Francis (2013), people with BPD have a lifetime suicide rate of around 10%. However, there seems to be improvement and mellowing out with middle age.

DSM-5 DIAGNOSTIC CRITERIA
for Borderline Personality Disorder

A pervasive pattern of instability of interpersonal relationships, self-image, and affects, and marked impulsivity, beginning by early adulthood and present in a variety of contexts, as indicated by five (or more) of the following:

1. Frantic efforts to avoid real or imagined abandonment. (**Note:** Do not include suicidal or self-mutilating behavior covered in Criterion 5.)
2. A pattern of unstable and intense interpersonal relationships characterized by alternating between extremes of idealization and devaluation.
3. Identity disturbances: markedly and persistently unstable self-image or sense of self.
4. Impulsivity in at least two areas that are potentially self-damaging (e.g., overspending money, sex, substance abuse, reckless driving, binge eating). (**Note:** Do not include suicidal or self-mutilating behavior covered in Criterion 5.)
5. Recurrent suicidal behavior, gestures, or threats, or self-mutilating behavior.
6. Affective instability due to a marked reactivity of mood (e.g., intense episodic dysphoria, irritability, or anxiety usually lasting a few hours and only rarely more than a few days).
7. Chronic feelings of emptiness.
8. Inappropriate, intense anger or difficulty controlling anger (e.g., frequent displays of temper, constant anger, recurrent physical fights).
9. Transient, stress-related paranoid ideations or severe dissociative symptoms.

From American Psychiatric Association. (2013). *Diagnostic and statistical manual of disorders.* (5th ed.). Washington, DC: APA.

VIGNETTE

Mrs. Kit is twice divorced and has been hospitalized several times for suicidal ideation. She is also prone to injuring herself by cutting her inner thighs and arms with a razor when anxious or experiencing feelings of abandonment. She has arrived for today's therapy session. Mrs. Kit's nurse therapist is leaving for a 2-week vacation and has been preparing Mrs. Kit for the separation for more than 2 months. The therapist has given Mrs. Kit the name and phone number of another therapist to call and see while she is away. Mrs. Kit arrives at the office with fresh razor marks on her arms and tells the nurse that she is quitting therapy because the nurse really does not like her anyway and she might as well kill herself: "Go, have a good time; I might not be here when you get back." Mrs. Kit then storms out of the office and refuses to answer her phone all day.

Narcissistic Personality Disorder
Pathological Personality Traits

Narcissistic personality disorder is a maladaptive social response characterized by a person's **grandiose sense of personal achievements.** People with this disorder consider themselves special and expect special treatment. Their demeanor is arrogant and haughty and their **sense of entitlement** is striking. They **lack empathy** for the needs or feelings of others and in fact **exploit others to meet their own needs.** If they are at fault in some way, they always blame others for the problems they themselves have caused. At times, people who have narcissistic PD are admired and envied by others for what appears to be a rich and talented life. However, they require this admiration in greater and greater quantities (**attention seeking**). On the other hand, narcissistic PD patients **often envy others' successes or possessions,** believing that they deserve the admiration and privileges more. Because of their fragile self-esteem, they are prone to depression, interpersonal difficulties, occupational problems, and rejection (Sadock et al., 2015). *They also use the defense mechanism of splitting, exhibit tantrums, and can be sadistic with paranoid tendencies.* Their relationships are shallow and superficial and based on what the other person can do for them. The diagnosis of narcissistic personality is often associated with anorexia nervosa and substance use disorders, with cocaine being highest on the list (APA, 2013).

VIGNETTE

Mr. Chad is the vice president of a successful business. He is very arrogant and always reminds people of what he has done for the company and where it would be without him. As an aside, he will say that it is he who really runs the company, and it is he who should be the president. When employees disagree with him or have a different or novel way to implement change or progress, he takes their ideas and plans and then "lets the employee go," later taking credit for the good idea. He is known to lose his temper on the slightest provocation such as having to wait for someone to start a meeting, but by the same token, he is usually late for meetings and appointments. His need for admiration is insatiable and he is preoccupied with fantasies of unlimited success, power, brilliance, and ideal love.

Histrionic Personality Disorder Traits

People with histrionic personality disorders **manipulate** others through their **dramatic, rapidly shifting, charming, flamboyant, and sexually seductive behaviors.** Their excessively emotional behavior is an attempt to be and remain the **center of attention,** love, and admiration that they require. They may act out with displays of temper, tears, and accusations when they are not getting the attention or praise they believe they deserve. Interactions are often characterized by a seductiveness or provocation to draw others into a relationship or work project, but their attention is usually short-lived since they are subject to constant, **sudden emotional shifts and emotional lability. Their relationships tend to be superficial and shallow and usually do not last long because of their constant need for attention and their insensitivity to the needs of others.** Histrionic people lack insight about their role in the failure of relationships. They may seek treatment for depression or another comorbid condition.

VIGNETTE

Ms. Miller, a 45-year-old woman, meets her therapist, Dr. Jim, for the first time dressed in a tight top and short skirt and wearing a lot of makeup. She becomes flirtatious with him and tells Dr. Jim that she wants extra time today because her story is so long and she is most likely more interesting than his other patients. Her speech is flamboyant and dramatic, but lacking in substance and facts. When the therapist reiterates the terms of the contract and reminds Ms. Miller that they have 20 minutes remaining in today's session to discuss her issues, she becomes angry and insulting and tells Dr. Jim he had better admit her to the hospital immediately or she will commit suicide.

CLUSTER C PERSONALITY DISORDERS

The main characteristics of cluster C disorders are the **experience of high levels of anxiety** and **outward signs of fear.** Individuals with cluster C personality disorders also show inhibitions, mostly in the sexual sphere (e.g., shy and awkward with potential sexual partners, impotence, or rigidity). They are often fearful and reluctant to express irritation and anger with others even when it is justified. People with these disorders (**avoidant, dependent, and obsessive-compulsive**) are inhibited and tend to internalize blame for the frustration in their lives, even when they are not to blame. This is directly opposed to individuals with paranoid, antisocial, borderline, and narcissistic personalities, who tend to blame others.

Avoidant Personality Disorder
Pathological Personality Traits

People with avoidant personality disorder have high levels of anxiety and outward signs of fear and **feelings of low self-worth.** They are **hypersensitive to criticism or rejection;** therefore they tend to **avoid situations that require socialization.** Even though they have a strong desire for affection and for relationships, they are fearful of rejection, disappointment, criticism, or ridicule. Therefore they can spend most of their time in self-imposed social isolation. They are inhibited and are fearful or reluctant to express irritation and anger with others even when it is justified. However, unlike a person with a borderline PD, they do not respond with anger to rejection, but rather withdraw. They **view themselves as personally unappealing or inferior to others** and consequently they have very low self-esteem. They are openly distressed by their isolation and their difficulty relating to others, as well as their low self-esteem, which adds to their inability to feel any joy or obtain any pleasure out of life. Because of their constant anxiety and feelings of low self-worth and inferiority to others, they are unable to feel empathy with others since they are consumed with their own self-deprecation. Virtually all people with avoidant PDs have social phobias.

> **VIGNETTE**
>
> Keith is a 32-year-old computer programmer. He is excessively shy, and rarely speaks with his coworkers other than perfunctory "hellos." He has never had a relationship with a woman, and tries to avoid situations in which he will be alone with any of the female employees. Sometimes the group goes out after work for a drink, and when Keith is asked he becomes very anxious and makes excuses for why he must decline. His sense of loneliness has become intolerable, and he finally seeks psychotherapy for depression, not knowing where else to turn.

Obsessive-Compulsive Personality Disorder
Pathological Personality Traits

People with obsessive-compulsive personality disorder (OCPD) are preoccupied with orderliness, stubbornness, perseverance, indecisiveness, and emotional constriction. The disorder is marked by a **pervasive pattern of perfection and inflexibility.**

These individuals are cautious and consider all choices in a methodical and inflexible manner. They are obsessed with rules and details and follow them rigidly, believing there is only one way to do things correctly. They have great difficulty incorporating new ideas or viewpoints (**rigid perfectionism**). They are often unable to make decisions and may have trouble completing tasks, since they persistently pursue tasks long after their actions have any consequence, and even in the face of repeated failures (**perseveration**). They are high achievers and do well in the sciences and intellectually demanding fields that require attention to detail, and they obtain their sense of self-worth from work and productivity, so much so that their devotion to work may exclude pleasurable activities and friendships.

They often have a very **formal demeanor,** lack a sense of humor, and have **limited interpersonal skills.** Although they are excessive in verbosity, these patients are miserly with material goods and emotions. They are uncomfortable with their feelings, relationships, and situations they cannot control or in which events are unpredictable. Even though they may have deep and genuine affection for others, their intimacy in *relationships is superficial* and rigidly controlled. People with obsessive-compulsive personality disorder are financially extremely **stingy,** and it is difficult for them to part with personal objects even if they are broken or worthless. Unlike people with obsessive-compulsive disorder (OCD) (refer to Chapter 11), people with this disorder do not display unwanted obsessions or compulsive ritualistic behavior. People with OCPD may come into therapy because their rigidity and need for control is causing problems in their intrapersonal or work relationships. Since this is a personality disorder, their behavior and personality traits do not fluctuate. Interestingly, many people with obsessive-compulsive personality disorder seem to be high functioning, with no difficulty in functioning.

People with OCPD often seek help because of psychological distress and inability to control their obsessions and their compulsive behaviors, and these obsessions and compulsions cause disruption in their ability to function in all areas of their life. Another difference is that the intensity of the obsessive-compulsive behaviors in people with OCPD can fluctuate at different times. Having said that, making a diagnosis between these two disorders can cause confusion in the clinical setting.

> **VIGNETTE**
>
> Mike is a 45-year-old middle manager for a microchip company. He works late and sometimes on the weekends, avoiding social and recreational activities. He has a need to get everything done to perfection, which has pushed back the deadline on many projects. He has experienced some heartburn now for a month, and his wife has been insisting he see a physician. He tells her when this project is finished he will go but hates to "waste" his money on physicians. In the physician's office he says he does not have time to take a treadmill test. When the physician tells Mike that he cannot make a diagnosis until he gets all the test results, Mike becomes very anxious.

Dependent Personality Disorder

People with dependent personality disorder traits **believe they are incapable of surviving if left alone** and have an excess need to receive care. They solicit caretaking by clinging and being perversely and excessively submissive. By early adulthood, these people perceive themselves as being unable to separate from others, work independently, or function at all on their own without constant support and guidance from others. If others do not initiate or take responsibility for them, their needs remain neglected. Their intense fear of separation and being alone is so great that they tolerate poor, even abusive treatment in order to stay in a relationship, and once a relationship ends there is an urgent need to get into another. They obsessively ruminate and fantasize about abandonment even when it is not threatened. Their high levels of anxiety intensify their inability to complete anything on their own; they are unable to make decisions without excessive advice and reassurance.

People with dependent personality disorder traits are at greater risk for anxiety and mood disorders, and this disorder often co-occurs with borderline, avoidant, and histrionic personality disorders. This condition commonly occurs in individuals who have a general medical condition or disability that requires them to be dependent on others.

VIGNETTE

Mr. Martin, 49 years old, has lived with his mother since high school. His mother cooks, cleans, and shops for him. He works as a shipping dock clerk and has had the job for 30 years. He even has to ask his mother's advice on what to wear each day for work. He has become extremely anxious and fearful because his mother has been scheduled for surgery and will be away from the home for 5 days. He is terrified that he cannot cope without her to care for him.

A POTENTIAL FUTURE PERSONALITY DISORDER

Passive-Aggressive Traits

Initially, the *Diagnostic and Statistical Manual of Mental Disorders (DSM-5)* was proposing passive-aggressive personality traits as a diagnosis under personality disorders. However, diagnosis was not felt to be fully developed at the time of the *DSM-5* publication. It is helpful, though, for nurses and others to be aware of these traits, because working with people who have passive-aggressive traits can be very confusing and disruptive to others.

People with passive-aggressive personality traits are **chronically irritable and unjustifiably blame others. They are verbally aggressive, hostile, and manipulative, and their interpersonal relationships are usually marked by ambivalence and conflict**. They resent being asked to do anything for anyone else either in work or in social situations, and their key traits are **negativism and obstructiveness and resentful when asked to do something.** Their demeanor is **usually sullen** and their work is often characterized by **procrastination and intentional inefficiency.** People with passive-aggressive behavioral traits are more likely to express their negative/hostile feelings indirectly such as being chronically late or "forgetting" to do something. Although they may openly agree to another's demands or requests, they rarely complete that demand or request. In fact, the actions of people with passive-aggressive personality traits are usually the opposite of their promises. **Therefore, a person with passive-aggressive traits often disrupts or sabotages other people's projects or plans.** Working with people who have passive-aggressive personality traits is usually very difficult.

VIGNETTE

A nursing instructor is perceived by her coworkers to be constantly complaining, extremely irritable, and avoiding responsibility in any way. The instructor was put in charge of one of the committees involved with an upcoming accreditation visit. As the months before the accreditation visit passed, it became more noticeable that this instructor had canceled many of the meetings for her committee, missed deadlines, and failed to complete her committee work. In fact, the day the draft was to be compiled, she called in sick. When one of the committee members suggested that the accreditation material was in her office, it was discovered that absolutely nothing had been done on the report. When this individual realized that others had been in her office, she became furious that anyone should invade her privacy. She then took the next 2 weeks off from work "sick," essentially jeopardizing the project.

ASSESSMENT

Primitive Defenses

People with personality disorders often exhibit outrageous and troublesome behaviors because they are unable to use higher level defense mechanisms to modulate painful feelings and to channel needs or aggression into creative outlets; ambivalence is poorly tolerated and impulse control is dismal (Groves, 2004). "Normal people," or at least those who live full and satisfying lives amid the inevitable personal crises and challenging circumstances that naturally constitute life, have at their disposal a variety of higher level defense mechanisms that they use to help them through such events and eventually continue with their lives. The "ego weakness" of people with PDs relies on more immature or primitive defenses (e.g., splitting, dissociation, psychotic thinking). (See Chapter 11 for definitions of immature or primitive defenses.)

These extreme and outrageous behaviors are thought to arise from intense affect, distorted cognitions, and inadequate or primitive defenses (Groves, 2004). Figure 13-1 identifies the unmodulated affects (rage, envy, shame), some of the challenging behaviors, and the cognitive processes that contribute to some of these behaviors. To add to the difficulties, personal boundaries are often blurred in many people with PDs. Closeness can seem like fusion, and the boundaries where one person begins and where another person ends are blurred. Needs are experienced as rage, and sexuality and dependency are confused with aggression (Groves, 2004).

The intense and inappropriate behaviors that characterize the lives of people with PDs tend to uproot their relationships in all settings and are no less disruptive in the health care setting. These primitive defenses are an attempt to control their inner chaos.

For nurses, clinicians, and other health care workers, much of the challenge is dealing with many of the PD defenses and behaviors. This is especially true with patients who have a borderline or antisocial (dyssocial) PD because nurses encounter these patients frequently in all medical settings.

As previously mentioned, people with PDs are difficult to diagnose, because they usually present with a co-occurring problem. Because of their comorbidity with other PDs and other complicated problems, their response to psychotherapy and medication is unpredictable.

It is observed that often many of the problematic symptoms and behaviors may decline over time. However, even when these individuals stop meeting the *DSM* criteria for a PD, their functional scores do not change. They continue to have serious problems.

Assessment Tools

Several structured interview tools are used to diagnose PDs. These tools are not used in all clinical settings because of the need for lengthy interviews (2 hours or longer) and evaluation.

Assessment of History

Taking a full medical history can help determine if the problem is psychiatric, medical, or both. Medical illness should never be ruled out as the cause for problem behavior until the data support this conclusion. Important issues in assessment for PDs include the following: a history of suicidal or aggressive ideation or actions, current use of medicines, substances use, ability to handle money, and legal history.

Important areas that should be investigated include current or past physical, sexual, or emotional abuse and level of current risk of harm from self or others. At times, immediate interventions may be needed to ensure the safety of the patient or others. Information regarding

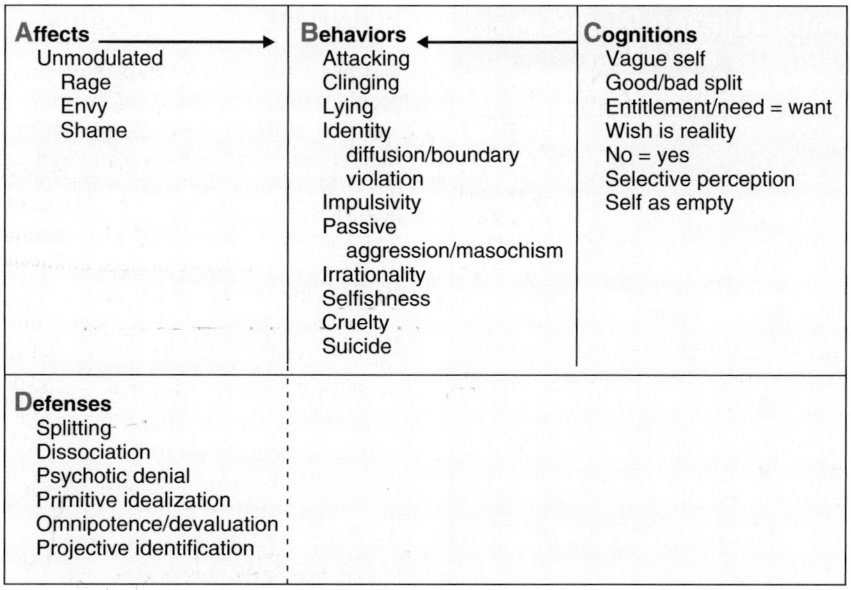

Affects	**B**ehaviors	**C**ognitions
Unmodulated	Attacking	Vague self
Rage	Clinging	Good/bad split
Envy	Lying	Entitlement/need = want
Shame	Identity	Wish is reality
	diffusion/boundary	No = yes
	violation	Selective perception
	Impulsivity	Self as empty
	Passive	
	aggression/masochism	
	Irrationality	
	Selfishness	
	Cruelty	
	Suicide	

Defenses
Splitting
Dissociation
Psychotic denial
Primitive idealization
Omnipotence/devaluation
Projective identification

FIGURE 13-1 ABCs of problem behaviors in difficult patients: how troublesome behaviors arise. (From Groves, J. E. [2004]. Personality disorders I: approaches to difficult patients. In T. A. Stern, J. B. Herman, & P. E. Slavin [Eds.], *Massachusetts General Hospital guide to primary care psychiatry.* [2nd ed.]. New York: McGraw-Hill.)

prior use of any medication, including psychopharmacological agents, is important. This information gives evidence of other contacts the patient has made for help and indicates how the health care provider found the patient at that time.

Assessment Guidelines
Personality Disorders

1. Assess for suicidal or homicidal thoughts. If these are present, the patient will need immediate attention.
2. Determine whether the patient has a medical disorder or another psychiatric disorder that may be responsible for the symptoms (especially a substance use disorder).
3. View the assessment of personality functioning from within the person's ethnic, cultural, and social background.
4. Ascertain whether the patient experienced a recent important loss. PDs are often exacerbated after the loss of a significant supporting person or as the result of a disruptive social situation.
5. Evaluate for a change in personality in middle adulthood or later, which signals the need for a thorough medical workup or assessment for unrecognized substance use disorder.
6. Be aware of the strong negative emotions these patients may evoke in you.

Self-Care for Nurses

Finding an approach for helping patients with PDs who have overwhelming needs can be daunting. The intense feelings evoked in the nurse/clinician often mirror the feelings being experienced by the patient. Health care workers may feel confused, helpless, angry, and frustrated. These patients are often hostile, calling the nurse inadequate or incompetent; many are abusive of authority and are often successful in using splitting behaviors with the staff—praising or disparaging the nurse to peers in such a way that the peers begin to react negatively toward one another. Usually this is the patient's attempt to defend against his or her own feelings of frustration and powerlessness, but when staff are split, the result is often substantial conflict within the treatment team.

Untrained and unsupported staff may easily regress or become vengeful in response to a difficult patient's sense of entitlement, manipulativeness, dependency, ingratitude, impulsivity, and rage (Zimmerman & Groves, 2010). *Frequent communication among staff and continuous availability of supervision and support are vital in times when the behaviors of these patients start to affect the confidence, feelings, behaviors, and effectiveness of staff members.*

Nurses and other health care workers should practice self-health management. This includes acknowledging and accepting their own emotional responses and attempting to ensure personal well-being.

DIAGNOSIS

As previously mentioned, people with PDs are usually admitted to psychiatric institutions because of presenting symptoms (medical or another psychiatric disorder), dangerous behavior, or a court order for treatment. People with both borderline personality disorders and antisocial personality disorders are the most challenging to work with and are most apt to be seen in any treatment setting. The behaviors central to these disorders often cause the most disruption in psychiatric and medical-surgical settings. The nursing care of BPD and antisocial behaviors and their behavioral manifestations are emphasized. Emotions such as anxiety, rage, and depression and behaviors such as withdrawal, paranoia, and manipulation are among the most frequent manifestations that health care workers need to address. See Table 13-1 for common potential nursing diagnoses.

OUTCOMES IDENTIFICATION

Realistic goal setting is based on the perspective that personality change involves one behavioral solution and one learned skill at a time. This can be expected to take much time and repetition. No matter how intelligent these patients may appear or how insightful they can be about themselves and others, PD patients find that change is slow and occurs via trial and error with the support of affect

TABLE 13-1   Potential Nursing Diagnoses for People with Personality Disorders

Signs and Symptoms	Nursing Diagnoses
Crisis, high levels of anxiety, unstable mood	Ineffective coping
	Labile, emotional control
	Risk for disturbed personal identity
Anger and aggression; child, elder, or spouse abuse	Impaired mood regulation
	Risk for other-directed violence
	Ineffective coping
	Impaired parenting
	Disabled family coping
	Risk for impaired attachment
	Ineffective impulse control
	Post-trauma syndrome
Withdrawal	Social isolation
Paranoia	Fear
	Disturbed sensory perception
	Disturbed thought processes
	Defensive coping
Depression	Hopelessness
	Risk for suicide
	Risk for self-mutilation
	Chronic low self-esteem
	Risk for spiritual distress
Difficulty in relationships, manipulation	Ineffective coping
	Impaired social interaction
	Defensive coping
Dysfunctional family processes	Interrupted family processes
	Disturbed personal identity
	Risk for loneliness
	Ineffective relationship
Failure to keep medical appointments, late arrival for appointments, failure to follow prescribed medical procedure or medication regimen	Ineffective self-health management
	Noncompliance (nonadherence)

Herdman, T.H. (Ed.) *Nursing Diagnoses-Definitions and Classification 2015-2017.* Copyright 2014, 1994-2014 NANDA International. Used by arrangement with John Wiley & Sons Limited. In order to make safe and effective judgments using NANDA-I nursing diagnoses it is essential that nurses refer to the definitions and defining characteristics of the diagnoses listed in this work.

management and much interpersonal reinforcement—there are no shortcuts. In terms of permanent change, learning is integrated at the cellular level. Often these patients may have already seen several caregivers, taking what they need from one nurse or counselor before moving on to the next. Their road to recovery is long and circuitous, and the nurse/counselor might be their most recent attempt to find healing.

Because larger steps are not realistic, outcomes need to be very modest and obtainable. For some individuals, overall outcome criteria might include the following:

- Minimizing self-destructive or aggressive behaviors
- Reducing the effect of manipulating behaviors
- Linking consequences to functional as well as dysfunctional behaviors
- Practicing the substitution of functional alternatives during a crisis
- Initiating functional alternatives to prevent a crisis
- Practicing ongoing management of anger, anxiety, shame, and happiness
- Creating a lifestyle that prevents regression

PLANNING

Basically, patients with PDs do not voluntarily seek treatment. Because people with antisocial and BPDs usually present to health care settings for other reasons, staff will benefit from in-service instruction and supervision regarding both acknowledging and coping with the behaviors of these disorders and learning techniques to prevent disruptions in the health care setting.

IMPLEMENTATION

It is often difficult to create a therapeutic relationship with individuals with PDs because most have experienced a series of interrupted therapeutic alliances, and their suspiciousness, aloofness, and hostility can be a setup for failure. The guarded and secretive style of many of these patients tends to produce an atmosphere of combativeness. When patients blame and attack others, the nurse needs to understand the context of their complaints; these attacks develop from feeling threatened, and the more intense the complaints, the greater the fear of potential harm or loss.

Lacking the ability to trust, patients require a sense of control over what is happening to them. Giving them choices—whether to come to a clinic appointment in the morning or afternoon, for example—may enhance compliance with treatment. Because these individuals are hypersensitive to criticism yet have no strong sense of autonomy, the most effective teaching of new behaviors builds on their own existing skills.

When people with PDs exhibit fantasies that attribute malevolent intentions to the nurse or others, it is important to orient them to reality. They need to know that even though they have insulted or threatened their caregiver, they will still be helped and protected from being hurt. When they are hurt by others, as naturally happens in everyday life, the nurse takes time to dissect the situation with them, asking when, where, and how it happened, and honestly describes for them how people, systems, families, and relationships work. It is important to be honest about their limitations and assets. The patient may already be aware of them, but acknowledging them demonstrates trustworthiness.

Ritter and Platt (2016) paraphrased Bateman (2012) who identified five common characteristics of evidence-based treatment for people with personality disorders:

- Provide patients with structured approach to problem-solving;
- Encourage patients to practice self-control;
- Help patients connect feelings to events and actions;
- Be active, responsive, invalidating the patient's; and
- Discuss countertransference issues with staff members.

Communication Guidelines

People with PDs may be excessively dependent, demanding, manipulative, or stubborn, or they may self-destructively refuse treatment. Nurses greatly enhance their ability to be therapeutic when they combine limit-setting, trustworthiness, manipulation management, and authenticity with their own natural style. People with borderline PD are impulsive (e.g., suicidal, self-mutilating), aggressive, manipulative, and even psychotic under periods of stress. People with antisocial PD most often are seen in the health care systems through court order. They are also manipulative, aggressive, and impulsive.

Refer to Table 13-2 for interventions for manipulative behaviors and to Table 13-3 for interventions for impulsive behaviors.

Milieu Therapy

Individuals with PDs may at times be treated within a therapeutic milieu. Short-term hospitalization may occur if an individual is assessed

TABLE 13-2   Interventions for Manipulation

Intervention	Rationale
1. Assess your own reactions toward patient. If you feel angry, discuss with peers ways to reframe your thinking to defray feelings of anger.	1. Anger is a natural response to being manipulated. It is also a block to effective nurse-patient interaction.
2. Assess patient's interactions for a short period before labeling as manipulative.	2. A patient might respond to one particular, high-stress situation with maladaptive behaviors, but use appropriate behaviors in other situations.
3. Set limits on any manipulative behaviors, such as • Arguing or begging • Flattery or seductiveness • Instilling guilt, clinging • Constantly seeking attention • Pitting one person, staff, group against another • Frequently disregarding the rules • Constant engagement in power struggles • Angry, demanding behaviors	3. From the beginning, limits need to be clear. It will be necessary to refer to these limits frequently because it is to be expected that the patient will test these limits repeatedly.
4. Intervene in manipulative behavior. • All limits should be adhered to by *all* staff involved. • Objective physical signs in managing clinical problems should be carefully documented. • Behaviors should be documented objectively (give time, dates, circumstances). • Provide clear boundaries and consequences. • Enforce the consequences.	4. Patients will test limits, and, once they understand the limits are solid, this understanding can motivate them to work on other ways to meet their needs. It is hoped that this will be done with the nurse clinician by following problem-solving alternative behaviors and learning new effective communication skills.
5. Be vigilant; **avoid:** • Discussing yourself or other staff members with the patient • Promising to keep a secret for the patient • Accepting gifts from the patient • Doing special favors for the patient	5. Patients can use this kind of information to manipulate you and/or split staff. Decline all invitations in a firm, but straightforward manner; for example: "I am here to focus on you." "I cannot keep secrets from other staff. If you tell me something I may have to share it." "I cannot accept gifts, but I am wondering what this means to you." "You are to return to the unit by 4 PM on Sunday, period."

TABLE 13-3   Interventions for Impulsive Behaviors

Intervention	Rationale
1. Identify the needs and feelings preceding the impulsive acts.	1. Identify triggers to impulsive actions.
2. Discuss current and previous impulsive acts.	2. Helps link pattern of thoughts or events that trigger impulsive action.
3. Explore effects of such acts on self and others.	3. Helps patients evaluate the results of their behaviors on self and others—may motivate change.
4. Recognize cues of impulsive behaviors that may injure others.	4. Once cues are recognized, planning alternatives to impulsive actions is possible.
5. Identify situations that trigger impulsivity, and discuss alternative behaviors.	5. Once aware of cause and effect, patient can make choices.
6. Teach or refer patient to appropriate place to learn needed coping skills (e.g., anger management, assertive skills).	6. Special skills training can potentiate positive change in behaviors.

to be suicidal. BPD patients requiring hospital admission for attempted suicide have an increased risk of adverse outcomes and require careful clinical monitoring. Classic psychiatric hospitalization is of unproven value for suicide prevention among BPD patients. A noteworthy study claims that short-term hospitalization at a general hospital may be the best alternative to psychiatric inpatient care (Berrino & Ohlendorf, 2011). Intensive treatment includes interventions with the family/friends to clarify communication processes, decrease acute conflicts, and teach the patient and family adapted coping behaviors. A combination of brief, intensive emergency-type treatment that readily connects to a comprehensive outpatient program may be a cost-effective alternative to inpatient hospitalization (Berrino & Ohlendorf, 2011).

The primary therapeutic goal of milieu therapy is affect management in a group context. Community meetings, problem-solving groups, coping skills groups, and socializing groups are all areas in which patients can interact with peers, consider relationship problems, delegate and take responsibility for certain tasks, discuss goals, collectively deal with problems that arise in the milieu, and learn problem-solving skills.

Through desensitization via social group experience, overwhelming and painful internal states can be felt and endured, even while the task of the group is accomplished. When a patient acts out unconscious thoughts and needs inappropriately, the therapeutic goal is to make those needs/thoughts conscious. Then the person can learn to verbally communicate more clearly his or her thoughts or needs to others, instead of acting them out in a socially unacceptable (e.g., antagonistic) manner.

Psychotherapy
Dialectical Behavior Therapy

Dialectical behavior therapy (DBT), a cognitive behavioral therapy, was developed by Marsha Linehan (1993) initially for the parasuicidal individual with borderline PD and is considered the most effective treatment for people with borderline personality disorder. Its theory and philosophy are borrowed from biological, social, cognitive behavioral, and spiritual orientations. Relaxation skills and mindfulness training are often initiated before a session with the intention to help the individual become less anxious and therefore more clearly focus on treatment. It is a four-stage treatment. In stage 1 the primary focus is on stabilizing the patient and achieving behavioral control, emotional regulation, distress tolerance skills, and constant crisis interventions. According to Blennerhassett and O'Raghallaigh (2005), the following are target behaviors:

- Decreasing life-threatening suicidal behaviors
- Decreasing therapy-interfering behaviors
- Decreasing quality-of-life–interfering behaviors
- Increasing behavioral skills

Dialectical behavior therapy involves replacing extremes of emotion and behavior with more moderate responses and has been widely successful. A new, effective strategy is the DBT Coach, which utilizes a smartphone application as an adjunct to standard DBT. The DBT Coach is designed to provide increased support in "opposite action" (OA). OA focuses on changing unwanted negative emotions in the moment by behaving in ways that are counter to the emotion's action urge. When users are experiencing a difficult emotion they are led to emotion-specific branching of possible responses by the DBT Coach. Next, users are asked if they are willing to work on changing the emotion. If they respond "yes," they are directed to specific coaching tools. If they respond "no," several screens help the user evaluate the pros and cons of changing the emotion. In cases where users are not willing to work on reducing the emotion, the program instructs them to call their therapist (Rizvi & Linehan, 2011).

Dialectical behavior therapy has been extremely effective in helping borderline individuals gain hope and quality of life. Advanced practice nurses are often specially trained in using these skills and techniques for use in their practice.

Systems Training for Emotional Predictability and Problem Solving (STEPPS)

This is a relatively new supplement approach in the treatment of borderline personality disorder. One approach to STEPPS is a 20-week manual-driven program, and the results of two studies demonstrated that this program was useful in reducing the intensity of core aspects of borderline personality disorder. Although it does not appear to reduce hospital utilization or suicidal ideation, it did seem to reduce the number of suicide attempts and emergency department visits (Ness, 2009).

APPLYING THE ART
A Person with Borderline Personality Disorder

Scenario

Maria is an 18-year-old female who has already met with me three times on the young adult unit. She always wore long sleeves even though the unit was warm. The last time we met, Maria shared her poetry, which expressed themes of loneliness amid the beauty of nature. Each time she seemed glad to see me while simultaneously disparaging the evening shift staff.

Therapeutic Goal

By the end of this interaction, Maria will choose to express her feelings using a nondestructive form of communication rather than through self-mutilating behavior.

Student-Patient Interaction	Thoughts, Communication Techniques, and Mental Health Nursing Concepts
Maria: "I wondered if you'd actually come back."	According to her chart, she has many reasons to mistrust, starting with her dad, who sexually abused her. She started self-mutilating in middle school when her parents divorced.
Student: "Hi, Maria. I came back as I said I would, but next Tuesday is my last day here." **Student's feelings:** Sometimes I feel guilty to enter my patients' lives only to leave again. I don't want to be one more person to let her down.	I give information reminding Maria of our original nurse-patient contract. Maria reacts with surprise, but avoids any discussion about termination of the nurse-patient relationship.

Student-Patient Interaction	Thoughts, Communication Techniques, and Mental Health Nursing Concepts
Maria: Avoids eye contact. "Read this." Hands me her poem. **Student's feelings:** I feel okay about her bossiness. I recognize that I'm in charge of my own boundaries. Actually I'm relieved that Maria and I get along. She gets in so much trouble with the staff. I've seen the staff get frustrated with Maria.	Maria says, "Read this" almost as a command. The abuse in her childhood left her feeling powerless. She needs to feel in charge of something.
Student: "Your poem describes the mother as 'daisy.' 'Daisy deigning to decorate my life.'" Maria nods. "The 'my life' person might feel lonely with such a powerful mother who drops by to decorate only." We make eye contact. "Is this about you, Maria?"	I reflect on feeling "lonely" and seek to clarify that the poem actually refers to Maria and her mother.
Maria: "She loves me, she loves me not." **Student's feelings:** I'm beginning to feel a little lost in the poetry. I need to pay better attention in my English classes!	Through the poem, Maria uses symbolism to safely express her thoughts and sad feelings.

APPLYING THE ART—cont'd

A Person with Borderline Personality Disorder

Student-Patient Interaction	Thoughts, Communication Techniques, and Mental Health Nursing Concepts
Student: "At first I didn't catch the meaning of 'daisy' in your poems. ' She loves me, she loves me not.' You're sharing about your mother."	
Student's feelings: *I feel so sad that she's so young yet still must battle this mental torment that so disrupts her life and her happiness. She shows so much talent in her writings.*	
Maria: "She says I can't come back to live with her! She's such a ____!"	Maria shows anger in her swearing. Fear and loss fuel her anger. Her mood changes so fast! *Emotional lability* that's the term.
Student: "You feel abandoned. Maybe thrown away like the daisy petals."	I use *reflection,* remembering that patients with *borderline personality disorder* vacillate between feeling *engulfed* by the person they move close to and needing to push that person away to *individuate* self again. Unfortunately, they often *devalue* the other person, get rejected, and then experience *abandonment depression* until once again they move too close.
Student's feelings: *I know from her history the chaos evident in her family. I also recognize that Maria pulls people close and then pushes them away. Still, I can't image not being able to turn to my family. I feel lonely at the thought.*	
Maria: "I don't feel anything. Just numb. I have to go to the bathroom."	Maria says she is numb, not *depressed.* The numbness *isolates* her feelings from awareness.
Student: "Okay." When Maria leaves, I tell my instructor and the nurse what just happened. The nurse immediately goes to find Maria.	I probably should have gone with her or asked if she felt like cutting when she said she felt numb. Self-mutilation breaks through the numbness that has its roots in Maria's past. As a child Maria had to *dissociate* to survive the sexual abuse.
Student's feelings: *I feel upset with myself for not immediately understanding that after this exchange Maria might cut herself!*	
Maria: *Standing in front of me.* "You told on me!" *Raises voice but sits down two chairs away.*	I understand her behavior; it will just take me a while to not take a patient's behavior so personally and look beyond the behavior to the patient's reason for the behavior.
Student's feelings: *I feel uncomfortable being yelled at, and my anxiety level begins to elevate some.*	
Student: "Maria, I told the nurse that you felt upset about your mom and maybe about my leaving. I was concerned that you would be okay."	When Maria confronts me, I *give truthful information.* When we *contracted* I said I would need to share important information with the *treatment team.*
Student's feelings: *I feel anxious, but I know that in reporting, I did the right thing. I want Maria to know I am concerned for her safety.*	

Student-Patient Interaction	Thoughts, Communication Techniques, and Mental Health Nursing Concepts
Maria: "I don't want to talk to you anymore."	
Student's feelings: *I feel sad as Maria rejects me. I know this isn't really about me, but still I feel sad.*	
Student: *Quietly.* "You're really upset at me and at your mother, yet you were still able to stop from cutting yourself."	I *reflect* feelings and make an observation and give *support* by identifying her nondestructive choice and that she has some control over not cutting herself.
Student's feelings: *I feel good that so far I'm able to contain my feelings in light of her angry and rejecting behavior toward me. I do know she needs me to stay calm and not be pushed away no matter how hard she tries.*	
Maria: "I'm so ____ at you. A fine nurse you'll be!" *Storms away.*	With the sarcasm, Maria *devalues* me. I remember devaluing as the other pole to *idealizing* others, also part of the disorder. Nevertheless, using words to express her anger shows some progress. She uses *withdrawal* in leaving me. The closeness threatens her safety by encroaching on her *ego boundaries.* Maria's deeper loss, which pertains to her mother, gets *displaced* into the anger at me.
Student: *I stay seated about 5 minutes. I notice Maria glancing over at me a few times before she leaves for lunch.*	Because I promised Maria that the 45 minutes we contracted was for her, I will make myself available to her for the contracted period of time.
Student's feelings: *Maria acts so very angry at me. I feel my heart rate pick up (guess it makes me anxious). Okay, I'll take some mindful breaths. It's hard to wait here but I want Maria to know she's worth waiting for.*	
Student: *I leave to debrief with my clinical group.*	Maria's self-esteem and even her sense of identify are fragile. She restores some kind of control or power by leaving me before I terminate with her.
Student's feelings: *I hope Maria will let me talk to her later today or at least on the last day I come.*	

Problem A 40-year-old female presents to the mental health clinic with a history of extreme mood swings and irritability. She is unable to keep a job or a relationship because of her frequent outbursts. She feels people are always abandoning her, and has a history of hitting herself on the head and legs as well as pulling out pieces of hair, to relieve emotional pain. She is diagnosed by the psychiatrist with borderline personality disorder (BPD) in addition to her other issues.

EBP Assessment

A. **What do you already know from experience?** People with BPD are difficult to treat because of feeling abandoned and being overly emotional. They tend to have tumultuous relationships and self-harm behaviors. They often have co-occurring diagnoses such as mood disorders or substance abuse, and a history of abuse or disrupted relationships with their caregivers in childhood.

B. **What does the literature say?** There is no medication to specifically treat a personality disorder, but SSRI antidepressants or mood stabilizers may be used for relief of symptoms that co-exist. The dysfunctional behaviors displayed helped the patient survive a chaotic childhood, but create difficulties in adult life. Dialectical behavior therapy (DBT) has been shown to be the most effective treatment for BPD. DBT is a form of cognitive behavioral therapy (CBT) that incorporates the acceptance of uncomfortable thoughts or feelings, and the development of coping skills and mindfulness practices.

C. **What does the patient want?** This patient states she wants to feel better, but has been resistant to medications or therapy, attending appointments but not following through with the recommendations. This response is common in patients with personality disorders, since the behaviors have been ingrained for most of their lives. Often, it will take a major loss or threat of a loss (such as a relationship or job) for the patient to accept that he or she needs to change.

Plan The psychiatrist has remained supportive throughout the fluctuations in patient mood and anger during appointments. Medications have been introduced slowly and in very small dosages because of resistance. The patient is in DBT therapy but feels the exercises assigned by the therapist are "really stupid." She has been encouraged to do them anyway. The patient is ashamed of her mental illness and does not want to pass on her behaviors to her children—this has been used therapeutically as an incentive to accept growth and change.

QSEN **QSEN Prelicensure Knowledge, Skills, and Attitudes (KSAs) Addressed:**

Informatics were used by the psychiatrist to provide quality online information for the patient, as the patient had been relying on inappropriate and inaccurate sources. **Team work** and **collaboration** occurred frequently between the psychiatrist and DBT therapist in this case, by email, phone, and in-person staffing.

National Alliance on Mental Illness. (2015). *Psychotherapy*. Retrieved from www.nami.org/Learn-More/Treatment/Psychotherapy; National Institute of Mental Health. (n.d.). *Borderline personality disorder* [website]. Retrieved from www.nimh.nih.gov/health/topics/borderline-personality-disorder/index.shtml.

Pharmacological, Biological, and Integrative Therapies

Each person with a personality disorder is unique in terms of behaviors and co-occurring needs (e.g., depression, anxiety). Generally, benzodiazepines for anxiety are not appropriate because the potential is great for abuse, as well as overdose. Many of these individuals present with co-occurring substance use disorders. Because people with PDs do not seek treatment for personality disorders, they are rarely seen in the health care system, with the exception of people with borderline PD (suicidal or self-harm behaviors) and antisocial PDs (remanded by the courts).

Because of their propensity for suicidal gestures and self-harm, medications with low toxicity are appropriate for patients with borderline PD. Because borderline PD patients may become psychotic under stress, a second-generation atypical antipsychotic can be helpful. Depression is highly comorbid in these patients; therefore the selective serotonin reuptake inhibitors (SSRIs) trazodone and venlafaxine are good choices because they are the least toxic in overdose (Preston et al., 2013). The SSRIs can also help borderline patients who have co-occurrence panic attacks. Carbamazepine (anticonvulsant) to help target impulsivity, uncontrolled behaviors, and self-harm has been useful. Some people with antisocial PD have problems with anger and acting-out. Lithium, anticonvulsants, or SSRIs may be helpful to minimize aggression. Anticonvulsants may be used with other PDs as well to help curb impulsive and aggressive behaviors.

People with schizotypal PD, although they rarely voluntarily seek treatment, may be helped with low-dose antipsychotic medications, which help ameliorate anxiety and the psychosis-like features associated with this disorder. Obsessive-compulsive PD is often helped with clomipramine (a tricyclic antidepressant) and SSRIs to ameliorate obsessional thinking and a comorbid depression.

EVALUATION

Evaluating treatment effectiveness in this patient population is difficult. Health care providers may never know the real results of their interventions, particularly in acute care settings. Even in long-term outpatient treatment, many patients find the relationship too intimate an experience to remain long enough for successful treatment. However, some motivated patients may be able to learn to change their behavior, especially if positive experiences are repeated. Each therapeutic episode offers an opportunity for patients to observe themselves interacting with caregivers who consistently try to teach positive coping skills. Perhaps effectiveness can be measured by how successfully the nurse is able to be genuine with the patient, maintain a helpful posture, offer substantial instruction, and still care for the patient. Specific short-term outcomes may be accomplished and, overall, the patient can be given the message of hope that quality of life can always be improved.

Neurobiology of Borderline Personality Disorder/Emotional Deregulation (EDR)

Borderline Personality Disorder (BPD) is actually a serious and disabling brain disease marked by impulsivity and dysregulation.

Serotonin: altered functioning of serotonin in the brain has been linked to depression, aggression and difficulty in controlling destructive urges. The serotonin transporter gene 5-HTT is thought to have shorter alleles in BPD which have been associated with lower levels of serotonin and greater impulsive aggression.

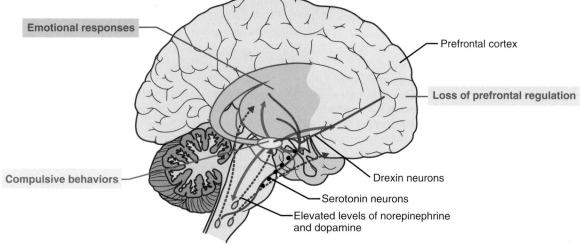

Emotional Dysregulation and the Brain

Emotional dysregulation: emotional responses that are poorly modulated e.g., angry outbursts, rage, marked fluctuation of mood, self-harm that can shift within seconds, minutes, or hours

Brain Imaging (fMRI) Supports:
Prefrontal cortex: in times of stress, this part of the brain helps us regulate emotions, restrain from inappropriate actions, helps with reality testing, and guides attention and thought. In people with BPD this part of the brain *doesn't respond*; instead there is an extreme perception and intensity of negative emotions.

Limbic system/ amygdala: in BPD, parts of the emotional center of the brain are overstimulated and take longer to return to normal. Also, it is believed that **certain neurotransmitters** that act as constraints in normal circumstances under-function in BPD, thus leaving a person in a prolonged state of the fight/flight response.

Medications/Therapy to Help Individuals Regulate Their Emotions

Method	What's Involved	What it Does
Dialectic behavioral therapy (DBT)	Mindfulness, deep breathing, relaxation techniques	Helps brain switch from sympathetic nervous system (arousal) to the parasympathetic (relaxation mode)
Medications	SSRIs, anticonvulsants, second-generation antipsy-chotics, lithium	Helps dampen angry, impulsive, labile behavior

Dialectical Living. Emotion Dysregulation. http://www. dialecticalliving.ca/emotion-regulation-disorder-dpd/

Neural correlates of negative emotionality in borderline personality disorder: an activation-likelihood-estimation meta-analysis (2013)

Ruocco, A. C., Amirthavasagam, S., Choi-Kain ,L. W.,, & McMain, S. S. Biological Psychiatry, 73(2)

Nauert, R. (2015). Brain scans clarify borderline personality disorder. Psych Central. Retrieved October 21, 2015, from http://psychcentral.com/news/2009/09/04/brain-scans-clarify-borderline-personality-disorder/8184.html

KEY POINTS TO REMEMBER

- People with personality disorders (PDs) present with the most complex, difficult behavioral challenges for themselves and the people around them.
- People with PDs have inflexible and maladaptive ways of handling stress; demonstrate disabilities in both work and intimate relationships; evoke strong, intense personal conflict with those around them; and have difficulty managing impulses.
- PDs often co-occur with other mental health disorders (e.g., depression, substance use disorder, somatization, eating disorders, PTSD, anxiety disorders), other personality disorders, and general medical conditions.
- It is unlikely there is any single cause for any of the personality disorders—most seem to have genetic and environmental risk factors.
- People with these disorders respond to stress (e.g., frustration, anger, loneliness) with more primitive defenses, resulting in outrageous behaviors unmodified by "normal" defenses.
- Needs are experienced as rage, and sexuality and dependency are confused with aggression.
- Self-assessment is an important part of assessment when working with a person with a PD. When personal feelings are not recognized or confronted, substantial interpersonal conflict will ensue.
- Determining if there is a history of suicide/homicide/self-mutilation, and if there are co-occurring disorders as well, is a vital part of the initial assessment interview.
- Nursing diagnoses are given and reflect the problematic behaviors of the PD at the time.
- Communication guidelines for manipulative and impulsive behaviors are outlined.

- Careful evaluation for antidepressants, anticonvulsants (for aggressive and impulsive behaviors), and antipsychotics (for stress-induced psychotic thinking) may offer the patient relief.
- Therapy has been used for patients with PDs; however, there is little evidence-based research comparing the efficacy of different therapies with different disorders, except for dialectical behavior therapy (DBT), which has been extremely effective in people with borderline PD.

APPLYING CRITICAL JUDGMENT

1. Ms. Pemrose is brought to the ED after slashing her wrist with a razor. She has previously been in the ED for drug overdose and has a history of addictions. Ms. Pemrose can be sarcastic, belittling, and aggressive to those who try to care for her. She has a history of difficulty with interpersonal relationships at her job. When the psychiatric triage nurse comes in to see her, Ms. Pemrose is at first adoring and compliant, telling him, "You are the best nurse I've ever seen, and I truly want to change." But when he refuses to support her request for diazepam (Valium) and meperidine (Demerol) for "pain," she yells at him, "You are a stupid excuse for a nurse. I want a physician immediately." Ms. Pemrose has borderline PD.
   A. What defense mechanism is Ms. Pemrose using?
   B. How could the nurse best handle this situation in keeping with setting limits and offering concern and useful interventions?
   C. When you research Ms. Pemrose's records, what might you expect to find in her history, including behavioral issues, family history, and potential comorbidities?
   D. In terms of safety, explain what you feel is the primary initial concern when planning care.
   E. If Ms. Pemrose agreed to accept treatment, describe the treatment regimen that has been determined to be most effective in people with borderline personality disorders.
   F. When Ms. Pemrose becomes manipulative, identify specific steps that can help minimize negative effects for manipulation.
   G. Identify the kinds of nursing interventions that might help when working with someone like Ms. Pemrose, who exhibits impulsive behavior.

CHAPTER REVIEW QUESTIONS

1. A person shoplifts merchandise from a community cancer thrift shop. When confronted, the thief replies, "All this stuff was donated, so I can take it." This comment suggests features of which personality disorder?
   a. Antisocial
   b. Histrionic
   c. Borderline
   d. Schizotypal
2. After a power outage, a facility must serve a dinner of sandwiches and fruit to patients. Which comment is most likely from a patient diagnosed with a narcissistic personality disorder?
   a. "These sandwiches are probably contaminated with bacteria."
   b. "I suppose it's the best we can hope for under these circumstances."
   c. "You should have ordered a to-go meal from a local restaurant for me."
   d. "I would rather wait to eat until the dietary department can prepare a meal."

3. A nurse plans care for a patient diagnosed with borderline personality disorder. Which nursing diagnosis is most likely to apply to this patient?
   a. *Ineffective relationships* related to frequent splitting
   b. *Social isolation* related to fear of embarrassment or rejection
   c. *Ineffective impulse control* related to violence as evidenced by cruelty to animals
   d. *Disturbed thought processes* related to recurrent suspiciousness of people and situations
4. The nurse assesses a new patient suspected of having a schizotypal personality disorder. Which assessment question is this patient most likely to answer affirmatively?
   a. "Do some types of situations frighten you?"
   b. "Do you often have episodes of prolonged crying?"
   c. "Is anyone in your family diagnosed with a mental illness?"
   d. "Is it ever very important for you to do everything correctly?"
5. A mental health nurse assesses a patient diagnosed with an antisocial personality disorder. Which comorbid problem is most important for the nurse to include in the assessment?
   a. Generalized anxiety
   b. Alcohol use and abuse
   c. Compulsions and phobias
   d. Dysfunctional sleep patterns

REFERENCES

American Psychiatric Association. (2013). *Diagnostic and statistical manual of mental disorders (DSM-5)* (5th ed.). Washington, DC: American Psychiatric Publishing.

Bateman, A. (2012). Treating borderline personality disorder in clinical practice. *American Journal of Psychiatry, 169*(6), 560–563.

Berrino, A., & Ohlendorf, P. (2011). Crisis intervention at the general hospital: an appropriate treatment of choice for acutely suicidal borderline patients. *Psychiatry Research, 186*, 287–292.

Black, D. W., & Andreasen, N. C. (2014). Personality disorders. In *Introductory textbook of psychiatry* (6th ed.). Washington, DC: American Psychiatric Publishing.

Blaise, M. A., Smallwood, P., Groves, J. E., et al. (2016). Personality and personality disorders. In Stern, et al.: *Massachusetts General Hospital comprehensive clinical psychiatry*. Philadelphia: Saunders/Elsevier.

Blennerhassett, R. C., & O'Raghallaigh, J. W. (2005). Dialectical behavior therapy in the treatment of borderline personality disorder. *British Journal of Psychiatry, 186*, 278–280.

Caligor, E., Yeomans, F., & Levin, Z. (2014). Personality disorders. In J. L. Cutler (Ed.), *Psychiatry* (3rd ed.). New York: Oxford University Press.

Dryden-Edwards, R. (2016). *Borderline personality disorder*. Retrieved January 20, 2016, from http://www.medicine.com/borderline_personality_ disorder/page9htm#how_can_borderline_ personality_ disorder_ be_ prevented.

Francis, A. (2013). *Essentials of psychiatric diagnoses: responding to the challenges of the DSM 5*. New York: Guilford Press.

Gordon, S. (2013). *The difficult patient*. Retrieved September 23, 2015, from http://susangordon.com/the-difficult-patient/.

Gregory, S., Ifytche, D., Simmons, A., et al. (2012). The antisocial brain: psychopathy matters. A structural MRI investigation of antisocial male violent offenders. *Arch Gen Psychiatry, 2012, 69*(9), 962–972.

Groves, J. E. (2004). Personality disorders I: approaches to difficult patients. In T. A. Stern, J. B. Herman, & P. E. Slavin (Eds.), *Massachusetts General Hospital guide to primary care psychiatry* (2nd ed.). New York: McGraw-Hill.

Linehan, M. M. (1993). *Understanding borderline personality disorder: a dialectical approach*. New York: Guilford.

Mayer, J. D. (2005). A tale of two visions: can a new view of personality help integrate psychology? *American Journal of Psychology, 60,* 294–307.

Ness, T. M. (2009). *STEPPS: a viable supplement to treatment of borderline personality.* Retrieved August 5, 2011, from www.psychiatrictimes.com/print/articles/10168/142-5290?printable=true.

Preston, J. D., O'Neal, J. H., & Talaga, M. C. (2013). *Handbook of clinical psychopharmacology for therapists* (7th ed.). Oakland, Calif: New Harbinger Publications.

Ritter, S., & Platt, L. M. (2016). What's new in treating in patients with personality disorders? Dialectical behavior therapy and old-fashioned, good communication. *Journal of Psychosocial Nursing, 54*(1), 38–45.

Rizvi, S., & Linehan, M. (2011). A pilot study of the DBT Coach: an interactive mobile phone application for individuals with borderline personality disorder and substance use disorder. *Behavior Therapy, 10,* 1016.

Sadock, B. J., Sadock, V. A., & Ruiz, P. (2015). *Kaplan & Sadock's synopsis of psychiatry: behavioral sciences/clinical psychiatry* (11th ed). Philadelphia: Wolters Kluwer.

Siever, L. J., & Weinstein, L. N. (2009). The neurobiology of personality disorders: implications for psychoanalysis. *Journal of the American Psychoanalytic Association, 57,* 361.

Verona, E., & Patrick, C. J. (2015). *Psychobiological aspects of antisocial personality disorder, psychopathy, and violence.* Retrieved November 2, 2016, from http://www.psychiatrictimes.com/special-reports/psychobiological-aspects-antisocial-personality-disorder-psychopathy-and-violence#sthash.oHFdg1Du.dpuf.

Zimmerman, D. J., & Groves, J. E. (2010). Difficult patients. In T. A. Stern, et al. (Eds.), *Massachusetts General Hospital handbook of general hospital psychiatry* (6th ed.). Philadelphia: Saunders/Elsevier.

Eating Disorders

Kathleen Ibrahim

ⓔ http://evolve.elsevier.com/Varcarolis/essentials

SELECTED CONCEPT: COGNITIVE DISTORTION—EATING DISORDER

People with eating disorders have cognitive distortions that are the result of processing errors in the brain. It is important to determine which cognitive distortions were present before the eating disorder, and which ones are the result of semistarvation.

Although the eating behavior is targeted, the underlying emotions of anxiety, dysphoria, and low self-esteem and the feelings of lack of control are also addressed through cognitive behavioral therapy.
(See www.anorexia-reflections.com/cognitive-distortions.html.)

OBJECTIVES

1. Compare and contrast the signs and symptoms of anorexia nervosa and bulimia nervosa.
2. Apply knowledge of patient safety needs when assessing for at least two life-threatening conditions that may develop for a patient with anorexia, and at least two for a patient with bulimia.
3. **QSEN** Identify examples of therapeutic interventions that are appropriate for the acute phase and those that are appropriate for the long-term phase of treatment when planning **patient-centered care** for a patient with anorexia nervosa.
4. **QSEN** Describe what you know about **evidence-based practice** in the optimal treatment of eating disorders.
5. **QSEN** Distinguish between effective treatments when planning **patient-centered care** for patients with acute bulimia and for individuals in long-term therapy for bulimia.
6. **QSEN** Discuss the **teamwork and collaboration** needed to effectively treat eating disorders.
7. Differentiate between the long-term prognosis of anorexia nervosa, bulimia nervosa, and binge eating disorder.

INTRODUCTION

For the majority of people, eating provides nourishment for the body as well as the soul. Families and friends gather around the table to break bread as they celebrate, mourn, laugh, cry, share, and demonstrate love. However, for some individuals, eating loses its communal value and becomes hidden and shrouded in secrecy and shame. People with eating disorders experience severe disruptions in normal eating patterns and a significant disturbance in the perception of body shape and weight.

Diagnostic categories included in this chapter are anorexia nervosa, bulimia nervosa, and binge eating disorders. Individuals with anorexia nervosa have intense irrational beliefs about their shape and weight, and they engage in self-starvation, express intense fear of gaining weight, and have a disturbance in self-evaluation of weight and its importance; females with anorexia often experience amenorrhea, although this is no longer a criterion for diagnosis (APA, 2013). There are two subtypes of anorexia: one in which the individual restricts his or her intake of food, and one in which the individual engages in binge eating and/or purging.

Individuals with bulimia nervosa engage in repeated episodes of binge eating followed by inappropriate *compensatory* behaviors such as self-induced vomiting; misuse of laxatives, diuretics, or other medications; fasting; or excessive exercise.

Individuals with eating disorders may display a mixture of anorectic and bulimic behaviors.

In the fifth edition of the *Diagnostic and Statistical Manual of Mental Disorders (DSM-5)*, eating disorders are now grouped under "Feeding and Eating Disorders," and the major change is the addition of binge eating disorder. Binge eating disorder is diagnosed when individuals engage in repeated episodes of binge eating, consuming large amounts of calories, after which they experience significant distress. These individuals do not regularly use the compensatory behaviors seen in patients with bulimia nervosa. Along with pica and rumination disorder, included in the *DSM-5*, is avoidant/restrictive food intake disorder (formerly: feeding disorder of infancy or early childhood") renamed to capture primarily children and adolescents with food preferences/restrictions that result in clinically significant medical complications (APA, 2013).

According to the Academy for Eating Disorders (AED, 2014), the most effective care involves a *multidisciplinary* team approach that enlists the expertise of various health care sectors, including medical physicians, psychologists, psychiatrists, nutritionists, and psychopharmacologists. In addition, families and spouses are always encouraged to participate.

PREVALENCE AND COMORBIDITY

Although anorexia nervosa and bulimia nervosa are fairly common predominantly in women, they are also among the most lethal of all psychiatric diseases. In fact, anorexia nervosa has the highest mortality rate of any mental illness (Hamilton, 2015). Reasons for death include starvation, substance abuse, and suicide. There also seems to be an increased rate of death from 'natural' causes, such as cancer. It is estimated that about 1 in 1000 women die from anorexia (Brown, 2013), and up to one-third of deaths related to all eating disorders are due to suicide (AED, 2012).

All eating disorders can contribute to "significant compromise in every organ system of the body, including the cardiovascular, gastrointestinal, endocrine, dermatological, hematological, skeletal, and central nervous system (AED, 2012).

Eating disorders are culturally influenced disorders with varying prevalence depending on the culture and its social norms. The actual number of individuals with eating disorders is not known because these disorders may exist for a long time before the person either willingly or unwillingly seeks help.

The estimated lifetime prevalence rate among women for developing anorexia nervosa is about 1% and the rate among men is 0.3%. For bulimia nervosa, the lifetime prevalence rate for women is 1.5% and for men it is 0.5% (Hudson et al., 2007). Female as well as male athletes demonstrate an increased incidence of eating disorders. Smink and colleagues (2013) have noted that with new *DSM-5* criteria lowering the threshold for anorexia nervosa and bulimia nervosa and the addition of binge eating disorder, the category of not otherwise specified is reduced. Therefore, the lifetime prevalence may be up to 4% for anorexia nervosa, 2% for bulimia nervosa, and 2% for binge eating disorder.

Anorexia nervosa has an average age of onset in early to middle adolescence, whereas bulimia nervosa more typically appears in late adolescence. The course for both anorexia nervosa and bulimia nervosa may be a single episode but more frequently the pattern is intermittent and often chronic in nature. Walsh (2013) notes the persistence of anorexia nervosa is rooted in dieting behavior, which is both highly rewarding and habit forming. There is a prevalent crossover pattern from anorexia nervosa restricting subtype, to anorexia nervosa binge/purge subtype, and then crossing over to bulimia nervosa (APA, 2013).

In the past decade there has been considerable research of disordered eating in older women. Mangweth-Matzek and colleagues (2014) found a preponderance of binge eating disorder and subthreshold anorexia and bulimia nervosa in middle-aged women. The range of emotional distress secondary to disordered eating and body image disturbances was comparable to their younger counterparts including specific concerns related to aging.

Eating disorders are almost always comorbid with other psychiatric illnesses. More than 50% of people with anorexia have one other concurrent psychiatric disorder, and almost 95% of people with bulimia have another psychiatric disorder. For example, anorexia nervosa is associated with social phobia (34% of cases), depression (65% of cases), bipolar disorder, and obsessive-compulsive disorder (26% of cases) (Sadock et al., 2015). There is a significant comorbidity with mood and anxiety disorders, substance abuse, body dysmorphic disorders, impulse control disorders, and personality disorders, especially borderline and obsessive-compulsive personality disorders. Kostro and colleagues (2014) note that rates of self-harm, suicide, and mortality are high among individuals with eating disorders and their relatives.

The *DSM-5* states that 1.6% of females and 0.8% of males have binge eating disorder and approximately one-third are obese (APA, 2013).

THEORY

The etiology of eating disorders is varied and complex. It appears that these disorders include a biological vulnerability or predisposition that is activated by genetic, psychological, environmental, and cultural factors.

Neurobiological and Neuroendocrine Models

Neuroendocrine abnormalities are noted in both anorexia nervosa and bulimia nervosa (Bailer & Kaye, 2011). It is not clear whether these abnormalities are preexisting or the result of disordered eating behaviors. There is some support for a primary pathology because people with active illness and people who have recovered have exactly the same abnormalities. Brain imaging studies demonstrate unusual activity in various regions of the brain including the frontal, cingulate, temporal, and parietal areas. In both anorexia nervosa and bulimia nervosa, serotonin pathways are abnormal. Researchers believe that this altered serotonin pathway may be key to anxiety responses, inhibition, and even distortions in body image. Brain scans also reveal altered serotonin receptors and transporters. This may be the basis for mood problems, reduced impulse control, and the motivation for eating and enjoying food. Trace and colleagues (2012) found an association between sleep problems and obesity and binge eating.

Genetic Models

Results of family, twin, and adoption studies of individuals with anorexia nervosa, bulimia nervosa, and binge eating disorder have shown that genetic factors contribute to the risk of developing an eating disorder (Thornton et al., 2011). For example, there is an approximately 70% concordance rate for identical twins, and only about 20% for nonidentical twins (Black & Andreasen, 2014). Female relatives of people with eating disorders are up to 12 times more likely to develop an eating disorder. Kaye and colleagues (2008) are conducting linkage analyses—studying pedigrees of individuals with multiply affected family members. These results (genetic markers) can be used to explore chromosomal regions that are known to contain genetic variation affecting risk. What is inherited is not clear. Both individuals with anorexia nervosa and individuals with bulimia nervosa have a characteristic phenotype—a constellation of personality traits that have been shown to be moderately heritable. Genetic vulnerability might stem from an underlying neurotransmitter dysfunction, or perhaps the vulnerability is one of inherited temperament, cognitive style, mood-regulating tendencies, and unique weight set point. Wade and colleagues (2013) note that many results from past studies exploring possible genetic factors have yielded nebulous results. While a genome-wide association analysis of eating disordered behavior in female twins did not reach significant levels, these researchers point to genome-wide association studies as the future direction in locating genetic risk for these serious illnesses.

Psychological Models

Although biology may create a predisposition for eating disorders, psychological determinants may play a role in activating them. Anorexia nervosa often results in amenorrhea in females and physiological changes that interfere with the development of an age-appropriate sexual role. Psychoanalytic theorists long believed that fear of sexual maturity and the need to maintain a childlike body were primary beliefs for people with anorexia. The "core psychopathology" in both anorexia and bulimia is thought to be low self-esteem and self-doubts about personal worth. These feelings produce harsh self-judgment focused solely on the issue of weight. The overvalued ideas about weight, shape, and control are critical to maintaining the eating-disordered behaviors (Fairburn, 2008).

Family theorists have long believed that specific dynamics converge to create individuals with eating disorders. For anorexia, these families are seen as controlling, emphasizing perfection, achievement, and compliance. Bulimic families are seen as chaotic and emotionally expressive, particularly in terms of conflict and negativity. Critics of these theories emphasize that these characteristics may not be the cause of the problem, but rather part of the genetic makeup related to the disorder. For example, the perfectionist and controlling qualities of anorectic families may be a result of obsessive genetic tendencies. However, the Academy for Eating Disorders has published a position paper based on current knowledge strongly opposing any theoretical model that states family dynamics are the primary cause of anorexia nervosa or bulimia nervosa (Le Grange et al., 2010). The Academy for Eating Disorders in a 2014 position statement emphasizes the importance of families as allies in treatment.

CULTURAL CONSIDERATIONS

The assumption that eating disorders are rare in non-Western countries and among ethnic minorities in the United States is no longer valid. Globalization has exposed minorities and non-Western societies to the value of the thin beauty ideal. Food refusal in non-Western societies may not be motivated by fat phobia but rather dieting may reflect personal meaning based on religious or ascetic values. In *DSM-5* the anorexia nervosa criterion of fear of weight gain has been expanded to include persistent behavior that interferes with weight gain to capture this subgroup of patients who do not endorse fear of gaining weight as motivation (APA, 2013).

SELF-CARE FOR NURSES

The nurse caring for the anorectic patient may find it difficult to appreciate the compelling force of this illness, regarding it as trivial (compared to a mental disorder such as schizophrenia), incorrectly believing that weight restriction, bingeing, and purging are self-imposed. Indeed, a patient may present his/her eating disorder as a lifestyle choice! The nurse may believe that the patient "chooses" to engage in behaviors that are risky and blame the patient for his or her health problems. In addition, the common personality traits of these clients—including perfectionism, obsessive thoughts and actions relating to food, and the need to control their therapy in such a way that they are in almost constant conflict with their caregivers—pose challenges to the nurse.

In the effort to motivate the patient and take advantage of the decision to seek help and be healthier, the nurse must take care not to cross the line toward authoritarianism and assumption of a parental role in the relationship. As the nurse struggles to build a therapeutic alliance and be empathetic, the patient's terror at gaining weight and resistance to nursing interventions may engender significant frustration. Nurses must guard against any tendency to be coercive in their approach and must be aware that one of the primary goals of treatment—weight gain—is the very outcome the client fears. Frequent acknowledgment of the situation for the client and of the constant struggle that so characterizes the treatment will help during times of extreme resistance. If countertransference/personal feelings are not recognized and examined, withdrawal may result to avoid feelings of frustration. Being supervised by a competent, supportive, more experienced clinician and sharing with peers help minimize feelings of frustration and can contribute to therapeutic growth in the nurse.

CLINICAL PICTURE

Anorexia nervosa and bulimia nervosa are two separate syndromes and as such they present two clinical pictures. Box 14-1 identifies the signs and symptoms of these disorders.

Eating disorders are serious and in extreme cases can lead to death. Box 14-2 identifies a number of complications that can occur and the laboratory findings that may result in individuals with eating disorders. Because the eating behaviors in these conditions are so extreme, hospitalization

---

BOX 14-1 Possible Signs and Symptoms of Anorexia Nervosa and Bulimia Nervosa

Anorexia Nervosa
- Terror of gaining weight
- Preoccupation with thoughts of food
- View of self as fat even when emaciated
- Peculiar handling of food:
  - Cutting food into small bits
  - Pushing pieces of food around plate
- Possible development of rigorous exercise regimen
- Possible self-induced vomiting; use of laxatives and diuretics
- Cognition is so disturbed that the individual judges self-worth by his or her weight
- Controls what he or she eats to feel powerful to overcome feelings of helplessness

Bulimia Nervosa
- Binge eating behaviors
- Often self-induced vomiting (or laxative or diuretic use) after bingeing
- History of anorexia nervosa in one fourth to one third of individuals
- Depressive signs and symptoms
- Problems with:
  - Interpersonal relationships
  - Self-concept
  - Impulsive behaviors
- Increased levels of anxiety and compulsivity
- Possible chemical dependency
- Possible impulsive stealing
- Controls/undoes weight after bingeing, which is motivated by feelings of emptiness

---

may become necessary. Box 14-3 identifies when an individual should be hospitalized; often hospitalization is via the emergency department (ED).

In treating patients who have been sexually abused or who have otherwise been the victim of boundary violations, it is critical that the nurse and other health care workers maintain and respect clear boundaries. Fundamental to the care of individuals with eating disorders is the establishment and maintenance of a therapeutic alliance. This will take time as well as diplomacy on the part of the nurse.

APPLICATION OF THE NURSING PROCESS

ANOREXIA NERVOSA

Assessment

The nurse assessing a patient with anorexia observes a cachectic (severely underweight with muscle wasting) male or female who may have lanugo (a growth of fine, downy hair on the face and back); mottled, cool skin on the extremities; and low blood pressure, pulse rate, and temperature readings. All of these findings are consistent with a malnourished and dehydrated state.

Cardinal symptoms for anorexia nervosa include dangerously low body weight measurements relative to the age and gender of the patient. Various standards help define significantly low body weight, including pediatric growth tables and Metropolitan Life Insurance tables. However, calculations based on body mass index (BMI) (weight in kilograms divided by height in meters squared) are more precise. Ideal BMIs are thought to be between 19 and 25. Automatic calculators of BMI are widely available on the Internet.

Individuals with the binge/purge type of anorexia nervosa may have prominent parotid glands—the largest of the salivary glands, located in each cheek in front of the ears—because of hyperstimulation from

---

BOX 14-2 Some Medical Complications of Anorexia Nervosa and Bulimia Nervosa

Anorexia Nervosa
- Bradycardia
- Orthostatic changes in pulse rate or blood pressure
- Cardiac murmur—one third with mitral valve prolapse
- Sudden cardiac arrest caused by profound electrolyte disturbances
- Prolonged QT interval on electrocardiogram
- Acrocyanosis
- Symptomatic hypotension
- Leukopenia
- Lymphocytosis
- Carotenemia (elevated carotene levels in blood), which produces skin with yellow pallor
- Hypokalemic alkalosis (with self-induced vomiting or use of laxatives and diuretics)
- Elevated serum bicarbonate levels, hypochloremia, and hypokalemia
- Electrolyte imbalances, which lead to fatigue, weakness, and lethargy
- Osteoporosis, indicated by low bone density
- Fatty degeneration of liver, indicated by elevation of serum enzyme levels
- Elevated cholesterol levels
- Amenorrhea
- Abnormal thyroid functioning
- Hematuria
- Proteinuria

Bulimia Nervosa
- Cardiomyopathy (rare occurrence due to diminished protein synthesis, malnutrition)
- Cardiac dysrhythmias
- Sinus bradycardia
- Sudden cardiac arrest as a result of profound electrolyte disturbances
- Orthostatic changes in pulse rate or blood pressure
- Cardiac murmur; mitral valve prolapse
- Electrolyte imbalances
- Elevated serum bicarbonate levels (although can be low, which indicates metabolic acidosis)
- Hypochloremia
- Hypokalemia
- Dehydration, which results in volume depletion, leading to stimulation of aldosterone production, which in turn stimulates further potassium excretion from kidneys; thus there can be an indirect renal loss of potassium as well as a direct loss through self-induced vomiting
- Severe attrition and erosion of teeth producing irritating sensitivity and exposing the pulp of the teeth
- Loss of dental arch
- Diminished chewing ability
- Parotid gland enlargement associated with elevated serum amylase levels
- Esophageal tears caused by self-induced vomiting
- Severe abdominal pain indicative of gastric dilation
- Russell's sign (callus on knuckles from self-induced vomiting)

BOX 14-3 Criteria for Hospital Admission of Individuals with Eating Disorders

Physical Criteria
- Weight loss more than 30% over 6 months
- Rapid decline in weight
- Inability to gain weight with outpatient treatment
- Severe hypothermia caused by loss of subcutaneous tissue or dehydration (body temperature lower than 36° C or 96.8° F)
- Heart rate less than 40 beats per minute
- Systolic blood pressure less than 70 mm Hg
- Hypokalemia (less than 3 mEq/L) or other electrolyte disturbances not corrected by oral supplementation
- Electrocardiographic changes (especially dysrhythmias)

Psychiatric Criteria
- Suicidal or severely irrepressible, self-mutilating behaviors
- Uncontrollable use of laxatives, emetics, diuretics, or street drugs
- Failure to comply with treatment contract
- Severe depression
- Psychosis
- Family crisis or dysfunction

- History of dieting
- Methods used to achieve weight control (restricting, purging, exercising)
- Value attached to a specific shape and weight
- Interpersonal and social functioning
- Mental status and physiological parameters

Assessment Guidelines
Anorexia Nervosa

1. Determine if medical or psychiatric condition warrants hospitalization (see Box 14-3).
2. Assess level of family understanding about the disease and where to receive support.
3. Assess acceptance of therapeutic modalities.
4. Perform a thorough physical examination with appropriate blood work.
5. Check for other medical conditions.
6. Determine the family's and the patient's need for teaching or information regarding the treatment plan (e.g., psychopharmacological interventions, behavioral therapy, cognitive therapy, family therapy, individual psychotherapy).
7. Assess the patient's and family's desire to participate in a support group.
8. The *DSM-5* uses body mass index (BMI) ranges derived from the World Health Organization to "gauge the level of severity, the degree of functional disability, and the need for supervision" (APA, 2013, p. 339). See the *DSM-5* box: Anorexia Nervosa for the specific BMI ranges.

VIGNETTE

Tina, a 16-year-old girl who is 60% of ideal body weight, is cachectic on admission to an inpatient psychiatric unit. She has lanugo over most of her body and prominent parotid glands. She is further assessed to be hypotensive (86/50 mm Hg) and dehydrated. In addition, she has a low serum potassium level and dysrhythmias that appear on an electrocardiogram (ECG). A decision is made to transfer her to the intensive care unit until she is medically stabilized. As an intravenous catheter is inserted, her severe weight phobia and fear of being overweight are underscored when she cries, "There's not going to be sugar in the IV, is there?" The nurse responds, "I hear how frightened you are. We need to do what's necessary to get you past this crisis."

---

repeated vomiting. Furthermore, they may present with severe electrolyte imbalance as a result of purging, which may be in the form of vomiting, abusing laxatives or diuretics, or using enemas. These individuals may be dangerously ill and often begin treatment in an intensive care unit.

As with any comprehensive psychiatric nursing assessment, a complete evaluation of biopsychosocial function is mandatory. The areas to be covered include the following patient characteristics:
- Perception of the problem
- Eating habits

DIAGNOSIS

Imbalanced nutrition: less than body requirements is usually the most compelling nursing diagnosis initially for individuals with anorexia. It generates further nursing diagnoses; for example, *Decreased cardiac output*, *Risk for injury* (electrolyte imbalance), and *Risk for imbalanced fluid volume*, which would have first priority when problems are addressed. Other nursing diagnoses include *Disturbed body image*, *Anxiety*, *Chronic low self-esteem*, *Deficient knowledge*, *Ineffective coping*, *Powerlessness*, and *Hopelessness* (see *DSM-5* box: Anorexia Nervosa).

DSM-5 DIAGNOSTIC CRITERIA

for Anorexia Nervosa

A. Restrictions of energy intake relative to requirements, leading to a significantly low body weight in the context of age, sex, developmental trajectory, and physical health. Significantly low weight is defined as a weight that is less than minimally normal or, for children and adolescents, less than that minimally expected.

B. Intense fear of gaining weight or becoming fat, or persistent behavior that interferes with weight gain, even though at a significantly low weight.

C. Disturbance in the way in which one's body weight or shape is experienced, undue influence of body weight or shape on self-evaluation, or persistent lack of recognition of the seriousness of the current low body weight.

Coding note: The ICD-9-CM code for anorexia nervosa is 307.1, which is assigned regardless of the subtype. The ICD-10-CM code depends on the subtype (see below).

Specify whether:

(F50.01) Restricting type: During the last 3 months, the individual has not engaged in recurrent episodes of binge eating or purging behavior (i.e., self-induced vomiting or the misuse of laxatives, diuretics, or enemas). This subtype describes presentations in which weight loss is accomplished primarily through dieting, fasting, and/or excessive exercise.

(F50.02) Binge-eating/purging type: During the last 3 months, the individual has engaged in recurrent episodes of binge eating or purging behavior (i.e., self-induced vomiting or the misuse of laxatives, diuretics, or enemas).

Specify if:

In partial remission: After full criteria for anorexia nervosa were previously met. Criterion A (low body weight) has not been met for a sustained period, but either Criterion B (intense fear of gaining weight or becoming fat or behavior that interferes with weight gain) or Criterion C (disturbances in self-perception of weight and shape) is still met.

In full remission: After full criteria for anorexia nervosa were previously met, none of the criteria have been met for a sustained period of time.

Specify current severity:

The minimum level of severity is based, for adults, on current body mass index (BMI) (see below) or, for children and adolescents, on BMI percentile. The ranges below are derived from World Health Organization categories for thinness in adults; for children and adolescents, corresponding BMI percentiles should be used. The level of severity may be increased to reflect clinical symptoms, the degree of functional disability, and the need for supervision.

Mild: BMI ≥17 kg/m²
Moderate: BMI 16-16.99 kg/m²
Severe: BMI 15-15.99 kg/m²
Extreme: BMI <15 kg/m²

From American Psychiatric Association. (2013). *Diagnostic and statistical manual of disorders* (5th ed., pp 338–339). Washington, DC: APA.

OUTCOMES IDENTIFICATION

Outcomes need to be measurable and include a time estimate for attainment (ANA, 2014). Some common outcome criteria for patients with anorexia nervosa include the following (fill in the appropriate time [e.g., within 3 weeks, by discharge]); the patient will:

- Refrain from self-harm.
- Normalize eating patterns, as evidenced by eating 75% of three meals per day plus two snacks.
- Achieve 85% to 90% of ideal body weight.
- Be free of physical complications.
- Demonstrate two new, healthy eating habits.
- Demonstrate improved self-acceptance, as evidenced by verbal and behavioral data.
- Address maladaptive beliefs, thoughts, and activities related to the eating disorder.
- Participate in treatment of associated psychiatric symptoms (defects in mood, self-esteem).
- Demonstrate at least one behavior and one interest that are appropriate to age.
- Participate in long-term treatment to prevent relapse.

PLANNING

Planning is affected by the acuity of the patient's situation. In the case of a patient with anorexia who is experiencing extreme electrolyte imbalance or whose weight is less than 75% of ideal body weight, the plan is to provide immediate stabilization, most likely in an inpatient unit (APA, 2006, 2012). Inpatient hospitalization is usually brief, attempts limited weight restoration, and addresses only acute complications (such as electrolyte imbalance and dysrhythmias) and acute psychiatric symptoms (such as significant depression). Some hospitalized patients experience refeeding syndrome, a potentially catastrophic treatment complication in which the demands of a replenished circulatory system overwhelm the capacity of a nutritionally depleted cardiac muscle, which results in cardiovascular collapse (APA, 2006, 2012).

Once a patient is medically stable, the plan begins to address the issues underlying the eating disorder. These issues are usually treated on an outpatient basis and will include individual, group, and family therapy as well as psychopharmacological therapy during different phases of the illness. The nature of the treatment is determined both by the intensity of the symptoms—which may vary over time—and by the experienced disruption in the patient's life.

The following are the three main goals for all eating disorders:

1. Restore the patient's nutritional state (APA, 2006, 2012).
   a. For anorexia nervosa this means restoring weight within normal range.
   b. For bulimia this means ensuring a balanced metabolic state.
2. Modify the patient's distorted eating behaviors.
3. Help change distorted and erroneous beliefs about weight loss and body image.

IMPLEMENTATION

See Table 14-1 for specific interventions regarding anorexia nervosa.

Acute Care

Patients with eating disorders may be admitted to intensive care, coronary care, and medical and special eating disorders units. Typically when an individual with an eating disorder is admitted to any of these units, the person is in a crisis state. The nurse is challenged to establish trust and monitor the eating pattern. Weight restoration and weight monitoring create opportunities to counter the distorted ideas that maintain

TABLE 14-1 Interventions for Anorexia Nervosa

Intervention	Rationale
1. Acknowledge the emotional and physical difficulty the patient is experiencing.	1. A first priority is to establish a therapeutic alliance.
2. Assess for suicidal thoughts/self-injurious behaviors.	2. The potential for a psychiatric crisis is always present.
3. Monitor physiological parameters (vital signs, electrolyte levels) as needed.	3. The life-threatening effect of weight restriction and/or purging needs to be monitored.
4. Weigh patient wearing only bra and panties/underwear on a routine basis (same time of day after voiding and before drinking/eating). Some protocol includes weighing with the patient's back to the scale.	4. Weights are a high-anxiety time. In the weight gain phase the patient is expected to gain ½ to ¾ lb at specified weigh-in intervals according to a set unit protocol. The underweight patient might try to manipulate the weight by drinking fluids or placing heavy objects in clothing before being weighed. Discussion of weight gain (or loss) may be postponed for the primary therapist.
5. Monitor patient during and after meals to prevent throwing away food and/or purging.	5. The compelling force of the illness makes it difficult to stop certain behaviors.
6. Recognize the patient's distorted image/overvalued ideas of body shape and size without minimizing or challenging patient's perceptions.	6. A straightforward statement that the nurse's perceptions are different will help to avoid a power struggle. Arguments and power struggles intensify the patient's need to control.
7. Educate the patient about the ill effects of low weight and resultant impaired health.	7. The treatment goal of gaining weight is what the patient most resists. Focus on the benefits of improved health and increased energy at a more normalized weight.
8. Work with patients to identify strengths.	8. When patients are feeling overwhelmed, they no longer view their lives objectively.

BOX 14-4 Cognitive Distortions Related to Eating Disorders

Overgeneralization: A single event affects unrelated situations.
- "He didn't ask me out. It must be because I'm fat."
- "I was happy when I wore a size 6. I must get back to that weight."

All-or-nothing thinking: Reasoning is absolute and extreme, in mutually exclusive terms of black or white, good or bad.
- "If I have one Popsicle, I must eat five."
- "If I allow myself to gain weight, I'll blow up like a balloon."

Catastrophizing: The consequences of an event are magnified.
- "If I gain weight, my weekend will be ruined."
- "When people say I look better, I know they think I'm fat."

Personalization: Events are overinterpreted as having personal significance.
- "I know everybody is watching me eat."
- "People won't like me unless I'm thin."

Emotional reasoning: Subjective emotions determine reality.
- "I know I'm fat because I feel fat."
- "When I'm thin, I feel powerful."

Adapted from Bowers, W. A. (2001). Principles for applying cognitive-behavioral therapy to anorexia nervosa. *Psychiatric Clinics of North America, 24*(2), 293–303.

symptoms, such as suicidal ideation, are addressed immediately. At the same time, a patient with anorexia begins a weight restoration program that allows for incremental weight gain. Based on the patient's height, a treatment goal is set at 90% of ideal body weight, the weight at which most women are able to menstruate.

In the effort to motivate the patient and take advantage of the decision to seek help and be healthier, the nurse must avoid authoritarianism and assumption of a parental role. As the nurse struggles to build a therapeutic alliance and be empathic, the patient's terror at gaining weight and resistance to nursing interventions may engender significant frustration. As previously stated, nurses must appreciate the compelling force of this illness and be aware that one of the primary goals of treatment—weight gain—is the very outcome the patient fears. Frequent acknowledgment of the difficulty of the situation for the patient and of the constant struggle that characterizes the treatment will help during times of extreme resistance.

Establishing a therapeutic alliance with a person with anorexia is challenging because the compelling force of the illness runs counter to therapeutic interventions. As patients begin to refeed, ideally they begin to participate in milieu therapy, in which the cognitive distortions that perpetuate the illness are consistently confronted by all members of the interdisciplinary team. Box 14-4 identifies some common types of cognitive distortion characteristic of people with eating disorders. Although the eating behavior is targeted, the underlying emotions of anxiety, dysphoria, and low self-esteem and feelings of lack of control are also addressed through counseling.

Health Teaching and Health Promotion

Self-care activities are an important part of the treatment plan. These activities include learning more constructive coping skills, improving social skills, and developing problem-solving and decision-making skills. The skills become the focus of therapy sessions and supervised food shopping trips. As patients approach their goal weight, they are encouraged to expand the repertoire to include eating out in a restaurant, preparing a meal, and eating forbidden foods.

Discharge planning is a critical component in treatment. Often family members benefit from counseling. The discharge planning process must address living arrangements and school and work plans, as well as the feasibility of independent financial status, applications for state and/or federal program assistance (if needed), and follow-up outpatient treatment.

the illness. Nurses and other health care providers provide milieu therapy, counseling, health teaching, and medication management. Within special eating disorder units and general psychiatric units, patient privileges may be linked to weight gain and treatment plan compliance.

The Royal Australian and New Zealand College of Psychiatrists released the first set of eating disorder guidelines that incorporate recommendations from the DSM-5 (Bernstein and Pataki, 2016):

- A multi-disciplinary treatment approach incorporating consideration of nutritional, medical and psychological aspects, family-based therapies in younger patients, and specialist therapist-led manual-based psychological therapy with long-term follow-up in all age groups should be used.
- In chronic anorexia nervosa, a harm minimization approach should be used.
- The approach to diagnosis and treatment should be culturally informed.

Communication Guidelines

The nurse on a behavioral health inpatient unit may have to operate as both primary nurse and group leader. The initial focus depends on the results of a comprehensive assessment. Interventions include milieu therapy, teaching, and psychotherapy. Any acute psychiatric

Milieu Therapy

Individuals admitted to an inpatient unit designed to treat eating disorders participate in a program provided by an interdisciplinary team and consisting of a combination of therapeutic modalities. These modalities are designed to normalize eating patterns and to begin to address the issues raised by the illness. The milieu of an eating disorder unit is purposefully organized to assist the patient in establishing more adaptive behavioral patterns, including normalization of eating.

APPLYING THE ART

A Person with an Eating Disorder: Anorexia

Scenario

I met 15-year-old Stacie on the eating disorders unit. A "straight A" student, Stacie was 5 feet 7 inches tall and weighed 90 pounds. Her mother was a physician and her father a college professor. Her older brother quarterbacked his college team. We had set up the contract that morning and she had just finished the post-lunch focus group.

Therapeutic Goal

By the end of this interaction, Stacie will express at least one painful feeling directly instead of acting out with self-destructive behavior.

Student-Patient Interaction	Thoughts, Communication Techniques, and Mental Health Nursing Concepts
Stacie: "They think we're going to all go and vomit after lunch so they keep us talking. Like that's going to help."	I should *clarify indefinite pronouns.* She used "they" a lot but I am guessing she means the staff. Her feelings take precedence right now.
Student's feelings: *I am feeling a bit overwhelmed. Where to start! She looks like a skeleton, and here I am always struggling with my own weight.*	
Student: "You sound pretty frustrated."	*Reflection* rarely fails to continue the interaction. I am aware of my own potential for *countertransference* in this situation.
Student's feelings: *Her thinness scares me.*	
Stacie: "I am! Sometimes I feel like a piece of taffy being pushed and pulled and stretched by everyone else."	Control sounds like a key issue. She is revisiting *autonomy versus shame and doubt.* I remember that adolescents re-encounter all of Erikson's earlier stages as part of *identity versus role confusion.*
Student's feelings: *I'm feeling some anxiety about being able to figure this out. She shares how controlled she feels by making an analogy to candy. Is her whole life about food?*	
Student: "Pushed and pulled?"	*Restatement* and *encouraging her to elaborate.* I hope this shows Stacie I am really listening by using her exact words.
Stacie: "Try being in that family of mine! You can't stay unless you're at the top of your game."	I wonder which carries the most emotional impact for her: achievement or staying in the family.
Student's feelings: *I am feeling drawn into her story. How overwhelming for her.*	

Student-Patient Interaction	Thoughts, Communication Techniques, and Mental Health Nursing Concepts
Student: "You feel a lot of pressure to excel ... at everything?"	I *restate* again. *Love and belonging to* precede *self-esteem needs.* Still, do I need to assess further with my *direct question* about how high she sets the bar for herself? If she sees herself as a constant failure and food becomes the only area she can control, then despair, even suicide, becomes a possibility.
Student's feelings: *I feel uncertain here. I probably should have focused first on the family part. Hope we can get back to her family stuff, too.*	
Stacie: "My mom would say, 'Honey, just be yourself,' but she'd really mean, 'as long as you get straight A's and make the family proud, like your brother does!'"	
Student's feelings: *I kind of feel intimidated by her straight A's. She accomplishes more than I do in my own studies. Why can't that be enough? I feel sad that she never feels good enough.*	
Student: "Somehow you never quite feel good enough." *Concerned look, leaning toward her.*	I reflect back her feelings. I hope to convey *empathy* with my nonverbal behavior.
Stacie: "That's it, exactly." *Eyes fill with tears. I pause to let her cry.*	When a person is crying, feelings are very close to the surface. Saying comforting things might help her push her feelings down. Expressing emotions directly is much healthier for her than using food to *displace* feelings.
Student's feelings: *I want to comfort her but I stop myself because the tears are healthy. She actually lets herself feel frustration and now sadness.*	
Stacie: *Crying.* "I can't tell you how long it's been since I actually cried."	
Student's feelings: *I'm glad she could unbottle some of her feelings and that she felt safe to do so with me.*	
Student: "Maybe crying is not such a bad thing."	I ask an *indirect question.* Maybe she will see that she can let out some of her painful feelings and that it is okay.

A Person with an Eating Disorder: Anorexia

Student-Patient Interaction	Thoughts, Communication Techniques, and Mental Health Nursing Concepts	Student-Patient Interaction	Thoughts, Communication Techniques, and Mental Health Nursing Concepts
Stacie: "It's not done in my family." **Student's feelings:** *Seems like she never lets go of the pressures she feels from her family. In some ways I understand that, with the way my family keeps me plugging through nursing; I feel like I'd really let them down if I failed.*	The family theme pervades her thoughts.	**Student:** "I wonder if a person can stay in the family yet still feel and do things a little differently than everyone else." **Student's feelings:** *I feel like Stacie really made some progress and we can build a foundation for the next time we talk. I feel more hopeful for her.*	Again, an *indirect question* asks Stacie to ponder without feeling interrogated. The work of *identity versus role confusion* means separating and *individuating* oneself as distinct from one's family.
		Stacie: "Maybe. I never thought of it that way." *Takes the tissue I offer, looking thoughtful.*	I'll report this to my instructor and chart about her being able to cry.

The highly structured milieu includes precise mealtimes, adherence to the selected menu, observation during and after meals, and regularly scheduled weigh-ins. Close supervision of patients includes monitoring of all trips to the bathroom after eating to ensure that there is no self-induced vomiting. Patients may also need monitoring on bathroom trips after seeing visitors and after any hospital pass. The latter is to ensure that the patient has not had access to and ingested any laxatives or diuretics.

Therapy groups are led by nurses and other interdisciplinary team members (especially dietitians) and are tailored to the issues of patients with eating disorders.

Psychotherapy

The patient may be involved in a variety of therapies as a multimodal approach to address different issues (APA, 2006, 2012). The following therapies are used in all of the eating disorders and are geared toward the recovery point of the patient:

- **Cognitive behavioral therapy** is used to diminish errors in the patient's thinking and perceptions that result in distorted attitudes and eating-disordered behaviors. The patient practices new ways of examining cognitions and self-monitors behaviors.
- **Dialectical behavioral therapy** is a form of cognitive behavioral therapy adapted to address problems associated with emotional dysregulation.
- **Interpersonal psychotherapy (ITP)** has proven especially effective and its focus is on finding appropriate community supports, and resolving interpersonal stressors that may trigger feelings of loss, bodily changes, interpersonal disputes, and/or isolation.
- **Group therapy** offers support to patients who feel isolated while offering an arena in which to explore the various issues and concerns inherent in eating disorders.
- **Family-based therapy (FBT)** is especially effective in early-onset and short-duration anorexia. It supports parent refeeding of children and identifies problematic family interactions that may be contributing to the problem.

Other therapies that have been found useful are motivational therapy, psychodynamic therapy after weight is more stable, and others (Bernstein and Pataki, 2016). These therapies may take place in a variety of settings, including a partial hospitalization program, community mental health center, psychiatric home care program, or more traditional outpatient treatment. Regardless of the setting, the goals of treatment remain the same: weight restoration with normalization of eating habits and initiation of the treatment of the psychological, interpersonal, and social issues that are integral to the experience of the patient.

Often the nurse and other health care workers might contract with the patient regarding the terms of treatment. For example, outpatient treatment can continue only if the patient maintains a weight that has been negotiated by both the patient and the health care team. If the patient's weight falls below the goal, other treatment arrangements must be made until the patient returns to the goal weight. This highly structured approach to treatment of patients whose weight is less than 75% of ideal body weight is essential. Techniques such as assisting the patient with a daily meal plan, reviewing a journal of meals and dietary intake, and providing for weekly weighing (ideally two or three times a week) are essential in order to reach a medically stable weight.

Families often report feeling powerless in the face of such mystifying behavior. For instance, patients are often unable to experience compliments as supportive and therefore are unable to internalize the support. They often seek attention from others but feel scrutinized when they receive it. Patients express that they want their families to care about them but are unable to recognize expressions of care. When others do respond with love and support, patients do not perceive this as positive. Consequently, families experience the tension of saying or doing the wrong thing and then feeling responsible if a setback occurs. Psychiatric nurse clinicians have an important role in assisting families and significant others to develop strategies for improved communication and to search for ways to be comfortably supportive to the patient.

Pharmacological, Biological, and Integrative Therapies

Numerous studies of fluoxetine have shown mixed results in maintaining weight and preventing relapse, and the summary of current data suggests fluoxetine is not an effective treatment for anorexia nervosa (Mitchell et al., 2013). Olanzapine, a second-generation antipsychotic, is increasingly being reported in the literature to positively affect weight gain and improve cognition and body image.

Long-Term Treatment

Anorexia nervosa is a chronic illness that waxes and wanes. Recovery is evaluated as a stage in the process rather than a fixed event. Factors that influence the stage of recovery include percentage of ideal body weight that has been achieved, the extent to which self-worth is defined by shape and weight, and the amount of disruption existing in the patient's personal life. The patient will require long-term treatment that might include periodic brief hospital stays, outpatient psychotherapy, and pharmacological interventions. The combination of individual, group, couples, and family therapy (especially for the younger patient) provides the anorectic patient with the greatest chance for a successful outcome.

As part of discharge planning the nurse needs to explore the patient's participation in social media. Websites such as Proud2BMe.org, an interactive online community for adolescents and young adults sponsored by the National Eating Disorder Association, may enhance empowerment and support. However, media messages and information provided by some websites (including those with a disclaimer that they do not contain self-harm content) may foster pro–eating disorder behavior. The use of "apps" may contribute to recovery especially if used in conjunction with a treatment provider (Fairburn & Rothwell, 2015).

EVALUATION

The process of evaluation is incorporated into the outcomes specified by the goals. Evaluation is ongoing, and short-term and intermediate goals are revised as necessary to achieve the treatment outcomes established. The goals provide a daily guide for evaluating success and must be continually re-evaluated for their appropriateness. Generally, the long-term outcome for anorexia nervosa in terms of symptom recovery is less favorable than that for bulimia nervosa.

APPLICATION OF THE NURSING PROCESS

BULIMIA NERVOSA

Assessment

People with bulimia nervosa may not initially appear to be physically or emotionally ill. They are often at or slightly above or below ideal body weight. However, as the assessment continues and the nurse makes further observations, physical and emotional problems become apparent. On inspection, the patient may demonstrate enlargement of the parotid glands and dental erosion and caries if the patient has been inducing vomiting. The history may reveal difficulties with impulsivity as well as compulsivity. Family relationships may be chaotic and reflect a lack of nurturing. These individuals' lives reflect instability and troublesome interpersonal relationships as well. It is not uncommon for patients to have a history of impulsive stealing of items such as food, clothing, or jewelry. Refer to Box 14-1 for a listing of the characteristics of bulimia nervosa and anorexia nervosa.

▶▶ Assessment Guidelines
Bulimia Nervosa

1. Medical stabilization is the first priority. Problems resulting from purging are disruptions in electrolyte and fluid balance and cardiac function. Therefore a thorough medical examination is vital.
2. Medical evaluation usually includes a thorough physical examination as well as pertinent laboratory testing of the following:
   - Electrolyte levels
   - Glucose level
   - Thyroid function tests
   - Complete blood count
   - Electrocardiogram (ECG)
3. Psychiatric evaluation is advised because treatment of psychiatric comorbidity is important to outcomes (depression and suicide are concerns).
4. Because of the frequency of coexisting disorders (e.g., depression, anxiety, substance use), always ask if the individual has any suicidal ideation.

5. Besides assessing for the use of diuretics, vomiting, or laxatives, ask patients if they are taking any diet pills, amphetamines, energy pills, or diet teas that claim to be all-natural.

VIGNETTE

I was a three-sport athlete throughout high school and then played volleyball in college. How did the bingeing and purging start, and how did it happen to me? I began to down thousands of calories at my parents' house and secretly go to the bathroom and purge, and then start all over again. By the time I went to college, I would go to several fast-food restaurants and order cheeseburgers, french fries, tacos, and milkshakes; consume them all by the time I got home; and then induce vomiting the minute I walked through the door. As time went by, the cycles became worse. I despised what I was doing and what it was doing to me, breaking blood vessels in my face, causing my eyes to swell, and causing me to deceive everyone. I hated it so much that each time I binged and purged, I swore to myself that it would never happen again. —Carly

---

DIAGNOSIS

Assessment of the patient with bulimia nervosa may reveal the need for multiple potential nursing diagnoses as a result of many disordered eating and weight control behaviors. Problems resulting from purging are a first priority because electrolyte and fluid balance and cardiac function are affected. Common nursing diagnoses include *Decreased cardiac output, Disturbed body image, Powerlessness, Chronic low self-esteem, Anxiety,* and *Ineffective coping* (substance abuse, impulsive responses to problems). (See *DSM-5* box: Bulimia.)

DSM-5 DIAGNOSTIC CRITERIA
for Bulimia Nervosa

A. Recurrent episodes of binge eating. An episode of binge eating is characterized by both of the following:
   1. Eating, in a discrete period of time (e.g., within any 2-hour period), an amount of food that is definitely larger than what most individuals would eat in a similar period of time under similar circumstances.
   2. A sense of lack of control over eating during the episode (e.g., feeling that one cannot stop eating or control what or how much one is eating).
B. Recurrent inappropriate compensatory behavior in order to prevent weight gain, such as self-induced vomiting; misuse of laxatives, diuretics or other medications; fasting; or excessive exercise.
C. The binge eating and inappropriate compensatory behaviors both occur, on average, at least once a week for 3 months.
D. Self-evaluation is unduly influenced by body shape and weight
E. The disturbance does not occur exclusively during episodes of anorexia nervosa.

Specify if:
   In partial remission: After full criteria for bulimia nervosa were previously met, some, but not all, of the criteria have been met for a sustained period of time.
   In full remission: After full criteria for bulimia nervosa were previously met, none of the criteria have been met for a sustained period of time.

Specify current severity:
   The minimum level of severity is based on the frequency of inappropriate compensatory behaviors (see below). The level of severity may be increased to reflect other symptoms and the degree of functional disability.
   Mild: An average of 1 to 3 episodes of inappropriate compensatory behaviors per week.

DSM-5 DIAGNOSTIC CRITERIA—cont'd

for Bulimia Nervosa

> **Moderate:** An average of 4 to 7 episodes of inappropriate compensatory behaviors per week.
>
> **Severe:** An average of 8 to 13 episodes of inappropriate compensatory behaviors per week.
>
> **Extreme:** An average of 14 or more episodes of inappropriate compensatory behaviors per week.

From American Psychiatric Association. (2013). *Diagnostic and statistical manual of disorders* (5th ed.). Washington, DC: APA; p 345.

OUTCOMES IDENTIFICATION

Some useful measurable outcome criteria for patients with bulimia nervosa follow (fill in the timeframe [e.g., in 1 week, by discharge]); the patient will:

- Refrain from binge/purge behaviors.
- Demonstrate at least two new skills for managing stress/anxiety/shame (triggers to binge/purge behaviors).
- Obtain and maintain normal electrolyte balance.
- Be free of self-directed harm.
- Express feelings in a non–food-related way.
- Verbalize desire to participate in ongoing treatment.
- State feels good about self and about who he or she is as a person.
- Name two personal strengths.

PLANNING

The criteria for inpatient admission of a patient with bulimia nervosa are included in the criteria for inpatient admission of a patient with an eating disorder, which is presented in Box 14-3. As with anorexia nervosa, the patient with bulimia may be treated for life-threatening complications, such as gastric rupture (rare), electrolyte imbalance, and cardiac dysrhythmias, in an acute care unit of a hospital. If the patient is admitted to a general inpatient psychiatric unit because of acute suicidal risk, only the acute psychiatric manifestations are addressed short term. Planning will also include appropriate referrals for continuing outpatient treatment.

IMPLEMENTATION

See Table 14-2 for intervention guidelines for a patient with bulimia nervosa.

Acute Care

A patient who is medically compromised as a result of bulimia nervosa is referred to an inpatient unit for comprehensive treatment of the illness. The cognitive behavioral model of treatment is highly effective and frequently serves as the cornerstone of the therapeutic approach. Inpatient units designed to treat eating disorders are especially structured to interrupt the cycle of binge eating and purging and to normalize eating habits. Therapy is begun to examine the underlying conflicts and distorted perceptions of shape and weight that sustain the illness. Evaluation for treatment of comorbid disorders, such as major depression and substance abuse, is also undertaken. In most cases of substance dependence, the treatment of the eating disorder must occur after the substance dependence is treated.

TABLE 14-2 Interventions for Bulimia Nervosa

Intervention	Rationale
1. Assess mood and presence of suicidal thoughts/behaviors.	1. Emotional dysregulation is at the core of bulimic behaviors and there is always the risk for self-destructive behaviors.
2. Monitor physiological parameters (vital signs, electrolyte levels) as needed.	2. The life-threatening effect of weight restriction and/or purging needs to be monitored.
3. Monitor the patient's weight as needed.	3. The weigh-in intervals are determined by the unit protocol for the bulimic patient depending on the percentage above or below ideal body weight.
4. Explore dysfunctional thoughts that maintain the binge/purge cycle.	4. Nonjudgmental reframing can balance and combat distorted thinking and challenge automatic behaviors.
5. Educate the patient that fasting can lead to continuation of bingeing and the binge/purge cycle, emphasizing its self-perpetuating nature.	5. The binge/purge cycle is maintained by the pattern of restricting, hunger, bingeing and purging accompanied by feelings of shame, then repetition of the cycle.
6. Monitor patient during and after meals to prevent throwing away food and/or purging.	6. A straightforward statement that the nurse's perceptions are different will help avoid a power struggle. Arguments and power struggles intensify the patient's need to control.
7. Acknowledge the patient's overvalued ideas of body shape and size without minimizing or challenging patient's perceptions.	7. Cognitive behavioral approaches can be very effective in helping the patient identify irrational beliefs about self and body image.
8. Encourage patient to keep a journal of thoughts and feelings.	8. A journal can provide information to identify irrational thinking and identify triggers that induce disordered eating behaviors. Reframing distorted beliefs and thinking can lead to healthier behaviors.

Communication Guidelines

Compared with the food-restricting patient with anorexia, the patient with bulimia nervosa often more readily establishes a therapeutic alliance with the nurse because the eating behaviors are so ego-dystonic, or against what the patient wants. The therapeutic alliance allows the nurse, along with other members of the interdisciplinary team, to provide counseling that gives useful feedback regarding the distorted beliefs held by the patient. See Box 14-4 for a list of common cognitive distortions.

In working with a patient who has bulimia, the nurse needs to be aware that the patient is sensitive to the perceptions of others. The patient may feel significant shame and totally out of control. In building a therapeutic alliance, the nurse needs to empathize with feelings of low self-esteem, unworthiness, and dysphoria (sadness or unease). The nurse may suspect dishonesty when the patient does not report bingeing or purging. An accepting, nonjudgmental approach, along with a comprehensive understanding of the subjective experience of the patient, will help to build trust.

Milieu Therapy

The highly structured milieu of an inpatient unit has as its primary goals the interruption of the binge/purge cycle and the prevention of the disordered eating behaviors. Interventions such as observation during and after meals to prevent purging, normalization of eating patterns, and maintenance of appropriate amounts of exercise are integral elements of treatment. The interdisciplinary team uses a comprehensive approach to address the emotional and behavioral problems that arise when the patient is no longer binge eating or purging. The interruption of the binge/purge pattern allows underlying feelings to surface and be examined.

Health Teaching and Health Promotion

Health teaching focuses not only on the eating disorder but also on the importance of meal planning, use of relaxation techniques, maintenance of a healthy diet and exercise, implementation of coping skills, and knowledge of the physical and emotional effects of bingeing and purging as well as the effects of cognitive distortions. This preparation lays the foundation for the second phase of treatment, in which there are carefully planned challenges to the patient's newly developed skills. For instance, the patient is expected to have a meal while on pass outside the hospital. On return to the unit, the patient can share the experience.

On discharge from the hospital, the individual is referred for long-term care to solidify the goals that have been achieved, address the attitudes and the perceptions that maintain the eating disorder, and deal with the psychodynamic issues that attend the illness. The patient and family could benefit from connecting with a national network that addresses eating disorders—Anorexia Nervosa and Related Eating Disorders (ANRED; www.anred.com), National Eating Disorders Association (NEDA; www.nationaleatingdisorders.org).

Psychotherapy

A cognitive behavioral approach is among the most effective treatment for bulimia nervosa. Patients with bulimia nervosa, because of possible coexisting depression, substance abuse, and personality disorders, often undergo various therapies. Although the specific eating-disordered behaviors may not be targeted in some therapies, it is those very behaviors that are responsible for much of the patient's emotional distress. It is imperative that irrational attitudes and perceptions of weight and shape be addressed. Therefore restructuring faulty perceptions and helping individuals develop accepting attitudes toward themselves and their bodies is a primary focus of therapy. When patients do not indulge in these bulimic behaviors, issues of self-worth and interpersonal functioning become more prominent (Fairburn, 2008).

Pharmacological, Biological, and Integrative Therapies

Fluoxetine (Prozac) has been approved by the Food and Drug Administration (FDA) for the treatment of bulimia nervosa and has been regarded as the gold standard in the treatment of this disorder. Either alone or in combination with other behavioral treatments, binge eating and purging behaviors are noted to be significantly decreased. Fluoxetine has a very favorable side effect profile compared to other pharmacological agents; however, as a selective serotonin reuptake inhibitor (SSRI), it contains the Black Box warning indicating increased risk of suicidal ideation (Mitchell et al., 2013).

EVALUATION

The process of evaluation is built into the outcomes specified by the goals. Evaluation is ongoing, and short-term and intermediate goals are revised as necessary to achieve the treatment outcomes established.

The goals provide a daily guide for evaluating success and must be continually reevaluated for their appropriateness.

BINGE EATING DISORDER

Although considerable controversy existed in *DSM-IV-TR* over whether this proposed diagnosis constituted a separate eating disorder, binge eating disorder is formally recognized as a specific disorder in *DSM-5*. Binge eating disorder is a variant of compulsive overeating. Although considerable controversy exists over whether this proposed diagnosis constitutes a separate eating disorder, 20% to 30% of obese individuals seeking treatment report binge eating as a pattern of overeating. These individuals report recurrent episodes of eating a large amount of food in a short period of time, and usually feeling guilty or shameful after bingeing. The pattern is not unlike bulimia nervosa; however, in binge eating disorder there are no compensatory mechanisms used (e.g., self-induced vomiting or inappropriate use of diuretics/laxatives). The *DSM-5* makes a distinction between binge eating disorder and obesity, stating that most obese individuals do not engage in recurrent binge eating behaviors, and, of note, the *DSM-5* does not include obesity as a mental disorder. Binge eating disorder usually exists with co-occurring psychiatric disorders such as bipolar disorder, depressive disorder, anxiety disorder, and, to a lesser extent, substance use disorders (APA, 2013).

Overeating is frequently noted as a symptom of a depression (i.e., atypical depression). High rates of mood disorders and personality disorders are found among binge eaters. Binge eaters also report a history of major depression significantly more often than non–binge eaters. They further report that binge eating is soothing and helps to regulate their moods. Although dieting is almost always an antecedent of binge eating in bulimia nervosa, in approximately 50% of a sample of obese binge eaters, no attempt to restrict dietary intake occurred before bingeing (APA, 2013). An effective program for those with binge eating disorder must integrate modification of the disordered eating with reported events and associated mood changes, working towards the ultimate goal of a more appropriate weight for the individual (Table 14-3) (Fairburn, 2008).

TABLE 14-3	Interventions for Binge Eating Disorder
Intervention	**Rationale**
1. Assess mood, psychosocial factors	1. Psychological distress frequently operates as a trigger and dysphoria is common.
2. Along with multidisciplinary team, determine treatment objectives.	2. Treatment focus may be primarily to interrupt binge eating with or without weight loss.
3. Provide nutritional counseling.	3. Approximately one-third of binge eaters are obese and are at risk for cardiovascular complications including diabetes mellitus type 2. In some patients a weight control program may trigger a resurgence of binge eating.
4. Provide psychosocial treatment.	4. Binge eating is associated with significant mood disturbance and psychosocial stress. There is evidence-based treatment for cognitive behavioral therapy and dialectical behavior therapy.

There is limited evidence to suggest that antidepressant, antiobesity, and other medications affect long-term improvement in the frequency of binge eating or in mood symptoms. Several studies of combination behavioral therapy and medication have yielded mixed results. Selective serotonin reuptake inhibitors have shown some efficacy in reducing binge eating behavior, and topiramate, an anti-epileptic drug, has shown a reduction in binge eating behavior with some weight loss in obese patients (Mitchell et al., 2013).

APPLYING EVIDENCE-BASED PRACTICE (EBP)

Problem A 47-year-old male is on a surgical unit after having bariatric surgery to promote weight loss. The RN brings him his first meal tray which consists of 15mL of clear liquid. The patient appears shocked and raises his voice in frustration, stating "this is not what I expected, get me some food!" The nurse sits down to talk with the patient, and discovers he had been binge eating large amounts up until the day before the surgery, and had not attended nutrition classes or counseling to prepare for the significant lifestyle changes post-surgery.

EBP Assessment

A. **What do you already know from experience?** Patients can be psychologically unprepared or lack education regarding the changes after bariatric surgery. Binge eating can be the result of a learned habit, metabolic or medical issues, or a response to past trauma or stress. The changes can be difficult and upsetting. Obese individuals experience prejudice and stigma.

B. **What does the literature say?** Protocol dictates that patients be referred for a psychiatric evaluation, and should be prepared by losing weight through dietary and other lifestyle changes prior to surgery. Obesity has a variety of contributing factors besides overeating in most cases. Severely obese individuals may not be able to lose weight in any other manner besides surgery. Most patients maintain most of their weight loss after bariatric surgery contrary to popular belief.

C. **What does the patient want?** The patient wants to feel better, but is very uncomfortable without eating his usual amounts. He wants to lose weight and be healthier but is distressed at this time. He is demanding food which would result in surgical complications.

Plan The RN reports the patient's response to the surgeon and his supervisor. He sits down with the patient to provide support and patient education. A nursing staff member is rotated to stay with the patient at all times for support during the initial stages of adjustment. Social services is notified to provide therapeutic support. The dietician begins to work with the patient to provide education he failed to obtain prior to his surgery by not attending his program. The RN administers a prn sedative as needed.

QSEN **QSEN Prelicensure Knowledge, Skills, and Attitudes (KSA's) Addressed:**
Safety was maintained through staying with the patient while distraught, to prevent surgical complications.
Team work and collaboration was displayed through consultation between the RN, surgeon, supervisor, social services, the dietician, and the patient.

Mayo Clinic. (1998-2015). *Gastric bypass surgery* [website]. Retrieved from: http://www.mayoclinic.org/tests-procedures/bariatric-surgery/basics/how-you-prepare/PRC-20019138
University of California Los Angeles Center for Obesity and Metabolic Health (COMET). (2015). *Post bariatric surgery guidelines*. Retrieved from: http://bariatrics.ucla.edu/workfiles/UCLA-Bariatric-postoperative-diet-instructions.pdf

KEY POINTS TO REMEMBER

- A number of theoretical models help explain risk factors for the development of eating disorders.
- Neurobiological theories identify an association between eating disorders, depression, and neuroendocrine abnormalities.
- Psychological theories explore issues of control in anorexia and affective instability and poor impulse control in bulimia, but these are not considered causes of eating disorders.
- Genetic theories postulate the existence of vulnerabilities that may predispose people toward eating disorders, and increasingly twin studies confirm genetic liability, which perhaps interacts with environmental mechanisms.
- Sociocultural models look both at our present societal ideal of being thin and at the ideal feminine role model in general.
- Families may serve as important allies in treatment.
- Eating disorders are now appearing in populations in which they had been rare. The dynamics—the stress of acculturation versus identification with the new culture—are being examined.
- Anorexia nervosa is a possibly life-threatening eating disorder that includes being severely underweight; having low blood pressure, pulse rate, and temperature measurements; being dehydrated; and having low serum potassium level and dysrhythmias. Anorexia

may be treated in an inpatient treatment setting—in which milieu therapy, psychotherapy (cognitive), development of self-care skills, and psychobiological interventions can be implemented.
- Eating disorders, thought to occur only in preteen or teen-age groups, are now being diagnosed in people ages 35 to 65.
- Long-term treatment is provided on an outpatient basis and aims to help patients maintain healthy weight; it includes treatment modalities such as individual therapy, family therapy, group therapy, psychopharmacology, and nutrition counseling.
- Individuals with bulimia nervosa are typically within the normal weight range, but some may be slightly below or above ideal body weight.
- Assessment of a patient with bulimia may show enlargement of the parotid glands, dental erosion, and dental caries if the patient has induced vomiting.
- Acute care may be necessary when life-threatening complications are present, such as gastric rupture (rare), electrolyte imbalance, and cardiac dysrhythmias.
- The primary goal of interventions for a patient with bulimia is to interrupt the binge/purge cycle.
- Psychotherapy as well as self-care skill training is included.
- Long-term treatment focuses on therapy aimed at addressing any coexisting depression, substance abuse, and/or personality

disorders that are causing the patient distress and interfering with quality of life. Self-worth and interpersonal functioning eventually become issues that are useful to target.

- Other specified feeding or eating disorder (OSFED), formerly eating disorder not otherwise specified (EDNOS) in *DSM-IV*, includes a variety of subthreshold patterns that do not meet full criteria as set forth in *DSM-5*.
- Binge eaters report a history of major depression significantly more often than non–binge eaters.
- Effective treatment for obese binge eaters integrates modification of the disordered eating, improvement of depressive symptoms, and achievement of an appropriate weight for the individual.

APPLYING CRITICAL JUDGMENT

1. Tom Shift, a 19-year-old model, has experienced a rapid decrease in weight over the past 4 months, after his agent told him he would have to lose weight or lose a coveted account. Tom is 6 feet 2 inches tall and weighs 132 pounds, down from his usual 176 pounds. He is brought to the emergency department with a pulse rate of 40 beats per minute and severe dysrhythmias. His laboratory workup reveals severe hypokalemia. He has become extremely depressed, saying, "I'm too fat … I won't take anything to eat. If I gain weight my life will be ruined. There is nothing to live for if I can't model." Tom's parents are startled and confused, and his best friend is worried and feels powerless to help Tom. "I tell Tom he needs to eat or he will die. I tell him he is a skeleton, but he refuses to listen to me. I don't know what to do."
   A. Which physical and psychiatric criteria suggest that Tom should be immediately hospitalized? What other physical signs and symptoms may be found on assessment?
   B. What are some of the questions you would eventually ask Tom when evaluating his biopsychosocial functioning?
   C. What are your feelings toward someone with anorexia? Can you make a distinction between your thoughts and feelings toward women with anorexia and toward men with anorexia?
   D. What are some things you could do for Tom's parents and Tom's friend in terms of offering them information, support, and referrals? Identify specific referrals.
   E. Explain the kinds of interventions or restrictions that may be used while Tom is hospitalized (e.g., weighing, observation after eating or visits, exercise, therapy, self-care).
   F. How would you describe partial hospitalization programs or psychiatric home care programs when asked if Tom will have to be hospitalized for a long time?
   G. What are some of Tom's cognitive distortions that would be a target for therapy?
   H. Identify at least five criteria that, if met, would indicate that Tom was improving.
2. You and your close friend Mary Alice have been together since nursing school and you are now working on the same surgical unit. Mary Alice told you that in the past she has made several suicide attempts. Today you accidentally come upon her bingeing while off the unit, and she looks embarrassed and uncomfortable when she sees you. Several times you notice that she spends time in the bathroom and you hear sounds of retching. In response to your concern, she admits that she has been bingeing/purging for several years but that now she is getting out of control and feels profoundly depressed.

   A. Although Mary Alice does not show any physical signs of bulimia nervosa, what would you look for when assessing an individual with bulimia?
   B. What kinds of emergencies could result from bingeing and purging?
   C. What would be the most useful type of psychotherapy for Mary Alice initially and what issues would need to be addressed?
   D. What kinds of new skills does a person with bulimia need to learn to lessen the compulsion to binge and purge?
   E. What would be some signs that Mary Alice is recovering?

CHAPTER REVIEW QUESTIONS

1. The school nurse assesses four adolescents, all of whom outwardly appear healthy. Which adolescent meets one criterion for anorexia nervosa with mild severity?
   a. 5'2" tall; weight 104 pounds
   b. 5'7" tall; weight 110 pounds
   c. 5'5" tall; weight 114 pounds
   d. 5'8" tall; weight 127 pounds
2. A nurse assesses four adolescents diagnosed with various eating disorders. Which comment would the nurse expect from the adolescent diagnosed with anorexia nervosa?
   a. "I look good because whenever I overeat, I purge myself."
   b. "I love sweets. I make myself throw up so I can eat more."
   c. "I've lost 60 pounds but I'm still a size 2. I want to be a size 0."
   d. "I've hidden my eating disorder from everyone, even my parents."
3. While weighing patients on an eating disorders unit, the nurse overhears a psychiatric technician say, "I wish I had an eating disorder; maybe I'd lose a little weight." What is the nurse's best action?
   a. Report the clinical observation to the nursing supervisor.
   b. Ask the psychiatric technician, "What did you mean by that comment?"
   c. Privately discuss the importance of sensitivity with the psychiatric technician.
   d. Immediately interrupt the interaction between the patient and psychiatric technician.
4. Shortly after hospitalization, an adolescent diagnosed with anorexia nervosa says to the nurse, "Being fat is the worst thing in the world. I hope it never happens to me." Which response by the nurse is appropriate?
   a. "You need to gain weight to become healthier."
   b. "Your world would not change if you gained a few pounds."
   c. "Tell me how your world would be different if you were fat."
   d. "Your attractiveness is not defined by a number on the scales."
5. A patient is hospitalized with a diagnosis of anorexia nervosa. The nurse reviews the patient's laboratory results below.
   Sodium 143 mEq/L
   Potassium 3.1 mEq/L
   Chloride 102 mEq/L
   Magnesium 2.2 mEq/L
   Calcium 8.4 mg/dL
   Phosphate 3.0 mg/dL
   The nurse should take which action next?
   a. Measure the patient's body temperature.
   b. Inspect the patient's skin and sclera for jaundice.
   c. Assess the patient's mucous membranes for erosion.
   d. Auscultate the patient's heart rate, rhythm, and sounds.

REFERENCES

Academy for Eating Disorders (AED). (2014). *Eating disorders: critical points for early recognition and medical risk management in the care of individuals with eating disorders* (3rd ed.). Academy for Eating Disorders (AED). http://www.aedweb.org/index.php/education/eating-disorder-information/eating-disorder-information-3.

American Nurses Association, American Psychiatric Nurses Association, & International Society of Psychiatric-Mental Health Nurses. (2014). *Psychiatric-mental health nursing: scope and standards of practice.* Silver Springs, Md: APA.

American Psychiatric Association. (2006). *Practice guidelines for the treatment of patients with eating disorders* (3rd ed.). Arlington, Va: APA.

American Psychiatric Association. (2012). *Guideline watch for the treatment of patients with eating disorders.* Arlington, Va: APA.

American Psychiatric Association. (2013). *Diagnostic and statistical manual of mental disorders (DSM-5)* (5th ed.). Arlington, Va: APA.

Bailer, U. F., & Kaye, W. H. (2011). Serotonin: imaging findings in eating disorders. *Current Topics in Behavioral Neurosciences, 6,* 59–79.

Bernstein, B. E. , & Pataki, C. (2016). Anorexia nervosa treatment and management. Retrieved from http://emedicine.medscape.com/article/912187-treatment.

Black, D. W., & Andreasen, N. C. (2014). *Introductory textbook of psychiatry* (6th ed.). Washington, DC: American Psychiatric Publishing.

Fairburn, C. G. (2008). *Cognitive behavior therapy and eating disorders.* New York: Guilford Press.

Fairburn, C. G., & Rothwell, E. R. (2015). Apps and eating disorders: A systematic clinical appraisal. *International Journal of Eating Disorders, 48*(7), 1038–1046.

Hamilton, G., Cullar, L., Elenback, R. (2015). Eating disorder hope: anorexia nervosa – highest mortality rate of any mental disorder: why? http://www.eatingdisorderhope.com/information/anorexia/anorexia-nervosa-highest-mortality-rate-of-any-mental-disorder-why.

Hudson, J. I., Hiripi, E., Harrison, G. P., et al. (2007). The prevalence and correlates of eating disorders in the national comorbidity survey replication. *Biological Psychiatry, 61,* 348–358.

Kaye, W. H., Bulik, C. M., Plotnicov, K., et al. (2008). The genetics of anorexia nervosa collaborative study: methods and sample description. *International Journal of Eating Disorders, 41*(4), 289–300.

Kostro, K., Lerman, J. B., & Attia, E. (2014). The current status of suicide and self-injury in eating disorders: a narrative review. *Journal of Eating Disorders, 2*(19), 1–9.

Le Grange, D., Lock, J., Loeb, K., et al. (2010). Academy for eating disorders position paper: the role of the family in eating disorders. *International Journal of Eating Disorders, 43*(1), 1–5.

Mangweth-Matzek, B., Hoek, H. W., Rupp, C. I., et al. (2014). Prevalence of eating disorders in middle-aged women. *International Journal of Eating Disorders, 47*(3), 320–324.

Mitchell, J. E., Roerig, J., & Steffen, K. (2013). Biological therapies for eating disorders. *International Journal of Eating Disorders, 46*(5), 470–477.

Sadock, B. J., Sadock, V. A., & Ruiz, P. (2015). *Kaplan and Sadock's synopsis of psychiatry* (11th ed.). Philadelphia: Wolters Kluwer/Lippincott Williams & Wilkins.

Smink, F. R., van Hoeken, D., & Hoek, H. W. (2013). Epidemiology, course and outcome of eating disorders. *Current Opinion in Psychiatry, 26*(6), 543–548.

Thornton, L. M., Mazzeo, S. E., & Bulik, C. M. (2011). The heritability of eating disorders: methods and current findings. *Current Topics in Behavioral Neuroscience, 6,* 141–156.

Trace, S. E., Thornton, L. M., Runfola, C. D., et al. (2012). Sleep problems are associated with binge eating in women. *International Journal of Eating Disorders, 45*(5), 695–703.

Wade, T. D., Gordon, S., Medland, S., et al. (2013). Genetic variants associated with disordered eating. *International Journal of Eating Disorders, 46*(6), 594–608.

Walsh, B. T. (2013). The enigmatic persistence of anorexia nervosa. *American Journal of Psychiatry, 170*(5), 477–484.

15

Mood Disorders: Depression

Elizabeth M. Varcarolis

http://evolve.elsevier.com/Varcarolis/essentials

KEY TERMS AND CONCEPTS

anergia, p. 199
anhedonia, p. 199
atypical antidepressants, p. 216
deep brain stimulation, p. 219
dual action reuptake inhibitor, p. 216
electroconvulsive therapy (ECT), p. 208
hypersomnia, p. 202
light therapy, p. 219

major depressive disorder (MDD), p. 197
mood, p. 197
persistent depressive disorder (PDD), p. 202
psychomotor agitation, p. 205
psychomotor retardation, p. 205
rapid transcranial magnetic stimulation
 (rTMS), p. 219
S-adenosylmethionine (SAMe), p. 220

selective serotonin reuptake inhibitor
 (SSRI), p. 197
St. John's wort, p. 220
tricyclic antidepressants (TCAs), p. 213
vagus nerve stimulation (VNS), p. 219
vegetative signs of depression, p. 205

SELECTED CONCEPT: SELF-ESTEEM

NANDA's definition of **self-esteem** is "a pattern of perceptions or ideas about the self that is sufficient for well-being and can be strengthened."

 Situational low self-esteem refers to a "negative perception of self-worth in response to a current situation," which may occur when our behavior is inconsistent with our values, when we fail at something, or when we experience a significant loss/rejection, for example.

 Chronic low self-esteem, however, "is long-standing negative self-evaluating/feelings about self or self-capabilities." These painful feelings often present in people with depression. Depression can be demoralizing, and painful levels of low self-esteem can erode a person's quality of life, and belief in self, which can dampen the spirit and contribute to hopelessness and helplessness for the future.

 Therapies that help biologically to lower depressive feelings and talking therapies that help change a person's perceptions of their self-concept have helped to decrease depression, increase quality of life, and increase functioning and productivity for many people.
 (NANDA, 2015 – 2017)

OBJECTIVES

1. Differentiate between major depressive disorder (MDD) and persistent depressive disorder (PDD).
2. Summarize the links between the stress model of depression and the biological model of depression.
3. **QSEN** Apply **patient-centered care** during an assessment of a depressed individual's behaviors in each of the following areas: (a) affect, (b) thought processes, (c) feelings, (d) physical characteristics, and (e) communication.
4. Apply communication strategies that are useful for depressed patients in a nursing care plan for a depressed individual.
5. **QSEN** Describe the **evidence-based practice** regarding the advantages versus the disadvantages of both the selective serotonin reuptake inhibitors (SSRIs) and the tricyclic antidepressants (TCAs).
6. Identify two atypical antidepressants and explain the unique advantages each attributes in specific circumstances.
7. Discuss at length, using a step-by-step approach, the role of monoamine oxidase (MAO) in our brain and explain why special dietary/medication restrictions have to be maintained when a monoamine oxidase inhibitor (MAOI) is prescribed.
8. Relate why the selegiline transdermal system (STS) is a breakthrough for the MAOIs.
9. **QSEN** Identify potential **safety issues** regarding the adverse reactions of the SSRIs, especially in older adults, and potential dangers during pregnancy.
10. **QSEN** Applying the knowledge of **evidence-based practice,** identify the attributes of a depressed individual for which electroconvulsive therapy (ECT) is most helpful.
11. **QSEN** Explain all the ways that **teamwork and collaboration** are useful in the treatment of depression.
12. **QSEN** There are a number of websites that enable individuals to perform a confidential screening test. Go to the Internet and find a screening test for depression (**informatics**).

INTRODUCTION

It is convenient for us to think of depression on a continuum since we have all had low moods and "blue" days, but according to Sadock and colleagues (2015), people with mood disorders describe a distinct quality to their pathological state. It is impossible to adequately convey the profound anguish that is experienced by an individual suffering a severe depressive episode unless we ourselves have had a similar experience.

The term depression is an umbrella term for a variety of disorders that range from mild, to moderate, to severely disabling. Depression is actually a syndrome rather than a disease. "While a disease is a specific condition characterized by a common underlying cause and consistent physical traits, a syndrome is a collection of signs and symptoms known to frequently appear together, but without a single known cause" (Chen, 2015). Clinical depressive syndromes can cause severe impairment in psychosocial functioning and increased mortality. Depressive disorders represent a group of syndromes that often share some common symptoms, but in fact have different etiologies, courses, and treatments (Preston et al., 2013). Research continues to try and identify markers in people with depression that can help predict how an individual might respond to a specific medication (APA, 2015). Treatments for depression do work, but unfortunately there is no one-size-fits-all, and finding the right combination of interventions may take time.

PREVALENCE AND COMORBIDITY

Depression is the most common mental illness seen in medical/psychiatric practice today. It is the leading cause of disability between the ages of 14 and 44 (Lliades, 2015). The World Health Organization (WHO) estimates that depression will soon be the number 2 cause of "lost years of healthy life" (Washington University, 2015). Studies indicate that the incidence of depression has been increasing over the past 50 years in the United States from 3.33% to 7.06% from 1991 through 2002 (Lliades, 2015). Women are 70% more likely than men to experience depression during the course of their lifetimes. Research has shown that this is in part due to hormones, such as with premenstrual dysphoric disorder. Also women are more likely to seek help for depression and men are more likely to self-medicate with alcohol/substances (Lliades, 2015).

Approximately 16.5% of people older than 18 years old in this country will have a major depressive episode in their lifetime. The 12-month prevalence of a major depressive disorder (MDD) is approximately 7% (APA, 2013).

A depressive syndrome frequently accompanies other psychiatric disorders such as anxiety disorders, posttraumatic stress disorder (PTSD), schizophrenia, substance use disorders, eating disorders, obsessive-compulsive disorders, and schizoaffective disorder. People with anxiety disorders (e.g., panic disorder, generalized anxiety disorder, phobic disorders) commonly present with depression, as do people with personality disorders (particularly borderline personality disorder), adjustment disorders, and brief depressive reactions. According to a 2010 study by the Centers for Disease Control and Prevention, African Americans have the highest rate of current depression (12.8%), followed by Hispanics (11.4%), and whites (7.9%).

People with chronic medical problems (e.g., hypertension, backache, diabetes, heart problems, arthritis, cancer) are at a higher risk for depression than those in the general population. Often depression may be the first symptom of a medical condition. Depression may be induced by substance abuse, such as alcohol, cocaine, marijuana, heroin, anxiolytics, and a host of prescription medications. The symptoms of a depression occur during bereavement and are expected as part of the normal process of mourning. *Mixed anxiety–depression* is perhaps

one of the most common depressive presentations. Symptoms of anxiety frequently co-occur with cases of MDD, persistent depressive disorder (PPD), or any other depressive syndrome. The anxious depression subtype accounts for about 45% of depressions according to the *Sequenced Treatment Alternatives to Relieve Depression (STAR*D) Project* (Fava et al., 2016). The presence of a co-occurring anxiety disorder with a depressive symptom has a negative effect on the course of the disease and these individuals are significantly less likely to benefit from an antidepressant than those without anxiety. Comorbidity has been shown to result in a higher rate of suicide, greater **severity of depression, and greater impairment in social and occupational functioning as well as including more coexisting illnesses, both medical and psychiatric.** Refer to Table 15-1 for different subtypes of depression.

Children and Adolescents

Children as young as 3 years of age have been diagnosed with depression. Depression in children and adolescents may present differently than depression in adults in that instead of a depressed mood, their mood may be irritable. Children with depression may not show classic signs of depression, but may complain of feeling unwell, refuse to go to school, complain of vague physical complaints, show aggression, and act clingy. Adolescents may mask depression through sulking, being negative or grouchy, getting into trouble at school, feeling misunderstood, withdrawing from others, or running away from the home or center (NIMH, 2010b).

- Major depressive disorder is said to occur in as many as 18% of preadolescents, which is perhaps a low estimate because depression in this age group is often underdiagnosed. At age 10 years, children have a 14% chance of suffering from a MDD in their lifetime; from ages 13 to 18, individuals have an 11.2% chance of being afflicted with a depressive disorder; and in those diagnosed between 18 and 24 years there is 10.9% rate of depression, and it is this age group that has the greatest risk for self-harm (Lliades, 2015; NIMH, 2010a).
- Major depression among adolescents is often associated with substance use disorder and antisocial behavior, both of which can obscure accurate diagnosis and lower levels of treatment response. The prevalence rate in individuals 18 to 29 years old is three times higher than in individuals 60 years old or older (APA, 2013).
- Children and adolescents with a major depressive disorder have a high rate of future reoccurrence. Those who have a very severe depression, and/or a sense of hopelessness, anxiety, and family conflict, are much less likely to achieve remission. However, early treatment with medication and cognitive behavioral therapy (CBT) in the first 12 weeks can help in achieving remission (NIMH, 2010a,b; Yellowlees, 2011a). Children in families with other depressed members seem to become depressed earlier (ages 12 to 13 years) than children in families with no other depressed members (16 to 17 years). Even before adolescence, girls are more vulnerable to depression than boys.

Older Adults

Depression among older adults (65 or older) has been declining; however, the suicide rate among elderly men is the highest of all age groups, perhaps related to unrecognized, untreated, or masked depression masquerading as another medical condition (Lliades, 2015). Depression can remain undiagnosed approximately 50% of the time in older adults. The good news is that efforts to improve recognition of depression and education have led to positive treatment response among older adults (Lowry, 2012b). However, research suggests that use of antidepressant medication in those 65 and older can be risky. Studies indicate that antidepressants in older adults are associated with falls, strokes, seizures, and other adverse outcomes. Those taking selective serotonin reuptake inhibitors (SSRIs) had more adverse events than older adults taking tricyclic antidepressants (TCAs). Therefore, SSRIs

TABLE 15-1 Specifiers for Major Depressive Disorder: Specify if Symptoms are Mild, Moderate, or Severe

Disorder	Symptoms
Major depressive disorder	Symptoms represent a change from usual functioning
	Associated with high mortality rate
	Significant in physical, social, and role functioning, as well as increased potential for pain and physical illness
Melancholic depression	Severe form of depression; complete loss of pleasure in life (anhedonia)* and inability to feel better
	Marked by early morning awakening, feels worse in the morning, movements are agitated or very slow, substantial weight loss, and/or extreme feelings of guilt
	Occurs in severe depressions and in those with psychotic features
Peripartum depression	Symptoms of a major depressive episode that occur either during pregnancy or within 4 weeks after childbirth
	Can present with or without psychotic features; psychotic features are common
	Severe ruminations or delusional thoughts about infant signify increased risk of harm to infant
	Disinterest in the infant; crying spells, severe anxiety, panic attacks, and suicidal thoughts can also be present
Seasonal depression	Indicates that episodes mostly begin in fall or winter and remit in spring
	Characterized by anergia, hypersomnia, overeating, weight gain, and craving for carbohydrates
	Responds to light therapy
Anxious depression	Significant amounts of anxiety along with depression; experiences of restlessness, difficulty concentrating, fear that something terrible may happen, fear of losing control
Catatonic depression	Characterized by abnormalities of movement behavior
	May present with echopraxia, echolalia, grimacing, stereotyped movements, posturing, negativism, stupor, waxy flexibility, agitation, mutism, mannerisms
Mixed depression	Presents with subthreshold manic or hypomanic symptoms
	Symptoms include elevated/expanded mood, inflated self-esteem, decreased need for sleep, for example
	Often poor response to medications, increased risk for suicide and substance abuse (lurasidone [Latudea])
Atypical depression	Rejection sensitivity (pathological sensitivity to perceived interpersonal rejection) that is present throughout life and results in functional impairment
	Other symptoms include hypersomnia, hyperphagia (overeating), leaden paralysis (feeling weighed down in extremities)
	Profound fatigue, low energy
	Personality and anxiety disorders are also co-occurring
	Mood may brighten in the event of positive events
Psychotic depression	Presents experience delusions (less frequently hallucinations)
	Psychotic features are mood congruent (consistent with the current mood)
	More common in bipolar disorder, risk factor for suicide
Persisting depressive disorder (dysthymic disorder)	A less severe but chronic depressed mood for most of the day, more days than not, lasting for at least 2 years
	Mood is not a change from usual behavior
Premenstrual dysphoric disorder	Up to one out of ten women have premenstrual symptoms that are so distressing and disabling that they warrant a diagnosis of premenstrual dysphoric disorder (PMDD). PMDD is characterized by severe depression, irritability, and other mood disturbances. Symptoms begin about 10 to 14 days before menses and improves within a few days

*Derives no pleasure from usual pleasurable activities or positive happenings.

are less likely to be given to older adults. Refer to Chapter 28 for more on depression in the older adult.

THEORY

Many theories attempt to explain the cause of depression; however, basically depression is thought to involve changes in **receptor-neurotransmitter relationships** in the following areas of the brain:

1. **Limbic system** (emotional alterations)
2. **Prefrontal cortex** (decreased mood, problems concentrating)
3. **Hippocampus** (memory impairments; feelings of worthlessness, hopelessness, and guilt)
4. **Amygdala** (anxiety and reduced motivation)

The primary neurotransmitters involved with depression are serotonin and norepinephrine, although dopamine is also related to depression.

It is becoming evident that depression is a heterogeneous, systemic illness involving an array of different neurotransmitters, neuronal pathways, hereditary processes, and/or traumatic life events.

BOX 15-1 Primary Risk Factors for Depression

- History of prior episodes of depression
- Family history of depressive disorder, especially in first-degree relatives
- History of suicide attempts or family history of suicide
- Member of the LGBT community (lesbian, gay, bisexual, transgender)
- Female gender
- Age 40 years or younger
- Postpartum period
- Chronic medical illness
- Absence of social support
- Negative, stressful life events
- Active alcohol or substance abuse
- History of sexual abuse

It is commonly accepted that genetic predisposition to the illness combined with childhood stress may lead to significant changes in the central nervous system (CNS) that may result in depression. However, there are common risk factors for depression that may signal the presence of this common and serious psychiatric illness (Box 15-1).

Biological Theories
Genetic Factors

Twin studies consistently show that genetic factors play a role in the development of depressive disorders. Various studies reveal that the average concordance rate for unipolar depression mood disorders among monozygotic twins (twins sharing the same genetic constitution) is 50%. That is, if one twin is affected, the second has a 50% chance of being affected. The percentage for dizygotic twins (different genetic constitution) is 20%. Thus identical twins (monozygotic) have a greater concordance rate than dizygotic twins. However, because concordance rates in monozygotic twins are not 100% it appears that other factors also must be involved.

Adoptive studies also have pointed to genetic contribution for the development of depression. For example, the risk for the development of depression in children born to parent(s) with a depressive illness is the same when these children are adopted by a nondepressive family.

Family studies are supportive of a genetic link, concluding that mood disorders are heritable for some people. Individuals who have a first-degree family member with depression are two to four times more likely to become depressed (APA, 2013; NIMH, 2015). Increased heritability is associated with an earlier age of onset, greater rate of comorbidity (especially alcoholism and psychosis), and increased risk of recurrent illness. However, any genetic factors that are present must interact with environmental and neurobiological preconditions for depression to develop.

Biochemical Factors

The brain is a highly complex organ that contains billions of neurons. There is much evidence to support the concept that depression is a biologically heterogeneous disorder; that is, many CNS neurotransmitter abnormalities can probably cause clinical depression. These neurotransmitter abnormalities may be the result of a variety factors that can result in neurotransmitter abnormalities, systemic biochemical, and/or hormonal changes that can affect the central nervous system (Preston et al., 2013). The most predisposing factors include genetic factors, environmental factors, medical conditions (such as cerebral infarction, hypothyroidism), severe stress, or medication or drug abuse. **Whatever the etiological contribution, depression is ultimately mediated through changes in the brain's neurochemistry and the circuitry involved in emotional regulations.**

Neurobiological investigations in depression have focused on the monoamine neurotransmitters (serotonin, noradrenaline, and dopamine). These neurons play a significant role in the functioning of the **limbic system** and the adjacent **hypothalamus** (Preston et al., 2013). These neurotransmitters in the brain are believed to be related to altered mood states.

Serotonin (5-hydroxytryptamine [5-HT]) **and norepinephrine (NE) are two major neurotransmitters involved in depression.** Serotonin is an important *regulator of sleep, appetite, and libido* (vegetative signs). A serotonin circuit dysfunction can result in *poor impulse control, low sex drive, decreased appetite, disturbed regulation of body temperature, and irritability*. Decreased levels of **norepinephrine** (NE) in the medial forebrain bundle (MFB) may account for anergia (reduction in or lack of energy), anhedonia (an inability to find meaning or pleasure in existence), *decreased concentration, and diminished libido in depression*.

The dopamine (DA), acetylcholine, and γ-aminobutyric acid (GABA) systems are believed to be involved in the pathophysiology of a major depressive episode. Dopamine neurons in the mesolimbic system are thought to play a role in the reward and incentive behavior processes, emotional expression, and learning processes that are disrupted in depression. This is particularly true in melancholic depression (severe MDD).

Some individuals with a **masked depression** present with severe pain (often pelvic, abdominal, or low back pain) and deny feelings of sadness, although they may suffer from the other symptoms of depression (Gananca et al., 2014). Serotonin and norepinephrine are also involved in the perception of **pain** by modifying the effects of substance P, glutamate, GABA, and other pain mediators (Narasimhan & Campbell, 2010). There is considerable overlap in the biological underpinnings of both major depression and chronic pain. For example, genetics and neurotransmitter functionality are similar in both (Narasimhan & Campbell, 2010). In some cases **chronic painful physical conditions (CPPCs)** such as backaches or headaches may be due to MDD rather than chronic pain, and in some cases these conditions may present as the only sign of depression (Hall-Flavin, 2015; Narasimhan & Campbell, 2010).

One theory to explain the dysfunction of the neurotransmitters NE, DA, and 5-HT is abnormalities in the number of receptor sites, which could increase or decrease the activity of neurotransmitters. It is important to keep in mind that the neurotransmitters specific to depression (norepinephrine, serotonin, and dopamine) have many subtypes, accounting for the complexity in treatment and varied patient responses to attempts to increase levels of these neurotransmitters through medications. The relationships among the serotonin, norepinephrine, dopamine, acetylcholine, and GABA systems are complex and need further assessment and study. However, medication that helps regulate these neurotransmitters has proved empirically successful in the treatment of many patients. Figure 15-1 shows a positron emission tomography (PET) scan of the brain of a woman with depression before and after taking medication.

PSYCHOSOCIAL THEORIES

The Stress-Diathesis Model of Depression

The stress-diathesis model of depression is a psychological theory that explains depression from an environmental, interpersonal, and life-events perspective combined with biological vulnerability or predisposition (diathesis). It is well known that psychosocial stressors and interpersonal events trigger certain neurophysical and neurochemical changes in the brain. Early life trauma may result in long-term hyperactivity of the corticotropin-releasing factor (CRF) and norepinephrine systems of the CNS with a consequent neurotoxic effect on the hippocampus that leads to neuronal loss. Because norepinephrine, serotonin, and acetylcholine play a role in stress regulation, when these neurotransmitters become overtaxed through stressful events, neurotransmitter depletion may occur and cause permanent neuronal damage, leaving the person vulnerable to depression later in life (Sadock et al., 2015). An analysis by Karg and colleagues (2011) of 54 studies published from 2001 to 2009 found there is evidence for a "depression gene." People who possess a "short" version of the serotonin transporter gene *(5-HTTLPR)* are at a higher risk of depression when they become stressed, especially if they have been maltreated as children and/or have unusually severe medical illness in childhood (WebMD, 2011). However, people with the "long" or protected version of the gene who underwent multiple life stressors experienced no more depression than people in the general population.

Therefore life events (psychosocial stressors and interpersonal events, especially in early life) may influence the development and recurrence of depression through the psychological and biological experience of stress in some people, which results in changes in the connections among nerve cells in the brain.

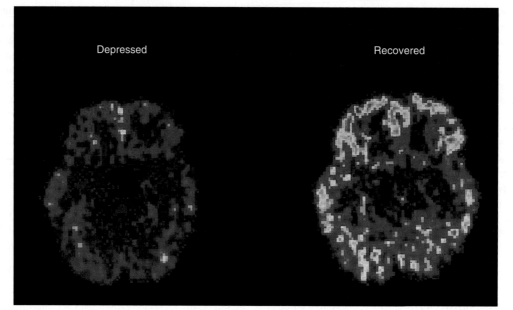

FIGURE 15-1 Positron emission tomography (PET) scans of a 45-year-old woman with recurrent depression. The scan on the left was taken when the patient was not taking medication and was very depressed. The scan on the right was taken several months later when the patient was well, after she had been treated with medication for her depression. Note that her entire brain, particularly the left prefrontal cortex, is more active when she is well. *(Courtesy Mark George, MD, Biological Psychiatry Branch, National Institute of Mental Health, Bethesda, Md.)*

Cognitive Theory

Aaron T. Beck, one of the early proponents of cognitive therapy, applied cognitive behavioral theory to depression. Beck proposed that people acquire a psychological predisposition to depression through early life experiences. These experiences contribute to negative, illogical, and irrational thought processes that may remain dormant until they are activated during times of stress (Beck & Rush, 1995).

Beck found that depressed people process information in negative ways, even in the midst of positive factors that affect the person's life. Beck believed that three automatic negative thoughts—called **Beck's cognitive triad**—are responsible for the development of depression:

1. *A negative, self-deprecating view of self:* "I really never do anything well; everyone else seems smarter."
2. *A pessimistic view of the world:* "Once you're down, you can't get up. Look around, poverty, homelessness, sickness, war, and despair are every place you look."
3. *The belief that negative reinforcement (or no validation for the self) will continue:* "It doesn't matter what you do; nothing ever gets better. I'll be in this stupid job the rest of my life."

The phrase *automatic negative thoughts* refers to thoughts that are repetitive, unintended, and not readily controllable. This cognitive triad seems to be consistent in all types of depression, regardless of clinical subtype.

The goal of CBT is to change the way a patient thinks, which will in turn help relieve the depressive syndrome. This is accomplished by assisting the patient in the following:

1. Identifying and testing negative cognition
2. Developing alternative thinking patterns
3. Rehearsing new cognitive and behavioral responses

Learned Helplessness

Martin Seligman's theory is that of learned helplessness. Seligman (1973) stated that although anxiety is the initial response to a stressful situation, anxiety is replaced by depression if the person feels no control over the outcome of a situation. People who believe that an undesired event is their fault and that nothing can be done to change it are prone to depression. The theory of learned helplessness has been used to explain the development of depression in certain social groups, such as older adults, people living in impoverished areas, and women.

CULTURAL CONSIDERATIONS

Depressive disorders among diverse cultures show substantial differences in symptom presentation, and in most countries, depressive disorders remain unrecognized because somatic symptoms often are the presenting complaint (APA, 2013).

According to the Cross-National Collaborative Group, the prevalence rate of depressive disorders in Asian Americans was the lowest in comparison to whites, African Americans, and Hispanics (Rihmer & Angst, 2009). Prevalence rates for MDD in whites are significantly higher than those in African Americans and Mexican Americans, although the opposite is true for persistent depressive disorder (PDD)/dysthymia (Riolo et al., 2005). It is truly hard to evaluate these kinds of statistics because people from minority groups often have a variety of presenting symptoms that differ in part from whites, often do not seek health care, and do not have the finances to afford health care. We know that, compared to men, women are twice as likely to be diagnosed with depression and also that divorced or single people are more vulnerable to depression than married individuals.

CLINICAL PICTURE

As mentioned, mood disorders range from mild to moderate to severe and are noted as such when making a diagnosis. There are distinct differences between the *DSM-5* diagnostic criteria for a MDD and those for a PDD (dysthymia), which are two of the most common depressive disorders seen in medical practice.

All forms of depression share common symptoms, which can make it difficult to make a correct diagnosis. Preston and Johnson (2015) and the *DSM-5* (APA, 2013) state that the following symptoms are most prevalent in **all** types of depression:

- Mood of sadness, despair, emptiness
- Negative, pessimistic thinking
- Loss of ability to experience pleasure in life (**anhedonia**)
- Low self-esteem
- Apathy, low motivation, and social withdrawal
- Excessive emotional sensitivity
- Irritability and low frustration tolerance
- Insomnia or hypersomnia
- Disruption (mild to severe) in concentration or ability to make decisions
- Suicidal ideation
- Excessive guilt
- Indecisiveness

Major Depressive Disorder (Single Episode or Recurrent)

People with a **major depressive disorder (MDD)** experience substantial pain and suffering, as well as psychological, social, and occupational disability. Basically, the individual is unable to function normally. A patient with MDD presents with a history of one or more major depressive episodes and no history of manic or hypomanic episodes. Many patients who are first diagnosed with a major depressive disorder will later prove to have a bipolar disorder (APA, 2013). In some cases, the patient's history of depression may include psychotic features. MDD with psychotic symptoms is a severe form of mood disorder that is characterized by delusions and/or hallucinations. For example, patients might have delusional thoughts that interfere with their nutritional status (e.g., "I am a terrible person so God put snakes in my stomach and told me not to eat."). This would be an example **of mood–congruent** delusion (e.g., I am a bad person; therefore I am being punished). The course of MDD often remits within 3 months for 20% and within 1 year for 80% of individuals. However, the occurrence of further episodes tends to be longer and more severe, and portends the risk for a continued cyclic occurrence (Fava et al., 2016). Comorbidity with medical illnesses or psychiatric disorders increases morbidity and mortality. Refer to Table 15-1 for a list of specifiers that may accompany an MDD. See the *DSM-5* box for specific symptoms.

VIGNETTE

Sally, a bright, successful, 34-year-old businessperson, finds her world is changing. Over the past few weeks she has become more and more withdrawn. Her life has become empty of meaning. She has great difficulty getting out of bed in the mornings, but finds it hard to sleep more than 3 to 4 hours a night, waking at 2 or 3 AM. She is constantly exhausted.

Sally finds it impossible to concentrate at work and has called in sick the past 2 days, unable to find the energy to dress, bathe, groom, or even eat. She has not eaten for 3 days except for some water and a few glasses of milk and a few crackers she found in a neglected box tucked away in the pantry. She has lost considerable weight.

When her best friend calls to find out why she has not shown up for work, Sally tells her, "I don't know. I just can't concentrate; I can't focus on anything. Nothing seems to be worth doing. I feel so heavy and empty inside. I don't see things getting any better." When her friend tries to coax her out of her mood, Sally snaps at her and tells her to mind her own business and leave her alone. Later, Sally is filled with remorse, telling herself she is a horrible person and does not deserve her friend's concern and loyalty. She wonders what it would be like if she no longer had to deal with all this pain; could she take this much longer?

DSM-5 DIAGNOSTIC CRITERIA
for Major Depressive Disorder

A. Five (or more) of the following symptoms have been present during the same 2-week period and represent a change from previous functioning; at least one of the symptoms is either (1) depressed mood or (2) loss of interest or pleasure.
   NOTE: Do not include symptoms that are clearly attributable to another medical condition.

1. Depressed mood most of the day, nearly every day, as indicated by either subjective report (e.g., feels sad, empty, hopeless) or observation made by others (e.g., appears tearful). (**NOTE:** In children and adolescents, can be irritable mood.)
2. Markedly diminished interest or pleasure in all, or almost all, activities most of the day, nearly every day (as indicated by either subjective account or observation).
3. Significant weight loss when not dieting or weight gain (e.g., a change of more than 5% of body weight in a month), or decrease or increase in appetite nearly every day. (**NOTE:** In children, consider failure to make expected weight gain.)
4. Insomnia or hypersomnia nearly every day.
5. Psychomotor agitation or retardation nearly every day (observable by others, not merely subjective feelings of restlessness or being slowed down).
6. Fatigue or loss of energy nearly every day.
7. Feelings of worthlessness or excessive or inappropriate guilt (which may be delusional) nearly every day (not merely self-reproach or guilt about being sick).
8. Diminished ability to think or concentrate, or indecisiveness, nearly every day (either by subjective account or as observed by others).
9. Recurrent thoughts of death (not just fear of dying), recurrent suicidal ideation without a specific plan, or a suicide attempt or a specific plan for committing suicide.

B. The symptoms cause clinically significant distress or impairment in social, occupational, or other important areas of functioning.
C. The episode is not attributable to the physiological effects of a substance or to another medical condition.
   NOTE: Criteria A through C represent a major depressive episode.
   NOTE: Responses to a significant loss (e.g., bereavement, financial ruin, losses from a natural disaster, a serious medical illness or disability) may include the feelings of intense sadness, rumination about the loss, insomnia, poor appetite, and weight loss noted by Criterion A, which may resemble a depressive episode. Although such symptoms may be understandable or considered appropriate to the loss, the presence of a major depressive episode in additional to the normal response to a significant loss should also be carefully considered. This decision inevitably requires the exercise of clinical judgment based on the individual's history and the cultural norms for the expression of distress in the context of loss.
D. The occurrence of the major depressive episode is not better explained by schizoaffective disorder, schizophrenia, schizophreniform disorder, delusional disorder, or other specific and unspecified schizophrenia spectrum and other psychotic disorders.
E. There has never been a manic episode or a hypomanic episode.
   Note: This exclusion does not apply if all the manic-like or hypomanic-like episodes are substance-induced or are attributable to the physiological effects of another medical condition.

From the American Psychiatric Association. (2013). *Diagnostic and statistical manual of mental disorders.* (5th ed.). Washington, DC: APA.

PERSISTENT DEPRESSIVE DISORDER

Persistent depressive disorder (PDD) (commonly known as **dysthymia or chronic depression**) is a less notably severe depression characterized by depressive symptoms that have been present for at least 2 years. Because PDD is more chronic in nature, PPD cannot be distinguished from the person's usual pattern of functioning: "I've always been this way. It's just the way I *am*." Although people with PDD suffer from social and occupational distress, it is not usually severe enough to warrant hospitalization unless an individual becomes suicidal. The age of onset is usually from early childhood and teenage years, although it can occur in adulthood after severe stress. The simultaneous presentation of a PDD and a MDD is referred to as a "double depression." Many individuals who are depressed may share a diagnosis of another psychiatric disorder.

Even though there are specific indicators for making a diagnosis between MDD and the more persistent depressive disorder, making a diagnosis can be difficult *because all forms of depression share similar core symptoms previously listed.* The major differences between MDDs and PDDs are the level of severity, duration, and persistence. In the severity of the symptoms, PDD is much less severe than an episode of MDD. In terms of duration, PDD (dysthymia) can endure for years. In addition to the core symptoms of depression just listed, there are other notable symptoms of PDD.

According to Preston and Johnson (2015) and Preston and colleagues (2013), the characteristics seen in an individual with persistent depressive disorder/dysthymia may include:

- Daytime fatigue
- Frequently but not always able to function at work and in social situations but not at optimal level
- Chronic low depressed/irritable mood
- Eating too much or too little
- Difficulty with sleeping; in PDD there is often difficulty getting to sleep and once asleep excessive sleeping (hypersomnia), and in MDD it is more common to find early-morning awakening.
- Loss of energy, fatigue, and chronic tiredness even for simple tasks
- Decreased capacity to experience pleasure, enthusiasm, or motivation
- Irritability
- Negative pessimistic thinking
- Low self-esteem

Shared symptoms between PPD and MDD include thoughts of death or self-harm/suicide; unexplained pain, feelings of worthlessness, helplessness, hopelessness, and low self-esteem

Refer to the following Assessment section for a more thorough discussion of the signs and symptoms in depression.

VIGNETTE

Sam had another bad week at work. He just cannot seem to perform the way he thinks he should—he never gets things right. Although his work seems acceptable to others, he constantly puts himself down. He wanted to take a class to improve his computer skills, but cannot seem to find the energy or the time. His weekends are filled with "hanging around" his apartment. "Nothing much going on ... there is never much going on. Life is dull; has it ever been otherwise?" His brother is always telling him that he has a face as long as a football field. "What's the matter with you, bro? You're good looking, smart. Go find a girl and have some fun in life. Why can't you just enjoy anything?" Sam just sighs. Who could be interested in him? He gets a cold beer from the fridge and continues watching reruns on TV.

ASSESSMENT

Undiagnosed and untreated depression is associated with more severe presentation of depression, greater suicidality, somatic problems, and severe anxiety or co-occurring anxiety disorders. Depression in older adults is often missed, especially if there are coexisting medical problems. As previously mentioned, depression in children and adolescents may remain undiagnosed when attention is focused on behavioral problems ("just a stage") or somatic complaints. Racial and economic disparities in health care, among other factors, lead to underdiagnosis and undertreatment of African Americans, Hispanics, and other minorities.

An older study identifying trends still relevant today, by Bijl and associates (2004), found that depressed individuals who sought treatment manifesting psychological symptoms were recognized as depressed about 90% of the time; in contrast, those who presented with only somatic symptoms (e.g., chronic pain, insomnia) were recognized as depressed around 50% of the time. In those who had a medical disorder, depression was identified only 20% of the time.

Assessment Tools

Numerous standardized screening tools can help the clinician assess the type of depression a person may be experiencing, for example, the Beck Depression Inventory (Beck & Rush, 1995), the Hamilton Depression Scale, the Geriatric Depression Scale, and Zung's Self-Rating Depression Scale. Refer to Figure 15-2 for an example of the signs and symptoms clinicians assess for before making a diagnosis of depression.

Assessment of Suicide Potential

A patient who appears depressed should always be evaluated for suicidal or homicidal ideation. White males complete more than 78% of all suicides (Andrew & Brenner, 2012). It is also the third leading cause of death among people ages 15 to 24 and the second leading cause of death in college students (Andrew & Brenner, 2012). Evaluation for suicidal potential might include the following statements or questions:

- "You have said you are depressed. Tell me what that is like for you."
- "When you feel depressed, what thoughts go through your mind?"
- "Have you ever thought about taking your own life in the past? Now? Do you have a plan? Do you have the means to carry out your plan? Is there anything that would prevent you from carrying out your plan?"

Refer to Chapter 23 for more on suicide prevention and intervention.

Areas to Assess
Mood

Nearly 97% of people with depression have **anergia** (lack of energy). **Anxiety,** a common symptom in depression, is seen in about 60% to 90% of depressed patients. Some feelings that may be inherent in a depressed mood are as follows:

- Feelings of **worthlessness** range from feeling inadequate to having an unrealistic evaluation of self-worth. These feelings reflect the **low self-esteem** that is a painful partner to depression. Statements such as "I am no good, I'll never amount to anything" are common. Themes of one's inadequacy and incompetence are repeated relentlessly.
- **Guilt** is a common accompaniment to depression. A person may ruminate over present or past failings. Extreme guilt can assume psychotic proportions: "I have committed terrible sins." "I have caused terrible pain and destruction to everyone I have ever known and now I'm paying for it."

The Hamilton Rating Scale For Depression

Patient's Name _____ Date of Assessment _____

To rate the severity of depression in patients who are already diagnosed as depressed, administer this questionnaire.
The higher the score, the more severe the depression.
For each item, write the correct number on the line next to the item. (Only one response per item)

1.   DEPRESSED MOOD (Sadness, hopeless, helpless, worthless)
_____ 0 = Absent
     1 = These feeling states indicated only on questioning
     2 = These feeling states spontaneously reported verbally
     3 = Communicates feeling states non-verbally—i.e., through facial expression, posture, voice, and tendency to weep
     4 = Patient reports VIRTUALLY ONLY these feeling states in his spontaneous verbal and non-verbal communication

2.   FEELINGS OF GUILT
_____ 0 = Absent
     1 = Self reproach, feels he has let people down
     2 = Ideas of guilt or rumination over past errors or sinful deeds
     3 = Present illness is a punishment. Delusions of guilt
     4 = Hears accusatory or denunciatory voices and/or experiences threatening visual hallucinations

3.   SUICIDE
_____ 0 = Absent
     1 = Feels life is not worth living
     2 = Wishes he were dead or any thoughts of possible death to self
     3 = Suicidal ideal or gesture
     4 = Attempts at suicide (any serious attempt rates 4)

4.   INSOMNIA EARLY
_____ 0 = No difficulty falling asleep
     1 = Complains of occasional difficulty falling asleep—i.e., more than 1/2 hour
     2 = Complains of nightly difficulty falling asleep

5.   INSOMNIA MIDDLE
_____ 0 = No difficulty
     1 = Patient complains of being restless and disturbed during the night
     2 = Waking during the night—any getting out of bed rates 2 (except for purposes of voiding)

6.   INSOMNIA LATE
_____ 0 = No difficulty
     1 = Waking in early hours of the morning but goes back to sleep
     2 = Unable to fall asleep again if he gets out of bed

7.   WORK AND ACTIVITIES
_____ 0 = No difficulty
     1 = Thoughts and feelings of incapacity, fatigue or weakness related to activities; work or hobbies
     2 = Loss of interest in activity; hobbies or work—either directly reported by patient, or indirect in listlessness,
        indecision and vacillation (feels he has to push self to work or activities)
     3 = Decrease in actual time spent in activities or decrease in productivity
     4 = Stopped working because of present illness

8.   RETARDATION: PSYCHOMOTOR (Slowness of thought and speech; impaired ability to concentrate; decreased
    motor activity)
_____ 0 = Normal speech and thought
     1 = Slight retardation at interview
     2 = Obvious retardation at interview
     3 = Interview difficult
     4 = Complete stupor

9.   AGITATION
_____ 0 = None
     1 = Fidgetiness
     2 = Playing with hands, hair, etc.
     3 = Moving about, can't sit still
     4 = Hand wringing, nail biting, hair-pulling, biting of lips

10.   ANXIETY (PSYCHOLOGICAL)
_____ 0 = No difficulty
     1 = Subjective tension and irritability
     2 = Worrying about minor matters
     3 = Apprehensive attitude apparent in face or speech
     4 = Fears expressed without questioning

FIGURE 15-2 The Hamilton Rating Scale for Depression. (From Hamilton, M. [1960]. A rating scale for depression. *Journal of Neurology, Neurosurgery and Psychiatry, 23,* 56–62.)

11.   ANXIETY SOMATIC: Physiological concomitants of anxiety (i.e., effects of autonomic overactivity, "butterflies," indigestion, stomach cramps, belching, diarrhea, palpitations, hyperventilation, paresthesia, sweating, flushing, tremor, headache, urinary frequency). Avoid asking about possible medication side effects (i.e., dry mouth, constipation).
_____ 0 = No difficulty
        1 = Subjective tension and irritability
        2 = Worrying about minor matters
        3 = Apprehensive attitude apparent in face or speech
        4 = Fears expressed without questioning

12.   SOMATIC SYMPTOMS (GASTROINTESTINAL)
_____ 0 = None
        1 = Loss of appetite but eating without encouragement from others. Food intake about normal
        2 = Difficulty eating without urging from others. Marked reduction of appetite and food intake

13.   SOMATIC SYMPTOMS GENERAL
_____ 0 = None
        1 = Heaviness in limbs, back or head. Backaches, headache, muscle aches. Loss of energy and fatigability
        2 = Any clear-cut symptom rates 2

14.   GENITAL SYMPTOMS (Symptoms such as: loss of libido; impaired sexual performance; menstrual disturbances)
_____ 0 = Absent
        1 = Mild
        2 = Severe

15.   HYPOCHONDRIASIS
_____ 0 = Not present
        1 = Self-absorption (bodily)
        2 = Preoccupation with health
        3 = Frequent complaints, requests for help, etc.
        4 = Hypochondriacal delusions

16.   LOSS OF WEIGHT
        A. When rating by history:
_____ 0 = No weight loss
        1 = Probably weight loss associated with present illness
        2 = Definite (according to patient) weight loss
        3 = Not assessed

17.   INSIGHT
_____ 0 = Acknowledges being depressed and ill
        1 = Acknowledges illness but attributes cause to bad food, climate, overwork, virus, need for rest, etc.
        2 = Denies being ill at all

18.   DIURNAL VARIATION
        A. Note whether symptoms are worse in morning or evening. If NO diurnal variation, mark none
_____ 0 = No variation
        1 = Worse in A.M.
        2 = Worse in P.M.

19.   DEPERSONALIZATION AND DEREALIZATION (Such as: Feelings of unreality; Nihilistic ideas)
_____ 0 = Absent
        1 = Mild
        2 = Moderate
        3 = Severe
        4 = Incapacitating

20.   PARANOID SYMPTOMS
_____ 0 = None
        1 = Suspicious
        2 = Ideas of reference
        3 = Delusions of reference and persecution

21.   OBSESSIONAL AND COMPULSIVE SYMPTOMS
_____ 0 = Absent
        1 = Mild
        2 = Severe

Total score: _____

FIGURE 15-2, cont'd

- **Helplessness** is evidenced by believing that everything is too difficult to accomplish (e.g., grooming, housework, working, caring for children). With feelings of helplessness come feelings of **hopelessness.** Even though most depressive states are usually time limited, during a depressed period people believe that things will never change, which leads some to consider suicide as a way to escape the constant mental pain. **Hopelessness is one of the core characteristics of depression and suicide, as well as a characteristic of schizophrenia, alcoholism, and physical illness.** Hopelessness results in negative expectations for the future and loss of control over future outcomes.
- **Anger** and **irritability** are natural outcomes of profound feelings of helplessness. Anger in depression is often expressed inappropriately. For example, anger may be expressed in destruction of property, hurtful verbal attacks, or physical aggression toward others. Anger may also be directed toward the self in the form of suicidal or self-destructive behaviors (e.g., alcohol abuse, substance abuse, overeating, smoking). These behaviors often result in feelings of low self-esteem and worthlessness.

Physical Changes—Clinical Symptoms

A person who is depressed sees the world through gray-colored glasses. Posture is poor, and the patient may look older than the stated age. Facial expressions convey sadness and dejection, and the patient may have frequent bouts of weeping. Conversely, the patient may say that he or she is unable to cry. Feelings of **hopelessness** and **despair** are readily reflected in the person's affect. For example, the patient may not make eye contact, may speak in a monotone, may show little or no facial expression (flat affect), and may answer with only yes or no responses. Frequent sighing is common.

People who are depressed often complain of lack of energy (**anergia**). Lethargy and fatigue can result in psychomotor retardation. Movements are slow, facial expressions are decreased, and gaze is fixed. The continuum in psychomotor retardation may range from slowed and difficult movements to complete inactivity and incontinence. At other times the nurse may note psychomotor agitation. For example, patients may constantly pace, bite their nails, smoke, tap their fingers, or engage in some other tension-relieving activity. At these times, patients feel fidgety and unable to relax.

Grooming, dress, and personal hygiene are markedly neglected. People who usually take pride in their appearance and dress may be poorly groomed and allow themselves to look shabby and unkempt.

Vegetative signs of depression are universal. Vegetative signs of depression are the somatic changes and alterations in those activities necessary to support physical life and growth (e.g., eating, sleeping, elimination, sex). For example, **changes in eating patterns** are common. About 60% to 70% of people who are depressed report having anorexia; overeating occurs more often in PDD.

Changes in sleep patterns are a cardinal sign of depression. Often, people have **insomnia,** waking at 3 or 4 AM and staying awake, or sleeping only for short periods. The light sleep of a depressed person tends to prolong the agony of depression over a 24-hour period. As mentioned, for some, sleep is increased (**hypersomnia**) and provides an escape from painful feelings. This is more common in younger depressed individuals or those with bipolar tendencies. In any event, sleep is rarely restful or refreshing.

Changes in bowel habits are common. Constipation is seen most frequently in patients with psychomotor retardation. Diarrhea occurs less frequently, often in conjunction with psychomotor agitation. **Interest in sex declines** (loss of libido) during depression. Some men experience impotence, and a declining interest in sex often occurs among both men and women, which can further complicate marital and social relationships.

Approximately 50% to 75% of people suffering from depression complain of **pain** with or without reporting psychological symptoms. People who suffer from **chronic pain** (e.g., back pain, headaches) need careful assessment for possible depression.

Cognition

When people are depressed, their thinking is slow and their memory and concentration are usually affected. Depressed people dwell on and exaggerate their perceived faults and failures and are unable to focus on their strengths and successes. As mentioned, identifying the presence of suicidal thoughts and suicide potential has the highest priority in the initial assessment. Approximately two thirds of depressed people contemplate suicide, and up to 10% to 15% of untreated or inadequately treated patients actually follow through with the suicide ideation (see Chapter 23).

When depressed, a person's ability to solve problems and think clearly is negatively affected. Judgment is poor, and **indecisiveness is common.** The individual may claim that the mind is slowing down. Evidence of delusional thinking may be seen in a person with major depression. Common statements of delusional thinking are "I have committed unpardonable sins," and "I am wicked and should die."

Self-Care for Nurses

People who are depressed often reject the presence, friendship, or interactions with others. Over time, family, friends, and health care workers can experience feelings of frustration, hopelessness, ineffectiveness, and annoyance and withdraw their concern and presence from the depressed individual. When working with depressed patients, nurses often experience the following:

- **Unrealistic expectations of self.** Often we have unrealistic expectations of ourselves or the depressed individual. Unmet expectations usually result in the nurse feeling anxious, hurt, angry and helpless, or incompetent. Identifying realistic expectations for oneself and for the patient is one way to decrease feelings of helplessness and can increase the nurse's self-esteem and therapeutic potential.
- **Becoming depressed while caring for a depressed patient.** We have all experienced a feeling of hopelessness or depression when around a person who is depressed, but once away from that person your mood is elevated and those feelings disappear. Some clinicians assume this is a diagnostic sign of patient depression—that is, feeling depressed around somebody who is depressed regardless of whether the person shows any symptoms. Often, however, we do not recognize that those feelings of hopelessness/helplessness/depression do not originate in us but rather we are experiencing what the other person/patient is experiencing via empathy. If the nurse is not able to identify that these feelings originate in the patient and are not the nurse's own feelings, the usual result is the nurse withdraws from the patient, and consequently experiences feelings of inadequacy, ineffectiveness, and increased anxiety. Once again, sharing your feelings with a more experienced clinician can help the nurse separate his or her feelings from the patient's feelings, allowing the nurse to provide optimal therapeutic care for the depressed individual.

In all cases it is extremely important for the nurse to share his or her negative feelings toward a patient, ideally with a mentor or a more experienced clinician. Sharing with a more experienced nurse or mentor can help you understand the source of your negative feelings, which will increase your ability to work with the patient and therapeutically grow as a nurse.

> **Assessment Guidelines**
> **Depression**

1. Always **evaluate the patient's risk of suicide or harm to others.** Overt hostility is highly correlated with suicide (see Chapter 23).
2. A thorough medical and neurological examination helps determine if the depression is primary or secondary to another disorder. Depression can be secondary to a host of medical or other psychiatric disorders, as well as medications or other substances. Essentially, evaluate the following:
   - If the patient is psychotic
   - If the patient has used drugs or alcohol
   - If co-occurring/comorbid medical conditions are present
   - If the patient has a history of a co-occurring psychiatric disorder (e.g., eating disorder, borderline personality disorder, anxiety disorder)
3. Assess history of depression. If the patient has a history, determine therapies used previously that were effective. Some of the following questions can be asked:
   - "Have you ever gone through or felt anything like this before?"
   - "What seemed to help you at that time?"
4. Assess support systems, family, and significant others and the need for information and referrals.
   - "With whom do you live?"
   - "Whom do you trust?"
   - "To whom do you talk when you are upset?"
5. Assess for any events that might have "triggered" a depressive episode.
   - "Has anything happened recently to upset you?"
   - "Have you had any major changes in your life?"
   - "Have you had any recent losses: job, divorce, loss of partner, child moving away, deaths?"
6. Include a psychosocial assessment that includes cultural beliefs and spiritual practices related to mental health and treatment. Determine if the depression is affecting the patient's beliefs and practice.
   - "How do you view depression?"
   - "Have you tried taking any over-the-counter remedies (e.g., herbs) to help with your depression?"
   - "Do you find solace in spiritual activities or a place of worship (e.g., church, temple, mosque)?"

DIAGNOSIS

Depression is complex; depressed individuals have a variety of needs and there are many nursing diagnoses. However, during the initial assessment, a high priority for the nurse is identification of the presence of suicide potential. Therefore the nursing diagnosis of *Risk for suicide* is always considered. Other key targets for nursing interventions are represented by the diagnoses of *Hopelessness, Impaired mood regulation, Ineffective coping, Social isolation, Spiritual distress,* and one or more of the *Self-care deficits (e.g., bathing/hygiene, dressing/grooming, feeding, toileting).* Table 15-2 identifies signs and symptoms commonly experienced in depression and offers possible nursing diagnoses.

TABLE 15-2 Potential Nursing Diagnoses for Depression

Signs and Symptoms	Nursing Diagnoses
Previous suicidal attempts, putting affairs in order, giving away prized possessions, suicidal ideation (has plan, ability to carry it out), overt or covert statements regarding killing self, feelings of worthlessness, hopelessness, helplessness	*Risk for suicide* *Risk for self-mutilation*
Lack of judgment, memory difficulty, poor concentration, inaccurate interpretation of environment, negative ruminations, cognitive distortions	*Decisional conflict* *Impaired memory* *Acute confusion*
Difficulty with simple tasks, inability to function at previous level, poor problem solving, poor cognitive functioning, verbalizations of inability to cope	*Ineffective coping* *Interrupted family processes* *Risk for impaired parent/infant/child attachment* *Ineffective role performance*
Difficulty making decisions, poor concentration, inability to take action	*Decisional conflict*
Feelings of helplessness, hopelessness, powerlessness	*Hopelessness*
Feelings of inability to make positive change in one's life or have a sense of control over one's destiny	*Powerlessness* *Ineffective coping*
Questioning meaning of life and own existence, inability to participate in usual religious practices, conflict over spiritual beliefs, anger toward spiritual deity or religious representatives	*Spiritual distress* *Impaired religiosity* *Risk for impaired religiosity*
Feelings of worthlessness, poor self-image, negative sense of self, self-negating verbalizations, feeling of being a failure, expressions of shame or guilt, hypersensitivity to slights or criticism	*Chronic low self-esteem* *Situational low self-esteem*
Withdrawal, noncommunicativeness, speech that is only in monosyllables, avoidance of contact with others	*Impaired social interaction* *Social isolation* *Risk for loneliness*
Vegetative signs of depression: changes in sleeping, eating, grooming and hygiene, elimination, sexual patterns	*Self-neglect (bathing/hygiene, dressing/grooming)* *Imbalanced nutrition: less than body requirements* *Disturbed sleep pattern* *Constipation* *Sexual dysfunction*

Herdman, T.H. (Ed.) *Nursing Diagnoses-Definitions and Classification 2015-2017.* Copyright 2014, 1994-2014 NANDA International. Used by arrangement with John Wiley & Sons Limited. In order to make safe and effective judgments using NANDA-I nursing diagnoses it is essential that nurses refer to the definitions and defining characteristics of the diagnoses listed in this work.

OUTCOMES IDENTIFICATION

Outcomes should include goals for safety. Even if the patient is not having self-destructive thoughts, one goal should be to name a person who the patient will contact if such thoughts arise. Goals for the outcomes of vegetative or physical signs of depression (e.g., *reports adequate sleep*) are formulated to show, for example, evidence of weight gain, return to normal bowel activity, sleep of 6 to 8 hours per night, or return of sexual desire.

PLANNING

The planning of care for patients with depression is geared toward the phase of depression the person is in and the particular symptoms the person is exhibiting. At all times the nurse and members of the health care team are cognizant of the potential for suicide, and assessment of risk for self-harm (or harm to others) is ongoing during the care of the depressed person. There is evidence that a combination of therapeutic (cognitive, behavioral, interpersonal psychotherapy [IPT]) and psychopharmacological interventions can be an effective approach in treating depression.

Nurses and clinicians need to assess and plan for any vegetative signs of depression, as well as changes in concentration, activity level, social interaction, or personal appearance, for example. Therefore the planning of care for a patient who is depressed is based on the individual's symptoms and attempts to encompass a variety of areas in the person's life. Safety is always the highest priority.

IMPLEMENTATION

Communication Guidelines

A person who is depressed may speak and comprehend very slowly. The lack of an immediate response by the patient to a remark does not mean that the patient has not heard or chooses not to reply; rather, the patient just needs a little more time to compose a reply. In extreme depression, however, a person may be mute.

Some depressed patients are so withdrawn that they are unwilling or unable to speak. Nurses may feel uncomfortable with silence and not being able to "do anything" to effect immediate change. However, just sitting with a patient in silence may be a valuable intervention. It is important to be aware that this time spent together can be meaningful to the depressed person, especially if the nurse has a genuine interest in learning about the depressed individual.

It is difficult to say when a withdrawn or depressed person will be able to respond. However, certain techniques are known to be useful in guiding effective nursing interventions. Some communication interventions to use with a severely withdrawn patient are listed in Table 15-3. Communication interventions to use when caring for depressed patients are offered in Table 15-4.

Health Teaching and Health Promotion

Teaching family/significant others and patient about depression. It is important for patients and their families to understand that depression is a legitimate medical illness over which the patient has no voluntary control. Depressed patients and their families need to learn about the biological symptoms of depression as well as the psychosocial and cognitive changes. Families must recognize the overt and covert signs of suicidal ideation and know precautionary measures to take if the warning signs of suicidal thinking or planning occur (see Chapter 23).

Medication teaching. Review of the patient's medications and their adverse reactions helps families evaluate clinical changes and maintain alertness for reactions that might affect patient compliance. Adverse effects of antidepressants and specific areas to be emphasized in patient and family teaching are presented later in this chapter. Written information should be provided. Often, patients have difficulty with a written list of instructions. It's helpful if after the nurse has gone over the information carefully with the patient/family to have them repeat the information back to you. Be cognizant of the patient's cultural background and ability understand and/or read English.

Teaching relapse prevention. Whenever possible, medication counseling should begin early and be carried out with the patient and the patient's significant others. One purpose of this is to identify interpersonal stresses and to discuss steps that can alleviate tension

---

VIGNETTE

Doris, a senior nursing student, was assigned to a depressed, suicidal, withdrawn woman who was admitted early this morning to the psychiatric unit for suicide observations. The instructor notices that Doris spends a lot of time talking with other students and their patients and little time with her own patient. The nursing instructor takes Doris aside and Doris acknowledges feeling threatened and useless and says that she wants a patient who will interact with her. After reviewing the symptoms of depression and its behavioral manifestations as well as the needs of depressed individuals, Doris turns her attention back to her patient. She spends short time periods sitting in silence, making observations, looking through a magazine, and offering to walk with her patient up and down the halls. Upon leaving for the day, the patient tells Doris "Thanks for spending time with me, it helped me focus on other things."

TABLE 15-3 Interventions for Severely Withdrawn Individuals: Communication

Intervention	Rationale
1. When a patient is mute, use the technique of *making observations*: "There are many new pictures on the wall" or "You are wearing your new shoes."	1. When a patient is not ready to talk, direct questions can raise the patient's anxiety level and frustrate the nurse. Pointing to commonalities in the environment draws the patient into, and reinforces, reality.
2. Use simple, concrete words.	2. Slowed thinking and difficulty concentrating impair comprehension.
3. Allow time for the patient to respond.	3. Slowed thinking necessitates time to formulate a response.
4. Listen for covert messages and ask about suicide plans: "Have you had thoughts of killing or harming yourself in any way?"	4. People often experience relief and decrease in feelings of isolation when they share thoughts of suicide.
5. Avoid platitudes such as, "Things will look up" or "Everyone gets down once in a while."	5. Platitudes tend to minimize the patient's feelings and can increase feelings of guilt and worthlessness because the patient cannot "look up" or "snap out of it."

TABLE 15-4   Interventions for Depression: Communication

Intervention	Rationale
1. Help the patient question underlying assumptions and beliefs and consider alternate explanations to problems.	1. Reconstructing a healthier and more hopeful attitude about the future can alter depressed mood.
2. Work with the patient to identify cognitive distortions that encourage negative self-appraisal. For example:	2. Cognitive distortions reinforce a negative, inaccurate perception of self and world.
a. Overgeneralizations	a. The patient takes one fact or event and makes a general rule out of it ("He always…"; "I never…").
b. Self-blame	b. The patient consistently blames self for everything perceived as negative.
c. Mind reading	c. The patient assumes others do not like him or her, and so forth, without any real evidence that assumptions are correct.
d. Discounting of positive attributes	d. The patient focuses on the negative.
3. Encourage activities that can raise self-esteem. Identify need for (a) problem-solving skills, (b) coping skills, and (c) assertiveness skills.	3. Many depressed people, especially women, are not taught a range of problem-solving and coping skills. Increasing social, family, and job skills can change negative self-assessment.
4. Discuss physical activities the patient enjoys (e.g., running, weightlifting). Explain that initially 10 to 15 minutes a day 3 or 4 times a week has short-term benefits.	4. Exercise can help reduce tension, alleviate depression and anxiety, improve self-concept, and shift neurochemical balance.
5. Encourage formation of supportive relationships, such as through support groups, therapy, and peer support.	5. Such relationships reduce social isolation and enable the patient to work on personal goals and relationship needs among people who share similar experiences.
6. Provide information referrals, when needed, for spiritual/religious information (e.g., readings, programs, tapes, community resources).	6. Spiritual and existential issues may be heightened during depressive episodes—many people find strength and comfort in spirituality or religion.

in the family/significant other system. Including significant others in counseling facilitates progress in the following ways:

- Increases the understanding and acceptance of the depressed family member.
- Increases understanding of symptoms that signal the need for relapse prevention.

Health teaching also may include teaching and interventions for self-care deficits. In addition to experiencing intense feelings of hopelessness, despair, low self-worth, and fatigue, the depressed person also may have physical deficits related to the depression.

It is believed that there is a potential mechanism linking diet, sleep and exercise to major depression. "These lifestyle factors influence a number of biological processes associated with major depression including neurotransmitter transmission, immuno-inflammation, oxidative and nitrosative stress, HPA balance, neuroprogression and mitochondrial health. Suffering from depression is also likely to lead to changes in diet, sleep and exercise, creating a vicious cycle of change" (Lopresti et al., 2013).

Some effective interventions targeting the physical needs of the depressed patient are listed in Table 15-5.

Milieu Therapy

When a person is acutely and severely depressed, the structure of the hospital setting may be necessary. The depressed person needs protection from suicidal acts in a supervised environment where antidepressant medications can be closely regulated. If a patient is thought to be suicidal, finding a safe environment may be the first action taken. Hospitals have protocols for suicidal observation and protection. If a patient is highly suicidal, refusing food, becoming debilitated, or exhibiting psychotic depression, then electroconvulsive therapy (ECT) may be the most effective treatment option.

Psychotherapy

Behavioral activation therapy (BA) is an evidence-based therapy and a core component of CBT, and it is one of the most effective treatments for depression. A recent study successfully used a "resting state

functional brain conductivity fMRI to predict therapeutic responses to talk therapy by identifying differences in brain wiring." Through imaging they were able to find which brain regions light up en masse before and after therapy. The therapy used is called behavior activation talk therapy, which focused on immediate behavior such as not getting to work on time or withdrawing in social situations (Derewicz, 2015).

CBT, interpersonal therapy (IPT), and behavioral therapy have been proven effective in the treatment of depression. However, only CBT and IPT demonstrate superiority in the maintenance phase. CBT helps people change a depressed person's negative styles of thinking and behaving, whereas IPT focuses on working through personal relationships that may contribute to depression. Outcome research has consistently found that CBT and medication are largely comparable. CBT helps guard against relapse, because people learn skills of how to reshape their thinking and behaviors. The benefits of adding CBT to antidepressant therapy for patients with treatment-resistant depression last long after the CBT sessions end (Brooks, 2016).

Some studies indicate that psychotherapy alone (CBT or IPT), especially in individuals with early life traumas (child abuse), is more effective than pharmacology alone. Actually, CBT combined with medications is proven effective in people with chronic depressions.

Mindfulness-Based Cognitive Therapy

There are increasing studies reported in the literature about the use of mindfulness-based cognitive therapy (MBCT) and its effectiveness in treating people who are experiencing relapse/reoccurrence of MDD. MBCT is a combination of CBT and mindfulness-based stress reduction (MBSR). Mindfulness is a form of meditation, and MBSR was developed by Kabat-Zinn at the University of Massachusetts in the early 1970s (Kabat-Zinn, n.d.). Mindfulness is a meditation technique that has been used successfully in patients coping with medical or mental health disorders; it shows promise as an effective tool to prevent relapse in patients with MDDs (Kuyken et al., 2008), as well as other disorders such as PTSD.

TABLE 15-5	Interventions Targeting the Physical Needs of the Depressed Patient
Intervention	**Rationale**

Nutrition—Anorexia

1. Offer small, high-calorie, and high-protein snacks frequently throughout the day and evening.

2. Offer high-protein and high-calorie fluids frequently throughout the day and evening.
3. When possible, encourage family or friends to remain with the patient during meals.
4. Ask the patient which foods or drinks he or she likes. Offer choices. Involve the dietitian.
5. Weigh the patient weekly and observe the patient's eating patterns.

1. Low weight and poor nutrition render the patient susceptible to illness. Small, frequent snacks are more easily tolerated than large plates of food when the patient is anorectic.
2. These fluids prevent dehydration and can minimize constipation.

3. This strategy reinforces the idea that someone cares, can raise the patient's self-esteem, and can serve as an incentive to eat.
4. The patient is more likely to eat the foods provided.

5. Monitoring the patient's status gives the information needed for revision of the intervention.

Sleep—Insomnia

1. Provide periods of rest after activities.
2. Encourage the patient to get up and dress and to stay out of bed during the day.
3. Encourage the use of relaxation measures in the evening (e.g., tepid bath, warm milk).
4. Reduce environmental and physical stimulants in the evening—provide decaffeinated coffee, soft lights, soft music, quiet activities.

1. Fatigue can intensify feelings of depression.
2. Minimizing sleep during the day increases the likelihood of sleep at night.
3. These measures induce relaxation and sleep.

4. Decreasing caffeine and epinephrine levels increases the possibility of sleep. Playing relaxing music can help the patient sleep.

Self-Care Deficits

1. Encourage the use of toothbrush, washcloth, soap, makeup, shaving equipment, and so forth.
2. When appropriate, give step-by-step reminders such as, "Wash the right side of your face, now the left."

1. Being clean and well groomed can temporarily increase self-esteem.

2. Slowed thinking and difficulty concentrating make organizing simple tasks difficult.

Elimination—Constipation

1. Monitor intake and output, especially bowel movements.

2. Offer foods high in fiber and provide periods of exercise.

3. Encourage the intake of fluids.
4. Evaluate the need for laxatives and enemas.

1. Many depressed patients are constipated. If the condition is not checked, fecal impaction can occur.
2. Roughage and exercise stimulate peristalsis and help evacuation of fecal material.
3. Fluids help prevent constipation.
4. These measures prevent fecal impaction.

APPLYING THE ART

A Person with Depression

Scenario

I met Nadia, a 39-year-old mother of three, in the mental health clinic where I was doing my psychiatric rotation. Her main complaint was severe fatigue, anhedonia, and inertia. She states she no longer has the energy to care for her children or her marriage, saying, "I am not fit to be a mother or wife."

Therapeutic Goal

By the conclusion of this interaction, Nadia will state she understands that depression is a treatable disorder and that it is her symptoms that are causing her despondent behavior.

Student-Patient Interaction	Thoughts, Communication Techniques, and Mental Health Nursing Concepts
Nadia: *Speaking slowly, eyes downcast.* "I couldn't face all those people."	
Student: "You're looking down like you are sad." *No response from Nadia.* "I wonder what facing the group means to you."	Depression slows everything: thoughts, feelings, and responses to others. I *make an observation* and *attempt to translate into feelings,* then shift to an *indirect question.* Because depression hinders Nadia's processing of information, I need to slow my pace. Allow more silence.
Student's feelings: *I should have stayed with "sad." I aimed for her feelings, then did not wait for her to share any feelings.*	
Nadia: *Slowly shakes her head back and forth. Silent for 3 minutes. No eye contact.*	
Student: *With a concerned look.* "You shake your head as if you are saying no."	I use *silence* along with attending behavior. I *make an observation* and then use *restatement.*

Continued

APPLYING THE ART—cont'd

A Person with Depression

Student-Patient Interaction	Thoughts, Communication Techniques, and Mental Health Nursing Concepts	Student-Patient Interaction	Thoughts, Communication Techniques, and Mental Health Nursing Concepts
Student's feelings: I know it's the right thing to do, but waiting during the silence makes me so anxious. I need to stay mindfully alert and attentive. I can endure the silence for Nadia's sake.		**Student:** *After waiting for 2 minutes.* "Nadia, I am here to be with you right where you are at this moment. No pressure."	I offer self and acceptance.
Nadia: "Everybody in group makes progress. I just keep sinking deeper."		**Nadia:** *Looking up.* "Thank you. You don't know how much that means. I do want to get better and not feel like depression consumes who I am."	
Student: "Sinking deeper?"	Nadia has just started taking antidepressant medication. Most affect *serotonin or norepinephrine neurotransmitter levels,* but therapeutic effectiveness takes 2 to 3 weeks. I use *restatement* to encourage Nadia to say more.	**Student:** *Nods.* "You want to get better. You were able to take the first courageous step. In deciding to get admitted, you acknowledge that your symptoms are a problem, and they are the symptoms of depression, a disorder."	I *give support.* Separating oneself as distinct from the disorder of depression restores some sense of control to Nadia.
Nadia: "Into depression. I can't pull it together even though I know my kids need me." *Makes eye contact.*	Depression erodes self-esteem, and low self-esteem in turn exacerbates depression.	*Student's feelings:* Nadia feels swallowed up (consumed) by the depression. I want her to know that depression need not be her life.	
Student's feelings: I know from experience that it's hard to pull anything together when you feel depressed.		**Nadia:** "Oh, I never thought of it that way … as a first step, not a sign of failure. My symptoms are from the depression."	
Student: "You care about your children." *She nods.* "Sounds like you find it difficult at this time to care about yourself very much."	I *attempt to translate into feelings* adding "at this time" to imply a temporary state (e.g., she will again find self-caring as she heals).	*Student's feelings:* As a nurse, my belief in Nadia's ability to battle the depression offers hope.	
Student's feelings: I've noticed that sometimes, like Nadia, nurses find it easier to care for others than take care of self, even basic self-care or prevention measures.		**Student:** *Nods.* "A treatable disorder." *I continue to sit with Nadia in silence for a short while.*	At some level, Nadia acknowledges a self not fully consumed by depression.
Nadia: *Sustaining eye contact.* "I can't do anything right. I have nothing to show for my life."		**Nadia:** "Yes, depression is a disorder, not all that I am."	Hope will grow as Nadia begins to take charge of her disorder through active investment in treatment.
Student: "Think about what you've accomplished! You have your children, your marriage, your teaching career." *Nadia shrugs, eyes downcast.*	I inadvertently minimized her feelings by giving *approval* and *advice,* which is *nontherapeutic.* Even though all the things I pointed out may be valid, none of it rings true for Nadia right now.		
Student's feelings: She has so much going for her. Why can't she see that? My response causes Nadia to pull away by withdrawing eye contact. When I deliver positives about Nadia before she feels more positive about herself, I discount her experience, which interferes with trust. I need to remember that support and nonjudgmental acceptance provide the foundation for the nurse-patient relationship.	One step that helps with depression would be for Nadia to problem solve and work through any cognitive distortions (e.g., "I can't do anything right"). *Cognitive behavioral therapy,* like antidepressant medication, takes time, but depression is a treatable disorder.		

Neurobiology of Depression and the Effect of Antidepressants

Imbalance of certain neurotransmitters (serotonin and norepinephrine) thought to contribute to depression in certain parts of the brain.
Prefrontal cortex (PFC): regulates role in executive functions and emotional control and memory.

Limbic system: (amygdala, hypothalamus, hippocampus) regulates activities such as emotions, physical and sexual drives, and the stress response (as well as processing, learning, and memory).

Anterior cingulate cortex (ACC): decreases motivation and ability to stay focused on a task, and disrupts ability to manage appropriate emotional reactions

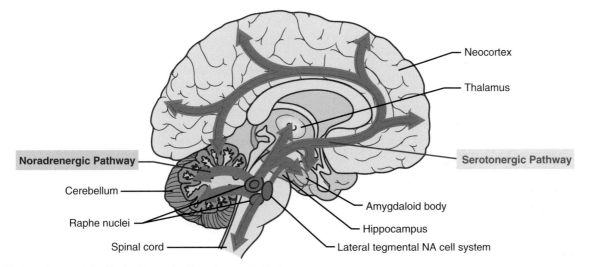

Various Parts of the Brain Along the Noradrenergic Pathway
The axons of these neurons project upward through the forebrain to the cerebral cortex, the limbic system, the thalamus, and the hippocampus.

Noradrenaline and the Noradrenergic System (NE): plays a major role in mood and emotional behavior as well as energy, drive, anxiety, focus, and metabolism.

Various Parts of the Brain Along the Serotonergic Pathway
The axons of serotonergic neurons originate in the raphe nuclei of the brainstem and project to the cerebral cortex, the limbic system, cerebellum, and spinal cord.

Serotonin and the Serotonergic System (5-HT): involved in the regulation of pain, depression, pleasure, anxiety, panic arousal, and sleep cycle, carbohydrate craving, PMS.

Medications for Depression
Medications for depression include the selective serotonin reuptake inhibitors (**SSRIs**), serotonin/norepinephrine reuptake inhibitors (**SNRIs**), noradrenergic and specific serotonergic antidepressants (**NaSSAs**), tricyclic antidepressants (**TCAs**), monoamine oxidase inhibitors (**MAOIs**), and atypical antidepressants.
They all work equally as well and are chosen by their safety profile and side effects.* All have a delayed response, a discontinuation syndrome, Black Box Warning-suicide.

Patient's Problem*	Side Effect Profile*	Example of Drug*
Fatigue	Stimulates the CNS	Fluoxetine (SSRI)
Insomnia	Substantial sedation	Mirtazapine (NaSSAs)
Sexual dysfunction	Enhances libido	Bupropion (atypical)
Chronic pain	Relieves pain	TCAs or duloxetine (SNRI)

*Adapted from page 341 *Lehne's Pharmacology for Nursing Care,* 9th Edition (2016) by Jacqueline Burchum DNSc APRN BC (Authors), Laura Rosenthal DNP ACNP (Author)

APPLYING EVIDENCE-BASED PRACTICE (EBP)

Problem An RN working with an obstetrics practice visits a new mother for a home visit to provide lactation and infant care support and education. This is the 19-year-old mother's first child. When the RN enters the home she finds the curtains drawn, and the new mother appears exhausted and unkempt. She begins crying while talking to the nurse, and expresses feelings of guilt that she does not feel closer to her baby or happy and excited. The RN suspects that the new mother has postpartum depression.

EBP Assessment

A. **What do you already know from experience?** Many new mothers experience depression or mood swings, or may have difficulties with bonding or learning to care for an infant. These feelings often cause the new mothers to feel guilty or abnormal. Mothers, especially first-time mothers, require support and education.

B. **What does the literature say?** Many women have mood swings after childbirth that can include feeling depressed, lacking concentration, sleeping poorly, and crying easily. If the mood changes last for longer than 10 days or are severe, they are considered postpartum depression. If the mother has hallucinations, delusional thinking (such as everything is contaminating the

baby), or thoughts to harm herself or the baby, the condition may be more serious—postpartum psychosis.

C. **What does the patient want?** The patient is open to any kind of help that would assist her in feeling better and being a good mom.

Plan The RN assessed the patient for thoughts of harming herself or the baby, which the mother denied having either now or in the past. The RN referred the mother for a psychiatric evaluation to see if therapy or medications would be appropriate. She helped the mother think of supportive friends and relatives that could help her with the baby, and allow her to get regular sleep. The RN provided lactation assistance and education as the mother was struggling with nursing. The RN and patient agreed to a weekly visit until she is feeling better, and was provided with resources to call in a crisis.

QSEN **QSEN Prelicensure Knowledge, Skills, and Attitudes (KSAs) Addressed:**

Safety was addressed through evaluation of suicidal or homicidal thoughts, and the provision of psychiatric resources.

Patient-centered care was provided by addressing the patient's pain and suffering, individual needs, and empowering the patient.

From the American College of Obstetricians and Gynecologists. (2013). *Frequently asked questions: postpartum depression.* Retrieved from www.acog.org/-/media/For-Patients/faq091.pdf?dmc=1&ts=20150906T1954007428; Epperson, N. (2014). *Postpartum depression.* Retrieved from http://familydoctor.org/familydoctor/en/diseases-conditions/postpartum-depression.printerview.all.html.

Group Therapy

Group therapy is a widespread modality for the treatment of depression; it increases the number of people who can receive treatment at a decreased cost per individual. Another advantage is that groups offer patients an opportunity to socialize and to share common feelings and concerns as well as provide patients with the opportunity to reach out and support others. Belonging to a group can help decrease feelings of isolation, hopelessness, helplessness, and alienation. Medication groups for patients and families can increase understanding of medications, including ways to handle various side effects and compliance and how to identify any side effects or any outside influences that may be keeping the patient nonadherent to his or her medications.

Pharmacological, Biological, and Integrative Therapies
Antidepressant Medication Therapy

Antidepressant therapy benefits about 65% to 80% of people with nondelusional unipolar depression. ECT has shown a 75% to 85% efficacy rate for those patients who are delusional or melancholic. It is believed by many that depressed individuals without psychotic features benefit most from a combination of specific psychotherapies (e.g., CBT, IPT, behavioral) and antidepressant medications, compared to either psychotherapy or psychopharmacological treatment alone. In fact, it is believed that the combination and continuation of at least two of these therapies may reduce the risk of recurrence or relapse of MDD and PDD. Essentially, the **core symptoms of depression improve with antidepressant therapy,** and **quality-of-life measures improve with certain psychotherapies.** Antidepressant drugs can positively alter poor self-concept, degree of withdrawal, vegetative signs of depression, and activity level. Target symptoms include the following:

- Sleep disturbance
- Appetite disturbance (decreased or increased)
- Fatigue
- Decreased sex drive
- Psychomotor retardation or agitation
- Diurnal variations in mood (often worse in the morning)

- Impaired concentration or forgetfulness
- Anhedonia (loss of ability to experience joy or pleasure in living)

One drawback to the use of antidepressant medication is that improvement in mood may take 1 to 3 weeks or longer. If a patient is acutely suicidal, this may be too long to wait. At these times, ECT may result in a safe and more rapid elevation in mood.

Safety. There is the possibility that children, adolescents, and young adults taking SSRIs may experience untoward side effects such as violent behavior, mania, or aggression, all of which can contribute to suicidal behavior. Now all antidepressants include a **Black Box warning** of increased risk of suicide in children and adolescents. A recent analysis of 70 trials of the most common antidepressants, involving more than 18,000 people, revealed that antidepressants could double the risk of suicide and aggressive behavior (Knapton, 2016). On further investigation, it was found that after comparing clinical trial information to actual patient reports, scientists found pharmaceutical companies had regularly misclassified deaths and suicidal events in people taking antidepressants to "favor their products" (Knapton, 2016).

Other studies warn against adults older than age 65 taking SSRIs because they are more prone to strokes, fractures, epilepsy, and even death. Therefore it should be concluded that all treatments have potential risks. The safest path is for clinicians to consider each patient individually when prescribing antidepressants. The Food and Drug Administration (FDA) recommends that all consumers of antidepressants be observed carefully for worsening of depression and suicidal thoughts.

Taking SSRIs during pregnancy is of concern. "Basically, serotonin is essential for embryogenesis, heart development, and the CNS and musculoskeletal system and so forth, and the fact of inhibiting serotonin during that critical period can result in multiple birth defects" (Davenport, 2016).

A recent study showed that antidepressant use during the second or third trimester of pregnancy can double the risk of a baby developing autism spectrum disorder (ASD) by age 7 years. The use of SSRIs appeared to be associated with the highest risk for a single drug, but the combination of two or more antidepressant drug classes was associated with the highest risk of a child developing ASD (Melville, 2015).

A Swedish study found that there was a link between use of SSRIs during pregnancy and lung hypertension in newborns (Lowry, 2012a) although more research is needed to ascertain safety in pregnant women. Caution should always be observed when prescribing any psychotropic agents to any individual, especially a pregnant woman.

Another area of concern is a potential link for those taking any kind of antidepressants and the occurrence of cerebral microbleeds. A longitudinal study of 2550 participants age 45 or older without a history of intracranial or extracranial bleeding in the brain, found an increased risk for microbleeds in antidepressant users both SSRIs or non-SSRIs.(Melville, 2016). This study supports previous cross-sectional results from other studies.

Classes of antidepressants. Although all antidepressants work equally well, they certainly do not all work well for all individuals. Because the complex interplay of neurotransmitters responsible for depression is unique for different individuals, a variety of antidepressants or a combination of antidepressants may need to be tried before the most effective regimen is found. Each antidepressant has adverse effects as well as cost, safety, and maintenance considerations. The following are some of the primary and secondary considerations when choosing a specific antidepressant:

Primary considerations:
- Previous response to antidepressants
- Ease of administration
- Safety and medical considerations (e.g., diabetes, cardiac disease)
- Associated symptoms of comorbidity (e.g., obsessive-compulsive disorder [OCD], PTSD, bipolar disorder, anxiety disorder, energy level)

Secondary considerations:
- Neurotransmitter specificity
- Family history of response
- Cost

The neurotransmitters and receptor sites in the brain are the targets of pharmacological intervention (Table 15-6). While reading the following section, and using Table 15-6 as a guide, see if you can identify potential side effects caused by the blockage of the given neurotransmitter.

Studies that compare the more recent SSRIs and dual action antidepressants to the TCAs fail to find support for one group over the other. The difference lies in the quality and quantity of adverse effects, complications, and patient compliance. Basic antidepressant classes include the following:

First-line agents:
- Cyclic antidepressants (e.g., TCAs)
- Dual action antidepressants (SSRIs, SNRIs, and NDRIs)
- Atypical antidepressants

Second-line agents:
- Monoamine oxidase inhibitors (MAOIs)

Tricyclic antidepressants. The tricyclic antidepressants (TCAs) inhibit the reuptake of norepinephrine and serotonin by the presynaptic neurons in the CNS. Therefore the amount of time that norepinephrine and serotonin are available to the postsynaptic receptors is increased. This increase in norepinephrine and serotonin levels in the brain is believed to be responsible for mood elevations when TCAs are given to depressed people.

The sedative effects of TCAs are attributed to antihistamine (H_1 receptor) actions and somewhat to anticholinergic actions. Patients must take therapeutic doses of TCAs for 10 to 14 days or longer before effectiveness is reached. The full effects may not be evident for 4 to 8 weeks. An effect on some symptoms of depression, such as insomnia and anorexia, may be noted sooner. A person who has shown a positive response to TCA therapy would probably be maintained on that medication for 6 to 12 months to prevent an early relapse. Choice of TCA is based on the following:

TABLE 15-6 Potential Effects of Receptor Blockade of Various Medications for Depression

	Receptor Blocked	Potential Effects
NE	Norepinephrine	Decreased depression
		Tremors
		Tachycardia
		Erectile and/or ejaculatory dysfunction
α_1	Specific receptor for epinephrine	Antipsychotic effect
		Postural hypotension
		Dizziness
		Reflux tachycardia
		Ejaculatory dysfunction and/or impotence
		Memory dysfunction
α_2	Specific receptor for norepinephrine	Priapism
5-HT	Serotonin	Decreased depression
		Antianxiety effects
		Gastrointestinal disturbance
		Sexual dysfunction
5-HT_2	Serotonin	Decreased depression
		Decreased suicidal behavior
		Antipsychotic effects
		Hypotension
		Ejaculatory dysfunction
		Weight gain and carbohydrate craving
DA	Dopamine reuptake blocked	Decreased psychosis
		Psychomotor agitation
		Parkinsonian effect
Ach	Acetylcholine	Anticholinergic effects
H_1	Histamine	Sedation
		Weight gain
		Cognitive impairment

- The drug that has proven effective for the patient or a family member in the past
- The drug's adverse effects

For example, a patient who is lethargic and fatigued may have the best results with a more stimulating TCA, such as desipramine (Norpramin) or protriptyline (Vivactil). If a more sedating effect is needed for agitation or restlessness, drugs such as amitriptyline (Elavil) and doxepin (Sinequan) may be more appropriate choices. **Regardless of which TCA is given, the dosage should always be low initially and should be increased gradually.** Caution should be used, especially in older adults because slow drug metabolism may be a problem. The accepted practice for older adults is always, **"Start low, go slow."**

Common adverse reactions. The chemical structure of TCAs is similar to that of antipsychotic medications. Therefore the **anticholinergic** effects (e.g., dry mouth, blurred vision, tachycardia, constipation, urinary retention, and esophageal reflux) are similar. These side effects are more common and more pronounced in patients taking antidepressants. These adverse effects are usually not serious and are often transitory, but **urinary retention and severe constipation warrant immediate medical attention.**

The α-adrenergic blockade of TCAs can produce postural orthostatic hypotension and tachycardia. Postural hypotension can lead to dizziness and increase the risk of falls.

Administering the total daily dose of the TCA at night is beneficial for two reasons. First, most TCAs have sedative effects and thereby aid sleep. Second, the minor side effects occur during sleep, which increases compliance with drug therapy. Table 15-7 reviews side effects of TCAs that are commonly prescribed.

TABLE 15-7   Characteristics of Specific Antidepressants*

Generic Name	Trade Name	Potential Side Effects	Advantages of Selective Drugs	Disadvantages of Selective Drugs
Selective Serotonin Reuptake Inhibitors (SSRIs): Most Popular Type of Antidepressants*				
Citalopram[†]	Celexa	• Headache, which usually dissipates in a few days	Minimal interaction with other drugs, minimal weight gain, sedation	Possible initial anxiety
Escitalopram[†]	Lexapro	• Nausea, which usually dissipates in a few days	Minimal interaction, low sedation, and weight gain	Possible initial anxiety 18 yr or older; 12-17 yr for MDD
Fluoxetine[†]	Prozac	• Sleeplessness and/or drowsiness during day, which usually dissipates in a few weeks	Activating (energizing)	Possible interaction with other drugs, initial anxiety 8 yr or older
Fluvoxamine	Luvox	• Tremors and/or dizziness		8 yr or older for OCD only
Paroxetine[†]	Paxil	• Sexual problems: reduces sexual drive, problems having and enjoying sex	Good antianxiety benefit	Weight gain, interacts with other meds, contraindicated in pregnancy
Sertraline[†]	Zoloft	• Agitation, feeling jittery and nervous; rare serotonin syndrome; rare activation of suicidal ideation	Not too sedating, nor prone to increased anxiety	Prone to gastrointestinal (GI) upset 6 yr and older only for OCD
Selective Serotonin Reuptake Inhibitor and Agonist (5-HT 1A receptor)				
Vilazodone	Vibyrd	Diarrhea, nausea, vomiting, insomnia, and sexual side effects	Helps to target comorbid anxiety	Caution in pregnancy, can cause weight gain, has withdrawal symptoms, and interacts with other drugs.
Norepinephrine and Serotonin Specific Antidepressants (NASSA)				
Mirtazapine	Remeron	Dry mouth, abnormal dreams, confusion, sedation, influenza-like symptoms, hypotension	Good for severe depression and elderly, less insomnia, less sexual dysfunction	High weight gain and sedation Rare: induction of mania, suicidal thoughts or behaviors
Norepinephrine Dopamine Reuptake Inhibitor (NDRI)				
Bupropion	Wellbutrin	Anxiety, insomnia, nausea, headache, dizziness, anorexia	Energizing, few sexual side effects, less weight gain	Rare seizures, doses over 400 mg; possible increased anxiety/insomnia
Serotonin Antagonist and Reuptake Inhibitors				
Nefazodone	Serzone	Nausea, headache, anxiety, sedation, dizziness	Good at reducing anxiety, fewer sexual side effects	*Has been associated with liver toxicity and has been discontinued in some countries for this reason. It is associated with many drug interactions.*
Buspirone	BuSpar	Anxiety, nausea, headache, dizziness	Mainly used in treatment of anxiety; can be antidepressant in higher doses Can act like an antidepressant in higher doses	Plus side: very useful augmenting drug for antidepressants
Dual Action Reuptake Inhibitors (Serotonin and Norepinephrine) (SNRIs)				
Duloxetine	Cymbalta	Nausea, diarrhea, anorexia, sexual dysfunction, hypertension, palpitations, increased blood pressure, urinary frequency/retention, inappropriate antidiuretic hormone, hyponatremia, sedation	Good for severe depression	Liver toxicity is a concern Seizures, thrombophlebitis, supraventricular dysrhythmia have occurred
Venlafaxine	Effexor	Headache, nervousness, insomnia, decreased appetite, sexual dysfunction, inappropriate secretion of antidiuretic hormone, hyponatremia	Good for severe depression, social anxiety disorder, generalized anxiety disorder	Possible high blood pressure, GI upset Rare: induction of hypomania Rare: activation of suicidal ideation
Desvenlafaxine	Pristiq	Nausea, insomnia, dry mouth, nervousness, anorexia, constipation, and increased blood pressure	Major depressive disorder (MDD)	Rare: induction of hypomania Rare: activation of suicidal ideation or behavior
Levomilnacipram	Fetzima	Nausea, constipation, increase heart rate, erectile dysfunction, tachycardia, hyperhidrosis	Major depressive disorder (MDD)	FDA-approved SNRI (July, 2013) Rare side effects too early to tell, dose-related adverse events include urinary hesitation and erectile dysfunction

TABLE 15-7 Characteristics of Specific Antidepressants—cont'd*

Generic Name	Trade Name	Potential Side Effects	Advantages of Selective Drugs	Disadvantages of Selective Drugs
Selective Norepinephrine Reuptake Inhibitors (Selective NRIs)				
Atomoxetine	Strattera	Not yet FDA approved for depression	Good for cognitive symptoms and anxiety, minimal sexual side effects	Possible sedation and/or anxiety; not FDA approved for depression
Reboxetine	Vestra	Not yet available in United States	Effective in improving energy and cognition Is targeted for unipolar depression and anxiety (e.g., panic attack)	Some U.S. studies do not find it useful in depression
Tricyclic Antidepressants (TCAs)				
Amitriptyline	Elavil	• Dry mouth		10 yr or older only for OCD
Clomipramine	Anafranil	• Constipation		
Desipramine	Norpramin	• Bladder problems (hard to empty bladder, weak		12 yr and older
Doxepin	Sinequan	urine stream, men with enlarged prostate may		6 yr and older (for bedwetting)
Imipramine	Tofranil	be more affected)		
Maprotiline	Ludiomil	• Sexual problems include reduced sex drive,		
Nortriptyline	Pamelor	problems having and enjoying sex		
Protriptyline	Vivactil	• Blurred vision, which usually dissipates quickly		
Trimipramine	Surmontil	• Drowsiness		
Amoxapine	Asendin			
Monoamine Oxidase Inhibitors (MAOIs)				
Isocarboxazid	Marplan	• MAOIs are always used as second-line	Most used‡	
Phenelzine‡	Nardil	treatment and only used in depressions that are	Most used‡	
Tranylcypro-mine‡	Parnate	resistant to other medications and treatments • MAOIs have high risk of hypertensive crisis		
Selegiline	Eldepryl, EMSAM Transdermal Patch	• If taken with any foods high in tyramine or any sympathomimetic drugs can lead to cerebral hemorrhage or death (refer to Table 15-9)	Inhibits type B MAO	Used in Parkinson's patients and FDA approved for depression

*Age FDA approved: all are 18 or older unless otherwise specified and stated in last column.
†Anticholinergic side effects include dry mouth, blurred vision, constipation, urinary retention, tachycardia, and possible confusion.
‡Most use MAO inhibitors.
From Preston, J. D., O'Neal, J. H., & Talaga, M. C. (2013). *Handbook of clinical psychopharmacology for therapists.* (7th ed.). Oakland, Calif: New Harbinger Publications; *Journal of Psychosocial Nursing and Mental Health Services.* (2011); Clip & save: drugs to treat depression. *Journal of Psychosocial Nursing and Mental Health Services, 49*(7), 15–16; National Institute of Mental Health (NIMH). (2011). *What medications are used to treat depression?* www.nimh.nih.gov/health/publications/mental-health-medications/what-medications; National Institute of Mental Health (NIMH). *Major depressive disorder among adults.* Downloaded February 26, 2011, at www.nimh.nih.gov/statistics/1MDD_ADULT.shtm1.

Potential toxic effects. The most serious side effects of the TCAs are cardiovascular in nature, including dysrhythmias, tachycardia, myocardial infarction, and heart block. Because the cardiac side effects are so serious, TCA use is considered a risk in patients with cardiac disease and in older adults. Patients should have a thorough cardiac workup before beginning TCA therapy. The risk of a lethal overdose with a TCA should always be taken into consideration when choosing an antidepressant.

Drug interactions. Individuals taking TCAs can have adverse reactions to numerous other medications. A few of the more common medications usually *not* given while TCAs are being used are listed in Box 15-2. A patient who is taking any of these medications along with a TCA should have a medical clearance beforehand because some of the reactions can be fatal.

Use of antidepressants may precipitate a psychotic episode in a person with schizophrenia. An antidepressant can precipitate a manic episode in a patient with bipolar disorder (BD). Depressed patients with BD often receive lithium along with the antidepressant.

Contraindications. Individuals who have recently had a myocardial infarction (or other cardiovascular problems), those with

---

BOX 15-2 Drugs to Be Used with Caution in Patients Taking a Tricyclic Antidepressant

- Phenothiazines
- Barbiturates
- Monoamine oxidase inhibitors
- Disulfiram (Antabuse)
- Oral contraceptives (or other estrogen preparations)
- Anticoagulants
- Some antihypertensives (clonidine, guanethidine, reserpine)
- Benzodiazepines
- Alcohol
- Nicotine

---

narrow-angle glaucoma or a history of seizures, and pregnant women should not be treated with TCAs, except with extreme caution and careful monitoring.

Patient teaching. Teaching patients and their significant others about medications is an expected nursing responsibility. Medication teaching is begun during the first encounter with the patient. The nurse or another qualified health care provider reviews the medications, possible side effects and necessary patient precautions. Areas for the nurse to discuss when teaching patients and their families about TCA therapy are presented in Box 15-3. Patients and significant others need to use an interpreter/ translator when needed and have written information for all medications that will be taken at home as well as phone numbers and emergency numbers when questions or problems arise

Selective serotonin reuptake inhibitors. The introduction of Prozac, the first **selective serotonin reuptake inhibitor (SSRI), in** 1988 heralded an important advance in pharmacotherapy. Essentially, the SSRIs selectively block the neuronal uptake of serotonin (e.g., 5-HT, 5-HT$_1$ receptors), thereby leaving more serotonin available at the synaptic site. (See Chapter 4 for detailed information on the mechanism of action of SSRIs.)

SSRI antidepressant drugs have a lower incidence of anticholinergic side effects (e.g., dry mouth, blurred vision, urinary retention), less cardiotoxicity, and faster onset of action than the TCAs. Patients are more likely to comply with a regimen of SSRIs than of TCAs because of the more favorable side effect profile, and compliance is a crucial step toward recovery or remission. The SSRIs seem to be effective in depression with anxiety features as well as in depression with psychomotor agitation.

Because the SSRIs cause fewer adverse effects and have low cardiotoxicity, they are less dangerous when they are taken in overdose. The SSRIs, serotonin-norepinephrine reuptake inhibitors (SNRIs), norepinephrine and dopamine reuptake inhibitors (NDRIs), and newer atypical antidepressants have a low lethality risk in suicide attempts compared with the TCAs, which have a very high potential for lethality with overdose. As mentioned previously, the SSRIs do have Black Box warnings that there may be an increase in suicidal thinking and/or behavior when taking the medication.

Indications. The SSRIs have a broad base of clinical use. In addition to their use in treating depressive disorders, the SSRIs have been prescribed with success to treat some anxiety disorders (e.g., panic disorder) in the obsessive-compulsive spectrum disorders (refer to Chapter 11). Fluoxetine (Prozac) has been found to be effective in treating some women who suffer from late luteal phase dysphoric disorder and bulimia nervosa.

Common adverse reactions. Agents that selectively enhance synaptic serotonin within the CNS may induce agitation, anxiety, sleep disturbance, tremor, sexual dysfunction (primarily anorgasmia), or tension headache. The effect of SSRIs on sexual performance may be the most significant undesirable outcome reported by patients.

Autonomic reactions (e.g., dry mouth, sweating, weight change, mild nausea, and loose bowel movements) also may be experienced with the SSRIs. See Table 15-7 for a general side effect profile of the SSRIs.

Potential toxic effects. One rare and life-threatening event associated with the SSRIs is **serotonin syndrome.** This is thought to be related to overaction of the central serotonin receptors, caused either by too high a dose or by interaction with other drugs. Symptoms include abdominal pain, diarrhea, sweating, fever, tachycardia, elevated blood pressure, altered mental state (delirium), myoclonus (muscle spasms), increased motor activity, irritability, hostility, and mood change. Severe manifestation can induce hyperpyrexia (excessively high fever), cardiovascular shock, or death.

The risk of this syndrome seems to be the greatest when an SSRI is administered in combination with a second serotonin-enhancing agent, such as an MAOI. For example, a person taking fluoxetine would have to discontinue this medication for **a full 5** weeks before starting an MAOI (5 weeks is the half-life for fluoxetine). If a person is already taking an MAOI, the person should wait **at least 2 weeks** before starting fluoxetine therapy. Other SSRIs have shorter periods

of activity; for example, sertraline and paroxetine have half-lives of 2 weeks, so there would need to be a 2-week gap between the administration of different medications.

Box 15-4 lists the symptoms of serotonin syndrome and gives emergency treatment guidelines. Box 15-5 is a useful tool for patient and family teaching about SSRIs.

Serotonin norepinephrine reuptake inhibitors (SNRIs) and norepinephrine dopamine reuptake inhibitors (SDRIs). These antidepressants are referred to as dual action reuptake inhibitors. Table 15-7 introduces **dual action reuptake inhibitors** and identifies

---

BOX 15-3 Patient and Family Teaching about Tricyclic Antidepressants

- The patient and family should be informed that improvement in mood may take from 7 to 28 days after initiation of treatment. Up to 6 to 8 weeks may be required for the full effect to be reached and for major depressive symptoms to subside. The family should reinforce this frequently to the depressed family member because depressed people have trouble remembering and respond to ongoing reassurance.
- The patient should be reassured that drowsiness, dizziness, and hypotension usually subside after the first few weeks.
- When the patient starts taking tricyclic antidepressants (TCAs), the patient should be cautioned to be careful working around machines, driving cars, and crossing streets because of possible altered reflexes, drowsiness, or dizziness.
- Alcohol can block the effects of antidepressants. The patient should be told to refrain from drinking alcohol.
- If possible, the patient should take the full dose at bedtime to reduce the experience of side effects during the day.
- If the patient forgets the bedtime dose (or the once-a-day dose), the next dose should be taken within 3 hours; otherwise, the patient should wait until the usual medication time the next day. The patient should *not* double the dose.
- Suddenly stopping TCAs can cause nausea, altered heartbeat, nightmares, and cold sweats in 2 to 4 days. The patient should call the physician or take one dose of TCA until the physician can be contacted.

BOX 15-4 Symptoms and Interventions for Serotonin Syndrome

Symptoms
- Hyperactivity or restlessness
- Tachycardia → cardiovascular shock
- Fever → hyperpyrexia
- Elevated blood pressure
- Altered mental status (e.g., delirium)
- Irrationality, mood swings, hostility
- Seizures → status epilepticus
- Myoclonus, incoordination, tonic rigidity
- Abdominal pain, diarrhea, bloating
- Apnea → death

Emergency Measures
1. Discontinue offending agent(s).
2. Initiate symptomatic treatment:
   - Serotonin receptor blockade: cyproheptadine, methysergide, propranolol
   - Cooling blankets, chlorpromazine for hyperthermia
   - Dantrolene, diazepam for muscle rigidity or rigors
   - Anticonvulsants
   - Artificial ventilation
   - Paralysis

BOX 15-5   Patient and Family Teaching about Selective Serotonin Reuptake Inhibitors

- Selective serotonin reuptake inhibitors (SSRIs) may cause sexual dysfunction or lack of sex drive. Inform nurse or physician.
- SSRIs may cause insomnia, anxiety, and nervousness. Inform nurse or physician.
- SSRIs may interact with other medications. Be sure physician knows other medications patient is taking (e.g., digoxin, warfarin). SSRIs should not be taken within 14 days of the last dose of a monoamine oxidase inhibitor (MAOI).
- No over-the-counter drug should be taken without first notifying physician.
- Common side effects include fatigue, nausea, diarrhea, dry mouth, dizziness, tremor, and sexual dysfunction or lack of sex drive.
- Because of the potential for drowsiness and dizziness, patient should not drive or operate machinery until these side effects are ruled out.
- Alcohol should be avoided. SSRIs may act synergistically, and people report increased effects of alcohol (e.g., one drink can seem like two). Alcohol is also a central nervous system (CNS) depressant that may work against the desired effect of the SSRI.
- Liver and renal function tests should be performed and blood counts checked periodically.
- Medication should not be discontinued abruptly. People report such effects as dizziness, nausea, diarrhea, muscle jerkiness, and tremors. If side effects from the SSRIs become bothersome, patient should ask physician about changing to a different drug. Abrupt cessation can lead to serotonin withdrawal.
- SSRIs should be used with caution in the elderly and in pregnant women. The physician should take into account the benefits versus the risk in these populations, as well as all patients taking SSRIs or any kind of antidepressant.
- Any of the following symptoms should be reported to a physician immediately:
  - Increase in depression or suicidal thoughts
  - Rash or hives
  - Rapid heartbeat
  - Sore throat
  - Difficulty urinating
  - Fever, malaise
  - Anorexia and weight loss
  - Unusual bleeding
  - Initiation of hyperactive behavior
  - Severe headache

TABLE 15-8   Common Adverse Reactions to and Toxic Effects of Monoamine Oxidase Inhibitors

Adverse Reactions	Comments
- Hypotension - Sedation, weakness, fatigue - Insomnia - Changes in cardiac rhythm - Muscle cramps - Anorgasmia or sexual impotence - Urinary hesitancy or constipation - Weight gain	Hypotension is the most critical side effect (10%); older adults, especially, may sustain injuries from falls.

Toxic Effects	Comments

Hypertensive crisis*
- Severe headache
- Stiff, sore neck
- Flushing; cold, clammy skin
- Tachycardia
- Severe nosebleeds, dilated pupils
- Chest pain, stroke, coma, death
- Nausea and vomiting
	1. Patient should go to local emergency department immediately—blood pressure should be checked.
	2. One of the following may be given to lower blood pressure:
	  - 5 mg of intravenous phentolamine (Regitine) or
	  - Oral chlorpromazine or
	  - Nifedipine (Procardia) (calcium channel blocker), 10 mg sublingually

*Related to interaction with foodstuffs and cold medication.

Unfortunately, the MAOIs also inhibit the breakdown of tyramine in the liver. Increased levels of tyramine can lead to high blood pressure, hypertensive crisis, and eventually cerebrovascular accident and death. Therefore people taking MAOIs must restrict their intake of tyramine so that their blood pressure does not rise to dangerous levels. See Table 15-9 for a list of foods that are high in tyramine.

Until 2006 the MAOIs commonly used in the United States were phenelzine (Nardil) and tranylcypromine sulfate (Parnate). In 2006 the FDA approved an MAOI that is delivered transcutaneously by way of a patch called the *selegiline transdermal system (STS)*. STS is able to inhibit monoamine oxidase in the central nervous system, increasing the availability of norepinephrine, serotonin, and dopamine, while at the same time avoiding the breakdown of tyramine in the liver and digestive tract. When STS is applied in doses of 6 mg over 24 hours by way of a skin patch, it does **not** require a tyramine-restricted diet. At higher doses (9 or 12 mg), dietary restrictions must be observed.

See Table 15-7 for an overview of MAOIs in current use and Table 15-8 for a description of their adverse effects. Patients who do not improve with initial therapy often show improvement when switched to another class of antidepressants or when a drug from another class is added to the therapy. Box 15-6 can be used as an MAOI teaching guide.

Contraindications. Use of MAOIs may be contraindicated when one of the following is present:
- Cerebrovascular disease
- Hypertension and congestive heart failure
- Liver disease
- Consumption of foods containing tyramine, tryptophan, and dopamine (see Table 15-9)
- Use of certain medications (Box 15-7)
- Recurrent or severe headaches

their strengths and side effect profiles. Each of these agents blocks different neurotransmitters and transmitter subtypes, which accounts for their strengths in targeting unique populations of depressed individuals as well as for their efficacy in treating other conditions.

Monoamine oxidase inhibitors. MAOIs are second-line medications but have proven benefits for patients who have not responded to other medications or to ECT treatment. They also have been found useful in re-refractory anxiety states. In particular, MAOIs have established efficacy in treatment of those with **atypical depression** (see Table 15-7).

In addition to being effective with atypical depression and MDD, MAOIs can be useful in treating other disorders such as panic disorder, social phobia, generalized anxiety disorder, obsessive-compulsive disorder, posttraumatic stress disorder, and bulimia. Essentially, MAOIs prevent the breakdown of norepinephrine, serotonin, and dopamine in the brain, thereby increasing the levels of these brain amines and resulting in elevated mood. (See Chapter 4 for detailed information on the mechanism of action of MAOIs.) Common adverse reactions and potential toxic effects of MAOIs are outlined in Table 15-8.

TABLE 15-9   Foods that Can Interact with Monoamine Oxidase Inhibitors

Category	Unsafe Foods (High Tyramine Content)	Safe Foods (Little or No Tyramine)
Foods that Contain Tyramine		
Vegetables	Avocados, especially if overripe; fermented bean curd; fermented soybean; soybean paste; broad beans (fava bean pods); sauerkraut	Most vegetables
Fruits	Figs, especially if overripe; bananas in large amounts (banana peel is extremely high in tyramine)	Most fruits
Meats	Meats that are fermented, smoked, cured, or otherwise aged; spoiled meats; liver, unless very fresh	Meats that are known to be fresh (exercise caution in restaurants; meats may not be fresh)
Sausages	Fermented varieties: bologna, pepperoni, salami, air-dried sausages, others	Nonfermented varieties
Fish	Pickled herring and smoked salmon negligible; lungfish row, sliced schmaltz herring in oil, salmon mousse; dried, pickled, or cured fish; fish that is fermented, smoked, or otherwise aged; spoiled fish	Fish that is known to be fresh; vacuum-packed fish, if eaten promptly or refrigerated only briefly after opening
Milk, milk products	Practically all cheeses, especially hard cheeses	Milk, yogurt, cottage cheese, cream cheese
Foods with yeast	Yeast extract (e.g., Marmite, Bovril)	Baked goods that contain yeast
Beer, wine	Some imported beers, tap (draft) beers, some wines, Chianti	Major domestic brands of beer; most white wines
Other foods	Protein dietary supplements; soups (may contain protein extract); shrimp paste; soy sauce	
Foods that Contain Other Vasopressors		
Chocolate	Contains phenylethylamine, a pressor agent; large amounts can cause a reaction	
Fava beans	Contain dopamine, a pressor agent; reactions are most likely with overripe beans	
Ginseng	Headache, tremulousness, and mania-like reactions have occurred	
Caffeinated beverages	Caffeine is a weak pressor agent; large amounts may cause a reaction	

From Burchum, J., & Rosenthal, J. (2015). *Lehne's pharmacology for nursing care* (9th ed.). St Louis: Elsevier/Saunders; Preston, J. D., O'Neal, J. H., & Talaga, M. C. (2013). *Handbook of clinical psychopharmacology for therapists* (7th ed.). Oakland, Calif: New Harbinger Publications.

BOX 15-6   Patient and Family Teaching about Monoamine Oxidase Inhibitors

- Tell the patient and the patient's family to avoid certain foods and all medications (especially cold remedies) unless prescribed by and discussed with the patient's physician (see Table 15-9 and Box 15-7 for specific food and drug restrictions).
- Give the patient a wallet card describing the monoamine oxidase inhibitor (MAOI) regimen.
- Instruct the patient to avoid Chinese restaurants (where soy sauce, sherry, brewer's yeast, and other contraindicated products may be used).
- Tell the patient to go to the emergency department immediately if he or she has a severe headache.
- Ideally, monitor the patient's blood pressure during the first 6 weeks of treatment (for both hypotensive and hypertensive effects).
- Instruct the patient that after the MAOI is stopped, dietary and drug restrictions should be maintained for 14 days.

BOX 15-7   Drugs that Can Interact with Monoamine Oxidase Inhibitors

Use of the following drugs should be restricted in patients taking monoamine oxidase inhibitors (MAOIs):
- Over-the-counter medications for colds, allergies, or congestion (any product containing ephedrine, phenylephrine hydrochloride, or phenylpropanolamine)
- Tricyclic antidepressants (e.g., imipramine, amitriptyline)
- Narcotics
- Antihypertensives (e.g., methyldopa, guanethidine, reserpine)
- Amine precursors (e.g., levodopa, L-tryptophan)
- Sedatives (e.g., alcohol, barbiturates, benzodiazepines)
- General anesthetics
- Stimulants (e.g., amphetamines, cocaine)

Brain Stimulation Therapies
Somatic Treatments

Electroconvulsive therapy (ECT). Brain imaging may help predict ECT response. New research demonstrates that brain scans can be predictive of those who will benefit most from ECT (Brooks, 2016). People with major depression who had been nonresponsive to at least two trials of medication were used in a controlled study. Those individuals with major depressive disorder who had reduced hippocampal volumes as shown on MRI scan showed significant change in the course of depression as well as in increased hippocampal and amygdalar volume after ECT. The hippocampus is involved with learning and memory, while the amygdala helps with emotional regulation, decision making, and memory.

Electroconvulsive therapy remains one of the most effective treatments for major depression with psychotic symptoms and for treatment of patients with life-threatening psychiatric conditions (e.g., self-harm). Today ECT is mostly reserved for people with treatment-resistant (TR)

- Surgery in the previous 10 to 14 days
- Age younger than 16 years

Ketamine (Ketalar) and ketamine-like N-methyl-D-aspartate receptor (NMDA) antagonists hold promise as a treatment for depression. Ketamine is derived from the hallucinogenic phencyclidine (PCP). So far, clinical trials have proved effective for single doses of ketamine that produce fast-acting results and last up to a week in both unipolar and bipolar depression as well as for those patients who have been treatment resistant (Howland, 2013). McMillan (2014) remarks that one cannot count on a single dose of ketamine to treat depression, however, ketamine might be a useful bridge for a highly suicidal patient to feel fast acting relief for the pain of depression while at the same time start working on other potential avenues for finding more lasting solutions.

depression, accounting for between 20% and 30% of depressed individuals. Treatment-resistant depression exists when pharmacological interventions fail or when the side effects are too uncomfortable.

Although stigmatized for many years, ECT is safe and effective and can achieve a 70% to 90% remission rate in depressed patients within 1 to 2 weeks. The following list describes when ECT may be indicated:

- There is a need for a rapid, definitive response when a patient is suicidal or homicidal.
- The patient is in extreme agitation or stupor.
- The patient develops a life-threatening illness because of refusal of foods and fluids.
- The patient has a history of poor drug response, a history of good ECT response, or both.
- Standard medical treatment has no effect.

ECT is useful in treating patients with major depressive and bipolar depressive disorders, especially when psychotic symptoms are present (e.g., delusions of guilt, somatic delusions, or delusions of infidelity). Patients who have depression with marked psychomotor retardation and stupor also respond well. However, ECT is not necessarily effective in patients with chronic depression, atypical depression, personality disorders, drug dependence, or depression secondary to situational or social difficulties. The usual course of ECT for a depressed patient is 2 or 3 treatments per week to a total of 6 to 12 treatments.

Procedure. The procedure is explained to the patient, and informed consent is obtained if the patient is being treated voluntarily. When informed consent cannot be obtained from a patient treated involuntarily, permission may be obtained from the next of kin, although in some states treatment must be court ordered. Use of a general anesthetic and muscle-paralyzing agents has revolutionized the comfort and safety of ECT. For an excellent article on ECT and thorough description of the procedure, go to *Electric Convulsive Therapy: Overview, Preparation, Technique* (2015) by Raj K. Kalapatapu at http://emedicine.medscape.com/article/1525957-overview.

Potential adverse reactions. On awakening from ECT, the patient may be confused and disoriented. The nurse and significant others may need to orient the patient frequently during the course of treatment. Many patients state that they have memory deficits for the first few weeks after treatment. Memory usually, although not always, recovers. ECT is not a permanent cure for depression, and maintenance treatment with TCAs or lithium decreases the relapse rate. Maintenance ECT (once a week to once a month) may also help to decrease relapse rates for patients with recurrent depression.

It should be noted, however, that about 50% to 60% of patients will respond to treatment, which includes available pharmacotherapies, cognitive behavioral therapies, and ECT (Scicurious, 2012). Therefore other methods are desperately needed to treat the 40% to 50% of depressed individuals who do not respond to available therapies.

Vagus nerve stimulation. Vagus nerve stimulation (VNS) was FDA approved in 2009 as an adjunctive, long-term treatment for patients with **treatment-resistant depression (TRD)** (those with chronic or recurrent MDD who have failed a minimum of four antidepressant medication trials or ECT, or both). ECT is considered by many the most effective acute intervention for TRD, but TRD patients often relapse during the first year following ECT.

The exact mechanism of action of VNS is not totally understood. VNS does affect blood flow to specific parts of the brain and affects neurotransmitters including serotonin and norepinephrine, which are implicated in depression. Vagus nerve stimulation does not seem to significantly relieve depression for most people; however, it does make a noteworthy difference for some individuals. The treatments are rather expensive and not covered by most insurance companies. VNS involves surgically implanting a device called a pulse generator into the upper left chest. The pulse generator is connected by a wire to the left vagus nerve; when the generator is stimulated electrical impulses are transmitted to areas of the brain that affect mood centers. When successful, there is an improvement of depressive symptoms. Because the vagus nerve affects many functions of the brain, VNS is being studied for other conditions as well (e.g., anxiety disorder, Alzheimer's disease, migraines, and chronic pain/fibromyalgia).

Rapid transcranial magnetic stimulation (rTMS). Rapid transcranial magnetic stimulation (rTMS), FDA approved in 2008, applies the principles of noninvasive electromagnetism to deliver an electrical field to the cerebral cortices, but unlike ECT, the waves do not result in generalized seizure activity. An electrical magnetic coil is placed on the scalp, not implanted. Pulsed high-intensity current passes through the coil, creating powerful magnetic fields that change the way brain cells function. Daily treatments last for approximately 40 minutes, resulting in very low incidence of side effects (Mrazek, 2010). rTMS demonstrated significant antidepressant effect in individuals with medication-resistant depression and those who cannot tolerate the side effects of standard antidepressants. Unfortunately, those with moderate depression did not show notable improvement and some individuals had no response at all (Mrazek, 2010). Other factors limiting the use of rTMS include that it can take several weeks to become effective and it is very expensive. rTMS may be a viable solution to those for whom antidepressants may be risky (e.g., pregnant women).

Deep brain stimulation. Deep brain stimulation (DBS) has been used in the treatment of Parkinson's patients for some time, followed by its utilization to treat patients with chronic pain. More recently, DBS has been used experimentally in patients with severe, treatment-resistant depression or obsessive-compulsive disorder (OCD) (NIMH, 2009; Scicurious, 2012). Therefore, the procedure has been employed and refined for many years. Implementation of DBS is considered major surgery because individual electrodes must be implanted into the chosen brain areas. In the treatment of depression the area of implantation is called the subcallosal cingulate (SCC). An insulated wire is connected to an impulse generator, which is connected to a battery-powered device that generates stimulation. The battery-powered device is usually placed under the skin, most often near the clavicle. Once implanted and activated the impulse generator can transmit signals that depolarize the local group of neurons near the implanted electrodes (Scicurious, 2012). A recent, though small, study provides positive data regarding DBS use in patients with treatment-resistant unipolar and bipolar depression (Holtzheimer et al., 2012). Currently people with resistant bipolar and unipolar depression do not improve, so this option offers some hope; however, it is risky and poses a danger of integrating hemorrhage.

Complementary and Integrative Therapies

Light therapy. Light therapy is the first-line treatment for seasonal affective disorder with or without medication (see Table 15-1). Full-spectrum wavelength light is the specific type of light used. People with seasonal affective disorder often live in climates in which there are marked seasonal differences in the amount of daylight. Seasonal variations in mood disorders in the Southern Hemisphere are the reverse of those in the Northern Hemisphere. Light therapy also may be useful as an adjunct to medications in treating chronic MDD or dysthymia PDD with seasonal exacerbations.

Light therapy is thought to be effective because of the influence of light on melatonin. Melatonin is secreted by the pineal gland and is necessary for maintaining and shifting biological rhythms. Exposure to light suppresses the nocturnal secretion of melatonin, which seems to have a therapeutic effect on people with seasonal affective disorder. Treatments consist of exposure to light balanced to replicate the effects of sunlight for 30 to 60 minutes a day.

St. John's wort. St. John's wort (*Hypericum perforatum*) is a whole plant product with antidepressant properties that is not regulated by the FDA. In numerous studies, St. John's wort demonstrated efficacy comparable with placebo and was generally comparable in effect to low-dose TCAs, and less so to SSRIs. The herb is not to be taken by certain patient populations, such as those who have MDD, women who are pregnant, or children. To date, any efficacy is found for people who have mild depression. St. John's wort poses potentially harmful drug interactions that can result in significant toxic effects on the liver. Some drugs that need to be avoided when taking St. John's wort are amphetamines or other stimulants, other antidepressants (MAOIs, SSRIs), warfarin, theophylline, digoxin, and other prescription and over-the-counter drugs. Because St. John's wort is not regulated by the FDA, there is no guarantee as to the amount of St. John's wort these over-the-counter products may contain.

S-Adenosylmethionine (SAMe). A study of *S-adenosylmethionine* (SAMe), an over-the-counter dietary supplement that is well tolerated and safe, was found to be effective as an adjunct treatment in people with MDD who are resistant to other treatment. There have been 40 previous studies, but the most recent study was a double-blind, placebo study conducted by Harvard Medical School and Massachusetts General Hospital. The administrators found that response rates and remission rates were higher for patients treated with medication and adjunctive SAMe (36.1% and 25.8%, respectively) than for those treated with adjunctive placebo (17.6% and 11.7%, respectively). Although the study warrants replication, SAMe may play a big role as adjunctive treatment for people with major depressive disorder who are nonresponsive to medications (Preston et al., 2013).

Peer support. We all experience positive results when talking to good friends regarding a problem or situation that is causing us difficulty; therefore it is no surprise that peer support/support groups can make a difference in people's lives. Studies seem to bear out that support groups are important in helping people with depression. Some reasons could be that support groups decrease feelings of isolation, provide a buffer against stressful events, increase health information, and offer role models

THE FUTURE OF TREATMENT

There is a great need for earlier detection and intervention, achievement of remission, prevention of progression, and integration of neuroscience and behavioral science in the treatment of depression. High-risk ages and groups, including the following, are in need of screening:

- Individuals in late adolescence and early adulthood
- Women in their reproductive years
- Adults and older adults with medical problems
- People with a family history of depression

There is also a need for education, particularly about the linkage between physical symptoms and depression. Psychopharmacological treatment should be augmented with cognitive behavioral therapies, and there is a need for more supplementary strategies, such as the following:

- Promotion of sleep hygiene
- Increase in exercise
- Better total health care

Continual research will result in more genetic screening tools and understanding of the pharmacogenetics of depression; the use of neuroimaging will become a common diagnostic tool and will not be restricted to research.

Brain imaging is already being used. A study from the University of Wisconsin–Madison (Johnstone et al., 2007) was perhaps the first study to use brain imaging, and it revealed a breakdown in normal patterns of emotional processing in people who are depressed. Using a functional magnetic resonance imaging scanner, the researchers found that healthy people are able to regulate their negative emotions through conscious efforts, such as envisioning a more positive outcome or reframing a negative situation.

The scan revealed that high levels of regulatory activity correlated with low levels of activity in the emotional response centers. They found that some depressed individuals lacked the ability to regulate emotions. In these individuals, high levels of regulatory activity did not change the levels of activity in the emotional centers, demonstrating that the neural circuits regulating emotion in some depressed individuals are dysfunctional.

EVALUATION

Short-term indicators and outcome criteria are frequently evaluated. For example, if the patient presents to the unit with suicidal thoughts, the nurse evaluates whether the patient still has suicidal thoughts, is able to state alternatives to suicidal impulses in the future, and is able to explore thoughts and feelings that precede suicidal impulses. Outcomes relating to thought processes, self-esteem, and social interactions are frequently formulated because these areas are often problematic in people who are depressed.

Physical needs also warrant nursing or medical attention. If a person has lost weight because of anorexia, is the appetite returning? If a person was constipated, is the bowel now functioning normally? If the person was suffering from insomnia, is he or she now getting 6 to 8 hours of sleep per night? If the indicators have not been met, an analysis of the data, nursing diagnoses, goals, and planned nursing interventions is made. The patient should be reassessed and the care plan reformulated when necessary.

▮ KEY POINTS TO REMEMBER

- Depression is the most commonly seen psychiatric syndrome in the health care system.
- There are a number of subtypes of depression and depressive clinical phenomena. Two primary depressive disorders are major depressive disorder (MDD) and chronic depressive disorder (dysthymic disorder). Bipolar disorder is the third major depressive disorder and is covered in Chapter 16.
- The symptoms in MDD are usually severe enough to interfere with a person's social or occupational functioning (inability to experience pleasure [**anhedonia**], significant weight loss, insomnia or hypersomnia, extreme fatigue [**anergia**], psychomotor agitation or retardation, diminished ability to think or concentrate, feelings of worthlessness, recurrent thoughts of death).
- A person with MDD may or may not have psychotic symptoms, and the symptoms a person usually exhibits during a major depression are different from the characteristics of the normal premorbid personality.
- In persistent depressive disorder (PDD) the symptoms last for at least 2 years and are usually considered mild to moderate. Usually, a person's social or occupational functioning is not as greatly impaired as they are in MDD, although they may cause significant distress or some impairment in these areas. The symptoms in a chronic/dysthymic depression (PDD) are often congruent with the person's usual pattern of functioning.
- Many theories exist about the cause of depression. The most accepted is the psychophysiological theory; however, cognitive theory, learned helplessness theory, and psychodynamic and life events issues help explain triggers to depression and maintenance of depressive thoughts and feelings.
- Nursing assessment includes the evaluation of affect, thought processes (especially suicidal thoughts), feelings, physical behavior, and communication. The nurse also needs to be aware of the symptoms that mask depression.
- Nursing diagnoses can be numerous. Depressed individuals are always evaluated for *Risk for suicide*. Some other common nursing diagnoses are *Anxiety, Hopelessness, Impaired social interaction, Chronic low*

self-esteem, Imbalanced nutrition, Constipation, Disturbed sleep pattern, Ineffective coping, Spiritual distress, Disabled family coping, and others.

- Interventions with patients who are depressed involve several approaches, including using specific principles of communication, planning activities of daily living, administering or participating in psychopharmacological therapy, maintaining a therapeutic environment, and teaching patients about the biochemical aspects of depression and medication teaching.
- Several short-term psychotherapies are effective in the treatment of depression, including IPT, CBT, and some forms of group therapy.
- Electroconvulsive therapy (ECT) is an effective treatment for people with major depression with psychotic features and for patient's refractory to other treatments. Vagus nerve stimulation (VNS) can be a valuable adjunctive treatment in treatment-resistant depression. Light therapy is the first line of treatment for seasonal affective disorder.
- Evaluation is ongoing throughout the nursing process, and patients' outcomes are compared with the stated outcome criteria and short-term and intermediate goals. The care plan is revised by use of the evaluation process when desired outcomes are not being met.

APPLYING CRITICAL JUDGMENT

1. You are spending time with Mr. Plotsky, who is being given a workup for depression. He avoids eye contact, he slouches in his seat, and his expression appears blank, but sad. Mr. Plotsky has suffered from numerous bouts of major depression in the past and says to you, "This will be my last depression. I will never go through this again."
   A. If safety is the first concern, what are the appropriate questions to ask Mr. Plotsky at this time?
   B. Give an example of the kinds of signs and symptoms you might find when you assess a patient with depression in terms of behaviors, thought processes, activities of daily living, and ability to function at work and at home.
   C. Mr. Plotsky tells you that he has tried every medication there is but that none have worked. He asks you about the herb St. John's wort. What is some information he should have about its effectiveness for severe depression, its interactions with other antidepressants, and its regulatory status?
   D. What might be some somatic options for a person who is resistant to antidepressant medications?
   E. Mr. Plotsky asks what causes depression. In simple terms, how might you respond to his query?
   F. Mr. Plotsky tells you that he has never tried therapy because he thinks it is for babies. What information could you give him about various therapeutic modalities that have proven effective for some other depressed patients?
2. When you are teaching Ms. Mac about her SSRI sertraline (Zoloft), she asks you, "What makes this such a good drug?"
   A. What are some of the positive attributes of SSRIs? What is one of the most serious, although rare, side effects of the SSRIs?
   B. Devise a teaching plan for Ms. Mac.

CHAPTER REVIEW QUESTIONS

1. A 28-year-old second-grade teacher is diagnosed with major depressive disorder. She grew up in Texas but moved to Alaska 10 years ago to separate from an abusive mother. Her father died by suicide when she was 12 years old. Which combination of factors in this scenario best demonstrates the stress-diathesis model?
   a. Cold climate coupled with history of abuse
   b. Current age of 28 coupled with family history of depression
   c. Family history of mental illness coupled with history of abuse
   d. Female gender coupled with the stressful profession of teaching
2. A patient tells the nurse, "No matter what I do, I feel like there's always a dark cloud following me." Select the nurse's initial action.
   a. Assess the patient's current sleep and eating patterns.
   b. Explain to the patient, "Everyone feels down from time to time."
   c. Suggest alternative activities for times when the patient feels depressed.
   d. Say to the patient, "Tell me more about what you mean by 'a dark cloud'."
3. A patient experiencing depression says to the nurse, "My health care provider said I need 'talk' therapy but I think I need a prescription for an antidepressant medication. What should I do?" Select the nurse's best response.
   a. "Which antidepressant medication do you think would be helpful?"
   b. "There are different types of talk therapy. Most patients find it beneficial."
   c. "Let's consider some ways to address your concerns with your health care provider."
   d. "Are you willing to give 'talk therapy' a try before starting an antidepressant medication?"
4. The nurse cares for a hospitalized adolescent diagnosed with major depressive disorder. The health care provider prescribes a low-dose antidepressant. In consideration of published warnings about use of antidepressant medications in younger patients, which action should the nurse employ?
   a. Notify the facility's patient advocate about the new prescription.
   b. Teach the adolescent about Black Box warnings associated with antidepressant medications.
   c. Monitor the adolescent closely for evidence of adverse effects, particularly suicidal thinking or behavior.
   d. Remind the health care provider about warnings associated with the use of antidepressants in children and adolescents.
5. Over the past 2 months a patient made eight suicide attempts with increasing lethality. The health care provider informs the patient and family that electroconvulsive therapy (ECT) is needed. The family whispers to the nurse, "Isn't this a dangerous treatment?" How should the nurse reply?
   a. "Our facility has an excellent record of safety associated with use of electroconvulsive therapy."
   b. "Your family member will eventually be successful with suicide if aggressive measures are not promptly taken."
   c. "Yes, there are hazards with electroconvulsive therapy. You should discuss these concerns with the health care provider."
   d. "Electroconvulsive therapy is very effective when urgent help is needed. Your family member was carefully evaluated for possible risks."

REFERENCES

American Psychiatric Association (APA). (2013). *Diagnostic and statistical manual of mental disorders (DSM-5)* (5th ed.). Washington, DC: APA.

American Psychiatric Association (APA). (2015). *International study brings researchers closer to personalize depression treatment.* Retrieved January 21, 2016, from http://psychnews.psychiatryonline.org/.

Andrew, L. B., & Brenner, B. E. (2012). *Depression and suicide.* Retrieved June 18, 2015, from emedicine.medscape.com/article/806779-overview.

Beck, A. T., & Rush, A. J. (1995). Cognitive therapy. In H. I. Kaplan, & B. J. Sadock (Eds.), *Comprehensive textbook of psychiatry/VI* (6th ed.) vol. 2. (pp. 1847–1856). Baltimore: Williams & Wilkins.

Bijl, D., van Marwijk, H. W., de Haan, M., et al. (2004). Effectiveness of disease management programs for recognition, diagnosis and treatment of depression in primary care. *European Journal of General Practice, 10*(1), 6–12 abstract.

Brooks, M. (2016). *Robust' evidence supports CBT for resistant depression.* Retrieved January 23, 2016, from http://www.medscape.com/viewarticle/857642.

Chen, J. (2015). *Why depression needs a new definition.* Retrieved January 22, 2016, from http://www.theatlantic.com/health/archive/2015/08/why-depression-needs-a-new-definition/399–9021.

Davenport, L. (2016). *Widely prescribed antidepressant linked to birth defects.* Retrieved January 23, 2016, from http://www.medscape.com/viewarticle/857244.

Derewicz, M. (2015). *Brain scans predict effectiveness of talk therapy to treat depression.* Retrieved September 15, 2015, from http://news.unchealthcare.org./2015/january/brain-scans-predict-effectiveness-of-talk-therapy-to–treat-depression.

Fava, M., Ostergaard, S. D., & Cassano, P. (2016). Mood disorders: depressive disorders (major depressive disorders). In T. A. Stern, M. Fava, T. E. Wilens, et al. (Eds.), *Massachusetts General Hospital comprehensive clinical psychiatry* (2nd ed.). China: Elsevier, Inc.

Gananca, L. A., Kahn, D. A., & Oquendo, M. A. (2014). Mood disorders. In J. L. Cutler (Ed.), *Psychiatry* (3rd ed). New York: Oxford University Press.

Hall-Flavin, D. K. (2015). *Pain and depression. Is there a link?.* Retrieved June 18, 2015, from http://www.MayoClinic.com/health/pain-anddepression/AN01449.

Holtzheimer, P. E., Kelley, M. E., Gross, R. E., et al. (2012). Subcallosal cingulate deep brain stimulation for treatment-resistant unipolar and bipolar depression. *Archives of General Psychiatry, 69*(2), 50–158 .

Howland, R. H. (2013). Ketamine for the treatment of depression. *Journal of Psychosocial Nursing Mental Health Services, 51*(1), 11–14.

Johnstone, T., van Reekum, C. M., & Urry, H. L. (2007). Failure to regulate: counterproductive recruitment of top-down prefrontal subcortical circuitry in major depression. *Journal of Neuroscience, 27*(33), 8877–8884.

Kabat-Zinn. (n.d.). *What is mindfulness-based stress reduction?* Retrieved June 18, 2015, from www.mindfullivingprograms.com/whatMBSR.php.

Karg, K., Burnmeister, M., Shudden, K., et al. (2011). The serotonin transporter promoter variant (5-HTTLPR), stress, and depression meta-analysis revisited: evidence of genetic moderation. *Archives of General Psychiatry, 68*(5), 444–454.

Knapton, S. (2016). *Antidepressants can raise the risk of suicide, biggest ever review finds.* Retrieved from http://www.telegraph.co.uk/science/2016/03/14/antidepressants-can-raise-the-risk-of-suicide-biggest-ever-revie/

Kuyken, W., Byrod, S., Taylor, R. S., et al. (2008). Mindfulness-based cognitive therapy to prevent relapse in recurrent depression. *Journal of Consulting and Clinical Psychology, 76*(6), 966–978.

Lliades, C. (2015). *Stats and facts about depression in America. Everyday health.* Retrieved June 18, 2015, from www.everydayhealth.com/health-report/major-depression/depression-statistics.aspx.

Lopresti, A. L., Hood, S. D., & Drummond, P. D. (2013). A review of lifestyle factors that contribute to important pathways associated with major depression: Diet, sleep and exercise. *Journal of Affective Disorders.*

Lowry, F. (2012a). *SSRIs in pregnancy linked to lung hypertension in newborns.* Retrieved January 25, 2012, from www.medscape.com/viewarticle/756875_print.

Lowry, F. (2012b). *Antidepressants safe, effective for all depression types.* Retrieved June 19, 2015, from www.medscape.com/viewarticle/765875.

McMillan, M. (2014). *Ketamine: the future of depression treatment?.* Retrieved January 23, 2016, from webmed.com/depression/news/2014.

Melville, N. A. (2016). *Antidepressant use linked to increase brain bleed risk.* Retrieved. January 22, 2016, from www.medscape.com/viewarticle/857102. print.

Melville, N. A. (2015). *Antidepressants in pregnancy linked to increase autism risk.* Retrieved January 22, 2016, from www.medscape.com/viewarticle/855915.

Mrazek, D. (2010). Transcranial magnetic stimulation can treat depression. *Psychiatric Clinics of North America, 30*(1), 51–68.

Narasimhan, M., & Campbell, N. (2010). A tale of two comorbidities: understanding the neurobiology of depression and pain. *Indian Journal of Psychiatry, 52*, 127–130.

National Institute of Mental Health (NIMH). (2010a). *Dysthymic disorder among children.* Retrieved June 19, 2015, from www.nimh.nih.gov/health/statistics/prevalence/dysthymic-disorder-among-children.shtml.

National Institute of Mental Health (NIMH). (2010b). *Early treatment decisions crucial for teens with treatment resistant depression.* Retrieved June 19, 2015, from www.nimh.nih.gov/news/science-news/2008/teens-with-treatment-resistant-depression-more-likely-to-get-better-with-switch-to-combination-therapy.shtml.

National Institute of Mental Health (NIMH). (2015). *Depression in Children and Adolescents Fact Sheet.* Retrieved June 18, 2015, from www.nimh.nih.gov.

National Institute of Mental Health (NIMH). (2009). *Women and depression: discovering hope/what are the different forms of depression?.* Retrieved June 19, 2015, from www.nimh.nih.gov/health/publications/women-and-depression-discovering-hope/index.shtml.

NANDA International. (2015). *NANDA International Nursing diagnoses: definitions and classification 2015-2017.* Hoboken, NJ: Wiley-Blackwell.

Preston, J., & Johnson, J. (2015). *Clinical psychopharmacology made ridiculously simple* (8th ed.). Miami, Fla: MedMaster.

Preston, J. D., O'Neal, J. H., & Talaga, M. C. (2013). *Handbook of clinical psychopharmacology for therapists* (7th ed.). Oakland, Calif: New Harbinger Publications.

Rihmer, Z., & Angst, J. (2009). Mood disorders: epidemiology. In B. J. Sadock, V. A. Sadock, & P. Ruiz (Eds.), *Kaplan and Sadock's comprehensive textbook of psychiatry* (9th ed.). vol. 1. Philadelphia: Wolters Kluwer/Lippincott Williams & Wilkins.

Riolo, S., Nguyen, T. A., & Greden, J. F. (2005). Prevalence of depression by race/ethnicity: findings from the National Health and Nutrition Examination survey. *American Journal of Public Health, 95*(6), 998–1000.

Sadock, B. J., Sadock, V. A., & Ruiz, P. (2015). *Kaplan & Sadock's synopsis of psychiatry: behavioral sciences/clinical psychiatry* (11th ed.). Philadelphia: Lippincott Williams & Wilkins.

Scicurious. (2012). *Deep brain stimulation for major depression: miracle therapy or just another treatment?.* Retrieved June 19, 2015, from www.google.com/?gws_rd=ssl#q=scicurious+2012+deep+brain+stimulation.

Seligman, M. E. (1973). Fall into hopelessness. *Psychology Today, 7*, 43.

Washington University, St. Louis, School of Medicine, Department of Psychiatry. (2015). *Depression facts.* Retrieved June 17, 2015, from www.psychiatry.wustl.edu/depression/depression_facts.htm.

WebMD. (2011). *Depressive gene link to response to stress.* Retrieved June 19, 2015, from www.webmd.com/search/search_results/default.aspx?query=Depression%20Health%20Center.

Yellowlees, P. (2011a). *Recurrence of major depression in adolescents.* Retrieved June 19, 2015, from www.medscape.com/viewarticle/747180.

Yellowlees, P. (2011b). *A closer look at suicide and antidepressants.* Retrieved June 19, 2015, from www.medscape.com/viewarticle/755801.

Bipolar Spectrum Disorders

Elizabeth M. Varcarolis

KEY TERMS AND CONCEPTS

acute phase, p. 232
antiepileptic drugs (AEDs), p. 238
bipolar I disorder, p. 224
bipolar II disorder, p. 224
bipolar disorder unspecified, p. 224
clang associations, p. 230
continuation phase, p. 232

cyclothymic disorder, p. 224
electroconvulsive therapy (ECT), p. 239
finger foods, p. 233
flight of ideas, p. 230
hypomanic, p. 224
lithium carbonate, p. 235
maintenance phase, p. 232

mania, p. 224
pressured speech, p. 230
psychoeducation, p. 239
rapid cycling, p. 235
seclusion protocol, p. 234

SELECTED CONCEPT: GENETIC FINDINGS POTENTIAL FOR NEW MEDICATIONS?

Increasingly, researchers are finding evidence that there is a genetic overlap on specific chromosomes among five different major mental illnesses that share the same common inherited genetic variations. For example, the genetic connection is strongest between schizophrenia and bipolar disorder; more moderate between bipolar disorder, depression, and attention-deficit/hyperactivity disorder (ADHD); and to a lesser extent between schizophrenia and autism.

These shared genetic roots are hoped to provide new insight into the cause of these chronic disabling disorders. Existing therapies for these groups of people are ineffective as long-term options. This information is hoped to lead to improved treatment and quality of life for these patients. These findings raise two questions for further research:

1. Do these shared genetic causes call into question the correctness of using two distinct diagnostic entities?

2. Can an understanding of these common genetic variants lead to future medications that will target these specific genes?

(Dallas, 2011; La Rose, 2015; Perlis & Ostacher, 2015)

OBJECTIVES

1. Discuss the progression of behaviors, speech patterns, and thought processes and thought content of a person escalating from hypomania to mania to delirious mania.

2. **QSEN** Apply best-known **evidence-based practice** to identify interventions for each of the progressions from hypomania to mania to delirious mania.

3. **QSEN** Describe in detail the **physical, safety**, personal, and legal considerations a nurse must be aware of during a patient's manic phase.

4. Discuss the rationale for at least five communication strategies that are effective with patients in acute mania.

5. **QSEN** Identify specific incidences when **teamwork and collaboration** are key for a patient in an acute phase of mania and those for a patient in delirious mania.

6. **QSEN** Apply knowledge of **safety** in establishing a milieu for a hospitalized patient in acute mania.

7. **QSEN** Using **informatics** identify expected side effects of lithium therapy.

8. Compare and contrast the differences between the signs and interventions for early and severe lithium toxicity.

9. **QSEN** Using **evidence-based knowledge**, identify the bipolar clinical subtypes that may respond better to anticonvulsant therapy as well as those that may respond better to lithium therapy. List the medications most appropriate for pregnant women with bipolar disorder.

10. **QSEN** Develop a **patient-centered teaching plan** for a patient with bipolar disorder who is in the continuation phase of treatment.

11. Compare and contrast the focus of treatment for a person in the acute manic phase and that for a person in the continuation or maintenance phase of a bipolar I disorder.

12. **QSEN** Describe how **teamwork and collaboration** are vital when working with people in a manic state and the responsibilities of the team and how their collaboration would be implemented.

INTRODUCTION

Bipolar disorders are a group of brain diseases that are marked by recurring depressed and elevated/irritable moods. These disorders are on a spectrum and are often referred to as bipolar spectrum disorders (BSDs). You may be familiar with the term *manic-depressive illness,* which is an older term for these disorders. BSDs can be disabling and impede a person's ability to function. These disorders are associated with severe morbidity both physically and mentally. Bipolar and related spectrum disorders are chronic, recurrent, and life-threatening illnesses that require lifetime monitoring. According to Brooks (2015) bipolar disorders are increasingly being diagnosed at younger ages, but there has been no drop in mortality rates. Unfortunately BSDs all too frequently go undiagnosed, with some individuals living 8 to 10 years before obtaining proper treatment if at all.

BSDs are characterized by two opposite poles. One pole is mania (or hypomania), which constitutes an exaggerated elevated, expansive, or irritable mood, accompanied by a persistent increase in activity and/or energy (APA, 2013). The other pole is a depressive episode, which adds to the morbidity. Bipolar brain diseases have many presentations and they all have different courses and treatments. Alternating mood episodes are characterized by mania, hypomania, depression, and even concurrent mania and depression (i.e., **mixed episode**s in which depressive symptoms occur during a manic attack). Periods of normal functioning may alternate with periods of illness (highs, lows, or mixed highs and lows).

Unfortunately, slightly less than half of individuals with BSDs regain full occupational, interpersonal, and/or social functioning even during remission. Individuals with BSDs have significant morbidity and mortality rates. It is estimated that between 25% and 50% of people with BSDs attempt suicide and the suicide rate of bipolar individuals is 15% to 20% (Perlis & Ostacher, 2015; Preston et al., 2013). BSDs are close to the top of disorders with the highest lifetime rate of completed suicide.

BIPOLAR SPECTRUM DISORDERS (BSDs)

Although it is now recognized that bipolar illness spans a wide spectrum of behaviors, we will focus on the most commonly identified disorders. The following are from the *DSM-5* (APA, 2013):

- Bipolar I disorder: At least one episode of "persistent or elevated, expansive or irritable mood" (mania), and at least one clearly recognizable episode of major depression. (Refer to Chapter 15 on depressive disorders.) There is marked impairment in social and occupational functioning. Psychosis may accompany the manic episode, and hospitalization may be warranted. The *DSM-5* uses specifiers to identify important sets of symptoms that may accompany a particular disorder. Specifiers for bipolar I disorder include such traits as anxious distress, mixed features, rapid cycling, melancholic features, atypical features, and peripartum onset.
- Bipolar II disorder: This disorder presents with recent severe and prolonged periods of depression that alternate with brief periods of hypomanic episode(s). Often these brief periods of hypomania may

be missed, however: *"A decreased need for sleep and a lot of daytime fatigue are the red flags for hypomania"* (Preston & Johnson, 2015, p. 21). **Hypomania** is essentially a less severe and less intense form of mania and may only last 2 to 4 days in most cases. These periods of hypomania alternate with depressive episodes that are more prolonged. Specifiers for bipolar II disorder include anxious to distress, mixed features, rapid cycling, mood congruent or mood incongruent, with peripartum onset, with catatonia, for example. Psychosis is not present in bipolar II. The hypomania of bipolar II tends to be euphoric and the depression tends to place the patient at particular risk for suicide. Bipolar II disorder is no less serious than bipolar I disorder, because both disorders are typically accompanied by serious impairment in work and social functioning (APA, 2013). Refer to Table 16-1 for the differences between hypomania and mania.

- Cyclothymic disorder: This disorder presents with hypomanic episodes alternating with persistent depressive episodes (dysthymia) for at least 2 years' duration, 1 year in children. Individuals with cyclothymia tend to have irritable hypomanic episodes.
- Bipolar disorder unspecified is a designation that includes disorders with bipolar features that do not meet criteria for any of the previously specified disorders. Although these disorders can cause distress and disruption in the individual's work, social, and private life, they are not a distinct bipolar disorder and are noted as "other specified" (APA, 2013).

All of these disorders are categorized as mild, moderate, or severe in terms of the symptoms.

Bipolar Disorder with Rapid Cycling Features

Rapid cycling consists of two or more distinct episodes of alternating episodes of both mania and depression (depression–mania–depression–mania) in a 12-month period. Rapid cycling usually indicates more severe symptoms such as poorer global functioning, higher recurrence risk, and greater resistance to conventional somatic treatments.

Mania or Hypomania with Mixed Features

The term *mixed features* is used when a patient in a full bipolar mania or hypomanic mood displays depressive symptoms at the same time—for example, increased activity or agitation and feelings of worthlessness or suicidal ideation at the same time (Preston & Johnson, 2015). The essential symptoms in mixed mania include the following (Preston & Johnson, 2015):

- Significant suicide risk
- Marked irritability
- Pessimism and unrelenting worry and despair
- Decreased need for sleep

Because rapid cycling can occur with either bipolar I or bipolar II disorder, the distinction between bipolar I and bipolar II diagnoses in conjunction with the rapid cycling or mixed mania is crucial. Each dictates specific treatment implications and appropriate medical interventions (Preston & Johnson, 2015).

DSM-5 DIAGNOSTIC CRITERIA

for Bipolar I Disorder

For a diagnosis of bipolar I disorder, it is necessary to meet the following criteria for a manic episode. The manic episode may have been preceded by and may be followed by hypomanic or major depressive episodes.

Manic Episode

A. A distinct period of abnormally and persistently elevated, expansive, or irritable mood and abnormally and persistently increased goal-directed activity or energy, lasting at least 1 week and present most of the day, nearly every day (or any duration if hospitalization is necessary).

B. During the period of mood disturbance and increased energy or activity, three (or more) of the following symptoms (four if the mood is only irritable) are present to a significant degree and represent a noticeable change from usual behavior:
 1. Inflated self-esteem or grandiosity.
 2. Decreased need for sleep (e.g., feels rested after only 3 hours of sleep).

DSM-5 DIAGNOSTIC CRITERIA—cont'd

for Bipolar I Disorder

3. More talkative than usual or pressure to keep talking.
4. Flight of ideas or subjective experience that thoughts are racing.
5. Distractibility (i.e., attention too easily drawn to unimportant or irrelevant external stimuli), as reported or observed.
6. Increase in goal-directed activity (either socially, at work or school, or sexually) or psychomotor agitation (i.e., purposeless non-goal-directed activity).
7. Excessive involvement in activities that have a high potential for painful consequences (e.g., engaging in unrestrained buying sprees, sexual indiscretions, or foolish business investments).

C. The mood disturbance is sufficiently severe to cause marked impairment in social or occupational functioning or to necessitate hospitalization to prevent harm to self or others, or there are psychotic features.

D. The episode is not attributable to the physiological effects of a substance (e.g., a drug of abuse, a medication, other treatment) or to another medical condition.

Note: A full manic episode that emerges during antidepressant treatment (e.g., medication, electroconvulsive therapy) but persists at a fully syndromal level beyond the physiological effect of that treatment is sufficient evidence for a manic episode and, therefore, a bipolar I diagnosis.

Note: Criteria A-D constitute a manic episode. At least one lifetime manic episode is required for the diagnosis of bipolar I disorder.

Hypomanic Episode

A. A distinct period of abnormally and persistently elevated, expansive, or irritable mood and abnormally and persistently increased activity or energy, lasting at 4 consecutive days and present most of the day, nearly every day.

B. During the period of mood disturbance and increased energy and activity, three (or more) of the following symptoms (four if the mood is only irritable) have persisted, represent a noticeable change from usual behavior, and have been present to a significant degree:
1. Inflated self-esteem or grandiosity.
2. Decreased need for sleep (e.g., feels rested after only 3 hours of sleep).
3. More talkative than usual or pressure to keep talking.
4. Flight of ideas or subjective experience that thoughts are racing.
5. Distractibility (i.e., attention to easily drawn to unimportant or irrelevant external stimuli), as reported or observed.
6. Increase in goal-directed activity (either socially, at work or school, or sexually) or psychomotor agitation.
7. Excessive involvement in activities that have a high potential for painful consequences (e.g., engaging in unrestrained buying sprees, sexual indiscretions, or foolish business investments).

C. The episode is associated with the unequivocal change in functioning that is uncharacteristic of the individual when not symptomatic.

D. The disturbance in mood and the change in functioning are observable by others.

E. The episode is not severe enough to cause marked impairment in social or occupational functioning or to necessitate hospitalization. If there are psychotic features, the episode is, by definition, manic.

F. The episode is not attributable to the physiological effects of a substance (e.g., a drug of abuse, a medication, other treatment).

Note: A full hypomanic episode that emerges during antidepressant treatment (e.g., medication, electroconvulsive therapy) but persists at a fully syndromal level beyond the physiological effect of that treatment is sufficient evidence for a hypomanic episode diagnosis. However, caution is indicated so that one or two symptoms (particularly increased irritability, edginess, or agitation following antidepressant use) are not taken as sufficient for diagnosis of a hypomanic episode, nor necessarily indicative of a bipolar diathesis.

Note: Criteria A-F constitute a hypomanic episode. Hypomanic episodes are common in bipolar I disorder but are not required for the diagnosis of bipolar I disorder.

Major Depressive Episode

A. Five (or more) of the following symptoms have been present during the same 2-week period and represent a change from previous functioning; at least one of the symptoms is either (1) depressed mood or (2) loss of interest or pleasure.

Note: Do not include symptoms that are clearly attributable to another medical condition.
1. Depressed mood most of the day, nearly every day, as indicated by either subjective report (e.g., feels sad, empty, or hopeless) or observation made by others (e.g., appears tearful). (Note: In children and adolescents, can be irritable moods.)
2. Markedly diminished interest or pleasure in all, or almost all, activities most of the day, nearly every day (as indicated by either subjective account or observation).
3. Significant weight loss when not dieting or weight gain (e.g., a change of more than 5% of body weight in a month), or decrease or increase in appetite nearly every day. (Note: In children, consider failure to make expected weight gain.)
4. Insomnia or hypersomnia nearly every day.
5. Psychomotor agitation or retardation nearly every day (observable or others; not merely subjective feelings or restlessness or being slowed down).
6. Fatigue or loss of energy nearly every day.
7. Feelings of worthlessness or excessive or inappropriate guilt (which may be delusional) nearly every day (not merely self-reproach or guilt about being sick).
8. Diminished ability to think or concentrate, or indecisiveness, nearly every day (either by subjective account or as observed by others).
9. Recurrent thoughts of death (not just fear of dying), recurrent suicidal ideation without a specific plan, or a suicide attempt or a specific plan for committing suicide.

C. The symptoms cause clinically significant distress or impairment in social, occupational, or other important areas of functioning.

D. The episode is not attributable to the physiological effects of a substance or another medical condition.

Note: Criteria A-C constitute a major depressive episode. Major depressive episodes are common in bipolar I disorder but are not required for the diagnosis of bipolar I disorder.

Note: Responses to a significant loss (e.g., bereavement, financial ruin, losses from a natural disaster, a serious medical illness or disability) may include the feelings of intense sadness, rumination about the loss, insomnia, poor appetite, and weight loss noted in Criterion A, which may resemble a depressive episode. Although such symptoms may be understandable or considered appropriate to the loss, the presence of a major depressive episode in additional to the normal response to a significant loss should also be carefully considered. This decision inevitably requires the exercise of clinical judgment based on the individual's history and the cultural norms for the expression of distress in the context of loss.

Bipolar I Disorder

A. Criteria have been met for at least one manic episode (Criteria A-D under "Manic episode" above).

B. The occurrence of the manic and major depressive episode(s) is not better explained by schizoaffective disorder, schizophrenia, schizophreniform disorder, delusional disorder, or other specified or unspecified schizophrenia spectrum and other psychotic disorder.

From the American Psychiatric Association. (2013). *Diagnostic and statistical manual of mental disorders* (5th ed.). Washington, DC: APA.

Studies indicate that there are striking differences between unipolar and bipolar depression.

- **Unipolar depression** (see Chapter 15) affects women more than men and appears later in life. Sleep disturbances manifest as general insomnia, difficulty falling asleep, or waking repeatedly at night. A loss of appetite and diminished interest in eating are common. Depression may be agitated (e.g., pacing and restlessness) and depressive episodes often last longer.
- **Bipolar depression** affects men and women more equally than unipolar depression. Onset is usually much younger, in the vicinity of 18 years old. Disturbances in sleep manifest as hypersomnia, excessive tiredness, and difficult morning waking. Changes in appetite occur (e.g., binge eating and cravings for carbohydrates), which may alternate with loss of appetite. Bipolar depression is more often marked by psychomotor retardation. Patients with bipolar depression are also at higher risk of drug abuse and suicide than those with unipolar depression.

PREVALENCE AND COMORBIDITY

The lifetime prevalence of bipolar disorders varies around the world but in the U.S. population it is estimated to be 4.4% with a lifetime prevalence of 1% for bipolar I disorder and 4% for bipolar II disorder (Preston and colleagues, 2013). Whereas major depression usually appears between 25 and 30 years of age, bipolar disorders emerge between childhood/adolescence and up to 60 or 70 years, with most cases of bipolar depression or mania manifesting at approximately 18 years (APA, 2013). Some recent studies reported that one third of the initial symptoms of BSD occurred before the age of 13 and another third occurred between the ages of 13 and 18 and predict greater comorbidity and functional impairment (Perlis & Ostacher, 2015). The male to female ratio for bipolar I is approximately 1:1 whereas for bipolar II it is 1:2. Men usually present with mania and females with depression.

Cyclothymia usually begins in adolescence or early adulthood and has a lifetime prevalence of 0.4% to 1%. There is a 15% to 50% risk that an individual with cyclothymia will subsequently develop bipolar I or bipolar II disorder (APA, 2013).

Comorbidity with other mental disorders is quite high and seems to occur in more than 50% of people with bipolar I and about 60% in bipolar II disorder, and with cyclothymia, substance use and sleeping disorders seem to be most prominent. Most common co-occurring disorders are anxiety disorders, behavioral disorders, personality disorders (e.g., borderline personality disorder), ADHD, and substance use disorder. Persons with bipolar disorder and co-occurring substance use problems seem to experience more rapid cycling and more mixed or dysphoric mania (anger and irritability) and report more hospitalizations. Co-occurring substance use and anxiety disorders worsen the prognosis and greatly increase the risk of suicide.

The bipolar spectrum disorders also have a high rate of *medical* comorbidity, especially cardiovascular, cerebrovascular, and metabolic diseases; endocrine disorders; type 2 diabetes; and obesity. There are also medical conditions that are associated with manic symptoms such as central nervous system (CNS) tumors or trauma, hyperthyroidism, seizure disorders, and some infectious diseases (e.g., human immunodeficiency virus [HIV]). Some drugs (like amphetamines) may mimic manic symptoms and use of antidepressants during a mixed or depressive phase of the illness without a mood stabilizer can trigger a manic episode in susceptible individuals.

THEORY

Because of increasingly sophisticated neuroimaging and genetic research methods, our knowledge of the neurobiology of bipolar disorder is one of complexity. It is a disorder involving complex disturbances in relationships and marked disruption in sleep patterns, linking environmental and genetic influences, neural systems and behaviors, and high rates of certain psychological and medical comorbidities. BSDs are now defined as a multisystem of disorders involving disturbances in all of these aforementioned domains.

Biological Findings
Genetic Factors

Twin, family, and adoption studies provide significant evidence to support the view that bipolar disorders have a strong genetic component. However, the inheritance of the bipolar disorders is not a matter of "one gene, one illness" but an expression of multiple genes and chromosomes. An early age of onset is associated with hereditability, which increases with the amount of shared genetic material. Identical twins have greater heritable risk, with up to 80% of the risk for BSD inherited (Perlis & Ostacher, 2015). First-degree relatives of a person with a bipolar disorder are between 7 and 10 times more likely to develop bipolar disorder than people in the general population (Perlis & Ostacher, 2015; Soreff & McInnes, 2011).

Increasingly, researchers are finding evidence that there is a genetic overlap on specific chromosomes that point to a susceptibility to bipolar disorder, schizophrenia, and major depressive disorder (MDD) (Perlis & Ostacher, 2015).

Neurobiological Factors

The interrelationships in the neurotransmitter system are complex. Mood disorders are most likely a result of complex interactions among numerous chemicals, including neurotransmitters and hormones. Neurotransmitters (norepinephrine, serotonin, and dopamine) have been implicated as causal factors in mania and depression. During a manic episode, patients with bipolar disorder demonstrate significantly higher plasma levels of norepinephrine and epinephrine, and people with depression have decreased levels of epinephrine and norepinephrine.

One study reported that people with bipolar disorder have about one third more neurotransmitters in two major areas of the brain, which may cause an overstimulation in the brain. Neuroreceptor oversensitivity also has been identified as a potential cause of bipolar disorder symptoms.

Neuroendocrine Factors

The hypothalamic-pituitary-adrenal (HPA) axis, which modulates the stress response and is involved in maintaining homeostasis, has been closely scrutinized in people with mood disorders for decades. The severity of manic episodes seems to be highly correlated to the degree of neuroendocrine alteration. A study suggested that disruption in the HPA axis and hormonal imbalances could also contribute to the clinical outcome of a BSD. This study offered evidence that hormonal exacerbations of mood symptoms in bipolar women may be a clinical marker of the severity of this disorder during their reproductive period (Dias, 2011).

Neuroanatomical Factors

Some studies with patients with severe recurrent bipolar disorders have identified ventricular enlargement, cortical atrophy, and sulcal widening. The higher resolution magnetic resonance imaging (MRI) scans identify reduced volumes in the hippocampus, medial orbital cortex, and anterior cingulum. Increased illness severity, bipolarity, and increased cortical levels are associated with diffuse and focal areas of atrophy. Brain pathways implicated in the pathophysiology of bipolar disorder are in subregions of the prefrontal cortex (PFC) and medial temporal lobe (MTL). Dysregulation in the neurocircuits surrounding these areas has been viewed through functional imaging (e.g., positron emission tomography, magnetic resonance imaging).

However, even though different studies have identified brain changes and neurochemical abnormalities, on imaging studies functional imaging in BSD is difficult to evaluate since there needs to be more evaluation of mood states at the time of imaging, and recognition of the practical difficulties in imaging a patient in full mania.

Preston and Johnson (2015) conclude that the neurobiology of bipolar spectrum disorders most likely includes both structural and functional abnormalities at multiple levels of the central nervous system. Presently, there seems to be no established neurochemical etiology of the bipolar spectrum disorders.

Psychological Influences

Although there is increasing evidence for genetic and biological vulnerabilities in the etiology of the mood disorders, stressful life events can trigger symptoms of bipolar disorder. Family atmosphere suggests an association between high expressed emotion and relapse. Bipolar individuals who suffered abuse as children revealed earlier onset of bipolar disorder, faster cycling frequencies, and an increase in comorbid disorders such as substance use and/or addictions.

CULTURAL CONSIDERATIONS

At the best of times, BSD diagnoses are often missed, especially in lower socioeconomic groups, and may remain untreated for years or for the patient's lifetime. Unipolar depression is a common misdiagnosis, as well as anxiety disorder or substance abuse disorder, which may or may not be co-occurring with a bipolar disorder. Cultural differences and beliefs can vastly complicate the issue. Spiritual/religious beliefs in many cultures or religions may include ghosts, spirits, or even the hearing of voices as a sign of divinity or being special. Clinicians not familiar with the culture often miss important cues and misinterpret the actuality of what is being reported. All too many times minority groups are misdiagnosed as having schizophrenia.

CLINICAL PICTURE

Mania may begin gradually over the course of a few weeks, but more typically it has an abrupt onset. Excessive activity over time can result in cardiac disorders and exhaustion. With effective treatment, the prognosis of any one manic episode is good. Unfortunately, reoccurrence is likely. A manic episode may last for a few days to months, and may be followed by a depressive episode that may occur suddenly. During this time there may be remorse for inappropriate behavior (marital infidelity, catastrophic business decisions, and financial ruin) during the manic episode; therefore the risk for suicide may be high. Suicide can occur in both manic and depressive phases of the bipolar disorder.

APPLICATION OF THE NURSING PROCESS

ASSESSMENT

Figure 16-1 presents the Mood Disorder Questionnaire (MDQ). This is *not* a diagnostic test; rather, it is a helpful screening device for assessment purposes.

Level of Mood

The euphoric mood associated with a bipolar illness is unstable and labile (continually fluctuating) (e.g., hypomania, depression, irritability, and euphoria). During euphoria patients may state they are experiencing "an intense feeling of well-being," are "cheerful in a beautiful world," or are becoming "one with God." This mood may change to irritation and quick anger when the elated person is thwarted. The irritability and belligerence may be short-lived, or it may become the prominent feature of a person's manic illness. When the person is elated, the overly joyous mood may seem out of proportion to what is occurring in the person's environment, and a cheerful mood may be inappropriate to the circumstances.

People in a manic state may laugh, joke, and talk in a continuous stream, with uninhibited familiarity. During mania people demonstrate boundless enthusiasm, treat everyone with confidential friendliness, and incorporate everyone into their plans and activities. "They know no strangers." Energy and self-confidence seem boundless.

Elaborate schemes to get rich and famous and acquire unlimited power may be frantically pursued, despite objections and realistic constraints. Excessive phone calls and emails are made, often to famous and influential people all over the world. People in the manic phase are busy at all hours of the day and night furthering their grandiose plans and wild schemes. To the manic person, no aspirations are too high and no distances are too far. No boundaries exist in reality to curtail the elaborate schemes.

In the manic state, a person often gives away money, prized possessions, and expensive gifts. When manic the person throws lavish parties, frequents expensive nightclubs and restaurants, and spends money freely on friends and strangers alike. This spending, excessive use of credit cards and high standards of living continue even in the face of bankruptcy. Intervention is often needed to prevent financial ruin. *As the clinical course progresses, sociability and euphoria are replaced by a stage of hostility, irritability, and paranoia.* The following vignette is how one patient describes this experience (Jamison, 1995a, p. 67).

VIGNETTE

At first when I'm high, it's tremendous ... ideas are fast, like shooting stars you follow until brighter ones appear. All shyness disappears; the right words and gestures are suddenly there. Uninteresting people and things become intensely interesting. Sensuality is pervasive; the desire to seduce and be seduced is irresistible. Your marrow is infused with unbelievable feelings of ease, power, well-being, omnipotence, euphoria ... you can do anything. But somewhere this changes.

The fast ideas become too fast and there are far too many. Overwhelming confusion replaces clarity. You stop keeping up with it—memory goes. Infectious humor ceases to amuse—your friends become frightened ... everything now is against the grain. You are irritable, angry, frightened, uncontrollable, and trapped in the blackest caves of the mind—caves you never knew were there. It will never end. Madness carves its own reality.

Refer to Table 16-1 for the characteristics of a person experiencing different phases of mania.

Behavior
During Mania

When in full-blown mania, a person constantly switches from one activity to another, one place to another and one project to another. Many projects may be started, but few, if any, are completed. Inactivity is impossible, even for the shortest period of time. Hyperactivity may range from mild to frenetic, wild activity. The writing of flowery

Mood Disorder Questionnaire

Instructions: Please answer each question as best you can.

1. Has there ever been a period of time when you were not your usual self and...

	Yes	No
you felt so good or so hyper that other people thought you were not your normal self or you were so hyper that you got into trouble?	☐	☐
you were so irritable that you shouted at people or started fights or arguments?	☐	☐
you felt much more self-confident than usual?	☐	☐
you got much less sleep than usual and found you didn't really miss it?	☐	☐
you were much more talkative or spoke much faster than usual?	☐	☐
thoughts raced through your head or you couldn't slow down your mind?	☐	☐
you were so easily distracted by things around you that you had trouble concentrating or staying on track?	☐	☐
you had much more energy than usual?	☐	☐
you were much more active or did many more things than usual?	☐	☐
you were much more social or outgoing than usual; for example, you telephoned friends in the middle of the night?	☐	☐
you were much more interested in sex than usual?	☐	☐
you did things that were unusual for you or that other people might have thought were excessive, foolish, or risky?	☐	☐
spending money got you or your family into trouble?	☐	☐

2. If you answered "Yes" to more than one of the above, have several of these ever happened during the same period of time?

3. How much of a problem did any of these cause you—like being unable to work; having family, money, or legal troubles; or getting into arguments or fights? Please select one response only.

   ☐ No problem   ☐ Minor problem   ☐ Moderate problem   ☐ Serious problem

4. Have any of your blood relatives (children, siblings, parents, grandparents, aunts, uncles) had manic-depressive illness or bipolar disorder?   ☐ ☐

5. Has a health care professional ever told you that you have manic-depressive illness or bipolar disorder?   ☐ ☐

Criteria for Results: Answering "Yes" to 7 or more of the events in question 1, answering "Yes" to question 2, and answering "Moderate problem" or "Serious problem" to question 3 are considered a positive screen result for bipolar disorder.

FIGURE 16-1 The Mood Disorder Questionnaire. (From Hirschfeld, R. M. A., et al. [2000]. Development and validation of a screening instrument for bipolar spectrum disorder: The Mood Disorder Questionnaire. *American Journal of Psychiatry, 157*[11], 1873–1875. Copyright ©2004 Eli Lilly and Co.)

and lengthy letters and the making of excessive long-distance telephone calls are accentuated. Individuals become involved in pleasurable activities that can have painful consequences. For example, spending large sums of money on frivolous items, giving money away indiscriminately, or making foolish business investments can leave a family penniless. Sexual indiscretion can dissolve relationships and ruin marriages.

During mania, individuals can be manipulative, profane, fault finding, and adept at exploiting others' vulnerabilities. They constantly push limits. These behaviors often alienate family, friends, employers, health care providers, and others. As mentioned earlier, mania may also present with dysphoria and irritability.

During *hypomania* individuals may experience voracious appetites for food as well as for indiscriminate sex. Although the constant activity of the hypomanic prevents proper sleep, short periods of sleep are possible. However, all persons experiencing mania sleep less, and some people may not sleep for several days in a row. The person is too busy to eat, sleep, or engage in sexual activity. **This nonstop physical activity and the lack of sleep and food can lead to physical exhaustion and even death if not treated and therefore constitutes an emergency**

Modes of dress often reflect the person's grandiose yet tenuous grasp of reality. Dress may be described as outlandish, bizarre, colorful, and noticeably inappropriate. Makeup may be garish or overdone.

TABLE 16-1 Mania on a Continuum

Hypomania	Acute Mania	Extreme Delirious Mania*
Communication		
1. Talks and jokes incessantly, is "life of the party," and gets irritated when not center of attention	1. May change suddenly from laughing to anger or depression; *mood is labile*	1. Totally out of touch with reality
2. Treats everyone with familiarity and confidentiality; often borders on crude	2. Becomes inappropriately demanding of people's attention, and intrusive nature repels others	—
3. Talk is often sexual—can reach obscene, inappropriate propositions to total strangers	3. Speech may be marked by profanities and crude sexual remarks to everyone (nursing staff in particular)	—
4. Talk is fresh; flits from one topic to the next; marked by *pressure of speech* (rapid talking, loud, and can be difficult to interrupt)	4. Speech marked by *flight of ideas,* in which thoughts race and fly from topic to topic; may have *clang associations*	4. Most likely has clang associations (stringing together of words because of their rhyming sounds, without regard to their meaning)
Affect and Thinking		
1. Persistently elevated, expansive, or irritable mood	1. Abnormally persistently elevated, expansive, or irritable mood	—
2. Full of pep and good humor, feelings of euphoria and sociability; may show inappropriate intimacy with strangers	2. Good humor gives way to increased irritability and hostility, short-lived period of rage, especially when not getting his or her way or when controls are set on behavior. May have quick shifts of mood from hostility to docility	2. May become destructive or aggressive—totally out of control
3. Feels boundless self-confidence and enthusiasm. Has elaborate grandiose schemes for becoming rich and famous. Initially, schemes may seem plausible.	3. Grandiose plans are totally out of contact with reality. Thinks he or she is a musician, prominent businessman, great politician, or religious figure, without any basis in fact	3. May experience undefined hallucinations and delirium
4. Judgment often poor. Gets involved with schemes in which job, marriage, or financial status may be destroyed.	4. Judgment is extremely poor.	—
5. May write large quantities of letters to rich and famous people regarding schemes or may make numerous worldwide telephone calls	—	—
6. Decreased attention span to internal and external cues	6. Decreased attention span and distractibility are intensified	
Physical Behavior		
1. Overactive, distractible, buoyant, and busily occupied with grandiose plans (not delusions); goes from one action to the next	1. Extremely restless, disorganized, and chaotic. Physical behavior may be difficult to control. May have outbursts, such as throwing things or becoming briefly assaultive when crossed.	1. *Dangerous state.* Incoherent, extremely restless, disoriented, and agitated. Hyperactive. Motor activity is totally aimless (must have physical or chemical restraints to prevent exhaustion and death).
2. Increased sexual appetite; sexually irresponsible and indiscreet. Illegitimate pregnancies in hypomanic women and venereal disease in both men and women are common. Sex used for escape, not for relating to another human being	2. No time for sex—too busy. Poor concentration, distractibility, and restlessness are severe.	2. Same as in acute mania but in the extreme
3. May have voracious appetite, eat on the run, or gobble food during brief periods	3. No time to eat—too distracted and disorganized	3. Same as in acute mania but in the extreme
4. May go without sleeping; unaware of fatigue. However, may be able to take short naps	4. No time for sleep—psychomotor activity too high; if unchecked, can lead to exhaustion and death	—
5. Financially extravagant, goes on buying sprees, gives money and gifts away freely, can easily go into debt	5. Same as in hypomania but in the extreme	5. Too disorganized to do anything

*Extreme mania is rarely seen today because short-acting antipsychotics and other medications are given for both manic and extreme mania.

During mania people are highly distractible. Concentration is poor, and individuals move from one activity to another without completing anything. Judgment is poor, and impulsive marriages and divorces often take place.

After Mania

People often emerge from a manic state startled and confused by the shambles of their lives. The following description conveys one patient's experience (Jamison, 1995a, p. 68).

> **VIGNETTE**
>
> Now there are only others' recollections of your behavior—your bizarre, frenetic, aimless behavior. At least mania has the grace to dim memories of itself … now it's over, but is it? Incredible feelings to sort through. Who is being too polite? Who knows what? What did I do? Why? And most hauntingly, will it, when will it, happen again? Medication to take, resist, resent, forget…but always to take. Credit cards revoked…explanations at work…bad checks and apologies overdue…memory flashes of vague men (what did I do?) …friendships gone, a marriage ruined.

Thought Content and Thought Processes

Thought content may include delusions or hallucinations. Approximately 50% of patients during the manic phase have psychotic symptoms (Black & Andreasen, 2014). Grandiose delusions are common. For example, a manic individual may think he or she has special powers and special abilities. At other times or concurrently, the delusions may be of a paranoid nature. Sensory perceptions may become altered as the mania escalates, and hallucinations may occur. However, in hypomania, no evidence of delusions or hallucinations is present. *Thought processes are revealed by the individual's speech.* Pressured speech reflects thought processes. Pressured speech is nonstop, usually loud, seemingly driven, and usually hard to interrupt. At times the attentive listener can keep up with the changes, even though direction changes constantly. Flight of ideas is a nearly continuous flow of accelerated speech with abrupt changes among topics that are usually based on understandable associations or a play on words (puns). Speech is rapid, verbose, and circumstantial (including minute and unnecessary details). When the condition is severe, speech may be disorganized and incoherent. The incessant talking often includes joking, puns, and teasing:

> *"How are you doing, kid, no kidding around, I'm going home … home sweet home…home is where the heart is…the heart of the matter is I want out, and that ain't hay…hey, Doc…get me out of this place."*

The content of speech is often sexually explicit and ranges from grossly inappropriate to vulgar. Themes in the communication of the manic individual may revolve around extraordinary sexual prowess, brilliant business ability, or unparalleled artistic talents (e.g., writing, painting, and dancing). The person may actually have only average ability in these areas.

Speech is not only profuse but also loud, bellowing, or even screaming. One can hear the force and energy behind the rapid words (pressured speech). As mania escalates, flight of ideas may give way to clang associations. Clang associations are the stringing together of words because of their rhyming sounds, without regard to their meaning:

> *"Cinema I and II, last row. Row, row, row your boat. Don't be a cutthroat. Cut your throat. Get your goat. Go out and vote. And so I wrote."*

Grandiosity (inflated self-regard) is apparent in both the ideas expressed and the person's behavior. People with mania may exaggerate their achievements or importance, state that they know famous people, or believe that they have great powers. The boast of exceptional powers and status can take delusional proportions in mania.

Cognitive Function

The onset of bipolar disorder is often preceded by comparatively high cognitive function. In fact, bipolar illness is often associated with creativity and high achievement (Black & Andreasen, 2014). However, there is growing evidence that about one third of patients who are bipolar display significant and persistent cognitive difficulties that include problems with verbal memory, sustained attention, and occasionally executive functioning as the disease progresses. These deficits often persist, even in remission. Cognitive impairment appears to be a core feature of bipolar disorder and a contributing factor to poor psychosocial outcomes.

The potential cognitive dysfunction among a large subgroup of patients with bipolar disorder has specific clinical implications:

- Cognitive function greatly affects overall function.
- Cognitive deficits correlate with a greater number of manic episodes, history of psychosis, chronicity of illness, and poor functional outcome.
- Early diagnosis and treatment **are** crucial to prevent illness progression, cognitive deficits, and poor outcome.
- Medication selection should consider **not only** the efficacy of the drug in reducing mood symptoms but also the cognitive effect of the drug on the patient.

⟫ Assessment Guidelines
Bipolar Disorder

1. **QSEN** Assess physiological safety (QSEN–Safety)
   - **Dehydration** – A person in acute untreated mania may easily become severely dehydrated, evidenced by poor skin turgor, dark and scant urinary output, and poor skin integrity.
   - **Cardiac Status** – Severe exhaustion and dehydration can lead to cardiac collapse.
   - **Poor Sleep** and constant activity lead to exhaustion.
   - **Need for Hospitalization** to physically stabilize the individual.
   - **Medical Exam** to determine whether mania is primary (bipolar disorder or cyclothymia) or secondary to a co-occurring condition (e.g., abuse of a drug or substance or toxin exposure) or a co-occurring medical condition (e.g., brain disease, certain infections including HIV, and endocrine disorders).
2. **QSEN** Other areas of safety (QSEN–Safety)
   - Assess whether the patient is a danger to self:
     - Manic behaviors can be exhaustive to the patient to the point of death.
     - Patients may not eat or sleep, often for days at a time.
     - Poor impulse control may result in harm to self or others.
     - Poor judgment.
     - Inappropriate sexual activity.
     - Uncontrolled spending. Protect the patient in mania from bankruptcy.
3. Assess the patient's and family's understanding of bipolar disorder, knowledge of medications, and knowledge of support groups and organizations that provide information on bipolar disorder and patient and family support.

DIAGNOSIS

Nursing diagnoses vary for a patient with a bipolar disorder. A primary consideration for a patient in acute mania is the prevention of exhaustion and death from cardiac collapse. Because of the patient's poor judgment, excessive and constant motor activity, probable dehydration, and difficulty evaluating reality, *Risk for injury* is a likely a primary diagnosis if the patient's activity level is dangerous to his or her health. *Impaired mood regulation* and *Labile emotional control* will most likely dominate during a full-blown manic phase. During the continuation phase, assessment of areas such as compliance to medication, risk for suicide, optimizing family support, and availability of social support can be invaluable in achieving relapse prevention. Refer to Table 16-2 for a list of potential nursing diagnoses for bipolar disorders.

OUTCOMES IDENTIFICATION

Phase I (Acute Mania)

QSEN   The overall goal during the acute manic phase is to **prevent injury**. Outcomes in phase I reflect physiological as well as behavioral issues (stated in measurable terms within realistic time frames). For example, the patient will: (QSEN–Safety)

- Be well hydrated within 24 hours—as evidenced by good skin turgor—and within normal limits of urinary output, concentration, and dilution.
- Maintain stable cardiac status, as evidenced by stable vital signs within normal limits (by *date*).
- Maintain or obtain tissue integrity, as evidenced by absence of infection or absence of untreated cuts or abrasions (by *date*).
- Get sufficient sleep and rest while in the hospital, as evidenced by 4 to 6 hours of sleep at night and 10-minute rest periods every hour.
- Demonstrate self-control with the aid of staff or medication, as evidenced by absence of harm to others *(state the behaviors)*.
- Make no attempt at self-harm with the aid of staff or medication, as evidenced by physical safety checked with regularity throughout period of acute mania.

Phase II (Continuation of Treatment)

The continuation phase lasts for approximately 2 to 6 months. Although the overall outcome of this phase is relapse prevention, many other outcomes must be accomplished to achieve **relapse prevention**. These outcomes include the following:

1. Patient and family will attend psychoeducational classes that discuss a variety of topics and give directions to patients and families to help prevent relapse
   - Knowledge of disease process
   - Knowledge of medication
   - Consequences of substance use for predicting future relapse
   - Recognizing early signs and symptoms of relapse
2. Support groups or therapy (psychoeducational groups and cognitive behavioral therapy [CBT], interpersonal social rhythm therapy [IPSRT], and family-focused therapy [FFT] are all evidence-based treatment modalities)
3. Communication and problem-solving skills training

Phase III (Maintenance Treatment)

The overall outcomes for the maintenance phase continue to focus on prevention of relapse and to limit the severity and duration of future episodes.

- Participation in learning interpersonal strategies related to work, interpersonal, and family problems
- Participation in psychotherapy group or other ongoing supportive therapy modality that has evidence-based support
- Knowledge of factors in relapse prevention
- Medication education and compliance

TABLE 16-2 **Potential Nursing Diagnoses for Bipolar Disorders**	
Signs and Symptoms	**Nursing Diagnoses**
Excessive and constant motor activity	*Risk for Injury*
	Impaired mood regulation
Poor judgment	*Imbalanced Nutrition: Less Than Body*
Lack of rest and sleep	*Requirements Deficient Fluid Volume*
Poor nutritional intake (excessive or relentless mix of above behaviors can lead to cardiac collapse)	
Loud, profane, hostile, combative, aggressive, demanding behaviors	*Risk for Self-Directed Violence*
Intrusive and taunting behaviors	*Labile Emotional Control*
Inability to control behavior	*Risk for Suicide*
Rage reaction	*Interrupted Family Processes*
	Ineffective Coping
	Ineffective Impulse Control
Manipulative, angry, or hostile verbal and physical behaviors	*Defensive Coping*
Impulsive speech and actions	*Ineffective Coping*
Property destruction or lashing out at others in a rage reaction	
Racing thoughts, grandiosity, poor judgment	*Disturbed Thought Processes*
	Ineffective Coping
Giving away valuables, neglecting family, making impulsive major life changes (divorce, career changes)	*Interrupted Family Processes*
	Caregiver Role Strain
Continuous pressured speech jumping from topic to topic *(flights of ideas)*	*Impaired Verbal Communication*
Constant motor activity, going from one person or event to another	*Impaired Social Interaction*
	Risk for Injury
Annoyance or taunting of others; loud and crass speech	
Provocative behaviors	
Failure to eat, groom, bathe, dress self because too distracted, agitated, and disorganized	*Self-Care Deficit (bathing/hygiene, dressing/grooming)*
Inability to sleep because too frantic and hyperactive (sleep deprivation can lead to exhaustion and death)	*Disturbed Sleep Pattern*
	Risk for Activity Intolerance
	Risk-Prone Health Behavior

- Family psychoeducation or therapy
- Increased social support
- Attendance at bipolar or substance use support groups
- Recovery groups

PLANNING

The planning of care for an individual with bipolar disorder usually is targeted toward the particular phase of mania (e.g., acute mania, continuation of treatment, or maintenance treatment); whether the symptoms are mild, moderate, or severe; and any other co-occurring issues identified in the assessment (e.g., risk of suicide, risk of violence to person or property, family crisis, legal crises, substance use disorder, risk-taking behaviors, issues surrounding medication compliance).

Acute Phase

During the acute phase (up to first 2 months), planning focuses on medically stabilizing the patient while maintaining safety. When mania is acute, hospitalization is usually safest for a patient. Nursing care is often geared toward decreasing physical activity, increasing food and fluid intake, ensuring at least 4 to 6 hours of sleep per night, alleviating any bowel or bladder problems, and intervening to see that self-care needs are met. Some patients may require seclusion or even electroconvulsive therapy, and they certainly need careful medication management.

Continuation Phase

During the continuation phase (2 to 6 months), planning focuses on maintaining compliance with the medication regimen and preventing relapse. Interventions are planned in accordance with the assessment data regarding the patient's interpersonal and stress reduction skills, cognitive functioning, employment status, substance-related problems, and social support systems, for example. During this time, psychoeducational teaching is a priority for patient and family. The need for referrals to community programs, groups, and support for any co-occurring disorders or problems (e.g., substance use disorder, family problems, legal issues, and financial crises) is evaluated.

Evaluation of the need for communication skills training and problem-solving skills training is important. People with bipolar disorders often have interpersonal problems that affect their work, family, and social lives, as well as other emotional problems. Residual problems resulting from reckless, violent, withdrawn, or bizarre behavior that may have occurred during a manic episode often leave lives shattered and family and friends hurt and distant. For many patients, specific psychotherapy (in addition to medication management) is needed to address these issues, although the focus of psychotherapeutic treatment will vary over time for each person.

Maintenance Phase

The maintenance phase begins at about 6 months, and planning focuses on preventing relapse and limiting the severity and duration of episodes. Patients with bipolar disorders require medications over long periods of time, if not a lifetime. Specific psychosocial therapies, support or psychoeducational groups, and periodic evaluations all help patients maintain their family and social lives in order to continue employment and minimize relapse rates.

IMPLEMENTATION

Self-Care for Nurses

During the manic phase, a patient can elicit numerous intense, unpleasant, and negative emotions in health care professionals. During mania, the patient is out of control and resists being controlled. The patient may use humor, manipulation, power struggles, or demanding behavior to prevent or minimize the staff's ability to set limits or control dangerous behaviors. The **consistent setting of limits**, followed by the whole staff, is the main theme in treating a person in mania since the patient will use a variety of ways to distract the staff, loosen the limits, and continue to escalate.

For example, the patient might get involved in power plays with the staff, by pointing out faults or oversights and drawing negative attention to one or more staff members. Alternatively, the patient may

become aggressively demanding, shouting to staff. This is done in a loud, shrill, and disruptive manner, provoking staff to become defensive, frustrated, and exasperated. When staff start losing control, it allows the manic behavior to go unchecked and escalate further.

OSEN Teamwork and collaboration are essential. Because consistent setting of limits by all staff is imperative for treatment to be effective, nurses, physicians, and all health care workers need to communicate with one another and reestablish limit setting in clear terms.

Patients with bipolar disorders are often ambivalent about treatment. They may minimize the destructive consequences of their behaviors or deny the seriousness of the disease. Some are reluctant to relinquish the increased energy, euphoria, and heightened sense of self-esteem of hypomania, before the devastating features of full-blown mania commence. Unfortunately, nonadherence to the regimen of mood-stabilizing medication is a major cause of relapse. Therefore establishing a therapeutic alliance with the bipolar individual is crucial.

Acute Phase

Hospitalization provides safety for a patient in acute mania (bipolar I disorder), imposes external controls on destructive behaviors, and provides medical stabilization.

Communication Guidelines

Communicating with a patient who is acutely manic can be challenging, but there are some specific and effective approaches for communicating with a person in the manic phase of bipolar disorder (Table 16-3). Essentially, the goal is to initially verbally engage the agitated individual, establish a collaborative relationship, and hopefully verbally de-escalate the patient out of the agitated state (Richmond et al., 2012).

Safety is a priority during the acute phase. Specific strategies can help maintain the safety of the patient during the hospitalized period. Staff members continually set limits in a firm, nonthreatening, and neutral manner to prevent further escalation of mania and to provide safe boundaries for the patient and others (Table 16-4).

Milieu Therapy

While hospitalized, the ideal setting for persons who are hyperactive and easily distracted is an atmosphere with decreased stimulation. Essentially, an effective milieu should be designed to decrease environmental stimulation, offer solitary or noncompetitive activities (e.g., writing, drawing, taking a walk with a health care worker, playing table tennis), and protect the patient from potentially embarrassing behaviors on the unit. However, when a patient's level of mood begins to escalate, the staff need to use their skills to employ other interventions.

Richmond and colleagues (2012) identify verbal de-escalation techniques that have proven in many cases to decrease the need for restraints or seclusion. When verbal de-escalation techniques do not work, seclusion may be necessary to prevent harm to self or others. Refer to Chapter 24 for verbal de-escalation techniques. Staff need to be well prepared and be knowledgeable about unit protocol regarding seclusion.

Seclusion. Control during the acute phase of hyperactive behavior almost always includes immediate treatment with an antipsychotic or a benzodiazepine. However, when a patient is dangerously out of control, and all other approaches have not proven successful, seclusion or restraints may be indicated. Seclusion provides comfort and relief to many patients who can no longer control their own behavior and serves the following purposes:

- Reduces overwhelming environmental stimuli
- Protects a patient from injuring self, others, or staff
- Prevents destruction of personal property or property of others

TABLE 16-3 Interventions for Acute Mania: Communication

Intervention	Rationale
1. Use firm and calm approach: "John, come with me. Eat this sandwich."	1. Structure and control are provided for patient who is out of control. Feelings of security can result: "Someone is in control."
2. Use short and concise explanations or statements.	2. Short attention span limits comprehension to small bits of information.
3. Remain neutral; avoid power struggles and value judgments.	3. Patient can use inconsistencies and value judgments as justification for arguing and escalating mania.
4. Be consistent in approach and expectations.	4. Consistent limits and expectations minimize potential for patient's manipulation of staff.
5. Have frequent staff meetings to plan consistent approaches and to set agreed-on limits.	5. Consistency of all staff is needed to maintain controls and minimize manipulation by patient.
6. With other staff, decide on limits, tell patient in simple, concrete terms with consequences; for example, "John, do not yell at or hit Peter. If you cannot control yourself, we will help you" or "The seclusion room will help you feel less out of control and prevent harm to yourself and others."	6. Clear expectations help patient experience outside controls as well as understand reasons for medication, seclusion, or restraints (if unable to control behaviors).
7. Hear and act on legitimate complaints.	7. Underlying feelings of helplessness are reduced, and acting-out behaviors are minimized.
8. Firmly redirect energy into more appropriate and constructive channels.	8. Distractibility is the nurse's most effective tool during the patient's manic phase.

TABLE 16-4 Interventions for Acute Mania: Safety and Physical Needs

Intervention	Rationale
Structure in a Safe Milieu	
1. Maintain low level of stimuli in patient's environment (e.g., away from bright lights, loud noises, and people).	1. Decreases escalating anxiety.
2. Provide structured solitary activities with nurse or aide.	2. Structure provides security and focus.
3. Provide frequent high-calorie fluids.	3. Prevents dangerous levels of dehydration.
4. Provide frequent rest periods.	4. Prevents exhaustion.
5. Redirect violent behavior through physical exercise (e.g., walking)	5. Physical exercise can decrease tension and provide focus.
6. When warranted in acute mania, use antipsychotics and seclusion to minimize physical harm via physician's order.	6. Exhaustion and death can result from dehydration, lack of sleep, and constant physical activity.
7. Observe for signs of lithium toxicity.	7. There is a small margin of safety between therapeutic and toxic doses.
8. Protect patient from giving away money and possessions. Hold valuables in hospital safe until rational judgment returns.	8. Patient's "generosity" is in fact a symptom of the disease and can lead to catastrophic financial ruin for patient and family.
Nutrition	
1. Monitor intake, output, and vital signs.	1. Adequate fluid and caloric intakes are ensured; development of dehydration and cardiac collapse is minimized.
2. Offer frequent high-calorie protein drinks and finger foods (e.g., sandwiches, fruit, milkshakes).	2. Constant fluid and calorie replacement are needed. Patient may be too active to sit at meals. Finger foods allow "eating on the run."
3. Frequently remind patient to eat. "Tom, finish your milkshake." "Sally, eat this banana."	3. During mania the patient is unaware of bodily needs and is easily distracted. Needs supervision to eat.
Sleep	
1. Encourage frequent rest periods during the day.	1. Lack of sleep can lead to exhaustion and death.
2. Keep patient in areas of low stimulation.	2. Relaxation is promoted and manic behavior is minimized.
3. At night, provide warm baths, soothing music, and medication when indicated. Avoid giving patient caffeine.	3. Promotes relaxation, rest, and sleep.
Hygiene	
1. Supervise choice of clothes; minimize flamboyant and bizarre dress (e.g., garish stripes or plaids and loud, unmatching colors).	1. The potential is decreased for ridicule, which lowers self-esteem and increases the need for manic defense. The patient is helped to maintain dignity.
2. Give simple step-by-step reminders for hygiene and dress. "Here is your razor. Shave the left side ... now the right side. Here is your toothbrush. Put the toothpaste on the brush."	2. Distractibility and poor concentration are countered through simple, concrete instructions.
Elimination	
1. Monitor bowel habits; offer fluids and foods that are high in fiber. Evaluate need for laxative. Encourage patient to go to the bathroom.	1. Fecal impaction resulting from dehydration and decreased peristalsis is prevented.

Seclusion is warranted when documented data collected by the nursing and medical staff reflect the following points:
- Substantial risk of harm to others or self is clear.
- The patient is unable to control his or her actions.
- Problematic behavior has been sustained (continues or escalates despite other measures).
- Other measures described (e.g., setting limits beginning with verbal de-escalation, using chemical restraints) have failed.

The use of seclusion or restraints is associated with complex therapeutic, ethical, and legal issues. Most state laws prohibit the use of unnecessary physical restraint or isolation. Most hospitals have well-defined protocols for treatment with seclusion. Seclusion protocol includes a proper reporting procedure through the chain of command when a patient is to be secluded. Refer to Chapter 24 for more on seclusion and restraint and accepted protocols and to Chapter 6 for more on the legal parameters.

APPLYING THE ART

A Person with Bipolar Disorder

Scenario
I approached Gloria, a 33-year-old woman who had seemed edgy and distracted when we talked earlier. She had been admitted to the hospital for the third time after becoming angry and threatening suicide over losing a job she loved—exercising and caring for the animals at a pet store. She is on suicide precautions.

Therapeutic Goal
By the end of this session, Gloria will show increased ability to problem solve as evidenced by insight that stopping medication exacerbates the disorder.

Student-Patient Interaction	Thoughts, Communication Techniques, and Mental Health Nursing Concepts
Student: *Smiling.* "Hi, Gloria. Would you talk some more about your feelings when you heard you were going to be fired from your job?"	I know that "could" or "would" acts like an *indirect question* rather than a *direct question*, meaning I will get more than a yes or no answer.
Gloria: "Get the _____ away from me! I'm sick of you people asking about that _____ job." *Clenching fists, practically yelling.*	
Student's feelings: *I forgot to tune in to Gloria as a person before I jumped in with questions. She's loud, but I'm okay. Her fear and loss fuel all that anger. Okay, self, mindfully breathe.*	I forgot to *assess* first! I must remember, she is afraid and *displacing* her frustration onto me. Each time she gets admitted means starting over. If only she had kept taking her Depakote and Abilify.
Student: *Quiet and concerned.* "Gloria, I'm _____, your nursing student. You've been through such a rough time. You feel upset at the job and anyone that asks you about it."	Using *reflection* makes sense because I hope that reflecting the feelings lets my *empathy* get through to her.
Student's feelings: *I can do this. I'll step back a little, slow things down, and keep telling myself that her anger is not really about me. I care about Gloria so I'm not going to be pushed away that easily.*	
Student's feelings: *I'm struggling with anxiety, too.*	I remember now. Anxiety is communicated interpersonally.
Gloria: "I need to walk." *Starts pacing quickly down the hall.*	Gloria is using walking as a healthy relief behavior for her anxiety.
Student's feelings: *I hope she'll let me walk with her. Walking will help my anxiety, too!*	

Student-Patient Interaction	Thoughts, Communication Techniques, and Mental Health Nursing Concepts
Student: "Good idea. Let's walk together. Tell me what's happening inside." *We quickly walk down the hall.*	I am offering myself by walking with her. Using an indirect question often helps the patient talk without feeling interrogated.
Student's feelings: *As she responds while we walk, I'm feeling calmer, too.*	
Gloria: "I feel like, why even try anymore? While I worked at the pet store, I felt like my life meant something. Then I go and stop taking my medicine. It's just so expensive. I'm such a loser." *Eyes fill with tears.*	
Student's feelings: *I feel so sad for her. She struggles so hard, and then seems to give in by quitting her medication. Sometimes I feel like a loser. Sometimes I feel like nursing school pressures me too much, especially when I bomb a test. I need to put my own "failure worries" on hold to handle later and refocus to fully tune in to Gloria.*	
Student: "Sounds like right now you're blaming yourself for what you've lost." *I pause, handing her a tissue.* "Gloria, I care about what happens to you. When you say, 'why even try' you mean…?"	By saying "right now" I plant the idea that she may not always choose to see herself as a failure. I must stay alert for countertransference. Using Gloria's name and reminding her who I am factor in that she is probably experiencing moderate anxiety, so her *perceptual field* of what she is able to take in decreases. I need to assess even a *covert reference* to *suicide*, especially with Gloria's history.
Gloria: "Don't worry. I don't want to kill myself anymore. But I just keep screwing up! I even let my animals down." *Glancing at me.*	When Gloria tells me not to worry she may be using *projection* in that she may still have some latent concern about her suicide potential. She is still on *15-minute checks*, which continues to be necessary, and I will report and chart about all this.
Student's feelings: *I wish she could see the survivor I see when I'm with her. I'm relieved Gloria recognizes she wants to live now. I have so much hope inside for her.*	

A Person with Bipolar Disorder

Student-Patient Interaction	Thoughts, Communication Techniques, and Mental Health Nursing Concepts	Student-Patient Interaction	Thoughts, Communication Techniques, and Mental Health Nursing Concepts
Student: "Talk some more about your animals."	By using a focusing approach, I remind her of what she values. She may also remember what she was able to do well, which may help her self-esteem. She said, "my animals," so I deliberately restated, "your animals" because they are so important to her.	**Gloria:** "I still get mad too easily, but I'm starting to think more clearly since my Abilify's been upped. I've been wondering if my boss would give me a second chance. I did well with the animals. My boss said so before I got sick again. My case manager made sure the beagle pup got back okay."	Gloria's actually able to problem solve now, so that means her anxiety has decreased to mild.
Gloria: "I loved caring for all of the animals, but especially the puppies. One little beagle had such sad eyes, I took him home. That's when I got in trouble. I know I wouldn't have done that if I'd kept taking my meds."	Was Gloria using identification? The beagle's "sad" eyes may have resonated with Gloria's own sadness.	**Student:** "I hear you reminding yourself that your skills in pet care endure even through this bout in the hospital."	I think the animals provide some of Gloria's love and belonging needs, which precede self-esteem needs. I validate with Gloria about her pet care skills.
Student: "So you recognize a link between stopping your meds and doing some things you wouldn't usually do when you take charge of your bipolar disorder by staying on your meds?" ***Student's feelings:*** *I feel kind of proud of myself for knowing to praise her about the meds.*	I am using the behavior modification technique of positive reinforcement by attending to Gloria's insight when she connects her impulsive behavior with stopping her psychotropics. I am also empowering her by deliberately associating taking her medications with taking charge of her disorder.	**Gloria:** "I really love those animals. I'm going to run this idea past the nurse and work out when and how to phrase things to call my boss." ***Student's feelings:*** *She's taking charge of this. Wow! I feel honored that Gloria trusted me. I'm beginning to trust myself some, too.*	The treatment team will be doing discharge planning.
		Student: "You are able to find a goal to work toward, maybe even begin to believe in yourself a little." **Gloria:** *Nods.*	I give Gloria support by naming her mentally healthy verbalizations as a goal. I am careful to add qualifiers—"maybe," "begin to," and "a little"—to insert the idea about believing in herself without overwhelming her.

Pharmacological and Biological Therapies

Unfortunately, relapse occurs in about 50% of treated patients within 2 years and in up to 70% to 90% within 5 years (Gitlin & Frye, 2012; Miklowitz & Gitlin, 2014). During the acute phase, medications are vital to bring the patient to a safe physical and psychological level of functioning. In fact, medications are pivotal and vital through all phases of treatment, and for many patients they are a lifelong protection and can mitigate against the number and severity of future episodes (relapse).

Bipolar Medications (Mood Stabilizers)

Individuals with bipolar disorder often require multiple medications. There may be times when an antianxiety agent (e.g., lorazepam, clonazepam) can help reduce severe agitation and anxiety or an antipsychotic agent (e.g., olanzapine) can help alleviate psychomotor activity and delusions or hallucinations. Anxiolytics or antipsychotics may be used for a limited time, but mood stabilizers are considered lifetime maintenance therapy for bipolar patients.

Most treatment guidelines advocate lithium and divalproex (Depakote) as first-line mood-stabilizing agents (Preston et al., 2013).

For individuals whose **recent episode was manic or hypomanic**, lithium and divalproex seem to have the largest body of evidence supporting their effectiveness as mood stabilizers. For those with **recent episodes of depression**, lamotrigine (Lamictal), olanzapine-fluoxetine combination (Symbyax), lurasidone (Latuda),

and quetiapine (Seroquel) are useful. For individuals who **present with rapid cycling**, lamotrigine or divalproex have proven effective (Preston & Johnson, 2015).

Lithium carbonate. Lithium carbonate ($LiCO_3$) is effective in the acute treatment of mania and depressive episodes and in the prevention of recurrent mania and depressive episodes. Once primary acute mania has been diagnosed, lithium is most often the first choice of treatment.

Lithium aborts 60% to 80% of acute manic and hypomanic episodes within 5 to 14 days. Lithium is less effective in people with mixed mania (elation and depression), those with rapid cycling, and those with atypical features. Lithium is particularly effective in reducing the following:

- Elation, grandiosity, and expansiveness
- Flight of ideas
- Irritability
- Anxiety
 To a lesser extent, lithium controls the following:
- Insomnia
- Psychomotor agitation
- Threatening or assaultive behavior
- Distractibility
- Hypersexuality
- Paranoia

Initially in the treatment of acute mania, an antipsychotic or benzodiazepine can help calm symptoms. Effective medications include

APPLYING EVIDENCE-BASED PRACTICE (EBP)

Problem A 63-year-old female is brought to the ED by ambulance. She is combative, hitting and grabbing at anyone within arm's length, and is speaking very loudly and rapidly. She is experiencing flight of ideas, where her speech flits from one topic to another without apparent connection. The topics range from people who are trying to hurt or kill her, to where is her cat Bubbles, to look how nice my hair looks don't touch it, to refusing to take medication, to thinking people are laughing at her. She has self-inflicted bleeding scratches on her face and arms. The EMT reports that the patient has not been taking her Depakote for 2 weeks as she ran out of medication and did not have transportation.

EBP Assessment

A. **What do you already know from experience?** The patient has been in the ED before and suffers from bipolar I disorder. Patients in manic states are often hyperverbal; combative; do not eat, drink, or sleep enough; and can even hallucinate or be delusional. Moods may be elevated, angry and irritable, or rapidly shifting. They may lash out at staff, family, or themselves.

B. **What does the literature say?** Seclusion and restraint (physical or chemical) were common practices for decades, used with agitated psychiatric patients. Newer research has shown these practices to be traumatizing to patients, and in some cases even dangerous. Best practice now dictates the use of alternative methods such as one-to-one staff, de-escalation techniques, walking, relaxation techniques, voluntary time out, prn medications, moving others away from the patient for safety, and more extensive therapeutic training for staff members. Seclusion and restraint are limited to situations of imminent danger to self or others, must have a physician or NP order, and have clear time and safety guidelines.

C. **What does the patient want?** The patient is unable to clearly articulate her needs since she is in a florid manic state. She is fearful, which can be interpreted as a need to feel safe and in control. She has been acting as a danger to herself and others, requiring intervention until she can competently make decisions for herself.

Plan The ED supervisor assigned an RN who this patient had a good rapport with in a prior ED visit to the case, and the supervisor assisted until the patient was calm and safe. Orders were obtained for Depakote and a prn benzodiazepine. The patient was allowed adequate time and communication with the RN to voluntarily take the medication, which she did, before a restraint and injection would have been considered. Staff walked with her, gently holding her hands so that she did not lash out at self or others, until the medication began to take effect. Small bites of food and sips of fluid were frequently offered. Psychiatry was called for a consult to determine further care.

QSEN **QSEN Prelicensure Knowledge, Skills, and Attitudes (KSAs) Addressed:**

Safety was considered, by having two staff with the patient, assigning an RN with good rapport, and avoiding the use of restraints.

Evidence-based practice was considered in this patient's situation, as the ED staff members had attended communication and de-escalation training, and used alternative methods instead of seclusion or restraint.

Susan L. Frost, Chyllia D. Fosbre, 2015

Duncan, S., Van der Merwe, M., Bowers, L., Simpson, A., & Jones, J. (2010). A review of interventions to reduce mechanical restraint and seclusion among adult psychiatric inpatients. *Issues in Mental Health Nursing, 31*, 413–424; Simpson, S., Joesch, J., West, I., & Jagoda, P. (2014). Risk for physical restraint or seclusion in the psychiatric emergency service (PES). *General Hospital Psychiatry, 36*(1), 113–118.
ED, Emergency department; *EMT,* emergency medical technician; *NP,* nurse practitioner; *prn,* as needed; *RN,* registered nurse.

---

antipsychotic agents such as olanzapine or haloperidol, or potent benzodiazepines such as lorazepam or clonazepam; however, *alprazolam (Xanax) is contraindicated because it can aggravate mania.* Antipsychotics act promptly to slow speech, inhibit aggression, and decrease psychomotor activity. The immediate action of the antipsychotic or benzodiazepine medication serves to prevent exhaustion, coronary collapse, and death until lithium reaches therapeutic levels.

The major disadvantage of lithium is that improvement is gradual. Antimanic effects begin slowly after the onset of treatment, but it can take up to 3 weeks to show improvement and up to months for stabilization. The other agents given in conjunction with lithium to help control the mania are then withdrawn when lithium reaches a therapeutic level (0.5 to 1.5 mEq/L) (Skidmore-Roth 2013). Lithium levels are best obtained approximately 12 hours after the administration of the last dose.

Blood levels are initially drawn weekly or biweekly until therapeutic levels are reached. For acute mania, a blood level of 0.6 to 1.2 mEq/L would be within the initial range (Hodgson & Kizior, 2013). For maintenance therapy, lithium levels should range from 0.4 to 1.0 mEq/L; however, levels of 0.6 to 0.8 mEq/L are effective for most. Levels higher than 1.5 mEq/L can result in significant toxicity. A typical maintenance dose is 300 mg of lithium carbonate three or four times daily. The window between therapeutic levels and toxic levels is very small with lithium, so plasma levels should be monitored routinely. In the beginning, levels should be monitored every 2 to 3 days to keep the levels within the therapeutic range. During maintenance therapy, drug levels should be monitored every 1 to 3 months.

Although lithium is an effective intervention for treating the manic phase of a bipolar disorder, it is not a cure. Many patients receive lithium with or without another mood stabilizer for maintenance indefinitely and experience manic and depressive episodes if the drug is discontinued.

The exact mechanism of how lithium normalizes the effects of bipolar disorder remains definitively unknown. It is known that lithium affects the storage, release, and reuptake of neurotransmitters. Antimanic effects result from an increase in neurotransmitter reuptake and an increase in serotonin receptors, producing antimanic and antidepressant effects. Besides the serotonergic properties and the effects on neurotransmitters, lithium is thought to stabilize calcium channels and to decrease neuronal activity via effects on the second messenger systems, all of which might add to its therapeutic profile.

Cases of severe lithium toxicity with levels of 2 mEq/L or greater constitute a life-threatening emergency. In such cases, gastric lavage and treatment with urea, mannitol, and aminophylline can hasten lithium excretion. Hemodialysis also may be used in extreme cases.

Adverse reactions. Refer to Table 16-5 for side effects, signs of lithium toxicity, and interventions.

For older adult patients, the principle of **"start low and go slow"** always applies. Levels are often monitored every 3 or 4 days. Some older adults may respond to a dose low enough to maintain a blood level of 0.3 to 0.4 mEq/L. As mentioned, toxic effects are usually associated with lithium levels of 1.5 to 2 mEq/L or higher, but they can occur at much lower levels (even within a therapeutic range).

TABLE 16-5 Lithium Side Effects and Signs of Lithium Toxicity

Level	Signs	Interventions
Expected Side Effects <0.4 to 1 mEq/L (therapeutic level)	Fine hand tremor, polyuria, and mild thirst Mild nausea and general discomfort Weight gain	Symptoms may persist throughout therapy. These symptoms often subside during treatment. Give with food to decrease nausea. Weight gain may be helped with diet, exercise, and nutritional management.
Early Signs of Toxicity <1.5 mEq/L	Nausea, vomiting, diarrhea, thirst, polyuria, slurred speech, muscle weakness	Medication should be withheld, blood lithium levels measured, and dosage re-evaluated.
Advanced Signs of Toxicity 1.5 to 2 mEq/L	Coarse hand tremor, persistent gastrointestinal upset, mental confusion, muscle hyperirritability, electroencephalographic (EEG) changes, incoordination	Interventions outlined above or below should be used, depending on severity of circumstances.
Severe Toxicity 2 to 2.5 mEq/L	Ataxia, serious EEG changes, blurred vision, clonic movements, large output of dilute urine, tinnitus, blurred vision, seizures, stupor, severe hypotension, coma; death is usually secondary to pulmonary complications	There is no known antidote for lithium poisoning. The drug is stopped, and excretion is hastened. If patient is alert, an emetic is administered. Otherwise, gastric lavage and treatment with urea, mannitol, and aminophylline hasten lithium excretion.
>2.5 mEq/L	Symptoms may progress rapidly; coma, cardiac dysrhythmia, peripheral circulatory collapse, proteinuria, oliguria, and death	In addition to the interventions above, hemodialysis may be used in severe cases.

Data from Burchum, J., & Rosenthal, L. (2016). *Lehne's pharmacology for nursing care* (9th ed.). St Louis, MO: Elsevier; Skidmore-Roth, L. (2008). *Mosby's nursing drug reference* (21st ed.). St Louis, MO: Mosby; Preston, J. D., O'Neal, J. H., & Talaga, M. C. (2013). *Handbook of clinical psychopharmacology for therapists* (6th ed.). Oakland, CA: New Harbinger Publications.

BOX 16-1 Patient and Family Teaching about Lithium Therapy

The patient and the patient's family should receive the following teaching. (They should be encouraged to ask questions and given the material in written form as well.)

- Lithium can treat your current emotional problem and helps prevent relapse. Therefore it is important to continue taking the drug after the current episode is over.
- Because therapeutic and toxic dosage ranges are so close, it is important to monitor lithium blood levels very closely—more frequently at first, then once every several months after that.
- Lithium is not addictive.
- It is important to eat a normal diet with normal salt and fluid intake (1500–3000 mL/day or six 12-ounce glasses of fluid). Lithium decreases sodium reabsorption in the kidneys, which could lead to a sodium deficiency.
- Watch sodium levels. A low sodium intake leads to a relative increase in lithium retention, which could produce toxicity.
- You should stop taking lithium if you have excessive diarrhea, vomiting, or sweating. All of these symptoms can lead to dehydration. Dehydration can raise lithium levels in the blood to toxic levels. **Inform your physician if you have any of these problems.**
- Do not take diuretics (water pills) while you are taking lithium.

- Lithium is irritating to the lining in your stomach. It helps to take lithium with meals.
- Lithium can cause renal damage. Kidney function should be assessed before treatment and once a year thereafter.
- Lithium can promote goiter (thyroid enlargement) and frank hypothyroidism. Plasma levels of T_3, T_4, and thyroid-stimulating hormone (TSH) should be measured before treatment and yearly thereafter.
- Do not take any over-the-counter medicines without checking first with your physician.
- If you find that you are gaining a lot of weight, you may need to consult your physician or nutritionist.
- Many self-help groups are available to provide support for people with bipolar disorder and their families. The local self-help group is (give name and telephone number).
- You can find out more information by calling (give name and telephone number).
- Keep a list of side effects and toxic effects handy (see Table 16-5), along with the name and number of a contact person.
- If lithium is to be discontinued, your dosage will be tapered gradually to minimize risk of early relapse.

Maintenance therapy. Lithium is unquestionably effective in preventing both manic and depressive episodes in patients with bipolar disorder. It has also shown up to a sevenfold reduction in suicide rates (Preston & Johnson, 2015). Both the person with a bipolar disorder and his or her significant other(s) should be given careful instructions about (1) the purpose and requirements of lithium therapy, (2) its adverse effects, (3) its toxic effects and complications, (4) situations in which the physician should be contacted, and (5) conditions that can increase the risk of toxicity, such as excessive sweating and dehydration, excessive diarrhea, or vomiting. The patient and family also should be advised that suddenly stopping lithium can lead to relapse and recurrence of mania. Box 16-1 outlines patient and family teaching regarding lithium therapy.

Patients need to know that **two major long-term risks of lithium therapy are hypothyroidism and impairment of the kidneys' ability to concentrate urine.** Therefore a person receiving lithium therapy must have periodic follow-ups to assess thyroid and renal function. Health care providers need to stress to patients with bipolar disorder and their families the importance of discontinuing maintenance therapy gradually.

Contraindications. Before lithium is administered, a medical evaluation is performed to assess the patient's ability to tolerate the drug. In particular, baseline physical and laboratory examinations should include assessment of renal function; determination of thyroid status, including levels of thyroxine and thyroid-stimulating hormone; and evaluation for dementia or neurological disorders, which presage a poor response to lithium. Other clinical and laboratory assessments, including an electrocardiogram, are performed as needed depending on the individual's physical condition.

Lithium therapy is generally contraindicated in people with cardiovascular disease and in those who have brain damage, renal disease, thyroid disease, or myasthenia gravis. Lithium also may harm a fetus and, whenever possible, is not given to women who are pregnant. Both the fear of pregnancy and the wish to become pregnant are major concerns for many bipolar women taking lithium. Lithium use is also contraindicated in mothers who are breast-feeding and in children younger than 12 years of age.

Drug interactions occur with some drugs and lithium therapy is contraindicated in those using, for example, nonsteroidal antiinflammatory drugs (NSAIDs), hydrochlorothiazide, angiotensin-converting enzyme (ACE) inhibitors, caffeine, alcohol, and diuretics.

Anticonvulsant Drugs

Approximately 20% to 40% of bipolar patients may not respond or respond insufficiently to lithium, or they may not tolerate it. Some subgroups of bipolar patients may not respond well to lithium but may do well when treated with anticonvulsant drugs.

Three anticonvulsants have demonstrated efficacy for the treatment of mood disorders—carbamazepine (Tegretol), divalproex (Depakote), and lamotrigine (Lamictal) (Preston et al., 2013)—and have been found to have other uses as well. A sustained-release form of carbamazepine (Equetro), Depakote, and Lamictal are all approved by the U.S. Food and Drug Administration (FDA) (Preston et al., 2013). Anticonvulsants used in bipolar and other disorders are especially effective in the following:

- Beneficial in controlling mania (within 2 weeks) and depression (within 3 weeks or longer)
- Superior in **dysphoric mania** (depressive thoughts and feelings during manic episodes)
- Superior in **rapid cycling** (four or more episodes a year)
- Drugs of choice for bipolar depression
- More effective when there is no family history of bipolar disease
- Effective at dampening affective swings in schizoaffective patients
- Effective at diminishing impulsive and aggressive behavior in some nonpsychotic patients
- Helpful in cases of alcohol and benzodiazepine withdrawal

Divalproex (Depakote). Valproic acid/valproate is useful in treating lithium nonresponders who are in acute mania, who experience rapid cycles, who are in dysphoric mania, or who have not responded to carbamazepine. It is also helpful in preventing manic episodes. As with carbamazepine, it is important to monitor liver function and platelet count periodically, due to the risk of blood dyscrasias, hepatotoxicity, and pancreatitis. A previous study demonstrates that women taking valproate may run the risk of developing polycystic ovarian syndrome and that valproate use may lead to birth defects and developmental delays in children exposed in utero (Wisner et al., 2011). Therefore, careful consideration by both the physician and the patient is mandatory for bipolar treatment in women during childbearing years.

Carbamazepine (Tegretol). Some patients with treatment-resistant bipolar disorder improve after taking carbamazepine and lithium or carbamazepine and an antipsychotic. Carbamazepine seems to work better in patients with rapid cycling and in severely paranoid and angry patients with mania than in patients with euphoric, overactive, and overfriendly manic behaviors. It is also thought to be more effective in patients who present with mixed bipolar disorders.

Blood levels of carbamazepine should be monitored at least weekly for the first 8 weeks of treatment because the drug can increase the levels of liver enzymes that accelerate its own metabolism. In some instances this can cause bone marrow suppression and liver inflammation.

Lamotrigine (Lamictal). Lamotrigine is a first-line treatment for bipolar depression and is approved for acute and maintenance therapy. It is generally well tolerated, but there are two concerns with this agent. One is a rare but serious dermatological reaction: a potentially life-threatening rash called Stevens-Johnson syndrome. Patients should be instructed to seek immediate medical attention if a rash appears, although in most cases rashes are benign (Preston et al., 2013). Another problem with lamotrigine is that in August 2010, the FDA announced that aseptic meningitis is another rare but serious side effect of lamotrigine (FDA, 2010).

Newer anticonvulsant drugs. Other popular anticonvulsants may be used in the treatment of refractory bipolar disorder. However, except for topiramate (Topamax) and oxcarbazepine (Trileptal), other anticonvulsants fail to demonstrate efficacy in practice and/or lack evidence-based studies to support their use (Preston et al., 2013). Topiramate is helpful in mania and does not appear to cause weight gain. Oxcarbazepine, a structural variant of carbamazepine, has the advantage of being better tolerated and has a more favorable drug interaction profile than other anticonvulsants (Preston et al., 2013). See Table 16-6 for commonly prescribed antiepileptic drugs (AEDs) and their adverse reactions.

Anxiolytics

Clonazepam (Klonopin) and Lorazepam (Ativan). Clonazepam and lorazepam are useful in the treatment of acute mania in some patients with treatment-resistant mania. These drugs are also effective in managing the psychomotor agitation seen in mania. They should be avoided, however, in patients with a history of substance use disorder.

Second-Generation Antipsychotics

In addition to showing sedative properties during the early phase of treatment, which may help with insomnia, anxiety, and agitation, the newer atypical antipsychotics seem to have mood-stabilizing properties. The four FDA-approved second-generation antipsychotics recommended as primary agents in the treatment of both acute mania and mixed mania are olanzapine (Zyprexa), risperidone (Risperdal), aripiprazole (Abilify), and ziprasidone (Geodon). Quetiapine (Seroquel) is FDA approved for acute mania but not for mixed mania. Of the aforementioned medications, only aripiprazole and olanzapine are FDA approved for maintenance therapy in bipolar disorders (Preston et al., 2013).

TABLE 16-6 Antiepileptic Drugs

Drug	Major Adverse Effects
Carbamazepine (Tegretol, Equerto, and others) FDA approved	• **Agranulocytosis** and **aplastic anemia** are most serious adverse reactions • Blood levels should be monitored throughout first 8 weeks because drug induces liver enzymes that speed its own metabolism. Dosage may need to be adjusted to maintain serum level of 6–8 mg/L. • Immediate action when severe adverse reactions appear (e.g., confusion, difficulty breathing, irregular heartbeat, skin rash or hives, jaundice) • Best use is for treatment and prevention of manic episodes. It is less effective for treatment and prevention of depression
Valproic acid (Depakene) **Valproic acid delayed reaction** (Stavzor) **Divalproex delayed release** (Depakote) Valproate injectable (Depacon) FDA approved	• **Baseline liver function tests should be performed and results monitored** at regular intervals • Bipolar disorder; bipolar depression • Hepatitis, although rare, has been reported, with fatalities in children. Symptoms include fever, chills, right upper quadrant pain, dark urine, malaise, jaundice/confusion, significant drowsiness • Best use for men and older women. Can cause birth defects in pregnant women • Lithium is more effective in reducing the risk of suicide and at preventing relapses. Divalproex has a more rapid onset and efficacy and is often chosen for first-line treatment; however, divalproex is effective in rapid cyclers and in mixed mania
Lamotrigine (Lamictal) FDA approved	• **Life-threatening** rash reported in 3 out of every 1000 individuals (Stevens-Johnson syndrome) • **Rare but potential** aseptic meningitis risk with lamotrigine • Use caution when renal, hepatic, or cardiac function is impaired • Often used in combination with other mood-stabilizing drugs, it is a good drug for long-term maintenance therapy • Bipolar depression; pain
Topiramate (Topamax)	• Used in acute mania or in combination with other drugs • Adverse effects include weight loss, cognitive side effects, fatigue, dizziness, and paresthesia • **Used off-label; not presently FDA approved** for bipolar disorder
Oxcarbazepine (Trileptal)	• Structural variant of carbamazepine • Thought to have better side effect profile and more favorable drug interaction profiles • **Used off-label; not presently FDA approved** for bipolar disorder

FDA, U.S. Food and Drug Administration.

Electroconvulsive Therapy

Electroconvulsive therapy (ECT) is used to subdue severe manic behavior. It is especially helpful in patients with treatment-resistant mania and patients with rapid cycling (i.e., those who experience four or more episodes of illness in 1 year). ECT is effective in patients with bipolar disorder who experience paranoid-destructive features (who often respond poorly to lithium therapy) and in those patients who are acutely suicidal (see Chapter 23).

Continuation Phase

The treatment continuation phase is a crucial one for patients and their families. The outcome for this phase is to prevent relapse. Community resources are chosen based on the needs of the patient, the appropriateness of the referral, and the availability of resources. Frequently, it is a case manager who evaluates appropriate follow-up care for patients and their families.

Medication adherence during this phase is perhaps the most important treatment outcome. This follow-up is frequently handled in a mental health center. However, adherence to the medication regimen is also addressed in day hospitals and in psychiatric home care visits. Some patients may attend day hospitals if they are not too excitable and are able to tolerate a certain level of stimuli. In addition to medication oversight, day hospitals offer structure, decrease social isolation, and help patients channel their time and energy. If a patient is homebound and unable to get to a mental health center or day hospital, then psychiatric home care is the appropriate modality for follow-up care.

Health Teaching and Health Promotion

Patients and families need information about bipolar illness with particular emphasis on the chronic and highly recurrent nature of the illness. They also need to be taught the symptoms of impending episodes. For example, changes in sleep patterns are especially important because they usually precede, accompany, or precipitate mania. Even a single night of unexplainable sleep loss can be taken as an early warning of impending mania. Health teaching stresses the importance of establishing regularity in sleep patterns, meals, exercise, and other activities.

Psychoeducation includes a rich combination of tools to improve functional outcomes for patients and their families (Box 16-2). At the very least, psychoeducation increases compliance by improving the regularity of daily life and sleep habits and by providing clear guidelines for both patients and families to follow.

Maintenance Phase

Maintenance therapy is aimed at preventing recurrence. Not only are some of the community resources cited earlier helpful, but patients and their families often greatly benefit from mutual support and self-help groups.

BOX 16-2   Psychoeducation for Patients with Bipolar Disorder and Their Families

Patients with bipolar disorder and their families need to know the following:

1. The chronic, cyclic, and episodic nature of bipolar disorder.
2. The fact that bipolar disorder is a long-term illness and that it requires maintenance treatment; therefore one or more mood-stabilizing agents may be taken for a long time.
3. The expected side effects and toxic effects of the prescribed medication, as well as whom to call and where to go in case of a toxic reaction.
4. The signs and symptoms of relapse that may "come out of the blue."
5. The role of family members and others in preventing a full relapse.
6. The phone numbers of emergency contact people, which should be kept in an easily accessed place.
7. The use of alcohol, drugs of abuse, even small amounts of caffeine, and over-the-counter medications can produce a relapse.
8. Good sleep hygiene is critical to stability. Frequently, the prodrome of a manic episode is lack of sleep. In some cases, mania may be averted by the use of sleep medications (e.g., temazepam [Restoril]).
9. Psychosocial strategies are important for dealing with work, interpersonal, and family problems; lowering stress; enhancing a sense of personal control; and increasing community functioning.
10. Group and individual psychotherapy is invaluable for gaining insight as well as skills in relapse prevention, providing social support, increasing coping skills in interpersonal relations, improving compliance with the medication regimen, reducing functional morbidity, and decreasing re-hospitalizations.

Health care workers need to remember the following:

1. Minimization and denial are common defenses that require gradual introduction of facts.
2. Anger and abusive remarks, although aimed at the health care provider, are symptoms of the disease and are not personal.

Adapted from Zerbe, K. J. (1999). *Women's mental health in primary care.* Philadelphia, PA: Saunders; Milkowitz, D. J. (2003). Bipolar disorder. In D. H. Barlow (Ed.), *Clinical handbook of psychological disorders* (pp. 523–560). New York, NY: Guilford Press.

Psychosocial Interventions

Pharmacotherapy and continuous psychosocial support are essential in the treatment of bipolar spectrum disorders. Individuals with bipolar spectrum disorders suffer from the psychosocial consequences of their past episodes and their vulnerability to experiencing future episodes. People who have bipolar disorder also have to face the burden of long-term treatments that may involve some unpleasant side effects.

During the course of their illness, many patients have sustained strained interpersonal relationships, marriage and family problems, academic and occupational problems, and legal or other social difficulties. Psychotherapy can help people work through these difficulties, which not only decreases some of the psychic distress but also increases self-esteem. Psychotherapeutic treatments in conjunction with psychopharmacology also can help patients improve their functioning between episodes and attempt to decrease the frequency of future episodes.

Psychotherapy

Psychotherapy is an important treatment in bipolar illness and results in greater compliance with the lithium regimen (Jamison, 1995b). Often patients receiving medication and psychotherapy place more value on psychotherapy than do clinicians. Moreover, patients treated with cognitive therapy are more likely to take their

medications as prescribed than patients who do not participate in therapy (Jamison, 1995a).

One patient describes her feelings about drug therapy and psychotherapy as follows (Jamison, 1995b):

VIGNETTE

I cannot imagine leading a normal life without lithium. From starting and stopping of it, I now know it is an essential part of my sanity. Lithium prevents my seductive but disastrous highs, diminishes my depressions, clears out the weaving of my disordered thinking, slows me, gentles me out, keeps me in my relationships, in my career, out of a hospital, and in psychotherapy. It keeps me alive, too.

But psychotherapy heals, it makes some sense of the confusion, it reins in the terrifying thoughts and feelings, it brings back hope and the possibility of learning from it all. Pills cannot, do not, ease one back into reality. They bring you back headlong, careening, and faster than can be endured at times. Psychotherapy is a sanctuary, it is a battleground, and it is where I have come to believe that someday I may be able to contend with all of this. No pill can help me deal with the problem of not wanting to take pills, but no amount of therapy alone can prevent my manias and depressions. I need both.

A large multicenter study showed increased rates of recovery from an acute episode using cognitive behavioral therapy (CBT), interpersonal and social rhythm therapy (IPSRT), and family focused therapy (Perlis & Ostacher, 2015).

Cognitive behavioral therapy. **Cognitive behavioral therapy,** an adaptation of Beck's cognitive therapy treatment for depression, is a skills-oriented form of therapy. CBT has been found valuable in helping patients with bipolar disorder accept their illness and the need for medical treatment. Some studies have pointed out that cognitive techniques have also been shown to be effective in decreasing affective symptoms, increasing social functioning, reducing the rate of relapse, and reducing the number of hospital admissions.

CBT focuses mainly on medication adherence, early detection and intervention, and stress and lifestyle management using a variety of CBT techniques. These interventions have been found most effective with patients who have bipolar I disorder. CBT is typically used as an adjunct to pharmacotherapy and involves identifying maladaptive cognitions and behaviors that may be barriers to a person's recovery and ongoing mood stability. It is also being used for bipolar disorder in children.

Interpersonal and social rhythm therapy. **Interpersonal and social rhythm therapy,** a formalized psychotherapy, is based on the idea that problems in interpersonal relationships and disruptions in daily routines can contribute to the recurrence of manic and depressive episodes in an individual with a bipolar disorder. IPSRT has been found effective in shortening a depressive episode in bipolar I patients. The interpersonal aspects of IPSRT derive from interpersonal psychotherapy (ITP) and focus on resolutions of interpersonal problems (e.g., unresolved grief, disputes, and role transitions) and prevention of further disputes. IPSRT is effective in the acute as well as the maintenance phases of treatment.

Family-focused therapy. Behavioral family management, family therapy, and psychoeducation help families stay together, lead to lower rates of rehospitalization, and improve family functioning. Family-focused therapy (FFT) combines many of the key target areas of CBT and IPSRT, including:

- Psychoeducation
- Relapse drill (prevention)
- Ways to make the diagnosis of bipolar disorder more acceptable to the patient

FFT is different from CBT and IPSRT in that it includes the family in therapy. FFT focuses on communication within the family, teaches communication skills, and prepares the entire family for relapse episodes.

Summary

To say that the pharmacological and psychological treatments that are currently available for bipolar disorder can improve the outcome and quality of life for people with bipolar disorders is valid. However, the access to such specialized treatments are concentrated in few reference centers around the globe, which can hardly cover the needs of a disease with a prevalence of almost 2% of the world population (Hidalgo-Mazzei et al., 2015). Newer electronic technologies (*informatics*) hope to increase access and bridge that gap. One of a variety of studies currently under way is aimed at combining a "signs and symptoms" monitoring system in a single smartphone application as an adjunctive intervention to medications and selected therapies. Hopefully this study will help determine the efficacy in preventing relapses, suicide attempts, and health resources consumption in bipolar patients improving their overall prognosis using interactive informatics.

Support Groups

Patients with bipolar disorder, as well as their friends and families, benefit from forming mutual support groups, such as those sponsored by the Depression and Bipolar Support Alliance (DBSA), the National Alliance on Mental Illness (NAMI), the National Mental Health Association, and the Manic-Depressive Association.

EVALUATION

Outcome criteria often dictate the frequency of evaluation of short-term and intermediate indicators. For example, does the patient have stable vital signs? Is the patient well hydrated within safe time limits? Is the patient able to control his or her own behavior or respond to external controls? Is the patient able to sleep for 4 or 5 hours per night or take frequent short rest periods during the day? Does the family have a clear understanding of the patient's disease and need for medication? Do the patient and family know which community agencies may help them?

If outcomes or related indicators are not achieved satisfactorily, the preventing factors are analyzed. Were the data incorrect or insufficient? Were nursing diagnoses inappropriate or outcomes unrealistic? Was intervention poorly planned? After the outcomes and care plan are reassessed, the plan is revised if indicated. Longer-term outcomes include compliance with the medication regimen; resumption of functioning in the community; achievement of stability in family, work, and social relationships and in mood; and improved coping skills for reducing stress.

KEY POINTS TO REMEMBER

- Biological factors appear to play a role in the etiology of the bipolar disorders. Strong genetic correlates have been revealed, especially through twin studies.
- Little doubt exists that an excess and/or imbalance in neurotransmitters is also related to bipolar mood swings, which supports the existence of neurobiological influences.
- Neuroendocrine and neuroanatomical findings support evidence for biological influences.
- Bipolar disorder often remains unrecognized, and early detection can help diminish co-occurring substance use disorders, suicide, and declines in social and personal relationships, and may help promote more positive outcomes.

- The nurse assesses the patient's level of mood (hypomania, acute mania, delirious mania), behavior, thought processes, and thought content and is alert to cognitive dysfunction.
- Some nursing diagnoses appropriate for a patient who is manic are *Risk for violence, Defensive coping, Ineffective coping, Impaired mood regulation, Labile emotional control,* and *Situational low self-esteem.*
- During the acute phase of mania, physical needs often take priority and demand nursing interventions. Therefore deficient fluid volume and imbalanced nutrition or elimination, as well as disturbed sleep pattern, are usually addressed in the nursing plan.
- Nurses and all staff need to use consistent limit-setting strategies using a neutral tone when a patient displays intrusive interpersonal behaviors and intervene quickly with impulsive and aggressive behaviors.
- The diagnosis *Interrupted family processes* is vital. Support groups, psychoeducation, and guidance for the family can greatly affect the patient's compliance with the medication regimen.
- Planning nursing care involves identifying the specific needs of the patient and family during the three phases of mania.
- Antimanic medications are available. Lithium has a narrow therapeutic index, which necessitates thorough patient and family teaching and regular follow-up. AEDs such as carbamazepine and valproic acid are useful, especially in treating people with disease refractory to lithium therapy; newer AEDs are also useful in treating patients who need rapid de-escalation and do not respond to other treatment approaches.
- Antipsychotic agents may be needed because of their sedating and mood-stabilizing properties, especially during initial treatment until antimanic medications kick in.
- For some patients, ECT may be the most appropriate medical treatment.
- Patient and family teaching takes many forms and is most important in encouraging compliance with the medication regimen and reducing the risk of relapse.
- Evaluation includes examining the effectiveness of the nursing interventions, changing the outcomes as needed, and reassessing the nursing diagnoses. Evaluation is an ongoing process and is part of each of the other steps in the nursing process.

APPLYING CRITICAL JUDGMENT

1. Kioshi Sung is taken into the emergency department after threatening in a loud voice to "Blow up the world to save the poor, and many more, where's the door? No more, no more. Let me loose." He had attacked a bartender who would not give him any more to drink. He has not eaten or slept for more than 1 week and only takes sips of fluids when offered. He talks nonstop, moving constantly, flailing his arms, and bumping into objects as he walks rapidly.
   A. Identify Mr. Sung's immediate needs (in terms of a nursing diagnosis). Describe the interventions you would plan for his physiological safety and his milieu (safe environment).
   B. Discuss the most appropriate communication techniques and approaches for Mr. Sung at this time. Give examples of what you would say and how you would say it.
   C. What possible medications would Mr. Sung most likely be given immediately? Long term?
   D. Write a medication treatment plan for Mr. Sung and his family.
   E. Describe at least four evidence-based therapeutic modalities for a bipolar patient.
   F. What symptoms would help you evaluate if a bipolar client was in hypomania, mania, or extreme mania?
   G. Name the most important interventions you would institute for each of the three phases of mania.

CHAPTER REVIEW QUESTIONS

1. A patient has a long history of bipolar disorder with frequent episodes of mania secondary to stopping prescribed medications. The patient says, "I will use my whole check next month to buy lottery tickets. Winning will solve my money problems." Select the nurse's best action.
   a. Educate the patient about the low odds of winning the lottery.
   b. Present reality by saying to the patient, "That is not good use of your money."
   c. Confer with the treatment team about appointing a legal guardian for the patient.
   d. Tell the patient, "If you buy lottery tickets, your money will run out before the end of the month."

2. Which comment by a patient diagnosed with bipolar disorder best indicates the patient is experiencing mania?
   a. "I have been sleeping about 6 hours each night."
   b. "Yesterday I made 487 posts on my social network page."
   c. "I am having dreams about my father's death 8 years ago."
   d. "My appetite is so robust that I've gained 4 pounds in the past 2 weeks."

3. A community mental health nurse counsels a group of patients about the upcoming flu season. What instruction does the nurse provide for patients who are prescribed lithium?
   a. "Stop taking your medicine and contact me if you have nausea, vomiting, and/or diarrhea."
   b. "Remember that lithium reduces your immunity, so you are more vulnerable to catching the flu."
   c. "The flu is contagious. Isolate yourself if you get the flu so that you avoid exposing others to it."
   d. "Because you take lithium, you may have flu symptoms that are not typically experienced by others."

4. A patient was diagnosed with bipolar disorder many years ago. The patient tells the nurse, "When I have a manic episode, there's always a feeling of gloom behind it and I know I will soon be totally depressed." What is the nurse's best response?
   a. "Most patients diagnosed with bipolar disorder report the same types of feelings."
   b. "Feelings of gloom associated with depression result from serotonin dysregulation."
   c. "If you take your medication as it is prescribed, you will not have those experiences."
   d. "Your comment indicates you have an understanding and insight about your disorder."

5. A patient diagnosed with bipolar disorder lives in the community and is showing early signs of mania. The patient says, "I need to go visit my daughter but she lives across the country. I put some requests on the Internet to get a ride. I'm sure someone will take me." What is the nurse's most therapeutic response?
   a. "I'm concerned about your safety when meeting or riding with strangers."
   b. "Have you asked friends and family to donate money for your airfare?"
   c. "You are not likely to get a ride. Let's consider some other strategies."
   d. "Have you asked your daughter if she wants you to come for a visit?"

REFERENCES

American Psychiatric Association. (2013). *Diagnostic and statistical manual of mental disorders (DSM-5)* (5th ed.). Washington, DC: Author.

Black, D. W., & Andreasen, N. C. (2014). *Introductory textbook of psychiatry* (6th ed.). Washington, DC: American Psychiatric Publishing.

Brooks, M. (2015). *Bipolar disorder recognized earlier, mortality remains high*. Retrieved May 23, 2015, from www.medscape.com/viewarticle/8454150.

Burchum, J., & Rosenthal, L. (2016). *Lehne's pharmacology for nursing care* (9th ed.). St Louis, MO: Elsevier.

Dias, R. (2011). Fluctuating hormones linked to more severe bipolar symptoms. *American Journal of Psychiatry, news release*. Retrieved March 12, 2011, from www.nih.gov/mrdlneplus/news/fullstory08850.html.

Gitlin, M., & Frye, M. A. (2012). Maintenance therapies in bipolar disorders. *Bipolar Disorders, 14*(Suppl 2), 51–65.

Hidalgo-Mazzei, D., Mateu, A., Reinares, M., et al. (2015). Self-monitoring and psychoeducation in bipolar patients with a smartphone application (simple) project: design, development and studies protocols. *BMC Psychiatry, 15*, 52.

Hodgson, B. B., & Kizior, R. J. (2013). *Saunders nursing handbook 2013*. St Louis, MO: Elsevier Saunders.

Jamison, K. R. (1995a). *An unquiet mind*. New York, NY: Knopf.

Jamison, K. R. (1995b). *Psychotherapy of bipolar patients*. New York: Paper presented at the U.S. Psychiatric and Mental Health Congress, November 18, 1995.

La Rose, L. (2015). The intersection of genetics, mental illness, and stigma. Retrieved September 6, 2015, from www.theravive.com/blog/post/2015/01/06/The-Intersection-of-Genetics-Mental-Illness-and-Stigma.aspx.

Miklowitz, D. J., & Gitlin, M. J. (2014). *Clinicians guide to bipolar disorder; Integrating pharmacology and psychotherapy*. New York, NY: Guilford Publications.

Perlis, R. H., & Ostacher, M. (2015). Bipolar disorder. In T. A. Stern, M. Fava, T. E. Wilens, & J. F. Rosenbaum (Eds.), *Massachusetts General Hospital comprehensive clinical psychiatry* (2nd ed.). St Louis, MO: Elsevier.

Preston, J., & Johnson, J. (2015). *Clinical psychopharmacology made ridiculously simple* (8th ed.). Miami, FL: MedMasters.

Preston, J. D., O'Neal, J. H., & Talaga, M. C. (2013). *Handbook of clinical psychopharmacology for therapists* (6th ed.). Oakland, CA: New Harbinger Publications.

Richmond, J. S., Berlin, J. S., Fishkind, A. B., et al. (2012). Verbal de-escalation of the agitated patient: Consensus statement of the American Association for Emergency Psychiatry Project BETA de-escalation workgroup. *Western Journal of Emergency Medicine, 13*(1), 17–25.

Skidmore-Roth, L. (2013). *Mosby's nursing drug reference* (26th ed.). St Louis, MO: Mosby.

Soreff, S., & McInnes, L. A. (2011). *Bipolar affective disorder*. Retrieved January 21, 2011, from http://emedicine.com.medscape.com/article/286342–overview.

S., Food U., & Drug Administration (FDA). (2010). *Lamictal (lamotrigine): label change—risk of aseptic meningitis*. Retrieved March 14, 2011, from www.fda.gov/Safety/MedWatch/SafetyInformation/Safety.

Wisner, K. L., Lockmen-Westin, E., Finnerty, M., et al. (2011). Valproate prescription prevalence among women of childbearing age. *Psychiatric Services, 62*, 218–220. Retrieved June 16, 2011, from psychservices.psychiatryonline.org/cgi/content/abstract/62/.

Zerbe, K. J. (1999). *Women's mental health in primary care*. Philadelphia, PA: Saunders.

Schizophrenia Spectrum Disorders and Other Psychotic Disorders

Elizabeth M. Varcarolis

http://evolve.elsevier.com/Varcarolis/essentials

KEY TERMS AND CONCEPTS

acute dystonia, p. 266
affect, p. 250
akathisia, p. 266
anosognosia, p. 245
associative looseness, p. 248
clang association, p. 249
cognitive symptoms, p. 247
concrete thinking, p. 248
delusions, p. 248
echolalia, p. 249
echopraxia, p. 249
extrapyramidal symptoms (EPS), p. 263
first-generation antipsychotics (FGAs)/
    conventional drugs, p. 263

hallucinations, p. 249
ideas of reference, p. 252
illusions, p. 249
negative symptoms, p. 247
neologisms, p. 248
neurocognitive symptoms, p. 251
neuroleptic malignant syndrome (NMS),
    p. 266
paranoia, p. 252
positive symptoms, p. 247
projection, p. 252
pseudoparkinsonism, p. 266
psychotic, p. 244
recovery model for schizophrenia, p. 260

second-generation antipsychotics (SGAs)/
    atypical agents, p. 263
stereotyped behaviors, p. 250
tardive dyskinesia (TD), p. 266
thought broadcasting, p. 248
thought insertion, p. 248
thought withdrawal, p. 248
waxy flexibility, p. 250
word salad, p. 249

SELECTED CONCEPTS: PSYCHOEDUCATION

An evidenced-based approach for patients and families with a schizophrenic member is a **psychoeducational approach.** Psycho-education brings educational and behavioral approaches into family treatment. The psychoeducational approach recognizes that families are secondary victims of a biological illness. In family therapy sessions, fears, faulty communication patterns, and distortions are identified. Improved problem-solving skills can be taught, and healthier alternatives to situations of conflict can be explored. A review of 44 studies showed that educating patients about the nature of their illness and treatment when added to standard care led to reduced admission and relapse as well as encouraged medication adherence. Teaching patients and families about the disease, need for medications, prodromal symptoms of relapse, and communication skills, resulted in increased satisfaction with mental health services, and improved quality of life (Xia et al., 2011)

OBJECTIVES

1. Describe the prodromal (early) symptoms that a person with schizophrenia may exhibit during the prepsychotic phase.
2. **QSEN** Identify **evidence-based** data that support the premise that schizophrenia is a neurological disease.
3. Compare and contrast the positive and negative symptoms of schizophrenia with regard to (a) their effect on quality of life, (b) their significance for the prognosis of the disease, and (c) their side effect profile.
4. Delineate ways that neurocognitive impairments affect a person who is struggling with schizophrenia; include prognosis and quality-of-life indicators.
5. **QSEN** Identify the numerous areas in which health care workers need to apply **safety** interventions for a person with schizophrenia during the different phases of treatment.
6. **QSEN** Demonstrate with classmates the best **evidence-based practice** we currently have for communicating with a person who is (a) hallucinating, (b) paranoid, and (c) experiencing delusions.

7. Teach a classmate, group, or friend the differences between the properties of first-generation antipsychotics (conventional) and those of second-generation (atypical) antipsychotic drugs regarding the following: (a) target symptoms, (b) indications for use, (c) adverse effects and toxic effects, (d) need for patient and family teaching and follow-up, and (e) potential for medical compliance.
8. **QSEN** Discuss **evidence-based** psychosocial therapies for patients with schizophrenia and their families.
9. Differentiate among the three phases of schizophrenia in terms of symptoms, focus of care, and intervention needs using Table 17-5 as a guide.
10. **QSEN** Identify specific times when **teamwork and collaboration** with other health care professionals are paramount for the implementation of safe and effective care for a person with schizophrenia.

OBJECTIVES—cont'd

11. **QSEN** Using **informatics**, search the web for available resources for patients and families coping with schizophrenia in your area (e.g., Mental Health America [www.nmha.org] or National Alliance on Mental Illness [NAMI] [www.nami.org/]).

12. **QSEN** Using **informatics**, search the web for a copy of the AIMS test for the detection of tardive dyskinesia (TD) (e.g., www.cqaimh.org/pdf/tool_aims.pdf).

13. Name and describe at least four other primary psychotic disorders.

INTRODUCTION

The schizophrenia spectrum disorders are devastating brain diseases that target young people in their teens or early twenties at the beginning of their productive lives. It is rarely evidenced in childhood. Schizophrenia profoundly disrupts an individual's ability to perceive reality accurately, to think clearly, to use language appropriately, to experience normal emotions, or to engage in normal social/occupational experiences. Schizophrenia spectrum disorders are a group of psychotic disorders. In a recent study of gene groups in people with schizophrenia, researchers were able to identify eight different gene profiles that indicate genetically different types of schizophrenia (Nauert, 2015).

Psychosis is not a diagnosis but a symptom. **Psychosis** refers to a total inability to recognize reality—for example, experiencing *delusions* (profoundly believing in ideas with no basis in fact, such as "I have the power to save the world") and *hallucinations* (experiencing sensory perceptions that are not based in reality, such as hearing voices that tell a person to jump in front of a train, or that they are a bad person).

Schizophrenia spectrum disorders affect people in different ways. Individuals diagnosed with schizophrenia vary widely in terms of their disabilities, presentations, and quality of life. Individuals with schizophrenia spectrum disorders have varying degrees of neurocognitive impairments, which are evidenced by disorganized thinking and disorganized speech. The neurocognitive aspects are perhaps among the most destructive features of schizophrenia. People with these disorders are usually socially isolated or alienated and have deep feelings of inadequacy, and it goes without saying that these disabilities ensure a poor quality of life. Other disruptive primary psychotic disorders are identified in Box 17-1.

Some individuals with schizophrenia function well with the aid of medications and social supports. Others are more disabled, and need a higher level of support in terms of housing, health maintenance, monetary aid, and more. Although schizophrenia is treatable, it is not curable and is a chronic and severe mental illness (SMI) (refer to Chapter 27, which outlines needs and supports for the severe mentally disabled in the community). Many individuals diagnosed with

BOX 17-1   Other Psychotic Disorders

Disorder and Incidence	Course	Description
Schizophreniform disorder Incidence 0.2%	Symptoms may last only a short time—from 1 to 6 months—and impaired social or occupational functioning is usually not apparent.	The essential features are exactly the same as those of schizophrenia (e.g., hallucinations, delusions, disorganized speech, grossly disorganized or catatonic behavior, and negative symptoms).
Brief psychotic disorder Not common	The episode is usually short-lived (1 day/no longer than a month) and the person returns to his or her premorbid level of functioning. Usually precipitated by extreme stress.	Brief psychotic disorder is characterized by a sudden onset of psychotic symptoms (delusions, hallucinations, disorganized speech) or grossly disorganized or catatonic behavior.
Schizoaffective disorder Incidence 0.3%	Better prognosis than schizophrenia, but significantly worse than a mood disorder.	Uninterrupted period of illness during which there is a major depressive, manic, or mixed episode, concurrent with symptoms that meet the criteria for schizophrenia. All other causes being ruled out.
Schizotypal (personality) disorder* (refer to Chapter 13) Incidence 0.2%	Relatively stable disorder with a few individuals progressing to schizophrenia.	A personality disorder considered by the *DSM-5* to be part of the schizophrenia spectrum disorders because it shares common genetics and neuropsychiatric characteristics.
Delusional disorder Incidence 0.2%	Ranges from remission without relapse to chronic waxing and waning.	Involves nonbizarre delusions (situations that occur in real life; e.g., being followed, infected, loved at a distance, or deceived by a spouse; having some great or unrecognized insight; or having a disease) for at least 1 month. The person's ability to function is not markedly impaired nor is the person's behavior obviously odd or bizarre. Delusions of persecution are the most common.
Substance/medication-induced psychotic disorder	This is an unfortunate everyday occurrence that is often fatal.	Caused by the ingestion or during withdrawal from a substance.

*Schizotypal personality disorder is discussed further in Chapter 13.

schizophrenia, even if given formal and informal supports, live with exacerbations and remissions of their active symptoms, and others have a chronic course of progressive deterioration (APA, 2013). Great progress in a person's functional ability and quality of life has been made even more possible with supports and methods through the Recovery Movement applied to schizophrenia and other psychotic disorders. Unfortunately, individuals with schizophrenia often don't believe that they are ill, which leads to complications in treatment. This condition is called anosognosia (the inability of a person to recognize that he or she has an illness because of the illness itself).

PREVALENCE AND COMORBIDITY

The lifetime prevalence of schizophrenia is said to be 1% worldwide with no differences related to race, social status, culture, gender, or environment (Sadock et al., 2015); according to the National Alliance on Mental Illness (2013), approximately 1.1% of American adults (about 2.6 million people) live with schizophrenia. A premorbid condition can be an indication of the potential complexity and eventual outcome for an individual who is later diagnosed with schizophrenia. For example, individuals with an early age of onset (18 to 25 years) are more often male and have poorer premorbid adjustment, more evidence of structural brain abnormalities, and more prominent negative symptoms. Individuals with a later onset (25 to 35 years) are more likely to be female, have less evidence of structural brain abnormalities, and have better outcomes. The younger the patient is at the onset of schizophrenia, the more discouraging the prognosis.

An abrupt onset of symptoms with good premorbid functioning is usually a more favorable prognostic sign. A slow, insidious onset over a period of 2 or 3 years is more ominous. Those whose prepsychotic personalities demonstrated good social, sexual, and occupational functioning have a greater chance for remission or complete recovery. A childhood history of withdrawn, reclusive, eccentric, and tense behavior is an unfavorable diagnostic sign.

Substance use disorders occur in more than 50% of individuals with schizophrenia (Sadock et al., 2015). Substance use is associated with a variety of negative outcomes, including incarceration, homelessness, violence, suicide, and infection with human immunodeficiency virus (HIV), and is linked with a poorer prognosis. **Tobacco use disorder** is very common in people with schizophrenia, and according to the *DSM-5*, more than 50% have a tobacco use disorder (APA, 2013). Smoking results in significant morbidity and mortality and is linked with a high rate of emphysema and other pulmonary and cardiac problems. These risks are even greater in people with schizophrenia because they tend to smoke two to three times more than the average smoker.

Depressive symptoms occur frequently in schizophrenia. **Suicide** is the leading cause of premature death in this population, accounting for about 6% to 10% of deaths in those who have schizophrenia (Sadock et al., 2015), and approximately 20% of those with schizophrenia attempt suicide during their lifetime (APA, 2013). The rates of co-occurring **anxiety disorders, obsessive-compulsive disorder, and panic attacks** are also significantly higher in this population than in the general population. Individuals diagnosed with **schizotypal or paranoid personality disorders** may later progress to full-blown schizophrenia (APA, 2013).

Obesity is significantly higher in schizophrenia, and perhaps in large part due to many of the antipsychotic medications, in particular the second-generation antipsychotics (SGAs)/atypical agents. Weight gain in turn often contributes to the development of comorbid **diabetes** and risk of **cardiovascular disease** (Sadock et al., 2015). **HIV** in schizophrenia is double the rate for the general population, associated with high-risk factors.

THEORY

Determining the causes of schizophrenia is clearly a complicated matter. What is known is that brain chemistry and brain activity are different in a person with schizophrenia than in a person without schizophrenia. The schizophrenias most likely occur as a result of a combination of **inherited genetic factors** and extreme **nongenetic factors** (e.g., virus infection, birth injuries, nutritional factors, head trauma early in life), which can affect the genes governing the brain or injure the brain directly. Both of these factors may eventually alter the structures of the brain, affect the brain's neurotransmitter system, and disrupt the neural circuits, resulting in impairment in cognition.

Neurochemical Contributing Factors

For many years the **dopamine hypothesis** was the most widely accepted explanation for the biochemical pathophysiology in schizophrenia. The dopamine hypothesis concluded there was a hyperactivity of the neurotransmitter dopamine in the limbic regions of the brain. This theory was derived from the study of the action of the first-generation antipsychotics (FGA)/conventional drugs that block the activity of dopamine (D_2) and, in doing so, reduce some of the symptoms of schizophrenia. This theory is enhanced by the fact that amphetamines, cocaine, methylphenidate (Ritalin), and levodopa are drugs that increase the activity of dopamine in the brain. These drugs can exacerbate the symptoms of schizophrenia in psychotic patients and simulate symptoms of schizophrenia with paranoid features in a person without schizophrenia.

With the development of the **SGAs**/atypical agents, which block serotonin (5-hydroxytryptamine, $5\text{-}HT_2$), it became apparent that **serotonin** might also play a role in causing some of the symptoms of schizophrenia. Another hypothesis postulates a role for other neurotransmitter systems in the pathophysiology of schizophrenia. One is glutamate or γ-aminobutyric acid (GABA). The glutamate hypothesis suggests that there is hypofunction in N-methyl-D-aspartate (NMDA) receptors in the glutamate system that leads to a combination of excitotoxicity and impaired neural plasticity (Black & Andreasen, 2014). Phencyclidine hydrochloride (PCP) induces a state that closely resembles schizophrenia. This observation led to sustained interest in the NMDA receptor complex and the possible role of **glutamate** in the pathophysiology of schizophrenia.

Genetic Factors

Numerous studies have substantiated over time that schizophrenia has a strong genetic component. Although most people with schizophrenia do not have a family history of the disease, schizophrenia and schizophrenia-like symptoms occur in about 10% of siblings of schizophrenic patients. A child who has one parent with schizophrenia has a 5% to 6% chance of developing the disease, whereas a child with two schizophrenic parents has a 46% likelihood of schizophrenia (Black & Andreasen, 2014). Numerous studies of twins (fraternal and identical) emphasize a significantly higher probability of a gene involvement, with close to 46% of identical twins versus 14% of fraternal twins being at risk for schizophrenia (Black & Andreasen, 2014). For identical twins reared apart the concordance rate for schizophrenia is similar.

Similar to gene involvement with bipolar spectrum disorders, schizophrenia is not a "one gene, one illness" disease, but rather caused by the involvement of multiple genes and other factors. Researchers have begun to identify many regions on chromosomes that are probably related to the development of schizophrenia spectrum disorders. In a recent study previously mentioned, researchers identified a group of eight genetically different types of schizophrenias. They found that there are different networks of 42 genes that work together to produce specific symptom profiles (e.g., positive symptoms, cognitive symptoms, disorganization) and that these symptom profiles reveal eight qualitative types of schizophrenias (Nauert, 2015).

Recent research has focused on a new schizophrenia risk gene called **C-4** which is responsible for a biological process called *synaptic pruning*. Synaptic pruning is the elimination of weak or redundant connections between neurons in the area of the brain associated with thinking and planning skills as the brain matures. This process occurs naturally in the teen years. The current hypothesis is that these genes go into overdrive and cause excessive or inappropriate "pruning" of neural connections that lead to the cognitive symptoms seen in schizophrenia. Therefore, individuals who acquire or inherit the mutated C-4 gene would have a higher risk of developing schizophrenia (Chavan, 2016; Rettner, 2016).

Neuroanatomical Factors

It is commonly accepted that schizophrenia has a neuroprogressive component that occurs after the onset of the disease and includes tissue volume decrease in both gray and white matter. Major emphasis is focused on the frontal lobes (Weinmann, 2015). Disruptions in the connections and communication within neural circuitry (communication pathways) are thought to be severe in schizophrenia. Therefore it is conceivable that structural cerebral abnormalities cause disruption to the entire circuitry of the brain. Numerous brain imaging techniques—such as computed tomography (CT), magnetic resonance imaging (MRI), functional MRI (fMRI), and positron emission tomography (PET)—provide substantial evidence that some people with schizophrenia have structural brain abnormalities. For example, MRI and CT scans demonstrate lower brain volume, larger lateral and third ventricles, atrophy in the frontal lobe, and more cerebrospinal fluid, among other findings, in some people with schizophrenia. PET scans show a low rate of blood flow and glucose metabolism in the frontal lobes of the cerebral cortex. The prefrontal cortex (PFC) plays a big role in cognitive functioning, which involves planning, abstract thinking, memory, social adjustment, decision making, and attention. Recently there has been evidence of faulty wiring between the PFC and other brain areas that are thought to cause cognitive disorders. In schizophrenia there seems to be disruption in the brain circuitry between the PFC and the thalamus (Cold Spring Harbor Laboratory, 2015). Other studies indicate that there is a decrease in cortical gray matter as well. Brain scans can disclose abnormalities of brain structure and function in schizophrenia. Although these studies are of interest for research, presently they have limited clinical relevance (Gerstein & Shlamovitz, 2015).

These are just a few of the many findings on brain imaging. Black and Andreasen (2014) state that the current thinking on the neuroanatomical findings of schizophrenia suggests a disease of multiple disturbed circuits in the brain.

Nongenetic Risk Factors

Infants for whom there is a history of perinatal complications (e.g., birth complications/injury) are at increased risk for developing schizophrenia as adults. Prenatal risk factors include viral infection (influenza, toxoplasmosis, and genital/reproductive infection), poor nutrition or starvation, or exposure to toxins. Lack of oxygen during birth is also considered a risk factor for the development of schizophrenia. Essentially, any early insult to the brain of a developing fetus or child (e.g., viral infections, environmental toxins, presence of certain genes) can lead to brain abnormalities. These brain abnormalities can be biochemical, structural, or functional and may lead to biological vulnerability.

Stress (social, psychological, and physical), although not a cause of schizophrenia, may precipitate the illness in vulnerable individuals and play a role in the severity and course of the disease. The use of street drugs such as cannabis, methamphetamine, and lysergic acid diethylamide (LSD) may also increase the risk of developing schizophrenia in vulnerable individuals, especially for those younger than age 21 whose brains are still developing.

These findings and others raise many questions. For example, is schizophrenia neurodevelopmental in origin, resulting from brain injury occurring early in life or in adolescence? If not, what causes these changes to occur? Why do brain changes progress as the disease progresses in some people and not in others? Why do some people show neuroanatomical changes and others do not?

CULTURAL CONSIDERATIONS

Although the developmental pattern of schizophrenia is fairly consistent across cultures, studies find that some symptoms of schizophrenia as well as prognoses are more severe in industrialized nations than in developing countries. Different cultural groups may view and interpret symptoms seen in schizophrenia in entirely different ways. What is considered normal or acceptable in one culture may be seen as pathological in another. In some subculture groups, "visions" or "voices" are an integral and expected part of various religious experiences (USDHHS, 1999). A study by Luhrmann and colleagues (2014) found that the cultural content of hallucinations in five different cultural groups (San Mateo, California; Accra, Ghana; and Chennai, India) identified interesting differences. While many of the African and Indian subjects registered predominantly positive experiences with their voices, Americans experienced their voices as violent and hateful. In India and Africa, the subjects were not as troubled by their voices. Those from India heard voices that emphasized playfulness and sex. The African experience more often involved the voice of God. Luhrmann and colleagues (2014) state, "One new approach claims it is possible to improve individuals' relationships with their voices by teaching them to name their voices and to build relationships with them, and that doing so diminishes their caustic qualities."

In Ireland, where religious piety is highly valued, delusions may include sainthood and religious content. In industrial advanced countries (e.g., the United States) that focus on surveillance and sinister uses of technology, delusions may assume a more paranoid flavor (e.g., being spied on by one's television or being under surveillance by the government). In Japan, one's honor and social conformity is prized; therefore delusions centering around slander or fear of being humiliated publicly are much more common (PBS, 2002). Therefore it would not be surprising in a culture that believes in ghosts, witches, or evil spirits for delusions to contain ancestral ghosts or witches.

It is important, therefore, to understand how family groups from different subcultures view a family member's "beliefs," "voices," or "visions." Knowing how the family views these symptoms and how they treat such phenomena in their cultural group can provide important information as to how mental health professionals can best approach and reframe treatment for the family and patient to make it more acceptable.

CLINICAL PICTURE

The signs and symptoms of schizophrenia are more numerous than presented here and not all symptoms apply to all individuals with schizophrenia. Each person with schizophrenia is a unique individual, although he or she shares common symptoms with others. These symptoms are discussed in more detail under the assessment section of Application of the Nursing Process in this chapter. The basic symptoms of schizophrenia, according to the National Alliance on Mental Illness (2009), Preston and colleagues (2013), and the APA (2013), are listed in Box 17-2.

APPLICATION OF THE NURSING PROCESS

ASSESSMENT

Course of the Disease

The course of schizophrenia usually includes recurrent acute exacerbations of psychosis. However, the previous belief of schizophrenia as a disease with an unalterable advancement to progressive deterioration might be inaccurate. A decade's worth of longitudinal studies demonstrated that early and aggressive treatment with antipsychotics may alter the course of the schizophrenias when given at the time of the first psychotic break. Prevention of relapse can be more important than the risk of side effects from medications because most side effects are reversible, whereas the consequences of relapse may be irreversible. *With each relapse of psychosis, there is an increase in residual dysfunction and deterioration* (Sadock et al., 2015).

The following are the phases in the course of the disease:

- **Prodromal phase:** Signs and symptoms that precede the acute, fully manifested signs and symptoms of disease. Prodromal symptoms occur in up to 80% to 90% of people with schizophrenia before the emergence of frank psychosis (acute phase). Early prodromal symptoms include social withdrawal and deterioration in function and depressive mood, followed by perceptual disturbances, magical thinking, and peculiar behavior, among others. Prodromal symptoms may appear a month to a year before the first psychotic break and represent a clear deterioration in previous functioning. Essentially, the symptoms include perceptual difficulties; increased stress, depression, anxiety, and sleep disturbances; and declined functional ability. Speech may be characterized by obscure symbolism. Late in the phase, words and phrases may become indecipherable. Frequently, the history of a person with schizophrenia reveals that during adolescence the person was withdrawn from others, lonely or perhaps depressed, and expressed vague or unrealistic plans regarding the future. If health care workers recognized the symptoms as possible prodromal symptoms of schizophrenia, early

treatment may help prevent full-blown psychosis and help diminish chronic symptoms.

- **Acute phase:** Periods of florid positive symptoms (more fully developed and flagrant) (e.g., hallucinations, delusions) as well as negative symptoms (e.g., apathy, withdrawal, lack of motivation) and cognitive symptoms.
- **Stabilization phase:** Period in which acute symptoms, particularly the positive symptoms, decrease in severity.
- **Maintenance phase:** Period in which symptoms are in remission, although there might be milder persistent symptoms (residual symptoms).

The *DSM-5* states that 20% of individuals diagnosed with schizophrenia have a favorable outcome, and, to a much lesser extent, some have recovered completely (APA, 2013). However, about two thirds of individuals diagnosed with schizophrenia have lives characterized by a marginalized existence, aimlessness, frequent hospitalizations, and poverty alienated from human contact (Sadock et al., 2015).

Treatment-Relevant Dimensions of Schizophrenia

The major symptoms of schizophrenia can be grouped into positive, negative, cognitive, and mood. For example, depression frequently occurs and can negatively affect the patient's long-term prognosis and increase the severity of emotional pain and confusion. Figure 17-1 presents an overview of these major symptom groups and the ways in which they can affect an individual's life.

1. **Positive symptoms** (e.g., hallucinations, delusions, bizarre behavior, paranoia) are referred to as *florid psychotic symptoms;* they are the ones that capture attention. Decades of analysis of treatment and study findings indicate that these florid psychotic symptoms may not be the core deficiency after all.
2. **Negative symptoms** (e.g., apathy, lack of motivation, anhedonia, poor thought processes) persist and are extremely destructive because they render a person inert and unmotivated. Refer to Box 17-3 for a list of positive and negative symptoms.
3. **Cognitive symptoms** are perhaps the most debilitating symptoms. Cognitive symptoms include impairment in memory; disruption in social learning; and inability to reason, solve problems, or focus attention. The greater the degree of negative and cognitive symptoms, the

---

*Numbers 1, 2, 3, and 4 are the major symptoms of schizophrenia.

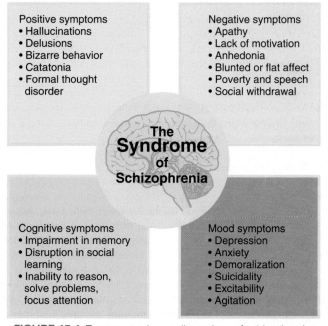

Positive symptoms	Negative symptoms
• Hallucinations • Delusions • Bizarre behavior • Catatonia • Formal thought disorder	• Apathy • Lack of motivation • Anhedonia • Blunted or flat affect • Poverty and speech • Social withdrawal

The **Syndrome** of **Schizophrenia**

Cognitive symptoms	Mood symptoms
• Impairment in memory • Disruption in social learning • Inability to reason, solve problems, focus attention	• Depression • Anxiety • Demoralization • Suicidality • Excitability • Agitation

FIGURE 17-1 Treatment-relevant dimensions of schizophrenia.

BOX 17-3   Positive and Negative Symptoms of Schizophrenia

Positive Symptoms

Hallucinations
- Auditory
  - Voices commenting
  - Voices conversing
  - Voices commanding
- Somatic-tactile
- Olfactory
- Visual
- Gustatory

Delusions
- Persecutory delusions
- Jealous delusions
- Grandiose delusions
- Religious delusions
- Somatic delusions
- Delusions of reference (events in the environment have special meaning)
- Delusions of being controlled
- Delusions of mind reading
- Thought broadcasting, insertion, withdrawal

Bizarre Behavior
- Clothing, appearance
- Social and sexual behavior
- Aggressive, agitated behavior
- Repetitive, stereotyped behavior

Positive Formal Thought Disorder and Speech Patterns
- Derailment
- Tangentiality
- Incoherence
- Illogicality
- Circumstantiality
- Pressure of speech
- Distractible speech
- Clang associations

Negative Symptoms

Affective Flattening
- Unchanging facial expression
- Decreased spontaneous movements
- Paucity of expressive gestures
- Poor eye contact
- Inappropriate affect
- Lack of vocal inflections

Alogia
- Poverty of speech
- Poverty of content of speech
- Blocking

Avolition, Apathy
- Impaired grooming and hygiene
- Lack of persistence at work or school
- Physical anergia

Anhedonia, Asociality
- Few recreational interests or activities
- Little sexual interest or activity
- Impaired intimacy and closeness
- Few relationships with friends or peers

Attention Deficits
- Social inattentiveness

more likely it is that the person will be unable to function on a job, engage in social activities, and care for self adequately and safely.

4. **Mood symptoms** include depression, anxiety, demoralization, dysphoria, and suicidology (Freudenreich et al., 2016).

Positive Symptoms

Positive symptoms—such as **hallucinations, delusions, bizarre behavior, and paranoia**—are associated with an acute onset, normal premorbid functioning, normal CT findings, normal neuropsychological test results, and favorable response to antipsychotic medications.

The positive symptoms appear early in the acute phase of the illness and often precipitate hospitalization. They are, however, the least important prognostically and, as mentioned, usually respond to antipsychotic medication. The positive symptoms are presented here in terms of alterations in thinking, speech, perception, and behavior.

Alterations in thinking

Delusions. Alterations in thinking can take many forms. Delusions are most often defined as false fixed beliefs that cannot be corrected by reasoning. They may be simple beliefs or part of a complex delusional system. In schizophrenia, delusions are often loosely organized and may be bizarre. Most commonly, delusional thinking involves the following themes: ideas of reference, persecution, grandiosity, somatic sensations, jealousy, and control. Table 17-1 provides definitions and examples of various delusions.

Approximately 75% of people with schizophrenia experience delusions at some time during their illness. The most common delusions are persecutory and grandiose, as well as those involving religious or hypochondriacal ideas. A person experiencing delusions is convinced that what he or she believes to be real *is* real. The person's thinking often reflects feelings of great fear and isolation: "I know the doctor talks to the FBI about ways to get rid of me without getting caught. They all want me dead."

At times, delusions hold a kernel of truth. One patient diagnosed with schizophrenia was brought to the hospital in an acutely psychotic state. He repeatedly told the staff that the mafia was out to kill him. Later, the staff learned that the patient had been selling drugs, had not paid his contacts, and gang members were trying to find him to hurt or even kill him.

Other common delusions observed in schizophrenia include the following:

- **Thought broadcasting**—belief that one's thoughts can be heard by others (e.g., "My brain is connected to the world mind. I can control all heads of state through my thoughts.")
- **Thought insertion**—belief that thoughts of others are being inserted into one's mind (e.g., "They make me think bad thoughts.")
- **Thought withdrawal**—belief that thoughts have been removed from one's mind by an outside agency (e.g., "The devil takes my thoughts away and leaves me empty.")
- **Delusion of being controlled**—belief that one's body or mind is controlled by an outside agency (e.g., "There is a man from darkness who controls my thoughts with electrical waves.")

Concrete thinking. Concrete thinking refers to an overemphasis on specific details and impairment in the ability to use abstract concepts. For example, during an assessment, the nurse might ask what brought the patient to the hospital. The patient might answer "a cab" rather than explaining the reason for seeking medical or psychiatric aid. When asked to give the meaning of the proverb "People in glass houses shouldn't throw stones," the person with schizophrenia might answer, "Don't throw stones or the windows will break." The answer is literal; the ability to use abstract reasoning is absent.

Alterations in speech (e.g., frequent derailment or incoherence)

Associative looseness. Associations are the threads that tie one thought to another and one concept to another. In schizophrenia, these threads are missing, and connections are interrupted. In associative looseness (or **looseness of association [LOA]**), thinking becomes haphazard, illogical, and confused. Zelda Fitzgerald wrote her husband, the writer F. Scott Fitzgerald, an account of going mad:

Then the world became embryonic in Africa—and there was no need for communication … I have been living in vaporous places peopled with one-dimensional figures and tremulous buildings until I can no longer tell an optical illusion from a reality … head and ears incessantly throb and roads disappear (Vidal, 1982).

Neologisms. Neologisms are made-up words that have special meaning for the person—for example, "I was going to tell him the *mannerologies* of his hospitality just won't do." "I want all the *vetchkisses* to leave the room and let me be." Children and creative

TABLE 17-1 Summary of Delusions*

Type of Delusion	Definition	Example
Ideas of reference	Misconstruing trivial events and remarks and giving them personal significance	When Maria saw the doctor and nurse talking together, she believed they were plotting against her. When she heard on the radio that a hurricane was coming, she believed this was really a message that harm was going to befall her.
Persecution	The false belief that one is being singled out for harm by others; this belief often takes the form of people in power conspiring against the person or following the person, or being persecuted by friends or colleagues	Sam believed that the Secret Service was planning to kill him. He believed that the Secret Service was poisoning his food. Therefore he would only eat food that he was certain was safe.
Grandeur	The false belief that one is a very powerful and important person, having special abilities, possessing great wealth or beauty	Sally believed that she was Mary Magdalene and that Jesus controlled her thoughts and was telling her how to save the world.
Somatic delusions	The false belief that the body is changing in an unusual way (e.g., rotting inside, heart is no longer beating)	David told the doctor that his brain was rotting away.
Jealousy	The false belief that one's mate is unfaithful; may have so-called proof	Harry accused his girlfriend of going out with other men, even though this was not the case. His "proof" was that she came home from work late twice that week. He persisted in his belief, even when the girlfriend's boss explained that everyone had worked late.
Erotomania	The false belief that another person, usually a stranger, high-class or famous person, is in love with him or her	Samantha is firmly convinced that Johnny Depp, the famous movie star, is madly in love with her. She imagines that callers who claim to have the wrong number are really Johnny. She sends him love letters and flowers through his agent. She tries repeatedly to get his home address.
Nihilistic	Exaggerated belief in the futility of everything; may deny his own existence, and believe that he or she is literally dead	Jason is becoming more preoccupied with the belief that the world will end soon. He questions his own existence, sometimes wondering if he is already dead.
Bizarre delusions	Clearly implausible and incomprehensible false beliefs that do not derive from ordinary experiences	Phoebe is obsessed with the idea that aliens are taking over her mind and are replacing parts of her brain with parts of an alien brain.

*A delusion is a false belief held and maintained as true, even with evidence to the contrary. This does not include unusual beliefs maintained by one's culture or subculture.

writers often make up their own words, but their creation of neologisms is imaginative, constructive, and adaptive. Neologisms in people with schizophrenia represent a disruption in thought processes.

Echolalia. Echolalia is the pathological repeating of another's words by imitation and is often seen in people with catatonia. Echolalia is the counterpart of echopraxia, mimicking the *movements* of another, which is also seen in catatonia.

Clang association. Clang association is the meaningless rhyming of words, often in a forceful manner ("On the track ... have a Big Mac ... or get the sack"), in which the rhyming is often more important than the context of the word. This form of speech pattern may be seen in individuals with schizophrenia; however, it may also be seen in people in the manic phase of a bipolar disorder or in individuals with a cognitive disorder, such as Alzheimer's disease or HIV-related dementia.

Word salad. Word salad is a term used to identify a jumble of words that is meaningless to the listener and perhaps to the speaker as well. It may include a string of neologisms. For example, "I sang out for my mother ... for this to hell I went. How long is road? These little said three hills hop aboard, share the appetite of the Christmas mice spread ... within three round moons the devil will be washed away."

Alterations in perception

Hallucinations. Hallucinations, especially *auditory hallucinations*, in people with schizophrenia are examples of alterations in perception. Hallucinations can be defined as sensory perceptions for which no external stimulus exists. When they occur, "they are vivid and clear, with the full force and impacts of normal perceptions, and not under

voluntary control" (APA, 2013, p. 87). The most common types of hallucination are the following:

- Auditory—hearing voices or sounds (most common hallucination in schizophrenia)
- Visual—seeing persons or things (possible, more probable in delirium or dementia)
- Olfactory—smelling odors (most common in temporal lobe epilepsy)
- Gustatory—experiencing tastes (rare, part of delusion of persecution, e.g., tasting poison in food)
- Tactile—feeling bodily sensations (common in cocaine/amphetamine/alcohol withdrawal)

Table 17-2 provides examples of these common types of hallucinations and describes the difference between hallucinations and illusions.

It is estimated that up to 90% of people with schizophrenia experience hallucinations at some time during their illness. Although the manner of manifestations of hallucination can be varied, auditory hallucinations are most common in schizophrenia. Voices may seem to come from outside or inside the person's head. The voices may be familiar or strange, single or multiple. Voices speaking directly to the person or commenting on the person's behavior are most common. A person may believe that the voices are from God, the devil, deceased relatives, or strangers. The auditory hallucinations may occasionally take the form of sounds like buzzing scratching, or banging.

Command hallucinations must be carefully assessed. The voices may command the person to hurt self or others. For example, a patient might state that "the voices" are saying "jump out the

TABLE 17-2   Summary of Hallucinations*

Type of Hallucination	Definition	Example
Auditory	Hearing voices or sounds that do not exist in the environment but are projections of inner thoughts or feelings	Anna "hears" numerous voices talking about how worthless she is.
Visual	Seeing a person, object, or animal that does not exist in the environment	Charles, who is experiencing alcohol withdrawal delirium, "sees" hungry rats hovering around him.
Olfactory	Smelling odors that are not present in the environment	Theresa "smells" her insides rotting.
Gustatory	Tasting sensations that have no stimulus in reality	Sam will not eat his food because he "tastes" the poison the FBI is putting in his food.
Tactile	Feeling strange sensations where no external objects stimulate such feelings; common in delirium tremens	Judy, who is a heavy cocaine user, screams that bugs are crawling under her skin.

*A hallucination is a false sensory perception for which no external stimulus exists. Hallucinations are different from illusions in that illusions are misperceptions or misinterpretations of a real experience. For example, a man sees his coat hanging on a coat rack and believes it to be a bear about to attack him. He does see something real but misinterprets it.

window" or "take a knife and kill your child." Command hallucinations are often terrifying for the individual. Command hallucinations may signal a psychiatric emergency. Patients who can give an identity to the hallucinated voice are at somewhat greater risk of compliance with the hallucinated command than are those who cannot.

Evidence of possible auditory hallucinatory behavior is turning or tilting of the head—as if the patient is listening to someone—or frequent blinking of the eyes and grimacing. Sometimes, patients verbally respond to "unseen others." Visual hallucinations occur less frequently in people with schizophrenia.

Personal boundary difficulties. People with schizophrenia often lack a sense of where their bodies end in relation to where others' bodies begin. Patients might say that they are merging with others or are part of inanimate objects. For example, depersonalization is a nonspecific feeling that a person has lost his or her identity; the self is different or unreal. People may be concerned that body parts do not belong to them, or they may have an acute sensation that the body has drastically changed. For example, a woman may see her fingers as snakes or her arms as rotting wood. A man may look in a mirror and state that his face is that of an animal. Derealization is the false perception by a person that the environment has changed. For example, everything seems bigger or smaller, or familiar surroundings have become strange and unfamiliar.

Alterations in behavior (grossly disorganized or catatonic). Bizarre and agitated behaviors are associated with schizophrenia and may have a variety of manifestations. **Bizarre behavior** may take the form of a stilted, rigid demeanor and eccentric dress, grooming, and rituals.

Many of the following behaviors are associated with schizophrenia with a catatonic specifier (rarely seen in schizophrenia today when properly medicated with an antipsychotic). However, catatonia may be seen in other conditions as well (e.g., brain damage, extreme manic phase of bipolar disorder, substance abuse).

- **Extreme motor agitation** is excited physical behavior, such as running about, in response to inner and outer stimuli, which can be harmful to self as well as to others.
- Stereotyped behaviors are motor patterns that originally had meaning to the person (e.g., sweeping the floor, washing windows) but are now mechanical and lack purpose.
- **Automatic obedience** is the performance by a catatonic patient of all simple commands in a robot-like fashion.

- **Waxy flexibility,** seen in catatonia, is evidenced by excessive maintenance of posture. Patients can hold unusual postures for long periods.
- **Stupor** refers to a state in which the catatonic patient is motionless for long periods and may even appear to be in a coma.
- **Negativism** is equivalent to resistance. In *active negativism,* the patient does the opposite of what he or she is told to do. When a person does not perform activities that are normal expectations, such as getting out of bed, dressing, and eating, the behavior is termed *passive negativism (catatonia).*

When patients with schizophrenia are acutely ill, impulse control is lacking. Frequently the lack of impulse control is expressed in socially inappropriate **agitated behaviors** such as grabbing another's cigarette or throwing food on the floor.

Negative Symptoms

Negative symptoms—such as apathy, anhedonia, poor social functioning, and poverty of thought—are most likely a result of the neurocognitive defects and are associated with an insidious onset, premorbid history of emotional problems, chronic deterioration, demonstration of abnormal findings on imaging scans, abnormal results on neuropsychological tests, and poor response to antipsychotic therapy.

The negative symptoms of schizophrenia develop over a long period of time. These are the symptoms that most interfere with the individual's adjustment and ability to survive. Because the presence of negative symptoms impedes the person's ability to initiate and maintain relationships and conversations, it affects the individual's ability to hold a job, make decisions, and maintain adequate hygiene and grooming.

The presence of negative symptoms contributes to the person's poor social functioning and social withdrawal. During an acute psychotic episode, negative symptoms are difficult to assess because the positive and more florid symptoms, such as delusions and hallucinations, dominate. Some of the negative phenomena are outlined in Table 17-3.

Affect is the observable behavior that expresses a person's emotions. In people with schizophrenia, affect may not coincide with inner emotions, and there is a prominent lack of emotional response. Affect can usually be categorized in one of three ways: flat or blunted, inappropriate, or bizarre. A **flat affect** (immobile facial expression or a blank look) or **blunted affect** (minimal emotional response) is commonly seen in schizophrenia. **Inappropriate affect** refers to an emotional response to a situation that is not congruent with the tone of the situation. For example, a young man breaks

TABLE 17-3 Negative Symptoms Observed in Schizophrenia

Phenomenon	Explanation
Affective blunting* (diminished emotional expression)	Severe reduction in the expression of emotions on the face, lack of eye contact, bland intonation of speech, etc.; often referred to as *flat affect* when no facial or other expressions of emotion are present
Anergia	Lack of energy: passivity, lack of persistence at work or school
Anhedonia	Inability to experience any pleasure in activities that usually produce pleasurable feelings; result of profound emotional barrenness
Avolition*	Lack of motivation: inability to initiate tasks, such as social contacts, grooming, and other aspects of activities of daily living
Poverty of content of speech	Speech that is adequate in amount but conveys little information because of vagueness, empty repetitions, or use of stereotypes or obscure phrases
Poverty of speech	Restriction in the amount of speech: answers range from brief to monosyllabic one-word answers
Thought blocking	May be signaled when a patient stops talking in the middle of a sentence and remains silent. After a patient stops abruptly: *Nurse:* "What just happened now?" *Patient:* "I forgot what I was saying. Something took my thoughts away."

*According to the *DSM-5*, avolition and affective blunting are the most prominent negative symptoms observed in schizophrenia.

into laughter when told that his father has died. **Bizarre affect** is especially prominent in the disorganized form of schizophrenia and includes grimacing, giggling, and mumbling to oneself. Bizarre affect is marked when the patient is unable to relate logically to the environment.

Neurocognitive Symptoms

Disruption in cognitive symptoms (inability to organize, plan, concentrate, etc.) is possibly the most damaging of all symptoms. Neurocognitive symptoms represent a third dimension and affect at least 40% to 60% or more of people with schizophrenia. Neurocognitive symptoms disrupt all aspects of the patient's life. Cognitive impairment destroys a patient's ability to hold a job, initiate or maintain a social support system, or live on his or her own. Cognitive impairment also causes difficulty with attention, memory, and executive functions (e.g., decision making and problem solving); impedes the person's ability to manage his or her own health care and/or participate fully in relapse prevention programs; and generally devastates the person's quality of life.

The degree of cognitive deficit is associated with the severity of negative symptoms; **disorganized thinking** reflects the degree to which disorganized speech, disorganized behavior, or inappropriate affect is present. The presence of good verbal memory is one cognitive indicator that the individual will eventually be able to function within the community because verbal memory is necessary to acquire psychosocial skills and retention of these skills.

Mood Symptoms

A fourth dimension involves variations in mood such as anxiety, suicidality, demoralization, and dysphoria. Co-occurring depressive symptoms increase the suffering of patients with schizophrenia and are all too common. A phenomenon known as *post psychotic depressive disorder* occurs in up to 25% of people after an acute psychotic episode and increases the risk of suicide. Recognition of depression during assessment is important. Depression increases the likelihood of suicide and substance use and impairs functioning.

Specifier: Catatonia

The *DSM-5* has added the specifier *catatonia* when symptoms of catatonia are present and may predominate. Symptoms of catatonia can exist in a number of other disorders, conditions, and situations, as mentioned earlier in "Alterations in Behavior." A person with a specifier of catatonia, although more rare today than in the past, might present with some of the following symptoms.

Catatonia. Although we tend to think of catatonia in terms of immobility, the essential feature of catatonia is *extreme abnormal motor behavior*. In fact, patients who exhibit either extreme motor agitation or extreme psychomotor retardation (with mutism, or even stupor) are rare when catatonia is present with a diagnosis of schizophrenia.

During the very withdrawn phase, the person does not move or eat, thus becoming vulnerable to pressure ulcers, contractures, and malnutrition. Patients may *exhibit bizarre posturing*, such as holding arms or legs rigid or bent at severe angles for a long period of time. Also, *waxy flexibility* may occur; for example, when a leg or arm is placed in an awkward position by someone else, the patient will hold that position for an uncomfortable length of time.

Another trait of catatonia is *stereotyped behavior* or following a routine obsessively, such as continually arranging and rearranging objects. Other characteristics of catatonia are *extreme negativism* and resistance. Speech patterns may include *echolalia* (persistently repeating the words of others), and *echopraxia* (mimicking the movements or gestures of others) may also be present.

During the extreme motor activity phase, the patient may run about ceaselessly and without purpose, leading to exhaustion, cardiac difficulties, or physical collapse. The onset of catatonia is usually abrupt, and the prognosis is favorable. Fortunately, with the advances in pharmacotherapy and improved individual management, severe catatonic symptoms are rarely seen today.

VIGNETTE

Mary has been motionless and has not spoken for days. When her husband raises her arm to dress her and take her to the hospital, her arm stays raised in the air until he lowers it *(waxy flexibility)*. When she starts to move, she does everything she is told to do (get up, sit down) and only moves on command *(automatic obedience)*. When he speaks to her, she repeats everything he says—for example, "Mary, drink this water." "Mary, drink this water" *(echolalia)*.

DSM-5 DIAGNOSTIC CRITERIA
for Schizophrenia

A. Two (or more) of the following, each present for a significant portion of time during a 1-month period (or less if successfully treated). At least one of these must be (1), (2), or (3):
   1. Delusions.
   2. Hallucinations.
   3. Disorganized speech (e.g., frequent derailment or incoherence).
   4. Grossly disorganized or catatonic behavior.
   5. Negative symptoms (i.e., diminished emotional expression or avolition).

B. For a significant portion of the time since the onset of the disturbance, level of functioning in one or more major areas, such as work, interpersonal relations, or self-care, is markedly below the level achieved prior to the onset (or when the onset is in childhood or adolescence, there is failure to achieve expected level of interpersonal, academic, or occupational functioning).

C. Continuous signs of the disturbance persist for at least 6 months. This 6-month period must include at least 1 month of symptoms (or less if successfully treated) that meet Criterion A (i.e., active-phase symptoms) and may include periods of prodromal or residual symptoms. During these prodromal or residual periods, the signs of the disturbance may be manifested by only negative symptoms or by two or more symptoms listed in Criterion A present in an attenuated form (e.g., odd beliefs, unusual perceptual experiences).

D. Schizoaffective disorder and depressive or bipolar disorder with psychotic features have been ruled out because either 1) no major depressive or manic episodes have occurred concurrently with the active-phase symptoms, or 2) if mood episodes have occurred during active-phase symptoms, they have been present for a minority of the total duration of the active and residual periods of the illness.

E. The disturbance is not attributable to the physiological effects of a substance (e.g., a drug of abuse, a medication) or another medical condition.

F. If there is a history of autism spectrum disorder or a communication disorder of childhood onset, the additional diagnosis of schizophrenia is made only if prominent delusions or hallucinations, in addition to the other required symptoms of schizophrenia, are also present for at least 1 month (or less if successfully treated).

Specify if:
The following course specifiers are only to be used after a 1-year duration of the disorder and if they are not in contradiction to the diagnostic course criteria.

First episode, currently in acute episode: First manifestation of the disorder meeting the defining diagnostic symptom and time criteria. An acute episode is a time period in which the symptom criteria are fulfilled.

First episode, currently partial remission: Partial remission is a period of time during which an improvement after a previous episode is maintained and in which the defining criteria of the disorder are only partially fulfilled.

First episode, currently in full remission: Full remission is a period of time after a previous episode during which no disorder-specific symptoms are present.

Multiple episodes, currently in acute episode: Multiple episodes may be determined after a minimum of two episodes (i.e., after a first episode, a remission and a minimum of one relapse).

Multiple episodes, currently in partial remission

Multiple episodes, currently in full remission

Continuous: Symptoms fulfilling the diagnostic symptom criteria of the disorder are remaining for the majority of the illness course, with subthreshold symptom periods being very brief relative to the overall course.

Unspecified

Specify if:
With catatonia (refer to the criteria for catatonia associated with another mental disorder, pp 119–120, for definition).

Coding note: Use additional code 293.89 (F06.1) catatonia associated with schizophrenia to indicate the presence of the comorbid catatonia.

Specify current severity:
Severity is rated by a quantitative assessment of the primary symptoms of psychosis, including delusions, hallucinations, disorganized speech, abnormal psychomotor behavior, and negative symptoms. Each of these symptoms may be rated for its current severity (most severe in the last 7 days) on a 5-point scale ranging from 0 (not present) to 4 (present and severe). (See Clinical-Rated Dimensions of Psychosis Symptom Severity in the chapter "Assessment Measure.")

Note: Diagnosis of schizophrenia can be made without using this severity specifier.

From American Psychiatric Association (APA). (2013). *Diagnostic and statistical manual of mental disorders* (5th ed.). Washington, DC: APA.

Other Presentations

Individuals who have a schizophrenic spectrum disorder have different neuroanatomical findings, distinct courses of disease development, individual responses to treatment, as well as different prognoses. Although not all patients will meet all *DSM-5* criteria for schizophrenia spectrum disorders, it is helpful to be aware of possible prominent presentations.

Although the *DSM-5* (APA, 2013) no longer includes certain previous subtypes, some individuals may present with severe paranoia, and others may present with severe disorganized symptomatology. Those with disorganized symptomatology are the people we often see on the street, in shelters, hidden away in parks, etc. People with schizophrenia with profound disorganization are discussed in full in Chapter 27.

The following presentations may be exaggerated, but they provide the reader with a visual picture of the person who presents with either paranoia or extremely disorganized symptoms.

Paranoia

Any *intense and strongly defended irrational suspicion* can be regarded as paranoia. Paranoid ideas cannot be corrected by experiences and cannot be modified by facts or reality. Projection is the most common defense mechanism used by people who are paranoid. For example, when paranoid individuals feel self-critical, they experience others as being harshly critical toward them. When they feel *angry,* they experience others as being unjustly angry at them, as if to say, "I'm not angry, you are!"

Because people who are paranoid are unable to trust the actions of those around them, they are usually guarded, tense, and reserved. Although patients may keep themselves aloof from interpersonal contacts, impairment in actual functioning may be minimal. To ensure interpersonal distance, they may adopt a superior, hostile, and sarcastic attitude. A common defense used by paranoid individuals to maintain self-esteem is to disparage others and dwell on the shortcomings of others. A paranoid individual misinterprets the messages of others or gives private meaning to the communications of others (ideas of reference). For example, a patient might see his wife talking to a man at a checkout counter at a supermarket and believe they are lovers and plotting to get rid of him. Minor oversights are often interpreted as personal rejection. It can be intimidating to be in the presence of an extremely paranoid individual.

People with prominent paranoia usually have a later age of onset of the disease (late twenties to thirties). In some cases, individuals who present with paranoid features often have a good outcome or recovery. Individuals with strong paranoid features often have intact cognitive abilities since psychotic paranoia usually appears later in life. When such a person is amenable to psychopharmacology, paranoid delusions are usually lessened to a great degree. Thus, they are often able to work, often in jobs that require a high degree of cognitive skills; however, they usually perform better in solitary pursuits and projects where their paranoia is less likely to be stimulated.

D.J. Jaffe, borrowing from the work of Weiden and Havens (1995), identified some helpful guidelines to use when working with an individual who is very paranoid (slightly modified from the verbatim original text taken from http://www.schizophrenia.com/family/mansymptoms.htm):

1. **Speak indirectly.** Avoid speaking directly to the person. Substitute pronouns such as "it," "he," "she" or "they" for the words "I" and "you." Like the body positioning, the purpose is to deflect the patient's paranoid projections away from one-on-one interactions with the clinician. Instead, paranoid symptoms are directed toward external and more general "real world" issues.

2. **Identify with, rather than fight, the patient.** Whenever possible, your attitudes and emotional expressions should parallel the patient's attitudes and expressions. The goal is to help the patient feel understood. Meet anger with reciprocal anger, frustration with frustration (i.e., you also express anger and frustration with the difficult circumstances). A paranoid individual is not thinking rationally and your attempts to rationalize will not likely be successful.

3. **Don't rationalize. Share mistrust.** The intuitive approach with a paranoid person is to try to persuade him or her to be more trusting. It is often better to do the opposite; that is, for you—along with the patient—to mistrust the world together. No attempt is made to correct or contradict the patient, or to test reality. Temporarily, the patient's account of reality is accepted as reality. The assumption behind this technique is that, in the midst of a paranoid state, the patient is overburdened and overwhelmed by a mixture of real-life stresses and distress from psychotic symptoms. While carefully avoiding collusion with the psychotic symptoms, you should attempt to find certain believable or credible aspects of the paranoid belief system. This allows you to agree with the patient on something. You then move on to a symptom area, attempt to substitute a less paranoid, more benign (and general) explanation for the more highly personalized paranoid one. The process of exchanging more malignant to benign paranoid beliefs is best done in a stepwise fashion, where the alternate explanation is only a notch less paranoid than the previous one. For example, rather than confront a patient's own behavior that led to her being arrested, the clinician agrees that some police are not trustworthy and goes on to talk about his own outrage at the Rodney King case .

See Table 17-7 for other interventions for paranoid individuals.

VIGNETTE

Sam stares at the nurse as she explains how to replace a bandage after minor surgery on his face. He frequently looks at the door and places himself near it. His general demeanor is condescending, and he becomes sarcastic when the nurse drops a bandage, asking, "Are you the best they could give me?" When the nurse answers the phone, he says, "So they got to you, too. You are all plotting against me" *(ideas of reference)*. He starts to mutter to himself and looks to his side as if he is talking to someone *(auditory hallucinations)*.

Paranoid states may occur in numerous mental or organic disorders, for example, people experiencing psychotic depression, a manic episode, or certain physical conditions (e.g., organic brain disease, drug intoxications) and most certainly paranoid personality disorder.

Disorganized

Disorganized components of schizophrenia represent the most regressed and socially impaired of all individuals with schizophrenia. People with schizophrenia who are severely disorganized are often homeless, which makes them easy targets for maltreatment. A person who presents with these symptoms of schizophrenia may have marked looseness of associations, grossly inappropriate affect, bizarre mannerisms, and incoherence of speech, and may display extreme social withdrawal and severe cognitive impairment. Although delusions and hallucinations are present, they are fragmentary and poorly organized. Behavior may be considered odd, and giggling or grimacing in response to internal stimuli is common.

Often, individuals with these symptoms have an earlier age of onset (early to middle teens), and the symptoms often develop insidiously. This syndrome is associated with poor premorbid functioning, a significant family history of psychopathological disorders, and a poor prognosis. Often, these patients can live in the community safely only in a structured and well-supervised setting. Unfortunately a large portion of the homeless population consists of people with this disorder. Families living with someone this vulnerable and disorganized need significant community support, respite care, and day hospital affiliations (refer to Chapter 27).

VIGNETTE

Pete pushes his grocery cart loaded with rags, bottles, bags, and such down the street. He appears disheveled, dressed in a dirty plaid shirt, a dirty baseball hat, and ragged jeans. He is giggling and laughing to himself. Once in a while he shouts out something, "Alms for the poor me … howdy to you all. … Where is it? Where is it?" *(looseness of association)*. He goes from garbage can to garbage can rummaging for food. He often sleeps under a bridge with a cardboard box as protection, and when the weather becomes too hot or too cold, he sometimes seeks help at a nearby shelter.

Assessment Guidelines
Schizophrenias and Other Psychotic Disorders

1. Determine if the patient had a medical workup; if so, was medical or substance-induced psychosis ruled out?
2. Verify whether the person uses alcohol or drugs.
3. Assess for command hallucinations (e.g., voices telling the person to harm self or another). If present, ask the patient:
   - Do you plan to follow the command?
   - Do you believe the voices are real?
   - Do you recognize the voices?
4. Review the patient's belief system. Is it fragmented? Is it poorly or well organized? Is it systematized? Is the system of beliefs unsupported by reality (delusion)? If yes, then find out if:
   - Delusions focus on someone trying to harm the patient
   - The patient is planning to retaliate against a person or organization
   - Precautions need to be taken
5. Assess for co-occurring conditions, including:
   - Depression
   - Suicidality
   - Anxiety
   - Substance use
   - History of violence

6. Inventory the patient's medications and assess whether the patient is adhering to the medication regimen.
   a. If the person is nonadherent with medications, ask what makes it difficult for him or her to follow this medication regime (fear of side effects, forgetting, lack of money?).
   b. Make clear notations of the reasons for nonadherence and what will be done to help the person to become more adherent (social services for monetary reasons, recovery group, medication group, etc.).
7. Determine the family's response to increased symptoms. Are they overprotective? Hostile? Suspicious? Overwhelmed?
8. Assess the manner in which family members and the patient relate.
9. Review the support system. Is the family well informed about the disease? Does the family understand the need for medication adherence? Is the family familiar with support groups available in the community or locations where respite and family support may be offered? Have family members received or been referred for psychoeducation?

DIAGNOSIS

People with schizophrenia have multiple disturbing and disabling symptoms that necessitate a multifaceted approach to care and treatment of the patient as well as the family. Table 17-4 lists potential nursing diagnoses for a person with schizophrenia. Unfortunately, *NANDA* (2015–2017) no longer includes ***Disturbed thought processes*** and ***Disturbed sensory perception: auditory or visual,*** which are precisely two areas for intervention for individuals suffering with psychotic symptoms. Hopefully, these nursing diagnoses will be reinstated in future editions of *NANDA*.

OUTCOMES IDENTIFICATION

Phase I (Acute)

During the acute phase of the illness, the overall goal is **patient safety and medical stabilization.** Therefore if the patient is at risk for violence to self or others, initial outcome criteria should address safety issues (e.g., *patient consistently refrains from inflicting serious injury to self or others*). Another outcome/goal might be *patient consistently refrains from acting on delusions or hallucinations.* Medication adherence is a vital outcome for all phases of recovery. Ideally, outcomes should focus on enhancing the patient's strengths and minimizing the patient's deficits.

Phase II (Stabilization) and Phase III (Maintenance)

Outcome criteria during the maintenance and stabilization phases focus on helping patients to adhere to medication regimens, understand their disease, and participate in available psychoeducational activities with their families.

During the stabilization phase, goals are directed toward continual recovery, improvement in functioning, and enhancement of the individual's quality of life. Improvement in functioning includes the ability to participate in social, vocational, or self-care skills training and involvement in social groups at various levels.

It is also important to include outcomes that address anxiety control and relapse prevention. Desired outcomes to reduce the patient's vulnerability to psychosis include the following: maintain a regular sleep pattern; reduce alcohol, drug, and caffeine intake; keep in touch with supportive friends and family; stay active (engage in exercise, hobbies, employment); have a routine daily and weekly schedule including enjoyable activities; and take medication regularly.

PLANNING

Phase I (Acute)

During the acute phase of schizophrenia, brief hospitalization is frequently indicated if the patient is considered a danger to self or others, refuses to eat or drink, or is too disorganized to provide self-care. Another indication for hospitalization is the need for specific observation, neurological workup, or other medically related tests or treatments for co-occurring disorders. The planning process focuses on the best strategies to ensure patient safety and provide symptom stabilization.

At this time the treatment team identifies aftercare needs for follow-up and support, as well as the appropriate referrals that will benefit the patient and family. Discharge planning considers not only external factors, such as the patient's living arrangement, economic resources, social supports, and family relationships, but also the internal factor of the patient's vulnerability to stress. Because relapse can be devastating to long-term functioning, vigorous efforts are made to connect the patient with community agencies that provide social supports and programs designed to help the patient remain well (see Chapter 5).

Phase II (Stabilization) and Phase III (Maintenance)

Planning during the stabilization and maintenance phases of treatment focuses on strategies to provide patient and family education and skills training (psychosocial education). **Relapse prevention skills are vital.** Planning identifies the social, interpersonal, coping, and vocational skills needed, as well as how and where these needs can best be met within the community. **Interventions are always geared toward the patient's strengths and healthy functioning as well as areas of deficiency.**

IMPLEMENTATION

Self-Care for Nurses

A person who is psychotic is intensely anxious, lonely, dependent, and distrustful. The intensity of these emotions often evokes similar emotions in others. Erlich and colleagues (2014) discuss that one's initial reaction to a psychotic patient may be one of anxiety, fear, and bewilderment. An individual who is extremely paranoid and hostile can be frightening and challenging even to staff. Supervision and support from more experienced nurses and staff should always be available in these situations.

Another challenge is trying to understand what the person is saying or means to say when his or her language is incomprehensible to you (e.g., looseness of associations [LOA]). Having to deal with people who are actively hallucinating or who have strong delusional systems (e.g., paranoid) can be very frightening for those who have not been exposed to this before or even to those who have. Usually the hallucinations and delusions are most pronounced when the individual is experiencing extreme levels of anxiety. Anxiety can be transferred to the nurse, clinician, and physician. Initially, students and nurses new to working with people with severe mental health problems need guidance and support. Without the support of more experienced staff to explore these reactions, the novice nurse may adopt defensive behaviors such as denial or withdrawal and avoidance. For nurses new to the psychiatric setting, especially for student nurses, supportive supervision must be available if learning is to occur. The student's part in the supervisory process is a willingness to discuss and identify personal feelings and problem behaviors. This can be, and often is, accomplished in group supervision; experienced psychiatric nurses call this peer group supervision.

TABLE 17-4 Potential Nursing Diagnoses for Schizophrenia

Symptoms	Nursing Diagnoses
Positive Symptoms	
Hallucinations	
Hears voices that others do not	***Disturbed sensory perception: auditory or visual†***
	Impaired environmental interpretation syndrome
	Fear
Hears voices telling him or her to hurt self or others *(command hallucinations)*	Risk for self-directed/other-directed violence
	Ineffective impulse control
Distorted Thinking Not Based on Reality	
Persecution: Thinks that others are trying to harm self	***Disturbed thought processes†***
Jealousy: Thinks that spouse or lover is being unfaithful, or thinks others are jealous of self when they are not	Defensive coping
Grandeur: Incorrectly thinks he or she has powers and talents or is someone powerful or famous	Disturbed personal identity
Reference: Believes that all events within the environment are directed at or hold special meaning for self	*Impaired environmental interpretation syndrome
Looseness of association: Shows loose association of ideas	Impaired verbal communication
Clang association: Uses words that rhyme in a nonsensical fashion	***Disturbed thought processes†***
Echolalia: Repeats words that are heard	(Disorganized or disturbed speech patterns in schizophrenia are evidence of disordered thought processes.)
Mutism: Does not speak	
Circumstantiality: Delays getting to the point of communication because of unnecessary and tedious details	
Concrete thinking: Unable to abstract; uses literal translations concerning aspects of the environment	
Negative Symptoms	
Uncommunicative, withdrawn, makes no eye contact	Social isolation
Preoccupied with own thoughts	Impaired social interaction
Expresses feelings of rejection or aloneness (lies in bed all day, positions back to door)	Risk for loneliness
	Ineffective relationship
Is stigmatized for diagnosis of schizophrenia	Risk for compromised human dignity
Talks about self as "bad" or "no good"	Chronic low self-esteem
Feels guilty because of "bad thoughts"; extremely sensitive to real or perceived slights	Risk for self-directed violence
	Risk for suicide
Shows lack of energy **(anergia)**	Ineffective coping
Shows lack of motivation **(avolition),** unable to initiate tasks (social contact, grooming, and other aspects of daily living)	Bathing self-care deficit
	Dressing self-care deficit
	Self-neglect
	Constipation
	Deficient diversional activity
Other	
Families and significant others become confused or overwhelmed, have lack of knowledge about disease or treatment, feel powerless in coping with patient at home	Compromised family coping
	Impaired parenting
	Caregiver role strain
	Deficient knowledge
	Deficient community health
Nonadherence to Medication and Treatment	
Patient stops taking medication (often because of side effects), stops going to therapy groups, family and significant others not aware of need for medications and treatments	Nonadherence

*Herdman, T.H. (Ed.) *Nursing Diagnoses-Definitions and Classification 2015-2017.* Copyright 2014, 1994-2014 NANDA International. Used by arrangement with John Wiley & Sons Limited. In order to make safe and effective judgments using NANDA-I nursing diagnoses it is essential that nurses refer to the definitions and defining characteristics of the diagnoses listed in this work.

†*Disturbed sensory perception: auditory or visual* and *Disturbed thought processes* are not included the 2015–2017 edition of *Nursing Diagnoses—Definitions and Classification.* However, because schizophrenia and so many other mental disorders are caused by disturbances in neurological functioning, *Disturbed sensory perception: auditory or visual* or *Disturbed thought processes* appears to be the most accurate nursing diagnosis to use for hallucinations and delusions. Also, because schizophrenia is known as a thought disorder, the diagnosis *Disturbed thought processes* seems to be ideal. Therefore they are included here but probably should not appear on your nursing care plan without instructors/professors understanding why you chose them.

Phase I (Acute)

Interventions are also geared toward the phase of schizophrenia (Table 17-5). During phase I the clinical focus is on crisis intervention, acute symptom stabilization (medication), and safety. Since hospitalization is used mostly for crises (e.g., suicide), alternatives such as partial hospitalization, halfway houses, and day treatment centers are frequently used as cost-effective alternatives to hospitalization. **Acute-phase interventions** include acute psychopharmacological treatment (psychobiological intervention); supportive and directive communications; limit setting (milieu management and counseling); and psychiatric, medical, and neurological evaluation.

Phase II (Stabilization) and Phase III (Maintenance)

Once the acute symptoms are somewhat stabilized, if the individual was hospitalized, he or she is discharged to the community, where appropriate treatment can be carried out during the maintenance and stabilization phases. Effective long-term care of an individual with schizophrenia relies on a three-pronged approach: medications, nursing interventions, and community support. **Family psychoeducation, as well as community support, is a key component of effective treatment.**

Phase II and phase III interventions include the following:
Health teaching includes teaching:
- Patient and family about the disease
- Patient and family about medication management
- Cognitive and social skills enhancement
- Strategies to minimize stress and to control anxiety levels

Health promotion and maintenance:
- Help patient and family identify signs of relapse and take preventive steps
- Improve deficits in self-care, social, and work functioning
- Encourage participation in nonthreatening activities
- Encourage social relationships
- Encourage family interaction

Communication Guidelines

Therapeutic strategies for communicating with patients with schizophrenia focus on lowering anxiety, decreasing defensive patterns, encouraging participation in therapeutic and social events, raising feelings of self-worth, and increasing medication compliance. Familiarity with the principles used for dealing with phenomena such as hallucinations, delusions, paranoia, and looseness of association (LOA) is helpful for establishing rapport and being effective.

Hallucinations

Because hearing voices is the most common hallucinatory experience reported by patients, the nurse initially should try to understand what the voices are saying or telling the person to do. Suicidal or homicidal messages necessitate initiation of safety measures for all members of the health care team. Does the person know whose voice he or she is hearing? Is the voice supportive or is it threatening in some way?

Hallucinations are real to the person who is experiencing them. Nurses should approach individuals who are hallucinating in a

TABLE 17-5 Treatment Focus at Different Phases of Schizophrenia

PHASE I		PHASE II	PHASE III
Acute: Onset, Exacerbation, or Relapse	**Subacute or Convalescent**	**Stabilization Phase Adaptive Plateau**	**Maintenance Phase Health Promotion**
Clinical Focus			
Crisis intervention	Social supports	Understanding and acceptance of illness	Social, vocational, and self-care skills
Safety	Stress and vulnerability assessment		Learning or relearning
Acute symptom stabilization	Living arrangements		Identification of realistic expectations
	Daily activities		Adaptation to deficits
	Economic resources		
Intervention			
Acute psychopharmacological treatment	Psychosocial evaluation	Support and teaching	Attention to details of self-care, social, and work functioning
Limit setting	Linkage with:	Medication teaching and side effect management	Direct intervention with family and/or employers
Supportive and directive care	• Social services	Direct assistance with situational problems	Cognitive and social skills enhancement
Psychiatric, medical, neurological evaluation	• Human services	Identification of prodromal and acute symptoms and signs of relapse	Medication maintenance
Meeting with family	• Community treatment agencies	Continued psychoeducational work with families as needed	Continued psychoeducational intervention with families as needed
	Psychoeducational interventions with families		Involvement with recovery groups and strategies
QSEN Professional Collaboration			
Inpatient treatment team	Social work department	Community support staff	Group therapists
Residential alternative to hospitalization	Health and human services	Family support groups	Social, vocational, and self-care providers
Community crisis intervention	Day treatment or a variety of community support services	Group therapists and self-help groups	Family, employer, community support staff
Internist		Practitioners of behavioral therapies using educational models and cognitive restructuring	
Neurologist			

Adapted from Gabbard, G. O. (2001). *Treatments of psychiatric disorders* (3rd ed.). Washington, DC: American Psychiatric Publishing.

nonthreatening and nonjudgmental manner. It is thought that when a person is hallucinating, he or she is experiencing anxiety, fear, loneliness, and low self-esteem, and the brain is not processing stimuli accurately.

During the acute phase of the illness, the nurse should maintain eye contact, call the patient by name, and speak simply.

Patient: "I hear my mother's voice saying terrible things about me. She says I am a horrible person and she wishes I had never been born."

Nurse: "That must be very upsetting, Tom. Are you feeling upset?" (*Nurse waits for a response.*)

Patient: "Yes, yes ... she makes me feel bad."

Nurse: "Tell your voice to go away. I hear you are very good at card games, let's you and I go over to the table and play a game of cards."

Here the nurse tries to identify the feelings the patient is experiencing, asks him to turn away from the voices, and distracts attention and focuses on something reality-based. Table 17-6 lists interventions for hallucinations.

Delusions

Delusions reflect the misperception of cognitive stimuli. When the nurse attempts to see the world as it appears through the eyes of the patient, it is easier to understand the patient's delusional experience.

Patient: "I see now ... you are an ISIS fighter in disguise who wants to drain my brain ... you all want me destroyed."

Nurse: "I don't want to hurt you, Tom. I am your nurse for the day. Thinking that others want to destroy you must be very frightening."

In this example, the nurse clarifies the reality of the patient's experience and empathizes with the patient's apparent experience and feelings of fear. The nurse avoids being drawn into the conversation regarding the content of the delusion but attempts to identify the feelings that the patient is experiencing. Talking about the person's feelings is helpful; talking about delusional material is not.

It is *never* useful to argue or try to "reason" with the patient regarding the content of the delusion. Doing so can intensify the patient's retention of irrational beliefs. However, it is helpful for the nurse to clarify misinterpretations of the environment.

Patient: "I see the doctor is here, and he is part of this plan to destroy me."

Nurse: "It is true the doctor wants to see you, but he wants to talk to you about your treatment and find out if the medication is helping you. Would you feel more comfortable talking to him in his office without people around?"

Interacting with the patient about concrete realities in the environment helps minimize the time available for the patient to focus on delusional thoughts. Performance of specific manual tasks within the scope of the patient's abilities is also useful in distracting the patient from delusional thinking. The more time the patient spends engaged in reality-based activities or with people, the more opportunity the patient has to become comfortable with reality. Table 17-7 lists interventions for a patient experiencing delusions.

Paranoia

A paranoid individual may make offensive yet accurate criticisms of the nurse or the unit policies. It is important that the staff not react to these criticisms with anxiety or rejection of the patient. Staff conferences, peer groups, and clinical supervision are effective ways of looking beyond the behaviors to the motivations of the patient. This provides the opportunity to reduce the patient's anxiety and increase staff effectiveness.

It is important to approach a patient who is paranoid in a nonjudgmental, respectful manner and use clear and simple language, which helps minimize the opportunity for the patient to misconstrue the meaning of a message. Be honest and consistent with the patient regarding expectations and in enforcing rules. Suspicious people are quick to discern dishonesty. Honesty and consistency increase stability and decrease tension. Explaining to the patient what you are going to do prepares the patient and minimizes the opportunity for misinterpreting your intent as hostile or aggressive. Avoid laughing, whispering, or talking quietly when the patient cannot hear what is being said. Suspicious patients will

TABLE 17-6 Interventions for Hallucinations

Intervention	Rationale
1. Watch patients for cues that they may be hallucinating (e.g., eyes darting to one side, muttering, or staring sideways; changes in facial expressions).	1. Patients are usually in high levels of anxiety at this time. Early intervention may help interrupt hallucinatory process and lessen patient's anxiety and potential for harm.
2. Ask patients directly if they are hallucinating. "Are you hearing voices?" "What are they saying to you?"	2. The content of the "voices" can help both you and the patient discover the patient's feelings (e.g., fear, anger, worthlessness). The nurse can then address the feelings.
3. If voices are telling patients to harm self or others (*command hallucinations*): a. Notify appropriate authority (e.g., police, physician, administrator according to unit protocols). b. If in the community, evaluate need for hospitalization.	3. People often obey hallucinatory commands to kill self or others. Early assessment and intervention could save lives.
4. **Document** what patients say, if they are a threat to self or others, who was contacted and notified and when.	4. If the patient threatens self or others, documentation shows that correct legal protocols were followed. Otherwise, nurses, physicians, and institutions can be held legally responsible.
5. Accept the fact that the voices are real to patients, but explain that you do not hear the voices. Refer to the voices as "your voices" or "the voices that you hear."	5. Validating that your reality does not include voices may help patients cast doubt on their voices.
6. Present a calm demeanor and stay with patients while they are hallucinating. At times you can tell patients to tell the "voices they hear" to go away.	6. When patients feel comfortable with a nurse, they can sometimes learn to push the voices aside when given repeated instruction.
7. Keep patients focused on simple, basic, reality-based topics. Help patients focus on one idea at a time.	7. Hallucinating patients are confused and disorientated; helps patients focus on people and happenings in reality.
8. Help patients identify times and situations when hallucinations are the most prevalent and intense.	8. Helps nurse and patients identify situations and times that are the most threatening and find ways to mitigate perceived threats.
9. Assess for signs of increase in anxiety, fear, or agitation and intervene as soon as possible.	9. The earlier intervention takes place, the easier it is to calm patients and prevent harm.

TABLE 17-7   Interventions for Delusions

Intervention	Rationale
1. Assess if external controls are needed: if patient is agitated and believes someone is going to harm him or her or if patient must harm someone else to survive; use safety measures.	1. Beliefs are real for the patient and delusional thinking might dictate a need for self-defense. Evaluate least restrictive alternatives (confer with others if helpful).
2. Be aware that the patient's delusions represent the way that he or she is experiencing reality.	2. Identifying the patient's experience helps the nurse to understand the patient's feelings.
3. Identify feelings: a. If belief is an attempt to "get" the patient, then the patient is experiencing *fear*. b. If belief is someone is controlling the patient's thoughts, then the patient is experiencing *helplessness*.	3. The nurse can focus on feelings, not delusional content. a. "If you believe the CIA is out to kill you, you must feel frightened; are you feeling frightened?" b. "If you believe your thoughts are being controlled, are you feeling helpless?"
4. Engage the individual in yoga, exercise, walking, etc.	4. Shift the focus from the delusions and engage the patient in reality-based activities.
5. Do not argue with the patient's beliefs or try to correct false beliefs with logic or facts.	5. Arguing will only increase the patient's defensive position, thereby reinforcing false beliefs.
6. Do not touch the patient; use gestures very carefully, particularly if the patient is paranoid.	6. Give a delusional patient a lot of space. Touching may be perceived as an aggressive or sexual attempt; gestures may be misconstrued to support delusional thinking.
Paranoid Individual	
1. Place yourself beside patient not face-to-face	1. Face to face can be interpreted by a paranoid individual as confrontational (either standing or sitting)
2. Avoid direct eye contact	2. This can be construed as confrontational or threatening.
3. A paranoid patient might not eat or drink, thinking the food is poisoned. Offer food and fluids in closed containers such as a can of soda, a carton of yogurt, unpeeled fruit, or a hardboiled egg	3. Food that has not "been tampered with" is "safe" to eat, and some nutritional intake is possible
4. After understanding the patient's underlying feelings (e.g., fear, helplessness), engage the patient in reality-based activities such as cards or crafts.	4. When the patient is focused on reality-based activities, feelings associated with delusions are momentarily lessened.
5. If the patient is paranoid, often intellectual functions are higher and may respond better to more intellectually taxing noncompetitive activities.	5. The more a person is focused in reality, the greater the delusions can be minimized during that time.
6. Observe for events that trigger delusions.	6. Essentially, observe for events that make the patient anxious and fearful. Problem solve ways to mitigate the effect of these situations or events.
7. If anxiety escalates and the patient loses control, use least restrictive interventions (e.g., one-to-one therapy, prn medications, last resort seclusion). Always follow unit protocol and provide detailed documentation.	7. Usually a calm, nonthreatening presence during high levels of anxiety helps lower anxiety levels.

prn, As needed.

automatically think that they are the target of the interaction and interpret it in a negative manner (*ideas of reference*). Refer to Table 17-7.

Associative Looseness

The symptom of associative looseness often mirrors the patient's autistic thoughts and reflects the person's poorly organized thinking. An increase in this type of communication often indicates that the patient is feeling increased anxiety and an inability to respond to internal and external stimuli. The patient's ramblings also may confuse and frustrate the nurse. The following communication guidelines are useful with a patient whose speech is confused and disorganized:

- Do not pretend that you understand the patient's communications when you are confused by words or meanings.
- Tell the patient that you are having difficulty understanding.
- Place the difficulty in understanding on yourself, *not* on the patient. For example, say, "I am having trouble following what you are saying," *not* "You are not making any sense."
- Look for recurring topics and themes in the patient's communications. For example, "You've mentioned trouble with your brother several times. Tell me about your brother and your relationship with him."

- Emphasize what is going on in the patient's immediate environment (here and now) and involve the patient in simple reality-based activities. These measures can help the patient better focus thoughts.
- Tell the patient what you do understand, and reinforce clear communication and accurate expression of needs, feelings, and thoughts.

Health Teaching and Health Promotion

The family needs to be included in any psychological strategies aimed at reducing exacerbation of psychotic symptoms. Education is an essential strategy and includes teaching the patient and family about the illness (causes, medications, medication side effects, prevention of relapse), helping the patient and family recognize the effect of stress, ensuring an understanding of the importance of medication to a good outcome, encouraging involvement in psychosocial activities, and identifying sources for ongoing support in dealing with the illness. Some hospitals and clinics offer medication groups for patients (and sometimes family members as well). Medication groups can help patients deal more effectively with troubling side effects, alert the nurse to possible adverse or toxic reactions, and increase adherence to the medication regimen.

A Person with Schizophrenia

Scenario

I noticed Aaron standing barefooted in the hallway with both shoes in his outstretched hand. He almost looked like a statue with his blank, unaware demeanor. He deliberately picked up each foot and then slowly rubbed the ball of each foot against the carpet.

Therapeutic Goal

By the end of the present encounter, Aaron will demonstrate increased comfort with the student nurse as evidenced by voluntarily walking together in the hallways of the psychiatric unit.

Student-Patient Interaction	Thoughts, Communication Techniques, and Mental Health Nursing Concepts
Student: "Aaron, I am _____, one of the nursing students. Aaron, I'm standing next to you, on your right side."	With *schizophrenia* it is important to say his name and say my own name to make clear our separateness.
Student's feelings: *I'm kind of nervous. How scary and lonely his world must be.*	
Aaron: *Quietly murmuring.* "Don't know left, right, right, correct. I can't quite gather first one, last one. Can't last long … long … long lost soul. Soul train."	He may have an *ego boundary* disturbance. He also holds his shoes far away from his body. What are the clues inside his *loose associations?* He looks stuck just standing there yet he holds his shoes like he is *ambivalent* about going somewhere.
Student's feelings: *I wonder why he rubs each foot against the floor like he really needs to feel where the floor is.*	
Student's feelings: *That part, "long lost soul," makes me feel sad. I felt lost when I first arrived here at school without a single friend. When I let myself know what I'm feeling, memories of the losses in my childhood begin to stir.*	I need to focus on Aaron and deal with potential *countertransference* later. His most intense words are "long lost soul." That phrase is near the end of his rambling associations. He may remember the last words he spoke at some level. I will *restate* and then use *reflection* of feelings.
Student: "Long lost soul. You're feeling kind of lost right now. It's hard to decide what to do next."	Maybe he wants to get away on his own "soul train." Is he an *elopement* risk? Probably not. He is too confused right now to plan anything, though he may follow easily. I'll give some structure to meet *safety needs.*
Student: "Aaron, it's _____. Come with me and we'll figure out how to help you." *I touch his arm to direct him toward the day area.*	

Student-Patient Interaction	Thoughts, Communication Techniques, and Mental Health Nursing Concepts
Aaron: *Abruptly tilts his head toward opposite wall. He begins mumbling like he's responding to an unseen other.*	The touch violated his precarious *ego boundary.* He's *hallucinating*—my touch must have increased anxiety. I need to speak in short sentences with many pauses to slow this down.
Student's feelings: *I'm so upset with myself. I acted without thinking about how threatening my touch would be without asking first. I so want to help him and now I've scared him. I want to say, "I'm sorry" but that's my need. I'll tell him later when he's able to process information. Okay, keep focused. He needs to feel safe more than anything.*	
Student: "Aaron, I'm here. I'll stay with you."	I *offer self.*
Aaron: *Mumbles.* "The mistop … don't … can't … ." *Looks panicked.*	He is approaching *panic level* anxiety. "Mistop." What is that? Is it a *neologism?*
Student: "Aaron, talk to me. What are the voices saying?"	
Student's feelings: *My first job is to stay calm myself. He looks terrified. I need to let him know he's safe. I am okay. Even if I don't say everything right, I do care.*	
Aaron: *Shakes his head.* "Soul train, blame, shame, going to the end of the line … supine … surprise … demise."	He is making *clang associations.* I hear covert references that may be to suicide. I will *restate* and then ask a *direct question* to assess suicide potential.
Student: "The end of the line; demise. Aaron, are the voices telling you to hurt yourself or someone else?"	He probably cannot *reality test* enough to tell me whether the voices tell him to kill himself. I must report this now, but I also do not want to leave him alone if there is the slightest potential for suicide. He needs *close constant observation.*
Student's feelings: *Overwhelmed, I can't do this alone. Maybe medication will help. I hope at some level he will feel safer.*	
Aaron: *Mumbles.*	Before he did not come with me. Now he is walking beside me. He feels more comfortable with me now.
Student: *Without crowding him, I position myself so he can see my face. Quiet and concerned.* "Let's go together to talk to the nurse."	
Aaron: *Slowly walks with me.*	

When people lack understanding of the disease and its symptoms, they may misinterpret a patient's apathy and lack of drive as laziness. This erroneous assumption can foster hostility by family members, caregivers, or others in the community. Thus further teaching about the negative and positive symptoms of schizophrenia can reduce these tensions.

It is vital that nurses, physicians, and social workers be aware of the community support resources and make this information available to discharged patients as well as to their families. Examples of such resources include community mental health services, home health services, work support programs, day hospitals, social skills and support groups, family educational skills groups, and respite care.

Milieu Therapy

Although hospital stays are usually short, effective hospital care involves more than protection from family, social, or work environments that are stressful or disruptive. Many patients need the structure provided by hospitalization. In fact, patients in the acute phase of schizophrenia improve more on a unit with a structured milieu than on an open unit that allows greater freedom. Partial hospitalization programs, halfway houses, and day treatment centers also provide a structured milieu. A therapeutic milieu provides safety, useful activities, resources for resolving conflicts, and opportunities for learning social and vocational skills.

Safety

An individual with schizophrenia or other related psychotic disorders, especially in the acute phase, may be prone to physical violence, often in response to hallucinations (*voices* telling them others are out to harm or kill them or telling them to jump out a window) or delusions (*believing* that another is out to harm or kill them). During this time, measures need to be taken to protect the patient and others. If verbal deescalation efforts and chemical restraints (antipsychotic medication) fail to lessen the patient's aggression, physical restraints and seclusion may be used as a very last resort (see Chapters 6, 15, and 23).

With the shifting of care for the seriously mentally ill (SMI) from inpatient to community-based treatment centers, the need for transitional care is heightened and the role of the nurse in providing a therapeutic milieu is broadened. Alternatives to hospitalization include partial hospitalization, halfway houses, and day treatment programs:

- **Partial hospitalization:** Patients sleep at home and attend treatment sessions during the day or evening.
- **Halfway houses:** Patients live in the community with a group of other patients, sharing expenses and responsibilities. Staff are present in the house 24 hours a day, 7 days a week.
- **Day treatment programs:** Patients live in a halfway house or on their own, sometimes with home visits, or in residential programs. Patients attend a structured program during the day.

Some of these programs may include group therapy, supervised activities, individual counseling, or specialized training and rehabilitation (see Chapter 5).

Psychotherapy
Program of Assertive Community Treatment

Program of Assertive Community Treatment (PACT) or Assertive Community Treatment (ACT) is designed for the most marginally adjusted and poorly functioning patients. Its aim is to prevent relapse, maximize social and vocational functioning, and keep the individual in the community. It emphasizes the patient's strengths in adapting to the community, provides support and assertive outreach, and involves almost all aspects of the patient's life (e.g., food, shelter, schooling, grooming, budgeting, and transportation). PACT/ACT programs provide mobile crisis intervention, supportive cognitive and behavioral therapy, and substance abuse treatment, to name a few features. These programs have been shown to reduce hospital admissions and improve quality of life for many of these patients (Black & Andreasen, 2014). PACT is a team approach available around the clock. Medication adherence is emphasized.

Family Therapy

All evidence-based approaches emphasize the value of family participation in treatment. Families with members who are struggling with schizophrenia often endure considerable hardships while coping with the psychotic and residual symptoms of the illness. Often these families become isolated from their relatives and communities. Families are perhaps the most consistent factor in patients' lives. More than half of patients discharged from a psychiatric facility return to their family of origin. The following example shows how a family came to distinguish between "Martha's problem" and "the problem caused by schizophrenia."

> **VIGNETTE**
>
> It was a good idea, us all meeting in the comfort of our own home to discuss my sister's illness. We were all able to say how it felt, and for the first time I realized that I knew very little about what she was suffering from or how much—the word *schizophrenia* meant nothing to me before but it's much clearer now. I used to think she was just being lazy until she told me in the meeting what it was really like (Gamble & Brennan, 2000).

Programs that provide support, education, coping skills training, and social network development are extremely effective. Medication and psychosocial treatments with family interventions have been shown to reduce relapse rates in the treatment of early schizophrenia. A popular approach with patients and families is a **psychoeducational approach.** It brings educational and behavioral approaches into family treatment. The psychoeducational approach recognizes that families are secondary victims of a biological illness. In family therapy sessions, fears, faulty communication patterns, and distortions are identified. Improved problem-solving skills can be taught, and healthier alternatives to situations of conflict can be explored. Family guilt and anxiety can be lessened, which facilitates change.

Multiple-family groups are beneficial for both families and to the family member with schizophrenia. Multiple-family groups have been found to be effective in reducing symptom relapses and rehospitalizations for individuals with schizophrenia (Jewell et al., 2009). Improvement seems to stem from an expansion of the social network available to the family and patient as well as an expansion in problem-solving capacity afforded by a group. Multiple-family groups also decrease emotional overinvolvement while increasing the overall positive tone, which is characteristic of such groups. Box 17-4 lists psychoeducational strategies for the patient and family.

Cognitive Behavioral Therapy

Data support the efficacy of cognitive behavioral therapy (CBT) in conjunction with medication for reducing the frequency and intensity of delusions and hallucinations (positive symptoms), promoting treatment resistance, improving insight and compliance, and alleviating aggression in patients with schizophrenia (Brauser, 2010; Rathod et al., 2010). People with schizophrenia or delusional disorders who seem to benefit most are usually chronic outpatients with treatment-resistant forms of the disease who often have distressing delusions or hallucinations. Usually several months are required, although treatment can last for years.

Social Skills Training

Social skills training (SST) can improve the level of social activity, foster new social contacts, improve quality of life, and help lower anxiety. Complex behaviors used in daily living are divided into discrete behavioral techniques (e.g., how to properly answer the phone and take a message, how to initiate a social dialogue, how to order a meal). SST has been shown to improve social competence in patients with schizophrenia (Brauser, 2010), especially in those newly diagnosed with the disease.

The Recovery Model Adapted for Schizophrenia

The recovery model for schizophrenia is based on the model used by the Substance Abuse and Mental Health Services Association (SAMHSA, 2012). According to the model, recovery has many pathways, each person is unique, and treatment needs to be personalized and holistic. The recovery model includes support by peers and family, as well as through relationships and social networks. Because we are all from different backgrounds and cultural subgroups, recovery must be culturally based.

The recovery model does not focus on symptoms as much as on fostering hope, rebuilding self-image, coping with life's challenges,

BOX 17-4 Psychoeducational Strategies for Patient and Family

1. Learn all you can about the illness.
   - Attend psychoeducational groups.
   - Attend support groups.
   - Join the National Alliance on Mental Illness (NAMI).
   - Contact the National Institute of Mental Health (NIMH).
2. Develop a relapse prevention plan.
   - Know the early warning signs of relapse (e.g., social withdrawal, trouble sleeping, increased bizarre or magical thinking).
   - Know whom to call and where to go when early signs of relapse appear.
   - Relapse is part of the illness, not a sign of failure.
3. Take advantage of all psychoeducational tools.
   - Participate in family, group, and individual therapy.
   - Learn new behaviors and cognitive coping skills to help handle intrafamily stress and interpersonal, social, and vocational difficulties. Get information from health care workers (nurse, case manager, physician), NAMI, community mental health groups, or a hospital.
   - Everyone needs a place to address their fears and losses, and to learn new ways of coping.

4. Comply with treatment.
   - Research has determined that people who do the best in coping with the disease comply with treatment that works for them.
   - Tell your health care worker (nurse, caseworker, physician, social worker) about troubling side effects (e.g., sexual problems, weight gain, "feeling funny"). Most side effects can be treated.
   - Keeping side effects a secret or stopping medication can prevent you from having the best quality of life. Share your concerns.
5. Avoid alcohol and drugs; they can act on the brain and precipitate a relapse.
6. Keep in touch with supportive people.
7. Keep healthy—stay in balance.
   - Self-care deficit is reflected in high rates of medical comorbidity.
   - Maintain a regular sleep pattern.
   - Maintain self-care (e.g., diet, hygiene).
   - Keep active (hobbies, friends, groups, sports, job, special interests).
   - Learn ways to reduce stress.

Patients and family members should be given telephone numbers and addresses of local support groups that are affiliated with NAMI (www.nami.org).

Data from Zerbe, K. J. (1999). *Women's mental health in primary care.* Philadelphia, PA: Saunders/Baillière Tindall; Tandon, R., et al. (2003). *Beyond symptoms control: Moving towards positive patient outcomes.* Paper presented at the American Psychiatric Association 55th Institute on Psychiatric Services, October 31, 2003, Boston, MA. Retrieved January 21, 2005, from www.medscape.com/viewprogram/2835_pnt

facilitating services leading to recovery, and helping the individual to have some control over his or her illness. The individual is a partner in planning his or her goals and formulating a treatment plan, not a "patient" (APNA, 2012). The clinician, nurse, or physician will set the primary goals—for example, the patient will no longer hear voices, the patient will keep appointments at the clinic, the patient will no longer think people are out to kill him or her. In addition, the individual with schizophrenia might set a goal to become more independent and socially involved. Taking medication and keeping

appointments will not by themselves help the individual to meet the goals.

Choosing any of the interventions mentioned above or the medications discussed below may be a part of the individual's treatment plan, which will also include many supports and treatment options. In the recovery model, the focus is on increasing the individual's abilities and functioning. Again, recovery is supported through relationships and social networks, encouraging internal empowerment through inclusion (SAMHSA, 2012). See Chapters 5 and 19 for more on the recovery model.

APPLYING EVIDENCE-BASED PRACTICE (EBP)

Problem A 52-year-old male with paranoid schizophrenia has been a patient at a community mental health clinic for about 10 years. Due to scarcity of psychiatric professionals in this rural area, he sees his psychiatric nurse practitioner (NP) via telemedicine. He has a history of being noncompliant with his appointments and medications, and as a result his symptoms have escalated. During the worst periods, the patient does not eat, drink, or sleep adequately, has vivid and terrifying hallucinations of bloody people and demons, and becomes very paranoid. He isolates in his home much of the time, and when he does come to town he appears disheveled and rants and raves loudly, which scares others. He has been arrested on several occasions as a result of his behaviors.

EBP Assessment

A. **What do you already know from experience?** This patient has a pattern of missing appointments and medications. Patients who adhere to their treatment plan have much better outcomes. This patient has complained frequently about the telemedicine appointments, although most of the clinic patients do not mind the setup. He says he doesn't like talking to a machine, and at times feels he is being recorded and his thoughts are being broadcast through the computer to the government.

B. **What does the literature say?** In general, telemedicine is cost effective, able to extend care to underserved areas, and used in numerous settings, including psychiatric clinics, emergency departments, nursing homes, home health, and correctional facilities. Patient perception varies, as some patients are satisfied with telemedicine appointments while others prefer face-to-face contact with

their provider. Nonadherence is an issue in up to 72% of patients with schizophrenia. The relationship between the primary care physician (PCP) and other staff and the patient is an important component in compliance with treatment.

C. **What does the patient want?** The patient does not like the telemedicine appointments. When taking his medications and thinking more clearly, he recognizes the need for treatment. While in an acute schizophrenic episode, he becomes extremely paranoid and it is difficult to reason with him.

Plan Due to the long-standing problems with this patient, the clinic devised an individualized plan of care. The patient was assigned a peer support person who visits him several times a week. Transportation was provided to a city about 75 miles away, where the patient can meet with his psychiatric NP face to face, accompanied by his peer support person for support. The patient became more compliant as he developed relationships with his caregivers, his symptoms were monitored more closely, and his paranoia was decreased. He eventually accepted telemedicine appointments part of the time.

QSEN QSEN Prelicensure Knowledge, Skills, and Attitudes (KSAs) Addressed:

Informatics was used to provide health care through telemedicine to the majority of patients in this rural setting.

Team work and collaboration was displayed as the clinic worked with the psychiatric NP and peer support to provide individualized care.

Susan L. Frost, Chyllia D. Fosbre, 2015

Acosta, F. J., Hernandez, J. L., Pereira, J., Herrera, J., & Rodriguez, C. J. (2012). Medication adherence in schizophrenia. *World Journal of Psychiatry,* 2(5), 74–82; American Telemedicine Association. (2012). Telemedicine case studies [website]. Retrieved from www.americantelemed.org/about-telemedicine/telemedicine-case-studies#.VfWZGBFViko

Neurobiology of Schizophrenia and the Effects of Antipsychotics

The antipsychotics affect a number of neurotransmitters including dopamine, noradrenaline/norepinephrine, serotonin, and GABA Excess of serotonin may contribute to both the positive and negative symptoms of schizophrenia. GABA regulates dopamine activity and in some people with schizophrenia, there is a loss of GABAergic neurons in the hippocampus, potentially causing hyperactivity of dopamine. However, since dopamine is the most studied and most prominent of the neurotransmitters (D1, D2, D3, D4, and D5) in schizophrenia, the role of dopamine is presented here.

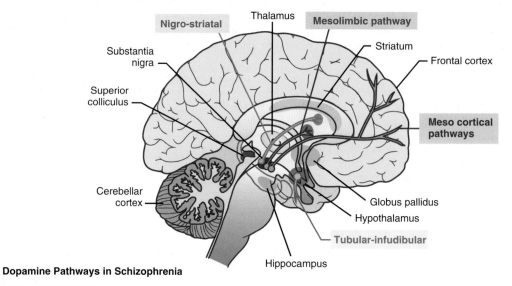

Dopamine Pathways in Schizophrenia

Mesolimbic pathway: reward motivation, emotions and positive symptoms of schizophrenia.

Meso cortical pathways: relevant to cognitive function and executive function and negative symptoms of schizophrenia

Nigro-striatal: normally responsible for purposeful movement.

Tubuler-infundibular: normally responsible for regulation of prolactin.

First generation antipsychotic (FGA) drugs are potent antagonists/blockers of D2.

Second generation antipsychotics (SGA) have less affinity for D2 receptors, and tend to bind with D3 and D4 receptors. Since the expression of D3 and D4 is limited to the neurons of the limbic system and cerebral cortex, the action of these drugs are limited to areas involved in the pathology of schizophrenia. Second generation drugs also inhibit the serotonin (5-HT) receptors. Since serotonin inhibits the release of dopamine, the dopaminergic transmission is affected.

The potential serious effects of the SGA's (metabolic effects: weight gain, diabetes, and dyslipidemia) come from the blockade of noradrenaline/norepinephrine (alpha-1), histamine, and acetylcholine.

Dopamine Pathways and Antipsychotic Responses

Dopamine Pathway	Abnormality in Schizophrenia	Responses to Antipsychotic Drugs
Mesolimbic pathway connects the VTA to the nucleus accumbens Associated with reward, motivation, and emotion	Hyperactive in schizophrenia Associated with positive symptoms (hallucinations, delusions, disorganized thought)	FGA—D2 blockage results in reduction in positive symptoms SGA—D3 and D4 antagonism results in reduction of positive symptoms
Mesocortical pathway made up of dopaminergic neurons that project from the ventral tegmental area to the prefrontal cortex Relevant to cognition, executive function, emotions, and affect	Hypofunction in schizophrenia results in cognitive impairment and negative symptoms (apathy, anhedonia, lack of motivation)	FGA—D2 blockage may result in a worsening of these symptoms SGA—Since there are more serotonin (5-HT) receptors than D2 receptors in this area, blockage of 5-HT is more profound. Blockage of 5-HT may help improve negative symptoms
Tuberoinfundibular pathway consists of dopaminergic projections from the hypothalamus to the pituitary gland Inhibits prolactin release	Unaffected	FGA (to a less degree SGA)—Blockade of D2 receptors increases prolactin levels resulting in hyperprolactinemia and lactation
Nigrostriatal pathway-substantial nigra to basal ganglia Responsible for purposeful movement	Unaffected	FGA (to a lesser degree SGA)—Long-term blockade of D2 receptors can cause upregulation (increase response to a stimulus) to those receptors, which may lead to extrapyramidal side effects e.g., tardive dyskinesia (TD).

Pharmacological, Biological, and Integrative Therapies

According to APNA (2012), there is greater focus on producing pharmacological treatments for schizophrenia that have fewer neurological side effects; mitigate medical concerns like diabetes, weight gain, and heart disease; target cognitive defects; and find strategies to better personalize treatments. This focus incorporates the recovery model for schizophrenia. Drugs used to treat psychotic disorders are called *antipsychotic medications.* Although they may alleviate many of the symptoms of schizophrenia, they cannot cure the underlying psychotic processes. Therefore when patients stop taking their medications, psychotic symptoms usually return. An additional concern is that with each relapse following medication discontinuation it takes longer to achieve remission after restarting medications. This leads to the possibility that the patient will eventually become unresponsive to treatment.

There are two basic groups of antipsychotic drugs: *first-generation antipsychotics* (FGAs)/conventional drugs, the dopamine antagonists (D_2 receptor antagonists); and *second-generation antipsychotics* (SGAs)/atypical agents, the serotonin-dopamine antagonists (5-HT$_{2A}$ and 5-HT$_{2C}$ receptor antagonists). In addition, some drugs are used to augment the antipsychotic agents for treatment-resistant patients.

All antipsychotic drugs are effective for most acute exacerbations of schizophrenia and for preventing or mitigating the occurrence of relapse. Two major government studies (in the United States and Great Britain) have established that both the first-generation antipsychotics (FGAs)/conventional drugs and the second-generation antipsychotics (SGAs)/atypical agents are equally effective at targeting the positive symptoms of schizophrenia (hallucinations and delusions), targeting the negative symptoms of schizophrenia (FGAs less so than SGAs), and improving neurocognition (Burchum & Rosenthal, 2016). "Therefore, the oversimplified distinction of antipsychotic drugs classes, in which FGAs are responsible for EPS [extrapyramidal side effects] and SGAs for metabolic side effects, though ingrained in clinical practice, is actually not supported by recent findings" (Divac et al., 2014). However, both first-generation and second-generation antipsychotic medications *should not* be used in older adults with dementia since they double the mortality risk (Burchum & Rosenthal, 2016).

The **atypical second-generation antipsychotics** have fewer disturbing EPS. However, the SGAs in general have a higher risk for metabolic syndrome (weight gain, diabetes, and dyslipidemia) than the first-generation antipsychotics. As well, the SGAs lead to more cardiovascular events and premature deaths than the first-generation antipsychotics (Burchum & Rosenthal, 2016). The SGAs are also considerably more expensive than the more traditional FGAs.

Although most individuals prefer oral medications, those who are nonadherent to medication therapy and are prone to frequent relapse, and/or would find it more convenient for their situation, are candidates for long-lasting injectable formulations (usually lasting 2 to 4 weeks). A 3-month injectable, paliperidone (Invega), is currently in development and will delay relapse with no increase in side effects (Melville, 2015).

Individuals may notice positive effects within 1 to 2 days, but it may take 2 to 4 weeks for more noticeable improvement, and several months for full effects (Burchum & Rosenthal, 2016). Most individuals with schizophrenia respond at least partially to antipsychotic drug therapy. However, without drug treatment, up to 70% to 80% of individuals will relapse within a year.

Because the SGAs/atypical agents (except for clozapine, which can cause agranulocytosis) are generally the treatment of choice for patients experiencing their first episode of schizophrenia, the second-generation antipsychotics are discussed first.

Second-Generation Antipsychotics/Atypical Agents

The second-generation antipsychotics first emerged in the early 1990s with clozapine (Clozaril). Unfortunately, clozapine produces agranulocytosis in 1% to 2% of people who take it. Agranulocytosis occurs when the bone marrow does not make enough of a certain type of mature white blood cells (neutrophils), exposing a person to increased infections and fever, and can be fatal. Clozapine also increases the risk for seizures. This drug is rarely used today except for treatment-refractory patients. The SGAs developed after clozapine do not share these same disadvantages.

Although there does seem to be increasing use of first-generation antipsychotics (FGAs), **the SGAs are still often chosen as first-line antipsychotics.**

Old second-generation antipsychotics (and some first-generation antipsychotics), with the exception of ziprasidone and aripiprazole, have a tendency to cause significant weight gain. Weight gain is a serious metabolic side effect and is associated with a cascade of additional side effects, including:

- Glucose dysregulation, which increases the propensity for diabetes
- Hypercholesterolemia, which increases the propensity for cardiovascular disease/stroke
- Hypertension
- Diminished self-esteem related to weight, which leads to problems in adherence to the medication regimen

There have been some cases in which the first indication of metabolic syndrome was discovered when the patient developed diabetic coma (Table 17-8).

First-Generation Antipsychotics/Conventional Drugs

The first-generation antipsychotics/conventional drugs were being less widely used because of their troubling side effects; however, the FGAs are being revisited because of the concern over the higher incidence of metabolic side effects with the SGAs and because FGAs are more cost-effective. The National Institute of Mental Health has conducted groundbreaking clinical antipsychotic trials of intervention effectiveness (CATIE) studies to compare continuation rates of the FGAs and SGAs. Important findings so far are that people quit taking older medications because of side effects, and that they quit taking the newer ones because of weight gain. Although there are many uncomfortable and some serious side effects with the FGAs, they are generally safe and when taken regularly can greatly reduce the rate of relapse.

"The FGAs block a variety of receptors within and outside the central nervous system (CNS) including *dopamine, acetylcholine, histamine,* and *norepinephrine* (Burchum & Rosenthal, 2016). Refer to Figure 4-13 for adverse effects related to the receptor blockage caused by antipsychotics. FGAs are effective in psychosis by blocking dopamine receptors in the mesenteric region of the brain, but they also affect the D_2 receptor sites in both the limbic and the motor centers. This blockage of D_2 receptor sites in the motor areas of the brain is responsible for some of the most troubling side effects of the FGAs, namely the extrapyramidal symptoms (EPS) of akathisia, dystonia, parkinsonism, and tardive dyskinesia (TD). TD is perhaps the biggest concern of all the EPS since it is irreversible and can be socially isolating. Other adverse reactions include anticholinergic effects, orthostasis, and lowered seizure threshold.

When the FGAs are used, the specific drug is often chosen for its side effect profile. For example, chlorpromazine (Thorazine), *a low potency* FGA, is the most sedating agent and has fewer EPS than do other antipsychotic agents, but it causes hypotension in large dosages. Haloperidol (Haldol), *a high potency* FGA, is the least sedating

TABLE 17-8 Second-Generation Antipsychotics (SGAs)/Atypical Agents

Drug Name, Generic (Trade)	Route(s)	Indication for Use	EPS	Ach	OH	Sed	Comments/Notable Adverse Reactions
Clozapine (Clozaril, Leponex)	PO ODT*: FazaClo	Treatment-resistant schizophrenia and schizophrenia-related suicide behavior	No	High	High	High	• **Not first line;** refractory cases only • Agranulocytosis in 0.8%-1%; scheduled WBC required • High seizure rate • Increased risk for diabetes • Significant weight gain (67%) • High lipid abnormalities • Excessive salivation • Tachycardia
Risperidone (Risperdal, Risperdal Consta)	PO ODT*: Risperdal M-TAB Consta Injection (long-acting)	Schizophrenia	High (dose-related)	Very low	Moderate	Low	• Hypotension/dizziness • Insomnia • Sedation • Rarely NMS, TD • Sexual dysfunction • Weight gain (18%) • Moderate lipid abnormalities • Increased risk for diabetes
Paliperidone (Invega) Invega Sustenna	Extended release Long-acting** intramuscular injection	Schizophrenia and schizoaffective disorder	Mild (dose-related)	Very low	Moderate	Low	• Has same side effects as risperidone • Better tolerated than risperidone • Not approved for elderly, especially those with dementia
Olanzapine† (Zyprexa Relprevv)	PO ODT*: Zyprexa Long-acting IM injection	Schizophrenia and agitation	Low	Moderate	Moderate	High	• Significant weight gain (34%) • High lipid abnormalities • Increased risk for diabetes • Drowsiness • Hyperprolactinemia • Agitation and restlessness • Insomnia • Hypotension • Seizures at initiation of therapy • Possibly akathisia or parkinsonism

Quetiapine† (Seroquel, Seroquel XL)	PO	Schizophrenia	Low	Mild	Moderate	Moderate	• Weight gain (23%)
							• Moderate lipid abnormalities
							• May increase risk for diabetes
							• **Serious side effects:**
							  • Cardiac dysrhythmias
							  • Syncope
							  • NMS
							  • Seizures

Generic (Trade) Name	Route/Form	Use					Serious side effects
Ziprasidone (Geodon), Injectable (short acting)	PO Short-acting IM injection	Schizophrenia and acute agitation	Low	Mild	Mild	Low	**Serious side effects:** • ECG changes‡ • QT prolongation; not to be used with other drugs known to prolong QT interval • Low propensity for weight gain • Diabetic ketoacidosis • Dyskinesia • NMS may occur
Iloperidone (Fanapt)	PO		Low (dose-dependent)	Low to mild	Low to moderate	Low to moderate	• Weight gain • May affect cardiac QTc interval • Not for use as first line in patients with cardiac conditions • May increase risk for diabetes and dyslipidemia • Severe EPS can cause NMS and TD
Asenapine (Saphris)	Sublingual tablets (ODT*)	Schizophrenia	Low to moderate (dose-dependent)	No	No	Moderate	• May increase risk for diabetes • Newer drug; at this writing, clinical use will tell; drug trials show favorable side effect profile • Severe EPS can cause NSM and TD
Lurasidone HCl (Latuda)	PO		High				• Take with food • Metabolic changes (high blood glucose and diabetes) • High cholesterol and triglycerides • Weight gain • Low WBC • More sensitive to heat; may take time to cool down • Most common reactions: sleepiness, inner restlessness (akathisia), movement abnormalities, muscle stiffness (Parkinson-like symptoms)
Brexpiprazole (Rexulti)							• FDA approved July 2015. • This atypical antipsychotic is approved in the treatment of schizophrenia, and as adjunct therapy for major depression.

*An orally disintegrating tablet (ODT) is a fast-disintegrating tablet or wafer that dissolves on the tongue.

**At this writing, researchers are working on paliperidone (Invega Sustenna), a long-term injectable that can be given once every 3 months.

†The safety of olanzapine at dosages >20 mg/day and quetiapine at dosages >800 mg/day has not been evaluated in clinical trials.

‡Ziprasidone use may carry a risk for QT prolongation in patients with preexisting cardiac disease, low electrolyte levels, or family history of QTc syndrome, or in patients taking other drugs that cause long QTc profiles.

Ach, Anticholinergic side effects (dry mouth, blurred vision, urinary retention, constipation, agitation); *ECG*, electrocardiogram; *EPS*, extrapyramidal symptoms; *IM*, intramuscular; *NMS*, neuroleptic malignant syndrome; *ODT*, orally disintegrating tablet; *OH*, orthostatic hypotension; *PO*, by mouth; *Sed*, sedation; *TD*, tardive dyskinesia; *WBC*, white blood cell count.

and is often used in large doses to reduce assaultive behavior, but it has a high incidence of EPS. The value of haloperidol for treating violent behaviors is its effectiveness in controlling hallucinatory phenomena with a low incidence of hypotension. People who are functioning at work or at home may prefer less sedating drugs; patients who are agitated or excitable may do better with a more sedating medication.

All of the conventional antipsychotic drugs can cause tardive dyskinesia, and should be used with caution in people who have seizure disorders because they can lower the seizure threshold. Table 17-9 identifies drugs according to low, medium, and high potency; gives dosages for treatment of acute symptoms and usual maintenance dosages; and lists other considerations.

Tardive dyskinesia (TD) is an EPS that usually appears after prolonged treatment, is more serious, and is not always reversible. Tardive dyskinesia consists of involuntary tonic muscular spasms that typically involve the tongue, fingers, toes, neck, trunk, or pelvis. This potentially serious EPS is most frequently seen in women and older patients. Tardive dyskinesia varies from mild to moderate and can be disfiguring or incapacitating.

Early symptoms of tardive dyskinesia are fasciculations of the tongue or constant lip smacking. These early oral movements can develop into uncontrollable biting, chewing, or sucking motions; an open mouth; and lateral movements of the jaw. In many cases, the early symptoms of tardive dyskinesia disappear when the antipsychotic medication is discontinued. In other cases, however, early symptoms are not reversible and may progress. No proven cure for advanced tardive dyskinesia exists. The National Institute of Mental Health developed a brief test for the detection of tardive dyskinesia referred to as the Abnormal Involuntary Movement Scale (AIMS). The AIMS test is one of the tools nurses and physicians can use to detect TD. The AIMS test can be obtained on the Internet.

Three of the more common EPS are acute dystonia (severe spasms of the muscles of the tongue, head, and neck; fixed upward deviation of the eyes; and severe back spasms that arch the trunk forward and thrust the head and lower limbs backward), akathisia (internal restlessness and external restless pacing or fidgeting), and pseudoparkinsonism (stiffening of muscular activity in the face, body, arms, and legs).

Neuroleptic malignant syndrome (NMS) is estimated to occur in about 0.2% to 1% of patients who have taken antipsychotic agents. It is believed that the acute reduction in brain dopamine activity plays a role in the development of NMS, which is fatal in about 10% of cases. It usually occurs early in the course of therapy but has been reported in people after 20 years of treatment.

Neuroleptic malignant syndrome is characterized by decreased level of consciousness; greatly increased muscle tone; and autonomic dysfunction, including hyperpyrexia, labile hypertension, tachycardia, tachypnea, diaphoresis, and drooling. Treatment consists of early detection, discontinuation of the antipsychotic agent, management of fluid balance, reduction of temperature, and monitoring for complications. Mild cases of neuroleptic malignant syndrome are treated with bromocriptine (Parlodel), whereas more severe cases are treated with intravenous dantrolene (Dantrium) and even with electroconvulsive therapy in some cases. See Table 17-10 for the side effects, onset, and nursing measures for EPS and NMS.

Agranulocytosis is also a serious side effect of the FGAs and can be fatal. Liver involvement also may occur. Nurses need to be aware of the prodromal signs and symptoms of these side effects and teach them to their patients and patients' families.

Side effects often appear early in therapy and can be minimized with treatment. Treatment usually consists of lowering the dosage or

prescribing antiparkinsonian drugs, especially centrally acting anticholinergic drugs. Commonly used drugs include trihexyphenidyl (Artane), benztropine mesylate (Cogentin), diphenhydramine hydrochloride (Benadryl), biperiden (Akineton), and amantadine hydrochloride (Symmetrel). However, treatment with antiparkinsonian drugs is not completely benign because the anticholinergic side effects of the antipsychotics may be intensified (e.g., urinary retention, constipation, failure of visual accommodation [blurred vision], cognitive impairment, and delirium).

Most patients develop tolerance to EPS after a few months. Effective nursing and medical management are important to encourage adherence with the medication regimen until the major side effects have been properly managed. Table 17-11 identifies some of the drugs most commonly used for the treatment of EPS.

A Caveat: How Antipsychotics Cause Brain Damage

There is recent concern that antipsychotics may be contributing to brain damage in people with schizophrenia and may be associated with, and even contribute to, the severity of cognitive symptoms seen in individuals with schizophrenia. It appears that the dosage, the duration of taking the drug, and the specific drug itself may play a part in the extent of brain damage (Mental Health Daily, 2015).

Prefrontal connectivity reductions. There is evidence derived from resting fMRI studies suggesting that connections in the prefrontal region of the brain are reduced as a result of antipsychotic treatment. A reduced number of connections may translate to reductions in complex thinking, planning, attention, emotional regulation, and memory.

Global brain volume loss. Studies have noted that antipsychotics reduce global brain volume. This means that the brain of a person with schizophrenia, who has undergone years of antipsychotic treatment (especially at high doses), may display signs of neurodegeneration. Reductions in global brain volume means that nearly every aspect of brain functioning has potential to become impaired.

White matter volume loss. White matter is tissue that allows your brain to communicate with the central nervous system. It is comprised of myelin and axons, both of which facilitate chemical messages within the brain. Since those taking antipsychotics experience reductions in white matter, the communication system within their brain becomes impaired.

Gray matter volume loss. Gray matter is known to include various regions of the brain responsible for sensory perception, emotions, self-control, speech, decision making, and muscle control. Individuals taking antipsychotics experience reductions in gray matter volume, making it tougher to perform certain functions. However, there seems to be more gray matter loss in patients taking higher mean daily doses of first-generation antipsychotics, and less gray matter loss in those patients taking only second-generation antipsychotics (Vita, et al., 2015).

Adjuncts to Antipsychotic Drug Therapy

Antidepressants. Antidepressants are added to antipsychotics when the symptoms meeting the criteria for major depression cause severe distress, including suicidal thoughts, or when depression is disabling. In fact, a study by Tiihonen and colleagues (2012) found that the use of antidepressants was associated with markedly decreased suicidal deaths.

Benzodiazepines. Although benzodiazepines have been used in the past as an adjunct to antipsychotics, a new study demonstrated that benzodiazepine use was associated with marked increase in morbidity (Tiihonen et al., 2012).

TABLE 17-9   First-Generation Antipsychotics/Conventional Drugs

Drug Name, Generic (Trade)	Route(s) of Administration	Indication for Use	Special Considerations
High Potency: Less histaminic effects (e.g., sedation), Less Ach*, More EPS			
Haloperidol (Haldol)	Tablet, oral concentrate, short-acting IM injection, long-acting IM injection (lasts 3-4 weeks)	Schizophrenia, acute agitation	• **Low** sedative properties; used in large doses with assaultive patients to avoid severe side effect of hypotension • Lessens chance of falls from dizziness or hypotension • **High** EPS • Can prolong the QT interval, leading to dysrhythmias • TD
Trifluoperazine (Stelazine)	Capsule, oral concentrate, short-acting IM injection	Schizophrenia	• **Low** sedative effect; good for symptoms of withdrawal or paranoia • **High** incidence of EPS and TD • NMS, convulsions, and agranulocytosis are rare but can occur • Ach
Fluphenazine (formally available as Prolixin)	Tablet, oral concentrate, short-acting IM injection, long-acting IM injection (every 2-4 weeks)	Schizophrenia and other psychotic disorders	• High EPS • Occasional sedation, orthostatic hypotension, Ach
Medium Potency			
Loxapine (Loxitane)	Capsule, oral concentrate, short-acting IM injection	Schizophrenia only	• EPS • Seizures • Confusion • NMS • Ach • Orthostatic hypotension, EEG changes, tachycardia, cardiac arrest
Perphenazine (formally available as Trilafon)	Tablet, oral concentrate, short-acting IM injection	Schizophrenia	• Side effects similar to fluphenazine • Can help control severe vomiting
Low Potency: Higher sedation, Higher Ach*, Fewer EPS			
Chlorpromazine (Thorazine)	Tablet, oral solution, suppository capsule, short-acting IM injection	Schizophrenia and other psychotic disorders Schizoaffective disorder Manic phase of bipolar disorder Intractable hiccups Control nausea and vomiting Control of severe behavior problems in children	• Increased sensitivity to sun (as with other phenothiazines) • Highest sedative and hypotensive effects • High Ach • Sedation • Lowers seizure threshold • Rare: agranulocytosis and NMS
Thioridazine (formally known as Mellaril)	Tablet, oral concentrate	Treatment-resistant schizophrenia only.	• **Not recommended as first-line antipsychotic** • Dose-related severe ECG changes (prolonged QTc intervals); may cause fatal cardiac arrhythmias

*Dosages vary with individual response to the antipsychotic agent used.
Data from Burchum, J. & Rosenthal, L. (2016). *Lehne's pharmacology for nursing care.* (6th ed.). St Louis, MO: Saunders; Skidmore, L. R. (2013) *Nursing Drug Reference* (26th ed.). St. Louis, MO: Mosby; Preston, J. D., O'Neal, J. H., & Talaga, M. C. (2013). *Handbook of clinical psychopharmacology for therapists* (7th ed.). Oakland, CA: New Harbinger Publications.
Ach, Anticholinergic side effects (dry mouth, dry eyes, blurred vision [especially near vision], urinary retention, constipation, agitation, tachycardia, sedation, and sexual dysfunction); *ECG,* electrocardiogram; *EEG,* electroencephalogram; *EPS,* extrapyramidal symptoms (Parkinsonian side effects, dystonia, akathisia); *IM,* intramuscular; *NMS,* neuroleptic malignant syndrome; *TD,* tardive dyskinesia.

TABLE 17-10   Nursing Measures for Extrapyramidal Symptoms and Neuroleptic Malignant Syndrome: First-Generation Antipsychotics/Conventional Drugs

Side Effect	Onset	Nursing Measures
All conventional antipsychotics share similar side effects, but differ in terms of potency as well as personal reaction to the drug. • Anticholinergic side effects (Ach) • Antiadrenergic side effect = orthostatic hypotension (drop in blood pressure on standing; may lead to falls and injury) • Lower seizure threshold • May raise prolactin levels, causing lactation • **Rarer: agranulocytosis, hyperthermia, neuroleptic malignant syndrome (NMS)**		

Extrapyramidal Symptoms (EPS)

Side Effect	Onset	Nursing Measures
1. **Pseudoparkinsonism:** masklike facies, stiff and stooped posture, shuffling gait, drooling, tremor, "pill-rolling" phenomenon	5 hours to 30 days	1. Alert medical staff. An anticholinergic agent (e.g., trihexyphenidyl [Artane] or benztropine [Cogentin]) may be used.
2. **Acute dystonic reactions:** acute spasms of tongue, face, neck, and back (tongue and jaw first) • **Opisthotonos:** tetanic heightening of entire body, head and belly up • **Oculogyric crisis:** eyes locked upward	A few hours to 5 days	2. Diphenhydramine hydrochloride (Benadryl) IM/IV or benztropine IM/IV. Relief occurs in minutes. Prevent further dystonias with any anticholinergic agent (see Table 17-11). Experience is very frightening. Take patient to quiet area and stay with him or her until medicated.
3. **Akathisia:** Distressing motor inner-driven restlessness (e.g., tapping foot incessantly, rocking forward and backward in chair, shifting weight from side to side).	2 hours to 60 days	3. Reduced dosage or switched to a low-potency antipsychotic. Treat with anticholinergic, benzodiazepine, or beta blockers.

4. **Tardive dyskinesia (TD)***
• **Facial:** protruding and rolling tongue, blowing, smacking, licking, spastic facial distortion, smacking movements
• **Limbs**
  • Choreic: rapid, purposeless, and irregular movements
  • Athetoid: slow, complex, and serpentine movements
• **Trunk:** neck and shoulder movements, dramatic hip jerks and rocking, twisting pelvic thrusts
	Months to years	4. No known treatment. Discontinuing the drug does not always relieve symptoms. Occurs in 15% to 20% of patients taking these drugs for more than 2 years. Eating difficulties; malnutrition can occur because of tongue and mouth involvement. Frequent screening with the AIMS test can help detect TD in early stages.

Neuroleptic Malignant Syndrome (NMS)

Side Effect	Onset	Nursing Measures
Somewhat rare, potentially fatal. • **Severe extrapyramidal:** severe muscle rigidity, oculogyric crisis, dysphasia, flexor-extensor posturing, cogwheeling • **Hyperpyrexia:** elevated temperature (>103°F [up to degrees 41°C])	Can occur in the first week of drug therapy but often occurs later. Rapidly progresses over 2 to 3 days after initial manifestation.	Stop neuroleptic. Transfer stat to medical unit. Bromocriptine (Parlodel) can relieve muscle rigidity and reduce fever. Dantrolene (Dantrium) may reduce muscle spasms.
• **Autonomic dysfunction:** hypertension, tachycardia, diaphoresis, incontinence • Level of consciousness from confused, mute, coma and/or seizures, even death.	**Risk factors:** • Concomitant use of psychotropics • Older age • Female gender (3:2) • Presence of a mood disorder (40%) • Rapid dose titration	Cool body to reduce fever. Maintain hydration with oral and IV fluids. Correct electrolyte imbalance. Dysrhythmias should be treated. Small doses of heparin may decrease possibility of pulmonary emboli. Early detection increases patient's chance of survival.

*Tardive dyskinesia (TD) is the most socially isolating of all the extrapyramidal side effects, which are all distressing and very uncomfortable for the individual.

Ach, Anticholinergic side effects (dry mouth, dry eyes, blurred vision [especially near vision], urinary retention, intestinal slowing [causing constipation], agitation, sedation, and sexual dysfunction); *AIMS,* Abnormal Involuntary Movement Scale; *IM,* intramuscular; *IV,* intravenous; *stat,* immediately.

TABLE 17-11   Treatment of Acute Extrapyramidal Side Effects

Drug	Chemical Type
Trihexyphenidyl* (Artane)	ACA
Benztropine mesylate* (Cogentin)	ACA
Biperiden* (Akineton)	ACA
Diphenhydramine hydrochloride (Benadryl)	Antihistamine
Bromocriptine mesylate (Parlodel)	D_2 dopamine agonist

*Antiparkinsonian drug.

ACA, Anticholinergic agent (after 1 to 6 months of long-term maintenance antipsychotic therapy, most ACAs can be withdrawn).

EVALUATION

Evaluation is always an important step in the planning of care and is especially important for people who have chronic psychotic disorders. Frequently, outcomes are too ambitious or do not include the patient's goals and serve only to discourage both the patient and the clinician. It is critical for staff to remember that change is a process that occurs over time; for a person diagnosed with schizophrenia, the period may be prolonged.

It is important to schedule regular evaluations for chronically ill patients so that new data can be considered and the patient's problems can be reassessed. Questions to be asked include the following:

- Is the patient not progressing because a more important need is not being met?
- Is the clinician/nurse using the patient's strengths and interests to achieve the outcomes?
- Are more appropriate interventions available for this patient to facilitate progress?
- If a newer antipsychotic agent is being tried, is there evidence of improvement or a regression in functioning?
- If the patient is nonadherent to medications, have the reasons for nonadherence been explored with the individual and the family, and have alternatives been implemented? As mentioned earlier in this text, noncompliance to medication is no longer sufficient to avoid lawsuits or civil court actions.
- Is the family involved? Are family members supportive? Do they understand the patient's disease and treatment issues?
- Are the patient and family aware of relapse issues (prodromal symptoms of relapse, medication compliance)?
- Are the patient and family working with effective community supports and treatments?

Active staff involvement and interest in the patient's progress communicate concern, help the patient to form and sustain interest, and prevent feelings of helplessness and burnout. Input from the patient can offer valuable information about why a certain desired behavior or situation has not occurred.

KEY POINTS TO REMEMBER

- Schizophrenia is a devastating brain disease. It is not one disorder but a group of disorders that appear on a spectrum along with other psychotic disorders. Psychotic symptoms in schizophrenia are more pronounced and disruptive than are symptoms found in other psychotic disorders. The basic differences are in the degree of severity of withdrawal, alteration in affect, impairment of intellect, and ability to function in the world.
- Neurochemical (catecholamines and serotonin), genetic, and neuroanatomical findings help explain the symptoms of schizophrenia. However, at present no one theory accounts for all phenomena found in schizophrenic disorders.
- When the nurse works with patients with schizophrenia, four specific groups of symptoms may be evident. No one symptom is found in all cases. The positive, negative, and cognitive symptoms of schizophrenia are three major categories of symptoms. Depression is almost always present.
- The positive symptoms are more florid (hallucinations, delusions, looseness of associations) and respond to antipsychotic drug therapy.
- The negative symptoms (poor social adjustment, lack of motivation, withdrawal) are more debilitating and do not respond as well to antipsychotic drug therapy.

- The cognitive degree of impairment is perhaps one of the most serious symptoms in the schizophrenic spectrum disorders and warrants careful assessment and interventions to increase the person's quality of life and ability to function in the community.
- Co-occurring moods (e.g., depression, anxiety, demoralization) need to be identified and treated to lower the potential for suicide, substance abuse, and relapse.
- Some nursing diagnoses are offered for positive symptoms (delusions and hallucinations), some are for negative symptoms (withdrawal, lack of energy), and some are family focused (see Table 17-4).
- Planning of outcomes proceeds by identifying the phase of schizophrenia and assessing the patient's individual needs based on functional ability, and involves identifying short-term and intermediate indicators.
- Interventions for people with schizophrenia include communication guidelines, family health teaching and psychoeducation, milieu management and strategies, psychotherapy, and pharmacological therapies.
- Specific communication strategies are necessary when dealing with a patient who is hallucinating, delusional, or paranoid.
- The recovery model is becoming more prevalent in the treatment of schizophrenia; when people have more control over their goals and the plan to meet those goals within a social networking system, the positive results look promising.
- Because antipsychotic medication is essential, the nurse must understand the properties, adverse effects, toxic effects, and dosages of the traditional, atypical, and other medications used to treat schizophrenia. This information must be shared with the patient and family.

APPLYING CRITICAL JUDGMENT

1. Differentiate between the short-term and long-term needs of people with schizophrenia. Identify the basic focus and interventions for the different phases.
2. Jamie, a 29-year-old woman, is being discharged in 2 days from the hospital after her first psychotic break, and she is extremely paranoid. Jamie is recently divorced and has been working as a legal secretary; recently, her work became erratic and her suspicious behavior was calling attention to herself at work. Jamie will be discharged in her mother's care until she is able to resume working. Jamie's mother is overwhelmed and asks the nurse how she is going to cope. "Jamie has become so distant, and she always takes things the wrong way. I can hardly say anything to her without her misconstruing everything. She is very mad at me because I called 911 and had her admitted after she told me she was going to get justice back in the world by blowing up evil forces that have been haunting her life and then proceeded to try to run over her ex-husband, thinking he was the devil. She told me there is nothing wrong with her, and I am concerned she won't take her medication once she is discharged. What am I going to do?"
3. Answer the following questions related to the case study just given. It is best if you can discuss and analyze responses to such situations with your classmates or instructor/professor.
   A. What are some of the priority concerns that the nurse could address in the hospital setting before Jamie's discharge?
   B. How would you explain to Jamie's mother some of the symptoms that Jamie is experiencing? What suggestions could you give her to handle some of her immediate concerns?

C. What issues could you raise to Jamie's nurse or clinician about Jamie's medication nonadherence? What strategies might help in this situation?

D. What are some of the community resources that might help support this family and increase the chances of continuity of care? Identify some useful community referrals that would be supportive for Jamie and her mother. Choose at least three and describe how they could be supportive to this family.

E. What do you think of the prognosis for Jamie? Support your hypothesis.

F. Discuss how you think the recovery model might help Jamie with some of her problems once she becomes less psychotic and paranoid.

G. Access the World Wide Web and search for the NAMI (National Alliance on Mental Illness) website (www.NAMI.org). List places in your community that are available to help people with severe mental illnesses (e.g., day care centers, respite centers, group homes).

H. Use the Internet to access www.samhsa.gov and read more about the recovery model with schizophrenia.

CHAPTER REVIEW QUESTIONS

1. A patient smiles broadly at the nurse and says, "Look at my clean teeth. I brushed them with scouring power because the label said, 'It brightens and whitens everything.'" Which term should the nurse include when documenting this encounter?
   a. Circumstantiality
   b. Concrete thinking
   c. Poverty of speech
   d. Associative looseness

2. A patient diagnosed with schizophrenia says, "I hear the voices every day. They always say bad things about me." Which action by the nurse has the highest priority?
   a. Assess the patient for suicidal thinking and plans.
   b. Review the patient's medication regime and compliance.
   c. Educate the patient about symptoms associated with schizophrenia.
   d. Suggest distracters for the patient to use when auditory hallucinations occur.

3. Three days after beginning a new regime of haloperidol (Haldol) 10 mg BID, the nurse observes that a hospitalized patient is drooling, has stiff and extended extremities, and has skin that is damp and hot to the touch. The patient has difficulty responding verbally to the nurse. What is the nurse's correct analysis and action in this situation?
   a. A seizure is occurring; place the patient in a lateral recumbent position and monitor.
   b. Serotonin syndrome has developed; place an intravenous line and rapidly infuse $D_5\frac{1}{2}$ NS.
   c. Neuroleptic malignant syndrome has developed; prepare the patient for immediate transfer to a medical unit.
   d. An acute dystonic reaction is occurring; promptly administer an intramuscular injection of diphenhydramine (Benadryl).

4. A patient diagnosed with schizophrenia complains to the nurse about persistent feelings of restlessness and says, "I feel like I need to move all the time." What is the nurse's next action?
   a. Add an activity group to the patient's plan of care.
   b. Assess the patient for other extrapyramidal symptoms.
   c. Perform a full mental status evaluation of the patient.
   d. Educate the patient about psychomotor agitation associated with schizophrenia.

5. A nurse begins a therapeutic relationship with a patient diagnosed with schizophrenia. The patient has severe paranoia. Which comment by the nurse is most appropriate?
   a. "Let's begin by talking about the goals you have for yourself."
   b. "I understand that you have problems with fear and suspiciousness of others."
   c. "As you get to know me better, I hope you will feel comfortable talking to me."
   d. "I am part of your treatment team. Our goal is to help stabilize your symptoms."

REFERENCES

American Psychiatric Association (APA). (2013). *Diagnostic and statistical manual of mental disorders (DSM-5)* (5th ed.). Washington, DC: APA.

American Psychiatric Nurses Association (APNA). (2012). *Shedding the label of schizophrenia through a recovery model.* A presentation made on December 14, 2012, sponsored by APNA, with speakers Mary Ann Nihart, Michael Rice, and Frederick J. Frese.

Black, D. W., & Andreasen, N. C. (2014). *Introductory textbook of psychiatry* (6th ed.). Washington, DC: American Psychiatric Publishing.

Brauser, D. (2010). *Better outcomes with antipsychotics plus psychosocial treatment for early schizophrenia.* Retrieved August 15, 2011, from www.medscape.com/viewarticle/728337.

Burchum, J., & Rosenthal, L. (2016). *Lehne's pharmacology for nursing care* (9th ed.). St Louis, MO: Elsevier Saunders.

Chavan, P. (2016). *Harvard & MIT scientists identify C4-A, the gene that causes schizophrenia.* Retrieved February 1, 2016, from http://www.thehealthsite.com/Harvard-MIT-scientists-identity-c-4-a-the-gene-that-courses-schizophrenia-poO116/.

Cold Spring Harbor Laboratory. (2015, April 7). Discovery of communication link between brain areas implicated in schizophrenia. ScienceDaily. Retrieved from www.sciencedaily.com/releases/2015/04/150407210901.htm

Divac, N., Prostran, M., Jakovcevski, I., & Cerovac, N. (2014). Second-generation antipsychotics and extrapyramidal adverse effects. *BioMed Research International, 2014.*

Erlich, Y., Williams, J. B., Glazer, D., et al. (2014). Redefining genomic privacy: trust and empowerment. *PLoS Biol, 12,* e1001983.

Freudenreich, O., Brown, H. E., & Holt, D. J. (2016). Psychosis and schizophrenia. In T. A. Stern, M. Fava, T. E. Wilens, & J. F. Rosenbaum (Eds.), *Massachusetts General Hospital comprehensive clinical psychiatry* (2nd ed.). St Louis, MO: Elsevier.

Gamble, C., & Brennan, G. (2000). Working with families and informed careers. In C. Gamble & G. Brennan (Eds.), *Working with serious mental illness: A manual for clinical practice.* London, England: Baillière Tindall.

Gerstein, P. S., & Shlamovitz, G. Z. (2015). *Emergent treatment of schizophrenia.* From http://e medicine.medscape.com/article/805988-overview#a4.

Jewell, T. C., Downing, D., & McFarlane, W. R. (2009). Partnering with families: multiple family group psychoeducation for schizophrenia. *Journal of Clinical Psychology, 65,* 868–878.

Lewis, F. (2011). *Older antipsychotics trump newer agents for schizophrenia: newer not necessarily better, researchers say.* Retrieved August 15, 2011, from www.medscape.com/viewarticle/744755_print.

Luhrmann, T. M., et al. (2014). Differences in voice-hearing experiences of people with psychosis in the USA. *India and Ghana: Interview-based study. British Journal of Psychiatry.*

Melville, N. A. (2015). *Long-term injectable antipsychotic cuts schizophrenia relapse.* Retrieved May 15, 2015, from http://www.medscape.com/viewarticle/842605.

Mental Health Daily. (2015). *Antipsychotics and brain damage: shrinkage & volume loss.* Retrieved from http://mentalhealthdaily.com/2015/07/03/antipsychotics-and-brain-damage-shrinkage-volume-loss/.

National Alliance on Mental Illness (NAMI). (2013). *Mental illness facts and numbers.* Reviewed March 2013, from www.NAMI.org/.

National Alliance on Mental Illness (NAMI). (2009). *Schizophrenia: PACT: Program of Assertive Community Treatment.* Retrieved March 18, 2011, from www.nami.org/template.CFM?Section=schizophrenia.

Nauert, R. (2015). *Eight different types of schizophrenia.* Retrieved May 2015 from http://psychcentral.com/news/2015/eight-different-types-of-schizophrenia/80805.html.

Nuechtrstein, K. H., & Green, M. F. (2013). *MCCB, MATRICS (Measurement and Treatment Research to Improve Cognition in Schizophrenia).* Retrieved August 28, 2013, from www.mhs.com/product.aspx?gr=cli&prod=mccb&id=overview.

PBS. (2002). *The secret life of the brain.* Retrieved March 22, 2011, from www.pbs.org/wnet/brains/episode3/cultures/index.html.

Peluso, M. J., Lewis, S. W., Barnes, T. R., et al. (2012). Extrapyramidal motor side-effects of first- and second-generation antipsychotic drugs. Retrieved June 6, 2012, from http://reference.Medscape.com/MEDLINE/abstract/22442101?src=nlbest.

Preston, J. D., O'Neal, J. H., & Talaga, M. C. (2013). *Handbook of clinical psychopharmacology for therapists* (7th ed.). Oakland, CA: New Harbinger Publications.

Rathod, S., Phiri, P., & Kingdon, D. (2010). Cognitive behavioral therapy for schizophrenia. *Psychiatric Clinics of North America, 33*(3). Retrieved March 20, 2011, from www.mdconsult.com/das/article/body/237614148-;2/jorg=c.

Rettner, R. (2016). *Schizophrenia gene discovery sheds light on possible cause; improper "pruning" of neural connections could lead to the development of mental illness.* Retrieved February 1 from www.scientificamerican.com/article schizophrenia-gene-discovery-sheds-light-on-possible-causes/.

Sadock, B. J., Sadock, V. A., & Ruiz, P. (2015). *Kaplan & Sadock's synopsis of psychiatry* (11th ed.). Philadelphia, PA: Wolters Kluwer/Lippincott Williams & Wilkins.

Substance Abuse and Mental Health Services Association (SAMHSA). (2012). *Recovery.* Retrieved August 20, 2013, from www.samsha.gov.

Tiihonen, J., Suokas, J. T., Suvisaari, J. M., et al (2012). *Polypharmacy with antipsychotics, antidepressants, benzodiazepines, and mortality in schizophrenia.* Retrieved June 13, 2012, from http://reference.Medscape.com/MEDLINE/abstract/22566579?src=nlbest.

U.S. Department of Health and Human Services (USDHHS). (1999). *Mental health: a report of the Surgeon General.* Rockville, MD: USDHHS, Center for Mental Health Services, National Institutes of Health.

Vidal, G. (1982). *The second American revolution and other essays (1976–1982).* New York, NY: Random House.

Vita, A., De Peri, L., Deste, G., et al. (2015). *The effect of antipsychotic treatment on cortical gray matter changes in schizophrenia: does the class matter? a meta-analysis and meta-regression of longitudinal magnetic resonance imaging studies.* Retrieved from http://www.ncbi.nlm.nih.gov/pubmed/25802081.

Weinmann, S., Aderhold, V., Haegele, C., et al. (2015). *Brain atrophy and antipsychotic medication—a systematic review.* Retrieved from http://www.europsy-journal.com/article/S0924-9338(15)30055-9/abstract?cc=y=.

Xia, J., Mirender, L. B., & Belgamwar, M. R. (2011). *Psychoeducation for schizophrenia.* Retrieved August 15, 2011, from http://medscape.com/viewarticle/735323.

18

Neurocognitive Disorders

Elizabeth M. Varcarolis

http://evolve.elsevier.com/Varcarolis/essentials

KEY TERMS AND CONCEPTS

agnosia, p. 280
agraphia, p. 282
Alzheimer's disease (AD), p. 279
aphasia, p. 280
apraxia, p. 280
cognition, p. 273
confabulation, p. 280
delirium, p. 273

dementia, p. 278
hallucinations, p. 274
hypermetamorphosis, p. 282
hyperorality, p. 282
hypervigilance, p. 275
illusions, p. 274
major neurocognitive disorder
 (dementia), p. 278

mild cognitive impairment (MCI), p. 277
mild neurocognitive disorders, p. 277
perseveration, p. 280
pseudodementia, p. 282
sundown syndrome, p. 273
tau protein, p. 279

SELECTED CONCEPT: COGNITION

Cognitive processing has a direct relationship to activities of daily living. Although primarily an intellectual and perceptual process, cognition is closely integrated with an individual's emotional and spiritual values. When human beings can no longer understand facts or connect the appropriate feelings to events, they have trouble responding to the complexity of life's challenges.

Major and mild neurocognitive disorders are based on degree of disturbances in the following six key cognitive domains (Black & Andreasen, 2014):

1) **Complex Attention:** The ability to maintain one's focus on persons, tasks, or happenings in the environment around one.
2) **Executive Functioning:** The ability to plan, make suitable decisions, rely on one's working memory, or respond appropriately to feedback, and mental stability.
3) **Learning and Memory:** The memory and recent memory (including free recall, acute recall, and recognition memory).
4) **Language:** Expressive language (including naming, fluency, grammar, and syntax) and receptive language.
5) **Social Cognition:** Recognition of emotions, theory of mind (i.e., ability to understand another person's mental state), and behavior regulation.
6) **Perceptual and Motor Ability:** Construction in visual perception

"Cognitive science in the 21st century is largely a multidisciplinary domain and the study of the brain, using an ever growing neuroimaging and neuroinvestigating technology, has allowed scientists to add important physiological knowledge to our understanding of the mental processes" (CogniFit, 2015).

OBJECTIVES

1. Using descriptive words, describe the behavior, cognitive abilities, clinical picture, and types of feelings a person with delirium might experience.
2. **QSEN** Discuss the critical **safety needs** of a patient with delirium and give examples of how you would meet them.
3. **QSEN** Demonstrate in a **patient-centered** nursing care plan interventions and rationales for the care of a person experiencing delirium.
4. Describe the four A's, the defense mechanisms, and the signs and symptoms occurring in each of the four stages of Alzheimer's disease (AD).
5. **QSEN** Identify **best evidence** with rationales for the various interventions for each of the following categories when caring for a patient with Alzheimer's disease or teaching family members: (a) communication, (b) health maintenance, and (c) safe environment.
6. **QSEN** Discuss the kinds of **teamwork and collaboration** needed in the community to support both patients with AD and their families (list at least four kinds of community service and different kinds of in-home service).
7. **QSEN** Applying **informatics,** find different types of family supports and individual supports for a patient with AD in your own community.

INTRODUCTION

Those disorders that affect the structural or functional areas of the brain and cause disturbances in normal cognition (memory, abstract thinking, or judgment) are referred to as neurocognitive disorders (NCD). The *DSM-5* (APA, 2013) categorizes the *neurocognitive disorders* into two broad categories based on level of severity: **major neurocognitive disorder** and **mild neurocognitive disorder**. Neurocognitive disorders affect the brain's ability to function intellectually, emotionally, socially, and occupationally. For example, a person might have a *"mild neurocognitive disorder – Alzheimer's"* disease in which the person can still function but at a lower level and meets the *DSM-5* criteria for mild neurocognitive disorder – Alzheimer's. Or a person may be diagnosed with a *"major neurocognitive disorder – Alzheimer's"* in which almost all aspects of brain function would be affected and eventually destroyed, in time leaving a shell of a once vital, functioning human being whose personality, life memories, and abilities are gone forever.

For our purposes here, we will discuss three main categories of the neurocognitive disorders/cognitive disorders: (1) *delirium*; (2) *mild neurocognitive disorder*; and (3) *major neurocognitive disorder* (using Alzheimer's disease as the example).

DELIRIUM

Delirium is a syndrome that is always *secondary to another condition*, such as a general medical condition or substance use (intoxication/ withdrawal), a medication, or a toxin exposure, or it may have multiple ideologies. Delirium is a transient disorder, and if the underlying physiological disturbances are corrected in a timely manner, complete recovery occurs. However, nurses and other health care workers need to be very cognizant of the fact that if the underlying etiologies are not addressed, dementia and even death may follow. It is also important to be aware that delirium may easily occur in a patient with dementia.

Delirium, one of the most commonly encountered medical disorders in medical practice, is often overlooked or misdiagnosed. It is a significant risk for all hospitalized older patients. Delirium is present in up to 15% to 53% of older individuals postoperatively, and in 70% to 87% of those who are in intensive care. Furthermore, 60% of nursing home residents and as many as 75% to 85% of people with a terminal illness develop delirium near death (APA, 2013).

Delirium presents with the following symptoms:

1. Mental confusion that develops quickly and usually fluctuates in intensity, and represents a change from the individual's normal attention and awareness.
2. Reduced awareness and responsiveness to the environment (disturbance in attention).
3. Disorientation and incoherency and severe memory disturbance.

Hallucinations and delusions are not uncommon, ideas of reference are frequent, and additional disturbances in cognition occur.

Nurses frequently encounter delirium on medical and surgical units in the general hospital setting, the emergency department (ED), the intensive care unit (ICU), etc. During certain phases of a hospital stay, confusion may be noted (e.g., after surgery or after the introduction of a new drug). The second or third hospital day may herald the onset of confusion and difficulty adjusting to an unfamiliar environment.

Delirium occurs more frequently in older patients. Surgery, drugs, urinary tract infections, pneumonia, cerebrovascular disease, and congestive heart failure are some of the most common causes. Delirium is also commonly seen in children with fever and in terminally ill patients.

Substance withdrawal delirium (SWD) and delirium are both a challenge to diagnose. Delirium is considered an emergency. A delayed or missed diagnosis can have serious implications because the longer the condition remains untreated, the greater the risk for permanent brain damage, dementia, or even death. Alcohol withdrawal delirium (delirium tremens [DT]) and its treatment are discussed in Chapter 19.

Depression often masquerades as a major neurocognitive disorder, delirium, and depression often co-occurs with dementia; therefore a clear definition of the three can be useful during assessment. Table 18-1 offers some guidelines for distinguishing among delirium, depression, and dementia.

The essential feature of delirium is a disturbance in consciousness coupled with cognitive difficulties listed above. Basically, it consists of **cognitive disturbances** (thinking, memory, disorientation, impairment, and perception [delusions, hallucinations]) and **attention disturbances** (inability to maintain focus and attention, and displaying confusion over situation and environment) (adapted from APA, 2013). The clinical manifestations of delirium develop over a short period (hours to days) and tend to fluctuate during the course of the day. Sundown syndrome, in which symptoms and problem behaviors become more pronounced in the evening and at night, may occur in both delirium and dementia.

Because delirium increases psychological stress, supportive interventions that lower anxiety and promote calm and security can foster a sense of control. Patients with delirium may appear withdrawn, agitated, or psychotic. Also, underlying personality traits often become exaggerated. For example, a person can become more paranoid or display more disinhibition.

Box 18-1 lists common causes of delirium.

APPLICATION OF THE NURSING PROCESS: DELIRIUM

ASSESSMENT

Generally the nurse suspects the presence of delirium when a patient abruptly develops a sudden disturbance in consciousness that is manifested in reduced clarity of awareness of the environment. An individual may have difficulty with orientation—first to time, then to place, and last to person. For example, a man with delirium may think that the year is 1972, that the hospital is home, and that the nurse is his wife. Orientation to person is usually intact to the extent that the person is aware of self-identity. *Level of awareness is disturbed and the ability to focus, sustain, or shift attention is impaired.* Questions need to be repeated because the individual's attention wanders, and the person might easily need to be refocused. Conversation is made more difficult because the person may be easily distracted by irrelevant stimuli.

Fluctuating levels of consciousness are unpredictable. Disorientation and confusion are usually markedly worse at night and during the early morning (sundowning). In fact, some patients may be confused or delirious only at night and may remain lucid during the day. Some clinicians use a mental status exam (MSE) to screen or follow the progress of an individual with delirium (see inside cover in back of text). Nursing assessment includes (1) cognitive and perceptual disturbances, (2) physical needs, and (3) moods and physical behaviors.

Cognitive and Perceptual Disturbances

It may be difficult to engage delirious individuals in conversation because they are easily distracted and display marked attention deficits, and because their memory is impaired. In mild delirium, memory deficits are noted on careful questioning. In more severe delirium,

TABLE 18-1 Comparison of Delirium, Dementia, and Depression

	Delirium	Dementia	Depression
Onset	Sudden, over hours to days	Slowly, over months to years	May have been gradual with exacerbation during crisis or stress
Cause or contributing factors	Hypoglycemia, fever, dehydration, hypotension; infection, other conditions that disrupt the body's homeostasis; adverse drug reaction; head injury; change in environment (e.g., hospitalization); pain; emotional stress	Alzheimer's disease, vascular disease, human immunodeficiency virus infection, neurological disease, chronic alcoholism, head trauma	Lifelong history, losses, loneliness, crises, declining health, medical conditions
Cognition	Impaired memory, judgment, calculations, attention span; can fluctuate throughout the day	Impaired memory, judgment, calculations, attention span, abstract thinking; agnosia	Difficulty concentrating, forgetfulness, inattention
Level of consciousness	Altered	Not altered	Not altered
Activity level	Can be increased or reduced, restlessness; behaviors may worsen in evening (sundown syndrome); sleep-wake cycle may be reversed	Not altered; behaviors may worsen in evening (sundown syndrome)	Usually decreased; lethargy, fatigue, lack of motivation; may sleep poorly and awaken in early morning
Emotional state	Rapid swings; can be fearful, anxious, suspicious, aggressive, have hallucinations and/or delusions	Flat; delusions	Extreme sadness, apathy, irritability, anxiety, paranoid ideation
Speech and language	Rapid, inappropriate, incoherent, rambling	Incoherent, slow (sometimes due to effort to find the right word), inappropriate, rambling, repetitious	Slow, flat, low
Prognosis	Reversible with proper and timely treatment	Not reversible; progressive	Reversible with proper and timely treatment

BOX 18-1 Common Causes of Delirium

Postoperative states

Drug intoxications and withdrawals
- Alcohol, anxiolytics, opioids, and central nervous system stimulants (cocaine, crack cocaine, and others)

Infections
- Systemic: pneumonia, typhoid fever, malaria, urinary tract infection, and septicemia
- Intracranial: meningitis and encephalitis

Metabolic disorders
- Dehydration
- Hypoxia (pulmonary disease, heart disease, and anemia)
- Hypoglycemia
- Sodium, potassium, calcium, magnesium, and acid-base imbalances
- Hepatic encephalopathy or uremic encephalopathy
- Thiamine (vitamin B_1) deficiency (Wernicke's encephalopathy)
- Endocrine disorders (e.g., thyroidism, parathyroidism)
- Hypothermia or hyperthermia
- Diabetic acidosis

Drugs
- Digitalis, steroids, lithium, levodopa, anticholinergics, benzodiazepines, central nervous system depressants, tricyclic antidepressants
- Central anticholinergic syndrome as a result of using multiple drugs with anticholinergic side effects

Neurological diseases
- Seizures
- Head trauma
- Hypertensive encephalopathy

Tumor
- Primary cerebral

Psychosocial stressors
- Relocation or other sudden changes
- Sensory deprivation or overload
- Sleep deprivation
- Immobilization
- Pain

memory problems usually take the form of obvious difficulty in processing and remembering recent events. For example, a mother might ask when her son is coming to visit, even though her son left a half hour earlier. Perceptual disturbances are also common. Perception is the processing of information about one's internal and external environment. Various misinterpretations of reality may take the form of illusions or hallucinations.

Illusions are errors in perception of sensory stimuli. For example, a person may mistake folds in the bedclothes for white rats or the cord of a window blind for a snake. The stimulus is a real object in the environment; however, it is misinterpreted and often becomes the object of the patient's projected fear. Illusions, unlike delusions or hallucinations, can be explained and clarified for the individual.

Hallucinations are false sensory stimuli (see Chapter 17 for guidelines in dealing with hallucinations). *Visual* hallucinations are common in delirium. *Tactile* hallucinations may also be present. For example, delirious individuals may become terrified when they "see" giant spiders crawling over the bedclothes or "feel" bugs crawling on their bodies. Auditory hallucinations occur more often in other psychiatric disorders, such as schizophrenia and psychotic depression.

The delirious individual generally has awareness that something is very wrong. For example, the delirious person may state, "My thoughts are all jumbled." When perceptual disturbances are present, the emotional response is one of fear and anxiety. Verbal and psychomotor signs of agitation should be noted.

Physical Needs
Physical Safety

A person with delirium becomes disoriented and may try to "go home." Alternatively, a person may think that he or she *is* home and may jump out of a window in an attempt to get away from "invaders." Wandering, pulling out intravenous lines and Foley catheters, and falling out of bed are common dangers that require nursing intervention.

An individual experiencing delirium has difficulty processing stimuli in the environment. Confusion magnifies the inability to recognize reality. The physical environment should be made as simple and as clear as possible. Objects such as clocks and calendars can maximize orientation to time. Eyeglasses, hearing aids, and adequate lighting without glare can maximize the person's ability to more accurately interpret the environment. The nurse should interact with the patient whenever the patient is awake. Short periods of social interaction help reduce anxiety and misperceptions.

Biophysical Safety

Autonomic signs, such as tachycardia, sweating, flushed face, dilated pupils, and elevated blood pressure, are often present. These changes must be monitored and documented carefully and may require immediate medical attention.

Changes in the sleep-wake cycle usually are noted, and in some cases a complete reversal of the night-day sleep-wake cycle can occur. The patient's level of consciousness may range from lethargy to stupor or from semicoma to hypervigilance. In hypervigilance, patients are extraordinarily alert and their eyes constantly scan the room; they may have difficulty falling asleep or may be actively disoriented and agitated throughout the night.

It is also important that the nurse assess all medications because the nurse is in a position to recognize drug reactions or potential interactions before delirium actually occurs.

Moods and Physical Behaviors

The delirious individual's behavior and mood may change dramatically within a short period. Moods may fluctuate from fear, anger, and anxiety to euphoria, depression, and apathy. These labile moods (quickly changing) are often accompanied by physical behaviors associated with feeling states. A person may strike out from fear or anger or may cry, call for help, curse, moan, and tear off clothing and then within a minute become apathetic or laugh uncontrollably. In short, behavior and emotions are erratic and fluctuating. Lack of concentration and disorientation complicate interventions. The following vignette illustrates the fear and confusion a patient may experience when admitted to an ICU. Read the following and analyze the nurse's approach.

VIGNETTE

A 55-year-old married man, Mr. Arnold, is admitted to the ICU after having cardiac surgery, a three-vessel coronary artery bypass graft. Mr. Arnold's surgery took longer than usual and has necessitated his remaining on a cardiac pump for 3 hours. He arrives in the ICU without further complications. On awakening from the anesthesia, he hears the nurse exclaim, "I need to get a gas." Another nurse answers in a loud voice, "Can you take a large needle for the injection?" During this period, Mr. Arnold experiences the need to urinate and asks the nurse very calmly if he can go to the bathroom. Her reply is, "You don't need to go; you have a tube in." He again complains about his discomfort and assures the nurse that if she will let him go to the bathroom, he will be fine. The nurse informs Mr. Arnold that he cannot urinate and that he has to keep the "mask" on so that she can get the "gas" and check his "blood levels." On hearing this, Mr. Arnold begins to implore more loudly and states that he sees the bathroom sign. He assures the nurse that he will only take a minute. In reality, the sign is an exit sign.

To prove to him that a bathroom does not exist in the ICU and that the sign does not indicate a bathroom, the nurse takes off the restraints so that Mr. Arnold's head can be raised to see the sign. He abruptly breaks away from the nurse's grasp and runs toward the entrance of the ICU. He discovers a door, which is the entrance to the nurses' lounge; Mr. Arnold barricades himself in the room and pulls out his chest tube, Foley catheter, and intravenous lines. He finds the bathroom that is connected to the lounge. Ten minutes later, the nurses and security personnel break through the barricade and escort Mr. Arnold back to bed.

When he becomes fully alert and oriented a day later, Mr. Arnold tells the nurses his perception of the previous day's events. Initially, he had thought he had been kidnapped and was being held against his will (the restraints had been tight). When the nurse yelled out about blood gas, he had thought she was going to kill him with noxious gas through his facemask (the reason he did not want to wear the facemask). All he could think about was escaping his tormentor and executioner. In this case, the nurse had not assessed the alteration in Mr. Arnold's mental status and allowed him to get out of bed. The medical jargon and loud voices had perpetuated his confusion and distortion of reality.

The nurses could have told Mr. Arnold where he was and that the nursing staff was caring for him, and oriented him frequently to time, place, and person; they could have better explained the function of his Foley catheter. What else could the nurses have done to help orient and comfort Mr. Arnold?

⏩ Assessment Guidelines
Delirium

1. **Patient safety**: Preventing physical injuries and self-harm as a result of confusion, aggression, or electrolyte and fluid imbalance
   a. Assess vital signs, level of consciousness, and neurological signs.
   b. Assess potential for injury (e.g., falls, wandering).
   c. Assess for fluctuating levels of consciousness and *monitor factors that worsen or improve symptoms.*
2. History and information gathering (get help from friends and family)
   a. Interview family or other caregivers to establish the patient's normal level of consciousness and cognition.
   b. Assess for past confusional states (e.g., prior dementia diagnosis, substance withdrawal/intoxication delirium).
   c. Identify any electroencephalographic, neuroimaging, or laboratory abnormalities documented in the patient's record.
3. Physical examination and a comprehensive nursing assessment to aid in identifying the cause
   a. Identify other disturbances in medical status (e.g., infection, dyspnea, edema, presence of jaundice).
   b. Perform a mental status exam.
   c. Assess the need for blood work, toxicology screening, x-rays, etc.
4. Assess the need for interventions to optimize comfort and orientation
   a. Assess the need for comfort measures (e.g., address pain or cold, improve positioning).
   b. Assess ways to increase patient's orientation (e.g., glasses, hearing aids, clocks, calendars, pictures from home, raising head of bed to increase reality-based environment).
   c. Remain nonjudgmental. Confer and ask for help from other staff when questions or acute unsafe situations arise.

DIAGNOSIS

Safety needs play a substantial role in nursing care so *Risk for injury* is always the greatest consideration. If fever and dehydration are present, fluid and electrolyte balance will need to be managed. If the underlying cause of the patient's delirium results in fever, decreased skin turgor, decreased urinary output or fluid intake, and dry skin or mucous membranes, then the nursing diagnosis of *Deficient fluid volume* is appropriate.

Any condition that alters brain activity, including metabolic imbalances, infections, altered sleep, intoxication/withdrawal, and medication use, can be viewed as a *Risk for acute confusion.* Perceptions are disturbed during delirium and may be acted on by the patient. For example, if feeling threatened or thinking that common medical equipment is harmful, the patient may pull off an oxygen mask, pull out an intravenous or nasogastric tube, or try to leave the health care facility. Hallucinations, distractibility, illusions, labile mood, disorientation, agitation, restlessness, and/or misperception are major aspects of the clinical picture. When some of these symptoms are present, *Risk for self-harm, Fear,* and *Acute confusion* are appropriate nursing diagnoses.

Because the sleep-wake cycle may be disrupted, the patient may be less responsive during the day and may become disruptively wakeful during the night. Therefore *Disturbed sleep pattern* related to impaired cerebral oxygenation or disruption in consciousness is a likely diagnosis.

Sustaining communication with a delirious patient is difficult. *Impaired verbal communication* related to cerebral hypoxia or decreased cerebral blood flow, as evidenced by confusion or clouding of consciousness, may be diagnosed.

Other nursing diagnoses include *Self-care deficit, Impaired environmental interpretation syndrome** (if delusions, illusions, or hallucinations are present), *Labile mood,* and *Impaired social interaction.* Table 18-2 identifies nursing diagnoses for any confused patient (delirium or dementia).

OUTCOME IDENTIFICATION

The predominant goal (outcome) is that a delirious patient will return to the premorbid level of functioning. Although the patient can demonstrate a wide variety of needs, *Risk for injury* is always present and foremost. Appropriate outcomes are as follows:

- Patient will remain safe and free from injury while in the hospital.
- During periods of lucidity, patient will be oriented to time, place, and person with the aid of nursing interventions, such as the provision of clocks, calendars, maps, and other types of orienting information.
- Patient will remain free from falls and injury while confused with the aid of nursing safety measures throughout the hospital stay.
- Patient's tubes (e.g., nasogastric [NG], intravenous [IV], oxygen [O$_2$]) will remain in place with aid of the nurse, family, and/or medication as needed.

Because levels of consciousness can change throughout the day, the patient needs to be checked for orientation (time, place, and person) frequently during different times of the day.

---

* *Impaired environmental interpretation syndrome* is no longer included in NANDA, however, it is one of the two nursing diagnoses that are appropriate for psychotic symptoms. The second is *Altered thought processes.* Hopefully these nursing diagnoses will be included in the next edition.

IMPLEMENTATION

Immediate medical interventions should be taken to identify the underlying cause of the delirium in order to prevent permanent damage. In very specific and infrequent situations, antipsychotic or anti-anxiety agents may be helpful in controlling behavioral symptoms.

A patient in acute delirium should never be left alone. In the past, often friends or family would sit with the patient. "However, with new

TABLE 18-2 Potential Nursing Diagnoses for the Confused Patient

Symptoms	Nursing Diagnoses
Wanders, has unsteady gait, acts out fear from hallucinations or illusions, forgets things (leaves stove on, doors open)	*Risk for injury* *Wandering* *Disturbed sleep pattern*
Awake and disoriented during the night *(sundown syndrome),* frightened at night	*Fear*
Too confused to take care of basic needs	*Acute confusion* *Bathing self-care deficit (specify)* *Bowel incontinence* *Dressing self-care deficit* *Feeding self-care deficit* *Functional urinary incontinence* *Imbalanced nutrition: less than body requirements* *Deficient fluid volume* *Ineffective self-health management*
Sees frightening things that are not there *(hallucinations),* mistakes everyday objects for something sinister and frightening *(illusions),* may become paranoid and think that others are doing things to confuse him or her *(delusions)*	*Fear* *Defensive coping* **Impaired environmental interpretation syndrome* *Ineffective impulse control* *Powerlessness*
Does not recognize familiar people or places, has difficulty with short- and/or long-term memory, forgetful and confused	*Impaired memory* *Acute* or *chronic confusion*
Has difficulty with communication, cannot find words, has difficulty in recognizing objects and/or people, incoherent	*Impaired verbal communication* *Ineffective relationship* **Altered thought processes*
Devastated over losing place in life as known (during lucid moments), fearful and overwhelmed by what is happening to him or her	*Spiritual distress* *Hopelessness* *Situational low self-esteem* *Grieving*
Family and loved ones overburdened and overwhelmed, unable to care for patient's needs	*Disabled family coping* *Interrupted family processes* *Impaired home maintenance* *Caregiver role strain* *Chronic sorrow* *Deficient community health*

* *Impaired environmental interpretation syndrome* is no longer included in NANDA, however, it is one of the two nursing diagnoses that are appropriate for psychotic symptoms. The second is *Altered thought processes.* Hopefully these nursing diagnoses will be included in the next edition. Herdman, T.H. (Ed.) *Nursing Diagnoses-Definitions and Classification 2015-2017.* Copyright 2014, 1994-2014 NANDA International. Used by arrangement with John Wiley & Sons Limited. In order to make safe and effective judgments using NANDA-I nursing diagnoses it is essential that nurses refer to the definitions and defining characteristics of the diagnoses listed in this work.

restrictions on restraint use and licensing and accreditation standards, it is no longer appropriate for family to be given the responsibility of watching or sitting with the confused patient. Even when family is visiting, they are not responsible for the patient safety; it remains the responsibility of the staff. Acute-care facilities utilize "sitters, who are trained to work with patients who are confused, demented, were delirious and may at times help prevent delirium" (Howard, 2015). The most cost-effective sitters are trained volunteers. Training for sitters includes teaching recognition of delirium and impending delirium and how to engage the patient through reading, conversation, playing music, and providing stimulation, rather than sitting mutely and passively by (Carr, 2013). Refer to Table 18-3 for guidelines in caring for a patient with delirium.

EVALUATION

Evaluation includes identifying if the long-term outcome criteria have been met. Long-term outcome criteria for a person with delirium include the following:
- Patient will remain safe.
- Patient will be oriented to time, place, and person by discharge.
- Underlying cause will be treated and ameliorated.

- Patient will return to premorbid level of functioning.

However, the short-term goals need constant assessment. Are the vital signs stable? Is the patient's skin turgor and urine specific gravity within normal limits?

MILD NEUROCOGNITIVE DISORDER

Mild neurocognitive disorders are disorders in which *mild* neurocognitive impairment exists, but this category excludes people with dementia or age-associated memory impairment. For example, a person older than 65 may have a cognitive decline greater than that typically experienced by others similar in age and education level. According to the *DSM-5*, cognitive declines "may present in one or more difficulties with complex attention, executive function, learning and memory, language, perceptual motor, or social cognition" (APA, 2013, p. 605). According to Knopman and Peterson (2014), there is a distinction between *mild cognitive impairment (MCI)* and **mild neurocognitive impairment dementia due to Alzheimer's.** Although both are characterized by cognitive impairment, in *mild neurocognitive impairment dementia due to Alzheimer's* more than one cognitive domain is affected and there is interference in the individual's ability to navigate daily life. In the case of *mild cognitive impairment* (MCI) memory

TABLE 18-3 Interventions for a Patient with Delirium

Intervention	Rationale
1. Work with treatment team to reduce or eliminate factors causing delirium.	1. Underlying factors can lead to dementia if not reversed.
2. Monitor neurological signs on an ongoing basis.	2. Track progression or reversal of neurological disequilibrium.
3. Introduce self and call patient by name at the beginning of each contact.	3. With short-term memory impairment, person is often confused and needs frequent orienting to time, place, and person.
4. Maintain face-to-face contact.	4. If patient is easily distracted, he or she needs help to focus on one stimulus at a time.
5. Use short, simple, concrete phrases.	5. Patient may not be able to process complex information.
6. Briefly explain everything you are going to do before doing it.	6. Explanation prevents misinterpretation of action.
7. Encourage family and friends (one at a time) to take a quiet, supportive role.	7. Familiar presence lowers anxiety and increases orientation.
8. Keep room well lit.	8. Lighting provides accurate environmental stimuli to maintain and increase orientation.
9. Keep head of bed elevated.	9. Helps provide important environmental cues and helps to strengthen orientation.
10. Provide clocks and calendars.	10. These cues help orient patient to time.
11. Encourage family members to bring in meaningful articles from home (e.g., pictures, figurines).	11. Familiar objects provide comfort and support and can aid orientation.
12. Encourage patient to wear prescribed eyeglasses or hearing aid.	12. Helps increase accurate perceptions of visual auditory stimuli.
13. Make an effort to assign the same personnel on each shift to care for patient.	13. Familiar faces minimize confusion and enhance nurse-patient relationships.
14. When hallucinations are present, clarify reality; for example, "I know you are frightened; I do not see spiders on your sheets. I'll sit with you for a while."	14. Person feels understood and reassured while reality is validated.
15. When illusions are present, clarify reality; for example, "This is a coat rack, not a man with a knife … see? You seem frightened. I'll stay with you for a while."	15. Misinterpreted objects or sounds can be clarified, once pointed out.
16. Inform patient of progress during lucid intervals.	16. Consciousness fluctuates: patient feels less anxious knowing where he or she is and who you are during lucid periods.
17. Ignore insults and name calling, and acknowledge how upset the person may be feeling. For example: *Patient:* "You incompetent jerk, get me a real nurse, someone who knows what they are doing." *Nurse:* "You are very upset. What you are going through is very difficult. I'll stay with you."	17. Terror and fear are often projected onto environment. Arguing or becoming defensive only increases patient's aggressive behaviors and defenses.
18. If patient behavior becomes physically abusive, first set limits on behavior. For example: *Nurse:* "Mr. Jones, you are not to hit me or anyone else. Tell me how you feel." *Nurse:* "Mr. Jones, if you have difficulty controlling your actions, we will help you gain control." Second, check orders for use of chemical or physical restraints.	18. Clear limits need to be set to protect patient, staff, and others. Often, patient can respond to verbal commands. Chemical and physical restraints are used as a last resort, if at all.

difficulty is the main symptom. In MCI an individual might forget things more often, such as important events or appointments, or have difficulty following a conversation or a plot in a book or movie. At the time, the person may have trouble finding his or her way around familiar places and often becomes overwhelmed by previously easy tasks. Therefore memory impairment is the predominant symptom.

Although mild cognitive impairment does not affect the individual's daily living and socialization, it might result in greater effort and time being required to perform tasks that used to be performed without a thought, and often the use of compensatory strategies are employed. The diagnosis is made when a trusted individual or clinician reports that there has been a mild decline in cognitive function in addition to evidence presented and documented, a standardized neuropsychological test shows there is modest impairment, or it is verified by a qualified clinical assessment. Noteworthy, however, it is estimated that "nearly half of all people who have visited a doctor about MCI symptoms will develop dementia in 3 or 4 years" (Alzheimer's Association, 2015).

In all disorders in which a patient experiences a change in cognitive functioning, a mental status exam (Figure 18-1) and a thorough medical workup are vital (e.g., history, physical, neurological exam, lab tests, scans, x-rays).

MAJOR NEUROCOGNITIVE DISORDER (DEMENTIA)

A major neurocognitive disorder (dementia) **is much more serious in nature than a mild neurocognitive disorder.** Dementia usually develops more slowly than delirium and is characterized by multiple cognitive deficits that include impairment in memory without impairment in consciousness. For a diagnosis of a *major neurocognitive disorder* there is evidence of "significant decline in the individual's previous levels of cognitive ability, such as complex attention, executive function, learning and memory, language, perceptual-motor, or social cognition" (APA, 2013, p. 602).

Major neurocognitive disorders can be classified as either primary or secondary. More than 80% of dementias are irreversible (primary dementias); those dementias that have a reversible component are **secondary** to other pathological processes (e.g., neoplasms, trauma, infections, toxin exposure). When the underlying causes are treated, the dementia often improves. However, most major neurocognitive disorders such as Alzheimer's disease are related to a **primary** encephalopathy. According to the *DSM-5*, Alzheimer's disease (AD) accounts for 60% to 90% of all dementias in the United States and in 2015 was the sixth leading cause of death in adults in the United States (Gatchel et al., 2016). "Every 67 seconds someone in the United States develops Alzheimer's" (Alzheimer's Association, 2015). **Primary neurocognitive disorders** have no known cause or cure; thus they are progressive and irreversible. In 2011 the Alzheimer's Association (AA) revised criteria and progression of Alzheimer's disease. The AA states that Alzheimer's disease begins long before symptom development and has basically three phases: *preclinical Alzheimer's, mild neurocognitive impairment dementia due to Alzheimer's,* and *major neurocognitive disorder due to Alzheimer's* (Alzheimer's Association, 2015). Examples of other major primary neurocognitive disorders include vascular dementia, Pick's disease, Huntington's disease, Creutzfeldt-Jakob disease, Lewy body disease, and Parkinson's disease.

Because Alzheimer's disease is the primary diagnosis for a major neurocognitive disorder (dementia) and the assessments and nursing interventions are primarily the same for all patients with dementia, this section focuses on AD.

Cultural Considerations

Although AD is not affected by ethnicity in terms of behaviors (e.g., wandering, insomnia, incontinence, and possibly aggression), there do seem to be differences regarding incidents of AD in different ethnic groups. For example, older African Americans are almost twice as likely to develop Alzheimer's disease as white Americans.

Notes on the Use of the Brief Neurocognitive Mental Status Exam

1. *Behavior observations*
   a. Look for signs of drowsiness or fluctuating degrees of alertness.
   b. This may be formally tested by administering a digit span test or by careful observation during the interview.
   c. Make note of slurred speech or word-finding problems.
   d. Watch for unsteady gait and poor gross motor coordination.

2. *Orientation* – Ask: "What is the date (month, day, year), and what time of day is it now?" "Can you tell me where you are right now? Please be specific." Ask the patient to identify relatives who have accompanied him or her.

3. *Recent memory* – Present three items and ask for immediate recall. Then after a period of five minutes, ask the patient to again recall the three items. Most normal adults should be able to recall three items. Inability to do so may suggest recent memory problems. A second trial may be conducted later in the interview.

4. *Calculations* – Ask the patient to begin with the number 100 and subtract 7 from this number, then subtract 7 again, and so forth. This test provides a rough measure of concentration.

5. *Reproduction of cross and cube* – Present stimulus illustrations shown below. You can copy them onto a 3-by-5-inch, unlined, white index card. Allow the patient to copy the designs one at a time onto a blank sheet of paper. Drawing performance can be compared to samples (see below) to derive rough estimates of the patient's constructional ability.

   Cross   Cube

6. *Thinking/Speech* – Note the presence of incoherent or irrelevant speech.

FIGURE 18-1 Neurocognitive mental status exam. (From Preston, J., O'Neal, J., & Talaga, M. A. [2010]. *Handbook of clinical psychopharmacology for therapists* [6th ed., pp. 301–302]. Oakland, CA: New Harbinger Publications.)

Hispanic Americans are about 1.5 times as likely to develop Alzheimer's disease as white Americans, although at this point there does not seem to be any genetic correlation (Alzheimer's Association, 2015). However, there are other correlations. African Americans and Hispanics are more prone to high blood pressure, cardiovascular disease, and diabetes, which are significant risk factors for Alzheimer's disease. Many African Americans and Hispanics live at lower economic levels and have less access to education and proper health care, which are also risk factors for AD (Alzheimer's Association, 2015).

Although the behaviors resulting from Alzheimer's disease are similar, attitudes and perceptions of such behaviors can vary greatly among cultural groups. The emotions of frustration, anger, guilt, anxiety, and conflict are closely tied to the cultural value placed on the ability to maintain control.

Native American cultures are more likely to accept their lack of control over the situation. Therefore they may be far more likely to respond to their family members' situation with a sense of *loss* that life with their loved one, and life as their loved one knew it, is gone forever. Among many in the white population, there is more of a belief that people should be able to alter or influence a situation, which results in stronger feelings of anger, guilt, anxiety, and conflict over having no impact on the course of AD.

Health care workers who are able to assess and understand the cultural aspects of caregiving behaviors may be able to offer services and training that are more congruent with the caregiver's culture. Health care workers have a long way to go to become more proficient in understanding the nuances of culture and how it relates to the quality of care that patients and families may ultimately accept. The issue is complicated by the fact that patients and families from a minority group may be composed of many different subcultural groups. A good example is the Hispanic population, which shares Spanish as a language; however, Hispanics comprise Mexicans, Cubans, Puerto Ricans, Salvadorans, and Nicaraguans, who all come from very distinct cultural backgrounds.

Risk Factors for Alzheimer's Disease
Age and Gender
Age seems to be the most important risk factor for AD. Women are much more susceptible to developing AD than men. Almost two thirds of individuals with Alzheimer's disease are women. The incidence of Alzheimer's disease doubles after the age of 65. For those under 65 years of age the incidence is about 4%. For those 65 to 74 years of age the risk is 15%, for individuals 75 to 84 years of age the incidence is 43%, and after 85 years of age the incidence is thought to be between 38% and 50% (Alzheimer's Association, 2015; Alzheimer's Organization, 2015a).

Other Common Risk Factors
People with Alzheimer's disease have much higher rates of diabetes, cardiovascular disease, and high blood pressure than do people who do not develop Alzheimer's disease. Also, it is noted that people at lower educational levels seem to have an increased risk for Alzheimer's disease than those at higher educational levels. Socioeconomic levels seem to affect the aforementioned statistics. Generally, people at lower socioeconomic levels appear to be more prone to AD than people with a higher standard of living. This may be explained in part by lack of adequate medical care (e.g., treatment of hypertension, diabetes) and poor dietary intake.

Risk factors also include a history of severe head injury, a first-degree relative with AD, a family history of AD (a genetic polymorphism on chromosome 19 apolipoprotein E gene [*APOE E4*]; discussed under "Genetic Theories" below), obesity, insulin resistance, vascular factors,

inflammatory markers, hypertension, and Down syndrome (Anderson & Hoffman, 2011). One study found that out of seven lifestyle factors, the following four had the highest correlation with AD risk: physical inactivity, depression, smoking, and midlife hypertension (Gatchel et al., 2016).

THEORY

To date, a single cause of AD has not been identified. Most likely, several genetic and nongenetic factors—that affect each person differently—may interact to cause AD.

Genetic Theories
One genetic risk factor consistently related to Alzheimer's disease is the cholesterol-carrying apolipoprotein E gene *(APOE E4)*. It is believed in the scientific community that *APOE E4* plays a part in 20% to 25% of Alzheimer's disease (Alzheimer's Organization, 2015a). There is evidence that the *APOE E4* genotype and the sex hormone estrogen have an interaction, which may explain higher rates of Alzheimer's in women (Alzheimer's Association, 2015).

Genetic factors associated with early-onset Alzheimer's disease consist of mutations in three genes. Early-onset AD is relatively rare, develops in people ages 30 to 60, and accounts for only 5% of people with the disease (Alzheimer's Association, 2015). Early-onset genetic defects that relate to Alzheimer's include the gene *APP* (amyloid precursor protein) on chromosome 21, the gene *PS-1* (presenilin-1) on chromosome 14, and the gene *PS-2* (presenilin-2) on chromosome 1.

Anatomical Pathology of Alzheimer's Disease
Alzheimer's disease (AD) is a complex disease that begins to damage the brain long before the symptoms appear, as mentioned above. AD affects processes that keep the neurons healthy, such as (1) communication pathways, (2) metabolism, and (3) repair. In a healthy brain neurons are supported by microtubules, which guide nutrients and molecules between the cell body and the axon terminals. A special protein called tau protein is responsible for the stability of the microtubules. In AD tau protein is subjected to chemical changes, which result in neurofibrillary tangles and cause disintegration of the microtubules, thus collapsing the neuron's transport system. This disintegration of the neuron transport system results in malfunction of communication between neurons, and eventually leads to neural cell death. It is the destruction and death of the cells that causes memory failure, personality changes, problems in carrying out daily activities, and other features of the disease (Anderson & Chawla, 2016; Anderson & Hoffman, 2011).

In the Alzheimer's brain (Alzheimer's Organization, 2015b):
- The **cortex shrivels up,** damaging areas involved in thinking, planning, speech, perception, and remembering.
- Early in the disease neuronal degeneration, along with severe shrinkage, occurs in the **hippocampus** (an area of the cortex that plays a key role in formation of new memories).
- **Ventricles** (fluid-filled spaces within the brain) grow larger.

The anatomical pathology of Alzheimer's disease includes senile plaques (SPs) and neurofibrillary tangles (NFTs). It is believed that the disease begins with the buildup of beta-amyloid protein, resulting in **senile plaques,** which are also called **beta-amyloid plaques.** These plaques are cores of degenerated neuron material that lie free of the cell bodies on the ground substances of the brain. The quantity of plaques has been correlated with the degree of mental deterioration.

The **neurofibrillary tangles** are the damaged remains of microtubules that allow the flow of nutrients through the neurons. These neurofibrillary tangles form in the hippocampus, which is the part of the brain responsible for recent (short-term) memory, as well as the medial temporal lobe that is the initial sites of tangle deposition and atrophy (Anderson & Chawla, 2016).

Granulovascular degeneration is another active process in the disease and it results in the filling of brain cells with fluid and granular material. Increased degeneration accounts for increased loss of mental function. **Brain atrophy** is observable with wider cortical sulci and enlarged cerebral ventricles, as demonstrated by computed tomography (CT) and magnetic resonance imaging (MRI) scans. Imaging techniques reveal significant loss of cells and volume in the regions of the brain devoted to memory and higher mental functioning.

APPLICATION OF THE NURSING PROCESS: DEMENTIA

ASSESSMENT

Overall Assessment

As we now know, AD is commonly characterized by progressive deterioration of cognitive functioning and changes in behavioral symptoms. Initially, deterioration may be subtle and insidious and may last for years. These brain changes probably start 10 to 20 years before any visible signs or symptoms appear, as previously mentioned. This period of time is referred to as the *prodromal phase* or *preclinical Alzheimer's disease.*

The cognitive symptom most often observed early in the development of AD is impairment in memory and learning. In the early stages of the disease, the affected individual may be able to compensate for loss of memory. Some people may have superior social graces and charm that give them the ability to hide severe deficits in memory, even from experienced health care professionals. This hiding is actually a form of **denial,** which is an unconscious protective defense against the terrifying reality of losing one's place in the world. Family members may also unconsciously deny that anything is wrong as a defense against the painful awareness that a loved one is deteriorating. As time goes on, symptoms become more obvious, and other defensive maneuvers become evident.

Another defense mechanism is confabulation—the making up of stories or answers to maintain self-esteem when the person does not remember. For example, the nurse addresses a patient who has remained in a hospital bed all weekend:

Nurse: "Good morning, Ms. Jones. How was your weekend?"
Patient: "Wonderful. I discussed politics with the president, and he took me out to dinner."

or

Patient: "I spent the weekend with my daughter and her family."
(*less grandiose*)

Confabulation is not the same as lying. When people are lying, they are aware of making up an answer; confabulation is an **unconscious** attempt to maintain self-esteem.

Perseveration (the repetition of phrases or behavior) is eventually seen and is often intensified under stress. The avoidance of answering questions is another mechanism by which the patient is able to maintain self-esteem unconsciously in the face of severe memory deficits. Therefore (1) denial, (2) confabulation, (3) perseveration, and (4) avoidance of questions are four defensive behaviors the nurse might notice during assessment.

Cognitive impairment involves the *four A's:*

- **Amnesia or memory impairment.** Initially, the person has difficulty remembering recent events. Gradually, deterioration progresses to include both recent and remote memory.
- Aphasia (loss of language ability), which progresses with the disease. Initially, the person has difficulty finding the correct word, then is reduced to a few words, and finally is reduced to babbling or mutism.

- Apraxia (loss of purposeful movement in the absence of motor or sensory impairment). The person is unable to perform once-familiar and purposeful tasks. For example, in apraxia of gait, the person loses the ability to walk. In apraxia of dressing, the person is unable to put on clothes properly (may put arms in trousers or put a jacket on upside down).
- Agnosia (loss of sensory ability to recognize objects). For example, the person may lose the ability to recognize familiar sounds (auditory agnosia), such as the ring of the telephone, a car horn, or the doorbell. Loss of this ability extends to the inability to recognize familiar objects (visual or tactile agnosia), such as a glass, magazine, pencil, or toothbrush. Eventually, people are unable to recognize loved ones or even parts of their own bodies.

There are also disturbances in executive functioning (planning, organizing, abstract thinking). The clumping of neurons in the brain results in the deterioration of working components in the brain. These cells contain memories, receive sights and sounds, activate hormone secretion, produce emotions, and command muscles into motion.

Assessing Stages of AD

AD has been classified according to the stage of the degenerative process. The number of stages defined ranges from three to seven, depending on the source. No matter the number of stages used as a guide, symptoms can fluctuate between each stage. Keep in mind brain changes start 10 to 20 years before any visible signs or symptoms appear during the preclinical/prodromal stage and occur before the diagnosis of AD is proposed. This section presents four stages of AD to help illustrate the progression of symptoms while they develop over the course of this deteriorating disease. Table 18-4 can be used as a guide to review these four stages of AD and highlight the deficits associated with each stage.

The rate of progression varies individually. The mean age of survival after diagnosis is approximately 3 to 10 years (Anderson & Chawla, 2016). Some individuals can live with AD for as long as 20 years (APA, 2013).

Stage 1: Mild Alzheimer's Disease

The loss of intellectual ability is insidious. The person with mild Alzheimer's disease loses energy, drive, and initiative and has difficulty learning new things. Because personality and social behavior remain intact, others tend to minimize and underestimate the loss of the individual's abilities. The individual may still continue to work, but the extent of the dementia gradually becomes evident in new or demanding situations. During the mild phases of AD, *apathy* is the most common behavioral problem to appear early and often persists throughout the course of the disease. *Depression* may also occur early on, especially if there is a family history of depression (Tampi & Tampi, 2014). Activities such as grocery shopping or managing finances are noticeably impaired during this phase.

VIGNETTE

Mr. Collins, a 60-year-old lineman for a telephone company, feels that he is getting old. He keeps forgetting things and writes notes to himself on scraps of paper. One day on the job, he forgets momentarily which wires to connect and connects all the wrong ones, causing mass confusion for a few hours. At home, Mr. Collins becomes very upset when his wife suggests that they invite the new neighbors for dinner. It is hard for him to admit that anything new confuses him, and he often forgets names (*aphasia*) and sometimes loses the thread of conversations. Once he even forgot his address when his car stopped working on the highway. He is moody and depressed and becomes indignant when his wife finds 3 months' worth of unpaid bills stashed in his sock drawer. Mrs. Collins is bewildered, upset, and fearful that something is terribly wrong.

TABLE 18-4   Stages of Alzheimer's Disease

Stage	Hallmarks
Stage 1 (Mild) Forgetfulness	Shows short-term memory loss; loses things, forgets Memory aids compensate: lists, routine, organization Aware of the problem; concerned about lost abilities Depression common—worsens symptoms Disease is not diagnosable from the symptoms
Stage 2 (Moderate) Confusion	Shows progressive memory loss; short-term memory impaired; memory difficulties interfere with all abilities Withdrawn from social activities Shows declines in instrumental activities of daily living (ADLs), such as money management, legal affairs, transportation, cooking, housekeeping Denial common; fears "losing his or her mind" Depression increasingly common; frightened because aware of deficits; covers up for memory loss through confabulation Problems intensified when stressed, fatigued, out of own environment, ill Commonly needs day care, or in-home assistance is needed at this time.
Stage 3 (Moderate to severe) Ambulatory dementia	Shows ADL losses: willingness and ability to bathe, grooming, choosing clothing, dressing, gait and mobility, toileting, communication, reading, and writing skills Shows loss of reasoning ability, safety planning, and verbal communication Frustration common; becomes more withdrawn and self-absorbed Depression resolves as awareness of losses diminishes Has difficulty communicating; shows increasing loss of language skills Shows evidence of reduced stress threshold; institutional care usually needed
Stage 4 (Late) End stage	Family recognition disappears; does not recognize self in mirror Nonambulatory; shows little purposeful activity; often mute; may scream spontaneously Forgets how to eat, swallow, chew; commonly loses weight; emaciation common Has problems associated with immobility (e.g., pneumonia, pressure ulcers, contractures) Incontinence common; seizures may develop Most certainly institutionalized at this point Return of primitive (infantile) reflexes

From Hall, G. R. (1994). Caring for people with Alzheimer's disease using the conceptual model of progressively lowered stress threshold in the clinical setting. *Nursing Clinics of North America, 29*(1), 129–141.

Stage 2: Moderate Alzheimer's Disease

Deterioration becomes evident during the moderate phase. Often the person with moderate AD cannot remember his or her address or the date. There are memory gaps in the person's history that may fluctuate from one moment to the next. Hygiene suffers, and the ability to dress appropriately is markedly affected. The person may put on clothes backward, button the buttons incorrectly, or not fasten zippers *(apraxia)*. Often, the person has to be coaxed to bathe.

Mood becomes labile, and the individual may have bursts of paranoia, anger, jealousy, and continued apathy. The occurrence of paranoia, aggression, and sleep-wake cycle disturbances cause great caregiver burden and caregiver depression (Tampi & Tampi, 2014). Activities such as driving are hazardous, and families are faced with the difficulty of taking away the car keys from their loved one. Care and supervision become full-time jobs for family members. Denial mercifully takes over and protects people from the realization that they are losing control, not only of their minds but also of their lives. Along with denial, people with AD begin to withdraw from activities and from others because they often feel overwhelmed and frustrated when they try to do things that once were easy. They may also have moments of becoming tearful and sad.

As important as it is to recognize all of the deficits during the progression to the moderate phase, it is helpful for caretakers to realize that the patient still retains abilities that influence care.

Stage 3: Moderate to Severe Alzheimer's Stage

At the moderate to severe stage, the person is often unable to identify familiar objects or people, even a spouse *(severe agnosia)*. The

> ### VIGNETTE
>
> Mr. Collins is transferred to a less complicated work position after his inability to function is recognized. His wife drives him to work and picks him up. Mr. Collins often forgets what he is doing and stares blankly. He accuses the supervisor of spying on him. Sometimes he disappears at lunch and is unable to find his way back to work. The transfer lasts only a few months, after which Mr. Collins is forced to take an early retirement. At home Mr. Collins sleeps in his clothes. He loses interest in reading and watching sports on television and often breaks into angry outbursts, seemingly over nothing. Often he becomes extremely restless and irritable and wanders around the house aimlessly.

person needs repeated instructions and directions to perform the simplest tasks *(advanced apraxia)*: "Here is the face cloth, pick up the soap. Now, put water on the face cloth and rub the face cloth with soap." Often the individual cannot remember where the toilet is and becomes incontinent. Total care is necessary at this point, and the burden on the family can be emotionally, financially, and physically devastating. The world is very frightening to the person with AD because nothing makes sense any longer. Agitation, violence, paranoia, and delusions are commonly seen. Another problem that is frightening to family members and caregivers is wandering behavior. It is estimated that about 60% of people with AD wander and are at risk for becoming lost.

Institutionalization may be the most appropriate recourse at this time because the level of care is so demanding, and violent outbursts and incontinence may be burdens that the family can no longer handle.

The following are some criteria that indicate the need for placement in a skilled nursing facility:

- Wandering
- Danger to self and others
- Incontinence
- Behavior affects the sleep and general health of others
- Total dependence on others for physical care

VIGNETTE

Mr. Collins is terrified. Memories come and then slip away. People come and go, but they are strangers. Someone is masquerading as his wife, and it is hard to tell what is real. Things never stay in the same place. Sometimes people hide the bathroom where he cannot find it. He in turn hides things to keep them safe, but he forgets where he hides them. Buttons and belts are confusing, and he does not know what they are doing there anyway. Sometimes he tries to walk away from the terrifying feelings and the strangers. He tries to find something he has lost long ago, if he could only remember what it is.

Stage 4: Late Alzheimer's Disease

Late in AD the following symptoms may occur: agraphia (inability to read or write), hyperorality (the need to taste, chew, and put everything in one's mouth), blunting of emotions, visual agnosia (loss of ability to recognize familiar objects), and hypermetamorphosis (manifested by touching of everything in sight). At this stage, the ability to talk, and eventually the ability to walk, is lost. If not already present, the individual may become incontinent at this time, have difficulty swallowing (dysphasia), may have seizures. Weight loss, increased sleeping, and moaning/grunting are also evident during the final stage. Toward the end of the late stage, stupor and coma may occur. Death frequently is secondary to infection or choking.

VIGNETTE

Mrs. Collins and the children keep Mr. Collins at home for a short while until his outbursts become frightening. Once, he is lost for 2 days after he somehow unlocks the front door. Finally, Mrs. Collins has her husband placed in a Veterans Administration (VA) hospital. When his wife comes to visit, Mr. Collins sometimes cries. He never talks and is always restrained in his chair when she comes to see him. The staff explains to her that although Mr. Collins can still walk, he keeps getting into other people's beds and scaring them. They explain that perhaps he wants comfort and misses human touch. They encourage her visits, even though Mr. Collins does not seem to recognize her. He does respond to music. His wife brings him a small CD player, and plays the country and western music he has always loved; at those times Mr. Collins nods and claps his hands.

Mrs. Collins is torn between guilt and love, anger and despair. She is confused and depressed. She is going through the painful process of mourning the loss of the man she has loved and shared a life with for 34 years. Three months after his admission to the VA hospital, and 8 years after the incident of the crossed wires at the telephone company, Mr. Collins chokes on some food, develops pneumonia, and dies.

DSM-5 DIAGNOSTIC CRITERIA

for Major or Mild Neurocognitive Disorder Due to Alzheimer's Disease

A. The criteria are met for major or mild neurocognitive disorder.
B. There is insidious onset and gradual progression of impairment in one or more cognitive domains (for major neurocognitive disorder, at least two domains must be impaired).

C. Criteria are met for either probable or possible Alzheimer's disease asfollows:
For major neurocognitive disorder:
Probable Alzheimer's disease is diagnosed if either of the following is present; otherwise, possible Alzheimer's disease should be diagnoses.
   1. Evidence of a causative Alzheimer's disease genetic mutation from family history or genetic testing.
   2. All three of the following are present:
      a. Clear evidence of decline in memory and learning at least one other cognitive domain (based on detailed history or serial neuropsychological testing).
      b. Steadily progressive, gradual decline in cognition, without extended plateaus.
      c. No evidence of mixed etiology (i.e., absence of other neurodegenerative or cerebrovascular disease, or another neurological, mental, or systemic disease or condition likely contributing to cognitive decline).
For mild neurocognitive disorder:
Probable Alzheimer's disease is diagnosed if there is evidence of a causative Alzheimer's disease genetic mutation from either genetic testing or family history.
Possible Alzheimer's disease is diagnosed if there is no evidence of a causative Alzheimer's disease genetic mutation from either genetic testing or family history, and all three of the following are present:
   1. Clear evidence of decline in memory and learning.
   2. Steadily progressive, gradual decline in cognition, without extended plateaus.
   3. No evidence of mixed etiology (i.e., absence of other neurodegenerative or cerebrovascular disease, or another neurological or systemic disease or condition likely contributing to cognitive decline).
D. The disturbance is not better explained by cerebrovascular disease, another neurodegenerative disease, the effects of a substance, or another mental, neurological, or systemic disorder.

From the American Psychiatric Association (APA). (2013). *Diagnostic and statistical manual of mental disorders* (5th ed.). Washington, DC: APA.

Diagnostic Tests for Dementia

A wide range of problems may masquerade as dementia and may be mistaken for AD. For example, depression and dementia in the older adult present with similar symptoms. It is important that nurses and other health care professionals be able to assess some of the important differences among depression, dementia, and delirium. Refer back to Table 18-1 for important differences among these three phenomena. It is important to emphasize that depression and dementia or depression and delirium can coexist in the same person. Therefore it is important that a complete and thorough medical exam (neurological, medical, psychiatric history, review of medications, and nutritional evaluation) be performed.

Other disorders that often mimic a major neurocognitive disorder (dementia) include drug toxicity, metabolic disorders, infections, and nutritional deficiencies. A disorder that mimics dementia is sometimes referred to as a pseudodementia. That is, although the symptoms may suggest dementia, a careful examination may reveal another diagnosis altogether, usually depression. This reinforces the importance of performing a comprehensive assessment (including laboratory tests) when symptoms of dementia are present to identify nondementia causes.

No definitive test presently exists to diagnose AD, although a recent imaging study may clear the way for diagnosing AD in those in the prodromal phase of AD (Ong et al., 2015). Preliminary evidence suggests that positron emission tomography (PET) and single photon emission computed tomography (SPECT) scans can aid in the diagnosis. Studies using magnetic resonance imaging (MRI) to measure the size of brain structures are illuminating; a recent study showed that about 12% of people with smaller brain structures and only mild minor cognitive symptoms will eventually progress to dementia (Black & Andreasen, 2014).

CT, PET, and other developing scanning technologies have diagnostic capabilities because they reveal brain atrophy and rule out other conditions, such as neoplasms. The use of mental status questionnaires such as the Mini-Mental State Examination (MMSE) in people older than 75 is sometimes recommended to increase earlier detection.

Assessment Guidelines
Dementia

1. Identify and treat any general medical conditions that might contribute to the dementia.
2. Evaluate potential of suicide or aggression toward others.
3. Explore how well the family is prepared for and informed about the progress of the patient's dementia (e.g., the phases and course of AD; vascular dementia; acquired immunodeficiency syndrome [AIDS]-related dementia; dementia associated with multiple sclerosis, Parkinson's disease, lupus erythematosus, or brain injury).
4. Review the medications the patient is currently taking, including over-the-counter (OTC) remedies, herbs, complementary agents, and recreational drugs.
5. Evaluate the patient's current level of cognitive functioning.
6. Discuss with family members how they are coping with the patient and their main issues at this time.
7. Assess evidence of neglect or abuse.
8. Review the resources available to the family. Ask the family members to describe the help they receive from other family members, friends, and community resources. Determine if caregivers are aware of community support groups and resources.
9. Determine the appropriate safety measures needed by the patient and arrange for them to be implemented.
10. Evaluate the safety of the patient's home environment (e.g., with regard to wandering, eating inedible objects, falling, engaging in provocative behaviors toward others).
11. Identify the needs of the family for teaching and guidance (e.g., how to manage catastrophic reactions; lability of mood; aggressive behaviors; nocturnal delirium and increased confusion and agitation at night, or sundown syndrome).

DIAGNOSIS

One of the most important areas of concern is the patient's *safety*. Many people with AD wander and may be lost for hours or days. Wandering, along with behaviors such as rummaging, may be perceived as purposeful to the patient. Wandering may result from changes in the physical environment, fear caused by hallucinations or delusions, or lack of exercise.

Seizures may occur in the later stages of this disease. Injuries from falls and accidents can occur during any stage as confusion and disorientation progress. The potential for burns exists if the patient is a smoker or is unattended when using the stove. Prescription drugs can be taken incorrectly, or bottles of noxious fluids can be mistakenly ingested, which results in a medical crisis. Therefore, *Risk for injury* is always present.

As the person's ability to recognize or name objects is decreased, *Impaired verbal communication* becomes a problem. As memory diminishes and disorientation increases, *Impaired environmental interpretation syndrome,** Impaired memory,* and *Chronic confusion* occur.

---

* *Impaired environmental interpretation syndrome* is no longer included in NANDA, however, it is one of the two nursing diagnoses that are appropriate for psychotic symptoms. The second is *altered thought processes.* Hopefully these nursing diagnoses will be included in the next edition.

During the course of the disease, people show personality changes, increased vulnerability, and often inappropriate behaviors. Common behaviors include hoarding, regression, and being overly demanding and aggressive. Therefore nurses and family members often intervene in behaviors that signal *Ineffective coping, Labile mood,* and *Harm to self and others.* Family caregivers often experience *Compromised* or *Disabled family coping.*

Additional family issues may emerge. Perhaps some of the most crucial aspects of the patient's care are support, education, and referrals for the family. The family loses an integral part of its unit. Family members lose the love, function, support, companionship, and warmth that this person once provided. *Caregiver role strain* is always present and planning with the family and offering community support are integral parts of appropriate care. *Anticipatory grieving* is also an important phenomenon to assess and may be an important target for intervention. Helping the family grieve can make the task ahead somewhat clearer and, at times, less painful. Refer back to Table 18-2 for potential nursing diagnoses for confused patients with dementia.

OUTCOMES IDENTIFICATION

Families who have a member with dementia are faced with an exhaustive list of issues that need to be addressed. Self-care needs, impaired environmental interpretation, constant confusion, ineffective individual coping, and role strain of the caregiver are just a few of the areas that nurses and other health care members will need to target (Box 18-2).

PLANNING

The planning of care for a patient with dementia is geared toward the patient's immediate needs. Figure 18-2 presents the Functional Dementia Scale, which can be used by nurses and families to plan strategies for addressing immediate needs and to track progression of the dementia.

Identifying level of functioning and assessing caregivers' needs help the nurse identify appropriate community resources. Does the patient or family need the following?
- Transportation services
- Supervision and care when primary caregiver is out of the home
- Referrals to day care centers
- Information on support groups within the community
- Meals on Wheels
- Information on respite and residential services
- Telephone numbers for help lines
- Home health aides
- Home health services
- The Alzheimer's Association's Safe Return program (http://www.alz.org/care/alzheimers-dementia-wandering.asp#ixzz3e0pQb-5Np)
- Additional teaching or psychopharmaceutical aids to manage distressing or harmful behaviors when appropriate and safe.

Because stress is a common occurrence when working with persons with cognitive impairments, the health care staff needs to be proactive in minimizing its effects as well as in teaching and providing guidelines to caregivers and loved ones. Reducing stress can be facilitated by the following measures:
- **Have a realistic understanding of the disease** so that expectations for the individual are realistic.
- **Establish realistic outcomes** for the person and recognize when they are achieved. These outcomes may be as minor as *patient feeds self with spoon,* yet it must be remembered that even the smallest

BOX 18-2 Suggested Outcome Criteria for a Major Neurocognitive Disorder (Dementia)*

Injury

- Patient will remain safe in all environments.
- With the aid of an identification bracelet and neighborhood or hospital alert, patient will be returned within 1 hour of wandering.
- Patient will remain free of danger during seizures.
- With the aid of interventions, patient will remain burn-free.
- With the aid of guidance and environmental manipulation, patient will not be hurt if a fall occurs.
- Patient will ingest only correct doses of prescribed medications and appropriate food and fluids.

Communication

- Patient will communicate needs.
- Patient will answer yes or no appropriately to questions.
- Patient will state needs in alternative modes when aphasic (e.g., will signal correct word on hearing it, will refer to picture or label).
- Patient will wear prescribed glasses or hearing aid each day.

Caregiver Role Strain

- Family members will have the opportunity to express "unacceptable" feelings in a supportive environment.
- Family members will have access to professional counseling.
- Family members will name two organizations within their geographical area that can offer support.
- Family members will participate in patient's plan of care, with encouragement from staff.
- Family members will state that they have outside help that allows them to take personal time for themselves each week or month.
- Family members will have the names of three resources that can help with financial burdens and legal considerations.

Impaired Environmental Interpretation: Chronic Confusion

- Patient will acknowledge the reality of an object or a sound that was misinterpreted (illusion), after it is pointed out.
- Patient will state that he or she feels safe after experiencing delusions or illusions.
- Patient will remain nonaggressive when experiencing paranoid ideation.

Self-Care Needs

- Patient will participate in self-care at optimal level.
- Patient will be able to follow step-by-step instructions for dressing, bathing, and grooming.
- Patient will put on own clothes appropriately, with aid of fastening tape (Velcro) and nursing supervision.
- Patient's skin will remain intact and free from signs of pressure.

*Not an exhaustive list.

FUNCTIONAL DEMENTIA SCALE

Circle one rating for each item:
1. None or little of the time
2. Some of the time
3. Good part of the time
4. Most or all of the time

Client: ______
Observer: ______
Position or relation to patient: ______
Facility: ______
Date: ______

1	2	3	4	1. Has difficulty in completing simple tasks on own (e.g., dressing, bathing, doing arithmetic).
1	2	3	4	2. Spends time either sitting or in apparently purposeless activity.
1	2	3	4	3. Wanders at night or needs to be restrained to prevent wandering.
1	2	3	4	4. Hears things that are not there.
1	2	3	4	5. Requires supervision or assistance in eating.
1	2	3	4	6. Loses things.
1	2	3	4	7. Appearance is disorderly if left to own devices.
1	2	3	4	8. Moans.
1	2	3	4	9. Cannot control bowel function.
1	2	3	4	10. Threatens to harm others.
1	2	3	4	11. Cannot control bladder function.
1	2	3	4	12. Needs to be watched so doesn't injure self (e.g., by careless smoking, leaving the stove on, falling).
1	2	3	4	13. Destructive of materials around him/her (e.g., breaks furniture, throws food trays, tears up magazines).
1	2	3	4	14. Shouts or yells.
1	2	3	4	15. Accuses others of doing bodily harm or stealing his or her possessions—when you are sure the accusations are not true.
1	2	3	4	16. Is unaware of limitations imposed by illness.
1	2	3	4	17. Becomes confused and does not know where he or she is.
1	2	3	4	18. Has trouble remembering.
1	2	3	4	19. Has sudden changes of mood (e.g., gets upset, angered, or cries easily).
1	2	3	4	20. If left alone, wanders aimlessly during the day or needs to be restrained to prevent wandering.

FIGURE 18-2 Functional Dementia Scale. (Rights were not granted to include this figure in electronic media. Please refer to the printed book.) (From Moore, J. T., et al. [1983]. A functional dementia scale. *Journal of Family Practice, 16,* 498.)

TABLE 18-5   Intervention Guidelines for Major Neurocognitive Disorders (Dementia): Communication

Intervention	Rationale
1. Always identify yourself and call the person by name at each meeting.	1. Patient's short-term memory is impaired; requires frequent orientation to time and environment.
2. Speak slowly.	2. Patient needs time to process information.
3. Use short, simple words and phrases.	3. Patient may not be able to understand complex statements or abstract ideas.
4. Maintain face-to-face contact.	4. Verbal and nonverbal clues are maximized.
5. Be near patient when talking, one or two arm-lengths away.	5. This distance can help patient focus on speaker as well as maintain personal space.
6. Focus on one piece of information at a time.	6. Attention span of patient is poor and patient is easily distracted; helps patient focus. Too many data can be overwhelming and can increase anxiety.
7. Talk with patient about familiar and meaningful things.	7. Self-expression is promoted and reality is reinforced.
8. Encourage reminiscing about happy times in life.	8. Remembering accomplishments and shared joys helps distract patient from deficit and gives meaning to existence.
9. When patient is delusional, acknowledge patient's feelings and reinforce reality. Do not argue or refute delusions.	9. Acknowledging feelings helps patient feel understood. Pointing out realities may help patient focus on realities. Arguing can enhance adherence to false beliefs.
10. If a patient gets into an argument with another patient, stop the argument and separate individuals. After a short while (5 minutes), explain straightforwardly to each patient why you had to intervene.	10. Escalation to physical acting out is prevented. Patient's right to know is respected. Explaining in an adult manner helps maintain self-esteem.
11. When patient becomes verbally aggressive, acknowledge patient's feelings and shift topic to more familiar ground (e.g., "I know this is upsetting for you, because you always cared for others. Tell me about your children.").	11. Confusion and disorientation easily increase anxiety. Acknowledging feelings makes patient feel more understood and less alone. Topics patient has mastery over can remind him or her of areas of competent functioning and can increase self-esteem.
12. Have patient wear prescription eyeglasses or hearing aid.	12. Environmental awareness, orientation, and comprehension are increased, which in turn increases awareness of personal needs and the presence of others.
13. Keep patient's room well lit.	13. Environmental clues are maximized.
14. Have clocks, calendars, and personal items (e.g., family pictures, Bible) in clear view of patient while he or she is in bed.	14. These objects assist in maintaining personal identity.
15. Reinforce patient's pictures, nonverbal gestures, X's on calendars, and other methods used to anchor patient in reality.	15. When aphasia starts to hinder communication, alternate methods of communication need to be instituted.

achievement can be a significant accomplishment for the impaired individual.

- **Maintain good self-care.** Nurses and caregivers need to protect themselves from the negative effects of stress by obtaining adequate sleep and rest, eating a nutritious diet, exercising, engaging in relaxing activities, and addressing their own spiritual needs.

IMPLEMENTATION

The needs of people with dementia are complex, change over time, and can take place in a variety of settings during various stages of the disease. Care settings include the emergency department, the general hospital, home settings, long-term care settings, and the community.

The nurse's attitude of unconditional positive regard is the single most effective tool in caring for individuals with dementia. It induces people to cooperate with care, reduces catastrophic outbreaks, and increases family members' satisfaction with care. A warm, empathic, and non-judgmental approach using calm, unhurried, clear communication can help allay confusion and agitation. The nurse and others should always introduce themselves with each encounter. Expectations should be clear and explained in simple, step-by-step instructions. To help patients maintain a sense of self-control, they should be given simple and appropriate choices in their care (e.g., "Do you want to wash your face before or after you brush your teeth?").

Because a considerable number of individuals with dementia have secondary behavioral disturbances (e.g., depression, paranoia, hallucinations, delusions, agitation, sleep-wake disturbances, wandering), there is an increase in the need for supervision. Many of these situations respond well to the interventions listed in Tables 18-5 and 18-6. For example, a woman who is 78 years old and believes that she is 23 and has babies at home would not be calmed by being told that she is 78 and has no babies. It is most helpful to reflect back to patients their feelings and to show understanding and concern for their plight. For example, "Mrs. Green, you miss your children, and this can be a lonely place."

Intervention with family members is critical. The effects of losing a family member to dementia—that is, watching the deterioration of a person who has had an important role within the family unit and who is loved and a vital part of his or her family's history—are devastating, exhausting, and painful. Nurses can teach families about the progression of the illness, give them guidelines for safely caring for their family member who lives at home (Tables 18-7 and 18-8), and find appropriate support for families who are grieving.

Communication Guidelines

How nurses choose to communicate with patients with dementia affects the patient's maintenance of self-esteem and ability to participate in care. People with dementia often find it difficult to express themselves. They:

- Have difficulty finding the right words
- Use familiar words repeatedly
- Invent new words to describe things (neologisms)
- Frequently lose their train of thought
- Rely on nonverbal gestures

See Table 18-5 for a variety of nursing interventions and guidelines integral for communicating with a cognitively impaired person. These interventions and guidelines also can be taught to family members.

TABLE 18-6 Intervention Guidelines for Dementia: Health Teaching and Health Promotion

Intervention	Rationale
Dressing and Bathing	
1. Always have patient perform all tasks within his or her present capacity.	1. Maintains patient's self-esteem and uses muscle groups; impedes staff burnout; minimizes further regression.
2. Always have patient wear own clothes, even if in the hospital.	2. Helps maintain patient's identity and dignity.
3. Use clothing with elastic, and substitute fastening tape (Velcro) for buttons and zippers.	3. Minimizes patient's confusion and eases independence of functioning.
4. Label clothing items with patient's name and name of item.	4. Helps identify patient if he or she wanders and gives patient additional clues when aphasia or agnosia occurs.
5. Give step-by-step instructions whenever necessary (e.g., "Take this blouse...put in one arm ... now the next arm ... pull it together in the front ... now ...").	5. Patient can focus on small pieces of information more easily; allows patient to perform at optimal level.
6. Make sure that water in faucets is not too hot.	6. Judgment is lacking in patient; patient is unaware of many safety hazards.
7. If patient is resistant to performing self-care, come back later and ask again.	7. Moods may be labile, and patient may forget but often complies after short interval.
Nutrition	
1. Monitor food and fluid intake.	1. Patient may have anorexia or be too confused to eat.
2. Offer finger foods that patient can take away from the dinner table.	2. Increases input throughout the day; patient may eat only small amounts at meals.
3. Weigh patient regularly (once a week).	3. Monitors fluid and nutritional status.
4. During periods of hyperorality, watch that patient does not eat nonfood items (e.g., ceramic fruit, food-shaped soaps).	4. Patient puts everything into mouth; may be unable to differentiate inedible objects made in the shape and color of food.
Bowel and Bladder Function	
1. Begin bowel and bladder program early; start with bladder control.	1. Establishing same time of day for bowel movements and toileting—in early morning, after meals and snacks, and before bedtime—can help prevent incontinence.
2. Evaluate use of disposable diapers.	2. Prevents embarrassment.
3. Label bathroom door as well as doors to other rooms.	3. Additional environmental clues can maximize independent toileting.
Sleep	
1. Because patient may awaken, be frightened, or cry out at night, keep area well lit.	1. Reinforces orientation; minimizes possible illusions.
2. Maintain a calm atmosphere during the day.	2. Encourages a calming night's sleep.
3. Medications are not recommended for sleep. The use of nonmedical interventions has proven most helpful in many cases. When medications have been prescribed, low-dose tricyclic antidepressants, neuroleptics with sedative properties (e.g., haloperidol [Haldol]), benzodiazepines, and others may be ordered.	3. Helps clear thinking and sedates. However, psychotic medications should be used with extreme care, and other methods should be applied first.
4. Avoid the use of restraints.	4. Can cause patient to become more terrified and fight against restraints until exhausted to a dangerous degree.

TABLE 18-7 Services for People with Major Neurocognitive Disorders (Dementia) and Their Families or Caregivers

Type of Service	Services Provided
Family or caregiver Some patients may live by themselves in the community; active case management is vital when this is the case.	Caregivers have a right to: • Easy access to services • Respite care • Full involvement in decision making • Assessment of the needs of the caregiver as well as those of the patient • Information and referral • Case management: coordination of community resources and follow-up
Community services	• Adult day care: provides activities, socialization, supervision • Physician services • Protective services: prevent, eliminate, and/or remedy effects of abuse or neglect • Recreational services • Transportation • Mental health services • Legal services

TABLE 18-7 Services for People with Major Neurocognitive Disorders (Dementia) and Their Families or Caregivers—cont'd

Type of Service	Services Provided
Home care	• Meals on Wheels • Home health aide services • Homemaker services • Hospice services • Occupational therapy • Paid companion or sitter services • Physical therapy • Skilled nursing • Personal care services: assistance in basic self-care activities • Social work services • Telephone reassurance: regular telephone calls to individuals who are isolated and homebound* • Personal emergency response systems: telephone-based systems to alert others that a person who is alone is in need of emergency assistance*

*Vital for those living alone.

TABLE 18-8 Interventions for a Safe Milieu in the Home

Intervention	Rationale
Safe Environment	
1. Gradually restrict use of the car.	1. Even mild cognitive impairment increases risk of vehicular accident.
2. Remove throw rugs and other objects in person's path.	2. Minimizes tripping and falling.
3. Minimize sensory stimulation.	3. Decreases sensory overload, which can increase anxiety and confusion.
4. If patient becomes verbally upset, listen briefly, give support, then change the topic.	4. Goal is to prevent escalation of anger. When attention span is short, patient can be distracted to more productive topics and activities.
5. Label all rooms and drawers. Label often-used objects (e.g., hairbrushes, toothbrushes).	5. May keep patient from wandering into other patients' rooms. Increases environmental clues to familiar objects.
6. Install safety bars in bathroom.	6. Prevents falls.
7. Supervise patient when he or she smokes.	7. Danger of burns is always present.
8. If patient has history of seizures, educate family on how to deal with seizures.	8. Seizure activity is common in advanced Alzheimer's disease.
Wandering	
1. If patient wanders during the night, put mattress on the floor.	1. Prevents falls when patient is confused.
2. Have patient wear MedicAlert bracelet that cannot be removed (with name, address, and telephone number). Provide police department with recent pictures.	2. Patient can easily be identified by police, neighbors, or hospital personnel.
3. Alert local police and neighbors about patient wandering.	3. May reduce time necessary to return patient to home or hospital.
4. If patient is in the hospital, have him or her wear brightly colored vest with name, unit, and phone number printed on back.	4. Makes patient easily identifiable.
5. Put complex locks on door.	5. Reduces opportunity to wander.
6. Place locks at top of door.	6. In moderate and late Alzheimer's-type dementia, ability to look up and reach upward is lost.
7. Encourage physical activity during the day.	7. Physical activity may decrease wandering at night.
8. Explore the feasibility of installing sensor devices and web-based GPS system.	8. Sensor provides warning if patient wanders. GPS can help locate patient.
9. Use a bed monitor.	9. Alerts staff if patient has left his or her bed during the night.
Useful Activities	
1. Provide picture magazines and children's books when patient's reading ability diminishes.	1. Allows continuation of usual activities that patient can still enjoy; provides focus.
2. Provide simple activities that allow exercise of large muscles.	2. Exercise groups, dance groups, and walking provide socialization as well as increased circulation and maintenance of muscle tone.
3. Encourage group activities that are familiar and simple to perform.	3. Activities such as group singing, dancing, reminiscing, and working with clay and paint all help to increase socialization and minimize feelings of alienation.

A Person with a Severe Neurocognitive Disorder (Dementia)

Scenario

I met 75-year-old Mr. Samson on our geriatric rotation. He had recently been moved to the Memory Disorder Unit of the nursing facility. His wife of 50 years, whom he called Darlin' (her name was Darlene), had resided on the assisted living side of the facility until her sudden death from a myocardial infarction 3 weeks earlier. Mr. Samson and I regularly used the pictures in the memory wallet that his wife and the staff had assembled to remind him about his life.

Therapeutic Goal

By the end of this encounter, Mr. Samson will focus on good times he and his wife shared together, and spend less time asking for her and wanting to know when she is coming to visit.

Student-Patient Interaction	Thoughts, Communication Techniques, and Mental Health Nursing Concepts
Student: "Mr. Samson, what's wrong?" **Mr. Samson:** *Crying.* "My Darlin', what's wrong with my Darlin'?" *He gestures toward the sign of the memorial service to be held for "Mrs. Darlene Samson" and one other resident who had died the previous month.*	I knew from the chart that Mr. Samson had attended his wife's funeral. I should have said my name and reminded him that we had talked a few times before, but I was worried because he was sitting in the lobby sobbing. He is crying like he just discovered "his Darlin'" died. How awful to not be able to hold on to your own life and what matters most in your memories.
Student: "Mr. Samson, I'm _____, your nursing student. You feel worried seeing your wife's name on the sign." *He nods.* "Let's use your memory wallet to remember together about your Darlin'." *I wait until he makes eye contact and takes the wallet out of his hip pocket.* **Student's feelings:** *I am feeling a little anxious now. I hope I did okay in calling Mrs. Samson Darlin' as he does. I hope he'll remember if I show him the picture the staff put in the wallet showing Mr. Samson standing and looking at his wife in the casket. Seems unkind in some ways.*	I *introduce* myself again and use *reflection.* Diverting to the task of looking through the memory wallet provides structure to help meet *safety needs.*
Student: *Smiling encouragingly.* "Tell me about the pictures." **Mr. Samson:** *No longer crying.* "This was our house. Darlin' keeps such a great garden. I used to love her tomatoes the best." *He points to the tall plants beside the house.* **Student's feelings:** *He's trying so hard. I admire him. I never knew either of my grandfathers.*	I know that the mental health focus needs to include helping with *reality orientation* for as long as his progressive *dementia* will allow. He uses the present tense "keeps ... garden," but the past tense for "was our house" and "used to love her tomatoes." He is having trouble sorting out the present from the past.

Student-Patient Interaction	Thoughts, Communication Techniques, and Mental Health Nursing Concepts
Student: "You still love tomatoes! I helped you make the tomato salad for lunch. None tastes as good as Darlin's did, I bet." **Student's feelings:** *I did well here by reminding him of still liking tomatoes.* **Mr. Samson:** "Right. I wonder if Darlin' picked the tomato salad. We meet in the solarium every day." **Student's feelings:** *I feel frustrated that he's talking about Darlin' like she's alive. Two days ago he talked like he remembered that Mrs. Samson died 3 weeks ago.*	I make an *observation.* I refer to Mrs. Samson's tomatoes in the past tense to *reinforce reality.*
Student: "Look at this next picture." *I wait as he absorbs the funeral home picture.* **Student's feelings:** *Was that too direct? I didn't know what to say when he talked about meeting her in the solarium.* **Mr. Samson:** "Oh God, oh God. She died. She's gone. When did she die? How can I go on without her?" *He buries his head in his hands, sobbing.* **Student's feelings:** *He's experiencing this as though for the first time. I feel ready to cry.*	How nontherapeutic. I sound like I am giving a command. I should have started with, "I have some sad news."
Student: "You must've loved her very much. It must be lonely without her. I am with you. May I hold your hand?" *He nods.* **Mr. Samson:** "We were married 50 years. She's the love of my life. Darlin' was my soul mate." **Student:** "You say, Darlin' was your soul mate. You miss her so much." **Student's feelings:** *I'll talk with the treatment team. He may need some extra support as his memory impairment grows and as he faces the memorial service.*	Touch communicates caring. I *validate* his feelings of longing. I ask permission before touching. I remain silent while he talks about his wife. I cannot imagine 50 years with one person. What an accomplishment. I use reflection. I also carefully restate to emphasize his use of the past tense. I wonder what effect the memorial service will have on him. When he comes to the point of grieving anew every time, we will have to take out the funeral picture and emphasize feelings using *validation therapy.*
Mr. Samson: "I do, every minute of every day." *He makes eye contact as we continue talking until he's calmer and no longer crying.* **Student's feelings:** *I like him and I feel so sad about his situation.*	
Student: "Are you ready to walk together back to your room so you can get ready for reminiscence group?" *He nods.*	Giving him a choice empowers him.

Health Teaching and Health Promotion

Educating families who have a cognitively impaired member is one of the most important areas for nurses. Families who are caring for a member in the home need to know about strategies for communicating and structuring self-care activities (see Table 18-6). According to Rabins and colleagues (2014), "Support programs for caregivers and patients with dementia significantly decreased the odds of institutionalization and improved caregiver well-being."

Therefore, families need to know where to get help and find support programs. Help includes professional counseling and education regarding the process and the progression of the disease. Families need to know about and be referred to community-based groups that can help bear this tremendous burden (e.g., day care centers, senior citizen groups, organizations providing home visits and respite care, family support groups). A list with definitions of some of the types of services available in the patient's community, as well as the names and telephone numbers of the providers of these services, should be given to the family.

1. The Alzheimer's Association is a national umbrella agency that provides various forms of assistance to people with the disease and their families. The Alzheimer's Association has launched Safe Return to help locate and return missing people with AD and other memory impairments. Wandering is a common behavior during the second and third stages of AD, and the Alzheimer's Association Safe Return program plus MedicAlert offer peace of mind to families (Alzheimer's Organization, 2015c).

2. Some communities are instituting small GPS systems that can be attached by a wristband or armband to help locate a person with AD or use of a "Comfort Zone Check-In®," which is a self-service web-based location management service.

Information regarding housekeeping, home health aides, and companions is also available through the Alzheimer's Association. Such outside resources can help prevent the total emotional and physical fatigue of family members. Types of resources that might be available in some communities are found in Table 18-7. When the nurse is unable to provide the relevant information, proper referrals by the social worker are needed. Information regarding advance directives, durable power of attorney, guardianship, and conservatorship should be included in the communication with the family.

Milieu Therapy

Interventions and guidelines for families in structuring a safe environment and planning appropriate activities are found in Table 18-8.

Agitation and aggression are especially distressing to patients, caregivers, and staff in memory units. Since there are no U.S. Food and Drug Administration (FDA) approved antipsychotics for behavioral symptoms in dementia, psychosocial interventions should always be tried first. Some interventions that are effective to reduce agitation and aggressive behavior are listed in Figure 18-3.

Sensory Interventions	Music therapy (listening) Light therapy Pet therapy Multisensory stimulation Hearing aids
Active Therapy/ Structured Activities	Dancing Exercise Social interation Music therapy (playing/singing) Art therapy Outdoor walks
Psychological/Therapy	Validation therapy Reality orientation Reminiscence therapy Psychosocial therapy Cognitive behavioral therapy Relaxation training Structured support groups

FIGURE 18-3 Interventions delivered directly to patients with dementia to reduce agitated and aggressive behavior. *(Retrieved from* http://effectivehealthcare.ahrq.gov/index.cfm/search-for-guides-reviews-and-reports/produced=1998pageaction=displayproduct*)*

APPLYING EVIDENCE-BASED PRACTICE (EBP) IN ACTION

Problem An 81-year-old female diagnosed with Stage 3 Alzheimer's is living in a Skilled Nursing Facility (SNF). She is a fall risk and frequently wanders away from the supervised area and outside. There are dangers in the uneven ground outside and traffic in the parking lot and nearby streets. She is no longer able to communicate verbally in a meaningful way.

EBP Assessment

A. **What do you already know from experience?** It is dangerous for Alzheimers patients to wander as they can be harmed in a number of ways. This patient has not responded to verbal redirection and staff is trying to avoid any type of restraint. Although the staff has caught her before she gets outside on most occasions, when several patient alarms are going off at the same time she has been able to make it further.

B. **What does the literature say?** "Alarm fatigue" can occur when many alarms such as front door buzzers, chair alarms, and monitors are going off constantly in a health care environment (Mitka, 2013). Alzheimers patients can be difficult to keep safe while providing a satisfying qualify of life and avoiding restraint use (Paiva, 2013).

C. **What does the patient want?** In this situation, the patient is no longer able to make her wishes known verbally in a meaningful way. The nurse called the patient's daughter to have a conversation about the patient's former life, interests, and enjoyments. During the conversation, the daughter revealed that her mother had grown up on a farm and spent as much time as possible in nature throughout the years. This information helped the nurse recognize how important being outside would be to her patient.

Plan Regular time outside was built into the patient's plan of care, including daily walks in the garden, and meals outside when weather permitted. The daughter also made the commitment to take her mother to nature settings during their outings rather than indoor events at least part of the time. When the nurse asked the patient if she would like to go outside, her facial expression changed, her eyes brightened, and she verbalized "yes".

QSEN **QSEN Prelicensure Knowledge, Skills, and Attitudes (KSA's) Addressed:**

Safety and **patient-centered care** were utilized by finding a way to keep the patient from wandering away while providing enjoyment.

Informatics was addressed in considering the issue of alarm fatigue.

Mitka, M. (2013). Joint commission warns of alarm fatigue: Multitude of alarms from monitoring devices problematic. *Journal of American Medical Association, 309*(221), 2315-2316.

Paiva, S., Peleja, R., Cunha, J., & Abreu, C. (2013). Preventing alzheimers wandering: The potential of involving communities. *International Journal of Healthcare Information Systems and Informatics, 8*(4).

▶ Neurobiology of Alzheimer's and the Effects of Medication on the Brain

Two essential neurotransmitters implicated in Alzheimer's disease are acetylcholine and glutamate.

Acetylcholine: is involved with learning, memory, and mood. As Alzheimer's disease progresses the brain produces less and less acetylcholine. What little acetylcholine is left is rapidly destroyed by the enzyme acetylcholinesterase.

Cholinesterase: inhibitors keep the acetylcholinesterase enzyme from breaking down acetylcholine, thereby increasing both the level and duration of action of the neurotransmitter acetylcholine.

Glutamate: is involved with cell signaling, learning, and memory. Glutamate binds to cells at the N-methyl-D-aspartate (NMDA) receptor and allows calcium to enter the cell. In Alzheimer's disease, excess glutamate from damaged cells leads to chronic overexposure to calcium.

NMDA: antagonists helps reduce excess calcium by blocking some NMDA receptors.

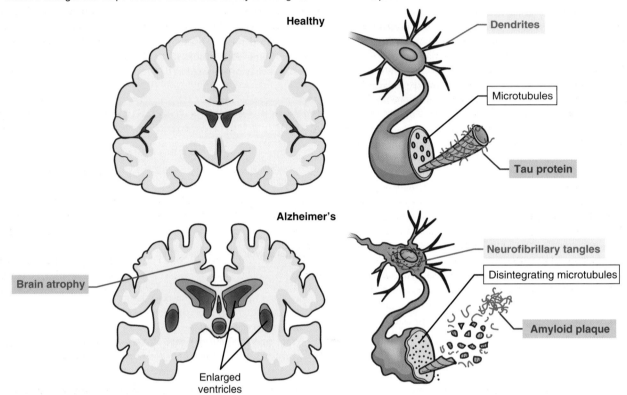

Brain Dysfunction

Amyloid plaques are sticky clumps found between nerve cells that may either cause or be the result of the disease. The clumps block communication at synapses that is normally protected by tau proteins and healthy microtubules. They may also activate immune system cells that trigger inflammation and devour disabled cells.

Neurofibrillary tangles are abnormal collections of protein threads inside nerve cells. They are comprised mainly of a protein called tau. Tangles disrupt the transport of food molecules, cell parts, and other key elements. This disruption results in cell death.

Brain atrophy is the cerebral cortex shriveling up, damaging areas involved in thinking, planning, and remembering. The hippocampus, an area of the cortex that is essential for memory, experiences severe shrinkage. Ventricles, the fluid-filled spaces within the brain, grow larger.

FDA Approved Drugs for the Treatment of Alzheimer's Disease

Drug name	Brand name	Classification	Approved For
galantamine	Razadyne	Cholinesterase inhibitor	Mild to moderate
donepezil	Aricept	Cholinesterase inhibitor	All stages
rivastigmine	Exelon	Cholinesterase inhibitor	All stages
memantine	Namenda	Namenda, an NMDA antagonist, helps reduce excess calcium by blocking some NMDA receptors	Moderate to severe
donepezil and memantine	Namzaric	Cholinesterase inhibitor and NMDA receptor antagonist combination	Moderate to severe

Pharmacological, Biological, and Integrative Therapies
Neurocognitive Impairment

Although there is no cure for Alzheimer's disease, there are four prescription drugs currently approved by the FDA for individuals with Alzheimer's disease. Because cholinesterase is well known to be low (up to 90%) in individuals with AD, medications called cholinesterase inhibitors can help delay or prevent symptoms from becoming worse for a limited time, and are useful in people with mild to moderate Alzheimer's disease. They work by preventing the breakdown of acetylcholine, and stimulate nicotinic receptors to release more acetylcholine into the brain. The FDA-approved cholinesterase inhibitors are *galantamine hydrobromide (Razadyne), rivastigmine tartrate (Exelon), and donepezil hydrochloride (Aricept)*. These FDA-approved agents demonstrate positive effects not only on cognition, but also on behavior and ability to function in activities of daily living for people with mild to moderate AD. All of these medications are effective in slowing down the progression of AD for a limited period (e.g., 3 months)—until the stores of acetylcholine have been depleted (Burchum & Rosenthal, 2016). At that point, the functioning of the individual may deteriorate drastically.

Memantine hydrochloride (Namenda), an *N*-methyl-D-aspartate (NMDA), works differently; it is an antagonist at the NMDA-glutamatergic receptor. This receptor is credited with mediating certain aspects of memory and learning (Black & Andreasen, 2014). The drug works by regulating glutamate and inhibiting the toxic effects of the excess influx of calcium that causes neurodegeneration (Burchum & Rosenthal, 2016). It is the first drug to target symptoms of AD during the moderate to severe stages of the disorder. Like the cholinesterase inhibitors, the benefits of memantine (Namenda) are time limited, and in many cases the results may be minimal.

A newer FDA-approved combination drug, Namzaric, is composed of both donepezil and memantine and is currently on the market and targeted to treat moderate to severe Alzheimer's disease (Table 18-9).

Targeting Behavioral Symptoms of Alzheimer's Disease/Dementia

Behavioral and psychological symptoms of dementia (BPSD) encompass a wide range of behaviors that are unsafe, cause disruptions that impair care, and lead to frustration for both staff and caregivers (e.g., agitation, hallucinations, disinhibition, labile mood) (Tampi & Tampi, 2014). These behaviors fluctuate over time.

Cognitive behavioral approaches and nursing interventions mentioned in this text are often helpful in lowering anxiety, dealing with physical agitation, and intervening with hallucinations and delusions (Tampi & Tampi, 2014). Rucci and Feinstein (2014) warn that signs of agitation or increasing anxiety may be caused by pain, urinary tract infections, dehydration, feeling lost and confused about one's surroundings, feeling frustrated by one's inability to communicate, among other factors, and that psychotropic interventions would be of no help in these types of situations.

The use of physical restraints is no longer sanctioned in those with cognitive deficits. The only restraints that do have some support if used occasionally and monitored closely are chairs with a laptop table (Kennard, 2015).

Medication to control disruptive behavior in patients with dementia is often associated with falls, worsening cognitive impairment, oversedation, and other adverse drug reactions. All

TABLE 18-9	Drugs Approved by the Food and Drug Administration for Alzheimer's Disease		
Drug Name	**Drug Type and Use**	**How It Works**	**Adverse Reactions**
Namenda® (memantine)	***N*-methyl-D-aspartate (NMDA) antagonist** prescribed to treat symptoms of *moderate to severe Alzheimer's*	Normalizes and regulates glutamate (a neurotransmitter) involved in learning and memory. Excess quantities are thought to contribute to neurodegeneration.	Dizziness, headache, constipation, confusion
Razadyne® (galantamine)	**Cholinesterase inhibitor** prescribed to treat symptoms of *mild to moderate Alzheimer's*	Prevents the breakdown of acetylcholine (ACh), increasing concentration of ACh in the hippocampus and neocortex areas in the brain that are important to memory and cognitive functions, and stimulates nicotinic receptors to release more acetylcholine in the brain.	Nausea, vomiting, diarrhea, weight loss, loss of appetite, syncope, gastrointestinal hemorrhage
Exelon® (rivastigmine)	**Cholinesterase inhibitor** prescribed to treat symptoms of *mild to moderate Alzheimer's* (patch is also for *severe Alzheimer's*)	Prevents the breakdown of acetylcholine and butyrylcholine (a brain chemical similar to acetylcholine) in the brain • start low and titrate upward • a.m. and p.m. dose with meals • patch once daily	Nausea, vomiting, diarrhea, weight loss, loss of appetite, muscle weakness, tremor, syncope bronchospasms, gastrointestinal hemorrhage
Aricept® (donepezil)	**Cholinesterase inhibitor** prescribed to treat symptoms of *mild to moderate, and moderate to severe Alzheimer's*	Prevents the breakdown of a chemical called acetylcholine in the brain • One daily dose at bedtime	Nausea, vomiting, diarrhea, insomnia, fatigue, muscle cramps, gastrointestinal hemorrhage
Namzaric	Combines **memantine hydrochloride extended-release (ER)** (also known as Namenda), and **donepezil hydrochloride** (also known as Aricept) to treat *moderate to severe Alzheimer's*	Donepezil improves the function of nerve cells in the brain by preventing the breakdown of acetylcholine. Memantine reduces the actions of chemicals in the brain that may contribute to the symptoms of Alzheimer's disease. • Twice-daily. • One daily dose at that time if **Namzaric ER**	• Same as Namenda • Same as Aricept

Adapted from National Institutes of Health. (2015). Alzheimer's disease medications fact sheet. Retrieved from http://www.nia.nih.gov/alzheimer's/publication/alzheimer's-disease-medications-fact-sheet#table; Gatchel, J. R., Wright, C. I., Falk, W. E., et al. (2016). Dementia. In T. A. Stern, M. Fava, T. E. Wilens, & J. F. Rosenbaum (Eds.), *Massachusetts General Hospital comprehensive clinical psychiatry* (2nd ed.); Burchum, J. R., & Rosenthal, L. D. (2016). *Lehne's pharmacology for nursing care* (9th ed.). St Louis, MO: Elsevier Saunders. Namzaric (updated February 1, 2016). Retrieved from www.drugs.com/pro/namzaric.html

antipsychotics have Black Box warnings: *"Treatment of behavioral disorders in elderly patients with dementia with antipsychotic medication is associated with increased mortality."* It is generally accepted that whatever modest benefit this classification of medication may provide is negated by the side effects. It is recommended that all antipsychotics be used sparingly for the few patients who benefit from them when behavioral interventions fail. However, anxiety, agitation, and delusional behaviors can often be tempered by timely, appropriate use of nursing interventions. The APA (2007) Guidelines for Treating Patients with Dementia (the most recent available) strongly suggest that nonpharmacological treatment should be tried first. Structural education programs for staff will help nurses, families, and others to manage disruptive behaviors through behavioral interventions and/or cognitive techniques in order to reduce the use of both medications and restraints. The APA Guidelines Watch for Alzheimer's and Dementia (Rabins et al., 2014; AHRQ, 2014) stated that updated systemic reviews and randomized controlled trials have increased the overall quality of evidence that *"psychosocial interventions improve or maintain cognition, function, adaptive behavior, and quality of life."* The use of antipsychotics in all settings (home, long-term care) should be limited.

When psychosocial interventions have failed, psychotropics may be necessary in managing behavioral symptoms of dementia, but these need to be used with extreme caution. Age alters the metabolism, absorption, and elimination of many medications, and older adults are more sensitive to these effects. The basic rule for older patients is **start low and go slow and monitor closely.** Targeting one core symptom (e.g., hallucinations) often helps with other symptoms such as agitation and fearfulness. And lastly, *weigh the risks carefully*.

In patients with coexisting depression, the choice of agents is usually based on the side effect profile. Selective serotonin reuptake inhibitors (SSRIs) have a low side effect profile and appear better tolerated, although the elderly and those with complex medical conditions may not be good candidates. Mirtazapine (Remeron) is also good because the side effects of weight gain and sedation may be desirable (Rucci & Feinstein, 2014). It should be noted, however, that the efficacy of these agents continues to be found negligible according to the APA Guidelines Watch (Rabins et al., 2014): "Clinical consensus still supports undertaking one or more trials of an antidepressant to treat clinically significant and persistent depressed mood in patients with dementia because of the increased rates of disability, impaired quality of life, and greater mortality associated with depression" (see Chapter 24).

Reducing the Risk for Alzheimer's

Although contracting dementia might be inevitable, there seems to be certain lifestyle changes that may either prevent or delay the onset of dementia. Modifiable risk factors include (Schnable, 2015):

* Staying physically active
* Stop smoking
* Avoid obesity, diabetes, hypertension, and vascular disease
* Drink moderately if at all
* Keep up your levels of vitamin D
* Reduce inflammation
* Get enough sleep, but not too much
* Avoid chronic stress and depression

Below is a recent study that demonstrated how certain lifestyle changes may reduce the risk of cognitive decline and dementia.

CAN WE SLOW PROGRESSION OF COGNITIVE DECLINE? POTENTIAL FOR THE FUTURE

The Finnish Geriatric Intervention Study to Prevent Cognitive Impairment and Disability (FINGER study) published in March 2015 is the first of its kind to demonstrate that specific lifestyle choices can reduce the risk of cognitive decline and dementia. This was a randomized controlled study that targeted lifestyle changes in the following areas: physical activity, diet, vascular risk factors, and brain training. The study included 1260 people aged 60 to 77 years. The intervention group underwent a program concentrated on four major areas (Hughes, 2015):

* *Physical exercise* based on international guidelines, guided by physiotherapists at the gym and consisting of individually tailored programs for progressive muscle strength training (one to three times per week) and aerobic exercise (two to five times per week).
* *Nutritional advice* based on the Finnish Nutrition Recommendations, delivered by study nutritionists (three individual sessions and seven to nine group sessions).
* *Cognitive training* (10 group sessions with a trained psychologist and individual sessions consisting of computer-based training) conducted in 2 periods of 6 months each, with each period including 72 training sessions (3 times per week, 10 to 15 minutes per session).
* *Management of metabolic and vascular risk factors* based on national guidelines. This included regular measurements of blood pressure, weight, body mass index, and hip and waist circumference; physical examinations; and recommendations for lifestyle management. Study physicians did not prescribe medication but strongly recommended participants to contact their own physician or clinic if needed.

Other studies are promising. A pilot study on deep brain stimulation (DBS) seems to have increased hippocampal volume and it is hypothesized that continuous stimulation was able to reactivate the memory circuits in the brain. A larger randomized double-blind study is presently being conducted (Anderson, 2015).

EVALUATION

Outcomes need to be stated in measurable terms, be within the capability of the patient, and be evaluated frequently. As the person's condition continues to deteriorate, outcomes need to be altered to reflect the person's diminished functioning. Frequent evaluation and reformulation of outcome criteria and short-term indicators also help diminish staff and family frustration, as well as minimize the patient's anxiety by ensuring that tasks are not more complicated than the person can accomplish. The overall outcomes for treatment are to promote the patient's optimal level of functioning and to retard further regression, whenever possible. Working closely with family members and providing them with the names of available resources and support sources may help increase the quality of life for both the family and the patient.

◼ KEY POINTS TO REMEMBER

* *Neurocognitive disorder* (NCD) is a term that refers to disorders marked by disturbances in orientation, memory, intellect, judgment, and affect, resulting from structural changes in the brain.
* Neurocognitive disorders (NCDs) are divided into mild and severe according to the *DSM-5*.
* Delirium, major neurocognitive disorders (dementia), and mild neurocognitive disorders/mild cognitive impairment encompass the cognitive disorders discussed in this text.

- Individuals with delirium and severe dementia are those who are most likely to be under care in hospital situations.
- Delirium is marked by acute onset, disturbance in consciousness, and symptoms of disorientation and confusion that fluctuate by the minute, hour, or time of day.
- Delirium is always secondary to an underlying condition; therefore it is temporary, transient, and may last from hours to days once the underlying cause is treated. If the cause is not treated, permanent damage to neurons can result.
- Dementia usually has a more insidious onset than delirium. There is global deterioration of cognitive functioning (e.g., memory, judgment, ability to think abstractly, orientation) that is often progressive and irreversible, depending on the underlying cause.
- Dementia may be primary (e.g., Alzheimer's disease, vascular dementia, Pick's disease, Lewy body disease). In this case, the disease is irreversible. Or it may be secondary to other causes and when treated may be reversed.
- Alzheimer's disease (AD) accounts for 60% to 90% of all cases of dementia; vascular dementia is the second leading cause and can account for up to 20% of all cases (APA, 2013).
- There is little known about the actual causes of AD. There are a number of risk factors, including advancing age, head trauma, obesity, diabetes, low socioeconomic status and educational levels, and the presence of apolipoprotein E4 (*APOE E4* allele), among others.
- There are four stages of Alzheimer's disease (these stages can overlap): stage 1 (mild), stage 2 (moderate), stage 3 (moderate to severe), and stage 4 (late).
- The behavioral manifestations of AD include confabulation, perseveration, aphasia, apraxia, agnosia, and hyperorality.
- No known cause or cure exists for AD, although a number of drugs that increase the brain's supply of acetylcholine (a nerve communication chemical) are helpful in slowing the progress of the disease for a limited period of time.
- People with AD have many unmet needs and present many management challenges to their families as well as to health care workers.
- Mild cognitive impairment (MCI) is a syndrome in which there is a decline in the previous level of cognitive functioning; it does not interfere with the person's ability to function and maintain independence in his or life, but the *DSM-5* states that mild NCD related to AD might make up a large contingent of those with MCI (APA, 2013).
- Knopman and Peterson (2014) make a distinction between mild cognitive impairment (MCI) and mild dementia.
- Specific nursing, psychosocial, cognitive, and behavioral interventions for neurocognitively impaired individuals can increase communication, safety, and self-care, as well as minimize confusion. The need for family teaching and community support is crucial.

APPLYING CRITICAL JUDGMENT

1. Mrs. Kendel is an 82-year-old woman who has progressive Alzheimer's disease. She lives with her husband, who has been trying to care for her in their home. Mrs. Kendel often wears evening gowns in the morning, places her blouse on backward, and sometimes wears her bra on backward outside her blouse. She often forgets the location of objects. She makes an effort to cook but often confuses frying pans and pots and sometimes has trouble turning on the stove. Once in a while, she cannot find the bathroom in time, often mistaking it for a broom closet. She becomes frightened of noises and is terrified when the telephone or doorbell rings. At times she cries because she is aware that she is losing her sense of her place in the world. She and her husband have always been close, loving companions, and he wants to keep her at home for as long as possible.

   A. Help Mr. Kendel by making a list of suggestions that he can try at home that might help facilitate (a) communication, (b) activities of daily living, and (c) maintenance of a safe home environment.

   B. Identify at least seven interventions that are appropriate to this situation for each of the areas cited in the question.

   C. Identify possible types of resources available for maintaining Mrs. Kendel in her home for as long as possible. Provide the name of one self-help group that you would urge Mr. Kendel to join.

   D. Share with your clinical group the name and function of at least three community agencies in your area that could be an appropriate referral for someone in your neighborhood who is living with a family member with AD.

CHAPTER REVIEW QUESTIONS

1. While interacting with a 62-year-old adult diagnosed with a progressive neurocognitive disorder, the nurse observes that the adult has slow responses and difficulty finding the right words. What is the nurse's best initial action?

   a. Suggest words that the adult may be trying to remember.

   b. Ask the adult, "Are you having problems saying what you mean?"

   c. Use silence to allow the adult an opportunity to compose responses.

   d. Discontinue the interaction to prevent further frustration for the adult.

2. An adult diagnosed with stage 2 Alzheimer's disease begins a new prescription for rivastigmine (Exelon). Which nursing diagnosis has the highest priority to add to the plan of care?

   a. *Risk for constipation*

   b. *Risk for altered sensory perception*

   c. *Risk for impaired oral mucous membranes*

   d. *Risk for imbalanced nutrition, less than body requirements*

3. Which newly hospitalized patient should the nurse monitor closely for development of delirium?

   a. 48-year-old who usually drinks a six-pack of beer daily

   b. 68-year-old who takes aspirin 650 mg twice daily for arthritic pain

   c. 72-year-old who says, "I have a glass of wine every evening to stimulate my appetite."

   d. 78-year-old diabetic whose blood glucose levels are consistently greater than 250 mg/dL

4. An 84-year-old tells the nurse, "I do four or five number puzzles every day to keep my brain healthy and sharp." When considering a holistic approach to maintaining mental health, the nurse should respond:

   a. "It is more important for you to have physical activity every day."

   b. "Let's think of some other activities we can add to your daily routine."

   c. "Repetition of the same activity is not helpful for keeping your brain healthy."

   d. "There are some herbal preparations that will also help keep your brain sharp."

5. A family member asks the nurse, "I know my uncle's Alzheimer's disease has progressed but is there any medication that can help him now?" Which response by the nurse is correct?
   a. "I'm sorry, but there are no medications that help with severe Alzheimer's disease."
   b. "Alzheimer's disease sometimes stabilizes. Let's hope that happens in this situation."
   c. "There are a few medications that may help. Let's discuss it with the health care provider."
   d. "It sounds like you're having difficulty accepting that your uncle's disease is irreversible. Would you like to talk about those feelings?"

REFERENCES

Agency For Healthcare Research And Quality (AHRQ). (2014). *Non-pharmacologic interventions for agitation and aggression in dementia.* Retrieved October 5, 2015, from http://www.effective-healthcare.ahrq.gov.

Alzheimer's Association. (2015). 2015 Alzheimer's disease facts and figures. *Alzheimer's & Dementia, 11*(3) 332+.

Alzheimer's Association. (2015). Alzheimer's disease facts and figures. *Alzheimer's & Dementia, 11*(3) 332+.

Alzheimer's Organization. (2015a). Risk factors. Retrieved June 2, 2015, from http://www.alz.org/alzheimer's_disease_causes_risk_factors. asp

Alzheimer's Organization. (2015b). Brain tour. Retrieved June 6, 2015, from http://www.alz.org/http://www.alz.org/brain-tour/healthy_vs_alzheimer's. asp

Alzheimer's Organization. (2015c). Wandering and getting lost. Retrieved June 8, 2015, from http://www.alz.org/care/demen-tia-medic-alert-safe-return.asp#ixzz3e0wHx9lg

American Psychiatric Association. (2013). *Diagnostic and statistical manual of mental disorders (DSM-5)* (5th ed.). Washington, DC: APA.

APA Work Group on Alzheimer's Disease and other Dementias (2007). American psychiatric association practice guideline for the treatment of patients with Alzheimer's disease and other dementias. 2nd ed. *American Journal of Psychiatry, 164*(12 Suppl), 5–56.

Anderson, H. S., & Chawla, J. (2016). *Alzheimer disease clinical presentation.* Retrieved January 30, 2016, from http://emedicine.med-scape.com/article/1134817-clinical #b3.

Anderson, H. S., & Hoffman, M. (2011). *Alzheimer's disease.* Retrieved April 9, 2012, from http://emedicine.medscape.com/arti-cle/1134817-overview.

Anderson, P. (2015). *DBS increases hippocampal volume Alzheimer's.* Retrieved June 20, 2015, from http://www.medscape.com/viewar-ticle/840108.

Black, D. W., & Andreasen, N. C. (2014). *Introductory textbook of psychiatry* (6th ed.). Washington, DC: American Psychiatric Publishing.

Burchum, J. R., & Rosenthal, L. D. (2016). *Lehne's pharmacology for nursing care* (9th ed.). St Louis, MO: Elsevier Saunders.

Carr, F. M. (2013). The role of sitters in delirium: an update. *Canadian Geriatrics Journal, 16*(1), 22–36.

CogniFit. (2015). *Cognition and the cognitive science.* Retrieved June 20, 2015, from http://www.cognifit.com/cognition.

Gatchel, J. R., Wright, C. I., Falk, W. E., et al. (2016). Dementia. In T. A. Stern, M. Fava, T. E. Wilens, & J. F. Rosenbaum (Eds.), *Massachusetts General Hospital comprehensive clinical psychiatry* (2nd ed., pp. 184–197). St. Louis: Elsevier.

Howard, K. (2015). *Personal communication with chapter reviewer, October* 2015.

Hughes, S. (2015). *Lifestyle changes can reduce cognitive decline.* Retrieved July 4, 2015, from http://www.medscape.org/viewarti-cle/842522.

Kennard, C. (2015). *Alternatives to restraint use in dementia care.* Retrieved from http://Alzheimer's.about.com/od/practicalcare/a/Re-straints 2htm.

Knopman, D. S., & Petersen, R. C. (2014). Mild cognitive impairment and mild dementia: a clinical perspective. *Mayo Clinic Proceedings 2014, 89*(10), 1452–1459.

Ong, K. T., Villemagne, V. L., Bahar-Fuchs, A., et al. (2015). *AB imaging with 18f-florbetben in prodromal Alzheimer's disease: a prospective study.* Retrieved July 1, 2015, from http://www.med-scap e.com/viewarticle/842447.

Rabins, P. V., Rovner, B. W., Rummans, T., et al. (2014). *APA 2014 guideline watch (October 2014): practice guideline for the treatment of patients with Alzheimer's disease and other dementias.* American Psychiatric Association (APA).

Rucci, J. M., & Feinstein, R. E. (2014). Neurocognitive disorders and mental disorders due to another medical condition. In J. L. Cutler (Ed.), *Psychiatry* (3rd ed. pp. 129–167). New York, NY: Oxford University Press.

Schnabel J. (2015). *How to reduce your risk of alzheimer's without taking rugs.* Retrieved from http://www.dana.org/alzrisk/.

Tampi, R. R., & Tampi, D. J. (2014). *Managing behavioral and psychological symptoms in the era of Black Box warnings.* Retrieved June 7, 2015, from http://www.psychiatrictimes.com/special-reports/managing-behavioral-and-psychological-symptoms-dimension-era-black-box-warnings.

Substance–Related and Addictive Disorders

Elizabeth M. Varcarolis

KEY TERMS AND CONCEPTS

SELECTED CONCEPT: SUBSTANCE-INDUCED COGNITIVE IMPAIRMENT AND YOUTH

The common denominator in all individuals with substance use disorders is changes in their brain circuits that may persist long after detoxification (American Psychiatric Association [APA], 2013). These changes are evidenced by common cognitive deficits in core executive functions. For example, all substance users have difficulty with planning, working memory, inhibition, and decision making. There are also alterations in selective attention, episodic memory, and difficulties with emotional processing.

The brain doesn't fully develop until early adulthood (early to mid-20s) therefore youth and teenagers are at risk for a "long-term impact on those whose brains are still busy building new connections and maturing in other ways" (National Institutes of Health [NIH], 2015).

OBJECTIVES

1. Identify the *Diagnostic and Statistical Manual of Mental Disorders, Fifth Edition (DSM-5)* basis for a substance use disorder, and name at least 5 of the 11 indicators needed for a diagnosis of a substance use disorder.
2. Describe the neurobiological process that occurs in the brain when a chemical substance of abuse enters the body. Include in your description neurotransmitters that enhance the progression of addiction.
3. Discuss the cognitive deficits that occur in all individuals with substance use disorders.
4. **QSEN** When planning **patient-centered care** for a person with a substance use disorder, identify four components of the assessment process discussed that you feel are most important.
5. Discuss the rationale for inclusion of motivation and spirituality for planning care and how that may affect your patient's progress toward sobriety.
6. **QSEN** Identify the **safety** issues for both patients and health care workers. How does reporting an impaired colleague to the proper authorities (a) protect the safety of patients and (b) affect the colleague's future ability to practice, physical health, and personal relationships (see Box 19-4)?
7. Describe two aspects of enabling behaviors that you have witnessed in friends, family, or others.
8. **QSEN** When planning **patient-centered care**, list the clinical manifestations you would find on assessment regarding the signs and symptoms of intoxication, overdose, and withdrawal for at least two substances of abuse.
9. **QSEN** Identify the signs and symptoms that would alert you to the need for **safety precautions** in a person who is withdrawing from alcohol, and describe the appropriate nursing care and pharmacological therapy needed.
10. **QSEN** Use an Internet search to retrieve the CIWA-Ar for Alcohol Withdrawal which objectifies alcohol withdrawal symptoms to help guide therapy (http://www.mdcalc.com/ciwa-ar-for-alcohol-withdrawal or http://www.regionstrauma.org/blogs/ciwa.pdf).
11. Apply the principles in the Recovery Paradigm that you would include in a nursing care plan for an individual with a substance use disorder.
12. **QSEN** Use an Internet search to determine the long-term effects of marijuana, amphetamines, and hallucinogenics (**informatics**).

INTRODUCTION

Mind-altering substances have been used since ancient times. There is evidence as early as 8000 BC that mead, a sort of honey wine, was brewed from fermented honey and perhaps was the first known alcoholic beverage. More recently, other drugs have been produced through modern chemistry, referred to as designer drugs or "bath salts" and their cousin, flakka. With the increased use of these designer drugs, so too have visits to the emergency department (ED) increased and in too many cases death has resulted.

Addiction is frequently referred to as an equal opportunity disease. Use and abuse of substances extends across social and economic boundaries. However, the degree to which the use of mind-altering substances is either accepted or condemned varies among cultures. For example, psychoactive substances like alcohol, nicotine, and caffeine are culturally accepted for adult use in most, but not all, segments of American society. Some cultures in the United States do not condone the use of alcohol or drugs as a social practice—for example, Muslim Americans and some religious groups that are considered Orthodox, such as Amish, Greek Orthodox, Hasidic Judaism, and others. To a lesser extent, marijuana use is accepted by other groups of individuals for both recreational and medicinal purposes. The use of psychoactive substances and the sequelae of prolonged, excessive use essentially alter the brain's function and structure, affecting mood, perception, and consciousness. For too many individuals, sustained psychoactive substance use can lead to psychological problems, psychosocial problems, medical problems, employment loss, legal issues, and difficulty or inability to participate in education (World Health Organization [WHO], 2010).

One unfortunate trend in the prevalence of substance use disorders is the increased arrests and incarceration in overcrowded facilities for nonviolent drug-related offenses. A more positive trend is that the disease concept of addiction is more prevalent and makes it easier for addicted individuals to obtain more humane and nonjudgmental treatment (Black & Andreasen, 2014). Unfortunately, appropriate treatment facilities are overcrowded; therefore, they are not readily available for many who seek help.

Substance use disorders are classified like all *DSM-5* (APA, 2013) disorders on a continuum from mild to moderate to severe. For the purposes of this chapter, the terms *abuse* and *addiction* are defined as follows.

> **Abuse** refers to the habitual use of a substance that falls outside of medical necessity or social acceptance and is used for the single purpose of altering one's mood, emotion, or state of consciousness.
>
> **Addiction** is a chronic, relapsing brain disease characterized by compulsive drug-seeking behavior motivated by cravings, despite harmful consequences, and by long-lasting changes in the brain. Tolerance and withdrawal are **no longer** mandatory for the definition of addiction in the *DSM-5* (APA, 2013); although within many classes of drugs they do occur and can be part of the criteria for making a diagnosis.

The *DSM-5* uses the term substance use disorder, which covers 10 classes of substances. The *DSM-5* defines *substance use* as "A problematic pattern of substance use leading to clinically significant impairment or distress, as manifested by at least 2 of 11 items, occurring within a 12-month period" (APA, 2013, p. 483). The 10 classes of psychoactive substances in the *DSM-5* are alcohol, caffeine, cannabis, hallucinogens (phencyclidine or similarly acting arylcyclohexylamines), other hallucinogens such as lysergic acid diethylamide (LSD), inhalants, opioids, sedatives, hypnotics, anxiolytics, stimulants (including amphetamine-type substances, cocaine, and other stimulants), tobacco, and other or unknown substances.

All of these substances have their own clinical picture of use, intoxication, and withdrawal (if withdrawal exists with the substance). Certain behaviors are characterized by compulsive and addictive-like qualities—for example, compulsive texting or sexting, compulsive overeating, compulsive shopping, sex addictions, compulsive gambling, and compulsive Internet use (e.g., porn, online gambling). These behaviors also excite the reward centers of the brain, releasing a rush of dopamine that reinforces the behavior. At present, only *pathological gambling* has a place in the *DSM-5* under substance use disorder.

PREVALENCE AND COMORBIDITY

Prevalence of Substance Use

The United States has one of the highest levels of substance abuse and addiction in the world. According to the CDC National Vital Statistics System Mortality File (2015), drug overdose is the leading cause of accidental death in the United States, with 47,055 lethal drug overdoses in 2014 (CDC, 2015). According to the results from the 2014 National Survey on Drug Use and Health, opioid use is driving this epidemic. Of the 21.5 million Americans 12 or older that had a substance use disorder in 2014, 1.9 million had a substance use disorder involving prescription pain relievers and 586,000 had a substance use disorder involving heroin addiction, with 18,893 overdose deaths related to prescription pain relievers, and 10,574 overdose deaths related to heroin in 2014 (SAMSHA, 2015). Adding to these alarming statistics is the increase in women who died from a heroin overdose which has tripled in the last few years (Hedegaard, et al., 2015). For those who start using drugs before the age of 14, their chance of becoming addicted is much higher than their older cohorts (Sadock, Sadock, & Ruiz, 2015). Since the brain is not fully developed until the mid-20s, early drug abuse negatively affects brain development.

Alcohol use disorder is the most common substance use problem in the United States. The prevalence of alcohol use in the United States is about 70% (Acharya & Issacs, 2015) and approximately 12% of

> **Who Is a Heavy Drinker?**
> When we really start to think about drinking, we need to know what "too much" actually looks like. Heavy drinking, which is often called "at risk" drinking, is alcohol consumption that exceeds the recommended daily limits:
> - **For men:** More than 4 standard drinks on any 1 day, or more than 14 standard drinks in any 1 week.
> - **For women:** More than 3 standard drinks on any 1 day, or more than 7 standard drinks in any 1 week.
>
> **What Does This Actually Mean?**
> **If you're a woman** and you drink two medium-sized glasses of wine (8 oz.) every night after work, you're over the limit before you even reach the weekend.
>
> **For men**, one night out with friends during which you drink three beers and a couple of shots would put you over the daily limit. Do this just twice in 1 week and you're probably drinking close to 10 to 14 standard drinks in just *2 days*, depending on the size and strength of the drinks (Aronson, M. (2015). Patient information: Alcohol use—when is drinking a problem? (Beyond the Basics) http://www.update.com/contents/alcohol-use-when-is-drinking-a-problem-beyond-the-basics. Michigan State University Physicians Office, (2010–2015). Thinking about drinking: what is "high risk" or heavy drinking? http://thinkingaboutdrinking.msu.edu/index.php?option=com_content&view=article&id=6&Itemid=16.

Americans are heavy drinkers (Black & Andreasen, 2014). According to the CDC fact sheet, "binge drinking" is the most common pattern of excessive alcohol use in the United States" (CDC, 2015a).

Marijuana is still the most commonly used illicit drug in the United States and is exceeded only by caffeine, alcohol, and nicotine as the most commonly used psychoactive substance by adults in the United States (Sadock, Sadock, & Ruiz, 2015). Cannabis is a major part of the youth culture and, as of 2012, 11.4% of eighth-graders, 28% of tenth-graders, and 36.4% of twelfth-graders use marijuana (Miech et al., 2015). A New Zealand study found that teenagers who were heavy users of marijuana were likely to lose 8 IQ points. During the time young users' brains are rapidly building new connections and maturing, marijuana is known to play a role in interfering with the connections between neurons. The damage to these connections is irreversible (NIH, 2015).

Nicotine addiction is high in all groups of people with substance dependence, as well as in those with psychiatric mental health issues. At least 20% of the U.S. population meet the criteria for tobacco use disorder, and nicotine causes 443,000 deaths a year (Burchum & Rosenthal, 2016). Nicotine is the psychoactive drug in tobacco, and nicotine dependence is considered the most common form of addiction in the United States today. In the United States, one in five deaths results from tobacco use and on average, smokers die 10 years earlier than nonsmokers (Jha et al., 2013). Although the rate of cigarette smoking among children, adolescents, and adults is tapering off, the use of electronic cigarettes (e-cigarettes) is exploding. E-cigarettes are advertised as safe, although they do contain nicotine. Many brands of e-cigarettes contain other health hazards as well. When tested, some brands of e-cigarettes contained toxic chemicals such as formaldehyde and acetaldehyde. One study found that "high-voltage use released enough formaldehyde-containing compounds to increase a person's lifetime risk of cancer five to 15 times higher than the risk caused by long-term smoking" (Thompson, 2015). Even though there is the consideration that e-cigarettes may help heavy smokers cut down or stop smoking, the concern is the nicotine in e-cigarettes that might become habit-forming for our youth and for young adults. In May of 2016, the FDA banned the sale of e-cigarettes to Americans under 18 and will require that many people buying e-cigarettes show photo identification.

Psychiatric Comorbidity

It seems that certain areas of the brain, such as the circuits in the brain that use the neurotransmitter dopamine, can affect both substance use disorders and other mental illnesses. The neurotransmitter dopamine is typically affected by addictive substances. This in part may explain the high rate of dual diagnoses (substance use disorders co-occurring with a psychiatric disorder). For example, psychiatric patients have about a 50% to 60% higher chance of having alcohol use disorder than those in the general population (Black & Andreasen, 2014). According to Sadock, Sadock, and Ruiz (2015), some studies indicate that up to 50% of addicts have a co-occurring psychiatric disorder. Other studies claim that 35% to 50% of individuals with a substance use disorder meet the criteria for antisocial personality disorder (Sadock, Sadock, & Ruiz, 2015). Among the highest percentage of people with psychiatric disorders with a co-occurring substance use disorder are those with schizophrenia and depression. Other common co-occurring psychiatric disorders include acute and chronic cognitive impairment disorders, attention deficit disorder, borderline personality disorder, and anxiety disorders.

Suicide is a high risk factor among individuals who abuse alcohol and/or drugs and is about 10% higher than in the general population and about 15% higher than in those who abuse or are addicted to alcohol (Sadock, Sadock, & Ruiz, 2015). Substance use increases the risk of suicide among children, adolescents, adults, and older adults.

Medical Comorbidity

A medical history, physical examination, and laboratory tests are used to gather data about drug-related physical problems. The extent of impairment depends on individual susceptibility as well as the amount of drug used and the route of administration. Numerous disorders affect the *gastrointestinal system* (e.g., esophagitis, gastritis, pancreatitis, alcoholic hepatitis, and cirrhosis of the liver). *Cardiovascular risks* are also significant. Alcohol can raise the levels of triglycerides in the blood. Excessive alcohol intake results in stroke, cardiomyopathy, cardiac dysrhythmia, and sudden cardiac death (American Heart Association [AHA], 2011). Also commonly associated with long-term alcohol use or abuse is tuberculosis, all types of accidents, suicide, and homicide.

Alcohol is the most prevalent of the substance use disorders; therefore, **alcohol-related medical problems** are the comorbidities most commonly seen in medical settings. The risks of health problems related to alcohol abuse are infinite. Excessive alcohol use damages the brain and most body organs. Especially vulnerable to alcohol-related damage is the **cerebral cortex**, which is responsible for higher brain functions, problem solving, and decision making. The **hippocampus**, which is the center of memory and learning, is also affected, as well as the **cerebellum**, which helps coordinate our movements. Specific disorders that involve the central nervous system include **Wernicke's encephalopathy** and **Korsakoff's psychosis**.

Specific disorders that involve the central nervous system include **Wernicke-Korsakoff's syndrome**, which is two separate entities but both are caused by thiamine (B_1) deficiency. In the Western world, thiamine deficiency is characteristically associated with chronic alcoholism, because chronic alcoholism affects thiamine uptake and utilization. Wernicke-Korsakoff's syndrome can also be caused by malabsorption syndrome, AIDS, or chronic infection, poor nutrition, eating disorders, or the effects of chemotherapy.

Wernicke's encephalopathy is a neurological disorder marked by *acute/subacute confusional states*, abnormal eye movements (nystagmus), and unsteady gait (ataxia). Wernicke's encephalopathy is a medical emergency that causes life-threatening brain disruption but if treated is often reversible. If not treated it can lead to chronic dementia and/or death.

Korsakoff's psychosis (Korsakoff syndrome) refers to *a chronic neurological condition* that usually occurs as a consequence of untreated Wernicke's encephalopathy. Korsakoff syndrome is marked by difficulty/inability to learn new information, remember recent events, and long-term memory gaps. Although memory problems are clearly evidenced, other thinking and social skills may be relatively unaffected.

Central Nervous System Stimulants

Cocaine users may experience extreme weight loss and malnutrition, myocardial infarction, brain damage, and stroke. *Methamphetamine* users are likely to suffer from hypothermia, seizures, brain damage, kidney damage, stroke, and death.

Nicotine in the form of cigarette smoking remains the greatest single cause of preventable illness and premature death (Burchum & Rosenthal, 2016). Smoking tobacco can cause chronic lung disease, coronary heart disease, chronic obstructive pulmonary disease (COPD), and stroke, as well as cancer of the lungs, larynx, esophagus, mouth, and bladder. Approximately 50% of Americans who do *not* smoke are exposed to secondhand smoke (SHS). A comprehensive scientific report concluded that there is no risk-free level of exposure to SHS. Secondhand smoke is responsible for heart disease and lung cancer in nonsmoking adults, is extremely harmful to infants and children (CDC, 2014b; U.S. Department of Health and Human Services [USDHHS], 2006), and is thought to be related to sudden infant death syndrome (SIDS). There is evidence that cigarette smoke contains more than 7000 chemicals, and about 70 of those cause cancer (American Cancer Society, 2015).

Anabolic-Androgenic Steroids

The effects of *anabolic-androgenic steroids (AASs)* can be serious and permanent if an individual does not stop taking these drugs (e.g., liver damage, renal failure, heart attack, elevated cholesterol levels, and serious depression, especially in withdrawal). Some of the untoward effects of steroid use in men are shrinking of the testicles, infertility, development of breasts, and increased risk for prostate cancer. Women often show male pattern baldness, changes in menstrual cycle, growth of facial hair, and a deepening of the voice. Stunting of growth attributable to premature skeletal maturation and accelerated pubertal changes can occur in adolescents using AASs (NIDA, 2012a). Research also suggests that users may experience paranoia, jealousy, delusions, and violent mood swings (NIDA, 2012a).

Route of Ingestion

The route of drug administration influences medical complications and affects addictive potential. For example, **intravenous drug users** have a higher incidence of infections, venous sclerosis, and testing positive for human immunodeficiency virus/acquired immunodeficiency syndrome (HIV/AIDS). **Intranasal users** may have sinusitis and a perforated nasal septum. Smoking a substance (e.g., marijuana, nicotine) increases the likelihood of respiratory tract problems. Both smoked and injected drugs enter the brain within seconds, producing a powerful rush of pleasure that lasts a short period of time, necessitating taking more of the drug more often to recapture the high. Refer to Table 19-1 for a description of physical complications associated with various classes of drugs and their routes of administration.

CONTRIBUTING FACTORS—SUBSTANCE-RELATED AND ADDICTIVE DISORDERS

The individual variation in a person's susceptibility to become addicted supports the premise that genetic/biological variations, psychological factors, and sociocultural influences all play a role in addiction.

TABLE 19-1   Physical Complications Related to Drugs of Abuse

Route	Physical Complications	Route	Physical Complications
Narcotics (e.g., Heroin), PCP, Cocaine or Crack, Methamphetamines		**Marijuana**	
Intravenous*	Human immunodeficiency virus (HIV)	Smoking, ingestion	Impaired lung structure
	Acquired immunodeficiency syndrome (AIDS)		Chromosomal mutation—increased incidence of birth defects
	Hepatitis		Micronucleic white blood cells—increased risk of disease as a result of decreased resistance to infection
	Bacterial endocarditis		Stroke
	Renal failure		Possible long-term effects on short-term memory
	Cardiac arrest		
	Coma	**Nicotine**	
	Seizures	Smoking, chewing	*Heavy, chronic use associated with:*
	Respiratory arrest		Emphysema
	Dermatitis		Cancer of the larynx and esophagus
	Pulmonary emboli		Lung cancer
	Tetanus		Peripheral vascular diseases
	Abscesses—osteomyelitis		Cancer of the mouth
	Septicemia		Cardiovascular disease
			Hypertension
Cocaine, Methamphetamines			
Intravenous,* intranasal, smoking	Perforation of nasal septum (when taken intranasally)	**Heroin**	
	Respiratory paralysis	Intravenous,* smoking	Constipation
	Cardiovascular collapse		Dermatitis
	Hyperpyrexia		Malnutrition
	Intracerebral hemorrhage		Hypoglycemia
			Dental caries
Caffeine			Amenorrhea
Ingestion	Gastroesophageal reflux		
	Peptic ulcer	**Inhalants**	
	Increased intraocular pressure in unregulated glaucoma	Sniffing, snorting, bagging (inhalation of fumes from a plastic bag), huffing (placing an inhalant-soaked rag over the mouth)	Tachycardia
	Tachycardia		Dysrhythmias
	Increased plasma glucose and lipid levels		Nervous system damage
			Hearing loss
PCP			Bone marrow damage
Ingestion	Respiratory arrest		Suffocation caused by displacing oxygen in the lungs, leading to respiratory depression/arrest

*The complications listed can result from any drug taken intravenously.
From Varcarolis, E. M. (2014). *Essentials of psychiatric mental health nursing.* (2nd ed. rev.) Philadelphia: Saunders.

The Neurobiology of Addiction

Three areas of the brain are necessary for life-sustaining functions and at the same time enhance the compulsive drug use that marks addiction (NIDA, 2014):

- **Brainstem**—controls basic functions such as heart rate, breathing, and sleeping.
- **Limbic system**—contains the brain's "reward circuit" that links brain structures controlling feelings of pleasure, thereby motivating us to repeat behaviors that cause pleasure and support survival (such as eating and sex), and stimulating creative pleasures such as viewing or participating in art and playing or listening to music. The limbic system is involved in the perception of both negative and positive emotions. Along with positive activation for feelings of pleasure, the limbic system is also activated by alcohol and drug use, explaining many of the negative moods common in those with addictions.
- **Cerebral cortex**—includes areas that process information from our senses (seeing, hearing, feeling, taste, and touch). One of the most important areas in the cerebral cortex is the forebrain, often referred to as the frontal cortex. The frontal cortex allows us to think, plan, solve problems, and make decisions.

Neurobiology and Neurotransmitters

There are many different chemicals in the brain that function as neurotransmitters, but a small handful do most of the work.

Neurotransmitter	Functions Affected	Drugs that Affect Functions
Inhibitory Neurotransmitters		
Gamma-aminobutyric acid (GABA)	Anxiety, memory, anesthesia	Sedatives, tranquilizers, alcohol
Serotonin	Mood (depression/anxiety/impulsivity), sleep quality, sexual desire, appetite	MDMA (ecstasy), LSD, cocaine
Acetylcholine	Formation of memories, verbal and logical reasoning, and the ability to concentrate. Involved in stimulation of muscles, memory, motivation, and attention	Nicotine
Endorphins and Enkephalin (Endogenous opioids)	Analgesia, sedation, substances involved with reward/punishment, mood	Heroin, morphine, prescription painkillers (oxycodone)
Excitatory Neurotransmitters		
Dopamine *Dopamine neurotransmitters can be both inhibitory or excitatory*	Pleasure and reward, movement, attention, memory, and energy. Dopamine is critical in the early stage of addiction	Virtually all drugs of abuse directly or indirectly augment dopamine (e.g., cocaine, PCP, opiates, marijuana, etc.)
Norepinephrine (noradrenaline)	Elevated levels can cause anxiety. Low levels associated with low energy, decreased ability to focus, and problems with sleep and memory.	Stimulants (e.g., cocaine, methamphetamine)

Neurotransmitter	Functions Affected	Drugs that Affect Functions
Epinephrine (also called adrenaline)	Excitatory neurotransmitter involved in arousal and alertness	Stimulants
Glutamate	Neuron activity (increased rate), learning, cognition, memory. It can also facilitate maintaining addiction and inducing its long-term effects.	Ketamine, phencyclidine, alcohol

Adapted from National Institute on Drug Abuse (NIH) (2007). Impacts of drugs on neurotransmission. Retrieved from http://www.drug-abuse.gov/news-events/nida-notes/2007/10/impacts-drugs-neurotransmission and other sources.

It has also been demonstrated that alcohol and drug use have specific effects on selected neurotransmitters. Dopamine is a neurotransmitter that plays a major role in all addictions, but the concepts that apply to dopamine can relate to other neurotransmitters as well. Dopamine is the brain chemical present in regions of the brain that regulate motivation, emotion, cognition or learning, and the ability to experience pleasure and pain.

All drugs (e.g., nicotine, stimulants, marijuana, caffeine, sedatives) directly or indirectly affect the **limbic (reward) system**. The reward system consists of the ventral tegmental area (VTA), the nucleus accumbens, and part of the cerebral cortex. These brain circuits allow us to feel pleasure, and they increase the response to dopamine as a reward from pleasurable activities (e.g., food, music, art, sex). However, the first time an individual uses a "substance," the neurons in the reward pathway release an unusually large amount of dopamine, resulting in unnaturally intense feelings of pleasure. The neurons in the reward pathway communicate through electrical signals that are passed from one neuron to another across a small gap called a synapse. Dopamine is then released into the synapse, crosses to the next neuron, and binds to that neuron's dopamine receptor (NIH, 2015). It is this binding that produces the initial intense feelings of pleasure.

As a result of this flood of neurotransmitters (e.g., dopamine), the neurons try to regulate the level of dopamine in the brain either by reducing the number of dopamine receptors or by synthesizing less dopamine. In the case of many drugs, eventually dopamine's ability to stimulate the reward center becomes very ineffective, and the individual is encouraged to increase the amount of the drug to raise dopamine levels to normal or higher levels; this vicious cycle of taking increasing amounts of the drug to even feel "normal" begins the cycle of tolerance to the drug and eventual addiction. Other nerve cells release γ-aminobutyric acid (GABA), which is an inhibitory neurotransmitter that helps moderate neuronal activity and protects the receptor nerve from becoming overstimulated.

Opioid drugs act on opioid receptors. Alcohol and other central nervous system (CNS) depressants act on GABA receptors. This finding helps explain the addictive and **cross-tolerance** effects that occur when alcohol use is combined with benzodiazepine use. Cross-tolerance occurs when one builds up a tolerance for one drug, while also building up a tolerance for another drug *in the same class of drugs*. Cocaine and amphetamines act on the dopamine and serotonin systems, producing the intense rush and resulting intense lows, reinforcing compulsive use. These two drugs also share the same receptors and are also cross-tolerant.

Genetic Contributions

Genetic factors are believed to account for between 40% and 60% of a person's vulnerability to addiction (Black & Andreasen, 2014). It is

▶ Neurochemistry of Addiction (e.g. Heroin Use An Epidemic), and the Role of Naloxone

When a person injects, smokes, or snorts heroin/opioid the drug travels quickly to the brain through the bloodstream. In the brain, the heroin is converted to morphine by enzymes. Morphine binds to opiate receptors in certain areas within the reward pathway including the VTA, nucleus accumbens, and cortex. Morphine also binds to areas involved in the pain pathway (including the thalamus, brainstem, and spinal cord).

The Reward Pathway

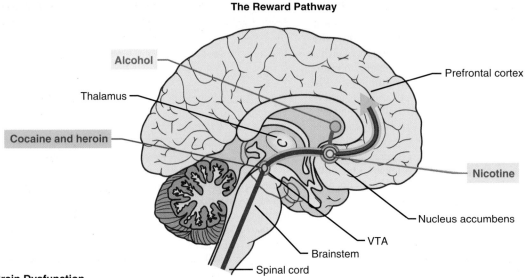

Brain Dysfunction

Tolerance: the analgesic (pain reducing) properties of heroin or morphine no longer respond to the drug in the initial way. Tolerance occurs in the pain passage pathway that includes the thalamus and the spinal cord. These areas are important in sending pain messages and are responsible for the analgesic effects of morphine. However a person does not develop tolerance to the respiratory depressive effects of heroin/morphine.
When morphine binds to opiate receptors, it inhibits an enzyme, adenylate cyclase, that coordinates the firing of impulses. After repeated opiate receptor activation by morphine, the enzyme adapts so that the morphine can no longer cause changes in cell firing.

Addiction: develops when the neurons adapt to exposure of the drug and only function normally in the presence of the drug. Many of the heroin or morphine withdrawal symptoms are generated when the opiate receptors in the thalamus and brainstem are deprived of morphine. Withdrawal can be very serious and the abuser will use the drug again to avoid the syndrome.

Naloxone's Reversal of Opioid Overdose: Overdose is particularly lethal due to respiratory depression. To reduce deaths from overdose naloxone (trade name Narcan) is being increasingly used by both health care providers and the general public. This drug is a pure opioid antagonist with no pharmacological properties. After intravenous, subcutaneous, and intramuscular injection it temporarily (1-2 hours) binds with them. Its binding ability is stronger than morphine's so it can push the morphine off and reverse the effects of morphine. A nasal spray formulation is currently available.

generally accepted that genetic factors are an important risk factor for psychoactive drug use. For example, alcoholism is three to four times more likely to occur in children of alcoholic parents than in children of nonalcoholic parents. Currently, molecular genetic techniques are being employed to define alcohol-related genes.

Recent research has identified specific gene alleles believed to be risk factors for cannabis dependence (Hand, 2016). There is also potential evidence for genetic factors that can link the comorbidity of cannabis dependence with major depression and risk of schizophrenia (Hand, 2016).

Psychological Observations

Although no known addictive personality type exists, associated psychodynamic factors, such as lack of tolerance for frustration and pain, lack of impulse control, lack of success in life, lack of affectionate and meaningful relationships, low self-esteem, lack of self-regard, and strong propensity for risk-taking behaviors, have been identified. These characteristics and perceptions are thought to contribute to the substance user's need to self-medicate in order to mitigate against uncomfortable feelings and emotional pain. Sadock, Sadock, and Ruiz

(2015) suggest that alcohol may be used to control panic, opioids to diminish anger, and methamphetamines to relieve depression.

Societal and Cultural Considerations

Societal and family values can be strong influences on whether a person's use of alcohol or illicit drugs becomes an addiction problem. If a person's family uses drugs, he or she is more likely to use these substances as well. If an individual's friends use drugs, peer pressure often prevails on an individual to use drugs as well. It has been found that youth and teenagers are more susceptible to peer pressure if they lack a close bond with parent(s), spend a large amount of time away from home, and have increased reliance on peers as opposed to parents (Black & Andreasen, 2014).

Women in general are diagnosed with substance use at lower rates than men although that trend may be changing. Unfortunately, girls and young women become addicted faster and are apt to suffer the consequences of substances of use more rapidly than boys and young men.

In Asian cultures, the prevalence rate for alcohol abuse is believed to be relatively low. This is partly because of their deficiency of aldehyde dehydrogenase, the chemical that breaks down alcohol to acetaldehyde. In approximately half of the Asian population, if the level of acetaldehyde increases in the blood, severe flushing and palpitations may occur. This reaction is thought to be effective in preventing many Asians from drinking.

According to Szalavitz (2015), addiction seems to hit people that are already hurting. It is generally accepted that there is a strong relationship between childhood trauma (adverse childhood experiences/ACE) and poor physical, mental, and behavioral outcomes later in life and the earlier the trauma, the higher potential for mental and/or physical sequelae. ACE includes: an alcohol and/or drug abuser in the household, one or no parents, being emotionally, physically, or sexually violated, experiencing a natural or man-made disaster, witnessing violence, incarcerated household member, family who is chronically depressed, mentally ill, institutionalized, suicidal, or households in extreme poverty. Therefore, it is unsurprising that mental health diseases such as addiction would be higher in this population as well. Szalavitz (2015) cites a study that found:

"one study of nearly 10,000 people found that those with four or more of these types of "adverse childhood experiences" (ACEs) have a risk of alcoholism that is seven times greater than those with none. Similarly, boys who have four or more ACEs are nearly five times more likely to inject drugs than those with none."

For a long time the American Indian has been unfairly stereotyped and stigmatized regarding the belief that they are biologically susceptible to alcohol, even in the absence of evidence. Studies as early as 2009, have found that "early exposure to adverse events was associated with early substance use and the subsequent development of substance-use disorders among American Indians" (Whitesell, et al., 2009).

EFFECTS OF SUBSTANCE USE IN PREGNANCY

Alcohol is the most teratogenic (toxic) of all substances of abuse during pregnancy. Drinking alcohol during pregnancy can have physical, mental, and behavioral consequences for the unborn child. If a pregnant woman takes a drink, the unborn child takes that same drink. Drinking alcohol during pregnancy can cause miscarriage, preterm birth, and stillbirth. Alcohol is extremely neurotoxic and interferes with the ability of the fetus to receive enough oxygen and nourishment for normal cell development in the brain as well as other organs. The American College of Obstetricians and Gynecologists and the Centers for Disease Control and Prevention stated there are no safe amount of alcohol to drink during pregnancy and call for total restriction of alcohol during the entire pregnancy (Cohen, 2015). A University of California study indicated that the end of the first trimester is the most vulnerable time for the fetus (Solomon, 2012). **Fetal alcohol syndrome (FAS)** is the most extreme example of the effect of alcohol on fetal development and has presently supplanted all other etiologies for mental retardation (Acharya & Issacs, 2015). Slightly less severe are the fetal alcohol spectrum disorders (FASDs).

The three basic criteria of FAS are mental retardation, delayed growth and development, and distinctive facial abnormalities. FAS and FASD are lifelong conditions that result in permanent physical disabilities (e.g., hearing, eyesight, facial abnormalities, organ deformities, cardiac defects, spinal defects, urogenital defects), mental disabilities (e.g., mental retardation, learning disabilities, memory impairment, CNS handicaps), and behavioral problems (e.g., hyperactivity, poor impulse control, criminal behavior) (Acharya & Issacs, 2015; CDC, 2015c; Meyer & Quenzer, 2013).

Nicotine

Women who smoke cigarettes prenatally have babies who are twice as likely to be low birth weight and who have increased risk of developmental issues (e.g., cerebral palsy, learning disabilities), congenital abnormalities,

and respiratory tract problems. Parental prenatal and postnatal smoking is believed to increase the risk for SIDS (sudden infant death syndrome). *Secondhand smoke* exposure is also thought to be a cause of SIDS, respiratory tract problems, ear infections, and asthma attacks in infants and children (American Cancer Society, 2015; CDC, 2014b).

Mothers who take **opiates** during pregnancy are more likely to experience intrauterine fetal deaths and are at a higher risk for infant death. Infants born to opiate-dependent mothers are addicted at birth and experience withdrawal symptoms.

PHENOMENA OBSERVED IN SUBSTANCE USE DISORDERS AND COMPULSIVELY ADDICTED BEHAVIORS

The nurse needs to be familiar with the following phenomena when working with patients with substance abuse problems.

- **Intoxication.** The *International Classification of Diseases (ICD)*-10 describes intoxication as "a transient condition following the administration of alcohol or other psychoactive substance, resulting in disturbances in the level of consciousness, cognition, perception, affect or behavior, or other psychophysiological functions and responses" (WHO, 2013).
- **Dual diagnosis** is the coexistence of substance use or abuse along with one or more other mental health disorders.
- **Tolerance** is the need for higher and higher doses of a substance to achieve the desired effect and/or to prevent withdrawal symptoms.
- **Withdrawal** symptoms occur after a long period of continued use and signifies a physical dependence. Withdrawal occurs "when blood or tissue concentration of a substance declines in an individual who has maintained prolonged heavy use of the substance" (APA, 2013, p. 484). For example, when a substance is stopped or reduced, drug-specific identifiable physical and psychological signs and symptoms occur.
- **Flashbacks** are transitory recurrences of a perceptual disturbance caused by a person's earlier *hallucinogenic drug use*; flashbacks occur during the person's drug-free state. Visual distortions, time expansion, loss of ego boundaries, and intense emotions are reported. Often flashbacks are mild and perhaps pleasant, but at other times individuals experience repeated recurrences of frightening images and/or terrifying thoughts. Flashbacks are common in individuals who suffer from posttraumatic stress disorder (PTSD) and are usually terrifying.
- **Co-dependent behavior** is overresponsible, dysfunctional helping behavior toward a person who exhibits compulsive/addiction behaviors (substance use, gambling, shopping, etc.). These behaviors essentially support and facilitate another person's addiction and encourage the addicted individual's irresponsibility, stunted growth, and disease progression. Under the guise of protection, the enabler helps to guarantee the need for the addicted person to be dependent on him or her at the expense of the individual who needs help. Refer to Box 19-1.
- **Cross-tolerance/synergistic effects**. When some drugs from the same class are taken together, the effect of either or both of the drugs is intensified or prolonged. For example, combinations of alcohol plus a benzodiazepine, alcohol plus an opiate, or alcohol plus a barbiturate produce synergistic effects. All of these drugs are CNS depressants and are cross-tolerant to one another. Therefore, taking two CNS depressants together results in a far greater degree of CNS depression than just the sum of the effects of each. Many unintentional deaths have resulted from taking alcohol along with another CNS depressant, causing a lethal drug combination.
- **Cross-dependence. Antagonistic effects** occur when one drug is taken to weaken or inhibit the effect of another drug. For example, cocaine is often mixed with heroin (speedball). The heroin (CNS depressant) is meant to soften the intense letdown of withdrawal from cocaine (CNS stimulant).

CLINICAL PICTURE AND PHARMACOLOGICAL TREATMENTS

A substance use disorder is diagnosed using the *DSM-5* criteria. If one substitutes the word alcohol with "substance," the criteria is the same for all substances with the exception of caffeine. One other exception is in the case of phencyclidine, other hallucinogens, and inhalants that presently have no specific *withdrawal symptoms* (APA, 2013).

DSM-5 DIAGNOSTIC CRITERIA

*for Alcohol Use Disorder**

A. A problematic pattern of alcohol use leading to clinically significant impairment or distress, as manifested by at least two of the following, occurring within a 12-month period.
1. Alcohol is often taken in larger amounts or over a longer period than was intended.
2. There is a persistent desire or unsuccessful efforts to cut down or control alcohol use.
3. A great deal of time is spent in activities necessary to obtain alcohol, use alcohol, or recover from its effects.
4. Craving, or a strong desire or urge to use alcohol.
5. Recurrent alcohol use resulting in a failure to fulfill major role obligations at work, school, or home.
6. Continued alcohol use despite having persistent or recurrent social or interpersonal problems caused or exacerbated by the effects of alcohol.
7. Important social, occupational, or recreational activities are given up or reduced because of alcohol use.
8. Recurrent alcohol use in situations in which it is physically hazardous.
9. Alcohol use is continued despite knowledge of having a persistent or recurrent physical or psychological problem that is likely to have been caused or exacerbated by alcohol.
10. Tolerance, as defined by either of the following:
    a. A need for markedly increased amounts of alcohol to achieve intoxication or desired effect.
    b. A markedly diminished effect with continued use of the same amount of alcohol.
11. Withdrawal, as manifested by either of the following:
    a. The characteristic withdrawal syndrome for alcohol (refer to Criteria A and B of the criteria set for alcohol withdrawal, pp 499–500).
    b. Alcohol (or closely related substance, such as a benzodiazepine) is taken to relieve or avoid withdrawal symptoms.

Specify if:

In early remission: After full criteria for alcohol use disorder were previously met, none of the criteria for alcohol use disorder have been met for at least 3 months but for less than 12 months (with the exception that Criterion A4, "Craving, or a strong desire or urge to use alcohol" may be met.

In sustained remission: After full criteria for alcohol use disorder were previously met, none of the criteria for alcohol use disorder have been met at any time during a period of 12 months or longer (with the exception that Criterion A4, "Craving, or a strong desire or urge to use alcohol," may be met).

Specify if:

In a controlled environment: This additional specifier is used if the individual is in an environment where access to alcohol is restricted.

From American Psychiatric Association (APA). (2013). *Diagnostic and statistical manual of mental disorders* (5th ed.). Washington, DC: APA.
*With exception of caffeine all other substances/behaviors follow these criteria. One other exception is in the case of phencyclidine, other hallucinogens, and inhalants where no specific withdrawal symptoms have been identified (APA, 2013).

BOX 19-1   Overresponsible (Co-dependent) Behaviors

Co-dependent individuals find themselves:
- Attempting to control someone else's drug use (behavior, compulsion, etc.)
- Spending inordinate time thinking about the addicted person
- Finding excuses for the person's substance use
- Covering up the person's drinking, drug taking, or lying
- Feeling responsible for the person's drinking or drug use
- Feeling guilty for the addicted person's behavior
- Avoiding family and social events because of concerns or shame about the addicted member's behavior
- Making threats regarding the consequences of the alcoholic's or drug abuser's behavior and failing to follow through
- Eliciting promises for change
- Feeling as if they are "walking on eggshells" on a routine basis to avoid causing problems, especially in relation to alcohol or drug use
- Allowing moods to be influenced by those of the addicted person
- Searching for, hiding, and destroying the abuser's drug or alcohol supply
- Assuming the alcoholic's or substance abuser's duties and responsibilities
- Feeling forced to increase control over the family's finances
- Often bailing the addicted person out of financial or legal problems

CENTRAL NERVOUS SYSTEM DEPRESSANTS

CNS depressant drugs include alcohol, benzodiazepines, and barbiturates. These drugs are cross-tolerant to one another. The signs and symptoms of intoxication are the same, but the treatments and withdrawal are different. The physical and psychological symptoms of intoxication, overdose, and withdrawal, along with possible treatments, are presented in Table 19-2.

Withdrawal reactions to alcohol and other CNS depressants are associated with severe morbidity and mortality, unlike withdrawal from most other drugs. The syndrome for alcohol withdrawal is the same as that for the entire class of CNS depressant drugs. Alcohol is used here as the prototype. The time intervals are delayed when other CNS depressants are the main drugs of choice or are used in combination with alcohol. In addition, as patients age their symptoms of withdrawal continue for longer periods and are more severe than those in younger patients.

Multiple drug and alcohol dependencies can result in simultaneous withdrawal syndromes that present a bizarre clinical picture and may pose problems for safe withdrawal. Family and friends may help provide important information that can assist in care planning.

Alcohol

Moderate use of alcohol is believed to have some positive qualities such as prolonging one's life, reducing the risk of dementia, and supplying some cardiovascular benefits (Burchum & Rosenthal, 2016).

However, when alcohol is habitually used to excess over a long period of time, the results are disastrous not only for the individual, but also for those who love and care for him or her. Disturbances in a person's life include physiological changes, psychological pain, disruptions in social and family life, and disruptions in education and work life.

Alcohol-related medical problems are the comorbidities most commonly seen in medical settings. As mentioned, the medical problems associated with excessive alcohol use are infinite. Risky drinking or

TABLE 19-2 Central Nervous System Depressants

Drugs	Intoxication Effects	Overdose Effects	Possible Overdose Treatments	Withdrawal Effects	Possible Withdrawal Treatments
Barbiturates	*Physical:*	Cardiovascular	*If awake:**	*Cessation of prolonged,*	Perform carefully
Benzodiazepines	Slurred speech	or respiratory	Keep awake.	*heavy use:*	titrated
Alcohol (EtOH)	Incoordination	depression	Induce vomiting.	Nausea and vomiting	detoxification
	Unsteady gait	or arrest	Give activated charcoal to aid absorption of drug.	Tachycardia	with similar
	Drowsiness	(mostly with	Check vital signs (VS) every 15 min.	Diaphoresis	drug.
	Decreased blood pressure	barbiturates)	*Coma:*	Anxiety or irritability	*Note:* Abrupt
	Psychological-perceptual:	Coma	Clear airway; insert endotracheal tube.	Tremors in hands, fingers,	withdrawal can
	Disinhibition of sexual or	Shock	Give intravenous (IV) fluids.	eyelids	lead to death.
	aggressive drives	Convulsions	Perform gastric lavage with activated charcoal.	Marked insomnia	
	Impaired judgment	Death	Check VS frequently for shock and cardiac	Grand mal seizures	
	Impaired social or occupational		arrest after patient is stable.	*After 5 to 15 years of*	
	function		Initiate seizure precautions	*heavy use:*	
	Impaired attention or memory		Possibly perform hemodialysis or peritoneal	Delirium	
	Irritability		dialysis.		
			Administer flumazenil (Romazicon) IV.		

From Varcarolis, E. M. (2014). *Essentials of psychiatric mental health nursing.* (2nd ed. rev.). Philadelphia: Saunders.
*These specific actions mostly apply for barbiturates, however, many apply to benzodiazepines as well.

"problem drinking" is described earlier as anything over 3 drinks in 1 day (or up to 7 drinks a week) for women, and over 4 drinks in 1 day (or up to 14 drinks a week) for men.

Cautions: For **babies,** the alcohol concentration in breast milk is equal to the alcohol concentration in the mother's blood. Alcohol intake during **adolescence** affects brain functioning in adulthood. **Older adults** have lower tolerance for alcohol and can't metabolize alcohol efficiently.

Alcohol Intoxication

Alcohol is the only drug for which objective measures of intoxication exist. The relationship between blood alcohol level (BAL) and behavior in a nontolerant individual is shown in Table 19-3. Knowledge of the BAL assists the nurse in determining the level of intoxication and the level of tolerance, and in ascertaining whether the person accurately reported recent drinking during the nursing history. These factors are also assessed by means of behavioral cues. As tolerance develops, a discrepancy is seen between BAL and expected behavior. A person with tolerance to alcohol may have a high BAL but minimal signs of impairment. *It should be noted that respiratory depression does not build up a tolerance. Therefore the higher the amount of alcohol ingestion, even though a tolerance might exist, the greater the risk for respiratory depression and respiratory arrest* (Burchum & Rosenthal, 2016).

VIGNETTE

Clarence comes to the emergency department with a blood alcohol level (BAL) of 0.31 mg %. He is stuporous and ataxic and has slurred speech. The fact that he is still alive indicates a high tolerance for alcohol. A nursing history conducted as Clarence sobers reveals an extensive drinking history. When the BAL is this high, assessing for withdrawal symptoms as well as the need for medical intervention are crucial.

Alcohol Withdrawal

Stages of Alcohol Withdrawal Syndrome

Stage	Symptoms
Minor	Anxiety, tremor, insomnia, headache, palpitations, gastrointestinal disturbances, diaphoresis, orientated to time, place, and person.
Moderate to Severe	Mild symptoms and diaphoresis, increased systolic blood pressure, tachypnea, tachycardia, confusion, mild hyperthermia, hallucinations (visual, tactile, and/or auditory) and illusions, although remains oriented to time, place, and person
DTs (delirium tremens)	Moderate symptoms and disorientation to time, place, and person, impaired attention, agitation, hallucinations (visual, tactile, and/or auditory), potential seizures

From Benzer DG. Management of alcohol intoxication and withdrawal. In: Miller NS, American Society of Addiction Medicine, eds. *Principles of Addiction Medicine*. Chevy Chase, Md.: The Society; 1994.

The early signs of withdrawal develop within a few hours after cessation or reduction of alcohol (ethanol) intake; they peak after 24 to 48 hours and then rapidly and dramatically disappear, unless the withdrawal progresses to alcohol withdrawal delirium. The person may appear hyperalert, manifest jerky movements and irritability, startle easily, and experience subjective distress often described as "shaking inside." Early symptoms of withdrawal appear 7 to 48 hours after cessation of alcohol intake and continue for 5 to 7 days. Early symptoms of withdrawal include intense tremors; cramps; vomiting; increases in heart rate, blood pressure, and temperature; and, in some individuals, grand mal seizures, particularly in people with a history of seizures. Careful assessment followed by appropriate medical and nursing interventions can prevent the more serious withdrawal reaction of delirium.

TABLE 19-3 Relationship Between Blood Alcohol Level and Effects in a Nontolerant Drinker

Blood Alcohol Level	Blood Alcohol Accumulation	Effects
0.05 mg %	1-2 drinks	Changes in mood and behavior; impaired judgment
0.08 mg %	5-6 drinks	Legal level of intoxication in most states. Clumsiness in voluntary motor activity
0.20 mg %	10-12 drinks	Depressed function of entire motor area of the brain, causing staggering and ataxia; emotional lability
0.30 mg %	15-19 drinks	Confusion, stupor
0.40 mg %	20-24 drinks	Coma
0.50 mg %	25-30 drinks	Death caused by respiratory depression

Alcohol Withdrawal Delirium

Alcohol withdrawal delirium (often referred to as delirium tremens or DTs) is considered a medical emergency and can result in death even if treated. Death is usually a result of sepsis, myocardial infarction, fat embolism, peripheral vascular collapse, electrolyte imbalance, aspiration pneumonia, or suicide. The state of delirium usually peaks 2 to 3 days (48 to 72 hours) after cessation or reduction of intake (although it can occur later) and lasts 2 to 3 days. Hallucinations are terrifying. In addition to anxiety, insomnia, anorexia, and delirium, features can include the following:

- Autonomic hyperactivity (e.g., tachycardia, diaphoresis, elevated blood pressure)
- Severe disturbance in sensorium (e.g., disorientation, clouding of consciousness)
- Perceptual disturbances (e.g., illusions, visual or tactile hallucinations)
- Fluctuating levels of consciousness (e.g., ranging from hyperexcitability to lethargy)
- Delusions (paranoid), agitated behaviors, and fever (temperatures of 100°F to 103°F)

Consistent and frequent orientation to time and place may be necessary. Encouraging the family or close friends (one at a time) to stay with the patient in quiet surroundings can help increase orientation and minimize confusion and anxiety.

The **visual/tactile hallucinations** and illusions are usually terrifying for the patient. **Illusions** are misinterpretations of objects in the environment, usually of a threatening nature. For example, a person may think that spots on the wallpaper are blood-sucking ants. However, illusions can be clarified, which reduces the patient's terror: "See, these are not spiders; they are just part of the wallpaper pattern."

Immediate medical attention is warranted in alcohol withdrawal delirium. The **CIWA-Ar (Clinical Institute Withdrawal Assessment for Alcohol)** is a validated instrument to assess alcohol withdrawal severity and can be downloaded through an Internet search at http://www.regionstrauma.org/blogs/ciwa.pdf. Refer to Table 19-4 for medical treatment during alcohol withdrawal delirium.

Psychopharmacology Used to Maintain Sobriety

Drugs used in helping individuals maintain sobriety are based on two strategies: making alcohol use unpleasant and reducing its reinforcing qualities. Presently, three drugs are approved for maintenance of sobriety (Burchum & Rosenthal, 2016):

TABLE 19-4 Alcohol Withdrawal Delirium*

Drug	Purpose
Sedatives	
Benzodiazepines[†]	
Chlordiazepoxide (Librium)	Provides *safe* withdrawal and has anticonvulsant effects; chlordiazepoxide and diazepam are cross-addicting
Diazepam (Valium)	Has anticonvulsant qualities
	Not metabolized in the liver
Seizure Control	
Carbamazepine (Tegretol), or valproic acid (Depakote)	Helps reduce withdrawal symptoms and the risk of seizures
Magnesium sulfate	Increases effectiveness of vitamin B₁ and helps reduce postwithdrawal seizures
Thiamine (vitamin B₁)	Given intramuscularly or intravenously before glucose loading to prevent *Wernicke's encephalopathy*
Alleviation of Autonomic Nervous System Symptoms (ANS)	
Beta blockers (propranolol) *or* alpha blockers (clonidine)	May help reduce ANS hyperactivity (e.g., tremor, tachycardia, elevated blood pressure, diaphoresis) but should only be used with benzodiazepine
	Most effective in short time

*__Supportive care__ includes making sure patient is well hydrated and positioned to prevent aspiration pneumonia or secondary substance use, and monitoring and replacing electrolytes as necessary, because calcium, magnesium, phosphorous, and potassium levels are low in people with alcoholism.
†Benzodiazepines should be gradually tapered and discontinued once detoxification is complete.
From Varcarolis, E. M. (2014). *Essentials of the Psychiatric Mental Health Nursing*, (2nd ed. rev.). Philadelphia: Saunders.

1. **Disulfiram (Antabuse)** is used after an individual has been alcohol free/sober for a number of months to demonstrate his or her ability to remain abstinent. This drug is used as a motivational aid for people who want to stay sober. **Patient teaching** includes explaining to the individual that when this drug is mixed with alcohol (as little as a quarter of an ounce) it can cause violent reactions such as pounding in the chest, a drop in blood pressure, nausea, vomiting, facial flushing, and potentially death. **It takes 14 days for the effects of the drug to leave the body.**

2. **Naltrexone (ReVia, Vivitrol)** reduces the desired pleasant feelings ("high") by blocking the release of endorphins related to alcohol/opioid intake. It also helps block drug cravings. An interesting finding regarding naltrexone is that it seems to be much more effective in those with a family history of alcoholism. The oral formulation of naltrexone is ReVia, and the dose is once a day.

3. **Acamprosate (Campral)** helps by reducing some of the unpleasant symptoms of abstinence such as anxiety, tension, and dysphoria, which can also cut down on the craving for the drug.

In a randomized clinical trial **gabapentin** was found to be effective in treating alcohol dependence and relapse-related symptoms of

TABLE 19-5 Pharmacotherapy in the Treatment of CNS Depressants*

Indications	Prescribing	Advantages	Risks
Disulfiram (Antabuse) ***Helps prevent relapse of alcohol abuse.*** Ingested in combination with alcohol, it will cause nausea, vomiting, headache, and flushing. **Must be alcohol-free for at least 14 days.**	**Induction:** 250-500 mg daily for 2 weeks **Maintenance:** 250 mg daily; range is 125-500 mg daily **Labs:** LFTs initially, then at 10-14 days, every 6 months thereafter	Useful in patients who have maintained sobriety but who have a history of relapse, current motivation, and a witnessed ingestion.	Metallic aftertaste; dermatitis; severe reaction or death could result from alcohol ingestion
Naltrexone (ReVia) ***Diminishes alcohol cravings***, possibly by reducing the reinforcing effects of alcohol. Also used to **block the effects of opiates.**	**Induction for opiate dependence:** Be sure patient is opioid-free for 7-10 days; confirm by UDS Start with 25 mg. If no withdrawal reaction, increase by another 25 mg; continue at 50 mg daily.	Very useful in the acute recovery phase of alcohol dependence (first 12 weeks).	Nausea, abdominal pain; constipation; dizziness; headache; anxiety; fatigue
Vivitrol (Naltrexone for Extended-Release, Injectable Suspension) Vivitrol is used **for alcohol abuse only** (should not be used if patient has opioid dependence).	**Induction for alcohol dependence:** Start at 50 mg daily. Continue at 50 mg daily. *Vivitrol (injection in buttocks):* Be sure patient is alcohol-free for at least 1 week: 380 mg/vial **Labs:** UDS, LFTs before; 6 months thereafter	Vivitrol may be easier for patients recovering from alcohol dependency to use consistently.	Vivitrol should not be used by a patient who is also using opioids, such as heroin
Acamprosate (Campral) **Diminishes alcohol cravings**, possibly by reducing intensity of prolonged withdrawal syndrome. Benefit emerges after 30-90 days.	**Induction:** Begin two 333-mg tablets, tid. Patients with renal impairment may need dosage reduction **Maintenance:** 666 mg tid **Labs:** BUN, creatine, creatinine clearance	Reasonably safe in patients with mild to moderate hepatic impairment (excreted via the kidneys). Need to have been abstinent at least 7 days.	Diarrhea and decreased libido
Buprenorphine Hydrochloride (Buprenex, Subutex); Buprenorphine Hydrochloride and Naloxone Hydrochloride (Suboxone) Treatment for **outpatient detoxification and maintenance** by specially trained and registered physicians.	**Induction:** Begin 8 mg SL on day 1, 16 mg day 2 **Maintenance:** Continue 16 mg SL daily thereafter; range is 4-24 mg daily **Labs:** UDS at induction, and monthly thereafter; LFTs on induction, and every 6 months thereafter	Buprenorphine can prevent symptoms of withdrawal in patients addicted to opiates; is an alternative to maintenance treatment with methadone.	Dizziness; nausea; respiratory depression

BUN, Blood urea nitrogen; *LFTs*, liver function tests; *SL*, sublingual (under the tongue); *tid*, three times daily; *UDS*, urine drug screen.
*Drug doses provided here are to be used as general guidelines. Results from current research, effects of specific doses, and "risk to benefit" changes should all be considered, along with physician preference, when determining the optimal dose for each patient.
Adapted from multiple sources.

insomnia, anxiety, dysphoria, craving, headaches, and/or pain in individuals with a co-occurring substance use disorder. Gabapentin has a favorable safety profile and is not harmful or lethal (Howland, 2014; Mason et al., 2014).

Refer to Table 19-5 for further information about pharmacotherapy for substance use disorders.

OPIATES

These drugs belong to the class of *narcotic analgesics*. Opioids build up tolerance and physical dependence and are taken over a prolonged period of time. The most common opiates of abuse are heroin, oxycodone, and meperidine (Demerol) (Burchum & Rosenthal, 2016). Other opiates include opium, codeine, fentanyl and its analogs, and methadone. Opiate use often starts with illicit social use, or can start when used for pain management. However, only a very small percentage of those who have been introduced to opiates for therapeutic reasons develop compulsive drug use (Burchum & Rosenthal, 2016). As mentioned earlier, heroin use is at epidemic proportions throughout the United States.

As the availability of the opioids (OxyContin, Vicodin, and Percodan) has become more difficult for addicted persons to obtain, the lower cost and availability of heroin has become the substitute.

Nonmedical use of prescription drugs may result in dangerous levels of tolerance, requiring withdrawal precautions during hospitalization, and increasingly results in overdose and death, as is the case with all opiate abuse. The presence of what is known as the triad of symptoms—*pinpoint pupils, depressed respiration,* and *coma*—is a strong indicator of opioid toxicity (Meyer & Quenzer, 2013). Immediate emergency care involves airway control and adequate oxygenation as the primary intervention.

Because of the devastating sequelae from opioid addiction mentioned earlier in this chapter, the CDC proposed guidelines for primary care physicians who prescribe opiates for chronic pain. These guidelines are not intended for cancer patients, palliative care, or end-of-life treatment. Essentially, the guidelines focus on *1) when to initiate or continue opioids for chronic pain; 2) opioid selection, dosage, duration, follow-up, and discontinuation;* and *3) assessing risk and addressing harms of opioid use* (CDC, 2016).

Psychopharmacology in the Treatment of Opiate Addiction

The first choice of treatment for **opioid toxicity** (coma, pinpoint pupils, respiratory depression) is usually **naloxone (Narcan)**, an opioid antagonist that can dramatically reverse the signs of overdose, essentially respiratory and central nervous system (CNS) depression. The disadvantages of naloxone are that it is short acting and must be readministered every few hours until opioid levels are nontoxic, which may take days (Burchum & Rosenthal, 2016). Although an individual may look symptom free, if administration of naloxone is not repeated until a nontoxic level is achieved, death may ensue (Burchum & Rosenthal, 2016). In November 2015, the U.S. Food and Drug Administration approved intranasal naloxone for the emergency treatment of known or suspected opioid overdose, as manifested by respiratory and/or CNS depression. The ready-to-use single-dose sprayer delivers a 4-mg dose by intranasal administration (Stephens & Tarabar, 2015). Because of the epidemic of overdose and deaths from heroin, this form of naloxone is being made more readily available to both health care providers and the general public.

Nalmefene (Revex) is another opioid antagonist with the advantage of a longer half-life, thereby decreasing the need for repeated dosing. However, a distinct disadvantage is that it puts the patient into prolonged withdrawal.

Detoxification is the first step in the treatment of opioid addiction. **Methadone,** which is a long-acting opioid, can be substituted for the opioid of addiction and then titrated downward to help ease the withdrawal symptoms.

Pharmacotherapy for Long-Term Management of Opioid Use Disorder

Methadone maintenance is probably the most effective treatment for heroin addiction and other illicit use of opioids. Methadone, an opioid agonist, exchanges one opioid for another, but methadone reduces the severe withdrawal effects, thus eliminating the craving for the drug. This eliminates the time spent in using and obtaining the drug, leaving more time for other things such as job training, education, and full-time work. Since methadone has a long half-life, dosing can increase up to 5 days at the same dose. Therefore careful monitoring and careful adjustments of the patient's dose must be made every 2 weeks and then less frequently (Meyer & Quenzer, 2013). Over time, since methadone is cross-tolerant with other opioids, the normal euphoric feelings that previously followed drug ingestion or injection are reduced or prevented and can block the effects of illicitly used opioids. However, methadone does pass the placental barrier like other opioids. Actual methadone maintenance therapy is limited to opioid treatment programs and requires daily clinic visits.

Buprenorphine Maintenance

Buprenorphine (Subutex) is an opioid partial agonist and is used for the same purpose as methadone maintenance. The advantage of buprenorphine is that it has weaker opioid effects, thus is less likely to result in overdose. It is longer acting and produces a milder withdrawal syndrome.

Since it has a longer duration of action, it requires less frequency of administration (one to three times a week). Prescriptions of buprenorphine can be given in a physician's office. Buprenorphine, when used in a maintenance program, alleviates cravings, reduces the use of illicit opioids, has a milder neonatal withdrawal, and increases retention in therapeutic programs (Burchum & Rosenthal, 2016; Meyer & Quenzer, 2013).

Buprenorphine has three formulations, all of which are taken once a day and sublingually. **Subutex** is buprenorphine only. **Suboxone** is buprenorphine combined with naloxone. Subutex is used for the first phase of treatment, and suboxone is later substituted for long-term treatment.

Naltrexone is used for maintenance after the patient has undergone detoxification. Naltrexone is an opioid antagonist that blocks the euphoric effects of the drug. ReVia is oral naltrexone and is taken once a day. Vivitrol is given intramuscularly (IM) once a month. Refer to Table 19-6 for the signs and symptoms of opiate intoxication, withdrawal, and overdose and possible treatments.

CENTRAL NERVOUS SYSTEM STIMULANTS

All stimulants (cocaine, amphetamines, and related compounds) accelerate the normal functioning of the body and affect the CNS. Psychomotor stimulants are known to increase alertness, heighten sexual arousal, increase behavioral excitement, increase well-being, increase energy, and diminish fatigue (Meyer & Quenzer, 2013). Severe effects include compulsive motor stereotypes; extreme energy or exhaustion; anorexia; possible extreme violence; rambling, incoherent speech; delusions of grandeur; irritability; hostility; anxiety; and fear. Common signs of stimulant use include dilation of the pupils, dryness of the

TABLE 19-6 Opiates*

Drugs	Intoxication Effects	Overdose Effects	Possible Overdose Treatments	Withdrawal Effects	Use in Withdrawal Treatments
Oxycodone	*Physical:*	Triad symptoms	Narcotic antagonist	Yawning	**Methadone** tapering and
Heroin	Constricted pupils	(coma, respiratory	(e.g., naloxone	Insomnia	can be used for mainte-
Meperidine (Demerol)	Decreased respiration	depression/arrest,	[Narcan]) to quickly	Irritability	nance therapy.
Morphine	Drowsiness	pinpoint pupils),	reverse central	Runny nose (rhinorrhea)	
Codeine	Decreased blood pressure	possible dilation of	nervous system	Panic	**Clonidine-naltrexone**
Methadone (Dolophine)	Slurred speech	pupils as a result of	depression	Diaphoresis	**Vivitrol (naltrexone**
Hydromorphone (Dilaudid)	Psychomotor retardation	anoxia		Cramps	for extended release
Fentanyl (Sublimaze)	*Psychological-perceptual:*	Cardiac arrest and		Nausea and vomiting	injectable suspension
Fentanyl analog	Initial euphoria followed by	death		Muscle aches ("bone pain")	over 1-month period)
Opium (paregoric)	dysphoria and impairment	Shock		Chills	**Buprenorphine:** for
	of attention, judgment,	Convulsions		Fever	treatment acts as an opioid
	and memory	Death		Lacrimation	substitute and can be used
				Diarrhea	for maintenance therapy or
					long-term treatment

*An opiate is a derivative or synthetic that affects the central nervous system and the autonomic nervous system. Medically it is used primarily as an analgesic (painkiller). Consistent use causes tolerance and distressing withdrawal symptoms.

From Varcarolis, E. M. (2014). *Essentials of psychiatric mental health nursing.* (2nd ed. rev). Philadelphia: Saunders.

nasal cavity, and excessive motor activity. Some of the consequences of high doses of CNS stimulants are seizures, heart failure, stroke, and integrative hemorrhage (Meyer & Quenzer, 2013). When a person who has ingested a stimulant experiences chest pain, has an irregular pulse rate, or has a history of heart trouble, the person should be taken to an emergency department immediately.

Cocaine and Crack

Cocaine is a naturally occurring stimulant extracted from the leaf of the coca bush. Crack is an inexpensive, widely available alkalinized form of cocaine. When crack is smoked, it takes effect in 4 to 6 seconds, producing a fleeting high (5 to 7 minutes) followed by a period of deep depression that reinforces addictive behavior patterns and guarantees continued use of the drug. Cocaine is classified as a schedule II substance—"high abuse potential with some recognized medical use."

Cocaine exerts two main effects on the body: anesthetic and stimulant. As an anesthetic, it blocks the conduction of electrical impulses within the nerve cells that are involved in sensory transmission, primarily pain transmission. It also acts as a stimulant for both sexual arousal and violent behavior. Cocaine produces an imbalance of neurotransmitters (dopamine and norepinephrine) that is most likely responsible for many of the physical withdrawal symptoms reported by heavy, chronic cocaine users: depression, paranoia, lethargy, anxiety, insomnia, nausea and vomiting, and sweating and chills—all signs of the body struggling to regain its normal chemical balance.

Methamphetamine

Methamphetamine is a highly addictive stimulant related to amphetamines, but it has a longer-lasting and more toxic effect on the CNS. Methamphetamines have neurotoxic (brain-damaging) effects, destroying brain cells that contain dopamine and serotonin. All amphetamines taken over a long period of time can result in visual hallucinations, delusions, and paranoia, and at the time of impairment symptoms can resemble schizophrenia.

As a result of the reduced levels of dopamine, Parkinson-like symptoms can develop. Prolonged use results in cracked teeth, skin infections, stroke, lung disease, kidney or liver damage, birth defects, and, in many cases, death.

Table 19-7 outlines the physical and psychological effects of intoxication from abuse of amphetamines and other psychostimulants, possible life-threatening results of overdose, and emergency measures for both overdose and withdrawal.

NICOTINE

Nicotine is highly addictive, highly toxic, and used worldwide. Nicotine can act as a stimulant, depressant, or tranquilizer. A high proportion of psychiatric outpatients are nicotine dependent, which makes them even more susceptible to the medical sequelae of cigarette smoking. High on the list of sequelae are lung cancer and other cancers, emphysema, and cardiovascular disease, as well as the adverse pregnancy outcomes discussed earlier. Nicotine can also be chewed (in smokeless tobacco), which adds mouth cancer to the long list of dangers.

Nicotine use results in dependence, and when users try to stop they experience an "abstinence syndrome." It is for that reason that individuals find it difficult to stop smoking. Major withdrawal symptoms include strong cravings, impaired concentration, nervousness, restlessness, irritability, impatience, and increased appetite, which usually leads to weight gain (Burchum & Rosenthal, 2016).

TABLE 19-7	**Central Nervous System Stimulants**					
Drugs	**Intoxication Effects**	**Overdose Effects**	**Possible Overdose Treatments**	**Withdrawal Effects**	**Withdrawal Treatments**
Cocaine, crack (*short acting*) *Note:* High obtained in 3 min snorted, 30 sec injected, 4-6 sec smoked (crack) Average high lasts 15-30 min for cocaine; 5-7 min for crack	*Physical:* Tachycardia Dilated pupils Elevated blood pressure Nausea and vomiting Insomnia *Psychological-perceptual:* Assaultiveness Grandiosity Impaired judgment Impaired social and occupational functioning Euphoria	Respiratory distress Ataxia Hyperpyrexia Convulsions Coma Stroke Myocardial infarction Death	Antipsychotics *Medical and nursing management for:* Hyperpyrexia (ambient cooling) Convulsions (diazepam) Respiratory distress Cardiovascular shock Acidification of urine (ammonium chloride for amphetamine)	Fatigue Depression ✓ Agitation Apathy Anxiety Sleepiness Disorientation Lethargy Craving	Antidepressants (e.g., desipramine) Dopamine agonist (e.g., bromocriptine)
Amphetamines (*long acting*) Dextroamphetamine Methamphetamine Ice (synthesized for street use)	Increased energy Increased wakefulness, increased respirations, increased hyperthermia, and euphoria *Severe effects:* State resembling paranoid schizophrenia Paranoia with delusions* Psychosis Visual, auditory, and tactile hallucinations Severe to panic levels of anxiety Potential for violence	Same as above	Same as above	Remains especially harmful, methamphetamine can cause cardiac and neurological damage	Same as above

*Paranoia and ideas of reference may persist for months afterward.
From Varcarolis, E. M. (2014). *Essentials the psychiatric mental health nursing.* (2nd ed. rev.). Philadelphia: Saunders.

There are currently seven pharmacological aids approved by the U.S. Food and Drug Administration (FDA) to help people decrease nicotine cravings and suppress symptoms of withdrawal. Five pharmacological aids to help in smoking suppression are nicotine-based: nicotine patches, nicotine gum, nicotine lozenges, nicotine nasal sprays, and nicotine inhalers. Nicotine-free products include varenicline (Chantix, Champix) and bupropion (Zyban, Buproban). The latter is the first choice for smokers with depression.

MARIJUANA

Marijuana (*Cannabis sativa*) is an Indian hemp plant in which tetrahydrocannabinol (THC) is the psychoactive ingredient. Psychoactive properties are found in all parts of the male and female plants (dry leaves, flowers, stems, and seeds), but the highest concentration of psychoactive substances is in the flowers of the female plant (Burchum & Rosenthal, 2016). The three subjective effects of marijuana are euphoria, sedation, and hallucinations.

Marijuana itself is a federally illegal drug, but state sanctioned in the states of Washington, Alaska, Oregon, and Colorado. Presently 23 states and the District of Columbia have approved the use of marijuana for medicinal purposes with a physician's prescription, and as of 2015 seven more states are pending approval for medicinal purposes.

The first cannabis-based prescription medication, Sativex, was released in the United Kingdom in 2010 as a mist spray approved to treat the spasticity (muscle tightness) in patients with multiple sclerosis. In the United States, the FDA has approved the use of two purified cannabinoids—dronabinol (Marinol) and nabilone (Cesamet)—for the intense nausea and vomiting as a result of chemotherapy, and dronabinol for patients with AIDS to combat physical wasting by increasing the individual's appetite and decreasing anorexia (Burchum & Rosenthal, 2016).

THC has mixed depressant and hallucinogenic properties. Marijuana is generally smoked, but it can be ingested. Desired effects include euphoria, detachment, and relaxation. Other effects include increase in appetite, talkativeness, slowed perception of time, inappropriate hilarity, heightened sensitivity to visual and auditory stimuli, and, in some cases, anxiety or paranoia. The untoward short-term effects cause memory loss, problems with balance and coordination, potential panic attacks, and psychosis. According to the NIH (2015), long-term effects from heavy use can cause mental problems, chronic respiratory problems, and loss of IQ points when used in adolescence. There has been great concern over chronic use of cannabis and the possibility that heavy use can produce persistent cognitive defects and/or an amotivational syndrome. An amotivational syndrome is characterized by apathy, loss of achievement motivation, decrease in productivity, difficulty with learning and memory, impaired concentration, lack of personal hygiene, and preoccupation with the drug. Overdose (psychosis in toxic doses) and withdrawal (other than strong cravings) rarely occur. There is also some preliminary data that postulates that heavy cannabis use in adolescents may be linked to premature death. More studies are needed to verify this link (Brooks, 2016).

CLUB DRUGS

Club drugs are a group of psychoactive drugs. They act on the central nervous system and can cause changes in mood, awareness, and how you act. These drugs are often abused by young adults (ranging from age 13 to young adults in their middle to late twenties) at all-night dance parties, dance clubs, and bars—places where young people gather to dance (E-medicine, 2015; NIDA, 2014). For a more detailed discussion go to https://www.nlm.nih.gov/medlineplus/clubdrugs.html. All-night dance parties are known for their electric music and the liberal use of club drugs such as ecstasy. Ecstasy (also called MDMA, Adam, Molly, and XTC) is a prototype of a class of substituted amphetamines that also includes MDA (methylenedioxyamphetamine, or "love") and MDE (3,4-methylenedioxy-*N*-ethylamphetamine, or "Eve"). These recreational drugs produce subjective effects resembling those of both stimulants and hallucinogens, and are classified in the *DSM-5* as "Other Hallucinogen Use Disorders."

MDMA primarily affects the neurons and neurotransmitters that increase the activity of three neurotransmitters—serotonin, dopamine, and norepinephrine. Serotonin is a regulator of mood, aggression, sexual activity, sleep, and sensitivity to pain and also releases oxytocin and vasopressin, which play important roles in love, trust, sexual arousal, and other social experiences (NIDA, 2013). MDMA acts to prolong the effects of serotonin in the brain as well as to increase the amounts of serotonin released from the neurons. It has similar effects on norepinephrine, which can cause an increase in heart rate and blood pressure. MDMA releases dopamine to a much lesser extent than the other neurotransmitters (NIDA, 2013).

Therefore, after taking MDMA individuals experience euphoria, increased energy, increased self-confidence, increased sociability, and a feeling of closeness to people. However, this surge of serotonin eventually leads to depletion of serotonin in the brain. This depletion of serotonin is responsible for the negative after effects of confusion, depression, sleep problems, drug craving, and anxiety that may occur soon after taking the drug or during the days or even weeks thereafter (NIDA, 2013). Because of their psychostimulant and psychedelic effects, ecstasy and the other drugs listed are increasingly abused. Adverse effects such as hyperthermia, heart failure, and kidney failure have occurred. Deaths from acute dehydration have been reported. Chronic heavy recreational use of ecstasy is thought to be responsible for sleep disorders, depressed mood, persistent elevation of anxiety level, impulsiveness, and hostility, as well as selective impairment of episodic memory and weakening of memory and attention.

Unfortunately, it is becoming more common for sellers of ecstasy (MDMA) to mix the drug with other substances, such as bath salts and other synthetic substances, which helps to explain the rise in ecstasy poisoning and ED visits.

BATH SALTS OR CATHINONES

A multitude of uncontrolled designer chemicals generally referred to as "bath salts" are flooding the market and are easily available to anyone through the Internet, health food stores, and drug stores. Among other things, they contain one or more synthetic chemicals related to cathinone, an amphetamine-like stimulant as well as to MDMA (ecstasy) (NIDA, 2012b, 2013),

Bath salts can contain a combination of the worst effects of several different drugs (e.g., hallucinogenic-delusional properties, dissociation, extreme agitation, and feelings of superhuman strength and combativeness) and have the hyperaddictive qualities of cocaine and methamphetamines.

Flakka is a "chemical cousin" to bath salts and perhaps the most dangerous. The most severe side effect is known as "excited delirium," which features violent behavior, hallucinations, and increases in body temperatures of up to 106°F. Internally there is muscle breakdown, which can lead to kidney failure. People who ingest flakka are also susceptible to risk of stroke or heart attack related to extreme tachycardia (NIH, 2015). All of these chemically manufactured drugs are available under many names and chemical mixtures, and strengths of ingredients vary. Trips to the ED are not uncommon after ingesting these compounds, and many deaths have occurred.

Table 19-8 lists the toxic effects of and treatments for these drugs, as well as withdrawal symptoms.

TABLE 19-8 Club Drugs

Club Drugs	Toxic Effects	Treatment	Withdrawal
Ecstasy (MDMA)	• Hyperthermia (elevated body temperature) and in rare conditions can lead to liver, kidney, or cardiovascular system failure or even death • Serotonin syndrome depletion • ↑ Water intake leads to hyponatremia • Neurological effects (confusion, delirium, paranoia)	No antidote Treat symptoms Cardiac monitoring Comprehensive chemistry panel identifies complications (e.g., hepatic or renal damage)	Profound depression secondary to serotonin depletion Confusion, sleep problems, anxiety, cravings that can last for weeks Repeated heavy use associated with cognitive impairment (potentially permanent memory loss)
Gamma-hydroxybutyrate (GBH) *Street names:* Fantasy GBH Liquid ecstasy Cherry meth (date rape drug)	Cheyne-Stokes respirations Seizures Coma Death	No antidote Treat symptoms Monitor cardiac status Comprehensive chemistry panel (to check renal, hepatic, or other complications) Antidote Flumazenil	Withdrawal symptoms include: • Anxiety • Insomnia • Tremors Like other benzodiazepines: • ↑ Seizure potential • Anxiety • Muscle pain • Photosensitivity • Headache • Lasting anterograde amnesia

From Varcarolis, E. M. (2014). *Essentials of psychiatric mental health nursing.* (2nd ed. rev). Philadelphia: Saunders.

DATE RAPE DRUGS

Flunitrazepam (Rohypnol) and Ketamine

The drugs most frequently used to facilitate a sexual assault (rape) are flunitrazepam (Rohypnol, or "roofies"), which is a fast-acting benzo-diazepine, and γ-hydroxybutyrate (GHB) and its congeners. They are odorless, tasteless, and colorless; mix easily with drinks; and can result in unconsciousness in a matter of minutes. Perpetrators use these drugs because they rapidly produce disinhibition and relaxation of voluntary muscle and cause the victim to have lasting anterograde amnesia.

Ketamine is a dissociative anesthetic that can also be slipped into an unsuspecting individual's drink without detection. Because it also induces amnesia, it is also used in the commission of sexual assault or rape. Alcohol potentiates the effects of these drugs. Refer to Chapter 22 for more on sexual violence and assault. Refer to Table 19-8.

HALLUCINOGENS

Lysergic Acid Diethylamide and Similar Drugs

LSD (acid), mescaline (peyote), and psilocybin (magic mushroom) are hallucinogens. Mescaline and the mushroom *Psilocybe mexicana* (from which psilocybin is isolated) have been used for centuries in religious rites by Native Americans living in the southwestern United States and northern Mexico. The hallucinogenic experience produced by LSD results in a dreamlike state of unreality, flashbacks and persistent perception disorders, as well as hallucinations. Refer to Table 19-9 for the signs and symptoms of hallucinogen intoxication and overdose.

DISSOCIATIVE DRUGS

Phencyclidine and Ketamine

Both phencyclidine (PCP) and ketamine were first used as anesthetic agents. Initially, PCP was considered promising because it didn't cause respiratory depression. Because of the sometimes violent side effects of PCP, ketamine was viewed as a safer alternative.

Both drugs produce a generalized anesthesia that lessens the sensations of touch and pain and makes staff interventions difficult. The dissociative effects of PCP and ketamine include feelings of being separate from one's body and environment. Both drugs also cause anxiety, tremors, numbness, memory loss, and nausea.

PCP, or 1-(1-phenylcyclohexyl) piperidine, is also known as angel dust, horse tranquilizer, and peace pill. The signs and symptoms of PCP intoxication range from acute anxiety to acute psychosis, as well as aggression, violence, and loss of coordination. Mood can be volatile and behavior bizarre. PCP can produce hypotension, coma, seizures, and muscular rigidity associated with the occurrence of hypothermia (Table 19-10). Chronic use of PCP can result in long-term effects such as dulled thinking, lethargy, loss of impulse control, poor memory, and depression.

Suicidal risk is always assessed, especially in cases of toxicity or coma. Refer to Chapter 23 for more information on suicide assessment.

Ketamine (cat valium, special K, vitamin K) shares many of the properties of PCP mentioned above. For the most part, the desired effects of ketamine are the dissociative effects of pleasantly floating in space. Others have described the out-of-body experiences as the feeling of rising above one's body. For some this sensation is pleasurable and peaceful, but for others it can be terrifying (Burchum & Rosenthal, 2016). Ketamine can also cause delirium and respiratory depression that can lead to respiratory arrest and death.

Salvia has hallucinogenic as well as dissociative effects on the CNS. It is a member of the mint family and traditionally used in religious rituals among Mexican Indians. Users may chew the fresh leaves, smoke dried and crushed leaves, or place a liquid extract under the tongue or inside the cheek. The Drug Enforcement Administration (DEA) considers it a "drug of concern." Young people in this country usually smoke the leaves. According to Meyer and Quenzer (2013), salvia produces vivid hallucinations, out-of-body experiences, and

TABLE 19-9   Hallucinogens*

Drugs	Intoxication Effects	Overdose Effects	Possible Overdose Treatments
Lysergic acid diethylamide (LSD) Mescaline (peyote) Psilocybin	*Physical:* Pupil dilation Tachycardia Diaphoresis Palpitations Tremors Incoordination Elevated temperature, pulse, respiration *Psychological-perceptual:* Fear of going crazy Paranoid ideas Marked anxiety, depression Synesthesia (e.g., colors are heard; sounds are seen) Depersonalization Hallucinations, although sensorium is clear Grandiosity (e.g., thinking one can fly)	Psychosis Brain damage Death	Keep patient in room with low stimuli—minimal light, sound, activity. Have one person stay with patient; reassure patient, "talk down" patient. Speak slowly and clearly in low voice. Give diazepam or chloral hydrate for extreme anxiety or tension.

*Hallucinogen produces *abnormal mental phenomena* in the cognitive and perceptual spheres; for example, distortion in space and time, hallucinations, delusions (paranoid or grandiose), and synesthesia may occur.
From Varcarolis, E. M. (2014). *Essentials of psychiatric mental health nursing.* (2nd ed. rev.). Philadelphia: Saunders.

TABLE 19-10   Dissociative Drugs

Drugs	Intoxication	Overdose/Toxic Effects	Potential Overdose Treatments
1-(1-Phenylcyclohexyl) piperidine (PCP)	*Physical:* May be impervious to pain Vertical or horizontal nystagmus Increased blood pressure, pulse, and temperature Ataxia Muscle rigidity Seizures Blank stare Chronic jerking Agitated, repetitive movements Belligerence, assaultiveness, impulsiveness Impaired judgment, impaired social and occupational functioning *Severe effects:* Hallucinations, paranoia Bizarre behavior (e.g., barking like a dog, grimacing, repetitive chanting speech) Regressive behavior Violent, bizarre behaviors Very labile behaviors	Psychosis Possible hypertensive crisis or cardiovascular accident Respiratory arrest Hyperthermia Seizures	*If alert:* *Caution:* Gastric lavage can lead to laryngeal spasms or aspiration. Acidify urine (cranberry juice, ascorbic acid); in acute stage, ammonium chloride acidifies urine to help excrete drug from body—may continue for 10-14 days. Put in room with minimal stimuli. Do not attempt to talk down patient! Speak slowly, clearly, and in a low voice. Administer diazepam. Haloperidol may be used for severe behavioral disturbance (*not* a phenothiazine). **Institute medical intervention for:** • Hyperthermia • High blood pressure • Respiratory distress • Hypertension
Ketamine	Experience varies from a pleasant floating sensation to out-of-body experiences that are described as either peaceful or terrifying	High doses can cause amnesia, elevation of blood pressure, and potentially fatal disruption of respiration	Medical treatment for hypertension and respiratory distress
Salvia	Similar to LSD but the dissociative experiences is a stark sense of unreality and loss of awareness of one's body or where he or she is. Some experiences mimic the sensations of traveling through space and becoming various objects.		

From Varcarolis, E. M. (2014). *Essentials for psychiatric mental health nursing.* (2nd ed. rev.). Philadelphia: Saunders.

feelings similar but not identical to those experienced with other hallucinogens and dissociative drugs. For example, a person might feel like he or she is turning into an object (a french fry, a pant leg, a ferris wheel), being pulled by some kind of force, losing his or her body and/ or identity, or traveling through time and space (Meyer & Quenzer, 2013). Refer to Table 19-10 for the signs and symptoms of intoxication, overdose, and effects, and potential medical interventions when appropriate.

TABLE 19-11 Inhalants

Drug	Intoxication Effects	Overdose Effects	Treatment
Volatile solvents (e.g., paint thinners, glues, gasoline, dry cleaner fluid) **Gases** (e.g., butane, propane, nitrous oxide) **Nitrates** (e.g., isoamyl, isobutyl, commonly known as "poppers") **Aerosols** (e.g., spray paint, hair or deodorant sprays, fabric protector sprays, vegetable oil sprays)	Similar to alcohol: Slurred speech, lack of inhibitions, euphoria, dizziness, drunkenness, violent behavior	Liver and brain damage, heart failure, respiratory arrest, suffocation, coma, death Capable of interfering with oxygen supply to vital organs by destroying oxygen-carrying ability of red blood cells; associated with fatal cardiac rhythm **Long-term use** can lead to deterioration of myelin sheath of nerve fibers, resulting in muscle spasms and tremors, or even permanent difficulty with basic movements such as walking, bending, and talking	Support affected systems Neurological symptoms may respond to vitamin B_{12} and folate

Data from National Institute on Drug Abuse. (Updated 2011). *Research report series: Inhalant use* (NIH Pub. No. 94-3819). Washington, DC: U.S. Department of Health and Human Services. Retrieved February 9, 2012, from http://www.drugabuse.gov/publications/infofacts/inhalants; Varcarolis, E. M. (2014). *Essentials of psychiatric mental health nursing.* (2nd ed. rev). Philadelphia: Saunders.

INHALANTS

For some early teenagers (ages 12 through 17), inhalants are often the first drugs of abuse because they may be found in the home or can easily be purchased. Inhalant use is also referred to as "huffing" or "backing." Inhalants include volatile solvents such as spray paint, glue, cigarette lighter fluid, and propellant gases used in aerosols. Inhalants starve the body of oxygen and force the heart to beat irregularly and more rapidly. Sudden death can occur from cardiac arrhythmia or arrest. Users can experience nausea and nosebleeds and lose their sense of hearing or smell. Chronic use can lead to muscle wasting and reduced muscle tone, and the poisonous chemicals gradually damage the lungs and the immune system. Long-term use also results in persistent medical and neurological problems (APA, 2013). Inhalant use may be an early marker of future substance abuse and should be the focus of increased preventive efforts and early diagnosis and treatment. Unfortunately, inhalants coexist with other substance use disorders, as well as other mental health disorders such as adolescent conduct disorder and antisocial personality disorders (APA, 2013). People with inhalant abuse or inhalant substance disorder often have a history of suicide attempts and suicide ideation. Types of inhalants, signs of inhalant intoxication, and side effects are listed in Table 19-11.

APPLICATION OF THE NURSING PROCESS

ASSESSMENT

Assessing use and abuse of substances is becoming more complex because of increased simultaneous use of multiple substances (**multiple drug use/polydrug use**) and new chemically engineered designer drugs. Accurate assessment becomes even more complicated in the presence of coexisting psychiatric disorders or physical illnesses, including HIV infection, AIDS, dementia, and encephalopathy.

Sensitivity to multicultural and racial issues is important in interpreting symptoms, making diagnoses, providing clinical care, and designing prevention strategies. Refer to Box 19-2 for areas to be covered in overall substance use assessment.

Initial Assessment

There is a consistent and significant association between alcohol or drug use and injury. Intracranial hematomas, subdural hematomas, and other conditions can remain unnoticed if the symptoms of acute alcohol intoxication and withdrawal are not distinguished from the symptoms of a brain injury. Therefore neurological signs (pupil size, equality, and reaction to light) should be assessed, especially in

BOX 19-2 Overall Assessment Guide for Substance Use

History of Patient's Substance Use*
1. What are the dates of first use, number of substances being taken, pattern of use, amount, frequency, periods of sobriety, time last taken?
2. Was patient treated previously for substance abuse? What was the outcome?
3. Is there a history of blackouts, delirium, or seizures?
4. Is there a history of withdrawal symptoms, overdoses, and complications from past substance use?
5. Is there a family history of drug or alcohol problems?

Medical History
1. Does the patient have any coexisting physical conditions (e.g., HIV infection)?
2. What medications does the patient presently take?
3. What is the patient's current medical status? Mental status?

Psychiatric History
1. Is there a history of comorbid psychiatric problems? Depression? Personality disorder? Conduct disorder? Schizophrenia?
2. Has the patient undergone treatment for a specific disorder? What medications were given and what was the outcome?
3. Is there a history of abuse (physical, sexual)? Family violence?
4. Is there a history of suicide? Violence toward others?
5. Is the patient having suicidal thoughts?

Psychosocial Issues
1. Does the patient have a poor work record related to substance use?
2. How has the patient's substance use affected his or her relationships with others?
   - Family
   - Friends
   - Professional relationships
   - Community involvement
3. How has the substance use affected the patient's ability to meet usual role expectations (e.g., parent, spouse, friend, employee)?
4. Is there a police or criminal record or legal problems related to substance use (e.g., vehicle accidents, driving while intoxicated, physical violence)?
5. Who does the patient identify as his or her support system? Who does the patient trust? Who cares for the patient? Who will help the patient if the patient asks for help?
6. Does the patient use coping styles that contribute to the maintenance of his or her drug or alcohol lifestyle?

*This information needs to be obtained immediately. It is vital to the evaluation of impending withdrawal, multiple withdrawals, impending overdose, and potential need for medical intervention

TABLE 19-12	Screening Instrument: The Alcohol Use Disorders Identification Test (AUDIT)					
	0	**1**	**2**	**3**	**4**	**Score**
How often do you have a drink containing alcohol?	Never	Monthly or less	2 to 4 times a month	2 to 3 times a week	4 or more times a week	
How many drinks containing alcohol do you have on a typical day when you are drinking?	1 or 2	3 or 4	5 or 6	7 to 9	10 or more	
How often do you have 5 or more drinks on one occasion?	Never	Less than monthly	Monthly	Weekly	Daily or almost daily	
How often during the last year have you found that you were not able to stop drinking once you had started?	Never	Less than monthly	Monthly	Weekly	Daily or almost daily	
How often during the last year have you failed to do what was normally expected of you because of drinking?	Never	Less than monthly	Monthly	Weekly	Daily or almost daily	
How often during the last year have you needed a first drink in the morning to get yourself going after a heavy drinking session?	Never	Less than monthly	Monthly	Weekly	Daily or almost daily	
How often during the last year have you had a feeling of guilt or remorse after drinking?	Never	Less than monthly	Monthly	Weekly	Daily or almost daily	
How often during the last year have you been unable to remember what happened the night before because of your drinking?	Never	Less than monthly	Monthly	Weekly	Daily or almost daily	
Have you or someone else been injured because of your drinking?	No		Yes, but not in the last year		Yes, during the last year	
Has a relative, friend, doctor, or other health care worker been concerned about your drinking or suggested you cut down?	No		Yes, but not in the last year		Yes, during the last year	
					Total Score	

Instructions to patient: Place an X in the box that best describes your answer to each question.
Scoring: Record the score (0, 1, 2, 3, or 4) for each response at the end of each line, and then add up the total score. The maximum possible is 40. A total score of 8 or more (for men up to age 60), or 4 or more (for women, adolescents, and men over 60) is considered a positive screen. For patients with totals near the cut-points, clinicians may wish to examine individual responses to questions and clarify them during the clinical examination.
Reprinted with permission from the World Health Organization. To reflect standard drink sizes in the United States, the number of drinks in the third question was changed from 6 to 5.

comatose patients suspected of having traumatic injuries. In addition, questions about alcohol or drug use should be asked as part of the assessment of any trauma victim and any family members or friends. A urine and/or blood toxicology screen or blood alcohol level (BAL) test should be performed. The legal limit in the United States is 0.08% blood alcohol content as measured by blood, urine analysis, or a breathalyzer test. Measurement can be useful for assessment purposes.

Assessment strategies must include collection of data pertaining to both the substance(s) of use and any psychiatric impairment or mental health disorder. Individuals with previously established psychiatric impairment may be experiencing substance use or addiction if they exhibit increasing frequency of symptoms, exacerbation of symptoms without obvious reason, or chronic nonadherence with treatment regimens. Self-medication or use of a substance in response to symptomatology secondary to psychiatric impairment (e.g., depression) is a common phenomenon when individuals are overwhelmed or dealing with psychic pain. Substance use disorders can remain undetected in those who are depressed, suicidal, or anxious unless a thorough history is taken. Similarly, the understanding and treatment of an individual with a substance use disorder are enhanced by inquiries about symptoms of depression and anxiety made with the patient, family, and friends.

Initial Interview Guidelines

Screening tests can be very helpful in identifying the problems and extent of the substance use.

Many standardized screening tools are available. The following are two good examples of screening tools for substance use disorders:
- **Alcohol:** The Alcohol Use Disorders Identification Test (AUDIT) (Table 19-12).
- **Other substances of abuse:** The B-DAST: Brief Drug Abuse Screening Test (Box 19-3). Each item counts as 1 point, and 6 or more points indicates a serious substance abuse problem.

Psychological Changes

Certain psychological characteristics are associated with substance use disorders, including *denial, depression, anxiety, dependency, hopelessness, low self-esteem,* and *various psychiatric disorders.* It is often difficult to determine which comes first—psychological changes or substance abuse. People who are addicted to substances are threatened on many levels.

Addicts establish a **predictable defensive style** to protect themselves against threats, such as disruptions in their lifestyle and the consequences of withdrawal. The elements of this style include various defense mechanisms (denial, projection, rationalization), as well as characteristic thought processes (all-or-none thinking, selective attention) and behaviors (conflict minimization and avoidance, passivity, manipulation). Refer to Chapter 11 for further discussion of defense mechanisms. The substance abuser is not able to relinquish these maladaptive coping styles until more positive and functional skills are learned.

⏩ Assessment Guidelines

1. Clarify that the presenting signs and symptoms are not due to a physical accident or condition (e.g., subdural hematoma from a fall).
2. Once substance use has been established, it is important to identify the **specific name of the drug, route, quantity, time of last use, and usual pattern of abuse.**
3. Assess for a severe or major withdrawal syndrome.
4. Assess for an overdose from a drug or alcohol that warrants immediate medical attention.
5. Assess the patient for suicidal thoughts or other self-destructive behaviors.
6. Evaluate the patient for any physical complications related to substance use disorders.
7. Explore the individual's interest in taking actions to address his or her drug or alcohol abuse/disorder.
8. Assess the patient and family for knowledge of community resources for alcohol and drug treatment.

BOX 19-3 **B-DAST: Brief Drug Abuse Screening Test**

Instructions: The following questions concern information about your involvement and abuse of drugs. Drug abuse refers to (1) the use of prescribed or over-the-counter drugs in excess of the directions and (2) any nonmedical use of drugs. Carefully read each statement and decide whether your answer is yes or no. Then circle the appropriate response.

YES NO 1. Have you used drugs other than those required for medical reasons?

YES NO 2. Have you abused prescription drugs?

YES NO 3. Do you abuse more than one drug at a time?

YES NO 4. Can you get through the week without using drugs (other than those required for medical reasons)?

YES NO 5. Are you always able to stop using drugs when you want to?

YES NO 6. Have you had blackouts or flashbacks as a result of drug use?

YES NO 7. Do you ever feel bad about your drug abuse?

YES NO 8. Does your spouse (or parents) ever complain about your involvement with drugs?

YES NO 9. Has drug abuse ever created problems between you and your spouse?

YES NO 10. Have you ever lost friends because of your use of drugs?

YES NO 11. Have you ever neglected your family or missed work because of your use of drugs?

YES NO 12. Have you ever been in trouble at work because of drug abuse?

YES NO 13. Have you ever lost a job because of drug abuse?

YES NO 14. Have you gotten into fights when under the influence of drugs?

YES NO 15. Have you engaged in illegal activities in order to obtain drugs?

YES NO 16. Have you ever been arrested for possession of illegal drugs?

YES NO 17. Have you ever experienced withdrawal symptoms as a result of heavy drug intake?

YES NO 18. Have you had medical problems as a result of your drug use (e.g., memory loss, hepatitis, convulsions, bleeding)?

YES NO 19. Have you ever gone to anyone for help for a drug problem?

YES NO 20. Have you ever been involved in a treatment program specifically related to drug use?

Items 4 and 5 are scored in the NO, or false, direction. Each item is 1 point. A score of 6 or more points suggests significant problems.

From Skinner, H. A. Addict Behav, 7:363.... Center for substance abuse treatment. Substance Abuse Treatment of Persons with Co-Occurring Disorders. Treatment improvement protocol (TIP) Series 42 DHHS publication NO (SMA) 05 – 3992. Rockville, Md., 2005. Substance Abuse and Mental Health Services Administration.

SELF-ASSESSMENT

"Patients struggling with addiction are some of the most difficult patients to treat, even for seemingly impenetrable physicians" (Ross, 2016). Unfortunately, stigma surrounding addiction persists and society, including health care workers, often view addicted persons as weak, self-indulgent, and lazy.

As a nurse, it is important to examine your own feelings and thoughts regarding how you feel about addicted individuals. Working with a more experienced clinician to help identify transference and countertransference issues can be invaluable. Some nurses may have extremely strong negative feelings, (e.g., feelings of disgust, loathing) while others may hold significant anger, others may feel sympathy, while others may practice avoidance. A further complication to compassionate care is that the helplessness, depression, and self-loathing in the addict gets transferred onto the nurse/health care worker, which will further distance people from the addicted individual (Ross, 2016). Although the disease theory of substance use and addiction is widely accepted, it does not always change people's feelings and prejudices.

Behaviors of a person who is addicted to a substance can raise a kaleidoscope of conflicting and intense emotions in all of us. Perhaps a family member is or was addicted, perhaps a friend of yours was hit by a drunk driver, or perhaps a rather brilliant and well-loved nursing colleague died of an overdose. Intense negative as well as intense positive personal emotions need to be examined before we can be effective with an individual, or even a coworker, with a substance use disorder.

Training programs are available to help health care workers obtain the tools and skills needed to treat the person behind the addiction, without which the task may be insurmountable (Ross, 2016).

Substance Use and Health Care Workers

It is believed that health professionals misuse alcohol and other drugs at about the same rate as the general population (10% to 15%). Nursing students are just as vulnerable to addictions. The American Nurses Association (ANA) estimates that 6% to 8% of nurses use alcohol or drugs to an extent that is sufficient to impair practice (WSNA, 2016). Other sources report an estimate of 10% to 15% of all nurses in the United States are addicted to some type of illegal or controlled substance. (See more at http://www.nursetogether.com/nurses-and-substance-abuse.) According to the National Council of the State Boards of Nursing many nurses with substance use disorder are unidentified,

unreported, untreated, and may continue to practice where their impairment may endanger the lives of their patients (NCSBN, 2014).

Often, the impaired nurse volunteers to work additional shifts to be nearer to the source of the drug. The nurse may leave the unit frequently or spend a lot of time in the bathroom. When the impaired nurse is on duty, more patients may complain that their pain is unrelieved by their narcotic analgesic or that they are unable to sleep, despite receiving sedative medications. Increases in inaccurate drug counts and vial breakage may occur.

A colleague may observe signs such as a tendency to isolate; preference for working alone to avoid being caught; irritability with peers; dramatic changes in mood, especially after bathroom breaks; decrease in productivity as the disease progresses; absence from and tardiness to work; arriving at work early and staying late (in order to attain drugs); odor of alcohol on breath; frequent intoxication at social functions; isolation from social functions to drink alone; slurred speech; and illegible writing charts when handwriting was usually neat.

If indicators of impaired practice are observed, they must be reported to the nurse manager. Intervention is the responsibility of the nurse manager and other nursing administrators. According to the American Nurses Association Code of Ethics, Provision 3.6 (ANA, 2015), "Nurses must be vigilant to protect the patient, the public, and the profession from potential harm when a colleague's practice, in any setting, appears to be impaired." "There is an ethical and legal responsibility to report if you feel a colleague is working while impaired." Puliti (2014) reported, "If a nurse suspects substance abuse in a colleague, he/she should not ignore the incident, enable the colleague, or lighten the suspected nurse's load. The colleague should be reported immediately to prevent any future incidents."

However, mandating punitive action makes it more difficult for impaired nurses to seek early intervention and assistance, which makes it more likely that the public will be endangered. It also makes it more difficult for colleagues to report a fellow colleague. "Helping colleagues and students recover from an addictive disorder by providing a non-punitive atmosphere is a life-saving first step for nurses, students, and those in their care" (Monroe & Kenaga, 2011).

Alternative-to-discipline (ADT) programs seem to be the answer for many impaired persons. The benefit of the ADT program is that it allows managers to remove nurses from the work environment quickly, unlike traditional disciplinary procedures that can extend for months to years. The approach of these programs provides nonjudgmental support and treatment that encourages the impaired colleague to stay in the profession.

Reporting an impaired colleague is not easy, even though it is our responsibility. Often he or she has high levels of denial and is not receptive to interventions. By the same token, the colleague of an impaired nurse may deny or rationalize what is happening, thus enabling the impaired nurse to potentially endanger lives while becoming sicker and more isolated.

Rehabilitative programs, either peer assistance programs or ADT programs, are offered by most, although not all, of the state boards of nursing. Some state boards of nursing allow impaired nurses to avoid disciplinary action if they seek treatment. Although the choices for action are varied (e.g., "alternative-to-discipline" or "peer assistance" programs), early intervention is essential, and the only choice that is wrong is for others to do nothing.

Our main responsibility is to our patients. Since most states now have programs in place to help addicted health care workers (doctors, nurses, pharmacists, etc.), impaired health care givers have options to protect their jobs and/or licenses while engaged in treatment and perhaps saving their own lives. Refer to Box 19-4.

DIAGNOSIS

Nursing diagnoses for patients with psychoactive substance use disorders are many and varied because of the large range of physical and psychological effects of drug abuse or dependence on the user and his or her family. Comorbid psychiatric problems also must be addressed. Potential nursing diagnoses for people with substance use disorders are listed in Table 19-13.

BOX 19-4 A Guide for Assisting Colleagues Who Demonstrate Impairment in the Workplace

Nurses and other health professionals impaired by alcohol or other drugs pose a serious risk of harm to patients, colleagues, and themselves. Employers have a duty to protect the patient as well as an ethical obligation to assist their employees. An employer should consider the following guidelines and/or ethical issues.

- **Confidentiality related to information concerning a chemical dependency problem is required by federal law.** Each employer should have a policy that includes:
  1. A cause for testing policy
  2. Identification of the person who will interact with the employee concerning their impaired practice
  3. A referral process for evaluation and treatment
  4. Clear consequences associated with refusing treatment
- **It is the obligation and responsibility of a colleague or coworker to document and report an impaired health professional's behavior to the employer or designated supervisor.** Such a worker should not be allowed to give patient care until he or she has been evaluated and received treatment.
- **A health care worker should be offered professional treatment in lieu of termination.** It is more cost effective; valuable expertise and service history may be lost if the health professional's employment is pre-emptively terminated, and the health professional is not afforded the opportunity to get treatment for what is a progressive medical illness.
- **It is important to note that the suicide risk is increased after an intervention or confrontation. It is necessary to ensure the health professional is not left alone after an intervention until a plan is in place.**
- **The health professional has the right to refuse treatment,** as it is each person's right to make that decision. The employer needs to make it clear that if evaluation and treatment are rejected, the health care worker's employment may be terminated.

Adapted from Washington State Nurses Association & Washington State Department of Health. (2013). *A guide for assisting colleagues who demonstrate impairment in the workplace.* Olympia, Wa.: Washington Health Professional Services.

APPLYING EVIDENCE-BASED PRACTICE (EBP)

Problem A registered nurse (RN) student was completing her psychiatric nursing rotation at a community hospital in California. The student's preceptor was an experienced RN with a history of alcohol addiction who had completed the Chemically Addicted Nurses Diversion Option (CANDO) program in Arizona several years earlier. The preceptor was open with her student about her experiences with addiction and recovery, and the student viewed her as a skilled and caring nurse. During the rotation, the preceptor had a grand mal seizure. The student called out for help, then knelt down to assist her preceptor. While in close proximity she smelled alcohol on her preceptor's breath. The student knows from class that she should report her preceptor, but a friend recently lost her job due to alcoholism and the student is torn and upset.

EBP Assessment

A. **What do you already know from experience?** Alcohol abuse contributes to poor judgment and errors in general, such as driving while intoxicated. It seems reasonable to this student that errors would also occur in caring for patients. The student has seen a nonsupportive response in the workplace to someone she cares about due to alcohol abuse, and does not want to hurt her preceptor.

B. **What does the literature say?** Most states have an intervention program for impaired nurses in lieu of discipline (Copp, 2009). The American Nurses Association estimates that 10% of nurses struggle with addiction (Copp, 2009), and other estimates range as high as 20% (Monroe & Kenaga, 2011), meaning most nurses will encounter this in their careers. The incidence of self-reporting is low, due to the nature of addiction and stigma, so most impaired nurses will be noticed first by colleagues. Addiction is a treatable disease, and the success rate in impaired nurse programs is good. Early intervention and a nonpunitive approach are essential for recovery (Monroe & Kenaga, 2011).

C. **What does the patient want?** The patient in this situation is really the impaired nurse. She seems to want sobriety due to several years remaining sober. She has been an excellent nurse and role model for the student during her psychiatric nursing rotation and values recovery.

Plan The student first approached her clinical instructor, who accompanied her to a meeting with the nursing supervisor. The nursing supervisor has had experience with the diversion program (California state impaired nursing program), and as a psychiatric nurse was supportive in the situation. States vary on acceptance to the program again after a relapse, and California is a state that allows this. The nursing supervisor planned to speak with the preceptor and offer her the diversion program as an option, once she recovers from her seizure. The preceptor would not be allowed to return to work until the issue was decided.

QSEN QSEN Prelicensure Knowledge, Skills, and Attitudes (KSAs) Addressed:

Safety was considered foremost for the patients, as the impaired nurse would be more prone to errors, and also for the nurse's health as well.

Evidence-based practice was used in understanding the nature of addiction and recovery, and programs available to the impaired nurse.

Copp, M. (2009). *Drug addiction among nurses: Confronting a quiet epidemic.* Retrieved from http://www.modernmedicine.com/modern-medicine/news/modernmedicine/modern-medicine-feature-articles/drug-addiction-among-nurses-con?page=full; Monroe, T., & Kenaga, H. (2011). Don't ask don't tell: Substance abuse and addiction among nurses. *Journal of Clinical Nursing, 20*(3–4), 504–509.

OUTCOMES IDENTIFICATION

When planning care for patients with substance use disorders, the patient's cultural background and values need to be reflected in the plan of care. The following are some examples of desired outcomes:

- Remaining free from injury while withdrawing from the substance
- Attending programs for treatment and maintenance of sobriety (e.g., self-help groups like Alcoholics Anonymous or group therapy, cognitive behavioral therapy, programs that follow the Recovery Paradigm)
- Attending a relapse prevention program during the active course of treatment
- Identifying cues or situations that pose increased risk of drug use
- Having a stable group of drug-free friends and socializing with them at least three times a week.
- By the same token, avoiding former substance-abusing friends and colleagues who trigger situations and the types of places related to former substance use.
- Demonstrating at least one or two new skills in dealing with troubling feelings (anger, loneliness, cravings, anxiety)

PLANNING

It cannot be stressed enough that planning care requires attention to the patient's social status, income, cultural and ethnic background, gender, age, substance use history, and current condition. It is safest to propose abstinence as a treatment goal for all individuals with substance use disorders. Abstinence is strongly related to good work

adjustment, positive health status, comfortable interpersonal relationships, and general social stability. Planning must also address the patient's major psychological, social, and medical problems, as well as the substance-using behavior. Involvement of appropriate family members is essential.

Unfortunately, a person's social status and social relationships often deteriorate as a result of addiction. Job demotion or job loss, with resultant reduced or nonexistent income, may occur. Meeting basic needs for food, shelter, and clothing is thereby hampered. Marriage and other close relationships deteriorate and fail, and the person is often left alone and isolated. The lack of interpersonal and social supports is a complicating factor in treatment planning for the addict.

IMPLEMENTATION

The aim of treatment is self-responsibility, not compliance. A major challenge is improving treatment effectiveness by matching subtypes of patients to specific types of treatment. Although individuals who are addicted to substances of use share some characteristics and dynamics, significant differences exist within the addict population with regard to physiological, psychological, and sociocultural processes. These differences influence the recovery process either positively or negatively.

Often the choice of inpatient or outpatient care depends on cost and the availability of insurance coverage. Outpatient programs work best for employed substance users who have an involved social support system. People who have no support and structure in their day often do better in inpatient programs when these programs are available.

TABLE 19-13 Potential Nursing Diagnoses for Substance Abuse

Signs and Symptoms	Nursing Diagnoses	Signs and Symptoms	Nursing Diagnoses
Vomiting, diarrhea, poor nutritional and fluid intake	*Imbalanced nutrition: less than body requirements* *Deficient fluid volume* *Risk for electrolyte imbalance*	**Family crises and family pain**, ineffective parenting, emotional neglect of others, increased incidence of physical and sexual abuse of others, increased self-hate projected to others	*Interrupted family processes* *Impaired parenting* *Risk for other-directed violence* *Dysfunctional family processes* *Ineffective relationship* *Ineffective impulse control*
Audiovisual hallucinations, impaired judgment, memory deficits, cognitive impairments related to substance intoxication or withdrawal (deficits in problem solving, ability to attend to tasks and grasp ideas)	*Impaired environmental interpretation syndrome** *Altered thought processes** *Risk for violence to self or others* *Ineffective impulse control* *Acute or chronic confusion* *Impaired mood regulation* *Risk for injury*	**Excessive substance abuse** affecting all areas of a person's life: loss of friends, poor job performance, increased illness rates, proneness to accidents and overdoses	*Defensive coping* *Impaired verbal communication* *Social isolation* *Risk for loneliness* *Anxiety* *Ineffective relationship* *Risk for suicide*
Changes in sleep-wake cycle, interference with stage 4 sleep, inability to sleep or long periods of sleeping related to effects of or withdrawal from substance	*Disturbed sleep pattern* *Insomnia* *Sleep deprivation*	**Increased health problems** related to substance used and route of use, as well as overdose	*Activity intolerance* *Ineffective airway clearance* *Ineffective breathing pattern* *Impaired oral mucous membrane* *Risk for infection* *Risk for decreased cardiac output* *Sexual dysfunction* *Risk for impaired liver function*
Lack of self-care (hygiene, grooming), failure to care for basic health needs	*Ineffective health management* *Self-neglect* *Bathing self-care deficit* *Feeding self-care deficit* *Nonadherence to health care regimen*	Total preoccupation with and majority of time consumed by taking and withdrawing from drug	*Risk-prone health behavior* *Ineffective impulse control* *Ineffective coping* *Impaired social interaction* *Dysfunctional family processes: Substance dependence*
Feelings of hopelessness, inability to change, feelings of worthlessness, feeling that life has no meaning or future	*Hopelessness* *Spiritual distress* *Situational low self-esteem* *Chronic low self-esteem* *Risk for suicide*		

*No longer included in NANDA for 2015–2017, but remains applicable for people experiencing hallucinations, delusions, and disorders of thought since there are no alternative nursing diagnoses.

Herdman, T.H. (Ed.) *Nursing Diagnoses-Definitions and Classification 2015-2017.* Copyright 2014, 1994-2014 NANDA International. Used by arrangement with John Wiley & Sons Limited. In order to make safe and effective judgments using NANDA-I nursing diagnoses it is essential that nurses refer to the definitions and defining characteristics of the diagnoses listed in this work.

In addition, neuropsychological deficits have been associated with long-term alcohol abuse as well as with other substances (e.g., methamphetamines). Impairment has been found in abstract reasoning ability, ability to use feedback in learning new concepts, attention and concentration spans, cognitive flexibility, and subtle memory functions. These deficits undoubtedly will have an impact on the process of treatment.

At all levels of practice, the nurse can play an important role in the intervention process by recognizing the signs of substance abuse in both the patient and the family and by being familiar with the community resources in their area.

Communication Guidelines

Communication strategies are designed to address behaviors that almost all substance abusers have in common, including dysfunctional anger, manipulation, impulsiveness, and grandiosity. Perhaps the best approach is to focus on developing warm, accepting relationships with addicted individuals so they may hopefully feel safe enough to start looking at their problems with some degree of openness and honesty. It is important to communicate in culturally appropriate ways. Nurses with advanced training have had extensive supervision in dealing with behaviors that are manipulative, hostile, impulsive, and grandiose. Individuals who are addicted to a substance will use any form of diversion or defense mechanism to sidetrack personal introspection and suppress psychological pain and self-loathing.

Health Teaching and Health Promotion
Relapse Prevention

Relapses are common during a person's recovery because of the chronic relapsing nature of substance use disorders and have both physiological and behavioral components. The goal of relapse prevention is to help individuals identify their "trigger situations" so that periods of sobriety can be lengthened over time and lapses and relapses are not viewed as total failures. Recovery is a lifelong process. Refer to Box 19-5.

APPLYING THE ART

An Individual with Substance Use Disorder

Scenario

During our previous two encounters, 34-year-old Kristen had repeatedly insisted she would "quit using and take my med." Now Kristen, a single mom, has just learned that her own mother has gained legal custody of Kristen's three preschool-aged children related to charges of child neglect. Before each of her two psychiatric hospitalizations in the past year, Kristen had chosen heroin over taking her psychotropic medication, and that decision then impaired taking care of her children.

Therapeutic Goal

By the end of this interaction, Kristen will show progress toward taking responsibility for acting-out behavior and acknowledge that choosing heroin when feeling out of control compounds her losses.

Student-Patient Interaction	Thoughts, Communication Techniques, and Mental Health Nursing Concepts
Kristen: *(Glances my way and motions "come on" as she rapidly paces the hallway.)*	
Student's feelings: *I'm surprised Kristen did not even stop to greet me.*	
Student: "Kristen, I'm having trouble keeping up with you. You seem really upset."	I had learned in the report about Kristen losing custody of her children. Initially she had cried, but her tears quickly turned to angry pacing. I offer to walk with Kristen.
Student's feelings: *Addiction makes me angry. Kristen shows such promise and then abandons everything when heroin calls. I know that some people at school see nothing wrong with "recreational" use of drugs. I look around the addictions unit and see pain everywhere.*	
Kristen: "Yes, I'm upset. My so-called mother stole my kids! I never injured my kids. I just asked my 5-year-old whether he wanted new shoes or wanted Mommy to feel better. It's not my fault. So my mother gets upset and bought the shoes. She thinks she can buy their love."	Kristen uses projection, blaming her mother for the loss of her children. I remember that clients with addiction use "stinking-thinking," which includes denial ("I'd never hurt my kids"), rationalization ("It wasn't me who chose heroin over shoes"), and projection.

Student-Patient Interaction	Thoughts, Communication Techniques, and Mental Health Nursing Concepts
Student: "Kristen, I'm concerned with what is happening with you, but I'm having trouble keeping up. Could you walk a little slower, so I can hear you clearly?"	I think Kristen may be ambivalent, not sure if she can tolerate me or anyone.
Student's feelings: *I really am concerned with her welfare, even though I feel frustrated that she totally denies her addiction.*	
Kristen: *(Kicks a chair, across the room, and yells in my face.)* "Get up here then if you care so much!"	She is escalating. I see staff on their way to help. Anxiety is communicated interpersonally. I need to talk her down.
Student's feelings: *I feel unnerved by this incident and want this behavior to stop.*	Okay. I am okay. I need to mindfully breathe and stay calm and in charge of myself.
Student: "Kristen, stop." *(Louder voice, then quieter.)* "Take a deep breath." *(Quietly concerned, trying to make eye contact.)*	I set limits and give information.
Kristen: *(Meets my eyes. Sarcastically:)* "Here comes the cavalry!" *(Three staff approach, but wait as I speak.)*	Though Kristen uses sarcasm, she nonetheless responds to the staff's arrival by backing away from me.
Student's feelings: *I feel kind of honored that the staff trust that I am doing well enough to wait to see if they're needed.*	
Student: "Kristen, I trust that you and I can get through this." *(Pauses.)* "Thank you for calming down and backing away from me." *(Looking concerned.)* "I know you're upset. Please back up." *(She does.)* "Thank you, Kristen." *(Staff step back, carefully watching as Kristen slowly walks to the chair. Kristen uprights the chair she kicked over, and then we both sit down.)*	I offer self and use reflection. I treat Kristen with respect as well as model socially appropriate interactions by saying please and thank you to Kristen for calming down and backing up.

An Individual with Substance Use Disorder

Student-Patient Interaction	Thoughts, Communication Techniques, and Mental Health Nursing Concepts	Student-Patient Interaction	Thoughts, Communication Techniques, and Mental Health Nursing Concepts
Student's feelings: *I made it through this with no one hurt. I feel more confident, but I'm also really relieved that the staff responded so quickly. I know the staff were ready to intervene if needed.*		**Kristen:** *(Nods.)* "I am gone. No more Kristen. I forget all the hassles. Then it all crashes down. I lose everything. I've screwed up everything again."	In choosing heroin, she also chooses "no more Kristen." The drug erodes her self-esteem and even her sense of self.
Kristen: "I don't know what got into me. I never meant to hurt you."		**Student's feelings:** *Some days I think how far I still have to go to be a nurse. Then I think of Kristen's long, long road to reach a drug-free life.*	
Student: *(Making eye contact.)* "It's frightening to see angry behavior and have you screaming in my face. I'm okay now. How about you?"	I assess and also let Kristen know my feelings. Her choices affect others. I nonjudgmentally accept Kristen, but not the hurtful behavior.	**Student:** "Everything?"	I use restatement, encouraging her to go on.
Kristen: *(Nods.)* "I'm sorry. Sometimes I feel so out of control."		**Kristen:** "Myself, my kids." *(Starts to cry.)*	Kristen shows partial insight but so far avoids attending Narcotics Anonymous.
Student's feelings: *Kristen tries to make things right by apologizing and fixing the chair.*		**Student:** *(Leans forward, waiting quietly.)*	I use attending behavior.
Student: "You kicked the chair and screamed in my face, but you were also able to say 'sorry.'"	I name the observed acting-out behavior but also give support by saying, "You were able to. . ."	**Student's feelings:** *I want to fill the silences, but I contain my anxiety.*	
Kristen: "I meant the 'sorry.' I always mean it. Then the pressure builds and. . ." *(Points to the needle tracks on her arms.)*	She uses heroin as a dysfunctional way to cope with anxiety. Unfortunately the heroin compounds her problems.	**Kristen:** "I miss them so much! They deserve better than me. I need to go lie down." *(Begins to turn away.)*	Kristen uses withdrawal by physically retreating to her room.
Student: "So, when you feel out of control, maybe even overwhelmed, you turn to heroin?"	I am so thankful I have other ways to cope and people who care about me.	**Student's feelings:** *I feel badly for so much she has lost because of heroin.*	Kristen feels exhausted by all of the emotions she's experienced.
		Student: "Okay, I'll check with you after lunch."	I give information and accept Kristen's decision to leave in order to give her control and build trust.
		Student's feelings: *I need to debrief in a clinical conference. I'm feeling exhausted too.*	
		Kristen: *(Nods, walking toward her room.)*	

VIGNETTE

Bill, 20 years old and single, is transported to the emergency department in a coma. He is accompanied by his mother, with whom Bill lives in a small apartment. Bill had been in his room at home. When his mother was not able to rouse him, she dialed 911 for an ambulance. A syringe and some white powder were found next to Bill. His breathing is labored, and his pupils are constricted. Vital signs are taken: his blood pressure is 60/40 mm Hg and his pulse is 132 beats per minute. Bill's situation is determined to be life-threatening.

Bill's mother is extremely distressed, but she is able to report to the staff that Bill has a substance use problem and had been taking heroin for 6 months before entering a methadone maintenance program. It is decided at this point to administer a narcotic antagonist, and naloxone is given intramuscularly. After this, Bill's breathing improves, and he responds to verbal stimuli. His mother later tells staff that Bill has been in the methadone maintenance program for the past year but has not attended the program or received his methadone for the past week. At their urging, she calls the program, which arranges to send an outreach worker, Mr. Rodriguez, to talk to her and Bill. An appointment is made with Mr. Rodriguez for the following Monday. Mr. Rodriguez knows that Bill's future ultimately rests with Bill and talks to him regarding how he perceives his situation, where he wants to go, and what he thinks he needs to get there.

After talking to Bill and reviewing Bill's history, the health care team decides that a self-help, abstinence-oriented recovery program might be the most helpful treatment. Bill has not been taking drugs for a long time, he has a job, and he appears motivated. Naltrexone (Trexan) will be given in conjunction with relapse prevention training, and Bill will regularly attend Narcotics Anonymous meetings.

General strategies for relapse prevention are cognitive and behavioral: recognizing and learning how to avoid or cope with threats to recovery; changing lifestyle; learning how to participate fully in society without drugs; and securing help from other people, or social support. Box 19-5 identifies relapse prevention strategies.

Principles and Awareness of Co-Occurring or Dual Disorders

The nurse needs to be aware of clinical practice guidelines that have been developed through research involving individuals with

BOX 19-5   Relapse Prevention Strategies

Basics

1. Keep the program simple at first; 40% to 50% of patients who abuse substances have mild to moderate cognitive problems while actively using.
2. Review instructions with health team members.
3. Use a notebook and record important information and telephone numbers.

Skills

Take advantage of cognitive behavioral therapy to increase your coping skills. Identify which important life skills are needed:

1. Which situations do you have difficulty handling?
2. Which situations are you managing more effectively?
3. For which situations would you like to develop more skills to act more effectively?

Relapse Prevention Groups

Become a member of a relapse prevention group. These groups work on:

1. Rehearsing stressful situations using a variety of techniques.
2. Finding ways to deal with current problems or ones that are likely to arise as you become drug free.
3. Providing role models to help you make necessary life changes.

Enhancement of Personal Insight

Therapy—group, individual, or family—can help you gain insight and control over a variety of psychological concerns. For example:

1. What drives your addictions?
2. What constitutes a healthy supportive relationship?
3. How can you increase your sense of self and self-worth?
4. What does your addictive substance give you that you think you need and cannot find otherwise?

Adapted from Zerbe, K. J. (1999). *Women's mental health in primary care* (pp. 94–95). Philadelphia, Pa.: Saunders.

co-occurring or comorbid diagnoses. The following six principles are applicable in inpatient and outpatient settings:

1. Expect a patient to have at least one co-occurring disorder.
2. Treatment success is increased when providers are empathic, hopeful, and work as a team.
3. Both addiction programs and mental health programs need a dual focus, which requires appropriate training for staff.
4. The substance use disorder and the psychiatric disorder are considered primary and need simultaneous treatment.
5. The Recovery Paradigm stresses that recovery occurs in stages, and treatment should be matched to the patient's needs and level of motivation and engagement.
6. Outcomes must be individualized to support progress in small steps over a long period.

Psychotherapy and Therapeutic Modalities

Achieving sobriety is only the first step toward what will be a long and complex recovery. In order to be successful, the treatment program has to focus on many aspects of the person's life that have been altered because of addiction. Examples include the individual's medical, social, vocational, legal, and psychological needs.

Recent guiding principles for the Recovery Paradigm for addictions as well as other mental health disorders include the following crucial components (Brauser & Barclay, 2012):

- Emerges from hope
- Is person-driven
- Occurs through many pathways
- Is holistic

- Is supported by peers and allies
- Is supported through relationships and social networks
- Is culturally based
- Is supported by addressing trauma
- Involves the individual, family, and community
- Is based on respect

Psychotherapy assists patients in identifying and using alternative coping mechanisms to reduce reliance on substances. Eventually, psychotherapy can assist recovering addicts to become increasingly comfortable with sobriety.

An important aspect of recovery in Alcoholics Anonymous and a host of other recovery modalities is **spirituality.** Spirituality levels and spiritual practices are related to improved outcomes (Slaymaker, 2009). There is a strong body of evidence that spiritual and religious beliefs could impact the use and abuse of substances (Lucchetti & Lucchetti, 2014). Higher spiritual levels often correlate with a sense of purpose, gratitude, and forgiveness, which are all aspects of spirituality (Slaymaker, 2009).

The following therapies or components of therapies have been found to be effective for people on the road to recovery:

- **Cognitive behavioral therapy** (**CBT**). CBT helps patients to recognize and avoid old triggers to using substances, and offers behavioral strategies to cope with situations that are most likely to induce cravings and abuse of drugs.
- Motivational incentives. Much like token therapy, positive reinforcements (such as privileges) are provided when a patient participates in counseling sessions, maintains a therapeutic drug regimen, or remains drug-free, for example.
- Motivational interviewing. Provides strategies to evoke rapid and internally motivated change to stop drug use and facilitate treatment. "Motivational interviewing strategies help resolve ambivalence by asking evocative questions that elicit change in thinking and behavior." (Tan et al., 2015, p. 29). Motivational interviewing is guided by four principles evoking change: (a) expressing empathy, (b) developing discrepancies, (c) rolling with resistance, and (d) supporting self-efficacy (Tan et al., 2015, p. 29).
- **Group therapy.** Group therapy is an extremely important element of recovery for most individuals with substance use disorders.

Many critical issues arise during the first 6 months of sobriety. These include the following:

- Physical changes take place as the body adapts to functioning without substances.
- Numerous signals occur in the patient's internal and external world that previously were cues to drinking and drug use. Different responses to these cues need to be learned.
- Emotional responses (feelings that were formerly diluted by substance use) are now experienced at full strength. Because they are so unfamiliar, they can produce anxiety.
- Responses of family members and coworkers to the patient's new behavior must be addressed. Sobriety disrupts a system, and everyone in that system needs to adjust to the change.
- New coping skills must be developed to prevent relapse and ensure prolonged sobriety.

Whatever therapy a person chooses, it needs to be directive, open and honest, and caring. The therapeutic process involves teaching the patient to identify the physical and emotional changes that are occurring at the present time. Confidentiality must be maintained throughout therapy *except* when it conflicts with requirements for mandatory reporting in certain circumstances (e.g., child abuse, danger to self or others).

Self-Help Groups for Patients and 12-Step Programs

Alcoholics Anonymous (AA) is the prototype for all of the 12-step programs that were subsequently developed for many types of addiction.

Caring for Patients Experiencing Psychiatric Emergencies

Ann Wolbert Burgess, DNS, RNCS, FAAN
Pioneer in Forensic Nursing

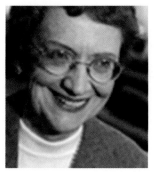

Dr. Ann Burgess is a clinical specialist in psychiatric nursing and sexual assault examiner who is an internationally recognized pioneer and researcher in the field of forensic nursing. Dr. Burgess is also a professor of psychiatric nursing at Boston College, where she teaches courses in victimology and forensic studies.

A prolific author, Dr. Burgess has authored textbooks in psychiatric nursing, crisis intervention, and the treatment of sexual assault victims and offenders. She has co-authored more than 150 professional articles and book chapters, including monographs for the U.S. Department of Justice on child sex trafficking and abduction, among other topics. Her research with victims of abuse began in 1972 when Dr. Burgess and Lynda Lytle Holmstrom cofounded one of the first crisis intervention programs for rape victims at Boston City Hospital. It was through their research that the diagnosis of rape-trauma syndrome established validity and has been admissible in court decisions. Her research has since included pornography, child eyewitnesses, ethics and sexual assault, exploitation of children, elder abuse, incarcerated women, and cyberstalking. Her work continues in the study of elder abuse in nursing homes, cyberstalking, and Internet sex crimes. She teaches courses in Victimology, Forensic Science, Forensic Mental Health, Case Studies in Forensics, and Forensic Science Lab.

In conjunction with the Federal Bureau of Investigation, Dr. Burgess studied serial perpetrators of sexual abuse and homicide, as well as the connection between child sexual abuse and delinquency, and future criminal behavior. She has frequently been an expert witness, including in high-profile cases, and her testimony has been described as "groundbreaking." She has received numerous awards, including Distinguished Professor (Uniform Services University), Inaugural Living Legend Award (American Psychiatric Nursing Association), and Inductee into the Sigma Theta Tau International Nurse Researcher Hall of Fame.

Crisis and Mass Disaster

Susan L. Frost, Chyllia D. Fosbre, Elizabeth M. Varcarolis

(e) http://evolve.elsevier.com/Varcarolis/essentials

KEY TERMS AND CONCEPTS

adventitious crisis/crisis of disaster, p. 326
crisis intervention, p. 325
Critical Incident Stress Debriefing
    (CISD), p. 330
maturational crisis, p. 326

National Incident Management
    System (NIMS), p. 326
phases of crisis, p. 327
primary care, p. 330
secondary care, p. 330

situational crisis, p. 326
tertiary care, p. 330
triage, p. 326

SELECTED CONCEPT: CRISIS

"The term crisis derives from the Greek words *krisis* (decision or judgment) and *krinein* (to decide)" (Harper, 2016).

A crisis is defined as a turning point at which time a crucial and decisive decision must be made. This crucial point can occur during an unstable political or economic situation or during a medical disease process, for example, with a turn toward either improvement or deterioration (Dictionary.com, 2015).

In real terms, a difficult and unsettling time in life provides a choice: to fall apart and decompensate, or to problem solve and grow through the process. Understanding this can help nurses to guide their patients experiencing crises toward positive and successful outcomes.
Retrieved from http://dictionary.reference.com/browse/crisis?s=t

Websites:
FEMA media library: www.fema.gov/media-library
National Incident Management System: www.fema.gov/national-incident-management-system
Video:
Red Cross assistance: www.youtube.com/user/AmRedCross
App:
Psychological first aid: https://play.google.com/store/apps/details?id=com.umnsph.pfa&hl=en

---

OBJECTIVES

1. **QSEN** Identify three principles of crisis intervention. How can these be used to provide **evidence-based care** to a patient in crisis?
2. Discuss what is meant by primary, secondary, and tertiary crisis intervention. Give a clinical example of the kinds of intervention needed for each phase of crisis intervention.
3. What is a triage team, why is it needed, and what are its responsibilities during an adventitious crisis/mass disaster?
4. **QSEN** Discuss the importance of **teamwork and collaboration** when identifying the initial needs of people facing an adventitious crisis/mass disaster.
5. **QSEN** Plan **patient-centered care** for a person who has experienced a situational crisis and identify the potential cognitive and emotional states likely to be present.
6. Identify the mental health safety needs that people may face if they do not obtain support during or after a crisis (refer also to Chapter 10).
7. Provide an overview of Critical Incident Stress Debriefing (CISD), including its purpose and process.

INTRODUCTION

A child is killed in a drive-by shooting; a husband announces to his wife of 30 years that he wants a divorce; tornadoes rip through the Southeast, leaving devastation, death, and homelessness in their wake. Each of these situations represents a crisis, an event that leaves individuals, families, or entire communities struggling to cope.

Everyone experiences crises. The experience itself is not pathological but rather represents a struggle for equilibrium and adjustment when problems seem unsolvable. A crisis presents both a danger to personality organization and a potential opportunity for personality growth. The outcome depends on how the individual, family, or community perceives and deals with the crisis and what outside supports are available.

Crises are acute, time-limited occurrences experienced as overwhelming emotional reactions to a stressful situational event, developmental event, or the person's perception of an event.

Crisis intervention is what nurses and other health professionals do to assist those in crisis to cope and assimilate the experience. Interventions need to be broad, creative, and flexible.

PREVALENCE AND COMORBIDITY

Many factors may limit a person's ability to problem solve or cope with stressful life events or situations. Some of these factors include the overwhelming presence of other stressful life events, mental illness, substance abuse, history of poor coping skills, diminished cognitive abilities, pre-existing physical health problems, limited social support network, and developmental or physical challenges. **Resiliency** learned through past successful experience with and resolution of crises and learned coping skills in the family are also germane factors.

THEORY

Erich Lindemann, an early crisis theorist, conducted a classic study in the 1940s on the grief reactions of close relatives of victims who died in the Coconut Grove nightclub fire in Boston. This study formed the foundation of crisis theory and clinical intervention. Lindemann was convinced that even though acute grief is a normal reaction to a distressing situation, preventive interventions could eliminate or decrease potentially devastating psychological consequences from the sustained effects of severe anxiety (Clark, 2015). He believed that the same interventions that were helpful in bereavement would prove helpful in dealing with other types of stressful events. Lindemann proposed a crisis intervention model as a major element of preventive psychiatry in the community.

In the early 1960s, Gerald Caplan (1964) further elaborated on crisis theory and intervention strategies. Since that time, our understanding of crisis and effective intervention has continued to be refined and enhanced by contemporary clinicians and theorists (James & Gilliland, 2013).

In 1961 a report of The Joint Commission on Mental Illness and Health addressed the need for community mental health centers throughout the country. This report stimulated the establishment of crisis services, which are now an important part of mental health programs in hospitals and communities.

Donna Aguilera and Janice Mesnick (1970) provided a framework for nurses for crisis assessment and intervention, which has grown in scope and practice. Aguilera (1998) continues to set a standard in the practice of crisis assessment and intervention.

Roberts's (2005) seven-stage model of crisis intervention is a more contemporary model useful in helping individuals who have suffered from an acute situational crisis as well as those who are diagnosed with acute stress disorder (Figure 20-1).

The devastating effects of the terrorist attacks on September 11, 2001, and the distressing lack of response to Hurricane Katrina in 2005 emphasized the need for crisis assessment and intervention by community mental health providers throughout the country to deal with all types of crises and the people who had been traumatized—victims, families, rescue workers, and observers (James & Gilliland, 2013; Kanel, 2015). Crisis theory defines specific aspects of crisis that are basic to crisis intervention (Box 20-1).

The ways of assessing crisis described in the following sections are derived from established crisis theory and constitute a sound knowledge base for the application of the nursing process to treatment of a patient in crisis. An understanding of three areas of crisis theory enables application of the nursing process: (1) types of crisis, (2) phases of crisis, and (3) aspects of crisis that have relevance for nurses.

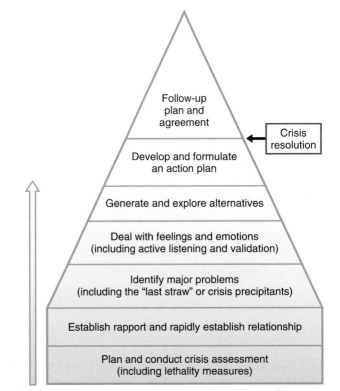

FIGURE 20-1 Roberts's seven-stage model of crisis intervention. *(From Roberts, A. R. (Ed.). (2005). Crisis intervention handbook [3rd ed.]. New York: Oxford University Press.)*

BOX 20-1   Foundation for Crisis Intervention

- A crisis is self-limiting and is usually resolved within 4 to 6 weeks.
- The goal of crisis intervention is to return the individual to the pre-crisis level of functioning. Resolution of a crisis may result in return to pre-crisis functioning, or to a higher or lower level.
- How a crisis is resolved is unique to the specific crisis, as well as how the individual responds and the interventions of others.
- During a crisis people are often more open to outside intervention than they are at times of stable functioning. When their normal coping methods have failed, the opportunity exists to learn different adaptive means of problem solving.
- A person in a crisis situation is assumed to be mentally healthy and to have functioned well in the past, but is presently in a state of disequilibrium.
- Crisis intervention deals with the person's present problem and resolution of the immediate crisis only, the "here and now." Addressing issues or needs not directly related to the crisis can take place at a later time, and referrals can be provided.
- A nurse must be willing to take a more directive role in intervention, especially initially, which is contrary to the usual therapeutic approach. As anxiety decreases, the patient can assist more in problem solving and planning.
- Early intervention increases the chances for a good prognosis.
- A patient is encouraged to set realistic goals and plan an intervention with the nurse that is focused on the current situation.

CLINICAL PICTURE

Types of Crises

There are three basic types of crises: (1) maturational, (2) situational, and (3) adventitious. It is possible to experience two types of crisis situations simultaneously. For example, a 51-year-old woman may be going through a midlife crisis (maturational) when her husband dies suddenly of cancer (situational). The presence of more than one crisis further taxes the individual's coping skills. People who have pre-existing mental health problems are prone to crisis and more vulnerable to its effects. Psychiatric emergencies are discussed in Chapters 21 through 24.

Maturational Crisis

A process of maturation through stages occurs throughout life. Erik Erikson (1902-1994) identified eight stages of growth and development in which specific tasks must be mastered to effectively reach maturity. Erikson postulated that each stage constitutes a maturational crisis.

When a person arrives at a new stage, previous coping styles are no longer appropriate, and new coping mechanisms have yet to be developed. For a time, the person is in transition. This often leads to increased anxiety, which may manifest as variations in the person's normal behavior until he or she establishes a new equilibrium. Marriage, the birth of a child, and retirement are examples of maturational crises.

Alcohol and drug addiction will interrupt an individual's progression through the maturational stages. As the patient escapes from stressors through the use of substances, he or she is not practicing communication and coping skills that contribute to maturity. When the individual gets clean and sober, he or she will discover that maturation has been halted at about the age that drugs or alcohol began to be used. The good news is that the developmental process can resume and progress through supportive treatment. If individuals do not receive treatment, their adult coping skills will be compromised. Successful resolution through maturational tasks leads to development of basic human qualities, according to Erikson. The way in which each developmental crisis is resolved becomes a foundation for the next stage, and thus affects the ability to pass through subsequent stages. If a person lacks adequate parenting, support systems, and role models, successful resolution of developmental tasks and emotional learning may be difficult or not occur. This can affect the individual throughout the life span. Conversely, successful progression sets the stage for continuing to adjust and mature. When a person is experiencing severe difficulty during a maturational crisis such as adjusting to retirement, professional intervention may be indicated.

VIGNETTE

A 65-year-old widower is asked to retire from his 40-year career as a city bus driver during company downsizing. Although he had been looking forward to the day when he could spend more time in leisure pursuits, he has spent the first year of retirement rarely leaving his house and becoming progressively more depressed. He finds himself feeling that he is worthless and not a contributing member of society. His sense of self has been damaged. Neighbors and friends encourage him to spend time with his grandchildren or volunteering, but he is unable to accept these activities as important or valuable, and rejects their suggestions or options. This gentleman is experiencing both a situational crisis (loss of job) and a maturational crisis (adjustment to retirement and a life stage).

Situational Crisis

A situational crisis arises from an external rather than an internal source and is frequently unanticipated. Examples of external situations that can precipitate a crisis include loss of a job, death of a loved one, unwanted pregnancy, a move, change of job, change in financial status, divorce, and severe physical or mental illness. Situational crises are somewhat common, and at least some of them will be experienced by all individuals during their lifetime. Response to the situation depends in part on the degree of support available from caring friends, family members, and groups; previous success in navigating life events (resiliency); and the overall physical and emotional health of the individual.

The stressful events that precipitate or constitute the crisis involve a loss or change that threatens a person's self-concept and self-esteem. Successful resolution of a crisis also depends on resolving the grief surrounding the loss.

Adventitious Crisis

An adventitious crisis (or crisis of disaster) is not a common part of everyday life. These types of crises are unplanned and tend to be catastrophic or violent in nature. Adventitious crises may result from natural disasters such as tsunamis, fires (Yarnell, Arizona where 19 firefighters lost their lives), hurricanes, flooding, or earthquakes (Japan); national disasters such as war (Iraq; Afghanistan); terrorist attacks, airplane or train crashes; or crimes of violence such as shootings in a public venue (numerous school shootings, rape, child abduction, or spousal abuse. The victim of an adventitious crisis can be an individual or a group. In situations such as a terrorist attack or other mass casualty incident (MCI), there are no guidelines for how to prepare or react (Portelli et al., 2011), and multiple organizations will be needed to respond and assist (Norman & Weiner, 2011). These types of incidents leave a wake of devastation in sheer number of casualties, roadways and utilities, and medical services, and overtax the abilities of first responders and governmental organizations. Victims are permanently changed and left to mourn, recover from the effects of severe trauma, and rebuild their lives and communities.

Recent studies confirm that natural and geophysical disasters taking place each year are noticeably skyrocketing. "Geophysical disasters include earthquakes, volcanoes, dry rock-falls, landslides, and avalanches. Climatic disasters are classified as floods, storms, tropical cyclones, local storms, heat/cold waves, droughts, and wildfires" (the Borgen Project, 2015).

Disaster Response

The National Incident Management System (NIMS) has been established to "provide a systematic approach to guide departments and agencies at all levels of government, nongovernmental organizations, and the private sector to work seamlessly" during disaster situations (Federal Emergency Management Agency [FEMA], 2015). The increase in natural disasters since 1990 has highlighted gaps and flaws in our ability to respond as a nation. There is still a need for better planning and clearer lines of communication among community, state, and federal disaster agencies in order to be effective in mitigating morbidity and mortality.

Efficient response to disaster requires a triage team and an ability to distribute casualties to the most appropriate facility for proper care. The underlying principle of triage is to separate those who need rapid medical care from those with more minor injuries. The triage process reduces the acute burden on medical facilities and finite resources, allowing responders to address the greatest number of casualties. The first needs during a disaster include rescue and evacuation efforts, food and shelter, medical attention, and physical safety (Roberts, 2005). Since 2002 the Department of Homeland Security has overseen a variety of agencies that focus on the safety and security of people during disasters in the United States. Nongovernmental agencies such as the International Medical Corps (IMC) and the American Red Cross (ARC) also provide medical care and relief efforts in the United States and around the world. After immediate needs are met, people need help to reconstruct and normalize their lives, including assistance with housing, jobs, and trauma counseling.

Victims of a disaster commonly experience *cognitive impairment* such as confusion, difficulty making decisions, and intrusive memories; *behavioral changes* such as using substances, difficulty functioning in work or daily routines, and sleep disturbances; or *emotional issues* such as fluctuating emotions, relationship strain, fear, or withdrawal. Posttraumatic stress disorder (PTSD) and depression are common diagnoses following a disaster. The importance of crisis intervention and psychological first aid in addition to physical healing cannot be overlooked. If individuals are not assisted early on, they are left vulnerable to stress-related disorders and chronic impairment. Disaster nursing is a growing field to address these needs. *Critical incident stress debriefing* is discussed later in this chapter.

Self-Care for Nurses

Nurses work with people in crisis frequently in all clinical settings—in the emergency department (ED) and on medical, surgical, psychiatric, obstetric, and pediatric units—and also experience crisis in their own lives and with family and friends. Nurses will encounter abused children, burn victims, gang shootings, loss of limbs, and numerous other painful situations with their patients. Nurses need to monitor their thoughts and feelings and learn to recognize when they need self-care, support, or professional help. This is especially true in the aftermath of a disaster or violence. Nurses often suppress their own feelings in order to effectively handle the immediate situation and may react at a later time with anxiety or shock.

When nurses are unaware of personal feelings or are suppressing them to cope, they may unknowingly prevent the expression of the painful feelings in their patients. Nurses have their own set of life experiences and wounds or sensitive areas. There may be times when the nurse, perhaps for personal reasons, feels he or she cannot deal effectively with a patient's situation. In these instances, it may be the more professional action to ask a colleague to care for the patient. It is crucial that supervision and guidance are available during the training process when working in the area of crisis intervention. The supervisor should be an experienced professional, such as a nurse counselor, nursing supervisor, or other health care expert. Nurses new to crisis intervention face common problems that must be addressed before they become comfortable and competent in the role. For example, nurses may set unrealistic goals and become frustrated or have difficulty dealing with certain issues such as suicide or child abuse. A number of schools of nursing now offer master's degrees in disaster nursing.

Even seasoned nurses and other health care workers exposed to disaster situations can become overwhelmed by witnessing catastrophic loss of human life or mass destruction of homes and communities. Disaster nurses need a supportive network and access to debriefing. Debriefing is an important step for staff in coming to terms with overwhelming violent or disastrous situations. Once the crisis is over, debriefing can help staff begin to heal themselves. Debriefing is discussed in more detail later in the chapter.

Phases of Crisis

Individuals experiencing a crisis will naturally use their normal coping skills to adapt. If the attempts are unsuccessful, the individual will try harder, and then expand his or her repertoire of coping skills. As efforts continue to be unsuccessful, the individual will become more frustrated, anxious, and disorganized. According to Erchul (2009) and Lowe and Galea (2015), Caplan identified four distinct phases of crisis:

- *Phase 1:* A person confronted by a conflict or problem that threatens the self-concept responds with increased feelings of anxiety. The increase in anxiety stimulates the use of problem-solving techniques and defense mechanisms in an effort to solve the problem and lower anxiety.
- *Phase 2:* If the threat persists and the usual defensive response fails, anxiety and discomfort continue to rise. Individual functioning becomes disorganized. Trial-and-error attempts at solving the problem and restoring a normal balance begin.
- *Phase 3:* If the trial-and-error attempts fail, anxiety can escalate to severe and panic levels, and the person mobilizes automatic relief behaviors such as withdrawal and flight. Some form of compromise such as redefining the situation or reevaluating needs may occur in this stage, in order to come to some sort of resolution. An example might be giving in on child visitation in order to end ongoing divorce proceedings.
- *Phase 4:* If the problem is not solved after considerable time and efforts, and coping skills have been ineffective and exhausted, anxiety can overwhelm the person. In this final phase of crisis, serious personality disorganization, depression, confusion, violence against others, or suicidal behavior can develop (Erchul, 2009; Lowe & Galea, 2015).

APPLICATION OF THE NURSING PROCESS

ASSESSMENT

A person's equilibrium may be adversely affected by an unrealistic or skewed perception of the precipitating crisis event, or inadequate supports and coping mechanisms (Aguilera, 1998; France, 2015). It is crucial to assess these factors when a crisis situation is evaluated. Data gained from the assessment can assist the nurse and the patient in setting realistic and meaningful goals as well as in planning possible solutions to the crisis situation.

After determining whether there is a need for safety interventions because of suicidal or homicidal ideation or gestures, the nurse then assesses three main areas: (1) the patient's perception of the event, (2) the patient's available supports, and (3) the patient's usual coping skills.

Assessing the Patient's Perception of the Precipitating Crisis Event

Whether an event is perceived as a crisis depends, in part, on the outlook and strengths of the patient. Having a physician's appointment canceled would be viewed as a trivial annoyance to most people, but for someone who is vulnerable from severe schizophrenia, the change could instigate a crisis and lead to worsening of symptoms (decompensation). Therefore it is important to view the event through the eyes of the patient. The nurse's initial task is to assess the individual's and possibly the family's perception of the problem. The more clearly the problem can be understood, the better the chance that an effective solution will be found and followed by the patient. Sample questions that may facilitate the assessment include the following:

- Has anything upsetting happened to you within the past few days or weeks?
- What was happening in your life before you started to feel this way?
- Has anything traumatic happened in the past that is still bothering you?
- What leads you to seek help now?
- Describe how you are feeling right now.
- How does this situation affect your life?
- How do you see this event as affecting your future?
- What would need to be done to resolve this situation?
- What kind of help do you think you need?

VIGNETTE

A 38-year-old female has gone back to nursing school as a second career. She is currently in her psychiatric nursing course. Normally an excellent student, she had missed two class periods and a clinical day and failed her last exam. Her psychiatric nursing professor calls her into the office to discuss the situation. The student begins crying and tells her professor that she had been dealing with the loss of her home due to a fire and subsequent relocation during the nursing program. Even with that severe stressor, she had been coping fairly well by keeping in touch with friends, doing yoga, praying, and focusing on her two young children. She had tried to see the relocation as a fresh start with some positive aspects. Recently, however, the student had been unable to complete her yoga routines due to muscle fatigue and pain. It was becoming difficult to even carry her textbooks to and from the car or blow-dry her hair. Her primary care provider (PCP) had initially diagnosed her with stress related to nursing school and the fire, but as the symptoms progressed she was given the diagnosis of myositis. Myositis is an autoimmune disorder that affects the muscles and produces symptoms of fatigue, weakness, and pain that may be progressive and at times fatal (United States National Library of Medicine, 2015). The student's normal coping mechanisms had failed with the addition of this diagnosis and she was now in a crisis situation. She was beginning to display relief behaviors such as panic attacks, and withdrawal from life events such as school or socializing with friends. These symptoms are indicative of phase 3 in the phases of crisis. This student is experiencing both situational (medical diagnosis, failing an exam) and adventitious (house fire) crises (Erchul, 2009; Lowe & Galea, 2015).

Assessing the Patient's Perception of the Precipitating Event(s)

The student spontaneously disclosed the upsetting events. What led her to seek help at this time was her failing coping mechanisms and an inability to function in nursing school, as well as the professor calling her in and expressing concern.

Nursing professor: "How are you feeling right now?"

Student: "So overwhelmed. I don't know much about myositis and I'm so scared. How can I finish school? How can I take care of my children? How bad is it going to get?"

Nursing professor: "What do you see happening in your life right now and in your future?"

Student: "I don't know if I can even finish school. The doctor says I need to start regular medication infusions, which will make me tired."

Nursing professor: "Let's talk and think through this situation together."

Assessing the Patient's Situational Supports

The patient's support systems are assessed to determine the resources available. Does the stressful event involve important people in the patient's life? Is the patient isolated from others, or are there family and friends who can provide vital support? Family and friends may be asked to aid the individual by offering material or emotional support. If these resources are not available, the nurse or other medical or psychiatric clinicians act as a temporary support system while relationships with individuals or groups in the community are established. The following are some sample questions to ask:

- With whom do you live?
- To whom do you talk when you feel overwhelmed?
- Who can you trust?
- Who is available to help you? Do you have a partner or significant other?
- Do you have spiritual beliefs or attend a place of worship?
- Do you attend school or any activities, groups, or clubs?
- During difficult times in the past, who was there to help you?

VIGNETTE

Assessing the Patient's Situational Supports

Nursing professor: "Do you have any family or friends to rely on right now?"

Student: "Yes, I have my best friend, my mother, and my yoga group."

Nursing professor: "Have you been talking to them?"

Student: "Not lately. I've been so overwhelmed and tired that I don't even want to answer my phone."

Nursing professor: "Would it be all right if we called some of your support people together, so that they can become more involved? You need to lean on these people again and not isolate so much."

Student: "Yes, I think that's good.... We can call my mom."

Once the student's mother was called, she agreed to come to the school and pick up her daughter. The student, professor, and mother all came up with a plan to help support the student during this time of crisis.

Assessing the Patient's Personal Coping Skills

In crisis situations it is important to evaluate the person's level of anxiety. Common coping mechanisms may be overeating, drinking, smoking, withdrawing, seeking out someone to talk to, crying, yelling, sleeping too much, praying, or engaging in other physical activity (Gil & Weinberg, 2015). The potential for suicide or homicide must be assessed. If the patient is thinking of harming self or someone else or is unable to take care of personal needs, hospitalization should be considered (Aguilera, 1998; France, 2015). Some sample questions to ask include the following:

- Have you thought of harming yourself?
- Have you been thinking that you don't want to be around or want to die? If yes, what have you been thinking about doing?
- Have you thought of hurting someone else? If yes, who do you want to harm? How would you do it?
- Do you have access to weapons?
- What do you usually do to feel better?
- Have you tried any of those coping mechanisms this time?
- What have you been doing to deal with the stress? How has it been working?

VIGNETTE

The nursing professor has learned that the student uses yoga, prayer, her children, and friends as support. She has been isolating and not using her support system, partly due to overwhelming stress and partly due to the muscle weakness related to the myositis.

Assessing the Student's Personal Coping Skills

Nursing professor: "Have you been thinking of killing yourself or anyone else?"

Student: "No, I would never do that. But I wish I could just disappear to get rid of all these problems."

Nursing professor: "What do you think we should do in this situation?"

Student's mother: "Maybe I could come and stay with her, or she could stay with me for a while. I could help with the children and driving her to doctor's appointments."

Student: (begins to cry) "That would be so wonderful, thank you!"

Nursing professor: "It sounds as if you need more information on your diagnosis as well. You are anticipating the worst scenario, and you need actual facts about what you will be dealing with."

The student, mother, and professor came up with the plan that the student would take a leave of absence from school for a semester, her mother would move in temporarily and help with the children, and the student would seek more information from her PCP about her new diagnosis. In addition, the professor gave the student a referral to a myositis website with information on support groups (www.myositis.org).

Assessment Guidelines
Crisis

1. Identify whether the patient's response to the crisis warrants psychiatric treatment or hospitalization (suicidal behavior, psychotic thinking, violent behavior, or inability to care for self).
2. Determine if the patient is able to identify the *precipitating event.*
3. Assess the patient's understanding of his or her present *situational supports.*
4. Identify the patient's usual *coping skills* and support system, and determine what coping mechanisms may help the present situation.
5. Determine whether there are certain religious or cultural beliefs that need to be considered in assessing and intervening in this person's crisis.
6. Assess whether this situation is one in which the patient needs primary intervention (education, environmental manipulation, new coping skills), secondary intervention (crisis intervention), or tertiary intervention (rehabilitation).

DIAGNOSIS

A person in crisis may exhibit various behaviors that indicate a number of problems. See Table 20-1 for signs and symptoms of people in crisis that may be used as a guide for developing nursing diagnoses.

Using the example in the preceding vignettes, the assessment of the nursing student's (1) perception of the precipitating event, (2) situational supports, and (3) personal coping skills provides the nurse with enough data to formulate two diagnoses and to work with the student in setting goals and planning interventions.

VIGNETTE

Nursing Diagnoses for the Student

The nurse formulates the following nursing diagnoses for the nursing student:
- *Ineffective coping* related to multiple stressors and new medical diagnosis, as evidenced by social withdrawal and missing school activities.
- *Powerlessness* related to overwhelming stress and physical weakness as evidenced by not using coping mechanisms and lack of knowledge about disease process.

OUTCOMES IDENTIFICATION

The planning of realistic patient outcomes is often done in conjunction with the patient or family. Realistic outcomes should consider the person's cultural and personal values. The nurse will document measurable goals that are realistic and include a time estimate (American Psychiatric Nurses Association [APNA] & International Society of Psychiatric–Mental Health Nurses [ISPN], 2013; Koenig, 2013). Without the patient's involvement, the outcome criteria may be irrelevant to the patient, leading to a lack of follow-through.

For example, a nurse who suggests that a woman leave her husband because he beats her may be surprised to find that the woman has different thoughts on what she wants as a solution. Thus goals and outcome criteria are always established with the patient and congruent with the patient's needs, values, and cultural expectations. They may also need to be reviewed and revised over the course of treatment.

VIGNETTE

The nursing student begins treatment in a community mental health clinic. She and her therapist set some outcome goals that were shared with the professor by the student.

1. She will attend a myositis support group meeting within 2 weeks.
2. She will learn more about her disorder within 2 weeks.
3. She will call one person daily for support.
4. She will take short walks and stop before reaching the point of fatigue.
5. She will begin medication treatments as prescribed by her PCP, scheduled to begin in 1 week.
6. She will attend counseling sessions every 2 weeks.
7. She will return to nursing school in the next semester.

PLANNING

Nurses may intervene through a variety of crisis intervention modalities, such as disaster nursing, mobile crisis units, group work, health education crisis prevention, victim outreach programs, and telephone hotlines. Crisis situations may present in any setting, including hospitals, clinics, and schools (as in the vignette).

The nurse may be involved in planning and intervention for an individual (physical abuse), for a group (students after a classmate's suicide), or for a community (train derailment). In planning after a crisis or disaster, the nurse considers the impact of the event on the patient's life. Is the patient able to continue functioning in work, school, or family responsibilities? Are others close to the patient also affected (Aguilera, 1998; France, 2015)? These questions will help guide immediate actions.

TABLE 20-1	Potential Nursing Diagnoses for Crisis Intervention	
Signs and Symptoms	**Nursing Diagnoses**
Overwhelmed, depressed, nothing in life worthwhile, hopeless, self-hatred	*Risk for self-directed violence* *Chronic low self-esteem* *Spiritual distress* *Hopelessness* *Impaired mood regulation* *Powerlessness*
Confused, highly anxious, incoherent, crying or sobbing, extreme emotional pain	*Anxiety (moderate, severe, panic)* *Acute confusion* *Labile, emotional control* *Sleep deprivation*
Difficulty with interpersonal relationships, isolated, has few or no social supports	*Social isolation* *Risk for loneliness* *Impaired social interaction*
Unable to function at work, school, or home; difficulty completing tasks or concentrating	*Ineffective coping* *Interrupted family processes* *Caregiver role strain*
Has experienced traumatic, emotionally overwhelming event or loss; feels depressed, insomnia, nightmares, crying, fear	*Risk for post-trauma syndrome* *Rape-trauma syndrome* *Dysfunctional grieving* *Chronic sorrow*

Herdman, T.H. (Ed.) *Nursing Diagnoses-Definitions and Classification 2015-2017.* Copyright 2014, 1994-2014 NANDA International. Used by arrangement with John Wiley & Sons Limited. In order to make safe and effective judgments using NANDA-I nursing diagnoses it is essential that nurses refer to the definitions and defining characteristics of the diagnoses listed in this work.

IMPLEMENTATION

Crisis intervention is within the scope of practice of all nurses. Initial goals are patient safety and anxiety reduction.

During the initial interview, the person in crisis first needs to gain a feeling of safety and security. Providing genuine support and hope will begin to decrease the patient's anxiety. The nurse assures the patient in crisis that help is available, and solutions will be found together. The patient's anxiety must be decreased to a level where the patient can hear and absorb potential ideas, before he or she will be able to actively problem solve with the nurse. False reassurance that everything will be all right damages trust and rapport. The nurse will need to be creative and flexible in helping the patient to solve his or her problems. Although the nurse helps guide the patient, it is important to remember that the patient is ultimately in charge of his or her own life and decision making.

See Table 20-2 for crisis interventions and corresponding rationales.

VIGNETTE

After making a plan with her counselor, the student decides that it is too soon to attend a support group. The patient's right to decide for herself is respected, and the plan is revised to include support groups at a later time.

TABLE 20-2   Interventions for Patients in Crisis

Intervention	Rationale
1. Assess for suicidal or homicidal thoughts or plans.	1. Safety is always the first consideration.
2. Take initial steps to make patient feel safe and to lower anxiety, such as providing a quiet environment, building rapport, and acknowledging the crisis experience.	2. When a person feels safe and anxiety decreases, the individual is able to participate in planning.
3. Listen carefully using eye contact and supportive body language, and provide feedback/summarization to ensure understanding.	3. When a person believes that someone is really listening, he or she feels cared about and supported, and this offers hope.
4. Crisis intervention calls for directive and creative approaches. Initially the nurse may make phone calls to help with tasks such as arranging babysitters and finding shelter.	4. Initially a person may be so confused and frightened that performing usual tasks is not possible.
5. Assess patient's support systems. Rally existing supports (with patient's permission) if patient is overwhelmed.	5. People in crisis are overwhelmed and nurses need to take a more active role.
6. Identify and mobilize needed social supports.	6. Patients may have concerns regarding shelter, child care, elder care, medical conditions, food, or psychiatric treatment and support.
7. Identify needed coping skills such as problem solving, relaxation, or job training.	7. Increasing existing coping skills and learning new ones can help with current crisis and minimize future effects.
8. Collaborate with the patient to plan interventions, as much as he or she is able at given time.	8. Patient's sense of control, self-esteem, and compliance with the plan are increased.
9. Plan regular follow-up to assess patient's progress through clinic appointments, phone calls, or home visits.	9. Plan is evaluated to see what works and what needs adjustment.

Levels of Nursing Care

There are three levels of nursing care in crisis intervention: (1) primary, (2) secondary, and (3) tertiary. As in all areas of nursing, psychotherapeutic nursing interventions in crisis are directed toward these three levels of care.

Primary

Primary care *promotes* mental health and reduces mental illness to decrease the incidence of crisis. On this level, the nurse can:

- Work with an individual to recognize potential problems by evaluating the stressful life events the person is experiencing.
- Teach individual specific coping skills, such as decision making, problem solving, assertiveness skills, meditation, and relaxation skills, to handle stressful events.
- Assist an individual in evaluating the timing or reduction of life changes to mitigate the effects of stress. This may involve working with the patient to plan environmental changes, make important interpersonal decisions, and rethink changes in occupational roles.

Secondary

Secondary care establishes intervention during an acute crisis to *prevent* prolonged anxiety from diminishing personal effectiveness and personality organization. The nurse's primary focus is to ensure the safety of the patient. After safety issues are addressed, the nurse works with the patient to assess the patient's problem, support systems, and coping styles. Desired goals are explored and interventions are planned. Secondary care lessens the time a person is mentally disabled during a crisis. Secondary-level care occurs in hospital units, emergency departments, clinics, or mental health centers.

Tertiary

Tertiary care provides support for those who have experienced a severe crisis and are now *recovering* from a disabling mental state. Social and community facilities that offer tertiary intervention include rehabilitation centers, sheltered workshops, day hospitals, and outpatient clinics. Primary goals are to facilitate optimal levels of functioning and prevent further emotional disruptions. People with severe and persistent mental problems are often extremely susceptible to crisis, and community outpatient and inpatient facilities provide the structured environment needed for recovery. See Chapter 27 for an extensive discussion of community supports for people with severe and persistent mental problems.

Critical Incident Stress Debriefing. Critical Incident Stress Debriefing (CISD) is an example of a tertiary intervention directed toward a group that has experienced a crisis such as a school shooting or natural disaster (Boscarino, 2015). A seven-phase group meeting offers individuals the opportunity to share their thoughts and feelings in a safe and controlled environment. The CISD process can also be effective for staff who have been exposed to a traumatic event such as a patient suicide (see Chapter 23) or community violence.

The phases of CISD are the following:

1. *Introductory phase*—The purpose and overview of the debriefing process is presented. Confidentiality is assured, team members are identified, and questions are answered.
2. *Fact phase*—Participants are assisted in discussing the facts of the incident from their perspectives.
3. *Thought phase*—All participants are asked to discuss their initial thoughts about the incident.
4. *Reaction phase*—Participants engage in freewheeling discussion about the worst, most painful parts of the incident.
5. *Symptom phase*—Participants describe cognitive, physical, emotional, or behavioral experiences at the time of the incident and ongoing.

6. *Teaching phase*—The feelings of the participants are affirmed. Guidance is provided regarding future symptoms and stress management techniques.

7. *Reentry phase*—The debriefing process thus far is reviewed, and any new topics are discussed. Team members provide encouragement and resources for additional help, and summarize the experience.

> **VIGNETTE**
>
> The student's ongoing counseling is really addressing all levels of crisis intervention: education and coping skills to prevent future problems, mitigation of symptom severity, and treatment of already established trauma related to the crisis.

EVALUATION

Ongoing evaluation will be performed until the crisis has resolved sufficiently to allow a return to normal pre-crisis functioning. As the patient's anxiety level reduces from severe to moderate to mild through successful interventions, the patient will need less support and return to independence. Appropriate questions to ask during evaluation(s) are as follows:

- Is the patient safe and feeling secure?
- Is the patient able to use existing coping skills? Has he or she learned new skills?
- Is the patient relying on his or her support system? Have new supports such as groups been put into place?
- Where is the patient's level of functioning in comparison to pre-crisis ability?
- Does the patient need or desire referrals for continued therapeutic work?

Once the process has been started, some patients may choose to explore other areas or issues in their lives.

> **VIGNETTE**
>
> During ongoing counseling, the patient's therapist makes evaluations of her functioning and support. At the end of 6 months, she has started meeting with a support group, her mother is able to move back to her own home, she is receiving regular medication and is feeling strong most of the time, and she is ready to return to nursing school. The patient's therapy frequency has gradually decreased to the current level of one session per month. It is decided to continue the monthly therapy sessions for support as the student returns to college.

APPLYING THE ART

A Person Needing Crisis Intervention

Scenario

A 30-year-old male has brought his young son to the free community health clinic for his allergy shot. The father asked the student nurse working at the clinic to spend some time talking. The father expressed gratitude for being able to obtain health care for his family, despite not having insurance. He also disclosed that his wife is pregnant, and he feels significant stress about caring for his family on a minimum wage income. He has been having regular panic attacks for the past few months.

Therapeutic Goal

By the end of this interaction, the father will have practiced a deep-breathing technique to use during panic attacks, and be aware of mental health resources available to those with a limited income.

Student-Patient Interaction	Thoughts, Communication Techniques, and Mental Health Nursing Concepts
Father: "How long can a person's heart pound really hard and fast before it gives out?"	I wonder where this is going and if I will know the answer to his question.
Student: "Are you experiencing this now?"	Exploring for more information.
Father: "No, just wondering because it happens a lot."	
Student: "Would you mind telling me what happens?"	Feeling relieved that his panic is not happening now.
Father: "I start breathing really fast, my heart pounds so I can feel it in my chest, and I feel really scared."	Using my assessment skills to observe his color, breathing, and affect.
Student: "How often does this happen and how long does it last?"	Continuing to explore, asking closed-ended questions for specific information.
Father: "Almost every day lately, and it lasts about a half an hour."	
Student: "What is happening before it starts?"	Hoping my instructor will come around before I run out of questions to ask.
Father: "It happens when I'm thinking about our bills and how I am going to take care of another baby."	

Student-Patient Interaction	Thoughts, Communication Techniques, and Mental Health Nursing Concepts
Student: "I can sure understand that, the worry about bills. Have you seen any type of health care provider for this yet?"	Clarifying symptoms
Father: "I've been to the emergency department a couple of times. They tell me my heart is fine and that it is just stress."	Offering self
	Relief that he has been examined and is okay
Student: "What have you tried to make it better?"	Leading question, open-ended question
Father: "I try to ignore it and watch TV. I did have some pills from the emergency department doctor but I ran out."	Teaching, modeling
Student: "Would you be willing to try a deep-breathing exercise that might help you calm down when you have a panic attack?"	Breathing out for one count longer than breathing in combats the tendency to hyperventilate. Deep breathing in this way balances the O_2-CO_2 ratio that is upset by hyperventilation.
Father: "Sure, anything!"	
Student: "Breathe along with me. Breathe in slowly and I will count one … two … three … hold it for a few seconds. Breathe out slowly and I will count one … two … three … four …. hold it for a few seconds." *(Student repeats this through several breathing cycles, also modeling by doing it along with the patient.)* "How do you feel now?"	Exploring
	Feeling really great that I was able to help him feel better!
Father: "Very calm and relaxed. Thank you, I think I can try that the next time."	Teaching, summarizing
Student: "Keep practicing even when you aren't anxious so you will be ready to use the breathing when you need it. May I give you some resources for counseling on a sliding income scale?"	Giving information
Father: "Yes, that would be appreciated."	

APPLYING EVIDENCE-BASED PRACTICE (EBP)

Problem A 62-year-old male presents to a mental health clinic after being referred by his endocrinologist for a psychiatric evaluation and treatment. The psychiatrist meets with the patient and his wife. The patient is tearful with symptoms of sadness, fatigue, oversleeping, and thoughts of wanting to die. He has recently lost a toe to surgery secondary to diabetes. Since the surgery his fear and anxiety have increased to a crippling level, and he is afraid of losing his entire leg. He also reports being overwhelmed by the number of doctor's appointments he must attend. The patient's fear is disproportionate to the realistic chance of a leg amputation and is interfering with his ability to manage his diabetes. His high anxiety contributes to forgetting his medications, refusing to exercise, and eating poorly for comfort.

EBP Assessment

A. **What do you already know from experience?** Patients display high anxiety in crisis situations that interferes with their ability to problem solve. Health care providers must take a more directive approach in care. The loss of one toe does not translate into a full leg amputation, especially with proper care. Patients may give up on taking care of themselves if they believe there is no hope or possibility of improvement.

B. **What does the literature say?** Diabetes is associated with increased diagnosis of anxiety disorders. A crisis depends on the patient's perception of the situation. The goal of crisis intervention is a return to at least pre-crisis functioning, but the result may also be a higher or lower level. Patients with depression are less likely to follow through with medical treatment.

C. **What does the patient want?** He wants to feel a lot less anxious and fearful. He wants assurance that his leg won't be amputated and that he will be able to function fully again. He wants to feel like himself and wanting to live again.

Plan The patient relies heavily on his wife, and she needs to be included for any plan to be successful. The patient is very spiritual so his minister was asked to visit for support with the patient's permission, and the patient was encouraged to use his usual coping method of prayer. Rapport is always important but was even more so in this case. The patient was prescribed medication temporarily to help reduce anxiety and depression to a level where other interventions would be possible. The patient was then open to diabetic education, which gave him more realistic information on the possibility of amputation and interventions he could do to prevent that. In the beginning stages, interventions were more directives, but as the crisis abated the patient was able to independently manage his care. The patient was assessed for suicidal thoughts. He was able to contract for safety not to harm himself, and was provided with a hotline number and regular counseling.

QSEN **QSEN Prelicensure Knowledge, Skills, and Attitudes (KSAs) Addressed:**

Team work and collaboration by interaction between endocrinologist and psychiatrist, as well as the inclusion of the patient's wife and spiritual leader.

Safety by assessing for suicidal thoughts and providing appropriate treatment and educating the patient to prevent further harm from uncontrolled diabetes.

From Conwell, W., Van Orden, K., & Caine, E. D. (2011). Suicide in older adults. *Psychiatric Clinics of North America, 34(2)*, 451–468; Kanel, K. (2015). *A guide to crisis intervention* (5th ed.). Stamford, Ct.: Cengage Learning; Koenig, H. G. (2013). *Spirituality in patient care.* West Conshohocken, Pa.: Templeton Press; Smith, K. J., Beland, M., Clyde, M., et al. (2012). Association of diabetes with anxiety: a systematic review and meta-analysis. *Journal of Psychosomatic Research, 74(2)*, 89–99.

KEY POINTS TO REMEMBER

- A crisis is not a pathological state but a struggle for emotional balance and equilibrium during a stressful event.
- Crises can lead to high anxiety, loss of functioning, and personality disorganization but can also offer opportunities for positive emotional growth and change.
- There are three types of crises: maturational (developmental stages), situational (external, unexpected), and adventitious (disaster, violence).
- The National Incident Management System (NIMS) is established to help governmental and private aid groups cooperate seamlessly during a crisis event.
- Situational and maturational crises are usually resolved within 4 to 6 weeks.
- Resolution of a crisis can result in a return to pre-crisis functioning, or a higher or lower level of functioning. The goal of crisis intervention is a return to at least pre-crisis functioning level.
- Social support and intervention can promote successful resolution.
- Crisis therapists take an active and directive approach with the patient in crisis, but as anxiety reduces the patient becomes more active in planning solutions.
- Crisis intervention is usually provided to a mentally healthy person who is temporarily overwhelmed and unable to function.
- A caring attitude, the ability to be flexible in planning care, the ability to listen, and an active approach help facilitate successful nursing interventions when a patient is in crisis.
- During a disaster, triage helps make the most efficient use of available and limited resources.
- Critical Incident Stress Debriefing (CISD) helps groups of patients or victims, as well as staff or first responders who have been exposed to a crisis situation, to make sense of the tragedy and to cope.

APPLYING CRITICAL JUDGMENT

1. List the three important areas of crisis assessment once safety concerns have been identified. Give examples of two questions in each area that need to be answered to assist in planning care.
2. A 21-year-old student shares with her college nurse that her father has lost his job. Her father has been drinking heavily for years and this trend has worsened since his job loss. The patient is having difficulty coping and wants to quit school due to stress and wanting to care for her ill mother and protect her siblings.
   A. How many different types of crises are occurring in this family? Discuss the crises from the viewpoint of each family member: the patient, father, mother, and siblings.
   B. If this family came for crisis counseling, what areas would you assess and what kinds of questions would you ask to evaluate individual and family needs (perception of events, coping styles, social supports)?
   C. Formulate some tentative goals you might set in conjunction with the family.
   D. Using informatics, identify by name appropriate referral agencies in your community that might be helpful to this family.
3. Identify an adventitious crisis that you have been aware of and that affected your life or emotions.
   A. If you are among a group of first responders, what would be the initial responsibility of your team?

B. Identify the needs of the people that would have to be met after safety concerns were addressed.

C. Discuss what could be done to protect against future mental health issues as a result of the disaster.

CHAPTER REVIEW QUESTIONS

1. While entering the building, an elementary school nurse observes a person in the distance emerging from a forest and approaching the school. The person is dressed in black from head to toe, wearing a backpack and carrying a long, narrow, dark object. Which action should the nurse take first?
   a. Move to a secure location
   b. Observe the intruder's features
   c. Take note of the intruder's location
   d. Activate the school code for an intruder

2. An adult has had long-term serious medical problems resulting in decreased libido and sexual performance. The adult's spouse privately says to the nurse, "I don't feel loved anymore. I feel sexual urges but my partner is not interested." Select the nurse's therapeutic response.
   a. "Tell me about how your partner shows love for you."
   b. "You're describing a scenario that many couples face."
   c. "Let's consider some other ways you can satisfy your needs."
   d. "I'm glad you are able to talk about and accept your situation."

3. The nurse in a high school meets with small groups of students the day after a school bus accident resulted in the death of five students. Which comment should the nurse use to begin the session?
   a. "Sometimes life is not fair. Yesterday's tragedy is an example of just how unfair it can be."
   b. "We're grateful that you are safe. Our discussion is to talk about feelings associated with yesterday's tragedy."
   c. "We've had a terrible loss. I also feel your pain. You need to talk about your feelings associated with the event."
   d. "Thank you for coming today. As school leaders, we know it is very important to respond to yesterday's tragedy."

4. A patient on an acute psychiatric unit removed the cap from the ceiling sprinkler, resulting in rapid flooding of the unit. After moving patients to a safe area, which action should the nurse take next?
   a. Conduct individual sessions with patients regarding the experience.
   b. Increase the volume of overhead music to distract patients from the event.
   c. Implement a psychomotor activity to reduce anxiety associated with the event.
   d. Lead a group session with patients to discuss feelings associated with the event.

5. Three weeks after being assaulted by a patient, a nurse develops headaches, insomnia, and gastrointestinal problems. The nurse has four absences from work over a 2-week period. Which action should the nursing supervisor employ?
   a. Refer the nurse for counseling and support.
   b. Ask the nurse about current personal problems.
   c. Direct the nurse to take paid vacation for the following week.
   d. Schedule the nurse for administrative tasks rather than patient care.

REFERENCES

Aguilera, D. C. (1998). *Crisis intervention: theory and methodology* (8th ed.). St Louis: Mosby.

Aguilera, D. C., & Mesnick, J. (1970). *Crisis intervention: theory and methodology*. St Louis: Mosby.

American Psychiatric Nurses Association (APNA) & International Society of Psychiatric–Mental Health Nurses (ISPN). (2013). *Psychiatric–mental health nursing: Scope and standards of practice* (2nd ed.). Washington, DC: American Psychiatric Nurses Association.

Borgen Project. (2015). Are Natural Disasters Increasing? Retrieved from http://borgenproject.org/natural-disasters-increasing/.

Boscarino, J. A. (2015). Community disasters, psychological trauma, and crisis intervention. *International Journal of Emergency Mental Health*, 17(1), 369–371.

Caplan, G. (1964). *Symptoms of preventive psychiatry*. New York: Basic Books.

Clark, E. J. (2015). *Bereavement care for the adult*. Retrieved from http://www.socialworkers.org/pressroom/events/911/clark.asp.

Erchul, W. P. (2009). Gerald Caplan (1917-2008). *American Psychologist*, 64(6), 563. Retrieved from http://psycnet.apa.org/index.cfm?fa=buy.optionToBuy&id=2009-13007-010.

Federal Emergency Management Agency (FEMA). (2015). *National Incident Management System*. Retrieved June 28, 2015, from https://www.fema.gov/national-incident-management-system.

France, K. (2015). *Crisis intervention: a handbook of immediate person-to-person help* (6th ed.). Springfield, Ill.: Thomas Books.

Fraser, R. (2010). *Why have natural disasters increased?* Retrieved May 3, 2011, from www.thetrumpet.com/?q=7020.5552.0.0.

Gil, S., & Weinberg, M. (2015). Coping strategies and internal resources of dispositional optimism and mastery as predictors of traumatic exposure and of PTSD symptoms: a prospective study. Psychological Trauma: Theory, Research, Practice, and Policy. *Advance online publication*.

Harper, D. (2016). *Crisis. Online Etymology Dictionary*. Retrieved from http://www.etymonline.com/index.php?term=crisis.

James, K. J., & Gilliland, B. E. (2013). *Crisis intervention strategies* (7th ed.). Pacific Grove, Calif.: Cengage Learning.

Kanel, K. (2015). *A guide to crisis intervention* (5th ed.). Stamford, Ct.: Cengage Learning.

Koenig, H. G. (2013). *Spirituality in patient care*. West Conshohocken, Pa.: Templeton Press.

Lowe, S. R., & Galea, S. (2015). The mental health consequences of mass shootings. *Trauma, Violence, & Abuse*, 1–21.

Norman, L. D., & Weiner, E. E. (2011). Emergency preparedness and response for today's world. In B. Cherry & S. R. Jacob (Eds.), *Contemporary nursing: issues, trends, & management* (5th ed.) (pp. 317–332). St Louis: Elsevier/Mosby.

Portelli, I., Fulmer, T., & Marr, M. C. (2011). Disaster nursing during terrorist events. In P. S. Cowen & S. Moorhead (Eds.), *Current issues in nursing* (8th ed.) (pp. 726–735). St Louis: Mosby/Elsevier.

Roberts, A. R. (2005). *Crisis intervention handbook: assessment, treatment, and research* (3rd ed.). New York: Oxford University Press.

United States National Library of Medicine. (2015). *Myositis*. Retrieved from http://www.nlm.nih.gov/medlineplus/myositis.html.

Child, Partner, and Elder Violence

Susan L. Frost, Chyllia D. Fosbre, Elizabeth M. Varcarolis

http://evolve.elsevier.com/Varcarolis/essentials

KEY TERMS AND CONCEPTS

Adult Protective Services (APS), p. 344
child abuse, p. 336
Child Protective Services (CPS), p. 334
cycle of violence, p. 340
elder abuse, p. 344

emotional abuse, p. 335
intimate partner violence (IPV), p. 338
neglect, p. 335
perpetrator, p. 334
physical abuse, p. 335

safety plan, p. 342
sexual abuse, p. 335
teen dating violence (TDV), p. 339
victim, p. 335

SELECTED CONCEPT: DOMESTIC VIOLENCE

Domestic violence (also called family abuse or battering) is prevalent among all ethnic, religious, age, social, and socioeconomic groups. Looking from the outside, a home that is meant to be a safe and secure haven can be an opulent mansion, a country ranch, a ghetto project apartment, and many other variations between. Although examples may be more visible in lower socioeconomic neighborhoods, violence and victimization in its various forms can occur in any of these homes. Types of abuse can include emotional, physical, sexual, neglect, spiritual, and economic. Domestic violence is most commonly thought of as occurring among family members, such as from a parent to a child, or between married partners. However, the concept of domestic violence expands to include abuse by trusted authority figures such as coaches, teachers, caregivers, and religious leaders. The wounds caused by domestic violence can leave lifelong scars and damage the fabric of society.

OBJECTIVES

1. Differentiate among the four types of family abuse and give two physical and behavioral indicators for each.
2. **QSEN** Consider how you would communicate with (a) a parent who is suspected of child abuse and (b) a woman who is the victim of intimate partner violence (IPV) while **providing patient-centered care.**
3. Identify at least five characteristics of an abusive parent.
4. Evaluate at least three red flags that a nurse might note during a family assessment that could indicate elder abuse is occurring.
5. **QSEN** Incorporating **evidence-based practice** and **safety**, identify the most dangerous time in a domestic violence relationship according to the literature.
6. **QSEN** Assess which various professions may be involved in **team work and collaboration** when obtaining forensic evidence from a child or adult victim of abuse.
7. **QSEN** Using a clinical example, describe the factors that make an older adult more vulnerable to abuse and in need of enhanced **safety** considerations.
8. **QSEN** Using **informatics**, research the resources and agencies related to elder abuse, intimate partner violence, and child abuse that are available in your community.

INTRODUCTION

Domestic violence (DV) is an extensive public health and criminal justice concern throughout the world. Domestic violence has widespread consequences that affect millions of women, men, and children. Physical and psychological trauma causes long-lasting damage in the lives of the victim, as well as in future generations and communities. In 2013 alone, 678,932 cases of child abuse were reported to Child Protective Services (CPS) in the United States (Centers for Disease Control and Prevention [CDC], 2015). The Adverse Childhood Experiences Study (ACES) found significant associations between childhood maltreatment and health and well-being in later life. The greater the number of adverse childhood events, the higher the probability of fetal death,

drug and alcohol use, depression and suicide attempts, heart disease, intimate partner violence, early sexual activity and adolescent pregnancy, sexually transmitted infections (STIs), and poorer quality of life (CDC, 2014a). Family violence is prevalent among all ethnic, religious, social, socioeconomic, and age groups. Although the home is supposed to be a safe and secure haven where love and support allow the family members to flourish, it can also be a place where abuse and fear occur. It doesn't matter whether the home is thousands of square feet and professionally decorated or a shanty in a poverty-stricken community; emotional, physical, sexual abuse, or neglect can and does occur (CDC, 2015). Domestic violence is normally thought of as occurring between more powerful (perpetrator) and less powerful (victim) family members. Examples of this include abuse of a child by a grandparent and abuse of a wife by a husband. However, this type of abuse can also be perpetrated by a trusted authority figure such as a religious leader, caregiver, health care provider, teacher, or coach.

The four main categories of abuse are emotional, physical, sexual, and neglect. All abuse can harm the victim's self-esteem and spirit, damaging the ability to form healthy emotional relationships and reach his or her full potential. Recovering from abuse takes a large amount of attention and energy that could better be spent in maturing and progressing through life. The nurse is often the first point of contact for people experiencing domestic violence and is in a position to contribute to prevention, detection, and effective intervention.

Emotional abuse includes name calling, excessive criticism, ignoring accomplishments, yelling and swearing, mocking, isolating, locking the victim in a room, threats and intimidation, and denying abuse and blaming the victim (Vancouver Coastal Health, 2015). *Physical abuse* usually encompasses emotional abuse in addition to physical damage. Types of physical abuse include kicking, hitting, pushing, choking, burning, using weapons, and shoving the victim down stairs. Some physical abuse victims are also tied or locked up for periods of time. Physical abuse has the potential for complications, including deformity, internal damage, fractures, and in some cases death. *Sexual abuse* can occur toward adults or child victims, and both genders can be victims of sexual abuse. Forms of sexual abuse include vaginal or anal rape, oral or manual touching, inappropriate comments, viewing the victim in the shower or while dressing, being made to watch or participate in pornography, and in the most extreme cases being sold to others for sexual favors.

Neglect as abuse includes the inconsistent provision of food, water, shelter, sanitation, or other basic needs. Neglect also encompasses lack of schooling, medical care, or supervision, and exposure to violent environments or substance abuse. Economic abuse is a form of neglect, when the dependent person has monetary resources withheld.

Sensitivity is required on the part of the nurse who suspects domestic violence. A person who feels judged or accused of wrongdoing is likely to become defensive, and any attempts to change coping strategies in the family will be thwarted. In some cases the nurse may be able to recommend resources for solving disagreements or methods of disciplining children, and in other cases the authorities may need to be contacted and involved. Avoiding inflammatory terms such as abuse while working with the individuals will be helpful in maintaining rapport and calm. While there are protective agencies for children and the elderly, in general most adults may choose to remain in an abusive situation. This can be difficult for the nurse to observe and accept. Potential indicators of domestic violence are listed in Box 21-1.

The victimization of lesbian, gay, bisexual, transgender, and questioning (LGBTQ) individuals is discussed in Chapter 22

THEORY

Most theories of intrafamily violence are related to psychology, sociology, or culture. Most conventional explanations of intrafamily violence are partial and incomplete. Experts advocate for a theory of violence that provides a comprehensive explanation that integrates interpersonal, institutional, and structural aspects of violence. Domestic violence is an extremely complex issue and is most likely an interaction of societal, cultural, and psychological factors and neurobiological influences.

Social Learning Theory

The social learning theory or the **intergenerational violence theory** of family violence purports that behaviors are developed through role modeling, identification, and human interaction (Sadock & Sadock, 2014; Widom & Wilson, 2015). According to this theory, a child who witnesses abuse or is abused in the family of origin learns that violence is an acceptable reaction to stress and internalizes the violent behavior as a behavioral norm. If the violent acting-out behaviors are condoned in the family or social milieu, the person is rewarded with a sense of power and control over others. Intergenerational abuse is considered a contributing factor in many cases of intimate partner violence (IPV), elder abuse, and child abuse.

Societal and Cultural Factors

According to the National Institute of Justice (NIJ, 2007), when abuse is seen in a family system, other correlates are often present, including:
- Poverty or unemployment
- Communities with inadequate resources and overcrowding
- Social isolation of families
- Substance abuse
- Early parenthood

The classic *frustration-aggression hypothesis* proposes that when frustration is high in response to negative societal situations, frustration may lead to aggression. Although these factors do correlate with family violence, they do not cause family violence, and not all frustrated individuals respond with violence. Some people respond to high levels of frustration with despair, depression, and resignation or attempts to change the situation (Sadock & Sadock, 2014; Widom & Wilson, 2015).

The *patriarchal theory* (often referred to as feminist theory) holds the view that male dominance in our political and economic structure exists to enforce the differential status of men over women. In many subcultures, women are viewed as the property of men, are subservient, and are kept relatively powerless in part through violence. The United Nations *Declaration on the Elimination of Violence Against Women* (General Assembly United Nations, 1993) states:

> Recognizing that violence against women is a manifestation of historically unequal power relations between men and women, which have led to domination of the discrimination against women by men and to the prevention of the full advancement of women, and that violence against women is one of the crucial social mechanisms by which women are forced into a subordinate position compared to men.

Psychological Factors

Psychological theories focus on the abuser having personality traits that cause abusive behaviors. According to psychological theories, the abuser has no control over his or her violence due to genetics, mental illness, or substance, and thus is not at fault. However, it is now known that many abusers and victims do not have a major mental illness according to the results of psychological testing, and many individuals with mental illness are not violent. The use of legal or illegal drugs coexists in some, but not all, cases of domestic violence (National Council on Alcoholism and Drug Abuse [NCADA], 2009; Smith & Fazel, 2015).

Some abusers argue that they are physically unable to control their anger and aggression, although this is not supported in all instances. For example, perpetrators of family violence may be able to refrain from

---

BOX 21-1   Indicators for Domestic Violence

- Recurrent emergency department (ED) visits for physical injuries attributed to being accident prone.
- Somatic symptoms reflecting anxiety or chronic stress, such as hyperventilation, gastrointestinal distress, hypertension, insomnia, nightmares, and even eczema or hair loss in some cases.
- Signs of depression, which can include sadness, tearfulness, sleep or appetite disturbance, irritability, loss of interest in usual activities, fatigue, and in some cases thoughts of suicide.

hitting their boss or a police officer, no matter how frustrated or angry they become. Abusers often plan where they will abuse their victims, at a time when no witnesses are around, and how to inflict damage without leaving visible marks or evidence (Minnesota Advocates for Human Rights [MAHR], 2006). See Chapter 24 for neurobiological factors related to violence and interventions for angry and aggressive patients.

Other psychological factors correlated with domestic violence include low self-esteem, poor problem-solving skills, history of impulsive behavior, hypersensitivity (sees self as victim), and narcissism (centers on self, lacks compassion for others). People with aggressive traits are usually immature, although some are able to present a mature facade to the outside world.

CHILD ABUSE

A report of child abuse is made every 10 seconds, and almost five children die every day as a result of child abuse (Childhelp, 2011). Child abuse takes place when a child is harmed physically, psychologically, sexually,

or through acts of neglect. It is generally believed that the number of child abuse cases is grossly underreported. The vast majority, about 80%, of deaths related to child abuse are in children under the age of 4, with the largest number being infants (CDC, 2015). Parents are the perpetrators in most cases, although siblings can also abuse one another. Each state is responsible for providing its own definition of child abuse. These definitions must meet the minimum standards established through the Child Abuse Prevention and Treatment Act (CAPTA), which read:

> Any recent act or failure to act on the part of a parent or caregiver, which results in death, serious physical harm, sexual abuse or exploitation, or act of failure to act which presents an immediate risk of serious harm (U.S. Department of Health and Human Services [USDHHS], 2010, p. 6).

Generally, most references recognize four different types of abuse: physical, emotional, sexual, and neglect. Table 21-1 provides definitions of different types of child abuse, as well as physical and behavioral indicators.

TABLE 21-1	**Types of Child Abuse and Physical and Behavioral Indicators**	
Type of Abuse	**Physical Indicators**	**Behavioral Indicators**
Physical Abuse		
Intentional physical injury inflicted by a caregiver	Bruises, wounds, injuries in differing stages of healing Patterning of abuse, such as marks in shapes such as coat hangers or cigarette burns, or hidden under clothing where they are harder to discern Bald patches on scalp Subdural hematoma (child younger than 2 years) Retinal hemorrhage	Excessive fear of parents or constant effort to please Wary of adult contact Nightmares or anxiety Obvious attempts to hide bruises or injuries Withdrawn, depressed, aggressive, or disruptive behavior at home or school Regressive behavior
Neglect		
Failure to provide for the child's basic needs	*Physical neglect:* Malnourished Underweight, poor growth pattern Inadequately supervised Poor hygiene Unattended physical problems Inappropriate dress *Educational neglect:* School problems or failure Not enrolled in mandatory school for age of child	Soiled clothing, poor hygiene Begging, stealing food Emaciated or has distended belly Arrives early or stays late at school Psychosomatic complaints Delinquency Alcohol or drug abuse Chronic truancy Special educational needs not being attended
Sexual Abuse		
Sexual abuse perpetrated by family or nonfamily member. Some types include exhibitionism; touching; oral, anal, or vaginal penetration; being forced to watch sex acts or pornography. In extreme cases, being sold for sexual favors.	Difficulty in walking or sitting Itching in private areas Urinary tract infections, painful urination Torn, stained, or bloody underclothing Bruises or bleeding in external genitalia, vaginal, or anal areas Sexually transmitted infection, especially in preteens Swollen private areas or discharge Objects or liquid in vagina, rectum, or urethra	Mistrust of adults Abnormal or distorted view of sex Advanced or unusual sexual behavior or knowledge for age Phobias: fear of the dark, men, strangers, leaving the house Delinquency or running away Self-injury or suicidal thoughts or behaviors Mental disorders may develop, including posttraumatic stress disorder, depression, dissociative disorder, eating disorders, conduct disorders, mood swings, and anxiety.
Emotional or Psychological Abuse		
Behaviors that convey to the child that he or she is worthless, flawed, unloved, or unwanted. These include constant criticism, threats, insults, yelling, ignoring, favoritism, and harsh demands.	Speech disorders Lag in physical development	Difficulty in learning and living up to potential Lack of self-confidence Inappropriate adultlike behavior or infantile behavior Poor social skills Dramatic behavior changes such as aggressiveness, drug use, change in friends or clothing, self-harm behaviors, compulsiveness, and a needy pursuit of attention.

The most commonly reported type of abuse is neglect, occurring in 59% of cases, with the next most common being physical abuse (USDHHS, 2009). Research conducted by the CDC (2015) states that one in four girls and one in six boys may be sexually abused before adulthood. More than one type of abuse can co-occur, and emotional abuse is always part of the picture.

An interesting problem in industrialized countries, where financial resources have increased and family size has decreased, is overindulgence of children. Overindulgence can be considered a type of neglect that can result in social and emotional impairment, lack of empathy, and physical problems related to inactivity and obesity. In years of economic recession, stress increases the incidence of child, partner, and elder abuse. Another modern form of emotional abuse is the public shaming of children by posting photos or descriptions on social media.

VIGNETTE: CHILD ABUSE

A 6-year-old Native American male falls on the school playground and goes to the school nurse to have minor abrasions on his knees cleansed and bandaged. While the nurse is taking care of him, she lightly touches his back and he quickly moves away from her. The nurse asks if it hurt and he quietly nods "yes." She asks a school counselor to come in and has the young boy pull up his shirt. There is a visible handprint and several welts across his back. The boy quickly starts to say he was bad and it was his fault for disrespecting the tribal elders, and that his father was teaching him. The nurse and school counselor know they are mandated reporters. The counselor stays with the child for support while the school nurse calls Child Protective Services (CPS) so an investigation can be done regarding signs of physical abuse. The counselor and nurse anticipate that the investigation may be taken over by tribal council leaders, and make sure that CPS is aware that the child is Native American.

APPLICATION OF THE NURSING PROCESS

ASSESSMENT

Child

Often the abused child appears timid or fearful of a parent or caregiver. The child may be disheveled or have a history of absenteeism from school. Even if a parent is abusive, children are very loyal to that parent. They may resist telling about the abuse out of attachment to the parent or fear of retribution later when they are alone. Children tend to believe that the abuse is their fault. If they had caused less trouble, or behaved better, they wouldn't have deserved the punishment or abuse. In general, parents are present for any questioning or examining of their child. In the case of suspected child abuse, however, after the initial interview with the parents, the child should be seen alone, giving him or her a chance to disclose mistreatment. Abusive parents will often find many excuses not to leave their child alone with the nurse. Children should be questioned gently and not pressured and may be better able to express themselves through drawing or playing with dolls. Do not suggest answers to the child. Reassure the child that the situation is not his or her fault. Sitting next to the child may feel supportive. Remember that children are concrete in their thinking. For example, if you ask a child if someone hit him or her, the child may say "no" because the injury occurred through being kicked, not hit. Open-ended questions such as "How did that happen to you?" "Where do you go after school?" or "What happens when you do something wrong?" may elicit a better response. Do not promise the child that everything said is confidential, as abuse must be reported. Avoid showing shock, no matter what the child discloses. The child's privacy must be maintained, including not forcing them to undress or be examined in front of a group (Ney, 2015).

Parent or Caregiver

Abusing parents vary by degrees of intelligence and education and come from all backgrounds. Specific characteristics are often found either singly or in combination among parents who abuse their children, including a history of being abused themselves, low self-esteem, social isolation or suspiciousness, drug or alcohol abuse, and rigid expectations of the child's behavior (Box 21-2). In interviewing a parent or guardian suspected of child abuse, ensure a private environment. Be direct, understanding, and professional. Be honest about the necessity to report the suspected abuse to CPS. Do not display horror, anger, or a judgmental attitude toward the parent. Again, open-ended questions will elicit the best, most descriptive response. Examples include: "What arrangements do you make when you have to leave your child alone?" "How do you punish your child?" "How do you get your infant to stop crying?" "How are things at home?"

DIAGNOSES AND OUTCOMES IDENTIFICATION

The most immediate concern is to ensure the child's safety and well-being. Primary nursing diagnoses that can be used to plan care in suspected child abuse include *Safety and risk for injury*. Other nursing diagnoses might include *Disabled family coping*, *Post-trauma syndrome*, *Anxiety*, *Fear*, *Impaired parenting*, *Acute pain*, *Delayed growth and development*, and *Imbalanced nutrition: less than body requirements*. The outcome of the care plan is that the physical, sexual, or emotional abuse or neglect has discontinued. Short-term goals could include receiving medical care within 1 hour, notification of the proper authorities, and maintaining the child's safety until appropriate arrangements have been made.

BOX 21-2   Characteristics of Abusive Parents

- A history of violence, neglect, or emotional deprivation as a child
- Low self-esteem, feelings of worthlessness, depression
- Poor coping skills
- Social isolation, may be suspicious of others
- Few or no friends, little or no involvement in social or community activities
- Involved in a crisis situation such as unemployment, divorce, financial difficulties, abusive relationship
- Rigid, unrealistic expectations of child's behavior
- Frequently uses harsh punishment
- History of severe mental illness, such as schizophrenia
- Violent temper outbursts
- Looks to child for satisfaction of needs for love, support, and reassurance
- Projects blame onto the child for his or her problems
- Lack of effective parenting skills
- Inability to seek help from others
- Perceives the child as bad or evil
- History of drug or alcohol abuse
- Feels little or no control over life
- Low tolerance for frustration
- Poor impulse control

Adapted from Boos, S. C., & Endon, E. E. (2015). *Physical abuse in children: diagnostic evaluation and management*. In J. F. Wiley (Ed.), UpToDate. Retrieved from http://www.UpToDate.com

IMPLEMENTATION

When child abuse is suspected, persons in authority, including nurses, teachers, spiritual leaders, coaches, counselors, and child care providers, are *legally* responsible for reporting to the appropriate child protective agency. Each state mandates that a report must be filed when suspected abuse or neglect is encountered. It is not necessary to have proof of the abuse. If there is a suspicion or if the child says something is happening, that is enough grounds to report. It is then up to the CPS agency to investigate and make a determination. For more on reporting child abuse and neglect, go to www.childwelfare.gov/ or call 1-800-422-4453.

The emergency department (ED) is usually where first contact is made with the abused child and family. Table 21-2 includes a list of nursing intervention guidelines to be used with the abused child and his or her family, with rationales for the interventions. The physician or nurse practitioner caring for an abused child should incorporate help from a variety of sources to ensure that the child is safe and cared for and that the family receives supportive help. Resources include the hospital social work department, mental health agencies, substance abuse treatment centers, and parenting classes. Counseling and supportive services have been shown to improve life outcomes for abused children. Just the presence of one supportive person and the act of being believed make a significant difference in the child's self-esteem and future success. Psychological and behavioral health was improved in 71% of children who participated in therapeutic interventions compared to those who did not (Trask et al., 2011).

Many factors exist in cases of child abuse, often including substance abuse by the parent(s). Additional factors that increase the rate of child abuse include single or teen parenthood, mental illness, a child with a medical or psychological disorder or handicap, and abuse of the parent in childhood or adult relationships.

Societal risk factors also play an important role. Poverty is thought to be among the most frequently and persistently noted risk factors for child abuse. Parents working full-time jobs for minimum wage are unable to cover the basic necessities for their families (Cowen & Cowen, 2011). In times of a downward economy such as that experienced in recent years, more families are affected and struggling (National Center for Children in Poverty, 2009). Families that live in lower socioeconomic neighborhoods lack health care and social support and are at risk for experiencing or witnessing violent crimes. A trend in today's society is that families are often separated by distance, even living across the country from each other. This type of family structure lacks the support of an extended family to help with child-rearing or the sharing of resources (National Center for Children in Poverty, 2009).

Early diagnosis of actual or potential child abuse and intervention correlates with a more positive prognosis. Interventions can include strengthening family ties and linking the family with community supports; coordinating services such as parenting skills, anger management, and coping skills; enhancing community awareness of child abuse and healthy parenting concepts; and providing emergency supports such as food and shelter for families.

INTIMATE PARTNER VIOLENCE

Intimate partner violence (IPV) is defined as "a pattern of assault and course of behaviors that may include physical injury, psychological abuse, sexual assault, progressive social isolation, stalking, deprivation, intimidation and threats" between current or former partners of an intimate relationship, regardless of gender or marital status (CDC, 2014b).

The majority of the victims of reported domestic violence are women (NIJ, 2015). Domestic violence is the number one cause of emergency department visits by women and is the primary cause of homelessness in women. However, a growing body of research is revealing the prevalence

---

TABLE 21-2   Interventions for the Abused Child and the Child's Family

Intervention	Rationale
1. Adopt a nonthreatening, nonjudgmental relationship with parents.	1. If parents feel judged, they may become defensive and leave without receiving care for the child.
2. Understand that the child does not want to betray his or her parents.	2. Even in an intolerable situation, the parents are the only security the child knows.
3. Provide a complete physical assessment of the child.	3. Allows health care worker to provide care and document evidence.
4. Use of dolls or drawing might help the child to tell how the injury or accident happened.	4. Young children might not have the vocabulary to explain what happened, or might be afraid of punishment.
Forensic Issues	
1. Be aware of your agency's and state's policy in reporting child abuse. Contact supervisor or social worker to implement appropriate reporting.	1. Health care workers are mandated to report any cases of suspected or actual child abuse. Suspicion or verbalization is enough to report; you do not have to prove the abuse happened.
2. Ensure that proper procedures are followed and evidence is collected.	2. Appropriate evidence helps protect the child's welfare.
3. Keep accurate and detailed records of incident: • Exact words of what the child or others involved say happened • A body map to indicate size, color, shape, areas, and types of injuries with explanation • Physical evidence, when possible, of sexual abuse Use of photos can be helpful. Check hospital policy. Police may be involved for photographing injuries.	3. Accurate records could help ensure the child's safety and supports the legal process.
4. Forensic examination of the sexually assaulted child should be conducted according to specific protocols: • Provided by law enforcement agencies • Follows state guidelines (www.childwelfare.gov)	4. Proper collection, handling, and storage of forensic specimens are crucial. Whenever available, a trained team or individual should perform this type of evidence collection for accuracy and sensitivity to the child victim.

Adapted from Varcarolis, E. M. (2015). *Manual of psychiatric nursing care plans: diagnoses, clinical tools, and psychopharmacology* (5th ed.). St Louis: Elsevier.

and significance of domestic violence by women against men (American Psychological Association [APA], 2011). Actual statistics are hard to ascertain since there is substantial underreporting of IPV by women and even more underreporting by men. Although the exact numbers of abused domestic partners are not known, it is estimated that up to 22% to 39% of all U.S. women experience physical assault by an intimate partner, with the worldwide rate reaching 69% (Weil, 2016; U.S. Preventive Services Task Force, 2013). Domestic violence by an intimate partner is the leading cause of female homicides and birth defects during pregnancy (CDC, 2014b). Attempting to leave the abuser was the precipitating factor in 45% of female murders by their intimate partner (Violence Policy Center, 2013). Because of this, it is especially important to educate women on being careful when planning to leave their abusers. Some hospitals provide cards with DV resources that are small enough to fit in a shoe, so as not to raise the suspicion of the abuser. Of the 2340 IPV-related deaths in 2007, 70% were females and 30% were males (CDC, 2014b). Domestic violence in intimate partnerships occurs in heterosexual, homosexual, bisexual, and transgendered individuals. Teen dating violence (TDV) is a disturbing trend, with approximately 25% to 33% of adolescents reporting verbal, physical, emotional, or sexual abuse from a dating partner each year (CDC, 2014c). Although women are usually the victims in adult partner abuse, in teen relationships girls and boys abuse each other about equally (CDC, 2014c). Violence is perpetrated by both past and current partners. About a quarter of all young women in high school and college have been physically or sexually abused by a dating partner (CDC, 2014c).

Teen abuse takes many forms, such as extreme possessiveness and jealousy, physical stalking or cyberstalking, manipulation and control of one's partner, demeaning one's partner in front of friends, threatening to commit suicide, or forced intimacy or sex. Depression, posttraumatic stress disorder (PSTD), anxiety disorders, and suicidal thoughts and attempts are potential sequelae to battering for all age groups (The President of the United States of America, 2016).

An abusive relationship is all about instilling fear and wanting to have power and control in the relationship. Anger is one way that the abuser tries to gain authority. He (or she) may also turn to physical, sexual, or psychological violence to maintain control. Psychological abuse may include threats to harm a child, pet, or loved one or displaying weapons. Violence against an intimate partner has effects on not only the victim, but children residing in the home as well. The children may experience feelings of guilt, depression, anxiety, behavioral acting-out including aggression, somatic symptoms, anxiety, nightmares, detachment from school and friends, and alcohol or drug abuse. In 30% to 61% of IPV cases, the children are also abused (Guy et al., 2013) and are unfortunately likely to carry the legacy forward into their adult lives as either the abuser or the abused.

VIGNETTE: TEEN DATING VIOLENCE/IPV

A 16-year-old male is brought to the emergency department after passing out at school. The boy admits to taking a handful of unknown pills he bought from another student. When discussing what had happened, the boy explains that 3 days ago his girlfriend posted a message on social media saying that she was breaking up with him because he was a terrible kisser, a horrible date, and worthless as a boyfriend and human being. Since the message was posted, classmates had continued to call him names and his friends were avoiding him. He tried to tell his parents, who just told him to "handle it like an adult" and "suck it up."

The Battered Partner

Women do not ask to be beaten, nor do they enjoy being battered. The battered partner lives in terror of the next beating. Women do not usually initiate the violence but may retaliate in self-defense. According to

Stockl et al., (2013), 67% to 75% of intimate partner homicides were associated with a reported history of intimate partner violence against the female.

The abused woman is often the subject of extreme and irrational jealousy, isolation, and verbal as well as physical abuse. Feelings of powerlessness and low self-esteem are common. After constant belittlement, insults, and degradation, the abused becomes so psychologically destroyed that she (or he) begins to believe her abuser's insults. This phenomenon is also seen in other cases of abuse, such as slavery or prisoners or war. Victims of abuse in general may eventually be brainwashed to the abuser's way of thinking and develop self-hatred. Because of the physical or sexual abuse and threats, the abused lives in a world of terror and fear for her life and the lives of her children. Isolation from family and friends, or even to a remote community, helps to perpetuate the abuse without detection or intervention. The violence and pain that exist inside the home remain secret through threats. Table 21-3 lists characteristics of the abused woman and violent partner.

TABLE 21-3   Behavioral Characteristics of Intimate Partner Violence

Characteristics of Violent Partner	Characteristics of Battered Partner
Denial and Blame: Denies that abuse occurs, shifts responsibility of abuse to partner. Makes statements that the victim caused the abuse, caused the abuser to react that way.	Eventually believes that if she does or says the right thing, the abuse will stop. If she does not do anything wrong, abuse will not occur. May be re-creating patterns from abuse during childhood that are familiar.
Emotional Abuse: Belittles, criticizes, insults, uses name calling, undermines	Becomes psychologically devastated and begins to believe partner's words. Lowered self-esteem. Unhealthy bond with the abuser.
Control through Isolation: Limits family or friends, controls activities and social events, tracks time or mileage on car and activities, stalks at work, takes to and from work or school, may demand permission to leave house	Gradually loses sight of personal boundaries for self, children. Over time becomes unable to accurately assess the situation without validation from a supportive network.
Control through Intimidation: Uses behaviors to instill fear, such as vile threats, breaking things, destroying property, abusing pets, displaying weapons, threatening children, threatening homicide or suicide, and increasing physical, sexual, or psychological abuse	Results in constant fear and terror that becomes cumulative and oppressive; contemplates suicide, contemplates homicide, occasionally completes suicide or homicide in self-defense. Posttraumatic stress symptoms develop.
Control through Economic Abuse: Controls money, makes partner account for all money spent; if partner works, calls excessively, forces partner to miss work; refuses to share money	Economic and emotional dependency may result in depression, high risk for secret drug or alcohol abuse. If she works, frequently loses job due to partner stalking and harassing. Is unable to save money to leave.
Control through Power: Makes all decisions, defines role in the relationship, treats spouse like a servant, takes charge of the home and social life	Continues to lose sense of self, becomes unsure of who she is, defines self in terms of partner, children, job, others; lacks personal power.

The Batterer

Violence is a learned behavior used by a person to control others. Frequently, violent partners were raised in a home where they themselves were beaten or where they witnessed parental beatings. Abusing someone less powerful or more vulnerable helps the violent partner feel more in control and powerful. Batterers may appear well adjusted from the outside but usually have only superficial relationships with others. They are extremely possessive, are pathologically jealous, believe in male supremacy in relationships, and often have a drug or alcohol problem, which is not a cause of the abuse but often an excuse or something that exacerbates the abuse. Without professional treatment, the behaviors almost always continue to escalate.

Cycle of Violence

Abuse toward a person in a partner relationship is not merely an exchange of blows on an isolated occasion, but rather a process that increases in intensity and escalates over time. The abusive relationship may start subtly. It may start by the abuser being critical of the way the partner dresses, disciplines the kids, or cares for the home. Or the abuser becomes unreasonably jealous, possessive, and watchful of the partner's activities. The abuse becomes more frequent, intense, and life-threatening over time. In Walker's classic study of 400 women in violent families (Walker, 1979), the cycle of violence was first operationally defined. The cycle of violence consists of three phases: (1) tension-building phase, (2) acute battering phase, and (3) honeymoon phase. Figure 21-1 shows behaviors that characterize the steps in the cycle.

The cycle of violence is a continuing cycle that is hard to break without help. Whatever pattern the violence follows, trust is broken, and shame and fear are constantly underneath the surface of the lives of the victims. Many women report that their partners never repent and enter the honeymoon phase, but rather that the violence is a constant presence in their lives.

Why Abused Partners Stay

There are many reasons women stay in violent domestic situations. Perhaps one of the *strongest* motives for staying is fear that the attacks will become even more violent or that the woman or her children could be murdered if they leave and are found by the batterer. This is a very real concern, and women are at the highest risk of further violence or even death when they threaten to leave or if they leave and are later found by their abuser. Women may end up in an abusive relationship if they were abused as children and abuse

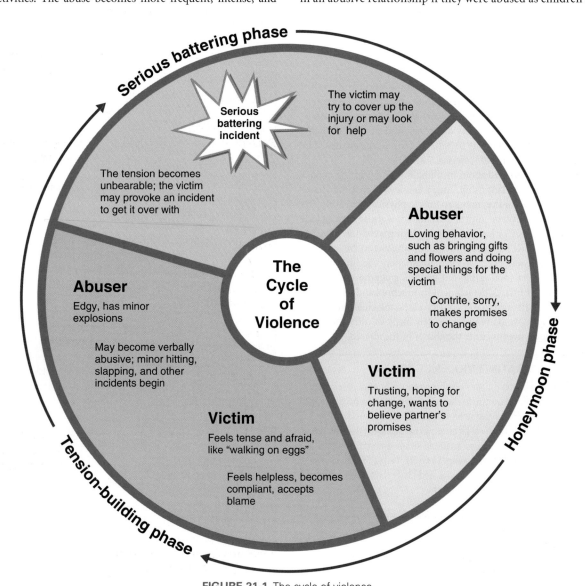

FIGURE 21-1 The cycle of violence.

seems familiar or normal. The abuse may also start later in the relationship and be slow or subtle. If women have not been exposed to IVP in their families, they may not have a frame of reference for early recognition.

Women may not leave an abusive relationship for many reasons. These include lack of financial support, lack of a support system after being isolated, fear or brainwashing developed through the abuse, depression or low self-esteem, religious values against divorce, belief that they deserved the abuse, and staying for the sake of the children. According to one third of homeless women, many with children, they are homeless as a direct results of DV. Until a woman has experienced a number of abuse cycles, she may believe the honeymoon phase will last and that the abuser has learned his lesson and changed.

APPLYING THE ART

A Person Experiencing Intimate Partner Violence

Scenario

During a clinical rotation in the emergency department (ED), a nursing student encountered a 28-year-old female on two separate occasions. The initial visit was for treatment of a dislocated shoulder sustained after falling down the basement steps per the patient. At the second visit, the patient was 3 months pregnant and complaining of abdominal cramping. Bruising around her left orbit was evident despite heavy makeup.

Therapeutic Goal

By the conclusion of this interaction, the patient will verbalize the intent to access her support system, decreasing her isolation.

Student-Patient Interaction	Thoughts, Communication Techniques, and Mental Health Nursing Concepts
Student: "Hello, I'm a nursing student working in the ED today. May I sit and talk with you while you wait for the nurse-midwife?"	Broad opening
Patient: "I don't really need to talk; I feel better now. The cramps barely hurt. I don't need that exam and I need to get home."	
Student's feelings: *I feel concerned about the patient's injuries—they seem suspicious or at least need to be explored.*	
Student: "You say you feel better, but you're still cramping. It's important for the safety of your pregnancy to be examined."	Restatement, presenting reality, giving information
Patient: "I know, but … never mind." *Patient gazes downward.*	
Student's feelings: *I'm worried for her. I need to work up the courage to ask her about abuse.*	
Student: "I'm concerned for you and your baby. Your injuries seem like they could be related to abuse. Are you being hurt at home?"	Exploring
Patient: "Oh no, my husband would never hurt me on purpose."	Restating, exploring
Student: "On purpose. Does he hurt you by accident sometimes?"	
Patient: "Well, I deserve it. I don't have the housework done or I am disrespectful to him."	Seeking information, suggesting collaboration
Student: "Do you have anyone, a friend or family member, you can talk to?"	

Student-Patient Interaction	Thoughts, Communication Techniques, and Mental Health Nursing Concepts
Patient: "My husband moved us here to Texas for his job. All my family is in Indiana. I haven't seen them in 3 years."	Offering self/support
Student: "I'm sure you miss them. That can be difficult to be far away when you are pregnant and going through a hard time"	
Patient: *Begins to cry.* "Yes, it is. I'm afraid for the baby. I have to keep calm."	Suggesting collaboration, formulating a plan of action
Student: "I would like to get the hospital social worker for you. She will have some resources for you, if you decide to get help or need to leave."	
Patient: "Oh no! I'm not going to leave. That would make him really angry, and a family should be together."	Offering self/support, presenting reality
Student: "You don't have to leave, that is your choice. I just want you to have help being so far away from everyone you know."	Giving information
Patient: "Yes, please, that would be good."	
Student: "I also want to talk to you about something important. When a woman goes to leave an abusive relationship, that is the most dangerous time to be seriously hurt or killed. It is important to do that carefully with a plan and help, and not to challenge the angry person. It is important not to leave flyers about women's shelters or counseling around the house where they can be found."	
Patient: "I understand, that makes sense."	Suggesting collaboration, formulating a plan of action, offering self/support
Student: "I'm going to let your midwife and the social worker know about your situation, so we can work together to support you."	
Patient: *(Softly)* "Thank you … don't say anything to my husband."	
Student's feelings: *I'm relieved that she is getting help, and glad I could be part of that.*	

APPLICATION OF THE NURSING PROCESS

ASSESSMENT

Abused women (or men) are most often seen in the ED, but they may be seen in a physician's office, clinic, or psychiatric setting (Zolotor et al., 2009). Although there has been greater recognition and response by the health care system to victims of intimate partner violence (IPV), there is room for continued education and improvement. The American Congress of Obstetricians and Gynecologists (ACOG, 2012) recommends screening for abuse at every visit. As much as we know, some nurses and other professionals still have an attitude of blaming the victim or a lack of understanding as to how the cycle occurs or continues. There has been expanded awareness of military sexual violence against women that was hidden in the past. The National Institute of Crime Prevention (NICP) is a company that offers training for professionals in law enforcement and health care on recognition and proper handling in IPV and sexual assault cases (NICP, 2011).

Some signs of probable IVP include a discrepancy between the injury and the explanation of how it occurred, minimization of the injury or abuse, and fearfulness regarding a partner or other individual. If IPV is suspected, a complete physical examination and appropriate testing need to be performed. Rape may be part of the abuse, so a gynecological exam including testing for sexually transmitted infections (STIs) and evidence collection should be performed. Administering the "morning-after pill" is a routinely offered treatment, as 5% of rapes result in a pregnancy according to Perry and colleagues (2015).

Signs of abuse in all ages or genders of victims may include burns; bruises; scars; wounds in various stages of healing, particularly around the head and neck; and fractures of limbs, ribs, or jaw. Physical examination includes assessing for signs of internal injuries such as bleeding, concussions, perforated eardrums, abdominal injuries, eye injuries, and strangulation marks on the neck. An examination might reveal burns from cigarettes, acids, scalding liquids, or appliances. Patterning of injuries can include bruises, lacerations, or contusions in the shapes of objects such as coat hangers, cords, irons, handprints, finger-grab prints, fly swatters, rope burns, bite or teeth marks, or belt buckles. Patterning can also refer to the location of the damage. Abusers often plan the location of abuse so that it cannot be easily noticed, such as on the torso, back, upper arms, and upper legs; inside body orifices; and under the hair. Examination should include attention to these hidden areas.

There are always psychological and emotional scars from abuse. The woman might present with signs of high anxiety and stress and complain of insomnia, chest pain, back pain, dizziness, stomach upset, trouble eating, or severe headache, for example. Signs of posttraumatic stress disorder (PTSD) are often present and should be part of an assessment. A brief history may reveal a series of falls, "accidents," and recent emergency department visits. The victim may be timid or vague in her explanations. A woman with any indication of IPV should always be seen alone, without her partner present, for at least part of the examination time. A reluctance on the part of the partner to leave the patient alone can be a red flag, although other reasons can account for a partner wanting to stay near. While alone, ask the potential victim if someone is hitting or otherwise hurting her—either a current or past partner, or anyone else—and if she feels safe in her current relationship. It is also important to ask if the children are also being harmed by the abuser in any way.

An assessment of the patient's support systems, suicide potential, and coping responses, including learned helplessness, substance abuse, denial, or self-harm, should be included in the assessment. Once the history of abuse has been ascertained, careful documentation such as verbatim verbal statements and physical findings should be recorded using a body map (Table 21-4). Ask the woman if she would allow photos to be taken. Although an adult victim has the right to refuse to report the assault, the nurse can document thoroughly and notify police. This will allow the patient to have contact with law enforcement for future support if needed, even if she chooses not to report at this time. Child Protective Services (CPS) must be notified if there are children in the home, as it would be assumed that the violence against the parent could also affect the children.

DIAGNOSIS AND OUTCOMES IDENTIFICATION

The threat to a woman's physical and psychological health, as well as to her life and possibly the lives of her children, as a result of IVP is the immediate concern. Nursing diagnoses that address these areas include *Risk for violence, Risk for injury, Acute/chronic pain, Risk for trauma,* and *Risk for self-directed or other-directed violence,* as well as *Social isolation, Disturbed sleep pattern, Powerlessness, Disturbed personal identity, Risk for post-trauma syndrome,* and *Disabled family coping.*

Unfortunately, women who are treated in the ED may admit to IPV but seldom return for treatment. Nurses often have strong reactions when children or women are treated violently. However, in the case of partner abuse, it is up to the abused partner to make the decision to stay in the battering situation or to leave. It is most helpful for the woman if the nurse can accept the woman's decision in a nonjudgmental way and support the woman in her decision.

The preferred outcome for health care personnel would be to see the woman opt for a safe environment for herself and her children in the form of safe houses, a caring relative, or a friend. Because that is not usually the woman's decision, the nurse can discuss options and provide the woman with referrals for safe houses and shelters, hotlines, support groups, and legal counseling as well as a safety plan. Box 21-3 contains an example of a basic IPV safety plan. Make sure the abused woman is warned not to leave any literature where the abuser can find it.

IMPLEMENTATION

Table 21-4 lists several interventions and their rationales related to the initial ED visit. It is important to help the battered partner begin to understand that no one deserves to be beaten, she did not cause the abuse, and it is not her fault. Years of conditioning that may have started in childhood can take considerable time to heal and relearn. While a woman may understand these concepts intellectually, it takes time to synthesize them into emotional and visceral understanding.

A Note on Programs for Batterers

Various types of programs have been set up across the country for men and women who batter their partners. Although the focus is on reducing or eliminating domestic violence through self-reflection and skill building, these programs also offer men options other than fines or incarceration. Programs vary in their strategies, but usually the first priorities are to protect the victims and to stress that the offender is accountable for the abuse in the relationship (Hayward et al., 2007). One study found that the programs help in some ways. For example, the women believed that communication had improved and that most of the men had developed alternate ways of dealing with their angry, impulsive urges other than in physical ways. However, even when the physical violence lessened or abated, the emotional, verbal, or sexual abuse remained or even increased (Hayward et al., 2007). The core problem with the aggressor is the need to exert constant and strict control. It is felt by many that in order to change the dynamics of abuse, the aggressor needs to work at changing his perceptions of himself and the world, which can reduce the need for violent control. In addition, abusers

TABLE 21-4 Interventions for Intimate Partner Violence: Emergency Department

Intervention	Rationale
1. Ensure that medical attention is provided to patient. Document injuries using body map. Ask permission to take photos.	1. If patient wants to file charges, photos boost victim's confidence to press charges now or in the future.
2. Set up interview in private and ensure confidentiality.	2. Patient might be terrified of retribution and further attacks from partner if she reveals abuse.
3. Assess in a nonthreatening manner information concerning: • Sexual abuse • Physical abuse • Emotional abuse • Abuse of children • Drugs of abuse • Thoughts of suicide or homicide	3. These are all vital issues in determining appropriate interventions for depression, anxiety, suicide prevention, and self-medication with alcohol or substances.
4. Encourage patient to talk about the battering incident without interruptions, in a kind and gentle manner, without judgment.	4. When patients share their stories, attentive listening is essential.
5. Ask how patient is faring with the children in the home.	5. In homes in which the mother is abused, children also tend to be abused or traumatized by what they witness.
6. Assess if patient has a safe place to go when violence is escalating. If she does not, include a list of shelters or safe houses with other written information. Some hospitals provide small cards that can fit in a shoe, so that the victim is not endangered by the abuser finding shelter and escape resources.	6. When abused patients are ready to leave their abusers, they need to go quickly. A plan is advised and it is better to leave when the abuser is not home unless the person is in danger and must flee immediately. Instruct the victim not to confront the abuser when leaving because this may worsen the rage. When a victim leaves, she is at the greatest risk for severe injury or being killed.

Legal Issues

1. Identity if patient is interested in pressing charges. If yes, give verbal and written information on: • Local attorneys who handle spousal abuse cases • Legal clinics • Battered women's advocates and shelters Call CPS if children are involved. Call law enforcement to make a report and assist the victim.	1. Often the spouse or partner is afraid of retaliation, but when ready to seek legal advice an appropriate list of lawyers well trained in this specialty area is needed.
2. Know the requirements in your state about reporting suspected spousal abuse.	2. Many states have or are developing laws or guidelines for protecting battered women.
3. Discuss with patient a safety and escape plan during escalation of anxiety before actual violence erupts (see Box 21-3).	3. Document escape plan and include shelter and referral numbers. This can prevent further abuse to children and patient.
4. Throughout work with battered spouses, emphasize that the beatings are not their fault.	4. When self-esteem is eroded, victims often believe that they deserved the beatings.
5. Encourage patient to reach out to family and friends whom they might have been avoiding.	5. Old friends and relatives can make helpful allies and validate that the patient does not deserve to be beaten. The victim will need a lot of support.
6. Know the psychotherapists in the community who have experience working with battered spouses or partners.	6. Psychotherapy with victims of trauma requires special skills.
7. If the patient is not ready to take action at this time, provide a list of community resources: a. Hotlines b. Shelters c. Battered women's groups and advocates d. Therapists e. Law enforcement f. Medical assistance or Aid to Families with Dependent Children (AFDC) g. Child Protective Services (CPS) has resources to support families, in addition to investigating allegations of abuse.	7. It can take time for patients to make decisions to change their life situation. People need appropriate information.

Adapted from Varcarolis, E. M. (2015). *Manual of psychiatric nursing care plans: diagnoses, clinical tools, and psychopharmacology* (5th ed.). St Louis: Elsevier.

often were abused or witnessed abuse in their families. Therapy to address the abuser's own personal wounds and emotional issues can also help to break the cycle of violence. Among batterers attending cognitive-behavioral therapy, almost 85% decreased or eliminated their behaviors of perpetrating physical or emotional abuse (Fernandez-Montalvo et al., 2015).

ELDER ABUSE

In the next decade and beyond there will be an overwhelming number of adults 65 years of age and older as the baby boom generation ages and people live longer and healthier lives, however, close to half (45%) of adults ages 65 and older had incomes below twice the poverty

BOX 21-3 Basic Intimate Partner Violence Safety Plan

It is important, whenever possible, to work with a domestic violence advocate to develop a safety plan that fits your needs.

- Move to a room with more than one exit, avoiding rooms with potential weapons such as kitchen knives or heavy objects.
- Know the quickest route out of your home.
- Know the quickest route out of your workplace. Determine resources the employer may have to protect employees, such as a security guard escort.
- Keep a bag packed with essentials: clothes, valuables, documents (such as passports, Social Security cards, medical records, bank cards, birth certificates), a list of phone contacts, a month's supply of medications, and money. Keep it hidden but make it easy to grab quickly, or consider keeping it with a friend, relative, or at work so it is not discovered by the abuser.
- Tell your neighbors about your abuse and ask them to call the police when they hear a disturbance.
- Have a code word to use with your children, family, and friends when you need help. Consider some of the new phone apps for alerting significant contacts in an emergency.
- Have a safe place selected in case you ever have to leave, such as a friend or relative's home or a shelter.
- Use your instincts, and do not provoke the abuser when considering leaving.
- Unless you are in danger at that moment, try to leave when the abuser is not at home or around you.
- You have the right to protect yourself and your kids.
- Call the National Domestic Violence Hotline at 1-800-799-7233 for further information and guidance.

Adapted from Goodman, P. E. (2006). The relationship between intimate partner violence and other forms of family and societal violence. *Emergency Medical Clinics of North America, 24*(4), 889–903; Office on Women's Health, U.S. Department of Health and Human Services. (2011). Violence against women: Safety planning for abusive situations. Retrieved from http://womenshealth.gov/violence-against-women/get-help-for-violence/safety-planning-for-abusive-situations.html

BOX 21-4 Five Kinds of Elder Abuse

1. **Physical abuse:** The infliction of physical pain or injury through slapping, hitting, kicking, pushing, restraining, overmedicating, or sexually abusing.
2. **Psychological abuse:** The infliction of mental anguish through yelling, name calling, humiliating, or threatening.
3. **Financial abuse or exploitation:** The misuse of someone's property and resources by another person, or refusal by a caregiver to provide needed resources.
4. **Neglect:** Failure to fulfill a caretaking obligation to provide nutrition, hydration, shelter, clothing, utilities, medical services, or other basic needs. This category may also include self-neglect.
5. **Sexual abuse:** Nonconsensual sexually molesting, touching, inappropriate comments or exposure to videos or acts, or actual rape.

Adapted from National Center on Elder Abuse Administration on Aging. (2016). Types of abuse. Retrieved from http://www.ncea.aoa.gov/FAQ/Type_Abuse/index.aspx

leaves many older adults who are mentally and physically healthy unprotected in a situation in which they are being abused or exploited by family members. Definitions of elder abuse and APS programs differ among states, resulting in a "patchwork of laws, definitions, and services throughout the country" (Quinn & Zielke, 2005, p. 451). These widely differing definitions and terminologies make it impossible to know the actual extent of the problem or to conduct sound research. There have been some recent movements at the national level to standardize the approach to the study of elder mistreatment.

CHARACTERISTICS OF ELDER ABUSE

The Abused Elder

Seniors can be especially vulnerable to abuse as well as to other crimes. Age-related syndromes often result in frailty and functional decline, making older adults less able to protect themselves. Abuse of seniors can include rape and sexual abuse. Elder abuse is most often diagnosed in older adults who have depression, alcohol or drug abuse, dementia, or a psychiatric illness, which compounds an older adult's vulnerability and draws attention to the person's situation.

It is estimated that 3% to 27% of the elderly experience some type of abuse or neglect, although the number is believed to be underreported (Halphen & Dyer, 2015). The risk of abuse rises as age advances, with women more often being the victims. People older than 80 years of age are two to three times more likely to suffer abuse and neglect than older adults in the 60- to 80-year-old age group, and victims of elder abuse are three times more likely to die than older adults who are not mistreated (Halphen & Dyer, 2015).

The Abuser

Early studies on elder abuse focused on the caretaker's stress and burden as causative factors in the abuse. More recent research indicates that the characteristics of the elder abuser more closely resemble the characteristics of the abuser in intimate partner violence (IPV). Most often the abuser is a middle-aged adult child or other family member. Often the caregiver is financially dependent on the older adult. Elder abusers may have a personality profile similar to abusers in other categories (intimate partner, child), such as being abused themselves or using substances. However, the family member inflicting the abuse may not be a cruel or insensitive person, but instead be a caring individual who is under extreme stress. In some cases the caregiver is grappling with a mental health issue or the overwhelming stress of his or her daily life

thresholds under the Supplemental Poverty Measure (SPM) in 2013 (Cubanski et al., 2015). As a result of the growing number of elderly persons, the incidence of elder abuse will also increase proportionally, which will translate to more responsibility for the health care system, including nurses. Fulmer and Blankenship (2011) estimate that approximately 6% of older adults are mistreated annually.

The World Health Organization (2015) considers elder abuse to be a violation of human rights as well as a significant cause of injury, isolation, and despair for the elderly population. As in other age groups, the elderly can be victimized through physical, sexual, or emotional abuse; neglect; and financial exploitation (Box 21-4). Abuse can occur by individuals and institutions such as skilled nursing facilities (SNFs) or even through self-neglect. Elder abuse is commonly known as "granny abuse" or as "granny dumping" when an elderly family member is left at a medical facility and not picked up by family members. It is estimated that 70% to 80% of elder abuse cases are not reported. The elderly may be loath to report family members for a variety of reasons, including intimidation and not wanting to be taken from the family. They may feel their situation is better than the alternatives.

All 50 states have established elder abuse prevention laws and reporting systems, and in all but 6 states reporting is mandatory (Halphen & Dyer, 2015). The Adult Protective Services (APS) division of each state receives and investigates reports of suspected elder abuse. To be eligible for APS help in most states, an older adult has to be deemed unable to care for himself or herself. This

(Fulmer & Blankenship, 2011). Relationship issues between the elderly parent and the child do not go away just because each person is older. Being thrust into close quarters together can exacerbate existing strain. It is partly the nurse's responsibility to assess and observe the family and determine their needs. Then the nurse and family must explore possible interventions to lessen family tension, including a change in living situation in some instances.

Abusers can also be staff members or residents in SNFs or other out-of-home living situations. Contrary to common belief, abuse in SNFs is most often perpetrated by residents toward other residents rather than by staff members (Halphen & Dyer, 2015).

APPLICATION OF THE NURSING PROCESS

ASSESSMENT

Nurse practitioners, physicians, nurses, and other health care professionals are often the only outside contact an older adult may have. In most states, health care workers are mandated to report elder abuse and neglect to APS (Halphen & Dyer, 2015).

Victims of abuse have twice as many physician and clinic visits as those not subjected to abuse. Because victims of abuse or neglect are most likely to be abused by family members, the abused are often afraid to reveal the abuse. There may be threats about disclosure or retribution, the victim may experience shame, or the abused may want to protect a loved one. There may be fear of being placed in a nursing home, and the known problems may be preferable to an unknown situation or leaving the home and family. It is important that family and friends are allowed to communicate about suspected abuse in a safe and nonjudgmental manner. Health care workers should make a routine evaluation for signs and symptoms of abuse when older adults visit health care facilities. Signs of elder abuse are very similar to those in child abuse or IPV. Some additional red flags more specific to elderly victims (Halphen & Dyer, 2015) include the following:

- Fear of being alone with the caregiver
- Malnutrition or begging for food, dehydration
- Bedsores, skin tears, bruises, swelling, or fractures
- In need of medical or dental care
- Left unattended for long periods
- Reports of abuse or neglect
- Passive, withdrawn, or emotionless behavior
- Appears overmedicated
- Vaginal or rectal pain, tears, or bleeding, or STIs
- Concern over finances
- Inability to pay for medications or needed services
- Transfer of property by an elder who lacks the mental capacity to consent
- Valuables missing

When patients with suspected abuse cannot leave the house, home visits may be warranted, allowing the nurse practitioner, physician, or clinician to assess the patient and environment.

DIAGNOSIS AND OUTCOMES IDENTIFICATION

Nursing diagnoses for abused older adults are much the same as with other cases of abuse. *Risk for injury, Acute or chronic pain, Fear, Anxiety, Risk for self-directed violence,* and *Risk for other-directed violence* have been discussed in prior sections. In addition, nursing diagnoses that relate to neglect and financial exploitation include *Impaired home maintenance, Self-care deficit, Caregiver role strain, Adult failure to thrive,* and *Powerlessness.*

TABLE 21-5 Interventions for Suspected Elder Abuse	
Intervention	**Rationale**
1. Check your state for laws regarding elder abuse.	1. All states have adopted laws to help protect elders and support their need for safety.
2. Involve Adult Protective Services (APS) if abuse is suspected.	2. APS can offer many sources to help guard the safety and well-being of abused elders.
3. Meet with other family members to identify stressors and problem areas, including caregiver strain.	3. Other family members may be unaware of the abuser's stress level or the lack of safety available for the abused family member.
4. If there are no other family members, notify other community agencies that might help stabilize the situation, such as: • Support group for elderly patient or for abuser and family members • Meals on Wheels • Day care for seniors • Respite services • Visiting nurse services • Assisted living	4. Minimizes family stress and isolation, and increases safety.
5. Encourage abuser to seek counseling.	5. Increases coping skills and social supports.
6. Suggest that family members meet on a regular basis for problem solving and support.	6. Encourages family to learn and solve problems together.

Successful long-term outcomes include the following:
1. Physical, emotional, or sexual abuse has ceased.
2. Neglect or financial exploitation has ceased.
3. Plans are in place to maintain safety.
4. The elder states that he or she feels more comfortable in the home.
5. Follow-up visits reveal less anxiety and tension between the caregiver and the elder.
6. Caregiver strain has been addressed through respite, sharing of responsibilities, and support.

Most hospitals and community centers have protocols that offer guidelines for nurses and other health care workers for suspected elder abuse. Immediate physical safety is always the first concern, as well as referring the patient to APS for evaluation. There are a number of services that APS can offer to address issues of patient neglect, abuse, and other forms of mistreatment. Potential services may include assistance with emergency housing, repairs, or modification for disabilities; help obtaining medical services; resources for food delivery or caretaker services; serving as a patient advocate; and legal referrals. These services are voluntary, and the patient has the right to accept or decline them (Halphen & Dyer, 2015). Greater social networking and supports could be a protective factor for the elderly in general (Fulmer & Blankenship, 2011).

IMPLEMENTATION

In addition to needed compassionate physical care, interventions include providing medical services, implementing APS or law enforcement interventions, and involving social services. Family or caregiver support may be needed, or in some cases alternative housing is necessary. Table 21-5 includes interventions for suspected elder abuse.

EVALUATION

Failures in interventions with abusive families not only are related to personal deficits of the individuals, but also involve inadequacies in the social, economic, and political systems in which we all live. Many disadvantaged individuals have limited access to needed services and experience inordinate stressors. Some of the societal attitudes that, in part, support abuse are the acceptance of corporal punishment to discipline children, the unequal caregiving burden placed on women, the lack of education and preparation for sexual activity and parenthood,

and the concept of "ageism" where the elderly are considered to have lesser value. Nurses can be instrumental in altering these perceptions through education in the course of their career duties.

Evaluation of interventions to stop elder abuse can include the willingness of the victim to acknowledge the abuse and to accept assistance, as well as the success of the plan. Because violence is a symptom of a family or health care organization in distress, intervention and evaluation will be a multidisciplinary approach. Follow-up is crucial in ensuring the ongoing safety of the elderly patient and support of the caregiving system, whether that be the family or the SNF.

APPLYING EVIDENCE-BASED PRACTICE (EBP)

Problem A 24-year-old female presents to the emergency department (ED) with complaints of abdominal pain. She is vague about her symptoms, and finally explains that she tripped and fell down her front porch steps while carrying groceries. Upon examination, it's discovered that she has bruising on her arms, torso, and left orbit in various stages of healing. Her records indicate several past ED visits for injuries, including a fractured arm. While she is in the examination room, her phone rings constantly with calls from her husband, and she is tense as she answers with short, cryptic responses. She explains that she has to hurry home, as she has two young children at home in addition to the toddler that has accompanied her to the ED. The toddler appears pale and shy, quietly holding on to her mother's clothing or hiding behind her.

EBP Assessment

A. **What do you already know from experience?** This patient has been to the ED with several injuries. She presents like other victims of intimate partner violence (IPV) the nurse has treated, being timid, vague, and tense on the phone with her husband. She may or may not be willing to admit the abuse.

B. **What does the literature say?** In cases of IPV the victim's injuries are often inconsistent with the explanation, and there may be a history of many injuries and ED visits. The victim may appear fearful or intimidated by the abuser. The victim may stay in the relationship for various reasons, including for the children or because they believe it will get better, they think they deserve the abuse, or they have nowhere to go. Many homeless women were domestic abuse victims. The highest risk of severe injury or being killed occurs when

the victim is trying to leave the abuser. Children may also be abused or traumatized by what they have witnessed.

C. **What does the patient want?** The nurse had another staff member take the toddler for a snack while gently questioning the mother. The patient broke down in tears and admitted she was a victim of IPV by her husband. She was fearful of being harmed and had little support in her life. She was agreeable to speaking with the police, although she was not sure she was ready to leave at this time.

Plan The patient was examined, including x-rays, and her injuries were treated. Social services was called and met with the patient to give her shelter and safety plan resources. The police took a report and photographs of the abuse. After speaking with everyone, the patient decided to take her children and go to a shelter. A shelter was called, and a representative was dispatched from the shelter to support and assist the patient. Child Protective Services (CPS) was called to remove the two children who were at home with the patient's husband, and to initiate an investigation into possible neglect or abuse of the children. The patient was terrified regarding her decision, and the nurse stayed with her during all interviews.

QSEN **QSEN Prelicensure Knowledge, Skills, and Attitudes (KSAs) Addressed:**

Safety by being aware of potential abuse and taking actions to keep the patient and her children safe.

Team work and collaboration by working with social services, law enforcement, an abuse shelter, and CPS to provide needed services for this family.

From Centers for Disease Control and Prevention. (2014b). *Understanding intimate partner violence: fact sheet.* Retrieved from http://www.cdc.gov/violenceprevention/pdf/ipv-factsheet.pdf

---

▮ KEY POINTS TO REMEMBER

- Physical and emotional trauma cause long-lasting damage to individuals and communities and are often passed down in a generational manner.
- Because the incidence of child, partner, and elder abuse is underreported, it is imperative that nurses learn to routinely assess for abuse.
- All states have mandatory guidelines for reporting child and elder abuse. However, in the case of IPV the victim is of a consenting and nonprotected age. Although nurses can provide resources, support, and guidance, it is ultimately their choice and responsibility to file any report of abuse.
- When a victim of IPV attempts to leave the abuser, the highest risk of severe harm or homicide exists.
- Abusive parents have characteristics that can be recognized by health care providers.
- Abuse often occurs in a cyclical pattern in which the tension grows, abuse occurs, then remorse and a honeymoon phase begin. The cycle will almost always continue and escalate without intervention.

- Responsibilities of the nurse and other health care team members in various cases of abuse are discussed.
- Nursing diagnoses, interventions, and outcomes are similar in all abuse cases, although each individual and age group has additional unique needs.

▮ APPLYING CRITICAL JUDGMENT

1. A 6-year-old boy is rushed to the emergency department by a neighbor who found him wandering in the street wearing only a dirty undershirt, seemingly dazed. He is covered in what appear to be cigarette burns, is cachectic, and has bruises on his wrists and ankles. He appears fearful and confused and does not respond to questioning except to say, "I hurt. I don't feel good."
   A. What is your first priority?
   B. What would you include in your documentation and on the body map?
   C. What else could you do to document his injuries besides note them on the body map?
   D. Who else would you need to involve or notify in this case?

CHAPTER REVIEW QUESTIONS

1. An emergency department nurse assesses a woman suspected of being abused by an intimate partner. Which assessment finding most clearly confirms the suspicion?
   a. Leathery facial tone
   b. Injuries in a bikini pattern
   c. Reluctance to be examined
   d. Lack of eye contact with the nurse

2. An emergency department nurse assesses a child with a fractured ulna. The nurse also observes yellow and purple bruises across the child's back and shoulders. Which comment by the parents should prompt the nurse to consider making a report to Child Protective Services?
   a. "We do not believe in immunization of our children."
   b. "This child is always creating problems for the family."
   c. "Our child would rather play alone than with other children."
   d. "We homeschool our children in order to include religious education."

3. A woman in a relationship characterized by a long history of battering and abuse tells the nurse, "We've had a rough time lately. I admit it: He beat me last night but then said he was sorry." Which event would the nurse expect to occur next in this relationship?
   a. Another beating by the abusive partner
   b. Love, gifts, and praise from the abusive partner
   c. A brief period during which the partners ignore each other
   d. The abusive partner leaves the relationship for a short time

4. The nurse assessed an elderly person who was abused by the caregiver. Afterward, which internal dialogue should prompt the nurse to seek guidance?
   a. "Sometimes I get so discouraged and frustrated with my job."
   b. "It's incredible that anyone could hurt a child or elderly person."
   c. "The abuser was probably a victim of abuse at some point in life."
   d. "I hope the abuser gets victimized so they know what it feels like."

5. A university football coach invites the campus nurse to talk to the team about healthy relationships in the community. Which topic has priority for the nurse to include?
   a. Appropriate behavior with intimate partners
   b. University resources for counseling and support
   c. The importance of role modeling for children and teens
   d. Public recognition of children with life-threatening illnesses

REFERENCES

American Congress of Obstetricians and Gynecologists. (2012). ACOG Committee Opinion No. 518: Intimate partner violence. *Obstetrics and Gynecology*, 119(2, Pt 1), 412–417.

American Psychological Association (APA). (2011). *Male victims of "intimate terrorism" can experience damaging psychological effects*. Retrieved from http://www.APA.org/news/press/releases/2011/04/intimate-terrorism.

Centers for Disease Control and Prevention (CDC). (2014c). *Understanding teen dating violence*. Retrieved from http://www.cdc.gov/violenceprevention/pdf/teen-dating-violence-factsheet-a.pdf.

Centers for Disease Control and Prevention (CDC). (2014b). *Understanding intimate partner violence: fact sheet*. Retrieved from http://www.cdc.gov/violenceprevention/pdf/ipv-factsheet.pdf.

Centers for Disease Control and Prevention (CDC). (2014a). *Adverse Childhood Experiences (ACE) Study*. Retrieved from http://www.cdc.gov/violenceprevention/acestudy/index.html.

Centers for Disease Control and Prevention (CDC). (2015). *Child maltreatment prevention*. Retrieved from http://www.cdc.gov/violenceprevention/childmaltreatment/index.html.

Childhelp. (2011). *National child abuse statistics*. Retrieved from http://www.childhelp.org/pages/statistics.

Cowen, J. A., & Cowen, P. S. (2011). Child maltreatment: nursing considerations. In P. S. Cowen & S. Morehead (Eds.), *Current issues in nursing* (8th ed.) (pp. 689–707). St Louis: Mosby/Elsevier.

Cubanski, J., Casillas, G., & Damico, A. (2015). Poverty among seniors: an updated analysis of national and state level poverty rates under the official and supplemental poverty measures. Kaser Family Foundation. Retrieved from http://kff.org/medicare/issue-brief/poverty-among-seniors-an-updated-analysis-of-national-and-state-level-poverty-rates-under-the-official-and-supplemental-poverty-measures/.

Fernandez-Montalvo, J., Echauri, J. A., Martinez, M., et al. (2015). Impact of a court-referred psychological treatment program for intimate partner batterer men with suspended sentences. *Violence and Victims*, 30(1), 3–15.

Fulmer, T., & Blankenship, J. L. (2011). Nursing care: victims of violence: elder mistreatment. In P. S. Cowen & S. Moorehead (Eds.), *Current issues and nursing* (8th ed.) (pp. 720–725). St Louis: Mosby/Elsevier.

General Assembly United Nations. (1993). *Declaration of the elimination of violence against women (Resolution 48/104)*. Retrieved from http://daccessdds.un.org/doc/UNDOC/GEN/N94/095/05/PDF/N9409505.pdf.

Guy, J., Feinstein, L., & Griffiths, A. (2013). *Early intervention in domestic violence and abuse*. Retrieved from http://www.eif.org.uk/wp-content/uploads/2014/03/Early-Intervention-in-Domestic-Violence-and-Abuse-Full-Report.pdf.

Halphen, J. M., & Dyer, C. B. (2015). *Elder mistreatment: abuse, neglect, and financial exploitation*. Retrieved from http://www.uptodate.com/contents/elder-mistreatment-abuse-neglect-and-financial-exploitation.

Hayward, K. S., Steiner, S., & Spould, K. (2007). *Women's perceptions of the impact of a domestic violence treatment program for male perpetrators*. Retrieved from http://www.Medscape.com/viewarticle/561278.

Minnesota Advocates for Human Rights (MAHR). (2006). *Stop violence against women: evolution of theories of violence*. Retrieved from http://www.stopvaw.org/Evolution_of_Theories_of_Violence.html.

National Center for Children in Poverty (NCCP). (2009). *Child poverty*. Retrieved from http://www.nccp.org/topic/childpoverty.html.

National Council on Alcoholism and Drug Abuse (NCADA). (2009). *Family violence and substance abuse*. Retrieved from http://www.ncada-stl.org-tml.

National Institute of Crime Prevention. (2011). *Domestic violence and sexual assault training conferences through NICP*. Retrieved from http://www.nicp.net/?page_id=12.

National Institute of Justice (NIJ). (2015). *Violence against women and family violence program*. Retrieved from http://www.nij.gov/topics/crime/violence-against-women/pages/welcome.aspx.

Ney, T. (Ed.). (2015). *True and false allegations of child sexual abuse: assessment and case management*. London: Routledge.

Perry, R., Zimmerman, L., Al-Saden, I., et al. (2015). Prevalence of rape-related pregnancy as an indication for abortion at two family planning clinics. *Contraception*, 91(5), 393–397.

President of the United States of America. (2016). *Presidential proclamation: national teen dating violence awareness and prevention month 2011*. Retrieved from https://www.whitehouse.gov/the-press-office/2016/01/29/presidential-proclamation-national-teen-dating-violence-awareness-and?platform=hootsuite.

Quinn, K., & Zielke, H. (2005). Elder abuse, neglect, and exploitation: policy issues. *Clinics in Geriatric Medicine*, 21(2), 449–457.

Sadock, B. J., & Sadock, V. A. (Eds.). (2014). *Kaplan & Sadock's synopsis of psychiatry: behavioral sciences/clinical psychiatry* (11th ed.). Philadelphia: Lippincott Williams & Wilkins.

Smith, E. N., & Fazel, S. (2015). Risk factors for violence and suicide in the general population: a meta-epidemiological study. *European Psychiatry, 30*(1), 28–31.

Stockl, H., Devries, K., Rotstein, A., et al. (2013). The global prevalence of intimate partner homicide: a systematic review. *Lancet, 382*(9895), 859–865.

Trask, E. V., Walsh, K., & DiLillo, D. (2011). Treatment effects for common outcomes of child sexual abuse: a current meta-analysis. *Aggression and Violent Behavior, 16*(1), 6–19.

U.S. Department of Health and Human Services (USDHHS). (2009). *Child maltreatment 2007.* Washington, DC: U.S. Government Printing Office.

U.S. Department of Health and Human Services (USDHHS). (2010). The Child Abuse Prevention and Treatment Act. Amended by P.L. 111–320. The CAPTA Reauthorization Act of 2010. Retrieved from http://www.acf.hhs.gov/sites/default/files/cb/capta2010.pdf.

U.S. Preventive Services Task Force. (2013). *Final recommendation statement: intimate partner violence and abuse of elderly and vulnerable adults: screening.* Retrieved from http://www.uspreventiveservicestaskforce.org/Page/Document/RecommendationStatementFinal/intimate-partner-violence-and-abuse-of-elderly-and-vulnerable-adults-screening#citation47.

Vancouver Coastal Health. (2015). *About adult abuse & neglect.* Retrieved from http://www.vchreact.ca/read_psychological.htm.

Violence Policy Center. (2013). *When men murder women: an analysis of 2011 homicide data.* Retrieved from http://www.vpc.org/studies/wmmw2013.pdf.

Walker, L. E. (1979). *The battered woman.* New York: Harper and Row.

Weil, A. (2016). Intimate partner violence: epidemiology and health consequences. In L. Park (Ed.), *UpToDate.* Retrieved from www.uptodate.com.

Widom, C. P., & Wilson, H. (2015). Intergenerational transmission of violence. In J. Lindert & I. Levav (Eds.), *Violence and mental health* (pp. 27–46). Netherlands: Springer Netherlands.

World Health Organization. (2015). *Ageing and life course: elder abuse.* Retrieved from http://www.who.int/ageing/projects/elder_abuse/en/.

Zolotor, A. J., Denham, A. C., & Weil, A. (2009). Intimate partner violence. *Primary Care: Clinics in Office Practice, 36*(1), 167–179.

Sexual Violence

Elizabeth M. Varcarolis

http://evolve.elsevier.com/Varcarolis/essentials

KEY TERMS AND CONCEPTS

acquaintance rape, p. 350

date rape, p. 350

date rape drug, p. 351

forensic evidence, p. 350

institutional protocol, p. 354

marital/partner rape, p. 350

rape, p. 350

rape kits, p. 354

rape-trauma syndrome, p. 355

sexual assault, p. 350

sexual assault nurse examiner (SANE), p. 353

sexual assault response team (SART), p. 353

survivor, p. 350

victim, p. 350

SELECTED CONCEPTS: THE VIOLENCE AGAINST WOMEN ACT: A TIMELINE AND SUPPORT FOR SURVIVORS

"In 1994 with the leadership by then-Sen. Joe Biden, Congress enacted Violence Against Women Act (VAWA). In 2000, *First* reauthorization creates dedicated funding for the prevention of sexual violence, including sexual assault and stalking, stressing the needs of an underserved population. In 2005, *Second* reauthorization creates dedicated funding for services for sexual assault survivors, prohibits the use of polygraphs with sexual assault victims, and requires that states pay for forensic examinations. In 2013, *Third* reauthorization broadens language to be inclusive of Native women, immigrant women and LGBTQ communities, plus expands housing protections for victims" (NSVRC, 2014, p .22).

All individuals, both men and women, who have been the recipient of sexual violence suffer severe, deep, long-lasting emotional scars, and besides potential physical trauma (e.g., sexually transmitted infections [STIs], pregnancy, vaginal/anal tearing) psychological consequences include depression, anxiety, difficulties with daily functioning, low self-esteem, eating disorders, self-destructive behaviors, substance abuse, and higher rates of suicide than in the general population, among others.

OBJECTIVES

1. **QSEN** Give examples of **teamwork and collaboration** by identifying the various functions and disciplines that constitute members of the sexual assault response team (SART).
2. **QSEN** Evaluate how sexual assault nurse examiners (SANEs) **promote safety** by describing the areas of expertise they provide to victims of sexual violence.
3. Prepare a mock **documentation** of your initial assessment of a victim of sexual assault (including objective and subjective data and a body map).
4. Summarize the characteristics of a perpetrator of sexual assault.
5. **QSEN** Incorporate **evidence-based practice** by identifying the specific data collected in the forensic component of the assessment that may be used as criminal evidence in court.
6. **QSEN** Promote safety by outlining the guidelines for emergency treatment of a woman or man who has been sexually assaulted.
7. **QSEN** Provide **patient-centered care** by delineating the symptoms of rape-trauma syndrome that you would include in your teaching to a victim of sexual assault to prepare him or her for the second phase.
8. **QSEN** Using **informatics**, write up a list of supports in your community that can be offered to an individual who has been sexually assaulted.
9. Identify individual vulnerabilities that might put a person at risk for sexual assault.
10. **QSEN** Using **informatics** search the Internet for the April 2013 A National Protocol for Sexual Assault Medical Forensic Examinations: Adults/Adolescents (2nd ed.).

INTRODUCTION

Sexual assault is an act of violence, power, and hate—not sex—and most often results in devastating severe and long-term trauma. It is often committed in the context of unequal power in order to demonstrate dominance and control. Sexual violence is related to teen pregnancy and the transmission of sexually transmitted infections (STIs), including human immunodeficiency virus (HIV).

In 2012 the U.S. Department of Justice (DOJ) updated the definition of sexual violence by adding: "The penetration, no matter how slight, of the vagina or anus with any body part or object, or oral penetration by a sex organ of another person, without the consent of the victim." Sexual violence occurs when a perpetrator commits sexual acts without a victim's consent, or when a victim is unable to consent (e.g., due to age, illness) or refuse (e.g., due to physical violence or threats) (Basile et al., 2014, p. 1). This updated definition is inclusive for either gender of victim and perpetrator, and recognizes that penetration with an object is as violent as penile/vaginal rape.

The term *sexual violence* encompasses any act from sexual harassment up to rape (Ybarra & Mitchell, 2013). Sexual violence is divided into the following categories (Centers for Disease Control and Prevention [CDC], 2014):

- **Completed or attempted forced penetration of a victim.** (Unwanted vaginal or oral penetration or an insertion through the use of physical force or threats to bring physical harm to the victim)
- **Completed or attempted alcohol- or drug-facilitated penetration of a victim.**
- **Completed or attempted forced acts in which a victim is made to penetrate a perpetrator or someone else.**
- **Completed or attempted alcohol- or drug-facilitated acts in which a victim is made to penetrate a perpetrator or someone else.**
- **Nonphysically forced penetration that occurs after a person is pressured verbally, or through intimidation or misuse of authority, to consent or acquiesce.**
- **Unwanted sexual contact.** (Intentional touching, either directly or through the clothing, of the genitalia, anus, groin, breast, inner thigh, or buttocks of any person without their consent. It includes having the victim touch a perpetrator.)
- **Noncontact unwanted sexual experiences.** (Does not include physical contact of a sexual nature between the perpetrator and the victim. It *does* include unwanted sexual violence such as exposure to pornography, verbal or behavioral sexual harassment, or exhibitionism, without consent or knowledge or to a person who is unable to consent or refuse.)

Sexual violence among children also includes:
- Coercing children to inappropriately touch the molester, often a trusted person
- Showing children pornographic photos and videos
- Initiating inappropriate conversations involving sexual topics

Sexual assault/sexual violence (SV) is an umbrella term encompassing the crimes of rape, date rape, acquaintance rape, gang rape (two or more perpetrators), marital/partner rape, sexual molestation, incest, statutory rape, and sexual assault of older adults.

Rape is a legal term rather than a medical diagnosis. Legal definitions of rape vary among states. For example, Ohio defines rape as (Cleveland Clinic Foundation, 2009):

> when sex is nonconsensual (not agreed upon), or a person forces another person to have sex against his or her will. It also occurs when the victim is intoxicated from alcohol or drugs.

Rape includes intercourse in the vagina, anus, or mouth and is a felony offense, which means it is among the most serious crimes a person can commit. Rape is a crime that can happen to men, women, or children.

Date rape is a form of acquaintance rape, but in the case of date rape (Cleveland Clinic Foundation, 2009): "The victim agreed to spend time with the attacker. Perhaps the victim even went out with the attacker more than once. Date rape is still rape."

All individuals who have been the recipient of sexual violence suffer severe, deep, emotional scars that may stay with them for the rest of their lives. Research has demonstrated that there is a long litany of other physical and mental health issues that are more prevalent in people who have been sexually assaulted. Beyond the physical trauma, such as risk of transmission of sexually transmitted infections (STIs) or human immunodeficiency virus (HIV), pregnancy, and various severe physical trauma related to rape, long-term psychological trauma can occur. Some of the painful consequences caused by sexual assault are depression, anxiety, difficulties with daily functioning, low self-esteem, eating disorders, self-destructive behaviors, substance abuse disorders, and higher rates of suicide than in the general population. Although the risk exists for both male and female rape victims, male rape victims are more likely to commit suicide and to become infected with HIV through anal tears than are women. Timely and age-appropriate interventions can greatly help to mitigate the devastating psychological sequelae and help victims become survivors; when emotional symptoms are confronted and addressed, the abused individual has a better chance of leading a full and productive life.

Presently, there is no mandated reporting for crimes of sexual assault unless they involve abuse of a minor or an elder. It is the responsibility of survivors of assault to make the decision to report the crime and it is the responsibility of health care workers to offer support, to provide information on obtaining legal counsel, and—with the patient's permission—to secure forensic evidence (evidence that can be used in court) by a qualified person for future prosecution.

PREVALENCE AND COMORBIDITY

Note that statistics on sexual violence and sexual assault are always approximate, are often varied, and only refer to reported cases. It is safe to infer that the actual numbers of sexual assaults are very much higher than the quoted statistics. *Both rape and child sexual molestation are among the most underreported crimes.* According to Ernoehazy (2013), best current estimates are that 1 in 6 women and nearly 1 in 33 men will be the victims of sexual assault at least once in their lives.

Children: Child Sexual Abuse and Incest

The statistics that we do have for the sexual assault of children are distressing. For example, some estimates indicate that one in four girls and one in six boys are sexually molested by the time they are 18 years old. According to a survey by Finkelhor and colleagues (2014), the proportion of participants who had experienced sexual assault by the age of 17 years was 26.6%.

It has been found that 30% of the cases of child sexual assault reported to Child Protective Services (CPS) involved children who at the time of the report were between the ages of 4 and 7 years (Parents for Megan's Law and The Crime Victims Center [PML], 2007a). The frightening statistic is that roughly 75% of these molestations are inflicted by family members. Abuse is likely to occur over a long-term, ongoing relationship and to escalate over time; it is estimated to last an average of 4 years or more. Even though strangers could be involved, the greatest percentage of molesters other than family members are persons the child trusts outside of the family, such as teachers, clergy/priests, babysitters, or family friends (TeenBreaks, 2011a).

The effects of **child sexual abuse** can last a lifetime. Sense of worth, distortion of self-concept, confusion about one's place in the world, and disruption in affective capabilities are common. Unfortunately, people who were sexually assaulted as children are approximately four to five times more likely to be sexually assaulted later in life. Abused children, compared to nonabused children, have higher rates of depression, substance abuse, dissociative disorders, other personality disorders, anxiety disorders, and post-traumatic stress disorder (PTSD) later in life. Child sexual violence that remains untreated may result in mental health issues, drug and alcohol abuse, criminal behavior, higher rates of suicide (either attempted or completed), and (not surprisingly) perpetuation of sexual abuse.

According to Women Organized Against Rape (WOAR, 2015), common reactions in children who have been sexually abused include:
- Fear of being alone, of going to sleep, or of strangers
- Outbursts of anger
- Increased isolation
- Physical symptoms such as headaches, stomach or genital discomfort, and skin rashes in the genital area
- Regression to early behaviors, such as a return to bedwetting or not wanting to sleep alone.
- Inappropriate sexual behaviors, such as sexually acting-out with other children or excessive masturbation

High School

The CDC (2011) states that 8% of high school students reported being forced to have sex; 11% of those were females and 5% were males. Date rape is also reported among high school students, as are physical and emotional abuse. Approximately 1 in 5 female high school students report being physically and/or sexually abused by a dating partner.

Young Adults

The U.S. Department of Justice (NSOPW) (updated 2014) statistics include:
- 35.8% of sexual assaults occur when the victim is between the ages of 12 and 17.
- 82% of all juvenile victims are female.
- 69% of the teen sexual assaults reported to law enforcement occurred in the residence of the victim, the offender, or another individual.
- Teens 16 to 19 years of age were 3 ½ times more likely than the general population to be victims of rape, attempted rape, or sexual assault.

Among college women, it is estimated that 20% to 25% will experience an attempted or completed rape by the end of their college career (CDC, 2011), and 90% of those women will know their attackers. According to Seaman (2015), data coming in from different campuses in different settings seem to support the hypothesis that one in five women in college (20%) will experience a sexual assault. Perhaps the majority of sexual assaults in young adults are **acquaintance rapes** or **date rapes.** Alcohol and other drugs often play a part in sexual assault, whether they are taken by the victim, the perpetrator, or both. Contrary to what some young men might think, intoxication by alcohol or drugs is not an excuse for sexual violence; sexual assault is still considered rape

under the law. Drugs are often used to facilitate sexual assault. Often these drugs are used for **gang rapes** (two or more sexual attackers). Although the number of rapes related to date rape drugs seems to be increasing, it is impossible to know the exact statistics. An assaulted woman may not report her abuse because the woman:
- Believes it is her fault
- Does not consider the incident sexual assault
- Does not want to report her abuser for fear of reprisal
- Does not want to get her "friend" or "date" in trouble
- Does not want others to know about the assault
- Cannot remember the incident clearly enough to feel she would be believed by others, especially if she had been drinking and/or taking other drugs

Another consideration is that date rape drugs are cleared from the body fairly quickly, and detecting them in the emergency department or other treatment center is often difficult. A urine sample must be obtained within a certain period of time to prove the existence of date rape drugs. The date rape drugs γ-hydroxybutyrate (GHB), flunitrazepam (Rohypnol), and ketamine are used mostly on college campuses (e.g., fraternity houses, bars, raves, clubs, nightclubs). Refer to Table 22-1 for more information on these drugs. Young men as well as women must be cautious about taking a drink that contains a date rape drug. See Applying Critical Judgment at the end of this chapter for ways to minimize ingestion of a date rape drug. However, it is important to remember that the most common drug used to facilitate the crime of rape is still alcohol.

According to WOAR (2015), common reactions to a sexual assault in adults are:
- Feelings of fear, anxiety, anger, and sadness
- Flashbacks or intrusive thoughts about the assault
- Outbursts of anger
- Eating and sleeping disturbances
- Depression
- Suicidal thoughts or self-harming behaviors
- Increased use of alcohol or drugs
- Changes in relationships with friends, family, and lovers
- Decreased desire for sex

Other common reactions after a sexual assault include "generalized pain throughout the body, and *emotional reactions* such as anger, fear, anxiety, guilt, humiliation, embarrassment, self-blame, and mood swings." This is true for males as well (American College of Obstetricians and Gynecologists [ACOG], 2014).

Male and LGBTQ Victims of Sexual Assault

LGBTQ stands for lesbian, gay, bisexual, transsexual, and questioning. Lesbian, gay, and bisexual, are sexual orientations, while transsexual is more gender identification. Sexual assault is usually committed by men against women, but it is also committed by women against men and between people of the same gender. The majority of perpetrators are male; however, women also sexually assault men. Women can force men to have sex, particularly if the male is younger and more vulnerable, and often through blackmail. Women also sexually assault other women, although the statistics are difficult to ascertain.

Men experience the same symptoms women do after being sexually abused. It is just as important for a man to receive counseling for sexual trauma as it is for a woman (WOAR, 2015). According to Roger Williams University (RWU, 2011a), crisis center statistics claim that in up to 10% of sexual assaults men reported being the victim, and most male rape victims reported being raped by other men. Gay men are victims of sexual assault slightly more often than heterosexual men, especially if they are the target of hate crimes. However, heterosexual

TABLE 22-1   Drugs Associated with Sexual Assault

Mechanism of Action	Effect	Additional Information
GHB (γ-hydroxybutyric acid)* Central nervous system depressant	Onset is within 10 to 20 minutes; duration is dose related and is from 1 to 4 hours *Lower doses:* Produces euphoria, amnesia, hypotonia, and depressed respiration *Higher doses:* Can cause seizures, unconsciousness, nausea and vomiting, coma, and death	GHB needs 12 hours to be excreted from the body Used to treat narcolepsy Rapidly metabolized; difficult to detect in emergency departments and other treatment facilities
Rohypnol (flunitrazepam)† Potent benzodiazepine; 10 times stronger than diazepam	Impact is within 10 to 30 minutes and lasts 2 to 12 hours Becomes more potent when combined with alcohol Causes dizziness, amnesia, lack of motor coordination, confusion, nausea and vomiting, respiratory depression, and blackout episodes lasting 8 to 24 hours	Not legal in United States Detected in urine for up to 72 hours
Ketamine‡ Anesthetic frequently used in veterinary practice; also hallucinogenic substance related to PCP (phencyclidine)	Onset is rapid, 20 minutes orally; duration is only 30 to 60 minutes Amnesia effects may last longer Usually administered as a powder that is snorted, smoked, injected, or dissolved in drinks Causes dissociative reaction with a dreamlike state leading to deep amnesia and analgesia and complete compliance of the survivor Later, survivor may be confused, paranoid, delirious, and combative with drooling and hallucinations	

*Street names include liquid ecstasy, salty water, scoop, homeboy, and grievous bodily harm.
†Street names include "forget" drug, roofies, club drug, roachies, rophies, and Mexican Valium.
‡Street names include special K, vitamin K, bump, kitkat, purple, and super C.

men are also raped in very large numbers. The vast majority of men who are sexually assaulted are assaulted by men who consider themselves heterosexual, although they may be bisexual. Although a great percentage of male rapes occur in prisons and the military, male rape can happen in cars, restrooms, colleges, and universities; at work; or in the home. The general statistics for male-on-male rapes often do not take into account the large number of unreported male-on-male rapes in prisons and in the military. The incidence of male-on-female rapes in the military has finally being acknowledged; however, male-on-male rapes most often remain unreported. When the number of male-on-male rapes unreported in the U.S. prison system is also considered, the extent and brutality of male-on-male sexual violence is revealed. Although laws addressing male-on-male rape have been established, they are often not acknowledged or enforced, and the culture of blaming the victim persists.

LGBTQ (Lesbian, Gay, Bisexual, Transgender, Questioning) Community

According to the CDC (2014), the LGBTQ community is at risk for violence in the form of bullying, harassment, physical assault, and increased suicide (attempted or completed) because of the negative way they are perceived and treated in many parts of society. Among gay and lesbian couples it has been reported that more than 50% of gay men and lesbians recounted at least one incidence of coercion by a same-sex partner. Gay and lesbian sexual survivors may not come forward for fear of facing homophobia and prejudice as well as making their personal lives more public (DC Rape Crisis Center, 2007). The CDC (2014) reported:

- Data from Youth Risk Behavior Surveys (YRBS) conducted during 2001 indicate that 19% to 29% of gay and lesbian students and 18% to 28% of bisexual students experienced dating violence in the prior year.
- 14% to 31% of gay and lesbian students and 17% to 32% of bisexual students had been forced to have sexual intercourse at some point in their lives.

Cultural Considerations

Sexual violence occurs in all socioeconomic groups; it occurs in the suburbs, in rural communities, and in large cities; and it occurs in well-educated upper-class families, in middle-class families, and in poor and disadvantaged families. Sexual violence occurs across all ages to men, women, and children.

Cultural and societal factors play a part in forming attitudes, for example, cultural and societal norms that maintain women's inferiority and support male superiority and sexual entitlement. In such groups, often weak laws and policies related to gender inequality and high tolerance for crimes of violence coexist. Some college fraternities reflect a societal context that could encourage violence toward women, and sexual assault on campus is thought to be increasing.

Male-on-male sexual violence in the military seems to be increasing and supports the theory that sexual assault is related to positions of power. Among women, the military is another example of a societal group in which sexual assaults of women result from gender inequality along with norms that support masculine dominance. Underreporting sexual assaults is rampant in all ages and all groups for both men and women. Mengeling and colleagues (2014) conducted a survey and found that among 205 servicewomen who experienced sexual assault in the military, only 25% reported their assault. The nonreporters stated reasons such as concerns about confidentiality and adverse treatment by peers, and the belief that nothing would be done. Interestingly, officers were less likely to report than were enlisted personnel.

Awareness of sexual assault in the military has captured the public's and Congress's attention over the past few years, and changes in military policy are in the process of being implemented. However, in order to instigate substantial change, strong, enforceable laws need to be established and rape must be recognized as a serious crime for which the perpetrator should be held responsible (Mengeling et al., 2014).

THEORY

Vulnerable Individuals

Sexual assault occurs in all age groups, genders, cultures, and socioeconomic backgrounds, but some groups appear to be more vulnerable and some situations are more conducive to sexual assault. Some of this has been previously stated; however, it all bears repeating.

- **Gender:** Women have a higher vulnerability rate than men (approximately 3 to 1). Both genders are more vulnerable if they are handicapped, have cognitive problems, or have mental disorders.
- **Age:** People ages 16 to 19 seem to have a higher rate of sexual victimization than any other age group. Children are most vulnerable between the ages of 8 and 12. One in three girls and one in six boys are sexually abused before the age of 18, which constitutes up to 44% of the total number of sexual assaults or rape.
- **Older adults:** Domestic violence against older adults includes physical and sexual abuse; the perpetrators are most often adult children, especially sons, but can also include spouses, caregivers, health care providers, and other relatives. Although statistics are difficult to ascertain, when an older adult is cognitively or functionally impaired, the likelihood of being sexually assaulted increases.
- **History of sexual violence:** Women who were raped before the age of 18 are two to three times more likely to be sexually assaulted as adults.
- **Drug and alcohol use:** Use of alcohol or drugs by the perpetrator, the victim, or both is related to increased rates of victimization.
- **High-risk sexual behavior:** High-risk sexual behavior is a vulnerability that is often a consequence of childhood sexual abuse.
- **Poverty:** Poverty can make women and children more vulnerable and place them in more dangerous situations. Poor women may be at risk when they need to support themselves or their children and trade sex for food, clothing, money, or other necessary items.
- **Ethnicity or culture:** Sexual violence against indigenous women in the United States is widespread. According to Amnesty International (2015), Native American and Alaskan Native women are more than 2.5 times more likely to be raped or sexually assaulted than other women in the United States. The majority of the perpetrators, up to 86%, were non-Native men according to the American Indian and Alaskan Native women survivors.

The Perpetrator of Sexual Assault

The causes of violence toward women are multifaceted and involve biological, psychological, and social factors.

Biological Factors

From a *biological* perspective, neurophysiological factors may be risk factors in violent behavior. Alterations in the functioning of neurotransmitters—such as serotonin, dopamine, norepinephrine, acetylcholine, and γ-aminobutyric acid—may interfere with cognition and behavior (see Chapter 24).

Psychosocial Factors

From a *psychosocial* perspective, studies have found a high incidence of psychopathology and personality disorders among sexual offenders. Antisocial personality disorder, in which people are viewed as objects, is one of the most prevalent. The act of rape involves a need for control, power, degradation, and dominance over others rather than sexual satisfaction. It is thought that some sexual offenders have difficulty finding willing sexual partners and resort to coercion or rape.

Many characteristics of perpetrators of sexual assault are the same as those found in perpetrators of child abuse, intimate partner violence, and elder abuse (see Chapter 21). Not surprisingly, most perpetrators of sexual abuse report being sexually assaulted as children. Some other characteristics include:

- Impulsive and antisocial tendencies
- Association with sexually aggressive and delinquent peers
- Preference for impersonal sex
- Hostility toward women
- Childhood history of sexual and physical abuse, or witnessing family violence as a child
- Membership in a gang
- Belonging to a societal group that often refuses to acknowledge acts of sexual assault (e.g., some parts of the military, prisons, and even parts of the Peace Corps to a smaller degree)

APPLICATION OF THE NURSING PROCESS

ASSESSMENT

Sexual assault response teams (SARTs) are available across the country, most notably in big cities. The purpose of SARTs is to help victims of sexual violence cope with the present and aftermath of sexual violence. These teams work in collaboration with a variety of resources, including (1) mental health agencies, (2) rape crisis advocates, (3) law enforcement personnel, (4) detectives or investigators, (5) emergency departments, (6) **sexual assault nurse examiners (SANEs)**, and (7) attorneys. SANEs are forensic nurses who have been certified to work with victims of sexual violence. Some of the functions of the SANE are to perform a physical examination of the survivor, collect forensic evidence, provide expert testimony regarding the forensic evidence collected, support the psychobiological needs of the survivor, be part of the SART, and work closely with law enforcement agencies and the prosecutor's office. Unfortunately, most rural counties don't have certified nurses trained to perform sexual assault kit examinations. Therefore facilities are charged with transferring the victim of sexual assault to the nearest hospital that has a trained forensic nurse or a SART. Unfortunately, having to travel an hour or two to go through a forensic exam might overwhelm a victim and ultimately allow rapists to reoffend.

Hotlines and Other Sources

If the sexually assaulted individual calls a hotline, a sexual assault and violence prevention center, the police, or a campus medical center, there is certain information the sexually assaulted person needs to

BOX 22-1   Information to Help a Recent Victim of Sexual Violence in the Aftermath of Rape (Either on the Phone or in Person)

1. Go to a safe place immediately.
2. Consider reporting the rape to the police or to the campus police if it happened on campus.
3. You can report the assault and later choose not to pursue criminal proceedings.
4. If you choose not to report the assault immediately, you can do so at a later time.
   Preserve evidence of the rape:
1. Do not wash your hands or face.
2. Do not shower or bathe.
3. Do not brush your teeth.
4. Do not change clothes or straighten up the area where the assault took place.
   Offer information regarding the location of a sexual assault response team (SART), a violence prevention resource center, a crisis center, or an emergency department in the area.
   Explain that even if the victim chooses not to press charges, the victim can still have a forensic examination without the rape being reported to the police.

Data from UC San Diego. (n.d.). *What to do if you are raped.* Retrieved May 23, 2011, from http://www.UCSD.edu/current-students/wellness/_organizations/sarc/if-you-are-raped.html

know. The assaulted person should have an advocate who can explain more about the person's options and rights (Box 22-1).

Emergency Departments

When an individual who has been sexually assaulted seeks treatment, he or she is most likely seen in the emergency department (ED). People who have been sexually assaulted often go to the ED to find emotional support, help in regaining a sense of control, and reassurance regarding their safety. *A sexual assault victim who arrives at the ED should not be left alone. The staff should provide privacy, and the victim should be a priority in triage.*

The nature of sexual assault carries with it complex implications, and the individual requires psychological support, medical care, documentation of pertinent history, a thorough physical examination, and collection of specimens for use as forensic evidence. Often the physical examination and the collection of evidence are performed by a gynecologist, an ED attending physician, or a SANE. The person who collects the evidence should be forensically trained in the collection of such data. Unfortunately, facilities differ widely in the kind of care they provide, and the ideal is not always the case—care is not always compassionate, comprehensive, or competent. Most hospitals have an institutional protocol for evidence collection and use "rape kits." Correct preservation of body fluids and swabs is essential because DNA (deoxyribonucleic acid; genetic mapping) can help identify the rapist. If a date rape drug is suspected, a urine sample should be collected.

The individual has the right to refuse legal help and medical examination. Sexual assault survivors need to know they have the right to refuse police assistance but still can choose to have forensic evidence collected. To collect evidence, a *consent form must be signed* to take photographs, perform a pelvic

examination, and carry out any other procedures necessary to collect evidence and provide treatment. The individual also needs to know that all documentation is confidential—that no one can access the information without permission, unless the case goes to court. Treatment and documentation need to be accurate and meticulous, because the documentation may constitute legal evidence if the individual chooses to prosecute.

Caution is advised about the use of pejorative language when documenting the history, findings, and verbatim statements. For example:

- Instead of "alleged," use *reported.*
- Instead of "refused," use *declined.*
- Instead of "intercourse," use *penetration.*
- Instead of "in no acute distress," *describe the behavior.*

After the immediate medical issues of the patient have been addressed, it is important that forensically trained personnel perform as many elements of the *forensic examination* as the individual will allow. Once the evidence is collected, it is imperative that providers maintain a "chain of custody" until it is turned over to the authorities.

⟫ Assessment Guidelines

Sexual Assault (Follow Unit Protocols)

1. Assess and document the circumstances of the event, including presence of threats (force, trauma, weapons, resistance, sexual acts), location of incident, and circumstances surrounding the assault. *Document in patient's own words* when possible.
2. Gather data that may be used as criminal evidence in court using the institution's protocol.
3. After consent forms have been signed, forensic evidence (debris) should be obtained from clothing, fingernail scrapings, head hair, and pubic hair; smears for sperm and/or acid phosphatase should be taken from any orifice involved. (*Note:* Elevated prostatic acid phosphatase levels are indicative of the presence of semen.) Permission for any photographs taken during the assessment also needs to be obtained. (Guidelines 3 through 8 are all considered forensic evidence that might be used in court at a later date and should be done by a forensically trained professional [e.g., SANE].)
4. Assess for evidence of any physical trauma (e.g., bites, stab wounds, contusions, gunshot wounds). Use drawings (body map) and photos to identify the areas and size of trauma.
5. Perform pelvic exam to identify vaginal and cervical trauma (perform anal exam in males and sodomized females). Culture for STIs.
6. Perform psychological assessment, noting reactions to the rape event (e.g., crying, fearfulness, agitation, preoccupation, detachment). Describe all behavior in writing.
7. Perform a mental status examination.
8. Determine drug use by either the assailant or the survivor. Assess situation for potential involvement of date rape drug if it occurred in a large gathering (e.g., college campus, bar, party). A urine sample might be useful if timing is correct. Emphasize to individuals that even if they were drinking, they are *not* at fault for being assaulted. (Refer to Table 22-1 for drugs associated with sexual assault.)
9. Identify the victim's support system (e.g., family, friends, others the person trusts), and ask for permission to involve them. Explain possible delayed reactions that might occur.

DIAGNOSIS

Rape-Trauma Syndrome

The nursing diagnosis *Rape-trauma syndrome* is a variant of posttraumatic stress disorder (PTSD) and is a common sequela of psychological trauma. Left untreated, psychologically traumatic events can have devastating effects.

There are two phases of rape-trauma syndrome. The acute phase begins immediately after the crisis, followed by the long-term phase, which may begin as long as 2 weeks after the rape and may last years if untreated. *Rape-trauma syndrome: compound reaction* is also a likely diagnosis and includes both the acute phase of disorganization and the long-term recovery phase.

The Acute Phase

Typical reactions to crisis often reflect cognitive, affective, and behavioral disruptions. The most common responses are shock, numbness, and disbelief. A person may appear self-contained and calm. At other times, cognitive function may be impaired, and the person may have difficulty making decisions, solving problems, or concentrating. Or the person may cry, become hysterical, be restless or agitated, or even smile or laugh. *The acute, or disorganization, phase* is characterized by physical reactions such as generalized pain throughout the body, eating and sleeping disturbances, and emotional reactions such as anger, fear, anxiety, guilt, humiliation, embarrassment, self-blame, and mood swings (ACOG, 2014). There is no "normal" response to a sexual assault.

The Long-Term Phase

The delayed, or organization, phase may not occur until months or even years after the events and is characterized by flashbacks, nightmares, and phobias as well as somatic and gynecological symptoms (ACOG, 2014). Emotional reactions may include depression, panic disorder, and suicidal ideation and attempts, and substance abuse is more prevalent among survivors of sexual assault. Therefore *Anxiety, Risk for injury to self, Low self-esteem, Helplessness, Acute confusion, Labile mood,* etc., may also be appropriate nursing diagnoses.

However, PTSD is the long-term consequence of sexual assault. It is important to teach individuals what to expect during this phase so they will be prepared and not feel as if they are "going crazy" or "losing their mind." It is also important to understand that all sexual assault survivors will deal with the event in their own manner. Common symptoms of PTSD related to sexual assault include the following:

- **Re-experiencing the trauma:** Recurrent nightmares about the rape, flashbacks, or uninvited, intrusive thoughts during the day or night
- **Social withdrawal:** Called "psychic numbing," involves not experiencing feelings of any kind
- **Avoidance behaviors and actions:** Avoidance of all places and activities, as well as thoughts or feelings, that could recall events about the rape
- **Increased psychological arousal characteristics:** Exaggerated startle response, hypervigilance, sleep disorders, or difficulty concentrating
- **Fears and phobias:** Fear of being alone, fear of sexual encounters, and fear of the indoors or outdoors are just some examples

- **Nightmares and difficulty sleeping:** Vivid nightmares of the event that wake the individual and cause terror, disturb sleep, and prevent sleep

OUTCOMES IDENTIFICATION

Short-Term Goals

The patient will:

- Have a short-term plan for handling immediate situational needs before leaving the ED.
- Have a written list of common physical, social, and emotional reactions that may follow a sexual assault before leaving the ED.
- State the results of the physical examination completed in the ED.
- Have written access to information on obtaining competent legal counsel and community supports (individual or group) before leaving the ED.
- Have a follow-up appointment with a rape counselor or crisis counselor.
- Have support from family and friends.
- Have a list with telephone numbers of clinics or rape crisis counselors.

Long-Term Goals

The ideal outcome is that the person eventually will be able to:

- Find ongoing support to help the individual deal with the many confusing and terrifying issues and thoughts regarding the event(s).
- Return to precrisis level of functioning with minimal or no residual symptoms (survivor).
- Experience hopefulness and confidence in going ahead with life plans.
- Have comfortable and enjoyable sex (for some, it may take many years for this to happen).

IMPLEMENTATION

- Ensure that exams are conducted at sites served by examiners with advanced education and clinical experience, if possible (U.S. Department of Justice Office on Violence Against Women, 2013).
- If a transfer from one health care facility to a designated exam site is necessary, use precautions to protect evidence (U.S. Department of Justice Office on Violence Against Women, 2013).
- These patients require compassionate care. **Follow the sexual assault protocol provided in your ED procedure manual. Most protocols will include the following guidelines:** treatment of all physical injuries, STI prophylaxis, pregnancy prevention (if patient agrees), forensic evidence collection, and counseling.
- **Compassionate care** involves approaching the person who has been sexually assaulted in a nonjudgmental and empathic manner. Patients need to hear and understand that the rape is *not* their fault, and confidentiality should be stressed repeatedly. It is important to help survivors and their significant others separate the issues of vulnerability from blame. Although individuals may have made choices that made them more vulnerable to assault, they are *not* to blame for the rape. See Table 22-2 for a list of interventions to be used for the victim of sexual assault.

TABLE 22-2 Guidelines for Sexual Assault

Intervention	Rationale
1. Have someone (friend, neighbor, sexual assault advocate, or staff member) stay with the patient while he or she is waiting to be treated in the emergency department (ED).	1. People in high levels of anxiety need someone with them until the anxiety level is down to moderate. *Never leave the individual alone.*
2. **Very important:** Approach patient in a nonjudgmental manner.	2. Nurses' attitudes can have an important therapeutic effect. Displays of shock, horror, disgust, or disbelief can increase anxiety and shame.
3. **Confidentiality is crucial.**	3. The patient's situation *is not to be discussed* with anyone other than medical personnel involved unless patient gives consent.
4. Explain to the patient the signs and symptoms that many people experience during the long-term phase, for example: a. Nightmares b. Phobias c. Anxiety, depression d. Insomnia e. Somatic symptoms	4. Many individuals think they are going crazy and are not aware that this is a process that many people in their situation have experienced.
5. Listen and let the patient talk. **Do not** press the patient to talk.	5. When people feel understood, they feel more in control of their situation.
6. Stress that the patient did the right thing to save his or her life.	6. Victims of rape might feel guilt or shame. Reinforcing that they did what they had to do to stay alive can reduce guilt and maintain self-esteem.
7. **Do not** use judgmental language: • Reported *not* alleged • Declined *not* refused • Penetration *not* intercourse • Instead of reporting "no acute distress," describe the behavior	7. Pejorative terms often reflect old myths and a lack of knowledge and understanding regarding the rape victim's experience and need for immediate intervention. Words like "alleged," "refused," and "intercourse" all minimize the devastation of the event.

Forensic Examination and Issues

1. Assess the signs and symptoms of physical trauma.	1. Most common injuries are to the face, head, neck, and extremities.
2. **Explain and get permission from patient to take photos/videos and specimens.**	2. Patient's consent is needed to collect and document evidence, which later may be used in court.
3. Make a body map to identify size, color, and location of injuries. Ask permission to take photos.	3. Accurate records and photos can be used as legal evidence in the future.
4. Carefully explain all procedures before doing them (e.g., "We would like to do a vaginal [rectal] examination and do a swab. Have you had a vaginal [rectal] examination before?").	4. The individual is experiencing high levels of anxiety. Explaining in a matter-of-fact way what you plan to do and why you are doing it can help reduce fear and anxiety.
5. Explain the forensic specimens you plan to collect; inform patient that specimens can be used for identification and prosecution of the rapist, for example: • Debris in head hair and pubic hair • Skin from underneath nails • Semen samples • Blood • Urine sample (if date rape drug is suspected)	5. Collecting body fluids and swabs is essential (DNA) for identifying the rapist.
6. Encourage patient to consider treatment and evaluation for sexually transmitted infections before leaving the ED.	6. Many survivors are lost to follow-up after being seen in the ED or crisis center and will not otherwise get protection.
7. Offer prophylaxis to pregnancy.*	7. Approximately 5% to 6% of women who are raped become pregnant.
8. All data must be carefully documented: • Verbatim statements • Detailed observations of physical trauma • Detailed observation of emotional status • Results from the physical examination • All lab tests should be noted	8. Accurate and detailed documentation is crucial legal evidence.
9. Offer support follow-up: • Rape counselor • Support group • Group therapy • Individual therapy • Crisis counseling	9. Many individuals can be burdened with constant emotional trauma. Depression and suicidal ideation are frequent sequelae of rape. The sooner the intervention, the less complicated the recovery may be.

*"A victim of sexual assault should be offered prophylaxis for pregnancy, subject to informed consent and consistent with current treatment guidelines. Conscience statutes will continue to protect health care providers who have moral or religious objections to providing certain forms of contraception. In a case in which a provider refuses to offer certain forms of contraception for moral or religious reasons, victims of sexual assault *must* receive information on how to access these services in a timely fashion." U.S. Department of Justice Office on Violence Against Women. (2013). *A national protocol for sexual assault medical forensic examinations: Adults/adolescents* (2nd ed., Section C, 9 – Pregnancy Evaluation and Care). Retrieved October 5, 2015, from http://www.njrs.gov/pdffiles1./ovw/241903.pdf

A Person Experiencing Sexual Assault

Scenario

A neighbor brought 40-year-old Margaret to the emergency department (ED) following her report of a sexual assault by a twenty-something male who gained access to Margaret's home by claiming the need to make a phone call because of car trouble. The ED called ahead to a nearby hospital that was set up for sexual assault victims and had a forensic examiner. Margaret was waiting for transportation. My student status enabled me to provide continuity of care so I could stay with Margaret, never leaving her alone in the ED. I established the contact, struggling to hear Margaret, who spoke in a whisper.

Therapeutic Goal

By the close of this interaction, Margaret will allow herself to acknowledge her survival and to express her concerns.

Student-Patient Interaction	Thoughts, Communication Techniques, and Mental Health Nursing Concepts
Margaret: (*Voice tense.*) "I don't want to be alone. Not now. Not ever." **Student's feelings:** *I would be afraid to be alone, too, if someone attacked me in my own home. But why did she trust a stranger? I struggle with countertransference. I have to be alert to not blame the victim as a way to distance myself; if I make this Margaret's fault, then rape cannot happen to me.*	Margaret started our interaction with a whisper, which makes me think she may be reacting with the *controlled style* in this *acute phase* of the *rape-trauma syndrome.* Yet her tense assertion of not wanting to be alone may indicate the *expressed style.*
Student: "I am staying right here with you. You've been through a terrible ordeal."	I *offer self* and *attempt to translate* into feelings.
Margaret: "I feel so ashamed."	Earlier Margaret asked for water and I had to say no until all the evidence is collected. I am staying alert and especially careful to follow the rape crisis protocol for this ED for Margaret's sake and for any legal ramifications.
Student: "What happened was not your fault. You don't have anything to be ashamed of." **Student's feelings:** *Without thinking, I immediately reassured Margaret that she has no reason to be ashamed. Even as I speak the words, I notice Margaret pulling away. I wonder now if I wasn't really reassuring myself.*	Reassurance seems supportive but actually discounts the patient's feelings. Margaret feels more alone now.
Margaret: "You don't understand. No one does." (*Looks downward.*)	
Student: "You're right. I don't understand what you went through. Margaret, I care about what happened to you and I want to understand."	I *offer self* and *give control* to Margaret, acknowledging that only she knows her experience.

Student-Patient Interaction	Thoughts, Communication Techniques, and Mental Health Nursing Concepts
Student's feelings: *I do care about Margaret.* **Margaret:** "I don't know how I will ever tell my husband." (*Eyes swell with tears, which she angrily brushes away, then proceeds to rub her temples.*)	
Student: "You feel worried about his reaction."	I *attempt to translate into feelings* by saying "worried." I assess Margaret's *anxiety* to be at least *moderate.* Physical signs arise at the *severe level* and Margaret is now rubbing her temples, as though she has a headache. Though she did not report a headache at the intake assessment, Margaret's stress and anxiety may be stimulating additional physiological responses.
Margaret: "Why would he even want to be with me—damaged goods."	
Student: "You feel damaged, unlovable." **Student's feelings:** *I feel sad that she has the added burden of dealing with the reactions of loved ones who might not be supportive.*	I use *restatement* and *attempt to translate into feelings.*
Margaret: "Unlovable." (*Eyes again fill with tears. Margaret presses her fists against her eyelids.*)	
Student: "Margaret, it's okay to cry." *Margaret shakes her head.*	I give permission to lend *support* and *acceptance.*
Student: "I wonder what it would mean to you to cry."	I ask an *indirect question* to assess underlying dynamics.
Margaret: (*Breathing deeply to suppress tears.*) "That I am a weak woman, so weak I couldn't stop that monster." **Student's feelings:** *It's kind of scary. This could be me at another time.*	She uses the word "monster." It must have been such a horrible violation of her personhood.
Student: "You had the strength to stay alive. You did what you had to do to survive. Your instincts acted properly to keep you alive."	I give *support* affirming that Margaret was, in fact, able to stay alive. She survived the assault.
Margaret: "I am alive. Damaged, but alive." (*Eyes water.*)	
Student: "You look close to tears." (*Margaret nods.*) "It's okay to grieve, to let your feelings out."	I *make an observation.* Sharing the pain and allowing the *grief* decrease the intensity of the pain.
Margaret: *Sobs, accepts a tissue, and holds on to my hand.* **Student's feelings:** *I feel Margaret's trust that she reaches for my hand.*	Just then the medical transportation arrived to take her to a hospital with a rape crisis counselor and sexual assault nurse examiner.

Pharmacological, Biological, and Integrative Therapies
Emergency Department

The updated U.S. Department of Justice Office on Violence Against Women (2013) protocol emphasizes the following:

- Consider sexual assault patients a priority.
- Perform a prompt, competent medical assessment.
- Then respond to acute injury, the need for trauma care, and safety needs of patients before collecting evidence.
- Alert forensic examiners (e.g., SANE) of the need for their services.
- Contact victim advocates so they can offer services to patients, if not already done.
- Assess and respond to safety concerns of victims upon arrival at the exam site (e.g., Are there threats to patient or staff?).
- Assess patients' need for immediate medical or mental health intervention prior to the evidentiary exam, following facility policy. Physical signs of sexual assault include (Ernoehazy, 2013):
- Presence of blood and/or sperm
- Contusions
- Lacerations
- Abdominal trauma
- Joint dislocation
- Mechanical back pain
- Lesions caused by forceful genital penetration
- Abruptio placentae

"In 2012, 346,830 women were raped. According to medical reports, the incidence of pregnancy for one-time unprotected sexual intercourse is 5%. By applying the pregnancy rate to 346,830 female survivors, RAINN estimates that there were **17,342 pregnancies** as a result of rape in 2012" (Rape, Abuse & Incest National Network [RAINN], 2015).

Emergency department treatment consists of the administration of prophylactic antibiotics for the most common STIs (chlamydia, gonorrhea, trichomoniasis, and bacterial vaginosis [BV]), with the victim's consent. Pregnancy prophylactics include the administration of Ovral tablets if pregnancy tests are negative. *Emergency contraception (EC) is a safe, effective medication that prevents pregnancy after sexual assault. It does not induce abortion or terminate a pregnancy.*

The guidelines also recommend updating the individual's tetanus if abrasions or open wounds are present and administration of the hepatitis B vaccine if not already immunized (Ernoehazy, 2013). The American College of Obstetricians and Gynecologists (ACOG, 2014)

states that "If the assailant's HIV status is unknown, clinicians should evaluate the risks and benefits of nonoccupational postexposure prophylaxis on a case-by-case basis."

Pharmacology

Short-term treatment with a benzodiazepine may help ameliorate the acute anxiety and agitation that follow a trauma. Antidepressants (selective serotonin reuptake inhibitors [SSRIs]) may be helpful for symptoms of PTSD such as hyperarousal, agitation, and insomnia, and in the treatment of depression and panic attacks.

Psychotherapy

Crisis counseling should always be available to any person who has been sexually assaulted, including referrals to the family physician, community psychologist, or community rape crisis line, for example. The nurse assesses the assaulted individual to ascertain if there are any thoughts of suicide or homicide. If no SART is available, information on support groups, therapists, and attorneys who work with sexual assault survivors should be provided before the person leaves the ED. A list of safe houses should also be available for those involved in intimate partner violence (IPV). Caring for survivors is not completed in a single visit. Their emotional state and other psychological needs should be assessed within 24 to 48 hours by phone after being treated and actual resolution may take years in some cases.

Group therapy or support groups can be beneficial for survivors. Sharing experiences with others who are going through the devastating physical and emotional aftermath of rape can be healing and break through feelings of isolation, shame, and guilt.

Therapy for Rapists

Alterations in thinking and behavior need to be undertaken in order to effect change. Unfortunately, most rapists do not acknowledge the need for change. No single method or program of treatment has been found to be totally effective.

EVALUATION

Most patients eventually will be able to resume their previous lives after supportive services and crisis counseling or therapy. If survivors are relatively free of signs of PTSD and their lifestyles are close to their lifestyles before the rape, the recovery is considered successful. Too often, without counseling of some kind various sequelae of the assault may remain for years or even a lifetime.

APPLYING EVIDENCE-BASED PRACTICE (EBP)

Problem A 19-year-old female presents to her college health center. When the RN is checking her in, the patient asks for the morning-after pill and begins to cry. As the nurse gently talks to her, the patient reveals she was raped while on a date the night before.

EBP Assessment

A. **What do you already know from experience?** Rape victims are often reluctant to talk about what happened, and may refuse treatment or to press charges. They may be embarrassed, hoping everything will just go away, or fearful of their attacker. It can be difficult as a nurse to support patient decisions when you feel a different action would be better.

B. **What does the literature say?** Rape is unfortunately more common that most people realize. Up to 29% of women will be raped in their lifetimes in the United States (Centers for Disease Control and Prevention [CDC], 2015; U.S. Department of Justice, 2015), and 32,000 rapes result in pregnancy annually. One in 71 men report being raped at some point in their lives (CDC, 2012). The majority of rapes are not reported, with college-age victims having the highest rate at 95% (U.S. Department of Justice, 2015). Sexual assault history should be elicited in a nonjudgmental and compassionate manner.

C. **What does the patient want?** The patient is requesting the morning-after pill. She is refusing a forensic examination or to speak with law enforcement.

APPLYING EVIDENCE-BASED PRACTICE (EBP)—cont'd

She initially does not want to even talk about the rape anymore with the nurse, but eventually accepts patient education and resources.

Plan The nurse supported the patient and followed her wishes. The patient was prescribed the morning-after pill by the clinic physician. The nurse told the patient that she could not and would not force her to do anything she did not want to do, but would like to give her some information. The nurse explained the forensic procedure, sexually transmitted infection testing, and time limits if the patient changes her mind. She discussed how reactions to trauma may appear later, as anxiety, depression, isolating, changes in relationships, decreased self-esteem, suicidal thoughts, flashbacks, or nightmares (CDC, 2015). The patient was given information on a rape support center, how to contact law enforcement, restraining orders, and counseling services. The clinic is engaged is improving outreach and rape prevention services at the college.

QSEN QSEN Prelicensure Knowledge, Skills, and Attitudes (KSAs) Addressed:

Quality improvement was addressed as the clinic worked to improve services.
Patient-centered care was practiced by the nurse, as she respected the individual's choices.

Centers for Disease Control and Prevention (CDC). (2015). *Sexual violence: Consequences.* Retrieved from www.cdc.gov/violenceprevention/sexualviolence/consequences.html; Centers for Disease Control and Prevention (CDC). (2012). *Sexual violence: Facts at a glance.* Retrieved from www.cdc.gov/violenceprevention/pdf/sv-datasheet-a.pdf; U.S. Department of Justice. (2015). *Rape statistics.* Retrieved from http://www.statistic-brain.com/rape-statistics/

KEY POINTS TO REMEMBER

- Sexual assault is an act of violence, control, and hate; it is a criminal offense that often results in severe long-term psychiatric trauma for the victim.
- To preserve forensic evidence, the victim should be aware of precautions to take before contacting the police, crisis center, or emergency facility.
- Contact with the sexual assault patient usually takes place in the ED. Only nurses with special training (e.g., sexual assault nurse examiners [SANEs]) assess the patient, collect data, and provide information and referrals (e.g., to therapists, legal counsel, support groups) for patients before they leave the ED.
- Permission is necessary for collecting forensic data, performing a pelvic examination, and taking photographs. Confidentiality is stressed.
- Following the sexual assault, a forensic examination is conducted and evidence is collected. The patient should be given medications to protect against STIs, evaluated for pregnancy, offered prophylaxis, and if warranted tested for HIV and syphilis. If abrasions are noted, a tetanus shot may be indicated if not updated in the past 5 years, and inoculation for hepatitis B is needed.
- Careful documentation of findings (diagrams and photos), observations of emotional status, and descriptions of the events surrounding the assault are documented using verbatim statements whenever possible.
- Assessment for date rape drugs should be included if the description of the event (loss of consciousness, vomiting) indicates they are a possibility. In such a case, a urine sample may be obtained.
- To help alleviate anxiety, explanations of all interventions or procedures are provided to the patient before they are performed.
- Before leaving the ED, sexually assaulted individuals are told what kinds of reactions are commonly experienced by sexually traumatized victims following a crisis.
- Follow-up counseling, support groups, and referrals to effective legal attorneys who specialize in sexual assault should always be given before discharge from the ED.

APPLYING CRITICAL JUDGMENT

1. Sally M. is brought by a friend to the emergency department (ED). She is dazed, and the friend explains that a few friends went to a bar and met some guy Sally had met at a party on campus. He bought them all drinks. Sally said that after a few drinks, "I felt funny and don't remember much except that I woke up outside the back of the bar with my underclothes off and a number of reddened marks and abrasions on my breasts and arms. I have so much pain and burning in my vagina. I feel like I'm going crazy, I am so frightened." Her friends found her semiconscious and brought her to the ED. Sally appears confused and alternates between crying uncontrollably and staring into space. She repeatedly says she wants to wash up and change clothes, but her friend wanted her to come into the ED as soon as possible.

   A. Chart the objective and subjective symptoms of Sally's physical and emotional trauma using the guidelines from this chapter and including a body map.

   B. After Sally consents to the forensic examination, how would you describe to her the procedures that will be performed during the forensic and pelvic examinations?

   C. Why might you ask Sally for a urine specimen at this time?

   D. Sally is afraid and does not want her parents or anyone on campus to know what happened, and especially does not want the event to be reported to the police. What information could you give her that may allay some of her concerns?

   E. Describe the emergency medical treatment that should be offered to all sexually assaulted individuals.

   F. If there is no SART in the ED, what actions should the hospital personnel take in a timely fashion?

   G. You know that Sally may experience devastating sequelae of her sexual assault that can take years to resolve. What kind of supports and referrals should Sally be given before she leaves the ED?

   H. Use the Internet to find resources available in your community to aid rape victims; print a handout with names, addresses, and phone numbers.

   I. Determine if there is a *sexual assault response team* (SART) in your community. Using the Internet, secure the phone number, address, and website address and share this information with your classmates.

   J. Determine if there is a sexual assault nurse examiner (SANE) in any of your community clinics or crisis centers and share this information with your classmates.

2. A friend calls you at 3 AM and tells you that she has been raped and has run out of the man's apartment to a nearby coffeehouse, not knowing what to do. You tell her you will meet her at the coffeehouse and then take her to the emergency department. You tell her

not to go home. What are some other things you would instruct your friend *not* to do to help preserve evidence?

3. Share among five different young people in separate situations the following guidelines for diminishing the risk of ingesting date rape drugs when at fraternity parties, large gatherings, raves, nightclubs, or rock concerts, for example:

   A. Do not accept open drinks (i.e., alcoholic or nonalcoholic beverages from strangers or others you do not know well or trust; this includes drinks that are in a glass).

   B. When in bars or nightclubs, always get your drink directly from the bartender and do not take your eyes off the bartender when you order; do not use the waitress or let somebody else go to the bar for you. At parties, only accept drinks in closed containers: bottles, cans, or Tetra Paks.

   C. Never leave your drink unattended or turn your back on your table.

   D. Do not drink from "resources like punch bowls, pitchers, tubs, or community water/juice bottles."

   E. Stay alert; if there is talk of date rape drugs or if your friends seem "too intoxicated" for what they have taken, leave the party or nightclub immediately and do not go back!

From U.S. Department of Health and Human Services, National Institutes of Health, National Institute on Drug Abuse, 6001 Executive Blvd., Washington, DC. Available at http://teenadvice.about.com/ Box.

CHAPTER REVIEW QUESTIONS

1. An elderly widow tells the nurse, "Since my sister-in-law's death, her husband has been making advances at me. He tried to come in my home with a bottle of wine. Even though he's family, I'm afraid of what might happen if I let him in." Which action should the nurse take first?

   a. Support the widow to clarify her thoughts and feelings about the situation.

   b. Explain to the widow how to obtain an order of protection (restraining order).

   c. Positively reinforce the widow for addressing the problem with a caring professional.

   d. Educate the widow about sexual assault and violence, including the importance of prevention.

2. An emergency department nurse talks with a newly admitted victim of reported rape. Which communication should the nurse offer to comfort this patient?

   a. "You are safe now. I will stay with you in this private room."

   b. "Would you like your friend to stay with you during your examination?"

   c. "You made a good decision to come to the hospital after you were raped."

   d. "What questions do you have about your examination by the sexual assault nurse examiner?"

3. A patient tells the nurse, "I was raped 8 years ago but never told anyone. Nevertheless, the memories haunt me every day. I should be over it by now." Which comment should the nurse offer next?

   a. "It sounds like you're judging yourself for continuing to struggle with your reaction."

   b. "Rape is criminal behavior. You should have reported the incident to law enforcement."

   c. "Are you now ready to engage in counseling to deal with your reactions to this experience?"

   d. "While it's important to learn from such life events, it's more important to put things in the past."

4. An emergency department nurse prepares to discharge a victim of reported rape. Which comment by the victim indicates that the nurse's teaching was effective?

   a. "I should bathe frequently over the next week."

   b. "I am required to follow up with law enforcement."

   c. "It's important for me to follow up with counseling."

   d. "I should delay any sexual activity for at least 3 months."

5. A victim of reported sexual assault tells the nurse, "This was entirely my fault. I should never have gone to that party alone." Which response by the nurse is most therapeutic?

   a. "This was a frightening experience for you."

   b. "What do you think you should have done differently?"

   c. "Would you like to tell me more about what happened?"

   d. "It sounds like you're blaming yourself for the assailant's behavior."

REFERENCES

American College of Obstetricians and Gynecologists (ACOG). (2014). *Sexual assault.* Retrieved July 11, 2015, from http://www.agog.org/Resources-And-Publications/Committees-on-Health-Care-for-Underserved-Women/Sexual-Assault.

Amnesty International. (2015). *Maze of injustice: A summary of Amnesty International's findings.* Retrieved July 6, 2015, from http://www.amnestyusa.org/our-work/issues/women-s-rights/violence-against-women/maze-of-injustice.

Black, M. C., Breiding, M. J., Smith, S. G., et al. (2011). *National intimate partner and sexual violence survey: 2010 summary report.* Retrieved July 6, 2015, from http://www.cdc.gov/Violence Prevention/pdf/NISVS_Report2010-a.pdf.

Breiding, M. J., Smith, S. G., Basile, K. C., et al. (2014). Prevalence and characteristics of sexual violence, stalking, and intimate partner violence victimization in the United States—National Intimate Partner and Sexual Violence Survey, United States, 2011. *Morbidity and Mortality Weekly Report, 63*(SS-8), 1–18.

Centers for Disease Control and Prevention (CDC). (2011). *Understanding sexual violence: fact sheet.* Retrieved May 16, 2011, from http://www.cdc.gov/violenceprevention.

Centers for Disease Control and Prevention (CDC). (2014). *LGBT youth: lesbian, gay, bisexual, and transgender.* Retrieved July 8, 2015, from http://www.cdc.gov/lgbthealth/youth. Htn.

Centers for Disease Control and Prevention (CDC). (2015). *Injury prevention and control: Division violence prevention.* Retrieved July 8, 2015, from http://www.cdc.gov/ViolencePrevention/index.html.

Cleveland Clinic Foundation. (2009). *Raising healthy infants, children and teens: rape and date rape.* Retrieved May 21, 2011, from http://my.clevelandclinic/healthy_living/violence/hic_rape_and_date_rape.aspx.

DC Rape Crisis Center. (2007). Retrieved February 10, 2007, from http://www.dcrcc.org/same-sex.htm.

Department of Justice (DOJ). (2012). *An updated definition of rape.* Retrieved July 5, 2015, from http://www.justice.gov/opa/blog/updated-definition-rape.

Ernoehazy, W. (2013). *Sexual assault practice essentials updated 2013.* Retrieved July 1, 2015, from http://emedicine.medscape.com/article/806120.overview-treatment.

Finkelhor, D, Shattuck, A., Turner, H.A., et al. The lifetime prevalence of child sexual abuse and assault assessed in late adolescence. Journal of Adolescent Health. Retrieved from http://www.unh.edu/ccrc/pdf/9248.pdf.

Mengeling, M. A., Booth, B. M., Tomer, J. C., et al. (2014). *Reporting sexual assault in the military: who reports and why most servicemen don't.* Retrieved July 9, 2015, from http://www.sciencedirect.com/science/article/pii/S0749379714001184.

National Sexual Violence Resource Center (NSVRC). The resource: the national sexual violence resource center' s newsletter. Retrieved from http://www.nsvrc.org/sites/default/files/publications_nsvrc-the-resource_fall-winter-2014.pdf.

Parents for Megan's Law and The Crime Victims Center (PML). (2007a). *Statistics: child sexual abuse.* Retrieved May 21, 2011, from http://www.parentsformeganslaw.org/public/statistics_childsexualabuse.html.

Rape, Abuse & Incest National Network (RAINN). (2015). *Who are the victims?* Retrieved July 10, 2015, from http://rainn.org/get-information/statistics/sexual-assault-victims.

Roger Williams University (RWU). (2011a). *Sexual assault: date rape drugs.* Retrieved May 22, 2011, from http://www.rwu.edu/studentlife/studentservices/counselingcenter/sexualassault/daterapedrug.

Seaman, A. M. (2015). *More evidence rape a significant problem on US college campuses.* Retrieved July 10, 2015, from http://bit.ly/1eg68zM. http://bit.ly/1Fovggq. J Adolesc Health 2015.

TeenBreaks. (2011a). *Incest, and sexual abuse.* Retrieved May 17, 2011, from http://www.teenbreaks.com/sexualabuse/incestsexualabuse.cfm.

U.S. Department of Justice Office on Violence Against Women. (2013). *A national protocol for sexual assault medical forensic examinations: adults/adolescents* (2nd ed.). Retrieved October 5, 2015, from. http://www.njrs.gov/pdffiles1./ovw/241903.pdf.

U.S. Department of Justice National Sex Offender Public (NSOPW). (updated 2014). Retrieved February10, 2016, from https://www.nsopw.gov/en

Women Organized Against Rape (WOAR). (2015). *Common reactions to sexual assault: long-term effects of sexual assault.* Retrieved July 5, 2015, from http://www.woar.org/resources/common-reactions-to-assault.php.

Women Organized Against Rape (WOAR). (2015). *Child sexual abuse and assault-reactions in children who have been sexually abused.* Retrieved July 5, 2015, from http://www.woar.org/resources/child-sexual-abuse.php.

Ybarra, M. L., & Mitchell, K. J. (2013). *Prevalence rates of male and female sexual violence perpetrators national sample of adolescents.* Retrieved July 2, 2015, from http://archpedi.jamanetwork.com/article. aspx? articleid=1748355.

Suicidal Thoughts and Behaviors

Elizabeth M. Varcarolis

http://evolve.elsevier.com/Varcarolis/essentials

KEY TERMS AND CONCEPTS

completed suicide, p. 362
Modified SAD PERSONS Scale, p. 365
physician aid in dying (PAD), p. 363
physician-assisted suicide (PAS), p. 363
postvention, p. 370

psychological postmortem
  assessment, p. 371
sub-intentioned suicide, p. 364
suicidal ideation, p. 362

Suicide Assessment Five-Step Evaluation
  and Triage (SAFE-T), p. 365
suicide, p. 362
suicide attempt, p. 362

SELECTED CONCEPT: THOUGHTS ON SUICIDE

"Suicide in its many forms has inspired everything from condemnation to romanticism, most focusing on the morality of taking one's own life and whether it can be justified as a reasonable option."

What happens when it hurts too much to live? Can it really be too painful to live one more moment with emptiness, depression, and despair? Not everyone who contemplates killing themselves is truly interested in ending their time on earth, often they just want to escape the pain or can't find a way out (Cholbi, 2013).

And what about an individual who is mentally competent, whose every moment involves suffering intractable pain from a terminal illness, and who wants to leave life with some dignity and control over when and how to say goodbye to loved ones (Vaughanbell, 2008).

OBJECTIVES

1. Explain the roles of culture, religion, and socioeconomic status as they relate to suicidal risk.
2. **QSEN** Provide **patient-centered care** by discussing the implications as well as the risk factors identified in the Modified SAD PERSONS Scale when determining risk for suicide potential.
3. **QSEN** Promote **safety** by discussing the kinds of safety procedures that are followed for an acutely suicidal individual who has been hospitalized.
4. Describe the need and rationale for postvention for family or friends of an individual who has completed suicide.
5. **QSEN** Discuss how staff psychological postmortem assessment postvention may contribute to improved coordination of care.
6. **QSEN** Identify the needed interventions that might provide **quality improvement** methods to help identify and prevent suicide for our returning war veterans.
7. Summarize the overt, covert, and behavioral clues and the steps in evaluating the lethality of a suicide plan for an individual who is contemplating suicide.
8. **QSEN** Using **informatics**, make a list of support groups within your community that might help people who are suicidal, such as support groups for veterans, suicide hotlines, crisis centers, and substance use groups (e.g., Alcoholics Anonymous, SMART Recovery).
9. **QSEN** Applying communication techniques, identify some of the most important dialogue and questions needed to **promote safety**.
10. Contrast and compare the pros and cons of "right to die" physician-assisted suicide (PAS) as outlined in the chapter.
11. **QSEN** Using **informatics** go to Suicide Assessment Five-Step Evaluation and Triage (SAFE-T): Pocket Card for Clinicians. http://store.samsha.gov/product/Suicide-Assessment-Five-Step-Evaluation-and-Triage-SAFE-T-Pocket-Card-for-Clinicians/SMA09-4432

INTRODUCTION

Suicide or completed suicide is the act of intentionally ending one's own life (intentional self-inflicted death). The act of intentionally taking one's own life arouses intense and complex emotions in others. Completed suicide leaves long-lasting emotional scars with family, friends, and even involved physicians nurses and staff. Suicide attempt includes all willful, self-inflicted, life-threatening attempts that have not led to

death. Suicidal ideation refers to the process of thinking about killing oneself. *Always* take an individual very seriously if he or she mentions some form of suicidal ideation. *Always* ask, "Are you thinking of killing yourself?" Listen very carefully to what the person does and does not say. Appropriate nursing interventions are outlined later in this chapter.

The more recent growth of the secular philosophy—the foundation of which is respect for an individual's will and basic human rights (death with dignity)—has influenced the perception of suicide in our society. This philosophy has led to a movement that supports the right of mentally competent adults to humanely end their own suffering. The natural extension of this perspective is the practice of physician-assisted suicide (PAS) or physician aid in dying (PAD) for the terminally ill, which operates under very strict guidelines. For example, Washington State, which passed the Death with Dignity Act in 2009, states that the following conditions must exist:

- The patient must not have any neuromedical or psychiatric conditions that impair capacity to reason and process information.
- The patient must be diagnosed as having less than 6 months to live.
- The patient must make a request orally and in writing, and have the agreement for PAS approved by two different physicians.
- After a 15-day waiting period, the patient must then make the request again.

The key difference between euthanasia and PAS/PAD is who administers the lethal dose of medication. Euthanasia entails the physician or another third party administering the medication, whereas PAD/PAS requires the patient to self-administer the medication and to determine whether and when to do this (Starks, 2013).

In the United States, as of February 2016, only four states have legalized PAS/PAD (death with dignity laws): Washington, Oregon, California, and Vermont. A number of states have bills pending legislation. It may be helpful to understand why some people are proponents of physician-assisted suicide. The following statement was made by Montana's State Justice John Warren when the law first passed, before it was contested by the Attorney General of Montana in 2011 (Kirkland, 2010):

> … a competent, incurably ill person (who is)… going through prolonged (terminal) suffering and shows excruciating physical deterioration to hang on to the last possible moment…. The state has not come close to showing that it has any interest, much less a "compelling" one in serving a competent, incurably ill individual's autonomous decision needs a licensed physician's assistance in dying so that she(he) may die with the same human dignity with which she(he) was born.

At present, other than the four U.S. states mentioned, only a few jurisdictions legally sanction PAS/PAD, including the Netherlands, Belgium, Switzerland, and Luxembourg (Dignitas, 2015). The "right to die with dignity" issue is very controversial and complex.

PREVALENCE AND COMORBIDITY

Suicide rates differ with **gender, age, race,** and **geography.** Suicide is the third leading cause of death among persons aged 10 to 14 years, the second among persons aged 15 to 34 years, the fourth among persons aged 35 to 44 years, the fifth among persons aged 55 to 64 years, and the 17th among persons 65 years and older (Centers for Disease Control and Prevention [CDC], 2015). Suicide completers are four times more likely to be men (Sadock, Sadock, & Ruiz, 2015). Suicide rates tend to increase with age. Most men are 45 years or older; white; separated, widowed, or divorced; and the suicide rate tends to peak after age 75 (Black & Andreasen, 2014). Among women, the suicide rate peaks after the age of 55 (Sadock, Sadock, & Ruiz, 2015). Whites are more likely to end their lives, and do so approximately two to three times more frequently than African Americans (Sadock, Sadock, & Ruiz, 2015). The suicide rate among Native Americans and Alaskan Native adolescents and young adults ages 10 to 34 is the second leading cause of death (CDC, 2015). Most suicide rates are higher in the western states and peak in the late spring and in the fall.

Epidemiological surveys have demonstrated that 90% of suicide completers had a diagnosable psychiatric condition at the time of the event (Black & Andreasen, 2014). "Mood disorders, especially major depressive disorder and bipolar disorder, are responsible for approximately 50% of completed suicides, alcohol and substance use disorders for 25%, psychosis about 10%, and personality disorders 5%" (Brendel et al., 2016, p. 590). Individuals with borderline personality disorders are often found to be chronically suicidal, and often this is one of the main focuses of their therapy. The Department of Veterans Affairs has been tracking the **suicide rate among Iraq and Afghanistan veterans** since 2008. Alarmingly, a recent calculation found that the number of deaths among active-duty U.S. soldiers by suicide was higher than that of all combat soldiers killed in Afghanistan (Rothberg & Feinstein, 2014). These statistics do not include the disproportionate rate of deaths of veterans returning to civilian life that psychologists speculate are most likely related to risky behaviors and that are more common among people with posttraumatic stress disorder (PTSD).

Traumatic brain injury (TBI) refers to any type of trauma to the head that affects brain functioning. It is estimated that between 15% and 23% of returning war veterans have experienced a TBI, which can have a severe impact on a person's functioning (Beck Institute Blog, 2010). It is believed that those who tested positive for TBI were more likely to be diagnosed with depression, anxiety disorders, PTSD, adjustment disorders, psychosis, and bipolar disorders (James et al., 2014). A 2011 study of veterans, consistent with other studies of people in the general population, found that individuals with TBI have an increased risk of dying by suicide compared with people without brain injuries (Voelker, 2012). Previous studies have found that military members who suffered more than one mild traumatic brain injury had "higher rates of suicide." A study of older veterans with mild brain injuries showed they were "more likely to develop Alzheimer's disease or other dementia-type diseases later in life" (Castillo, 2014).

Physical illnesses may also play a role in increasing suicide risk. It is estimated that 5% of suicide completers had a serious medical condition at the time of their suicide (Black & Andreasen, 2014). For example, people with TBI, terminal epilepsy, and/or painful diseases such as acquired immunodeficiency syndrome (AIDS), cancer, multiple sclerosis, Huntington's chorea, and Parkinson's disease are at an increased risk for suicide. For those in extreme pain or those with little if any quality of life, intentional death—either physician-assisted or self-inflicted—may be a means of escaping from intolerable pain and the extreme limitations imposed by illness.

Certain medications may also contribute to symptoms of depression; these include antihypertensives, benzodiazepines, calcium channel blockers, corticosteroids, hormonal medications, and medications to treat pain. Depression and substance use disorder (benzodiazepines, opioids) contribute to higher rates of suicide. Multiple medications have the adverse effect of inducing suicide ideation, and many come with Black Box warnings. This is why the U.S. Food and Drug Administration (FDA) requires all new drugs to be assessed for precipitating suicidal feelings.

Nurses are likely to encounter individuals with suicidal thoughts or active intent in outpatient settings, intensive care units, nursing homes, or medical-surgical units; during home visits; or even among one's own family and friends.

THEORY

Sigmund Freud (1856–1939) developed some of the first psychological theories of suicide in the early 1900s. Freud described suicide as a murderous attack on an ambivalently loved, internalized significant person, often referred to as "murder in the 180th degree." Building on Freud's theory, **Karl Menninger** (1893–1990) suggested that all individuals who commit suicide experience three interrelated emotions: revenge, depression, and guilt.

Edwin Shneidman (1918-2009) proposed that victims of suicide suffer unbearable psychological pain, a sense of isolation, and the perception that death is the only solution to their situation. In essence, an individual feels that "there is no way out." Shneidman identified self-destructive behaviors (compulsive use of drugs, hyperobesity, gambling, self-harmful sexual behaviors, medical noncompliance, and other high-risk behaviors) as sub-intentioned suicide.

Herbert Hendin, medical director of the American Foundation for Suicide Prevention, states that Shneidman was the first person in the United States to call public attention to the problem of suicide. Hendin goes on to say that "however, the biggest advances in the field of suicide prevention in the last 15 years have been in the field of biology and the pharmacology of depression and suicide; it borders on malpractice for a doctor not to prescribe medication for seriously depressed individuals" (Curwen, 2004).

Contributing Risk Factors for Suicide

Many risk factors may be involved, but there is no single theory that explains suicide. There are, however, some commonalities. Commonalities include aggressive/impulsive traits, hopelessness or pessimistic traits, substance use disorders and alcoholism, a history of physical or sexual abuse during childhood, a history of head injury or neurological disorder, and cigarette smoking.

Other factors often involved in individuals who attempt or complete suicide are poor critical thinking skills, troubled emotional lives (anger, anxiety, guilt, boredom), and a low threshold for emotional pain. However, note that a person may experience one or more risk factors and not be suicidal.

Poland (2009) cites assessment of markers for youth suicide that involve family and developmental background:

- Children or teens who lost a parent to suicide (three times more likely to commit suicide)
- Childhood maltreatment
- Problematic family relations
- History of bullying and victimization
- Family history of suicide
- Socioeconomic problems
- Parental psychopathology
- Peer problems
- Legal and/or discipline problems

Refer to Figure 1-1 for a clinical algorithm for the suspicion of suicide risk.

Neurobiological Aspects of Suicide

Low levels of 5-hydroxyindoleacetic (5-HIAA) in cerebral spinal fluid (CSF) have long been associated with impulsive suicide-like violence. For example, people who have attempted suicide have lower levels of 5-HIAA serotonin functioning, and those who completed suicide have the lowest levels of 5-HIAA. In fact, low levels of 5-HIAA in the CSF can predict future attempts and future completed suicides (Brendel et al., 2016). **Serotonin (5-hydroxytryptamine; 5-HT)** is an important neurotransmitter as it pertains to completed suicide. Studies of the brains of those who have completed suicide show abnormalities of the serotonin system in an area of the brain called the *ventral medial prefrontal cortex*. Changes in both presynaptic and postsynaptic serotonin receptors in the prefrontal cortex are present in some but not all suicide completers (Brendel et al., 2016; Mathews et al., 2013).

Biological responses to *stress* may also constitute a risk factor for many people. The **noradrenergic system** is a mediator of acute stress responses, and overactivity of that system has been associated with both severe anxiety or agitation and higher suicidal risk, according to Mathews and colleagues' (2013) research of the literature. The **hypothalamic-pituitary-adrenal (HPA) axis** is another major stress response system. The HPA axis is associated with major depression, and suicide victims often exhibit HPA axis abnormalities (Mathews et al., 2013).

Genetic Factors

Suicide has long been shown to cluster in some families; therefore family history is pertinent. A striking example is the family of novelist Ernest Hemingway, in which five members in four generations completed suicide (a number of Hemingway's family members suffered from mental illness and/or substance use disorders). Several lines of research involving twin and adoption studies found links to suicide behavior independent of psychiatric disorders (Black & Andreasen, 2014). For example, concordance rates are higher in monozygotic twins (same genetic makeup) than in dizygotic twins (two separate genetic makeups). When identical twins (monozygotic) are adopted out to separate homes, the suicide concordance rate is significantly higher than in fraternal twins (dizygotic) who are adopted out to separate homes. To date, no specific gene has been isolated; however, research is looking at a genetic link between serotonin-related genes and suicidal behavior and impulsive aggression (Black & Andreasen, 2014; Mathews et al., 2013).

Societal Factors

Societal factors that may increase the potential for suicide include loss or lack of social supports, negative life events, and severe life stress. Therefore suicide potential is apt to be higher among individuals facing these circumstances, including those who are impoverished; are recently divorced, separated, or bereaved; are childless or homeless; live alone; have few to no supports; and are grappling with recent negative life events. Suicide also seems to be higher among the unemployed and during economic turndowns. During economic expansions the suicide rate seems to fall (Black & Andreasen, 2014).

Psychological Factors

People who are psychotic, especially those who experience command hallucinations telling them to kill themselves or who have delusions that they must die, are at a high risk for suicide. A trio of psychological-emotional factors is often present when people become suicidal: hopelessness, helplessness, and feelings of worthlessness. **Hopelessness** refers to lack of purpose in life, **helplessness** refers to lack of social support, and **worthlessness** refers to low self-esteem or lack of love for self. According to Brendel and colleagues (2016), extreme hopelessness appears to be a key predictor of suicide. Often this type of thinking is precipitated or intensified by a negative and overwhelming event. In other words, people may contemplate suicide when they feel trapped and that "there is no way out."

Age
Adolescents and Young Adults

Suicide rates are increasing most rapidly in the 14- to 24-year-old age group in the United States. Those under the age of 30 show increased rates of alcohol/drug use or antisocial personality disorder (Black & Andreasen, 2014). Native American and Alaskan Native youth have suicide rates at crisis levels and have the highest suicide rate of all youths (CDC, 2015).

Indigenous populations in the U.S. have been suffering from a youth suicide epidemic for decades. The epidemic and risk factors associated with it can be connected to the mistreatment of Native Americans throughout history which has caused their communities to suffer from numerous inequalities such as poverty, inadequate housing, loss of land, and destruction of culture (Yurasek, 2014).

Other strong risk factors for youth are aggression, disruptive behaviors, depression, and social isolation. The following additional factors are related to youth suicide:

- Frequent episodes of running away
- Frequent expressions of rage
- Family loss or instability
- Frequent problems with parents
- Withdrawal from family and friends
- Expression of suicidal thoughts or talk of death or the afterlife when sad or bored
- Difficulty dealing with sexual orientation
- Unplanned pregnancy
- Perception of school, work, or social failure

Older Adults

Surprisingly, although previously much higher, the latest CDC (2015) statistics show that suicide is the seventeenth cause of death of those over 65 years of age.

However, after saying that, nurses need to know the risk factors for potential suicide. Risk factors to be assessed among older adults include social isolation, solitary living arrangements, widowhood, lack of financial resources, poor health, and feelings of hopelessness.

Most older adults who complete a suicide have visited their primary care physician in the month before the suicide, sometimes on that very day. Recognition and treatment of depression in the medical setting can prevent suicide in older adults.

CULTURAL CONSIDERATIONS

The meaning of suicide has traditionally reflected the religious beliefs of a culture. For example, in cultures with a Judeo-Christian tradition, life is considered a gift, and to take away one's life is a sin. Cultures historically steeped in Roman Catholic teachings (South America, Spain, Italy, Ireland) often have lower rates of suicide. To the contrary, people who practice the Shinto religion believe in reincarnation; therefore suicide may be seen as an *honorable* solution to life's problems. According to the World Health Organization (WHO, 2014), Japan has a suicide rate 60% higher than the global average. The WHO (2014) also expressed growing concern over the high suicide rates globally among vulnerable groups that experience discrimination, such as refugees and migrants; indigenous peoples; and lesbian, gay, bisexual, transgender, and questioning (LGBTQ) persons. Higher suicide rates are also seen among those who are incarcerated and those who live through war. By far the strongest risk factor for suicide is a previous suicide attempt.

Protective factors exist in many cultures or subcultures. Protective factors for African-American men and women include religion and the extended family. African-American women have the lowest suicide rate. Among Hispanic Americans, the Roman Catholic religion (in which suicide is considered a sin) and the importance given to the extended family decrease the risk for suicide. Among Asian Americans, suicide rates are noted to increase with age. Beliefs that reduce suicide include adherence to religions that tend to emphasize interdependence between the individual and society wherein self-destruction is seen as disrespectful to the group, or as selfish.

APPLICATION OF THE NURSING PROCESS

ASSESSMENT

There are a number of tools for ascertaining risk factors when assessing for potential suicidal behaviors. However, it is very difficult to predict suicide. An acronym that can stimulate the health care worker's recall when in a crisis situation is the Modified SAD PERSONS Scale (Box 23-1). The SAD PERSONS Scale is commonly used in emergency departments and helps staff to quickly evaluate the urgency of referral to mental health sources or protective care (Wyatt et al., 2012).

The Suicide Assessment Five-step Evaluation and Triage (SAFE-T) **for Mental Health Professionals** is also very popular (Box 23-2). SAFE-T drew upon the American Psychiatric Association Practice Guidelines for the Assessment and Treatment of Patients with Suicidal Behaviors. The five steps include:

1. **IDENTIFY RISK FACTORS** Note those that can be modified to reduce risk
2. **IDENTIFY PROTECTIVE FACTORS** Note those that can be enhanced
3. **CONDUCT SUICIDE INQUIRY** Suicidal thoughts, plans behavior and intent

---

BOX 23-1 Modified SAD PERSONS Scale*

SAD PERSONS can be modified to remedy the omission of an **available lethal plan**. This modification reminds the clinician to ask about lethal means when assessing suicidality. *If lethal means are available, the clinician can then take whatever action is reasonably indicated to reduce the likelihood of a suicide.*

S	Sex	1 male
A	Age	1 if <19 or >45 years, or*
D	Depression or hopelessness†	2
P	Previous attempts or psychiatric care	1
E	Excessive alcohol or drug use	1
R	Rational thinking loss (psychotic or organic illness)	1
S‡	Separated, widowed, divorced	1
O	Organized plan or serious attempt	2
N	No social support	1
A	Availability of lethal plan	
S‡	Stated future intent (determined to repeat or ambivalent)	1

Guidelines for Action

Points	Clinical Action
0-5	May be safe to discharge (depending on circumstances). (If sent home, have follow-up appointment arranged and discharge patient with family or friend.)
6-8	Probably requires psychiatric consultation.
>8	Probably requires hospital admission, voluntary or involuntary. (Would need agreement of two psychiatrists for involuntary admission.)

*Attempt (A) also in this modified scale.
†Two points are given for the combination of depression (hopelessness) and previous attempt.
‡The original SAD PERSONS Scale had *social supports lacking* for the first *S* and *sickness* for the second *S* (which is also a risk factor). In this version, the second *S* stands for *stated future intent*.
Data from Patterson, W. M., Dohn, H. H., Bird, J., et al. (1983). Evaluation of suicidal patients: The SAD PERSONS Scale. *Psychosomatics, 24,* 343–349; Wyatt, J. P., Illingworth, R. N., Graham, C. A., et al. (2012). *Oxford handbook of emergency medicine* (4th ed., p. 609). Oxford, England: Oxford University Press. There has been more than one modification to the SAD PERSONS Scale by Patterson et al.

4. **DETERMINE RISK LEVEL/INTERVENTION** Determine risk. Choose appropriate intervention to address and reduce risk
5. **DOCUMENT** Assessment of risk, rationale, intervention, and follow-up

Verbal Clues

Always take a suicide threat seriously. Whether a person makes one or a thousand threats, take the threats seriously. Assessing verbal clues includes the following:

Overt statements
- "I can't take it anymore."
- "Life isn't worth living anymore."
- "I wish I were dead."
- "Everyone would be better off if I died."

Covert statements
- "It's okay now. Everything will be fine."

- "Things will never work out."
- "I won't be a problem much longer."
- "Nothing feels good to me anymore, and probably never will."
- "How can I give my body to medical science?"

Behavioral Clues

Sudden behavioral changes may be noticed, for example:
- Giving away prized possessions
- Writing farewell notes
- Making out a will
- Putting personal affairs in order
- Having global insomnia
- Exhibiting a sudden and unexpected improvement in mood after being depressed or withdrawn
- Neglecting personal hygiene

BOX 23-2 SAFE-T

Suicide Assessment Five-Step Evaluation and Triage for Mental Health Professionals

Suicide assessments should be conducted at first contact, with any subsequent suicidal behavior, increased ideation, or pertinent clinical change; for inpatients, prior to increasing privileges and at discharge.

Risk Factors

Suicidal behavior: history of prior suicide attempts, aborted suicide attempts or self-injurious behavior

- Current/past psychiatric disorders: especially mood disorders, psychotic disorders, alcohol/substance abuse, ADHD, TBI, PTSD, Cluster B personality disorders, conduct disorders (antisocial behavior, aggression, impulsivity). Co-morbidity and recent onset of illness increase risk
- Key symptoms: anhedonia, impulsivity, hopelessness, anxiety/panic, insomnia, command hallucinations
- Family history: of suicide, attempts or psychiatric disorders requiring hospitalization
- Precipitants/Stressors/Interpersonal: triggering events leading to humiliation, shame or despair (e.g., loss of relationship, financial or health status—real or anticipated). Ongoing medical illness (esp. CNS disorders, pain). Intoxication. Family turmoil/chaos. History of physical or sexual abuse. Social isolation.
- Change in treatment: discharge from psychiatric hospital, provider or treatment change
- Access to firearms

Protective Factors

Protective factors, even if present, may not counteract significant acute risk
- *Internal*: ability to cope with stress, religious beliefs, frustration tolerance
- *External*: responsibility to children or beloved pets, positive therapeutic relationships, social supports

Suicide Inquiry

Specific questioning about thoughts, plans, behaviors, intent
- *Ideation*: frequency, intensity, duration—in past 48 hours, past month and worst ever
- *Plan*: timing, location, lethality, availability, preparatory acts
- *Behaviors*: past attempts, aborted attempts, rehearsals (tying noose, loading gun), vs. non-suicidal self-injurious actions
- *Intent*: extent to which the patient (1) expects to carry out the plan and (2) believes the plan/act to be lethal vs. self-injurious
- *Explore ambivalence:* reasons to die vs. reasons to live
  - For Youths: ask parent/guardian about evidence of suicidal thoughts, plans, or behaviors, and changes in mood, behaviors or disposition
  - Homicide Inquiry: when indicated, esp. in character disordered or paranoid males dealing with loss or humiliation. Inquire in four areas listed above.

Risk Level/Intervention
- Assessment of risk level is based on clinical judgment, after completing steps 1-3
- Reassess as patient or environmental circumstances change

Risk Level	Risks/Protective Factor	Suicidality	Possible Interventions
High	Psychiatric disorder with severe symptoms of acute precipitating event protective factors not relevant	Potentially lethal suicide attempt or persistent ideation with strong intent or suicide rehearsal	Admission generally indicated unless a significant change reduces risk. Suicide precautions
Moderate	Multiple risk factors, few protective factors	Suicidal ideation with plan, but no intent or behavior	Admission may be necessary depending on risk factors. Develop crisis plan. Give emergency/crisis numbers
Low	Modified risk factors, strong protective factors	Thoughts of death, no plan, intent or behavior	Outpatient referral, symptom reduction. Give emergency/crisis numbers

Document
- Risk level and rationale; treatment plan to address/reduce current risk (e.g., setting, medication, psychotherapy, E.C.T., contact with significant others, consultation); firearm instructions, if relevant; follow-up plan. For youths, treatment plan should include roles for parent/guardian.

ADHD, Attention-deficit hyperactivity disorder; *ECT,* electroconvulsive therapy; *PTSD,* posttraumatic stress disorder; *TBI,* traumatic brain injury.

▶▶ Assessment Guidelines

Sommers-Flanagan and Sommers-Flanagan (2015) suggest listening to the patient's suicidal thoughts and impulses without judgment because "they represent your client's unique efforts to cope with their interpersonal life problems" (p. 306).

Suicide Risk

1. **Identify current feeling states:** feelings of depression, hopelessness, helplessness, anxiety or panic, lack of interest or pleasure, and difficulty sleeping. For example: "Sometimes when I feel ___ (fill in the feeling state identified by the patient), I think about suicide."

2. **Ask directly.** Always ask: "Are you thinking of, or have you been thinking of, killing yourself?" If yes, evaluate for (Sommers-Flanagan & Sommers-Flanagan, 2015):
   a. Frequency: How often do these thoughts occur?
   b. Duration: Once they have begun, how long do they persist?
   c. Intensity: On a scale from 0 to 10, how likely are you to act on these thoughts?

3. **Ask if the person has a plan.** "When you think about suicide, do you have a way that you might do this?"

4. **Determine the lethality of the plan** in terms of risk.
   - How detailed is the plan? (The more detailed, the greater its lethality.)
   - How lethal is the proposed method?
     - Guns, hanging, carbon monoxide, and staging a car crash are extremely lethal.
     - Slashing wrists, inhaling natural gas, and ingesting pills are lower risk.
     - A plan that doesn't allow for a last-minute reversal of the action is consider more lethal.
   - Availability of means. Does the person have a gun? Access to a tall building?

5. **Gather information about risk factors**—patient's age, sex, medical problems, psychiatric problems or emotional distress, excessive use of drugs or alcohol, a recent significant loss, unemployment, lives alone, etc.—that would put the patient at higher risk.

6. **If there is a history of a suicide attempt, assess:**
   - Intent: Was there a high probability of being discovered?
   - Lethality: Was the method used highly lethal or less lethal?
   - Injury: Did the patient suffer physical harm (e.g., was the patient admitted to an intensive care unit)?

7. **Consult with one or more professionals and collaboratively develop a safety plan** with the patient. The patient thinks through and writes down ways to cope when feeling suicidal, who can be called, etc.

8. **If the patient is to be managed as an outpatient, also assess** the following:
   - Social supports: Is there someone who can stay with the patient?
   - Significant other's knowledge of the signs of potential suicidal ideation (e.g., increasing withdrawal, preoccupation, silence, remorse).
   - Provision of safety resources (knowledge of community resources, telephone numbers).

DIAGNOSIS

Risk for suicide is the most immediately important nursing diagnosis, and self-restraint from suicide is the ideal outcome. Other nursing diagnoses include *Ineffective coping, Hopelessness, Social isolation, Spiritual distress, Chronic low self-esteem, Post-trauma syndrome,* and *Anxiety.*

OUTCOMES IDENTIFICATION AND PLANNING

Interventions during the crisis that attempt to accomplish both short-term and long-term outcomes include:

Short-term outcomes
- Will have a family member or friend stay with the suicidal individual overnight
- Will have a follow-up appointment with a counselor or therapist
- Will have a list of telephone numbers of self-help groups, hotlines, organizations, and therapists in the area where the individual lives

Longer-term outcomes
- Optimizes events and environmental factors to help minimize further self-destructive acts
- Is able to explore alternatives and increase problem-solving skills
- Has shown evidence of increased coping skills
- States that feelings of isolation and loneliness are fewer and not as hurtful
- Is engaged in treatment for co-occurring mental health issues (e.g., depression, substance abuse, PTSD)

IMPLEMENTATION

Unfortunately, there seems to be a lack of evidence that supports any particular approach to prevention. Often, people who later complete suicide have made their intentions known to a health care worker or physician shortly before the event or have sought nonspecific help. Although restriction of access to means, treatment of depression, assistance with problem-solving skills and other therapies, and prescription of psychotropic medications may be effective, none of these interventions has been systematically investigated.

Some interventions are considered to support a person's resilience and act as protective factors:
- Family and community support
- Effective and appropriate clinical care for mental, physical, and substance abuse disorders
- Restricted access to highly lethal methods of suicide
- Cultural and religious beliefs that discourage suicide and support self-preservation instincts
- Acquisition of learned skills for problem solving, conflict resolution, and nonviolent management of disputes
- Cognitive behavioral therapy

Nursing interventions during the crisis are outlined in Table 23-1. Nursing interventions after the crisis period are outlined in Table 23-2.

Communication Guidelines

Nurses and other health care providers use communication skills and counseling techniques as one of their most important tools. Communication and counseling skills used by the nurse working with a suicidal person are practiced (1) in the community, (2) in the hospital, and (3) on telephone hotlines. During a suicidal crisis, the following information should be conveyed to the patient in all settings:
- The crisis is temporary.
- Unbearable pain can be survived.
- Help is available.
- The patient is not alone.

The nurse remains nonjudgmental and listens attentively.

APPLYING THE ART

A Person with Suicidal Behaviors

Scenario

I met 55-year-old Raymond on the adult psychiatric unit following a suicide attempt from a self-inflicted gunshot would. Raymond had damaged the right side of his neck and face, and part of his right ear, but missed every vital vessel and somehow lived. He had shown improvement by participating more actively in group therapy and had progressed from one-to-one observation (no farther than an arm's length away) to close constant observation within continuous visual range. I was meeting with him for the third time.

Therapeutic Goal

By the conclusion of this encounter, Raymond will feel comfortable enough with me to reveal his suicide attempt.

Student-Patient Interaction	Thoughts, Communication Techniques, and Mental Health Nursing Concepts
Student: "Raymond, I'm here after lunch as agreed."	I *offer self.* Being back when I said I would be builds trust.
Raymond: *(Avoids eye contact.)* "You can stay if you want. I don't feel like talking much." *(Glances up briefly, then stares at the floor.)*	Although I need to *evaluate* my *nursing practice,* Raymond's behavior change most likely came from his *mood disorder. Depression* influences his perception of just about everything.
Student's feelings: *While reserved, earlier Raymond's voice had more animation. He also made eye contact. Did I do something wrong to impair the relationship?*	
Student: "I'll stay here with you." *(Leans toward him with a concerned expression.)*	I offer *self* with words and with attending behavior. My silence shows nonjudgmental acceptance.
Student's feelings: *I have the hardest time waiting. I keep wanting to fill the silence. I sit on the left because Raymond has hearing loss on the right from the gunshot wound.*	
Raymond: *(Silent for 4 minutes.)* "My wife wants a divorce."	Does this increase his suicide risk further? Such a lethal method...to shoot yourself. I remember that sometimes when a suicide fails the patient sees self once again as a failure.
Student's feelings: *Divorce. Another loss. I am beginning to pick up his feelings of hopelessness.*	
Student: "How devastating. How hurtful."	*Reflection* communicates empathy because I have to really connect to be able to discern his probable feeling.
Student's feelings: *Sometimes when I use reflection, I worry that it sounds fake. Maybe because I'm still having to think about how to ask things. Even if I'm wrong about his feelings, I hope he senses that I care, because I do.*	
Raymond: *(Nods.)* "She said she can't take it anymore."	

Student-Patient Interaction	Thoughts, Communication Techniques, and Mental Health Nursing Concepts
Student: "You say she can't take it anymore?"	*Restatement* helps him elaborate.
Raymond: "My depression. Doing this." *(Touches the dressing on his ear, carefully shakes his head from side to side, then stares downward.)*	*Suicide* acts as a two-edged sword, hurting the survivors as well as the patient. I remember reading that suicide also acts as an *attempt* to *communicate,* but communicate what?
Student's feelings: *I wonder what his marriage was like before this. When I have trouble with the people I love I often feel bad about myself too.*	
Student: "You shake your head, like you feel regret."	I *make an observation* and use *reflection.*
Raymond: "About so many things. At my age I should be able to readily name my accomplishments but all I see are my failures. I can't believe she had an affair. Then I look at how I've screwed up and it's no wonder. I can't even kill myself right."	At the root of all this rests low self-esteem paired with depression. Was his suicide attempt a way to punish his wife as well as himself for being as he says a "screw-up"?
Student's feelings: *Where do I start? His despair makes me feel down too.*	His age puts him into *generativity vs. stagnation.* To feel he has no accomplishments sounds like stagnation rather than meeting the generativity task.
Student: "You're having trouble finding any reason to choose to live."	The 3-month period after an attempt remains high risk for another suicide attempt. I need to actively assess his suicide potential.
Student's feelings: *I should have checked the chart to see if he has attempted suicide before.*	
Raymond: "Some days more than others."	He feels *ambivalent.* I double-check that the staff member assigned to the close constant observation is indeed watching him.
Student's feelings: *I'm feeling worried that he may attempt again.*	
Student: "So, sometimes you are able to find something in you worth saving."	I give *support.* Using the words, "you are able to" reinforces his *self-esteem.*
Student's feelings: *I feel hopeful that he lets himself experience "some days" when he finds a reason to choose life. I need to help him get the feelings out, both the despair and the hope.*	
Raymond: "I guess so, but not today. Not with divorce papers in my hand."	In report this morning, the nurse indicated that Raymond's antidepressant and therapies may be starting to help. I remember that as *depression lifts,* the patient may experience the energy needed to carry through the *suicide plan.*
Student's feelings: *He sounds unsure. It's painful to struggle with depression. I know what depression feels like.*	

A Person with Suicidal Behaviors

Student-Patient Interaction	Thoughts, Communication Techniques, and Mental Health Nursing Concepts	Student-Patient Interaction	Thoughts, Communication Techniques, and Mental Health Nursing Concepts
Student: "Today you're feeling pretty hopeless." *(He nods.)* "So hopeless you're thinking about suicide again?" **Student's feelings:** *My anxiety skyrockets. Okay. I am right here in the chair next to him. He and I are both safe right now. I can do this.* **Raymond:** *(Nods.)*	His *suicide risk* suddenly increased with the impact of the divorce papers. He does not have a weapon but he could rip out his stitches. I stay alert and watch his hands.	**Student:** "Raymond, I care about you. Have you done or are you planning to do something to yourself right now?" **Raymond:** *(Mumbles.)* **Student:** *(Moving closer.)* "Raymond, I need your help with this. Please. Did you do something?" **Student's feelings:** *Part of me prays he will answer me!* **Raymond:** "I saved up all my pills and took them all."	I assess suicidality with a *direct question*. Communicating caring gives support. A *caring relationship* deters suicide.
Student: "Do you have a plan right now?" **Student's feelings:** *My heart rate is increasing but I'm keeping my voice calm.*	I ask a *direct question* to *assess suicide risk*. I need to tell staff as soon as I can. He needs to be on one-to-one observation with staff only an arm's length away.	**Student:** "When? What? How many?" **Student's feelings:** *I feel frantic. Okay, self, breathe mindfully.* **Student:** *I stop asking questions. I call and motion to staff. The nurse comes over to assess and begin emergency intervention with Raymond.* **Student's feelings:** *I feel relieved to get help.*	Too many *questions* at once. I will overload him. I need help now. The whole *treatment team* on the psychiatric unit works together. *Confidentiality* always includes the explanation that danger to self or others is always reported.
Raymond: "It'd be easier at home." **Student's feelings:** *He's given a lot of thought to this. I'm doing okay with connecting with Raymond.*	Raymond continues to talk and that is so much healthier than hurting himself.	**Student:** *(As Raymond is transported off the unit, I walk alongside and I hold out my hand.)* "Raymond, you were able to tell me about overdosing. That's a beginning of caring about yourself." **Student's feelings:** *By holding out my hand, I nonverbally ask permission to touch.*	My words and nonverbals give *support*.
Student: "So you've thought of suicide while in the hospital, too." **Raymond:** *(Looks down.)* **Student's feelings:** *Is Raymond avoiding eye contact? I don't want to lose the connection.*	The *current risk* takes precedence over thoughts of suicide at home. I *validate* with him. He uses *avoidance*. What is he hiding?	**Raymond:** *(Squeezes my hand.)* **Student's feelings:** *I needed to know that he knows that I care.*	

TABLE 23-1 Interventions during the Crisis Period

Intervention	Rationale
Inpatient	
1. **Follow institutional protocol** for suicide regarding creating a safe environment (taking away potential weapons—belts, sharp objects; checking what visitors bring into patient's room).	1. Provides safe environment during time patient is actively suicidal and impulsive; self-destructive acts are perceived as the only way out of an intolerable situation.
2. Keep accurate and thorough records of patient's behavior—both verbal and physical—as well as all nursing and physician actions: • Establish frequent rapport with the person. • Assess patient for his or her ability to seek out staff when struggling with suicidal thoughts. If patient is unable to do this, place on close observation.	2. These might become court documents. If patient's needs or requests are not documented, they do not exist in a court of law.
3. *Suicide precaution* (one-on-one monitoring at arm's length away) or *suicide observation* (15-minute visual check of mood, behavior, and verbatim statements), depending on level of suicide potential.	3. Protection and preservation of the patient's life at all costs during crisis is part of medical and nursing staff responsibility. **Follow institutional protocol.**
4. Keep accurate and timely records and document patient's activity—usually every 15 minutes—including what patient is doing, with whom, etc. **Follow institutional protocol.**	4. Accurate documentation is vital. The chart is a legal document regarding patient's "ongoing status" and interventions taken.
5. If accepted at your institution, construct a *no-suicide contract* with the suicidal patient. Use clear, simple language. When contract expires, it is renegotiated.	5. The *no-suicide contract* helps patients know what to do when they begin to feel overwhelmed by pain (e.g., "I will speak to my nurse/counselor/support group/family member when I first begin to think of harming myself").
6. Encourage patients to talk about their feelings and problem solve alternatives.	6. Talking about feelings and looking at alternatives can minimize suicidal acting-out.

TABLE 23-2 Interventions after the Crisis Period

Intervention	Rationale
1. Arrange for patient to stay with family or friends. If no one is available and the person is highly suicidal, hospitalization must be considered.	1. Relieves isolation and provides safety and comfort.
2. Weapons and pills are removed by friends, relatives, or the nurse.	2. Helps ensure safety.
3. Encourage patients to talk freely about feelings (anger, disappointments) and help plan alternative ways of handling anger and frustration.	3. Gives patients alternative ways of dealing with overwhelming emotions and gaining a sense of control over their lives.
4. Encourage patient to avoid decisions during the time of crisis until alternatives can be considered.	4. During crisis situations, people are unable to think clearly or evaluate their options.
5. Contact family members; arrange for individual or family crisis counseling.	5. Re-establishes social ties and mobilizes family support to deal with precipitating event(s) or overwhelming situation.
6. Activate links to social supports in the community (e.g., self-help groups).	6. Diminishes sense of isolation and provides contact with individuals who care about the suicidal person.
7. If anxiety is extremely high or patient has not slept in days, an antianxiety or antidepressant might be prescribed. **Only a 1- to 3-day supply of medication should be given. Family member or significant other should monitor pills for safety.**	7. Relief of anxiety and restoration after sleep loss can help the patient think more clearly and might help restore some sense of well-being. SSRIs are most commonly given, but they have Black Box warnings and patient and family/friends need to be educated.*

SSRI, Selective serotonin reuptake inhibitor.

*The FDA approved two antidepressants for the treatment of depression in children and teenagers — fluoxetine (Prozac) for age 8 or older, and escitalopram (Lexapro) for age 12 or older. Mayo Clinic (2013). Antidepressants for children and teens. Mayo Foundation for Medical Education and Research.

TABLE 23-3 Interventions for Follow-Up Psychotherapy

Intervention	Rationale
1. Identify situations that trigger suicidal thoughts (define the precipitating event).	1. Identifies targets for learning more adaptive coping skills.
2. Assess patient's strengths and positive coping skills (talking to others, creative outlets, social activities, problem-solving abilities).	2. Identifies areas to build on and draw from when planning alternatives to self-defeating behaviors.
3. Assess patient's coping behaviors that are not effective and that result in negative emotional sequelae: drinking, angry outbursts, withdrawal, denial, and procrastination.	3. Identifies areas to target for teaching and planning strategies for supplanting negative behaviors with more effective and self-enhancing behaviors.
4. Encourage patients to look into their negative thinking, and reframe negative thinking into neutral objective thinking.	4. Cognitive reframing helps people look at situations in ways that allow for alternative approaches.
5. Point out unrealistic and perfectionistic thinking.	5. Constructive interpretations of events and behavior open up more realistic and satisfying options for the future.
6. Spend time discussing patient's dreams and wishes for the future. Identify short-term goals that can be set for the future.	6. Renewing realistic dreams and hopes can give promise to the future and meaning to life.
7. Identify things that have given meaning and joy to life in the past. Discuss how these things can be reincorporated in the present lifestyle (e.g., religious or spiritual beliefs, group activities, creative endeavors).	7. Reawakens in patient abilities and experiences that tapped areas of strength and creativity. Creative activities give people intrinsic pleasure and joy, and a great deal of life satisfaction.

Psychotherapy

See Table 23-3 for interventions to be used during follow-up psychotherapy.

Postvention

Intervention for family and friends ("survivors") of a person who has completed a suicide—called a postvention—should be initiated within 24 to 72 hours after the death. Natural feelings of denial and avoidance predominate during the first 24 hours (Thompson, 1996). Mourning the death of a loved one who has completed suicide is always painful. Family and friends are often faced with the process of mourning without the normal social supports; unfortunately, neighbors, acquaintances, and even family and friends are often confused and may blame the family for the death. Families with members who have completed suicide are often stigmatized and isolated.

Survivors often feel that they are "going crazy" and need to be told that these feelings are normal. Survivors also need outlets for the undercurrent of anger toward the deceased, who is responsible for the trauma, confusion, and pain inflicted on them. Unfortunately, few friends or family members of a person who has completed suicide seek counseling. Pronounced feelings of anger and guilt are common reactions. Within 6 months of the suicide, 45% of survivors report mental deterioration, with symptoms of depression or posttraumatic stress disorder.

People exposed to traumatic events, such as family and friends of persons who have completed suicide or persons who have experienced the sudden death of a family member or friend, often manifest the following posttraumatic stress reactions: irritability, sleep disturbances, anxiety, exaggerated startle reaction, nausea, headache, difficulty concentrating, confusion, fear, guilt, withdrawal, anger, and reactive depression. The particular pattern of the emotional reaction and the type of response differ with each survivor depending on the relationship to the deceased, circumstances surrounding the death, and the coping mechanisms of the survivor. The ultimate goal of intervention is to reduce the trauma associated with the sudden loss. *Posttrauma loss debriefing* can help initiate an adaptive grief process and prevent self-defeating behaviors.

Self-Care for Nurses

All health care workers who provided care for a suicide victim are similarly traumatized by suicide, including medical staff, nursing staff, and ancillary staff. Staff may also experience symptoms of posttraumatic stress disorder, including guilt, shock, anger, shame, and decreased self-esteem. Other patients on the unit who may have suicidal tendencies need to be closely monitored as well. The first 24 hours after inpatient suicide is crucial for both safety and crisis management reasons.

Among the tasks for staff and administrators is a thorough psychological postmortem assessment. The event is carefully reviewed by all members of the treatment team to identify the potential overlooked clues or faulty judgments, as well as to determine changes that are needed to agency protocols. Most facilities have a clear policy about interventions with families after suicide. Although some lawyers advise all health care personnel who had contact with the family to secure legal counsel, others recommend designating a spokesperson who can follow up and provide family and friends with support without discussing the details of the client's care. Referrals need to be made available to family members and friends to assist them in dealing with and addressing the many emotional reactions and problems that may easily develop, especially among children and adolescents.

With regard to *documentation*, all staff need to ensure that the record is complete and entries are completed in a timely fashion. Legal cases have shown that the client should be evaluated periodically for suicide risk, that the treatment regimen should provide high-level security, and that staff members should be informed of the individual's treatment.

An excellent article, "Aftermath of Suicide in the Hospital: Institutional Response" (Ballard et al., 2008), was first published in *Psychosomatics* and can be found on the Internet (http://www.ncbi.nlm.nih.gov/pmc/articles/PMC2857997/).

Self-help groups are extremely beneficial for survivors of a suicidal family member or friend. Many people join self-help groups, even if the suicide took place 25 to 30 years ago. Self-help groups for the survivors of a family member or friend who completed suicide are similar to all other self-help groups. Essentially, these groups are operated by people who have lost someone through suicide.

Box 23-3 gives some guidelines for coping with a suicide loss. Also, the American Foundation for Suicide Prevention (www.afsp.org) can provide helpful information.

BOX 23-3 Guidelines for Survivors of Suicide

- Know you can survive. You may not think so, but you can.
- Know you may feel overwhelmed by the intensity of your feelings, but all your feelings are normal.
- Anger, guilt, confusion, and forgetfulness are common responses. You are not crazy; you are in mourning.
- Having suicidal thoughts is common. It does not mean that you will act on these thoughts.
- Find a good listener with whom to share. Call someone if you need to talk.
- Do not be afraid to cry. Tears are healing.
- Give yourself time to heal.
- Remember, the choice was not yours. No one is the sole influence in another's life.
- Give yourself permission to get help.
- Be aware of the pain of your family and friends.
- Steer clear of people who tell you what or how to feel.
- Know that there are support groups that can be helpful. If you cannot find one, ask a professional to help start one.
- Call on your personal faith to help you through.
- It is common to experience physical reactions to your grief, such as headaches, loss of appetite, and inability to sleep.
- Wear out all of your questions, anger, guilt, or other feelings until you can let them go. Letting go does not mean forgetting.
- Know that you will never be the same again, but you can survive and go beyond just surviving.

Modified from Dunne, E., McIntosh, J., & Dunne-Maxim, K. (1987). *Suicide and its aftermath: understanding and counseling the survivors.* New York, NY: Norton.

APPLYING EVIDENCE-BASED PRACTICE (EBP)

Problem A nurse working on a suicide crisis line receives a call late at night from a 33-year-old male. He reports thoughts of wanting to die, and has a plan to shoot himself. As the nurse talks to the patient, she writes down the phone number from caller ID, and messages a colleague to dispatch a crisis team. The patient tells the nurse that his father shot and killed himself almost a year ago. He expressed anger that the physician prescribed Valium for his depressed and alcoholic father, and that he did not receive mental health treatment. The patient also expresses guilt that he had not been aware of his father's despair.

EBP Assessment

A. **What do you already know from experience?** People who have a family member or friend who has committed suicide have increased risk for suicide, especially around anniversary dates. Surviving family members experience a lot of guilt and pain. Depressants such as alcohol and benzodiazepines contribute to depression and suicidal thoughts.

B. **What does the literature say?** Survivors of suicide experience guilt, anger, abandonment, denial, helplessness, and shock (Centers for Disease Control and Prevention [CDC], 2015). Suicide is the tenth leading cause of death among Americans, and 800,000 people worldwide die from suicide each year—more than from war and homicide combined. The key to suicide

prevention is a collaborative approach (World Health Organization [WHO], 2015).

C. **What does the patient want?** The patient is reaching out for help. Although his suicidal feelings are very strong, he is asking for assistance to control them. He is currently receiving help at a mental health center. He wants the pain to "just go away."

Plan The nurse immediately obtained contact information from caller ID and the patient, and dispatched a crisis team. This procedure was developed in response to quality improvement recommendations, after some callers hung up before help could be sent. The nurse obtained the patient's permission to notify his mental health center of his current crisis. The crisis team arrived on scene, and after assessing the patient's level of suicidality as being high, transported him for admission to a psychiatric facility.

QSEN **QSEN Prelicensure Knowledge, Skills, and Attitudes (KSAs) Addressed:**

Quality improvement measures were taken in response to callers hanging up before receiving help.

Informatics was involved by obtaining the patient's information through caller ID, messaging a colleague for help electronically, and emailing the mental health center through a secure portal.

Centers for Disease Control and Prevention (CDC). (2015). *Suicide: Risk and protective factors.* Retrieved from http://www.cdc.gov/vioenceprevention/suicide/riskprotectivefactors.html

World Health Organization (WHO). (2015). *Suicide* (Fact sheet no. 298). Retrieved from http://www.who.int/mediacentre/factsheets/fs398/en/

KEY POINTS TO REMEMBER

- People who attempt or complete suicide often share many risk factors, but people who have experienced the same risk factors are not always suicidal.
- Psychosis, substance use disorders, poor problem-solving skills, impulsivity, a low threshold for pain, and feelings of hopelessness place people at high risk for suicide when overwhelmed.
- Adolescents, older adults, white males, Native Americans, and Alaskan Natives have the highest rates of completed suicide. Some cultures play a protective role.
- Always try to identify the precipitating event for clues to areas of intervention.
- Assessment should include verbal clues, behavioral clues, and lethality of the plan as evaluation of the risk factors.
- The Modified SAD PERSONS Scale gives a quick overview of major risk factors.
- If suicidal risk is assessed, always ask directly: "Are you thinking of killing yourself?"
- During the crisis period when a person is acutely suicidal, specific interventions can prove helpful (in or out of the hospital) and many save lives (see Table 23-1).
- After the crisis period is over, other interventions can prove helpful in increasing coping skills, enhancing problem solving, and minimizing isolation and loneliness (see Table 23-2).
- Recall that intervention for family and friends of a person who has completed suicide is called *postvention*. Postvention can help lessen the guilt, anger, grief, pain, and myriad emotions that can stay with survivors for years.

APPLYING CRITICAL JUDGMENT

1. Sam T. is a 62-year-old man whose wife recently died of leukemia. His only son moved to California 2 years ago with his two daughters. Sam had been caring for his wife for 3 years before her death and has become withdrawn and despondent since her death. He is now in the emergency department after a "fender bender" and is getting two stitches on his ear; his blood alcohol level is 0.6. He does admit to being very depressed after losing his wife. You ask Mr. T. if he has thought about killing himself and he says, "Well, there is always a last resort, isn't there?" When you question him about the lethality of his plan, he admits to having a gun in the house for protection.
   A. How many risk factors does Mr. T. have using the Modified SAD PERSONS Scale?
   B. Do you think he needs hospitalization? If not, what should be put in place before he returns home? Explain the rationale behind your answer.
   C. What are Mr. T.'s needs? What kinds of referrals do you think would help him deal with this crisis?
   D. What do you think about the "fender bender"?
   E. Name at least three groups in your community to which you could refer Mr. T.
2. Have you ever known anyone who has completed a suicide? Contemplated suicide? If so, looking back at the risk factors, do you think there were any options open to these individuals? If so, what might have been available for an effective intervention?

CHAPTER REVIEW QUESTIONS

1. A parent tells the nurse about the death of a child 2 years ago. Which comment by this parent warrants the nurse's priority attention?
   a. "I still have some of my child's toys and clothes."
   b. "A parent should never live longer than their child."
   c. "I never returned to church again after the death of my child."
   d. "My child has been dead a long time, but it seems like only yesterday."
2. A patient diagnosed with major depressive disorder was hospitalized for 2 weeks on an acute psychiatric unit. One day after discharge, the patient completed suicide. Recognizing likely reactions among staff, which action should the nursing supervisor implement first?
   a. Assess each staff member individually for suicidal intent and/or plans.
   b. Provide a private setting for staff members to talk about feelings associated with the event.
   c. Remind staff members that suicide is a risk for the patient population and they are not at fault.
   d. Invite a guest speaker to conduct an educational session for staff members about suicide risk factors.
3. On the sixth anniversary of her spouse's death a widow says, "Sometimes life does not seem worth living anymore. I wish I could go to sleep and never wake up." Which response by the nurse has priority?
   a. "Are you considering suicide?"
   b. "You still have so much to live for."
   c. "Grief can sometimes last for many years."
   d. "Why do you continue to grieve something from long ago?"
4. A patient who had a stroke 3 days ago tearfully tells the nurse, "What's the use in living? I'm no good to anybody like this." Which action should the nurse employ first when caring for a patient demonstrating hopelessness?
   a. Implement the institutional protocol for suicide risk.
   b. Support the patient to clarify and express feelings of grief.
   c. Educate the patient about the success of stroke rehabilitation.
   d. Offer the patient an opportunity to confer with the pastoral counselor.
5. A single adult says to the nurse, "Both of my parents died several years ago and my only sibling committed suicide 2 weeks ago. I feel so alone." After determining that the adult has no suicidal ideation, the nurse should:
   a. Explore the adult's feelings of survivor's guilt.
   b. Assess the adult's cultural beliefs and spirituality.
   c. Refer the adult for cognitive behavioral therapy (CBT).
   d. Refer the adult to a self-help group for suicide survivors.

REFERENCES

American Foundation for Suicide Prevention. http://www.afsp.org.

Ballard, E. D., Pao, M., Horowitz, L., et al. (2008). Aftermath of suicide in the hospital: institutional response. *Psychosomatics*, *49*(6), 461–469.

Beck Institute Blog. (2010). *Veterans with TBI and suicidality*. Retrieved July 20, 2015, from http://www.beckinstituteblog.org/?category_name=suicide.

Black, D. W., & Andreasen, N. C. (2014). *Introductory textbook of psychiatry* (6th ed.). Washington, DC: American Psychiatric Publishing.

Brendel, R. W., Brezing, C. A., & Lagomasino (2016). This suicidal patient. In T. A. Stern, M. Fava, T. E. Wilens, et al. (Eds.), *Massachusetts General Hospital comprehensive clinical psychiatry* (2nd ed.).

Castillo, M. (2014). *Traumatic brain injury triples risk for early death, study says. CBS news.* Retrieved from http://www.cbsnews.com/news/traumatic-brain-injury-early-death-risk/.

Centers for Disease Control and Prevention (CDC). (2015). *Suicide: facts at a glance.* Retrieved from http://www.cdc.gov/violenceprevention/pdf/suicide-datasheet-a.pdf.

Cholbi, M. (2013). Suicide. In E. N. Zalta (Ed.), *Stanford encyclopedia of philosophy.* Retrieved April 20, 2016, from http://plato.stanford.edu/archives/sum2013/entries/suicide/.

Curwen, T. (2004). *His work is still full of life.* Retrieved July 20, 2015, from http://articles.latimes.com/2004/jun/05/entertainment/et-shneidman5.

Dignitas. (2015). *Life help.* Retrieved July 18, 2015, from http://www.dignitas.ch/index.php?option=com_content&view=article&id=54&lang=en.

James, L. M., Strom, T. Q., & Leskela, J. (2014). Risk-taking behaviors and impulsivity among veterans with and without PTSD and mild TBI. AMSUS. *The Society of Federal Health Professionals, 179*(4), 357–363.

Kirkland, M. (2010). *US Supreme Court: the right to die vs. the value of life.* Retrieved July 18, 2015, from http://www.upi.com/Top_News/US/2010/03/21/US-Supreme-Court-The-right-to-die-vs-the-value-of-life/43371269156600/.

Mathews, D. C., Richards, E. M., Niciu, M. J., et al. (2013). Neurobiological aspects of suicide and suicide attempts in bipolar disorder. *Translational Neuroscience, 4*(2), 203–216.

Poland, S. (2009). *Youth suicide prevention: physicians can make the difference.* Retrieved July 20, 2015, from http://www.medscape.com/viewarticle/588917.

Rothberg, B., & Feinstein, R. E. (2014). Suicide. In J. L. Cutler (Ed.), *Psychiatry* (3rd ed.). New York, NY: Oxford University Press.

Sadock, B. J., Sadock, V. A., & Ruiz, P. (2015). *Kaplan and Sadock's synopsis of psychiatry: behavioral sciences/clinical psychiatry.* Philadelphia, PA: Wolters Kluwer/Lippincott Williams & Wilkins.

Sommers-Flanagan, J., & Sommers-Flanagan, R. (2015). *Clinical interviewing* (5th ed.). Hoboken, NJ: Wiley.

Starks, H., Dudzinski, D., & White, N. (2013). *Physician aid-in-dying. Ethics. Medicine.* University of Washington School of Medicine.

Thompson, R. (1996). *Post-traumatic loss debriefing: Providing immediate support for survivors of suicide and sudden loss.* Ann Arbor, MI: Erie Clearinghouse on Counseling and Personal Services.

Vaughanbell. (2008). *The philosophy of suicide.* Retrieved August 23, 2011, from http://mindhacks.com/2008/05/18/the-philosophy of suicide/.

Voelker, R. (2012). Exploring the link between suicide and TBI. *American Psychological Association, 43*(11), 38.

World Health Organization (WHO). (2014). *Suicide (Fact sheet No. 398).* Washington, DC: WHO.

Wyatt, J. P., Illingworth, R. N., Graham, C. A., et al. (2012). *Oxford handbook of emergency medicine* (4th ed.). Oxford, England: Oxford University Press.

Yurasek, E. (2014). *Native American and Alaskan native youth suicide.* A thesis submitted in partial fulfillment of the requirements for the Honors in the Major Program in Anthropology in the College of Sciences and in the Burnett Honors College at the University of Central Florida.

Anger, Aggression, and Violence

Elizabeth M. Varcarolis

ⓔ http://evolve.elsevier.com/Varcarolis/essentials

KEY TERMS AND CONCEPTS

aggression, p. 375
anger, p. 374
bullying, p. 375
catastrophic reaction, p. 384

comfort rooms, p. 382
critical incident debriefing, p. 383
de-escalation techniques, p. 378
lateral bullying, p. 375

restraint, p. 380
seclusion, p. 380
violence, p. 375

SELECTED CONCEPT: BULLYING

Bullying is an intentional display and use of *violence*, as subtle as it might appear in some instances. Bullying can be defined as an offensive, intimidating, malicious, condescending behavior designed to humiliate and terrorize. Bullying takes place in all environments. It takes place in politics, the workplace, in schools, the home, in the military, prisons, in communities, nursing homes and medical facilities etc. All kinds of bullying behaviors create a toxic environment. Bullying is usually persistent, systematic, and ongoing.

OBJECTIVES

1. Discuss the interplay of neurobiology, medical history, past history, and sociological/demographic issues that contribute to risks for violence.
2. **QSEN** **Promote safety** by demonstrating the physical indicators of a patient who is beginning to escalate out of control.
3. **QSEN** Provide **patient-centered care** by comparing and contrasting interventions for a patient who is angry and loud in the pre-escalation phase with those for a patient who is escalating to a more aggressive phase.
4. **QSEN** Identify specific **safety measures** you would take when engaged in de-escalating an aggressive individual.
5. **QSEN** Plan **patient-centered nursing** care for a patient who is in seclusion.
6. **QSEN** Incorporate **evidence-based practice** by describing the use of communication and procedures implemented when placing an individual in restraints.
7. **QSEN** Discuss how **teamwork and collaboration** are vital to applying seclusions or restraints to a patient who is a danger to self or others.
8. **QSEN** Discuss how **quality improvement** methods can develop from the process of critical incident debriefing.
9. Document an example of the areas for which the nurse must provide written information when violence was averted or actually occurred.
10. **QSEN** Incorporate **evidence-based practice** by identifying calming and reassuring communications and the optimum milieu in managing a patient whose behaviors are escalating.

INTRODUCTION

Violence is harmful to the health of both victim and aggressor. The recipient of violence is susceptible to changes in the brain related to depression, anxiety, and immune-related diseases. Aggressors may suffer the same effects (Society for Neuroscience, 2014).

This chapter discusses how nurses in a variety of health care settings can recognize cues for escalating anger and aggression, and how they can learn to de-escalate and intervene with individuals whose anger is escalating and/or out of control.

ANGER, AGGRESSION, AND VIOLENCE

Universal differentiation among the terms *anger, aggression*, and *violence* is difficult or almost impossible because of cultural perceptions and social backgrounds. **Anger** is a normal—and not always

logical—human emotion, and no judgment needs to be passed on it. Anger varies in intensity from mild irritation to intense fury and rage.

Anger is usually a response to something that is happening or has happened. Anger may arise as a response to feelings of vulnerability and uneasiness because of a frustration of desire; feelings of hurt, fear, or vulnerability; a threat to one's needs (emotional or physical); or a challenge. Simply put, anger is an unplanned reaction to a stressor. Although we are all familiar with the feelings of anger, not everyone responds to anger with aggression or violence in the same way. When anger is channeled in a constructive manner (e.g., assertive communication, critical reasoning), individual needs can be met in a safe manner. Anger becomes unhealthy if it gets in the way of a person's functioning or relationships or puts others at risk. When anger is left unchecked and escalates, the results often lead to negative forms of aggression or violence. The acting out of anger may meet immediate needs, but at the expense of causing emotional or physical harm to ourselves or others.

Aggression is not the same as violence. Aggression may be appropriate or self-protective—as in protecting oneself, one's family, or a person being bullied. Or, aggression can be defined as "forceful goal directed action that may be verbal or physical; the motor counterpart of the effect of rage, anger, or hostility" (Sadock, Sadock, & Ruiz, 2015, p. 1407). Bresin and Gordon (2013) conducted two research studies based on the catharsis theory of aggression which implies there is a healing and anger-reducing affect that occurs through aggression. Bresin and Gordon's definition of aggression in these studies was the "act of participants verbally retaliating against negative feedback." These studies revealed that "Although some forms of aggression are maladaptive, such as abuse, physical violence, and verbal abuse, adaptive forms of aggression appear to not only create a calming effect, but also empower participants with the tools necessary to regulate anger emotions in the future." Essentially aggression is used as an attempt to regain control over a stressor or flee the situation.

Violence does not always have anger as its origin, but it does have the discrete intention of doing harm to a specific person or group. Violence is the unjust, unwarranted, or unlawful display of verbal threats, intimidation, or physical force with the intent of causing property damage, personal injury, or even death to another individual (Feinstein & Rothberg, 2014). Acts of violence lead to significant physical and psychological harm to others. *Bullying* is an all too common form of unchecked acts of violence in our schools, workplaces, and health care systems, and throughout cyberspace.

BULLYING AND VIOLENCE

Bullying is an intentional display and use of *violence*, as subtle as it might appear in some instances. Bullying can be defined as offensive, intimidating, malicious, condescending behavior designed to humiliate and to terrorize. Bullying involves persistent, systemic violence toward an individual or group.

Bullying occurs between persons with different levels of authority (e.g., supervisor or manager to staff nurse, boss to employee, teacher to student, parent to child). Lateral bullying refers to bullying among those of equivalent status (e.g., employee to employee, nurse to nurse, child to child, teenager to teenager, sibling to sibling, political opponent vs. political opponent).

Bullying in Health Care Environments

In an ongoing ANA survey of nurses' health and safety, 21 percent reported they were at a "significant level of risk" for violence at work, and 25% to 50% reported experiencing various instances of bullying in their workplace. Specifically, 50% said they had experienced verbal or non-verbal aggression from a peer and 42 percent from a person in a higher level of authority (American Nurses Association [ANA], 2015).

Robbins (2015) states the incidence of bullying in nursing is staggering. Researchers estimate at least 85% of nurses have been verbally abused by a fellow nurse, and one in three nurses quits her job because of bullying and that "bullying—not wages—is the major cause of a global nursing shortage. In the United States, the Bureau of Labor Statistics projects that by 2022, there will be a shortfall of 1.05 million nurses."

A partial list of bullying behaviors among nurses in the health care setting is consistent with most types of bullying that take place in other workplace environments:

- Providing unwanted or invalid criticism, excessively monitoring another's work
- Gossiping, spreading lies or false rumors, assigning derogatory nicknames
- Taking credit for another person's work without acknowledging his or her contribution, blocking career pathways and other work opportunities

- Publicly making derogatory comments about staff members or their work, including use of body language (eye rolling, dismissive behavior), often in front of others
- Using sarcasm or ridicule, making someone the target of practical jokes
- Blaming someone without factual justification
- Allocating unrealistic workloads and not supporting colleagues
- Being condescending or patronizing
- Using physical or verbal innuendo or abuse, using foul language, raising one's voice and shouting or humiliating someone in front of colleagues
- Breaking confidences

Bullying takes place in all environments. It takes place in politics, workplace, schools, the home, in the military, prisons, and on and on. In the medical community, all kinds of bullying behaviors create a toxic environment for staff, families, workplace employees, or those in any other setting in which either lateral violence or bullying takes place. School environments, workplace environments, and health care environments should ideally have a system whereby those who are bullied are given alternatives and support, and policies should be established to help eliminate an atmosphere in which bullying and/or violence exists. Those who are bullied are prone to negative feelings about self, humiliation, poor self-concept, and great emotional pain, and many can suffer severe reactions that may last a lifetime, such as depression, posttraumatic stress disorder (PTSD), anxiety disorders, and even attempted or completed suicide.

PREVALENCE AND COMORBIDITY

Anger, aggression, and violence are common aspects of social interaction, occur in all environments, and have become a major public health problem. The incidence of workplace violence in the health care system is notably higher than that found in private sector industries and is not confined to the United States. Workplace-related violence against nurses is a major international occupational health problem. Violence can occur anywhere in the hospital, but is most frequent in psychiatric units, emergency departments (EDs), waiting rooms, and geriatric units. Nurses in EDs experienced the highest rate of on-the-job violence.

Specific **medical and neurocognitive disorders** can result in agitated, aggressive, or violent behavior. For example, certain brain tumors, Alzheimer's disease, delirium, temporal lobe epilepsy, and traumatic brain injury (TBI) to certain parts of the brain can cause changes in personality that include increased aggression or violence. Other medical conditions that may affect an individual's control of violence are infections, subdural hematomas, Tourette's syndrome, degenerative disorders, endocrine-metabolic imbalances, and intoxication.

People with **mental health disorders** are often perceived as potentially aggressive or violent. It is important to know that psychiatric patients are 2.5 times more often the recipients of violence (e.g., raped, mugged, attacked) than people in the general population (Feinstein & Rothberg, 2014). However, individuals with a chronic psychotic condition (e.g., schizophrenia, mania, substance intoxication/withdrawal) are at a higher risk of perpetrating violence than those who are not psychotic (Black & Andreasen, 2014). Some individuals with personality disorders (e.g., narcissistic, antisocial, and borderline personality disorders) are also more prone to violent behavior.

THEORY

Environmental and Demographic Correlates of Violence

Probably the strongest predictor of adult violence is *childhood aggression*. Behaviors such as setting fires or performing acts of animal cruelty during childhood, or being diagnosed with conduct disorder, are red flags (Black & Andreasen, 2014). Many violent adults also suffered violence in childhood (e.g., physical, sexual, and emotional abuse) and are perpetuating the cycle of violence.

One of the strongest contributing factors to violent behavior in clinical settings is the *abuse of alcohol and other substances* (intoxication or withdrawal), such as amphetamines, cocaine, hallucinogenic drugs, sedative-hypnotics, and other substances that lower inhibitions and impair judgment.

Demographic correlates include risk factors such as male gender, young age (15 to 24 years), and family history of violence. Persons of **lower socioeconomic status** are more likely to be perpetrators as well as victims of violence. Poorer populations are more apt to experience discrimination, family breakdown, alienation, and constant fight for survival (Black & Andreasen, 2014). Socially, angry reactions are learned and reinforced through the family and societal norms.

Neurobiological Factors
Brain Structure
There is no one site in the brain responsible for anger, aggression, and violence, although there are many areas of the brain that are believed to contribute in some way to either increasing or decreasing these emotions. The neurobiology of aggression and violence is complex and our knowledge is as yet incomplete, and much of it comes from animal studies.

As we already know, the limbic system is responsible for our emotional life and plays a role in storing our memories. The limbic system is composed of the hypothalamus, hippocampus, amygdala, septum, cingulate, and fornix. Essentially, the *limbic system* mediates primitive emotions and behaviors that are necessary for survival, has a role in regulating the behavior of aggression in humans and animals, and judges events as either aversive or rewarding. Specific areas of importance include the hippocampus and *amygdala*. It is thought that the "amygdala is a vital nexus in the neural network supporting aggression and violence" (Victoroff, 2009, p. 2675) and that the amygdaloid cells respond to perceived threats (e.g., emotional facial expressions).

Anger biologically stimulates the *hypothalamus*, causing the body to react to the anticipation of harm (fight or flight response). The *temporal lobe* of the brain receives messages from both the limbic system and the hypothalamus. In the temporal lobe, memory is thought to be integrated; memory of previous insults is important in the cognitive appraisal of threat in the face of new stimuli. This lobe is also the source of complex partial seizures, which may lead to aggressive behavior. The prefrontal cortex receives messages from both the limbic system and the hypothalamus and appears to play a role in modulating the aggressive impulses in a social context and making judgments of these impulses (Gerken et al., 2016). Both magnetic resonance imaging (MRI) studies and positron emission tomography (PET) scans in the prefrontal cortex show changes in violent individuals. MRIs show a reduction in the volume of the prefrontal gray matter. PET scans reveal decreased prefrontal blood flow and metabolism (Gerken et al., 2016).

Neurotransmitters
It seems that most of the neurotransmitters have some connection to or play some part in aggression and violence. However, to date the presence or absence of a single neurotransmitter has not been conclusively identified as a contributing factor for violence, although there have been studies and theories.

In numerous studies, low central *serotonin (5-HT, 5-hydroxytryptamine)* function has been correlated with impulsive aggression as well as an impulsive history of suicide, and with low levels of 5-hydroxyindoleacetic acid (5-HIAA), a metabolite of serotonin, in cerebrospinal fluid (CSF). Serotonin is thought to act as a modulator in the central nervous system to lessen impulsive and violent behaviors (Black & Andreasen, 2014). It is unclear, however, if low levels of 5-HIAA in CSF are a marker for impulsivity or a certain kind of aggression.

As complicated as the catecholamines *(norepinephrine [NE] and epinephrine)* are, they are thought to play a role in preparing the body for the fight-or-flight response, both on a peripheral level (preparing muscles and cardiac status for fight) and on a cognitive level. NE may enhance vigilance and play a role in impulsivity and episodic violence in humans (Gerken et al., 2016). The exact effects of NE on violence and aggression are unclear at the present time.

It is pretty well accepted that the dopaminergic system is involved in behavioral activation, motivated behavior, and reward processing. It has also been established that dopamine plays an active role in the modulation of aggressive behaviors (Jalain, 2014). A study by Schluter and colleagues (2013) found that higher degrees of dopamine storage in the striatum and midbrain correlated with lower degrees of aggressive responses as identified in PET scans.

Genetic Factors
Twin studies, adoption studies, studies of twins reared apart, and family and molecular genetic studies have long suggested that there is a genetic component in the etiology of violence. However, as yet no specific chromosomal abnormality has been associated with increased risk for aggression (Gergen et al., 2016). Although there seem to be genetic contributions to aggression, most scientists agree that genetic characteristics alone do not account for the complexities of human behavior.

Most likely the study of the neurobehavioral aspect of violence—particularly frontal lobe dysfunction, altered serotonin metabolism, and the influence of heredity—will lead to a deeper understanding of factors in the genesis of violence. There is little doubt that social and evolutionary factors most likely play a role.

CULTURAL CONSIDERATIONS

Violence is a complex issue. As mentioned previously, socioeconomic issues as well as medical and psychiatric issues are all contributing factors. The different rates of violent crime among societies and within subcultures emphasize the importance of social factors in the genesis of violence. For example, race *or* ethnicity may be a factor.

Males in general are far more violent than females. Individuals with the highest prevalence of violence appear to be of lower economic class, be male, have substance abuse disorders, and/or have psychotic or organic medical disorders. A subculture that supports the use of intimidation and aggression as an acceptable way of problem solving and achieving social status can reinforce the use of violence as acceptable behavior. This is particularly true in an environment where healthy, appropriate, and effective ways of dealing with frustration, anger, and aggression are not modeled.

APPLICATION OF THE NURSING PROCESS
ASSESSMENT

Subjective Data
On admission, the nurse completes a comprehensive history of the patient gathered from a variety of sources (using informatics to obtain the patient's history, both medical and psychological), including family, friends, and the patient when appropriate. It is important for the nurse to take an accurate history of the patient's background and usual coping skills, as well as to determine the patient's perception of the issue (if possible). For example, does the patient have a history of previous violence, substance abuse, or psychotic behavior?

The patient should be asked the following questions (Black & Andreasen, 2014):

1. Have you ever thought of harming someone else?
2. Have you ever seriously injured another person?
3. What is the most violent thing you have ever done?

Objective Data

Expressions of anxiety and anger generally look similar. Both may involve increased demands, irritability, frowning, redness of the face, pacing, twisting of the hands, or clenching and unclenching of the fists. Changes in mood and behavior from quiet to talkative and loud, from talkative to silent and withdrawn, from calm to angry, or from depressed to elated also may occur. Box 24-1 identifies signs and symptoms that indicate the risk of escalating anger, which may in turn lead to aggressive behavior. Simple observation of these signs, however, does not provide the information necessary to determine the appropriate intervention. Recent history can be invaluable.

VIGNETTE

A male abuser has been admitted to the unit for spousal and child abuse. He is considered at high risk for violent acting-out behaviors. Violence can be anticipated to be toward female authority figures and female staff members. Therefore male staff is assigned to this patient. He is placed in a secure room until behavior can be assessed more fully regarding violence toward others. The male nurse conducts the interview with appropriate and unobtrusive staff for backup.

VIGNETTE

An intoxicated, homophobic male is admitted to the unit for detoxification. Violence can be anticipated if an all-male team is brought together to escort the patient to a quiet room. Therefore a female staff member is chosen as the spokesperson, once again with appropriate and unobtrusive staff available for backup.

BOX 24-1   Some Predictive Factors for Violent Outcomes*

1. Signs and symptoms that usually *(but not always)* precede violence:†
   a. Angry, irritable affect
   b. Hyperactivity: most important predictor of imminent violence (e.g., pacing, restlessness, slamming doors)
   c. Increasing anxiety and tension: clenched jaw or fist, rigid posture, fixed or tense facial expression, mumbling to self (patient may have shortness of breath, sweating, and rapid pulse rate)
   d. Verbal abuse: profanity, argumentativeness
   e. Loud voice, change of pitch, or very soft voice forcing others to strain to hear
   f. Intense eye contact or avoidance of eye contact
2. Recent acts of violence, including property violence
3. Stone silence
4. Suspiciousness or paranoid thinking
5. Alcohol or drug intoxication (withdrawal)
6. Possession of a weapon or object that may be used as a weapon (e.g., fork, knife, rock)
7. Milieu characteristics conducive to violence:
   a. Loud
   b. Overcrowding
   c. Staff inexperience
   d. Provocative or controlling staff
   e. Poor limit setting
   f. Staff inconsistency (e.g., arbitrary revocation of privileges)

*Violent outcomes include screaming, cursing, yelling, spitting, biting, throwing objects, hitting, and punching at self or others.
†Sometimes violence may be perceived to come from "out of the blue."

⏩ Assessment Guidelines
Anger, Aggression, and Violent Acting-Out

1. *A history of violence is the single best predictor of future violence.*
2. Paranoid ideation and frank psychosis (e.g., command hallucinations) are indicators of possible aggression or violence.
3. Patients who are hyperactive, impulsive, or predisposed to irritability are at higher risk for violence.
4. Assess the patient's risk for violence:
   • Does the patient have a wish or intent to harm?
   • Does the patient have a plan?
   • Does the patient have means available to carry out the plan?
   • Does the patient have demographic risk factors, including male gender, ages 14 to 24 years, low socioeconomic status, and low support system?
5. Aggression occurs most often in the context of limit setting by the nurse.
6. Patients with a history of inability to control anger and limited coping skills, including lack of assertiveness or use of intimidation, are at higher risk of using violence.
7. Assess self for personal triggers and responses likely to escalate the individual's violence.
8. Assess personal sense of competence when in any situation of potential conflict; consider asking for the assistance of another staff member.
9. Assess any personal negative thoughts or feelings you may hold toward the patient that could escalate both your anxiety and the anxiety of the patient.
10. Draw on previous knowledge of the policies and procedures for providing care to potentially violent patients.

DIAGNOSIS

The safety of patients and others is always the first priority. When anxiety escalates to levels at which there is a threat of harm to self or others, *Ineffective impulse control, Risk for self-directed violence,* and *Risk for other-directed violence* are primary diagnoses. If a patient's anxiety is escalating and not amenable to early nursing interventions, and if de-escalating techniques are not effective, psychopharmacological means or restraints may be necessary to ensure the safety of patients and staff.

Initially, when anxiety begins to escalate and there is a potential for aggression, *Ineffective coping* (overwhelmed or maladaptive) is a likely nursing diagnosis. Patients may have coping skills that are adequate for daily events in their lives but are overwhelmed by the stresses of illness or hospitalization. Therefore *Risk for stress overload* might be an appropriate diagnosis. A more long-term nursing diagnosis for patients who have a pattern of maladaptive coping that is marginally effective and consists of a set of coping strategies that has been developed to meet unusual or extraordinary situations (e.g., abusive families) would be *Ineffective family coping.*

Nurses can teach patients methods of coping that will decrease anxiety and distress. However, patient behavior may escalate quickly, or the patient may mask early signs of distress. Nurses may be distracted and may miss those early signs, even when they are visible. Other nursing diagnoses may include *Confusion, Disturbed thought processes,** and *Disturbed sensory perception.**

---

*These nursing diagnoses are no longer included in NANDA (2015-2017). However, it is hoped that these nursing diagnoses will be included in future versions of NANDA.

TABLE 24-1   Interventions for the Pre-assaultive Stage: Use of De-escalation Techniques

Intervention	Rationale
1. Pay attention to angry and aggressive behavior. Respond as early as possible (see Box 24-1).	1. Minimization of angry behaviors and ineffective limit setting are the most frequent factors contributing to the escalation of violence.
2. Emphasize that you are on the patient's side (e.g., "We want to help you, not hurt you.") and that "this is a safe place and you are safe." The clinician should stand at an angle to the patient so as not to appear confrontational.	2. Establish yourself as an ally who wants to help the patient gain control. Never provoke or use threats.
3. Assess personal safety and provide for self-care.	3. Pay attention to the environment. • Leave door open or use hallway. Choose a quiet place, but one that is visible to staff. • Have a quick exit available. • If you are uncomfortable, have other staff nearby. • The more angry the patient, the more space is needed to feel comfortable. • Never turn your back on an angry patient. • If on *home visit*, go with a colleague. • Leave immediately if there are signs that behavior is escalating out of control.
4. Appear calm and in control.	4. The perception that someone is in control can be comforting and calming to an individual who is beginning to lose control.
5. Do not try to speak while the aggressive person is yelling.	5. Loudly arguing with the patient will only escalate anger and violence.
6. Speak softly in a nonprovocative, nonjudgmental manner.	6. When the tone of voice is low and calm and words are spoken slowly, anxiety levels in others may decrease.
7. Demonstrate genuineness and concern. • Do not treat the individual in a humiliating manner. • Ask, "What will help now?"	7. Even the most psychotic schizophrenic individual may respond to nonprovocative interpersonal contact and expressions of concern and caring.
8. Set clear, consistent, and enforceable limits on behavior (see Box 24-2) (e.g., "It's okay to be angry with Tom, but it is not okay to threaten him. If you are having trouble controlling your anger we will help you.").	8. Gives patient understanding of expectations and consequences of not adhering to those behaviors.
9. If patient is willing, both nurse and patient should sit at a 45-degree angle. Do not tower over or stare at the patient.	9. Sitting at a 45-degree angle puts you both on the same level but allows for frequent breaks in eye contact. Towering over or staring can be interpreted as threatening or controlling by paranoid individuals.
10. When patient begins to talk, listen. Use clarification.	10. Allows patient to feel heard and understood, helps build rapport, and energy can be channeled productively.
11. Acknowledge the patient's needs regardless of whether the expressed needs are rational or irrational, possible or impossible to meet.	11. Contributes to individual's perception that the nurse is trying to understand the core of the aggression. Determine how some of the patient's needs can be met in a productive way.

OUTCOMES IDENTIFICATION

Short-term or intermediate outcome goals may include the following:
• The patient will display nonviolent behaviors toward self and others *(by date)*.
• The patient will recognize when anger and aggressive tendencies begin to escalate and employ at least one new tension-reducing behavior at that time (e.g., time out, deep breathing, talking to a previously designated person, employing an exercise such as jogging) *(by date)*.
• The patient will make plans to continue with long-term therapy (individual, family, group, anger management, medication management) to work on violence prevention strategies and increase coping skills *(by date)*.

Long-term outcome goals may include the following:
• The patient and others will remain free from injury.
• Hostile and abusive behavior toward others, property, animals, and so on will cease.
• Use of assertive and cognitive reasoning behaviors to replace aggressive behaviors is in constant evidence.
• A variety of healthy anxiety reduction techniques to keep anger in check are used.
• Aggressive and violent impulses are controlled.

PLANNING

Planning interventions necessitate conducting a sound assessment, including history (previous acts of violence, comorbid disorders), present coping skills, and willingness and capacity of the patient to learn alternative and nonviolent ways of handling angry feelings. However, one of the most important aspects of planning is consistency of approach by staff. A clear management approach to deal with violent situations and individuals includes staff well versed in unit protocols and well trained in de-escalation techniques. De-escalation techniques are outlined and discussed under "Implementation" below and in Table 24-1. *Teamwork and cooperation* are paramount in protecting other patients, staff, and particularly the individual who is losing control. The following questions help determine appropriate planning.

Does the patient have:
• Good coping skills but is presently overwhelmed?
• Marginal coping skills?
• A tendency to use anger or violence as a way to cover other feelings and gain a sense of mastery or control?
• A neuropsychiatric or chronic psychotic disorder?
• A tendency toward violence?
• Cognitive deficits (in the form of misinterpretation of environmental stimuli) that predispose to anger?

Does the situation call for:
- Psychotherapeutic approaches to teach the patient new skills for handling anger?
- Immediate intervention to prevent overt violence (de-escalation techniques, restraints or seclusion, or medications)?

Does the environment provide:
- A safe, therapeutic milieu?
- Privacy for the patient?
- Enough space for patients, or is there overcrowding?
- A healthy balance between structured time and quiet time?

Do the skills of the staff call for:
- Additional education in verbal de-escalation techniques?
- Counseling interventions because of punitive and arbitrary approaches to patients?
- Additional training in restraint techniques?

Planning also involves attention to the number of personnel who are available to respond to a potentially violent situation.

IMPLEMENTATION

Ensuring Safety

Promoting safety is always a first consideration. **Ensure your safety first.** You must feel safe to be able to communicate in a calm manner. Staff and other personnel should be alerted in case reinforcement is needed. The goals are that no one will become hurt and the patient will experience the least restrictive interventions. The following is a list of specific interventions for working with a potentially angry, aggressive, or violent patient:

1. Move the individual to a calm and quiet place.
2. All patients should be searched for contraband and dangerous objects when admitted to the unit and after visits.
3. Give the patient space. Always minimize personal risks. Stay at least one arm's length away from patient. Use more space if patient is anxious or if you want more space. *Always trust your instincts.*
4. Provide adequate space for the patient and staff to ensure easy withdrawal from an escalating situation.
5. Know where panic buttons or alarms are located to be able to call for assistance from other staff quickly if necessary. Sometimes it is necessary to wear a body alarm to ensure safety.
6. Exit strategies apply to both the nurse and the patient. The nurse should be positioned between the patient and the door, but not directly in front of the patient or in front of the doorway. Facing the patient can be interpreted as confrontational, and it can also make the patient feel trapped. It is better to stand off to the side and encourage the patient to have a seat.
7. Set limits at the outset using these de-escalation techniques (Box 24-2).
   - Direct approach: "Violence is unacceptable." Describe the consequences (medications, restraints, seclusion). Best for confused or psychotic patients.
   - Indirect approach: Use the indirect approach if patient is not confused or psychotic. Give patient a choice. "You have a choice. You can take this medication and go into the interview room (or hallway, for example) and talk, or you can sit in the seclusion room until you feel less anxious."
8. When interviewing a patient whose behavior begins to escalate:
   - Provide feedback about what you observe: "You seem to be very upset." Such an observation allows exploration of the patient's feelings and may lead to de-escalation of the situation.
   - If the patient's behavior continues to escalate, end the interview and assure the patient that the staff will provide for the patient's safety (as well as everyone else's safety); then leave the patient.

> **BOX 24-2 Setting Limits**
>
> 1. Set limits in only those areas in which a clear need exists to protect the patient or others.
> 2. Establish realistic and enforceable consequences of exceeding limits.
> 3. Make patient aware of limits and the consequences of not adhering to the limits before incidents occur. The patient should be told in a clear, polite, and firm manner what the limits and consequences are, and should be given the opportunity to discuss any feelings or reactions to them.
> 4. All limits should be supported by the entire staff, written in the care plan, and communicated verbally to all involved.
> 5. When a decision to discontinue the limits is made by the entire staff, the decision is based on consistent desired behavior, not promises or sporadic efforts.
> 6. The staff should formulate their own plan to address their own difficulty in maintaining consistent limits.
>
> Adapted from Chitty, K. K. & Maynard, C. K. (1986). Managing manipulation. *Journal of Psychosocial Nursing and Mental Health Services*, 24(6), 8–13.

9. Having enough staff is essential for a show of strength and is often enough to avert confrontation. One person is chosen as spokesperson and is the only one who talks to the patient, but staff needs to maintain an unobtrusive and nonthreatening presence in case the situation escalates.
10. Give the patient the opportunity to walk to the quiet room voluntarily without assistance when team interventions seem appropriate.
11. Do not touch the patient unless the team is with you and you are ready for a possible restraint situation.
12. In the event of a restraint or seclusion situation, the team functions as a single unit, with each member assigned a limb or a function as previously practiced according to unit protocols and policy.
13. Avoid wearing dangling earrings, necklaces, or ponytails. The patient may become focused on these and grab at them, causing serious injury. This is a serious danger.

Stages of the Violence Cycle

When interventions to prevent or deal with patient violence are considered, sometimes it is helpful to identify the stage of violence. These stages include the *pre-assaultive stage, the assaultive stage, and the post-assaultive stage.* See Chapter 11 for nursing interventions for moderate levels of anxiety that escalate to severe and panic levels.

Pre-assaultive Stage: De-escalation Approaches

During the pre-assaultive stage, the patient becomes increasingly agitated. **Staff members require training in both verbal techniques of de-escalation and physical techniques to restrain without harm. The better trained the staff, the less chance that either staff or the patient will be injured.** Frequently verbal interventions are sufficient during this stage. Interventions at this stage are listed in Table 24-1.

Throughout these procedures, maintain the patient's self-esteem and dignity. Linehan (1993) states that respect can be maintained if the nurse operates from the following assumptions:
- Patients are doing the best they can.
- Patients want to improve.
- Patients' behaviors make sense within their world view.

The use of empathic statements such as "It sounds like you are in pain and confused," "You're here to get help, and we're going to try to figure out what's going on," and "Let us help you, don't be afraid" can aid in reducing anxiety and anger. These statements reinforce the feeling that the person is in a safe environment and that everyone is there to help in his or her treatment and that staff have an idea of what the person is going through.

VIGNETTE

A 24-year-old male who was in an automobile accident is bedridden with a pelvic fracture. During his first day of admission, he yells at each nurse who walks by his room, using expletives in his demands that the nurse enter the room.

Intervention

The nurse who is assigned to the patient for the evening stops in his doorway after he yells at her. She asks in a calm, nonsarcastic manner, showing mild disbelief, "Is this working for you? Do nurses really come in here when you yell at them that way?" The patient responds sullenly, justifying his behavior by complaining about his care. The nurse responds by saying, "It seems to me that you need to feel you can get care when you need it." The patient responds in a loud voice that he has been waiting 20 minutes for a bedpan and how would she like it? The nurse gets him his bedpan, and he has calmed down somewhat. The nurse's challenge has caught his attention. The nurse then goes on to suggest (i.e., teach) alternative strategies for contacting her and other nurses. The strategies are immediately put into use by the patient.

When health care personnel can teach patients alternate strategies and healthier ways to meet their needs, patients have more choices and thus more control over their situation.

Assaultive Stage: Medication, Seclusion, and Restraint

The American Psychiatric Nurses Association's (APNA, 2000, rev. 2007, rev 2014) *Seclusion and Restraint Standards of Practice* states:

> **Standard: Any staff providing care to persons at risk for harming themselves or others and who participate in seclusion and restraint shall have received training and demonstrate current competency in all aspects of dealing with behavioral emergencies.**

> **Be sure to know the unit and hospital protocol for seclusion and restraint in whatever part of the hospital you choose to work.**

If the patient progresses to the assaultive stage, the staff must respond quickly. Generally, a team approach with at least five staff members is advisable to restrain a resistant patient, but the team may be larger if the patient requires it. One person is chosen as the spokesperson or leader and is the only one who speaks to the patient and instructs members of the team. The following interventions include the use of medications and seclusion and/or physical restraints.

Seclusion "is the involuntary confinement of a person alone in a room or an area where the person is physically prevented from leaving. It may only be used for the management of violent or self-destructive behavior" (APNA, 2000, rev 2007, rev 2014). Restraint refers to (1) any manual method or physical or mechanical device, material, or equipment that immobilizes or reduces the ability of a person to move his or her arms, legs, body, or head freely; or (2) a drug or medication when it is used as a restriction to manage the person's behavior or restrict the person's freedom of movement and is not a standard treatment or dosage for the person's condition (APNA, 2000, rev. 2007, rev. 2014).

The least restrictive means of restraint is *always* tried first and seclusion or restraint is used *only after* alternative interventions have been attempted (e.g., trauma-informed approach, verbal interventions, medications, decrease in sensory stimulation, removal of a particular problematic stimulus, presence of a significant other, frequent observation, use of a sitter who provides 24-hour one-to-one observation of the patient).

Seclusion or restraint is used in the following circumstances (APNA, 2000, rev. 2007, rev. 2014):

- The patient presents a clear and present danger to self or others.
- The patient has been legally detained for involuntary treatment and is thought to pose an escape risk.
- The patient requests to be secluded or restrained.

When deciding on whether to use restraints or seclusion, Zeller and Wilson (2015) suggest: "If the patient is an immediate danger to others, restraint is indicated. Yet if a patient is only disruptive and uncooperative, but is not a danger to others, seclusion should be considered. If the patient seems willing to sit in a quiet room, then an unlocked seclusion room may be attempted. If not, then a locked seclusion is indicated. However, if the patient could or does become a danger to self while in seclusion, restraint is appropriate. Even when restrained, a patient will engage."

Before the development of psychotropic medications, seclusion and restraint were extremely common methods of managing aggressive behavior. In the past half-century their use has decreased dramatically as a result of effective medications. *All facilities that use seclusion and restraint have strict regulatory policies that should follow state, federal, and regulatory agency guidelines. Students as well as all staff members should be familiar with their institution's policies.*

APPLYING THE ART

A Person with Anger and Aggression

Scenario

I'd just attended a group therapy session on the forensic unit, during which the group leader had to set limits with 24-year-old Hector. During our initial one-to-one Hector had been almost overly polite, in contrast to his abrasiveness with some of the other patients in group. I followed Hector out of the group room.

Therapeutic Goal

By the end of this interaction, Hector will identify at least one incident where a person can demonstrate an act of kindness or caring toward another and still see himself as masculine.

Student-Patient Interaction	Thoughts, Communication Techniques, and Mental Health Nursing Concepts
Hector: *(In harsh, loud voice.)* "Bunch of losers."	He went from being friendly with me this morning to this abrupt outburst of anger.
Student's feelings: *I was taken aback and intimidated by how lightning-fast Hector's anger arose when some other guys took the seats that Hector had chosen for us during group.*	

A Person with Anger and Aggression

Student-Patient Interaction	Thoughts, Communication Techniques, and Mental Health Nursing Concepts	Student-Patient Interaction	Thoughts, Communication Techniques, and Mental Health Nursing Concepts
Student: "You're talking about what just happened in group." *(I walk toward the seating area closest to the nurses' station, where I can be observed by the staff, and signal them for help if need be.)* **Student's feelings:** *After Hector's bullying episode in group, I feel safer in plain view.* **Hector:** *(In a loud and angry voice.)* "Just because I made those guys get out of those seats. What did you think? You think that's such a big deal?"	I *validate* to make sure I understand his reference. I am beginning to realize that Hector's earlier politeness and charm might have to do with his *personality disorder*.	**Student:** "You are able to say how your dad taught lessons with his fists. I'm guessing any little boy would feel enormous pressure when interacting with others in the context of either you win or you get pounded." **Student's feelings:** *I'm beginning to see how powerless Hector must feel somewhere inside all that bravado. I am beginning to feel some compassion for him.* **Hector:** "He was just teaching me how to be a man."	I give *support* by using the words "you are able to" in order to encourage Hector to recognize a link between his current responses and past abusive experiences. He justifies his father pounding on him. A *history of violence* is the best *predictor of violence*. Hector defines how to be a man in the same way his father did. Does he know other ways exist?
Student: "But why did you have to yell and scream at them? I remember some yelling and swearing." **Student's feelings:** *I didn't think this through with all his anger coming out. I am reacting defensively, and I'm feeling like I am in way over my head. I feel like I need a break.*	Asking a *why question* is nontherapeutic for sure. He will take it as criticism. I hope he does not get any angrier.	**Student:** "I wonder if a person can be a man in other ways besides winning or losing. This morning I saw you help when someone bumped the patient carrying breakfasts back for those who eat on the unit." **Student's feelings:** *My belief in my nursing self fluctuates. But I do feel some rapport exists between us.*	I use an *indirect question* and make an *observation* of his recent behavior. I know that when a person feels comfortable with you, even if one uses "nontherapeutic techniques," a person will often understand the intent behind the words.
Student: "What were you feeling when you saw they were in the seats you wanted?" **Student's feelings:** *I hope he focuses on his feelings rather than my accusatory "why" question.*	I attempt to *translate* into feelings. When in doubt, always go for feelings.	**Hector:** "What a mess." **Student:** "And you helped anyway. Then, when the patient apologized so much, you told him, 'It's okay. Accidents happen.'"	I *make observations* describing Hector's healthier behaviors, like spontaneously helping another.
Hector: "Look, I always get a raw deal. The leader likes those guys better than me."	After all this, I do not think I will be going with him to *occupational therapy*. That way, I will get to consult my instructor to check if I am on the right track.	**Hector:** "Others helped too."	Hector excels at generating *negative attention*. He does not know what to do with *positive feedback*.
Student: "But when this happened, you were feeling…what?" **Student's feelings:** *It really is okay to take care of myself. Knowing I can access my teacher and staff readily if need be allows me to refocus and attend to Hector's needs.*	I again ask him to *focus* on his feelings.	**Student:** "You also spoke kindly to him." **Hector:** *(Shrugs.)*	Again I *make an observation* and give my attention to *positively reinforcing* his kind act.
Hector: "Nothing. Never mind."	I wonder what makes Hector unable to look at his feelings at all. He refers to the leader like he is competing for attention. Almost like *sibling rivalry*. Perhaps all that macho talk hides *low self-esteem*.	**Student:** "Sometimes it seems manliness and kindness might coexist in one person." **Hector:** *(Nods slightly.)* "I need a drink of water." *(Goes to water fountain.)* **Student's feelings:** *I feel glad that he nods even slightly. I find it difficult to make even small changes, like regularly flossing my teeth. What must Hector's world be like? I have people who care about me. Who does he have for support…especially since he's an expert at pushing others away?*	I deliberately link Hector's kind words with his earlier idea of manhood. His *intermittent explosive disorder* is most likely connected to his repeated abusive "lessons" equating any vulnerability or even a kindness as weakness. Hector nods, showing *partial understanding* that demonstrating kindness is okay for a man, although it appears to make him anxious as he uses physical withdrawal (getting a drink) to protect himself (fight-or-flight response).
Student: "I think I'd feel frustrated when directed to give the other patients their original chairs back. Maybe even a little embarrassed." **Hector:** *(Avoids eye contact.)* "My dad would've pounded the _____ out of me for letting those guys win."	I *give information* about self but really the intent serves to *reflect* Hector's possible feelings.		

A patient may not be held in seclusion or restraint without a physician's order (verbal, written, or telephone order). Sometimes this is not possible, and the decision is made by a qualified staff member to initiate seclusion or restraint because of a behavioral emergency. However, either way, the patient must be evaluated within 1 hour by a physician or licensed independent practitioner (LIP). Restraints may be preferred when staff believe that continued verbal and calming strategies would allow the patient to de-escalate and that restraints could be removed at the earliest possible time. Mechanical restraints are avoided in individuals who have a history of sexual abuse and trauma, and they also are contraindicated in patients who may be at risk for positional asphyxia, sudden cardiac collapse, or other physical and medical conditions.

Once in restraints, a patient must be protected from all sources of harm. *Each team member is trained in the correct use of physical restraining maneuvers as well as in the use of physical restraints.* The team is organized before approaching the patient so that each team member knows his or her individual responsibility regarding limb securing. The spokesperson explains to the individual in a straightforward and calm manner exactly what the team is about to do and why. If restraints are to be used, the person is informed at this point of the team's intent and the reason for the team's actions. Sometimes the patient is ready to cooperate and moves to the seclusion room on his or her own.

VIGNETTE

A 19-year-old male has a 2-year history of quadriplegia. This patient also has a history of drug abuse that began in grade school, an inability to set or work toward long-term goals, and a primary coping style of anger and intimidation. The patient is admitted to an inpatient psychiatric unit because of increasing suicidal ideation. He clearly communicates to staff that his preferred means of coping with anger is to "cuss people out" and run into them with his wheelchair. However, in the hospital, the consequence of wheelchair assaults is that the patient is secluded in his room, which he finds intolerable. The patient asks the staff to help him manage his anger.

Intervention
The nurse assigned to this young man sets aside time to interview him regarding the triggers for his anger. He identifies several issues that "make him angry." These typically relate to feeling unheard and controlled by the staff. Together, the nurse and patient examine alternative ways for him to deal with these situations, such as telling the staff that he does not feel that they are listening to him and letting them know that he needs to be involved in the planning of his care to increase his sense of control. The patient and nurse role-play a situation in which the patient is told by a staff member that he must attend a group session. Such a situation would usually result in the patient becoming angry and aggressive, but in the role-played situation he is willing to "try out" alternative communication techniques to communicate his feelings to the staff member and thus to handle his anger. In addition, the patient is willing to enter into a behavioral contract with the nurse, stating that he will not curse at staff or assault anyone with his wheelchair. Instead, he will let the staff know when he is feeling angry and what the triggering issue is so that a nonaggressive resolution can be found.

Response
Because this patient is motivated to gain increased personal control, he responds positively to these suggestions. In addition, once it becomes clear that feeling unheard and out of control underlies most episodes of anger, the patient is able to target these issues for problem solving. He rapidly develops effective and appropriate ways to make himself heard and understood. He also becomes adept at communicating when he feels out of control and at finding ingenious ways of negotiating control on issues that are particularly important to him. The patient's suicidal impulses, which occur when he is frustrated, also diminish.

Once the patient is restrained, the nurse might administer an intramuscular injection of a barbiturate, antihistamine, or antipsychotic depending on the individual's underlying condition and the physician's order. The nurse's role is to provide an explanation to the person for the medication and to make sure that the individual is properly restrained so that the medication can be administered safely. Throughout this time, the spokesperson continues to relate to the person using a calm, steady voice, communicating decisiveness, consistency, and control.

While the patient is restrained and in seclusion, staff closely monitor the patient to determine the person's ability to reintegrate into unit activities. Usually every 15 minutes, face-to-face observation is made through the locked door window. A person 14 years of age or younger should have constant face-to-face observation. Reintegration is gradual and is geared toward the patient's ability to handle increasing amounts of stimulation. If the reintegration proves to be too much for the patient and results in increased agitation, the patient is returned to the room or to another quiet area.

Generally a structured reintegration is the best approach. For instance, reintegration can begin by reducing four-point restraints to two-point restraints. Once the patient no longer requires the locked seclusion room, the patient may be given specified time-out periods to leave the room and move slowly into the milieu of the unit. The time-out periods are gradually lengthened until the person is able to maintain control within the part of the unit that is quiet, dimly lit, and/or has fewer patients.

Better Alternatives to the Use of Seclusion and Restraint: The Recovery Model. Sivak (2012) points out that there is no evidence to support the therapeutic value of seclusion and restraint and reports that 150 people die each year as a result of these practices with the mentally ill and that others are left psychologically harmed, physically injured, or traumatized (Substance Abuse and Mental Health Services Administration [SAMHSA], 2011). New approaches that focus on the recovery model are being researched and developed to reduce the use of seclusion and restraint. One potential intervention that came out of the recovery movement is the use of comfort rooms, where the psychiatric facility sets aside a "special room" to which a person can go voluntarily to self-manage anxiety and distress (Sivak, 2012).

The use of recovery model approaches and the "trauma-informed approach" has been reported as helpful to reduce the use of seclusion and restraint (Psychiatric News Alert, 2015; APNA, 2000, rev. 2007, rev. 2014). A trauma-informed approach and trauma-specific interventions address reducing the trauma's consequences and facilitate healing (SAMHSA, 2015): "A program, organization, or system that is trauma-informed:

1. *Realizes* the widespread impact of trauma and understands potential paths for recovery;
2. *Recognizes* the signs and symptoms of trauma in clients, families, staff, and others involved with the system;
3. *Responds* by fully integrating knowledge about trauma into policies, procedures, and practices; and
4. Seeks to actively resist *re-traumatization*."

"A *trauma-informed approach* reflects adherence to six key principles rather than a prescribed set of practices or procedures. These principles may be generalizable across multiple types of settings, although terminology and application may be setting- or sector-specific.

1. Safety
2. Trustworthiness and Transparency
3. Peer support

4. Collaboration and mutuality
5. Empowerment, voice and choice
6. Cultural, Historical, and Gender Issues"

Post-assaultive Stage

Once the patient no longer requires seclusion or restraints, the staff should review the incident with the patient as well as among themselves. Discussion with the patient is an important part of the therapeutic process. Reviewing the incident allows the patient to learn from the situation, identify the stressors that precipitated the out-of-control behavior, and plan alternative ways of responding to these stressors in the future.

Critical Incident Debriefing

Staff analysis of an episode of violence, referred to as critical incident debriefing, is crucial for a number of reasons. *First,* a review is necessary to ensure that quality care was provided to the patient. Staff members need to critically examine their response to the patient. Questions to be answered include the following:

- Could we have done anything that would have prevented the violence?
- If yes, then what could have been done, and why was it not done in this situation?
- Did the team respond as a team? Were team members acting according to the policies and procedures of the unit? If not, why not?
- Is there a need for additional staff education regarding how to respond to violent patients?
- How do staff members feel about this patient? About this situation? Feelings of fear and anger must be discussed and handled. Otherwise, the patient may be dealt with in a punitive and nontherapeutic manner.

Second, the profound effects of workplace violence unfortunately do not disappear after the incident is over, and the harm is not only to the individual assaulted. At times some nurses and staff may internalize (depression, avoidance, withdrawal) or externalize (anger, outbursts, fluctuating mood) their emotional and behavioral responses to the event. These are normal responses to an abnormal event. However, agencies need to provide support and debriefing to prevent long-term psychological sequelae for all types of workplace violence. Employee morale, productivity, use of sick leave, transfer requests, and absenteeism are affected by patient violence, especially if a staff member has been injured. Staff members must feel supported by their peers as well as by the organizational policies and procedures established to maintain a safe environment.

Documentation of a Violent Episode

Most facilities provide standardized seclusion and restraint records. There are a number of areas for which the nurse *must* provide documentation in situations where violence either was averted or actually occurred:

- Reason for seclusion or restraint
- Assessment of behaviors that occurred during the pre-assaultive stage *(time)*
- Nursing interventions and the patient's responses *(time)*
- Evaluation of the interventions used
- Detailed description of the patient's behaviors during the assaultive stage
- All nursing interventions used to defuse the crisis
- Patient's response to those interventions
- Name(s) of person(s) called to assess the patient and order any medications, seclusion, and/or restraints *(time)*
- Time patient put in restraints or seclusion

- Observations of and interventions performed while the patient was in restraints or seclusion (food, toileting, vital signs, verbatim statements, and general behaviors) (15 to 30 minutes depending on state law)
- Any injuries to staff or patient
- The way in which the patient was reintegrated into the unit milieu *(time and behavior)*
  See Chapter 6 for more definitive legal and procedural guidelines.

Anticipating Increased Anxiety and Anger in Other Hospital Settings

Hospitals can be lonely, scary places for many people. Patients often feel that they are not being heard, and they may feel vulnerable, discounted, frightened, out of control of their situation, and tired. Some patients may have specific vulnerabilities for responding to their increasing anxiety and loss of autonomy with the use of violence. Therefore some patients with poor coping skills or mental or neurological problems may resort to anger, intimidation, or violence to obtain their short-term goals of feeling control or mastery. For others, the anger occurs when limited or primitive attempts at coping are unsuccessful and alternatives are unknown. For these patients, anger and violence are particular risks in inpatient settings.

This is especially true for hospitalized patients with chemical or alcohol dependency who may be anxious about not having access to their substance of choice; they may have well-founded concerns that any physical pain will be inadequately addressed. Those individuals with marginal coping skills may also have personality styles that externalize blame. That is, they see the source of their discomfort and anxiety as being outside themselves; relief must therefore also come from an outside source (e.g., the nurse, medication).

Interventions begin with attempts to understand and meet the patient's needs. For instance, baseline anxiety can be moderated by the provision of comfort items before they are requested (e.g., decaffeinated coffee, deck of cards); this can build rapport and acts symbolically to reassure the patient. Anxiety also can be minimized by reducing ambiguity. This strategy includes clear and concrete communication. An interaction providing clarity about what the nurse can and cannot do is most usefully ended by offering something within the nurse's power to provide (i.e., leaving the patient with a "yes").

Interventions for anxiety might also include the use of distractions, such as magazines, action comics, and video games. Generally, distractions that are colorful and do not require sustained attention work best, although this varies according to the patient's interests and abilities. Finally, patients with a high level of baseline anxiety and limited coping skills are helped when their interactions with the treatment team are predictable; this might include speaking with the physician at a specific time each day or having the patient see a single spokesperson from the treatment team each day.

Because some patients have limited coping skills, once anxiety is moderated, nursing interventions include teaching alternative behaviors and strategies. With increased tools to deal with anxiety and frustration, patients have the opportunity to have choices and an increased sense of control over their behaviors.

Often, anger may be communicated via verbal abuse directed at the nurse. If attempts to teach alternatives have not been successful, three interventions can be used:

1. The first intervention is to leave the room as soon as the abuse begins; the patient can be informed that the nurse will return in a specific amount of time (e.g., 20 minutes) when the situation is calmer. This is said in a straightforward manner. If the nurse is in the middle of a procedure and cannot leave immediately, the nurse can discontinue conversation and eye contact, completing the procedure quickly and efficiently before leaving the room. Note that the nurse avoids chastising, threatening, or responding punitively to the patient.

2. Withdrawal of attention to the abuse is successful only if a second intervention is also used. This step requires attending positively to, and thus reinforcing, nonabusive communication by the patient. Interventions can include discussing non–illness-related topics, responding to requests, and providing emotional support.

3. Patients who are regularly verbally abusive may respond best to the predictability of routine, such as scheduled contacts with the nurse (e.g., every 30 minutes or every 60 minutes) as long as the patient's behavior is not abusive. Such a contract works only to the extent that the nurse maintains the scheduled contacts as agreed on, and other staff members must be informed of the contract and remain consistent so that they do not inadvertently sabotage it by responding to incidental requests by the patient. If the patient's illness or injury requires nursing care outside the scheduled contact times, these visits can be carried out in a calm, brief manner. This contract is negotiated with the patient and addresses the patient's anxiety about getting needs met and being heard.

Implementing appropriate interventions can be difficult when the nurse is feeling threatened. Remaining matter-of-fact with patients who habitually use anger and intimidation can be difficult because these people are often skillful at making personal and pointed statements. It is important for the nurse to remember that patients do not know their nurses personally and thus have no basis on which to make accurate judgments. Nurses can also vent their own responses elsewhere, with other staff or family members, or via critical incident debriefing.

Interventions for Patients with Neurocognitive Deficits

Patients with cognitive deficits are particularly at risk for acting aggressively. Such deficits may result from delirium, dementia (e.g., Alzheimer's disease, multi-infarct dementia), or brain injury. Traditional approaches to disorientation and to the agitation that it can cause have relied heavily on reality orientation and medication. Reality orientation consists of providing the correct information to the patient about place, date, and current life circumstances. For some patients, orientation does not work. Because of their cognitive disorder, they can no longer "enter into our reality," and they become frightened and agitated and may become aggressive. Sedating medication may calm agitation, but in some cases the risks may outweigh the benefits. *Sedation only further clouds a patient's sensorium, which makes disorientation worse and increases the risk for falls and injuries. It is better to examine alternative interventions.*

Sometimes the patient with a cognitive disorder experiences such severe agitation and aggression that it is referred to as a **catastrophic reaction**. The patient may scream, strike out, or cry because of overwhelming fear. Adopting a calm and unhurried manner is the best response. The steps for making contact with a patient who is experiencing a catastrophic reaction are listed in Box 24-3.

Patients who misperceive their setting or life situation may be calmed by validation therapy. Some disoriented patients believe that they are young and feel the need to return to important tasks that were a significant part of their earlier years. For example, an older woman may insist that she must go home to take care of her babies. Telling the patient that her babies have grown up and that she no longer has a home is not only cruel but also nontherapeutic and will result in increased agitation. It is often more helpful to reflect back to the patient the feelings behind her demand and to show understanding and concern for her worry.

Rather than attempting to reorient the patient, the nurse asks the patient to further describe the setting or situation referenced by the patient (e.g., the need to return home). During the conversation the nurse can comment on what appears to be underlying the patient's distress, thus validating it. For example, the woman who believes that she

---

BOX 24-3 Cognitive Deficits and the Catastrophic Reaction: Making Contact

Cognitive deficits result in:
- A decreased ability to interpret sensory stimuli
- A decreased ability to tolerate sensory stimuli

Striking out represents fear or the feeling that the environment is out of control.

The presence of a second agitated person (e.g., staff member) leads to increased agitation; therefore:

1. Face the patient from within 2 feet, remaining as calm and unhurried as possible.
2. Say the patient's name.
3. Gain eye contact.
4. Smile.
5. Repeat steps 2 through 4 several times if necessary, to gain and maintain eye contact.
6. Use gentle touch and keep voice soft (the person often matches this tone and lowers his or her voice also).
7. Ask the patient if there is a need to use the bathroom.
8. Help the patient regain a sense of control—ask what is needed.
9. Validate the patient's feelings: "You look upset. This can be a confusing place."
10. Use short, simple sentences. Complex explanations just represent more noise.
11. Decrease sensory stimulation.
12. Get the patient to use rhythmic sources of self-stimulation (e.g., humming, a rocking chair).

Adapted from Rader, J., Doan, J., & Schwab, M. (1985). How to decrease wandering, a form of agenda behavior. *Geriatric Nursing, 6*(4), 196–199.

---

needs to return home to care for her children is asked to tell the nurse more about her children. The nurse may note that the patient misses her children and may be lonely: "Mrs. Green, you miss your children, and the hospital can be a lonely place."

As the nurse shows interest in aspects of the patient's life, the nurse establishes himself or herself as a safe, understanding person who can be trusted. In turn, the patient often becomes calmer and more open to redirection. When patients reminisce in this fashion, they often reorient themselves: "Of course, they're all grown and doing well on their own now." See Chapter 18 for a more extensive discussion of interventions for people with cognitive impairments.

Psychotherapy

Management of chronic aggression requires comprehensive neuropsychological testing and cognitive behavioral assessment to establish the appropriate treatment approach for each individual. Besides psychopharmacological treatment, individual therapies may include behavioral management, cognitive behavioral techniques, family interventions, and psychosocial supports (Gerken et al., 2016). The cognitive behavioral assessment includes determining the psychotherapeutic approach most appropriate for a chronically aggressive patient. Data are obtained regarding the type of aggressive behavior, psychiatric diagnosis, and patient's intellectual ability. Behavioral techniques include limit setting, distraction and redirecting techniques, relaxation, and biofeedback. These techniques have met with limited success.

Gerken and colleagues (2016) suggest that the trauma-informed approach, and trauma-informed therapies in combination with medication, is much more successful for diminishing the need for restraint and seclusion.

APPLYING EVIDENCE-BASED PRACTICE (EBP)

Problem A 60-year-old male diagnosed with schizoaffective disorder had an appointment at a mental health clinic for an outpatient nursing visit. As the patient entered the office, he was gazing downward and seemed tense. He sat down briefly in the chair, then stood up rapidly and jumped on the desk just a few inches away from the registered nurse (RN), shouting, "You all are practicing Voodoo, trying to kill me with the lithium. I'm going to smash your face in!" The RN backed away and stated calmly and firmly, "No, you are not; you are going to leave or I will call security." The patient rushed out the door and yelled, "I'll leave, you don't have to call security, but when I kill my wife it's on you!"

EBP Assessment
A. **What do you already know from experience?** Patients with mental illness are not all violent, but there are times when violence and threats occur. Mental health professionals are involved with patients during acute phases of their disorders and must be prepared to react in a safe manner.
B. **What does the literature say?** Duty to warn was developed after a psychiatric patient revealed his plan to kill a young woman to a psychology intern, and followed through with killing her. Duty to warn places limits on confidentiality and requires action on the part of the professional. In some states duty to warn is mandatory, and in others it is optional or not required at all (National Conference of State Legislatures, 2013). Forty to fifty percent of psychiatric residents will be attacked by a patient during the 4 years of their program (Anderson & West, 2011).
C. **What does the patient want?** When the patient initially came to the clinic, he stated that he wanted to control his anger and was tired of people becoming scared of him. In this moment of acute psychosis the patient is lashing out. Safety always takes precedence.

Plan The RN is required in her state to perform a duty to warn. She called the police to report the patient's threat against his wife. Next, she called the patient's wife to let her know a threat had been made against her. The RN also called security to watch the premises for the agitated patient. The police found the patient and completed a report. Eventually, the patient returned to the clinic for future services but was required to have his case manager with him at all times while at the facility.

QSEN **QSEN Prelicensure Knowledge, Skills, and Attitudes (KSAs) Addressed:**

Safety was addressed in handling the acute situation and by acting on duty to warn guidelines.

Team work and collaboration occurred between the RN, police, security, and the case manager in handling the outburst and threat.

Anderson, A. & West, S. G. (2011). Violence against mental health professionals: when the treater becomes the victim. *Innovation in Clinical Neuroscience*, 8(3), 34–49; National Conference of State Legislators. (2016). *Mental health professionals duty to warn*. Retrieved from http://www.ncsl.org/research/health/mental-health-professionals-duty-to-warn.aspx

Pharmacological Therapies

Aggression, hostility, and violent behaviors are usually a result of the underlying psychiatric or medical disorder (Gerken et al., 2016; Preston et al., 2013).

Medications for Acute Aggression

If treating the underlying condition doesn't work, or if the underlying condition is unknown, the medication prescribed should be the most benign. Benzodiazepines are often the first choice for acute aggressive episodes, especially in episodic dyscontrol and incipient rage episodes.

Benzodiazepines are safe but may have paradoxical reactions in individuals with certain personality disorders (Gerken et al., 2016). Second-generation antipsychotics, particularly ziprasidone (intramuscular) or olanzapine (intramuscular or orally disintegrating), can be useful in emergency situations (Gerken et al., 2016).

Medications for Chronic Aggression

Chronic aggression is a common problem in psychiatry, and aggression can be diminished only after a therapeutic dose of the appropriate medication once a provisional diagnosis is made. Treatment should be geared toward the underlying psychiatric or medical condition. Preston and colleagues (2013) outlined the most effective medications for specific underlying conditions (Table 24-2).

EVALUATION

Evaluation of the care plan is essential for patients who are angry and aggressive. A well-considered plan has specific outcome criteria. Evaluation provides information about the extent to which the interventions have achieved the outcomes. If the outcomes have not been achieved, the plan must be revised. Revision focuses on all aspects of the nursing process:
- Was the assessment accurate and thorough?
- Were the nursing diagnoses applicable to the assessment data?

TABLE 24-2   Medications for Chronic Aggression

Medication	Associated Features
Anticonvulsants (e.g., carbamazepine)	Labile mood, poor impulse control, organicity e.g., dementia
Antipsychotics	Disorganized behavior
Beta blockers (propranolol)	Organicity e.g., dementia
Buspirone	Organicity
Clonidine	Anxiety, agitation
Lithium	Labile mood, impulsivity
Selective serotonin reuptake inhibitors (SSRI's)	Anger "attacks"

From Preston, J. J., O'Neal, J. H., & Talaga, M. C. (2013). *Handbook of clinical psychopharmacology for therapists*. Oakland, CA: New Harbinger Publications, p. 169.

- Did the nursing diagnoses accurately drive nursing interventions?
- Was the plan comprehensive and individualized?
- Were interventions appropriate?
- Were interventions carried out properly?
- If restraint or seclusion was needed, was the protocol followed correctly and was safety for staff as well as the patient maintained?
- Were guidelines to improve quality improvement methods found for future use?

For instance, the initial plan may have included assessment of the environmental stimuli that precede a patient's agitation. Once these are identified, the plan provides interventions that are specific to those stimuli. However, the plan will work only if staff members evaluate the effectiveness of the approach by noting the extent to which agitation is decreased. Evaluation may reveal that the patient's agitation has decreased except in specific situations. The plan is then revised to include these situations.

KEY POINTS TO REMEMBER

- Angry emotions and aggressive actions are difficult targets for nursing intervention.
- Nurses benefit from an understanding of how the angry and aggressive patient should be approached.
- Understanding patient cues to escalating aggression, appropriate intervention goals for individuals in a variety of situations, and helpful nursing interventions is important for nurses in any setting.
- The roles of sociocultural influences and neurobiological vulnerabilities are intertwined in a person's propensity for violence.
- Cues to assess when anger is escalating (verbal and nonverbal, including facial expressions, breathing, body language, and posture) are provided.
- Assess the patient's history. A patient's past aggressive behavior is the most important indicator of future aggressive episodes.
- Many approaches are effective in helping patients de-escalate and maintain control.
- The general hierarchy of interventions for coping with aggression is verbal intervention, trauma-specific interventions, psychopharmacology, seclusion, and then restraint.
- Different interventions are used depending on the patient's level of anger.
- Guidelines for de-escalation of patient behavior are given.
- Specific medications such as barbiturates, antipsychotics, lithium, selective serotonin reuptake inhibitors (SSRIs), and anticonvulsants may prove useful for short- or long-term therapy.
- As a last resort, seclusion or restraints may be needed to ensure the safety of the patient as well as the safety of other patients and the staff.
- Each unit has a clear protocol for the safe use of restraints and for the humane management of care during the time the patient is restrained, as well as clear guidelines for understanding and protecting the patient's legal rights.
- Careful documentation of any incidence of escalating violence, especially any violence leading to seclusion or restraints, must be made according to the laws of your state.

APPLYING CRITICAL JUDGMENT

1. Mr. Arnold, a 24-year-old man, is currently in the manic phase of bipolar disorder. He is admitted to an inpatient unit. Staff note that the patient is agitated and irritable and has a history of assault. He shouts at the nurse in a loud, piercing voice, yelling that she is a "slut, a mut, tut-tut." He is pacing anxiously, invading the staff's personal space, and pointing his finger in the faces of some staff.
   A. What would be some appropriate nursing diagnoses for Mr. Arnold at this time?
   B. Describe how you would document his behavior.
   C. What are some of the interventions you and your colleagues might try first? What interventions might you try next? Explain the rationale for your decision.
   D. Describe the kinds of objective and subjective data you would document as well as the frequency of documentation according to the protocols of your hospital.
   E. List the various aspects of interventions of patient care for someone who is in seclusion.
   F. Role-play verbal techniques you could use during any other interventions being initiated at this time.
2. In the morning 2 days later, Mr. Arnold comes to the nurses' desk and asks for a pass. When told that the physician needs to write an order for his pass and the physician will not be on duty until the afternoon, Mr. Arnold becomes verbally loud, demanding that the nurse phone the physician "right this minute to get that pass."
   A. What interventions by you and your colleagues would be most appropriate to start at this time?
   B. Role-play your verbal techniques.
   C. What are the personal safety measures you and your colleagues would take when treating a patient with escalating aggression?
3. Write a summary of the protocols for intervening with irate patients as found in the hospital procedure manual.
4. Describe a time in your life when you have witnessed bullying or have been bullied by others.
   A. If you were the one being bullied, describe how you felt. What could be some long-term effects?
   B. If you were watching a coworker being bullied by a staff member in charge, how might you react today?
   C. Have you ever witnessed or been involved in a student-to-student, nurse-to-nurse, or colleague-to-colleague incidence of bullying? What would you do today?

CHAPTER REVIEW QUESTIONS

1. Select the completion of this sentence that demonstrates an adult is coping in a healthy way: "I am feeling so angry right now…
   a. I'm afraid I'm going to cry."
   b. I would like to punch something."
   c. I want to talk to someone about it."
   d. I want to curl up and sleep for a long time."
2. In a hostile voice, a patient experiencing mania yells at the nurse: "You WILL listen to me and not interrupt. I have some really important stuff to say. I'm tired of you nurses and doctors acting like you have all the answers." To facilitate effective communication, which initial response should the nurse provide?
   a. "You are our patient, so we always listen to you."
   b. "I can talk with you better if you use a calm voice."
   c. "It's our job to help you get through this manic episode."
   d. "Patients have an important role in treatment planning."
3. A female nurse is appointed to a committee with seven men. At the beginning of the meeting, the chairman asks the nurse to be the secretary. The nurse responds, "No. You're just asking me to be secretary because I'm the only the woman here." Which response would have been more effective?
   a. "There are others more qualified than I am to be secretary."
   b. "I would be glad to perform another role for our committee."
   c. "I'm probably overreacting, but I find your request offensive."
   d. "Thank you for asking, but your request is sexually discriminatory."
4. An 8-year-old tells a parent, "I like to scare kids at school by showing them pictures of clowns. Some kids are terrified." How should the nurse counsel the parents regarding this behavior?
   a. Recommend family therapy for the child, siblings, and parents.
   b. Suggest the parents enroll the child in an anger management program.
   c. Educate both parents about bullying, including possible origins and long-term effects.
   d. Teach the parents about the developmental phase and tasks for an 8-year-old child.
5. A woman experienced a double mastectomy yesterday. Now she cheerfully says to the nurse, "I didn't need those things anyway. No more wet T-shirt contests for me!" How should the nurse interpret this comment?
   a. The patient is realistically accepting her loss.

b. The comment is sarcastic, which may reflect anger.
c. The patient is experiencing a distorted body image.
d. The comment suggests guilt regarding prior behavior.

REFERENCES

American Nurses Association (ANA). (2015). *ANA panel aims to prevent violence, bullying in health care facilities*. Retrieved July 25, 2015, from http://www. nursingworld.org/MainMenuCategories/WorkplaceSafety/Healthy-Nurse/bullyingworkplaceviolence/ANA-Panel-Aims-to-Prevent-Violence-Bullying.

American Psychiatric Nurses Association (APNA). (2000, rev. 2007, rev. 2014). *Seclusion and restraint standards of practice*. Retrieved July 12, 2015, from http://www.apna.org.

American Psychiatric Association: Psychiatric News Alert. (2015). *Recovery model helps reduce use of seclusion, restraint and large hospital system*. Retrieved from http://alert.psychnews.org/2014/11/recovery-model-helps-reduce-use-of.html

Black, D. W., & Andreasen, N. C. (2014). *Introductory textbook of psychiatry* (6th ed.). Washington, DC: American Psychiatric Publishing.

Bresin, K., & Gordon, K. H. (2013). Aggression as affect regulation: extending catharsis theory to evaluate aggression and experiential anger in the laboratory and daily life. *Journal of Social and Clinical Psychology, 32*(4), 400–423.

Claffey, C. (2011). ED nurses continue to be victims of workplace violence according to new report. *American Nurse Today, 6*(11).

Feinstein, R. E., & Rothberg, B. (2014). Violence. In Janice L. Cutler (Ed.), *Psychiatry* (pp. 403–417). New York: Oxford: University Press.

Gerken, A. T., Gross, A. F., & Saunders, K. M. (2016). Aggression and violence. In T. A. Stern, M. Fava, T. E. Wilens, et al. (Eds.), *Massachusetts General Hospital comprehensive clinical psychiatry* (2nd ed.) (pp. 709–717). China: Elsevier.

Jalain, C. I. (2014). The impact of serotonin and dopamine on human aggression: a systematic review of the literature. *Master's Theses, Paper 6*. Retrieved from http://aquila.usm.edu/masters_theses/6.

Linehan, M. (1993). *Cognitive-behavioral treatment of borderline personality disorder*. New York, NY: Guilford Press.

Preston, J. D., O'Neal, J. H., & Talaga, M. C. (2013). *Handbook of clinical psychopharmacology for therapists* (7th ed.). Oakland, CA: New Harbinger Publications.

Robbins, A. (2015). *Mean girls of the ER: the alarming nurse culture of bullying and hazing*. Marie Claire, May.

Sadock, B. J., Sadock, V. A., & Ruiz, P. (2015). *Glossary Kaplan & Sadock's synopsis of psychiatry* (11th ed.). Philadelphia, PA: Lippincott Williams & Wilkins.

Schluter, T., Winz, O., Henkel, K., et al. (2013). The impact of dopamine on aggression: an [18F] FDOPA Penn study and healthy males. Retrieved July 20, 2015, from http:www.ncbi.nlm. nih.gov-/pubmed/24155295.

Sivak, K. (2012). Implementation of comfort rooms to reduce seclusion, restraint use, and acting out behaviors. *Journal of Psychiatry & Neuroscience, 50*(2), 24–34.

Society for Neuroscience. (rev. 2014). *Aggression on the brain*. Retrieved July 17, 2015, from http://www.brainfacts.org/sensing-thinking-behaving/mood/articles/2008/aggression—the-brain/.

Substance Abuse and Mental Health Services Administration (SAMHSA). (2011). A seclusion and restraint overview. Retrieved February 14, 2012, from http://www.samhsa.gov/matrix2/seclusion_matrix.aspx.

Substance Abuse and Mental Health Services Administration (SAMHSA). (2015). *Trauma-informed approach and trauma-specific interventions*. Retrieved July 15, 2015, from http://www.samhsa.gov/nctic/trauma-interventions.

Victoroff, J. (2009). Human aggression. In B. J. Sadock, V. A. Sadock, & P. Ruiz (Eds.), *Kaplan and Sadock's comprehensive textbook of psychiatry* (9th ed.) (pp. 2671–2702). Philadelphia, PA: Wolters Kluwer/Lippincott Williams & Wilkins.

Zeller, S. L., & Wilson, M. P. (2015). Management of aggression. *Paradigm, 19*(3), 12–15.

Care for the Dying and Those Who Grieve

Carol O. Long

ⓔ http://evolve.elsevier.com/Varcarolis/essentials

KEY TERMS AND CONCEPTS

acute grief, p. 390
anticipatory grief, p. 390
bereavement, p. 390
burnout, p. 397
caring presence, p. 396
compassion, p. 397
compassion fatigue, p. 397

complicated grief, p. 390
disenfranchised grief, p. 390
end of life conversations, p. 395
FICA, p. 395
Four Gifts, p. 396
Four Tasks of Mourning, p. 391
grief, p. 390

grief work, p. 390
hospice care, p. 389
loss, p. 389
meaning reconstruction, p. 390
mourning, p. 390
palliative care, p. 389
uncomplicated grief, p. 390

SELECTED CONCEPT: COMPASSION

Compassion is the ability to be with someone who is suffering. Compassion begins with understanding suffering. Through silence, expressive compassion, listening to stories, and the compassionate voice of one's own, the nurse is transformed from witnessing suffering to making changes to relieve it (Ferrell & Coyle, 2008; Reich, 1989).

OBJECTIVES

1. Discuss and differentiate between palliative care and hospice in terms of (a) purpose, (b) philosophy and goals, (c) settings, and (d) various supports available to families.
2. Compare and contrast the terms *loss, grief, mourning,* and *bereavement.*
3. Identify the behavioral outcomes that indicate healthy bereavement.
4. Delineate at least five symptoms of complicated grief.
5. Discuss and give examples of the various phenomena experienced during the normal grief process (e.g., sensations of somatic distress, changes in behavior).
6. Describe three short-term interventions that can be used to help a person experiencing complicated grief come to terms with his or her loss.
7. Describe and discuss the Four Tasks of Mourning as identified in this chapter
8. Select at least two patient-centered goals of care at end of life, and discuss how you would address these issues.
9. Identify key communication interventions that support patient-centered goals of care.
10. Explain the interventions you would take to help grief-stricken caregivers in the following areas:
    a. Helping the bereaved caregivers come to terms with their feelings
    b. Helping people say goodbye
    c. Helping families maintain "hope"
    d. Establishing presence
11. Describe the importance of self-care interventions for nurses.

INTRODUCTION

Dying in America

Over the past 30 years, there have been tremendous advances in end of life and palliative care in the United States. The National Palliative Care Registry survey report estimates that more than 6 million Americans are receiving formal palliative care from palliative care teams in 1734 fifty-bed hospitals, achieving 61% of all hospitals of this size (Center to Advance Palliative Care [CAPC], 2014). Teno and colleagues (2013) examined Medicare claims that listed the site of death, place of care, and health care transitions of older adults in 2000, 2005, and 2009 as a quality measure for end of life care. Results indicated

that deaths in acute care hospitals have decreased and the use of hospice has increased. However, patients were likely to be in the intensive care unit (ICU) or experience burdensome transitions of care in the 30 days prior to death. Thus lack of palliative care teams in some hospitals, short lengths of stay in hospice, and aggressive and life-preserving measures at end of life indicate that more can be done.

A recent Institute of Medicine (IOM, 2014) study and report challenges practitioners and the health care system to improve the quality and availability of palliative care services to support quality of life through the end of life. Five recommendations specify that (1) more and better comprehensive care is needed for people with advanced serious illness along with (2) improved client-patient communication that includes advance care planning, (3) professional education and ongoing development in palliative care, (4) improved financing to provide quality end of life care, and (5) public education and engagement about advance care planning and informed choices.

What is palliative care and how does it improve care for patients with serious life-threatening illnesses? The National Consensus Project's *Clinical Practice Guidelines for Quality Palliative Care*, Third Edition (2013), which is sanctioned by leading hospice and palliative medicine and nursing organizations, endorses the Centers for Medicare and Medicaid Services (CMS) and National Quality Forum (NQF) definition: "Palliative care means patient and family-centered care that optimizes quality of life by anticipating, preventing, and treating suffering. Palliative care throughout the continuum of illness involves addressing physical, intellectual, emotional, social and spiritual needs to facilitate patient autonomy, access to information and choice." These standards and guidelines emphasize collaborative and coordinated care by an interdisciplinary team, services that are available concurrently or independent of curative or life-prolonging care, and support of patient and family hope for peace and dignity until death. Hospice care is provided at the end of life and is a part of the palliative care trajectory. A sample of these standards is listed in Box 25-1.

Hospice care is a model for compassionate, holistic, and medically managed end of life services. The Medicare hospice benefit was enacted in 1982 and is largely available across all insurance plans. A recent National Hospice and Palliative Care Organization (2014) report indicates that approximately 5800 hospices provided care to 1.5 to 1.6 million patients. Most patients (34.5%) die or are discharged within 7 days of admission. Cancer diagnoses accounted for 36.5% of deaths, followed by dementia (15.25%), heart disease (13.4%), lung disease (9.9%), and debility unspecified (5.4%). Most of the care (66.6%) is provided in the patient's place of residence (e.g., home, nursing home, or residential facility), with 26.4% in a hospice inpatient facility and 7.0% in an acute care hospital.

Hospice care is delivered by an interdisciplinary team of physicians, nurses, chaplains, social workers, certified nursing aides, volunteers, and bereavement counselors. All medications and supplies related to the terminal diagnosis are covered by Medicare reimbursement, and many other insurance providers mimic the Medicare benefit. Individuals are perceived as living fully until they die; their choices and preferences are respected and incorporated in the plan of care. The patient and family is considered the unit of care and receives counseling support around the tasks of anticipatory grief and mourning as well as spirituality and finding meaning and purpose at the end of life. Hospice services will continue to evolve, subject to increasing regulatory measures to report quality of care in the future (Box 25-2).

This chapter focuses on nursing care for those who are dying, care for family members and others who grieve, and self-care for nurses.

LOSS, GRIEF, AND MOURNING

Loss is part of the human experience, and grief and mourning are the normal responses to loss. We grieve on a recurring basis as we face the commonplace losses in our lives, such as the loss of a relationship (e.g., divorce, separation, death, abortion), health (e.g., a body function or part, mental or physical capacity), friendship, status, prestige, or security (e.g., occupational, financial, social, cultural). Some losses may be even more intangible, such as the loss of a projected future or dreams. Normal losses include changes in circumstances, such as retirement, a promotion, marriage, and the aging process.

It could be said that the course of our lives depends on how we adapt to losses and how we use change as a vehicle for growth. Understanding how to support healthy grieving and mourning in oneself and for others is a vital life skill. Unfortunately, contemporary mainstream U.S. culture perpetuates many damaging **myths about grief and mourning,** such as:

- Grief and mourning are the same experience and the same for everyone.
- There is a predictable and orderly stage-like progression to grieving.
- It is best to move away from grief rather than toward it.
- Following the death of someone important to you, the goal is to "get over it."
- Tears are an expression of weakness.

BOX 25-1   Selected National Consensus Project Clinical Practice Guidelines, 2013

Domain 3: Psychological and Psychiatric Aspects of Care
  Guideline 3.1 The interdisciplinary team assesses and addresses psychological aspects of care based upon the best available evidence to maximize patient and family coping and quality of life.
  Guideline 3.2 A core component of the palliative care program is a grief and bereavement program available to patients and families based on assessment of need.
Domain 7: Care of the Patient at the End of Life
  Guideline 7.1 The interdisciplinary team identifies, communicates, and manages the signs and symptoms at the end of life to meet the physical, psychosocial, spiritual, social and cultural needs of patients and families.
  Guideline 7.4 An immediate bereavement plan is activated post-death.

National Consensus Project (NCP) for Quality Palliative Care. (2013). *Clinical practice guidelines for quality palliative care* (3rd ed.). Retrieved February 13, 2015, from https://www.hpna.org/multimedia/NCP_Clinical_Practice_Guidelines_3rd_Edition.pdf

---

BOX 25-2   Quality Improvement Measures in Hospice and Palliative Care

With the implementation of the Patient Protection and Affordable Care Act (Section 3004) and Social Security Act [Section 1814(i)] and attention to palliative care and hospice by the NQF, CMS has mandated the Hospice Item Set and quality measure to ensure patients' quality of life needs are being met. These data will be publicly reported and tied to the hospice payment system in the future. Selected measures are featured:

NQF #1641. Treatment Preferences
The medical records of seriously ill patients enrolled in hospice or receiving specialty palliative care in an acute hospital setting will have documentation of life-sustaining practices.

Modified NQF #1647 Beliefs/Values Addressed (if desired by the patient)
The medical record of hospice patients will show documents of a discussion of spiritual/relations concerns or documentation that the patient/caregiver/family did not want to discuss.

CMS, Centers for Medicare and Medicaid Services; *NQF,* National Quality Forum.
National Quality Forum. (n.d.). *National voluntary consensus standard: palliative and end of life care—A consensus report/final report.* Retrieved from http://www.qualityforum.org/Publications/2012/04/Palliative_Care_and_End of life_Care%E2%80%94A_Consensus_Report.aspx

Grief is the individualized response to a loss that is perceived, real, or anticipated. Grief is a normal response to loss at the time of death. It is experienced emotionally, cognitively, physically, socially, and spiritually. Normal grief is known as uncomplicated grief. *Uncomplicated grief is anything but uncomplicated* but it is described as a normal progression through the grief process, as defined by cultural and societal values, and includes reactions such as depressed mood, insomnia, anxiety, poor appetite, loss of interest, guilt, dreams about the deceased, confusion, and poor concentration. Psychological states may include shock, denial, anger, and yearning and searching for the deceased. Socially, grievers may experience isolation and disappointment as their friends and families fail to understand what they are facing. Spirituality is frequently either shaken or strengthened by the experience of profound loss. Acute grief, a term coined by Dr. Erich Lindemann (1994), is the result of an unexpected death of a family member and can result in an exacerbation of any pre-existing medical or psychiatric problems. A history of depression, substance abuse, or posttraumatic stress disorder (PTSD) can complicate grief.

The term anticipatory grief, though far from a perfect term, helps people recognize that grief is a part of the complex process of living with a terminal prognosis. During anticipatory grieving, the dying individual and family may display primary emotions such as anger (e.g., protesting that this is happening, anger at the patient for not fighting harder, anger at the medical system, displaced anger at others because of helplessness in the face of suffering, anger at God), sadness (e.g., sorrow and regret for the present and the future), hurt (e.g., pain over what the patient is enduring, the pain of being unable to protect each other, the pain of loss), fear and anxiety (e.g., a pervasive sense that something more should or could be done, dread of what is coming next, loss of control, a sense that time is running out), and bridled grief (e.g., experiencing hits or bursts of grief but keeping it in check as long as the patient is alive) (Ayalon & Green, 2012). From the moment of diagnosis, patients and families begin to both experience and anticipate losses, and it does **not** become any easier when death occurs.

Disenfranchised grief is a term coined by Dr. Kenneth Doka (1989) to acknowledge losses that are not socially sanctioned, openly acknowledged, or publicly mourned. Grief may be disenfranchised because of the relationship of the griever (e.g., life partner, health care worker, defense attorney, divorced spouse), the nature of the loss (e.g., miscarriages, abortions, war heroes), the type of death (e.g., executions, homicides, suicides, human immunodeficiency virus/acquired immunodeficiency syndrome [HIV/AIDS]), or the grieving style related to gender differences or stage in life. In such situations mourners may not have the opportunity to publicly grieve the loss. Once losses are recognized as disenfranchised, it becomes easier to support them within and among individuals sharing the same experience.

Complicated grief essentially means that the grief work is unresolved and occurs when individuals have difficulty coming to terms with their loss and experience phenomena outside the normal grief reaction, which impairs the individual's ability to function in social or occupational situations, or resume previous roles. Thoughts may be intrusive, involving preoccupation with the deceased long after what is felt to be a normal period of mourning coupled with an inability to get away from persistent and painful yearning for the loved one. The bereaved may want to die in order to rejoin their loved one: "Life is empty. I have no interest in anything. I am only half a person now." Complicated grief may be chronic or grief that extends for at least a year after the death; delayed, when normal grief reactions are postponed or suppressed; or exaggerated, when the individual takes drastic measures that are self-destructive (e.g., suicide) or masked, or be present when the survivor is unaware that behaviors that are interfering with normal activities are a result of the loss. The *Diagnosis and Statistical Manual of Mental Disorders (DSM-5)* (American Psychiatric Association [APA], 2013) identifies criteria that define complicated grief as a disorder called *persistent complex bereavement disorder.*

Mourning refers to all the ways in which a person outwardly expresses grief and the efforts taken to manage grief. This includes culturally determined practices such as wakes, funerals, sitting shiva (a ritual specific to Jewish mourners), or decorating the gravesite. Mourning is influenced by culture, religious or spiritual practices, family traditions, and one's own personality and beliefs. The passage of time alone does not always heal grief; it is what we do with the time that seems to help. Sharing our grief with others seems to relieve some of its effects and allows us to move through it. Social media sites provide outlets for grievers to find understanding and meaningful connections with others. Attending grief support groups and seeing a counselor are also activities of mourning. It is mourning that gradually releases us from the pain of loss.

Bereavement is the state of having lost a significant other and the corresponding social experience (Corless, 2015). It refers to the event of losing an important person to death and is derived from the Old English word *berafian,* meaning "to rob." Most cultures provide symbols and contexts for bereavement, such as wearing black or a black armband. Bereaved people experience themselves as being set apart from the current of ordinary life. Contemporary society in the United States has left behind the visible symbols of bereavement, with the result that those in mourning often feel isolated and alone. Bereavement services for 12 months after the death are part of the hospice insurance benefit.

THEORY

Some of the most widely known early grief theorists describe commonly experienced psychological and behavioral phenomena experience by those who are grieving a loss. Erich Lindemann (1994), in his classic study about the survivors of Boston's Coconut Grove nightclub in 1942, coined the term grief work, which is used to describe the process of grief recovery or how a person adjusts to the loss. Others postulated various phases of bereavement that proceed in orderly sequences within certain time frames, the best known from Elisabeth Kübler-Ross's (1969) book *On Death and Dying.* The various frameworks for grieving and phases of grief are useful for helping people to normalize the deeply felt and disturbing phenomena they experience when they confront profound loss. However, these frameworks do not provide the focus of care during the grieving process nor do they typify the predictability of a person moving through stages. The process of grief work derives from the details of a person's unique experience and the emotions felt do not always follow a pattern of response. The griever constructs and reconstructs the world around him or her through the experience as a survivor of loss known as meaning reconstruction (Neimeyer et al., 2010). The following are common phenomena a person may experience at some point in the grief process:

1. Shock and disbelief
2. Denial
3. Sensation of somatic distress
4. Preoccupation with the image of the deceased
5. Guilt
6. Anger
7. Change in behavior (e.g., depression, disorganization, panic, restlessness)
8. Reorganization of behavior directed toward a new object or activity
9. Acceptance

While emotional responses vary from one individual to the next, a common first response is that of **denial.** The person is emotionally unable to accept his or her painful loss. Denial functions as a buffer against intolerable pain and allows the person slowly to acknowledge the reality of death. The mourner may appear to be functioning like a robot. Often, the bereaved person feels numb. A death may be accepted intellectually during this stage—"It's just as well, she was suffering"—although the emotional responses are still repressed. Denial is a needed defense that lasts for a few hours or a few days. Denial can also be thought of as disbelief, and may recur over the early course of bereavement ("This morning I picked up the phone to call her and dialed her number before I remembered that she is gone"). However, persistent denial suggests that the mourning may be complicated, making it difficult to move through the process of mourning.

As denial fades, painful feelings begin to surface. The finality of the loved one's death becomes more of a reality. Waves of anguish and pain are experienced and may be localized in the chest or the epigastric area. **Anger** may surface at this time. Physicians and nurses are often the objects of blame. Awareness by staff that anger is often displaced onto people in the health care environment may decrease defensive staff behaviors. **Guilt** is often experienced, and the bereaved blames himself or herself for taking or for failing to take specific actions. The griever may need to be supported patiently as he or she gradually comes to terms with a past that cannot be changed by hindsight. Guilt often indicates profound regret that things could not have been different than they were.

Crying is a common phenomenon early on (and often within cultural norms) with intense suffering and despair. Crying can afford a welcome release from pent-up anguish and tension. Assessment of cultural patterns is important in understanding crying. Failing to cry can be the result of cultural influences or environmental restraints. The person may cry in private. Inability to cry, however, may be the result of a high degree of ambivalence toward the deceased. A person who is unable to cry may have difficulty in successfully completing the work of mourning. Grievers as well as those around them have bought into a belief that they should not surrender to mourning.

Since these pioneering scholars, other models describing how we grieve and the relationship to mourning have emerged. Self-control is valued and the dominant cultural and familial message is usually "Shape up and get on with your life." In reality, mourning demands that who we are and the world we live in be reconstructed and remodeled in major ways. This requires much talking, working, engaging, writing, feeling, experimenting, and risk taking, supported by others who do not try to fix or rush the griever. Instead of "getting over it" as soon as possible, successful mourning asks us to engage in a complex process of finding a new and durable connection to who we are now and to the person who died. J. William Worden (2009) describes this process as the Four Tasks of Mourning:

1. Accept the reality of the loss
2. Process the pain of grief while caring for the self
3. Adjust to a world without the deceased
4. Find an enduring connection with the deceased in the midst of embarking on a new life

These tasks indicate a natural movement that results when people actively engage in mourning, rather than fitting one's own experience into someone else's framework. When people "hang in there" with their mourning over time, they instinctively progress toward the final task. Finally, they are able to remember the loved one without so much pain. They have the energy to engage in life and be open to new relationships and activities. They sense that they now carry that departed person with them in an enduring way that no longer requires a physical presence. They are able to love again.

Other research focuses on issues such as the relationship between grief and trauma, the grieving process during various developmental periods of life, the advantages of resiliency and adaptability in

mourning, interventions appropriate for specific populations, definition of complicated or intractable grief and its treatment, and many more topics. According to Bonanno (2009), resilient people show no grief and the absence of grief is a healthy outcome. These individuals have the ability to "bounce back" from adversity and regain health (van Kessel, 2013).

Stroebe and Schut (1999) describe mourning as "dual processes," both of which derive from models of stress and coping. The bereaved individual oscillates between **loss-oriented** and **restoration-oriented** tasks. The loss-oriented processes are those that deal with recognizing the loss, whereas the restoration-oriented processes aim at re-creating a new life. A person's ability to oscillate, or move between these spheres, is an indication of his or her coping and inner resources. One contribution of this model is that it normalizes distraction from the loss experience as an integral part of successful mourning. Mourners are encouraged to take breaks, experience positive emotions, delay or defer some of the pain of grieving, and essentially control the amount of grief they are able to bear. Various phenomena experienced during bereavement are described in Table 25-1.

PATIENT AND FAMILY-CENTERED GOALS OF CARE

No one spends as much time at the bedside of those who are dying and with their families than nursing professionals. Thus caring for individuals with serious or life-threatening illness through death and supporting their families require special skills, personal awareness, and ongoing self-care. Because of their daily, hands-on care and the mandate of the profession to comfort the patient, nurses have a heightened proximity to the experiences and feelings of their patients. Nurses are affected by cultural myths about grief and mourning in the same way the rest of society is; when they are faced with a person who is grieving or dying, nurses may feel uncomfortable and unequipped to face the loss. They often feel acutely uncomfortable when witnessing expressions of deep grief and pain and try to "fix it" with an intervention. Normal activities of mourning, such as weeping, protesting, or expressing anger or despair, are perceived as "meltdowns" or signs of "losing it," and nurses may feel inadequate in the face of such "breakdowns" and leave the griever, consider medicating the griever, or request a counselor for the griever. This reflects our societal misunderstandings about grief and mourning, but may also be a response to the nurse's unmourned losses, difficult memories, and unresolved feelings that are awakened. The following competencies, skills, and interventions assist nurses in understanding their own feelings about loss and grief and ways to enhance caring for terminally ill patients and their families, both of whom may be grieving.

Communication Skills

Communication skills are vital in connecting with dying individuals and their family members and are an essential competency in palliative care (Dahlin & Wittenberg, 2015). To be comfortable in caring for the terminally ill requires addressing barriers, such as fear of one's own mortality, lack of experience in caring for the dying, the desire to foster hope, and unrealistic societal expectations for cure. Family system changes, financial uncertainties, compromised educational or mental health capacity, physical limitations, and the impact of culture and spirituality are factors that influence communication (Wittenberg-Lyles et al., 2010, 2013). Becoming proficient in effective nonverbal and verbal communication is directed at overcoming these barriers and instituting methods or practices that support the patient and family members.

Allow yourself to be genuinely interested without feeling that you have to be an expert or have the answers. Ask open-ended questions

TABLE 25-1   Phenomena Experienced during Bereavement

Symptoms	Examples
Sensations of Somatic Distress The bereaved may experience tightness in the throat, shortness of breath, sighing, mental pain, or exhaustion; food tastes like sand; things feel unreal. Pain or discomfort may be identical to the symptoms experienced by the deceased. Normally, symptoms are brief.	A woman whose husband died of a stroke complains of weakness and numbness on her left side.
Preoccupation with the Image of the Deceased The bereaved introduces into conversation, thinks about, and talks about numerous memories of the deceased. The memories are positive. This process continues with great sadness. The idealization of the deceased lets the bereaved relive the gratifications associated with the deceased and helps resolve any guilt the bereaved feels concerning the deceased. The bereaved may also assume many of the mannerisms of the deceased through identification. Identification serves the purpose of holding on to the deceased. Preoccupation with the deceased can continue for many months before it lessens.	A man whose wife has very recently died states, "I just can't stop thinking about my wife. Everything I see reminds me of her. We picked up this seashell on our honeymoon. I remember every wonderful moment we had together. The pain is so great, but the memories just keep coming." His friends notice that when he talks, his hand gestures and expressions are very like those of his recently deceased wife.
Guilt The bereaved reproaches himself or herself for real or imagined acts of negligence or omissions in the relationship with the deceased.	"I should have made him go to the doctor sooner." "I should have paid more attention to her, been more thoughtful."
Anger The anger the bereaved experiences may not be toward the object at its source. Often the anger is displaced onto the medical or nursing staff. Often it is directed toward the deceased. The anger is at its height during the first month but is often intermittent throughout the first year. The overflow of hostility disturbs the bereaved, resulting in the feeling that he or she is "going insane."	"The doctor didn't operate in time. If he had, Mary would be alive today." "How could he leave me like this…how could he?"
Change in Behavior: Depression, Disorganization, Restlessness A person may exhibit marked restlessness and an inability to organize his or her behavior. A depressive mood during routine activities is common, decreasing as the year passes and the intensity of the grief declines. Absence of depression is more abnormal than its presence. Loneliness and aimlessness are most pronounced 6 to 9 months after the death. Reorganization of behavior directed toward a new object or activity gradually occurs. The person renews his or her interest in people and activities. The grieving thus releases the bereaved from one interpersonal relationship, and new ones are free to take its place.	Six months after her husband died, Mrs. Faye states, "I just can't seem to function. I have a hard time doing the simplest tasks. I can't be bothered with socializing. I feel so down…so, so empty." Twenty months after her husband's death, Mrs. Faye tells a friend, "I'll be away this weekend. I am going fishing with my brother and his friend. This is the first time I've felt like doing anything since Harry died."

and listen in a spirit of seeking to understand the dying individual, not to "fix" him or her. This is the person's story. Avoid using the lens of your own belief system. This is the patient's and family's framework of values. You are there to learn and support, not to change their spirituality or faith, or lack thereof. Seek to hear unspoken questions. Sometimes a patient's existential issues are not communicated in words. These may be unspoken questions, such as: "Do you know what I am hoping for today?" "Can you tell if I am feeling despair?" "Do you know what brings me courage and peace?" "Can you help calm my fears?" *Possessing good listening skills is cited as the most important characteristic needed by a health care worker when talking with a dying individual and his or her family.* Sometimes, by listening to a patient's dreams, these unspoken emotional or spiritual states can also be explored and addressed.

One of the most important skills necessary in caring for the dying and their family members is to be "in the moment." Demonstrate presence and caring behaviors. Allow for a review of successes in the patients' lives and their lasting legacy; discuss any suicidal thoughts using a nonjudgmental approach and make appropriate referrals for care; allow time for patients to express their feelings and give them as

BOX 25-3   Dignity in Caring

"Patient care and caring about patients should go hand in hand. Caring implicates our fundamental attitude towards the dying, and the ability to convey kindness, compassion and respect. Yet all too often, patients and families experience health care as impersonal, mechanical; and quickly discover that patienthood trumps personhood. …Caring is the gateway to disclosure; without it, patients are less likely to say what is bothering them, leading to missed diagnoses, medical errors and compromised patient safety."

From Chochinov, H. M. (2013). Dignity in care: Time to take action. *Journal of Pain and Symptom Management, 46*(5), 756–759.

much control over their care as possible; assist in supporting the family in repairing conflicts; help to make the most of things they enjoy (e.g., visits with friends, foods and music, storytelling, living in the moment); and assist with spiritual comfort—finding solace in spiritual beliefs and achieving a peaceful death (Brown & Johnston, 2011). Convey caring, sensitivity, and compassion. Listen. Be patient; be present (Box 25-3).

A Person Experiencing Grief

Scenario

I met 19-year-old Monica during her brief hospitalization to stabilize her insulin-resistant (type 1) diabetes. Under her veneer of sarcasm, I sensed depression as she talked about her pledging a sorority, too much partying, failing grades, and her diabetes raging out of control.

Therapeutic Goal

By the conclusion of this interaction, Monica will make at least one decision to break out of her self-destructive cycle and deal with the issue(s) and feelings she is pushing down.

Student-Patient Interaction	Thoughts, Communication Techniques, and Mental Health Nursing Concepts
Monica: "You're back again. Couldn't find anything better to do?"	
Student's feelings: *Monica's sarcasm tends to disconcert me until I remind myself that fear and loss fuel her anger.*	
Student: "Hi, Monica. I will be working with you again today. How are you?"	I ignored her comment, which *non-reinforces* the sarcasm. I am willing myself to not take it personally.
Monica: "Fine. The doctor just yelled because my right heel has a sore on it that I've ignored. If I fail one more class, I go on academic probation and finals start next week. Yeah, I'm doing just great."	I forgot that using a social greeting like "How are you?" typically elicits an automatic "fine." Using a *broad opening* like "What's been happening with you since we talked yesterday?" would better let Monica know that I really want her to share.
Student: *(Leaning in.)* "Somehow your 'just great' doesn't sound so great."	I make an observation and then use *attending* body language to show empathy.
Student's feelings: *I feel overwhelmed listening to her. Because I carry a heavy academic load, I identify with her struggles. Yet I feel some frustration that Monica does not seem to take charge of her life.*	Is that countertransference? Is that my own fear that I will lose control of all the pieces I juggle?
Monica: "No use worrying." *(Leaning in and speaking quietly.)*	
Student: "And yet somehow the worry creeps back in. Sometimes the worry looks like sadness or even anger. Sometimes it shows up as a blood sugar that refuses to stabilize."	I refer to "the worry" and "a blood sugar" to depersonalize the reference, yet still allow Monica to choose insight, if possible.
Student's feelings: *I hope I'm not pushing her too much. We have some rapport and she lets herself vent with me.*	

Student-Patient Interaction	Thoughts, Communication Techniques, and Mental Health Nursing Concepts
Monica: *(Nods.)*	
Student: "You feel overwhelmed."	
Monica: "The doctor yelling about my foot! Wish I could hide in some hole where no one could ever find me or tell me what I should be doing."	In *crisis terms* the doctor "yelling" likely acted as the *precipitating event*.
Student: "I wonder what pressures you the most."	I ask Monica an indirect question to help her identify stress. Should I have instead attempted to translate into feelings? For example, "You're discouraged and having a hard time believing in yourself."
Monica: "The feeling that no matter what I do, it isn't enough. It isn't good enough. I'm not good enough."	
Student: "You say you aren't good enough—for who?"	I am assessing a *balancing* factor in *crisis* when I help Monica talk about her *perception of the event* and most significantly, her perception of self.
Monica: "Since I was diagnosed when I was 6, my mother insisted I was the same as everybody else. 'The diabetes doesn't change anything, Monica. You can do anything!' So I pledge a sorority, go with the flow, ignoring what I should or shouldn't eat or drink. Then I stay out late and screw up my sleep and my blood sugar goes haywire. I feel bad, so I don't study."	Monica *projects* the blame for her trouble onto her mother. *What must it be like for a person to deal with diabetes since 6 years old?*
Student: "So in trying to prove the diabetes does not matter, it ends up influencing major areas of your life. What does your mother say now?"	I *clarify* to try to understand Monica's meaning. I also *gather information*.
Monica: "Nothing. She doesn't know I'm in here."	Monica independently brought up the subject of her mother, so I will listen to see if her mother is a *situational support*, a second balancing factor in crisis.
Student: "She doesn't know?"	I *restate* to say, "Go on."
Monica: "I thought I could put it off until after finals, but my life is falling apart."	

Continued

APPLYING THE ART—cont'd

A Person Experiencing Grief

Student-Patient Interaction	Thoughts, Communication Techniques, and Mental Health Nursing Concepts	Student-Patient Interaction	Thoughts, Communication Techniques, and Mental Health Nursing Concepts
Student: "Put what off, Monica?" ***Student's feelings:*** *Did I do this the right way? I probably should have helped her talk about her life falling apart but I am also curious about what she has put off.*	I still do not understand about "put off," so I ask an *indirect question.*	***Student's feelings:*** *Helping Monica look at saying goodbye makes me think about telling the people I love how much they mean to me.*	
Monica: *(Sobbing.)* "She's dying. My mother is dying. She's survived the cancer so long that I never thought she'd actually die. She has maybe 2 months."	She has been grieving losing her mother.	**Monica:** "I haven't gone home all semester. I barely talk when she calls. I guess if I go home I can't pretend that it's not happening anymore."	Monica uses the word *pretend*. The *denial* stage of grief plays a part, too.
Student: "Oh! I'm so sorry. You've been holding this pain inside, trying to put off…?" ***Student's feelings:*** *My feelings of sorrow came out without my thinking first.*		**Student:** "It's natural to feel afraid. It's scary to let yourself experience this pain of saying goodbye." *(She nods.)* "I wonder what you think might happen." ***Student's feelings:*** *I feel good that Monica is working with me to think through how she will handle talking to her mother.*	I give *support* and ask an *indirect question.*
Monica: "No one knows. My friends don't even know." ***Student's feelings:*** *I feel compassion for her. She must feel so alone.*		**Monica:** "Maybe I won't be strong. I'll break down."	
Student: "I wonder what telling others would mean to you."		**Student:** "And then?"	I help Monica *problem solve* by anticipating what will likely happen with each step, in order to decrease her *anxiety*. Being able to predict meets *safety needs.*
Monica: "That I can't make it by myself. That it's real. She's going to die. I can't do my life without her." *(Crying.)* ***Student's feelings:*** *I am picking up some of her feelings of aloneness and powerlessness with the impending death of her mom. I have to watch that I don't get sucked into these feelings but rather focus on Monica's feelings and thoughts.*	I wonder if *unconsciously* Monica's nonadherence with her diabetic regimen and doing poorly at school has to do with *acting out* her belief that "I can't do my life without her." I know how devastated I would be to lose my mother.	**Monica:** "My mom will cry, too." **Student:** "You will cry together." *(Monica nods.)* **Monica:** "I need to talk to her. Will you stay with me while I call?" **Student:** "Yes." ***Student's feelings:*** *I am honored that Monica is reaching out to me and has at least made a decision to be with her mom and share their losses together.*	Our talking together highlighted the third crisis *balancing factor,* namely, *situational support.* Before we terminate today, I want to help Monica think about who can lend support as she juggles school, her diabetes, and the *grief* of losing her mother.
Student: "Monica, what are you saying, that you don't want to live?"	Is she saying she cannot live without her mother? Is this a covert message about suicide?		
Monica: "I wouldn't do anything to hurt myself, but I already feel so lonely, like she's gone already." ***Student's feelings:*** *I feel relieved that she chooses to not hurt herself, though her lifestyle choices aren't healthy.*	She describes *anticipatory grief.* However, Edwin Shneidman might refer to her behavior as subintentional suicide.		
Student: "You feel lonely. You miss her already. In what ways have you been able to let your mother know what she means to you?"	I validate to be sure I understand. Again, I need to assess for counter-transference and keep the pace at Monica's comfort level, not my own.		Monica's decision to call her mother means she is *working through the denial stage* of the grief process and she is ready to go through the painful process of saying goodbye.

Assess and Address Spirituality

Nurses can strengthen their comprehensive care-planning skills by giving additional attention to spirituality and cultural determinants of care near the end of life (Baird, 2015; Long, 2011). Spirituality goes beyond religious affiliation and practices and can be an important component of how an individual defines hope and healing. Spirituality encompasses questions about how our lives relate to the rest of creation without requiring a specific religious affiliation; for example: What energizes our lives? What will survive our personal death, if anything? How do we explain to ourselves the things that happen in life? When do we feel most peaceful? How have we surmounted life's hardest challenges? Using the FICA tool, nurses can learn about the patient's spirituality and provide a means for augmenting strengths and decreasing distress (Box 25-4). Nurses have a unique opportunity to integrate spirituality into patient care through assessment, planning, and interventions that support the patient and family experiencing life-threatening illness or at end of life (Puchalski et al., 2009; Puchalski & Ferrell, 2010).

Advance Care Planning

Nurses have an ethical duty to help their dying patients and their families through conversations regarding advance care planning (American Nurses Association [ANA], 2014). There are many documented barriers to **advance care planning** and having end of life conversations. Although awareness of the need to communicate our end of life choices is steadily growing in the United States, the 2004 National Nursing Home Survey and 2007 National Home and Hospice Care Survey reported that hospice patients were most likely to have completed advance directives (88%), followed by nursing home residents (65%); the least likely to have completed these directives was home health patients (Jones et al., 2011). Patients and families may create barriers by concealing the extent of their worry and grief, by feeling confused and fearful about dying, and by adhering to cultural preconditions. Physicians may fear bearing bad news, not fully understand advance directives, view death as the enemy, have medical-legal concerns, and lack training in interpersonal relational processes. Nurses can assist dying patients in clarifying goals and wishes for end of life care by exploring values, beliefs, and priorities.

Advance directives provide a person with the right to self-determination and specificity in everyday clinical decisions and actions, and affirm choices for treatment options such as cardiopulmonary resuscitation, tube feedings, internal cardiac devices, and comfort care. These written instructions identify the patient's wishes when the patient is no longer able to speak on his or her own behalf. Living wills, durable power of attorney for health care, and programs such as the Five Wishes and POLST (Physician Orders for Life-Sustaining Treatment) specify these decisions; however, when there are no advance directives, these decisions are unknown. Thus interdisciplinary teamwork is vital to ensure that decisions are documented and that patients have the conversation about their wishes with their durable health care power of attorney to ensure their rights are upheld (Prince-Paul & Daly, 2015).

Interdisciplinary Teamwork

Interdisciplinary teamwork is essential in the care of the dying and their family members. **Collaboration among colleagues of different disciplines joins members together to create a holistic person and family-centered plan of care.** Collaboration requires team member flexibility, collective ownership of goals, and sharing with one another to create tasks and responsibilities (Wittenberg-Lyles et al., 2013). Similarly, effective teams must learn to overcome conflicts within the team or in patient care. This requires openness, joint ownership, and respect for one another. For the person who is dying and the family members, this is essential in executing a plan of care that meets the needs of the individual and contributes to a "good death" (Box 25-5).

CARING FOR THOSE WHO GRIEVE

"Endings matter, not just for the person but, perhaps even more, for the ones left behind" (Gawande 2014, p. 232).

Needs of family members are a constant focus in palliative care. The transition from thoughts of the person living to thoughts of the person dying or "fading away" evolves during the end of life journey.

BOX 25-4 FICA: Taking a Spiritual History

F: Faith and Belief "Do you consider yourself spiritual or religious" or "Do you have spiritual beliefs that help you cope with stress?" If the patient responds "no," the physician might ask, "What gives life meaning?" Sometimes patients respond with answers such as family, career, or nature.

I: Importance "What importance does your faith or belief have in your life? Have your beliefs influenced how you take care of yourself in this illness? What role do your beliefs play in regaining your health?"

C: Community "Are you a part of a spiritual or religious community? Is this of support to you and how? Is there a person or group of people you really love or who are really important to you?" Communities such as churches, temples, and mosques, or a group of like-minded friends can serve as strong support systems for some patients.

A: Address "How would you like me, your health care provider, to address these issues in your health care?" Often it is not necessary to ask this question but to think about what spiritual issues need to be addressed in the treatment plan. Examples include referrals to chaplains, pastoral counselors, or spiritual directors, journaling, and music or art therapy. Sometimes the plan may be simple—to listen and support the person in his or her journey.

From Puchalski, C. M., & Romer, A. L. (2000). Taking a spiritual history allows clinicians to understand patients more fully. *Journal of Palliative Medicine, 3*(1), 129–137. Reprinted with permission, C. Pushalski, MD, 2015.

BOX 25-5 How Do Nurses Learn about Caring for End of Life Patients?

Sponsored by the American Association of Colleges of Nursing and the City of Hope, the End-of-Life Nursing Education Consortium (ELNEC) has been in existence for 15 years. The ELNEC curriculum and supportive materials are evidence-based and targeted at improving end of life education in nursing schools and continuing education of practicing nurses employed in health care organizations. To date, more than 19,500 nurses across the globe have learned about palliative care nursing and the care of patients from young to old; pain and symptom management; loss, grief, and bereavement; ethics and goals of care; cultural and spiritual considerations in palliative care; communication methods; and care of the patient and family during the final days and hours. Core themes across all curricula include (1) care of the dying patients and their family members as a unit of care, (2) the importance of culture, (3) the role of the nurse as advocate, (4) the critical need for attention to special populations, (5) end of life issues that affect systems of care, (6) critical financial issues that influence end of life care, and (7) interdisciplinary care for quality care at the end of life.

Data from End-of-Life Nursing Education Consortium (ELNEC). (2015). *ELNEC fact sheet.* Retrieved from http://www.aacn.nche.edu/elnec/about/fact-sheet; End-of-Life Nursing Education Consortium (ELNEC). (2012). *History, statewide efforts and recommendations for the future: Advancing palliative care nursing.* Retrieved from http://www.aacn.nche.edu/elnec/publications/ELNEC-Monograph.pdf

Adjustments to a "new way of life" redefine family identities and roles. Increasing physical and emotional burden may ensue and change in everyday life may occur daily. A continual search for meaning spawns personal growth, and preparation for death includes meeting the patient's final wishes (Steele & Davies, 2015). Thus nurses can help families during this time with the following caring interventions.

Helping Bereaved Caregivers Make Sense of Their Feelings

Once a distressing symptom has been identified as grief, there are many activities of mourning that can bring some relief and improve coping. Actively mourning includes talking about feelings, journaling or writing, emoting, expressing what needs to be said, resolving and forgiving things that hurt, recognizing differences in grieving styles and abilities, using simple ritual, seeking support outside the family, and planning for a changed life. People often rehearse important events in life, such as becoming a parent, moving to a new home or job, or getting married or divorced. It can also help people to rehearse life as it may be after loved ones decline further and ultimately die. One wife caring for her husband with advanced dementia who was dying at home confessed that she frequently imagined herself at her husband's viewing and funeral. She thought this was probably an unloving and disloyal thing to do while he was living, and was relieved to find out that perhaps it was primarily a means of coping with her anticipatory grief. She visualized herself having survived the thing she most feared (his death) and having a role and identity beyond (his funeral) to give herself the strength to go through what was coming. Thus families during these transition phases can be supported by the nurse.

Clinical interventions related to anticipatory grieving can be facilitated by helping family members normalize feelings, active listening, and the development of supportive relationships. A nonjudgmental stance, ongoing education, advocacy, and monitoring for complications or a maladaptive state such as functional decline of the family caregiver can help with proactive attention to anticipatory grieving (D'Antonio, 2014).

VIGNETTE

Naming Something Gives Us Options

Julie was the wife, younger by 20 years, of a hospice patient dying of lung cancer. Julie cared for Edward in their home with help from the hospice team. During each home visit, the hospice social worker noticed that Julie seemed more drawn and fatigued. That was understandable, since Edward was getting weaker, thinner, and more confined to his room. The social worker asked Julie what was most distressing to her at this time. In tears, she said that Edward was no longer looking fondly at her or wanting to spend time together. She thought he no longer loved her, and this was deeply painful to her. The social worker described the phenomenon of anticipatory grieving, and talked about the many losses they were both experiencing. "You mean Edward is grieving?" Julie said, with amazement. "Yes," replied the social worker. "You are too. Just think of all that he will soon be forced to leave, most of all you, the love of his life. One way to deal with that is to withdraw early, to avoid some of the pain of parting." Julie's relief was obvious. She easily grasped that, while she wanted to grow closer as she anticipated his death, Edward might need to shut her out. Thereafter, she began to act on her mourning needs by being with him more, even as she supported Edward's needs by letting him know she understood how hard this was for him. Of course, Julie was grief-stricken when he died, but she had been able to express her love, reminisce about their life together, reflect the value of Edward's life back to him, and say goodbye. In addition, she had been spared needless suffering before his death due to prematurely pulling apart from each other.

Helping People Say Goodbye

It is helpful for a nurse to understand the experience of families caring for a terminally ill patient. When bereaved caregivers were asked about their main challenges in a series of interviews (Clukey, 2007), they identified the following:

- *Adjusting to caregiving demands.* This challenge becomes all-consuming and includes physical, emotional, and practical stressors. With the patient getting so much attention, you can help by inquiring of caregivers how they are doing and what they are feeling. Listen and ask open-ended questions. Ask how you can help them.

- *Gathering information.* Most caregivers have a need to understand everything they can about the diagnosis, treatment options, and medical care for their loved ones. Anxiety usually surrounds these topics, and obtaining information may buttress a sense of control. You can help by communicating acceptance of their need to understand things. Encourage them to ask questions, as often as necessary. Slow down, repeat instructions, and check in frequently to see if they would like anything clarified.

- *Finalizing the connection to the dying person.* This is often done by spending time with the patient and enjoying things together. Reminiscing, looking at photographs, and visiting are all ways to show appreciation for the person's life. Barriers to this process may be the tendency to protect each other by pretending that time will never run out; loss of energy, alertness, and focus; the effects of medications; and resistance to feeling the pain of grief.

Dr. Ira Byock provides a simple structure to this process in the **Four Gifts** of resolving relationships (Byock, 2004). In essence, they invite the movement through four phases of communication:

- Forgiveness (I forgive you, please forgive me.)
- Love (I love you, I know you love me.)
- Gratitude (Thank you, and I receive your thanks.)
- Farewell (We will have an enduring connection.)

Each emotional movement opens into the next. Think of these as simple, natural, spontaneous, and creative. When they have taken place, people report a sense of peace and gratification. Encourage family members to express what is important to them, provide a caring presence, and understand that successful bereavement includes a sense that one was able to say goodbye. For example, out-of-town family members can speak to a nonresponsive patient through a telephone held to the patient's ear; a card or letter can be read to a dying patient and placed in his or her hands on behalf of a family member who cannot be at the bedside. These simple interventions help satisfy the need to finalize the connection with the loved one.

Helping Families Maintain Hope

Families seem to need to have hope as long as the dying person is present. *Do not think of hope as a form of denial of reality.* Hopefulness can coexist with knowledge that recovery or longevity is not a realistic goal. Forms of hope include the hope that the loved one knows how important he or she is to them; the hope that the caregivers are not falling short in their efforts at providing comfort; and the hope that the dying person knows how much he or she will be missed. Sources of hope for terminally ill patients and families include humor, uplifting memories, setting goals, and maintaining independence and the love and support of family members and friends (Cotter & Foxwell, 2015). Additional ways to foster hope and connectedness can be achieved through reminiscence, encouraging life review for patients, and legacy-building.

VIGNETTE
Guiding the Family in Saying Goodbye

The plan was for John to move from the ICU to home with hospice care, have his ventilator removed at that time, and die peacefully surrounded by his family. A hospice bereavement counselor was consulted to help prepare John's four teenage grandchildren for his death. When the counselor arrived at the hospital late on the afternoon of his impending transfer home, she discovered that John was too fragile to be moved and would be extubated in the ICU instead. His wife, two adult children, and the four grandchildren were gathered in a waiting room, restless and worried. The counselor worked closely with the ICU nurse to help the family with the task of finalizing the relationship. They were invited to gather around John to touch him, tell him what he meant to them, share stories, and connect with him as each one preferred. While he was not able to respond, the nurse suggested that he might be able to hear them anyway. Gradually the family relaxed and expressed many things, crying, laughing, and holding hands. Then the staff asked if anyone wanted time alone with John. His wife immediately stepped forward. After her, each one requested private time. Finally, they were asked to leave the room so he could be medicated and extubated in private. Each step was carefully explained by the nurse and counselor. Finally, the whole family circled his bed, weeping or silent, as he gradually stopped breathing. The two staff members kept vigil with them in a corner of the room. His death was peaceful and quiet. So was the family, as each person gave him a final kiss before leaving the room.

The message: The dying person, if cognitively intact, often has preferences about where he or she will die, with what level of consciousness, with which people around, and with what level of comfort. Each family member will usually have a sense of how it will be at the time of the death. Some know they want to be present. Others prefer to remember the patient alive. When the hopes of the survivors are not met, people usually need to reconcile themselves with their disappointment during the period of bereavement. You can help by understanding the function of hope during the time of anticipatory mourning. You can listen carefully when hopes are being abandoned or reformulated as conditions change. Be sensitive to the fact that each member of the family, including the dying person, will have differing hopes. Assess hopes by asking open-ended questions such as "How would you like her to feel about that?" or "Ideally, how would you like this to work out?"

Therapeutic Presence

When survivors of terminally ill loved ones describe what was most helpful to them, high on the list is the presence of people who could just "be there" (Clukey, 2007). For the health care practitioner, this means that the art of presence needs to be seen as a preferred treatment intervention, and not simply as the absence of being able to "do something for them." Effective presence requires that the care provider accept the reality of suffering, helplessness, mourning, and mortality itself. It asks one to slow down, put other demands aside for a while, and simply be there. Watch and listen, tolerate pauses and silences, and use open-ended questions. *People going through intense life experiences report that they do not remember what others said to them, but only what the others made them feel. The intentional presence of another person makes people feel seen, valued, and important.*

SELF-CARE FOR NURSES

One of the hazards and challenges of becoming a professional care provider is that of practicing self-care. First, we must understand why this is so important. Then we must establish habits of good self-care. Finally, we must continually return to these habits as they are pushed into the background by the necessities of life and work. Nursing requires many skills and much knowledge, but also a great deal of compassion. Compassion is the ability to be with someone who is suffering. Thus compassion is a relational phenomenon. It is less like a feeling and more like a human capacity that is developed and sustained in relationship to others. Even brief and fleeting expressions of compassion nourish this quality in our self and in others. Truly hearing the suffering of others puts us in touch with our own needs and vulnerabilities, and we may feel like protecting ourselves from that vulnerability. One way to do that is to engage in our own thoughts rather than deeply listening to another's need. Many in helping professions worry that they are not as compassionate as they would like to be, and tell themselves that they are "failures." Burnout, decreased work performance due to negative behaviors and thoughts, and compassion fatigue, or the emotional pain or cost of working traumatized persons, may result in stress responses for nurses (Vachon et al., 2015). Think of compassion and self-care as a practice or a habit of thought and action that connects us meaningfully with others. Discover what practices keep refilling your reservoir of compassion and make them habitual, which will augment job satisfaction.

Sometimes nurses need to mourn the death of a person for whom they have provided care and developed fondness. An entire staff may need to mourn the death of a particular patient or an overload of recent deaths. After patients die, nurses may be faced with managing their own tasks of mourning, such as making sense of the death, dealing with mild to intense emotions, and realigning relationships. Support groups, debriefing sessions, and the ability to attend memorial services are just a few ways that health care organizations can support nursing staff and diminish the potential for compassion fatigue.

To balance a work life that centers on others, create habits that reconnect you with your own life, your well-being, your commitment to work, and your enjoyment of the larger world. Find people you can trust at work and support one another. Accept one another's failings, successes, vulnerabilities, and intentions. Work for systemic changes at your place of employment that will enhance self-care, such as exercise programs and periodic debriefings and memorials when patients die. Review key ethical standards regularly (ANA, 2015). They express the highest and best goals of nursing care. Continue to increase your knowledge base and seek professional certifications. Ask your supervisor to email inspiring or appreciative messages to the staff. Take a few moments to thank and appreciate one another. Use your spiritual belief system to provide a sustaining context for human suffering and human kindness.

APPLICATION OF THE NURSING PROCESS

ASSESSMENT

Often the history of an individual can alert health care personnel to signs or symptoms of potential difficulty that a person may encounter during a time of mourning. The following questions identify risk factors that may complicate the successful completion of mourning:

1. Do any of the following factors relate to the bereaved?
   - Was the bereaved heavily dependent on the deceased?
   - Were there persistent, unresolved conflicts with the deceased?
   - Was the deceased a child? (Perhaps the most profound loss of all)
   - Does the bereaved have a meaningful relationship or support system?
   - Has the bereaved experienced a number of previous losses?
   - Does the bereaved have sound coping skills?

2. Was the deceased's death associated with a cultural stigma (e.g., AIDS, suicide, homicide)?
3. Has the bereaved had difficulty resolving past significant losses?
4. Does the bereaved have a history of depression, drug or alcohol abuse, or other psychiatric illness?
5. If the bereaved is young, are there indications for special interventions?
6. Was the deceased a veteran or victim of war?

Prolonged depression is the most common response to unresolved grief. Disturbances in mood are associated with biological changes in the body during stress-related depressive illness. Some examples include electrolyte disturbances, nervous system alterations, and faulty regulation of the autonomic nervous system. Always assess the potential for suicide. Someone who is having difficulty negotiating the work of mourning and is suffering can benefit from counseling, as mentioned earlier.

►► Assessment Guidelines
Grieving and Complicated Grieving

1. Identify whether the individual is at risk for complicated grieving (see assessment history).
2. Identify the bereaved person's cultural and spiritual beliefs, length of typical grieving, and mourning rituals.
3. Evaluate for psychotic symptoms, agitation, increased activity, alcohol or drug abuse, and extreme vegetative symptoms (e.g., anorexia, unintended weight loss, insomnia).

4. Do not overlook people who do not express significant grief in the context of major loss. These individuals might have an increased risk of subsequent complicated or unresolved grief reactions.
5. Complicated grief reactions require significant interventions. Suicidal or severely depressed people might require hospitalization. Always assess for **suicide** with signs of depression or other dysfunctional signs.
6. Assess support systems. If support systems are limited, find bereavement groups in the community.
7. When grieving is stalled or complicated, a person is at high risk for major depression or other mental illnesses. There are a variety of therapeutic approaches that have proved beneficial. Make referrals.
8. Grieving can bring with it severe spiritual anguish. Assess whether spiritual counseling or a specific counselor would be useful for the bereaved.

Table 25-2 presents a comparison between the symptoms of a "normal" mourning process and those of a complicated grief reaction.

DIAGNOSIS

Four nursing diagnoses that apply to grief are *Grieving, Complicated grieving, Risk for complicated grieving,* and *Chronic sorrow.* During the time of grief, especially if the grieving process is prolonged or

TABLE 25-2 Common Responses and Pathological Intensification during Grief	
Typical Response	**Pathological Intensification**
Dying Emotional expression and immediate coping with the dying process	Avoidance; feeling of being overwhelmed, dazed, confused; self-punitive feelings; inappropriately hostile feelings
Death and Outcry Outcry of emotions with news of the death and turning for help to others or isolating self with self-soothing	Panic, dissociative reactions, reactive psychoses, suicidal ideation
Warding Off (Denial) Avoidance of reminders and social withdrawal, focusing elsewhere, emotional numbing, not thinking of implications to self or of certain themes	Maladaptive avoidance of confronting the implications of death through drug or alcohol abuse, promiscuity, fugue states, phobic avoidance, feeling of being dead or unreal
Reexperience (Intrusion) Intrusive experiences, including recollections of negative experiences during relationship with the deceased, bad dreams, reduced concentration, compulsive reenactments	Flooding with negative images and emotions; uncontrolled ideation, self-impairing compulsive reenactments, night terrors, recurrent nightmares, distraught feelings resulting from the intrusion of anger, anxiety, despair, shame, or guilt; physiological exhaustion resulting from hyperarousal
Working Through Recollection of the deceased and a contemplation of self with reduced intrusiveness of memories and fantasies and with increased rational acceptance, reduced numbness and avoidance, more "dosing" of recollections, and a sense of working it through	Feeling of inability to integrate the death with a sense of self and continued life; persistent warding-off themes that may manifest as anxious, depressed, enraged, shame-filled, or guilty moods; self-injurious behaviors; and psychophysiological syndromes
Resolution Reduction in emotional swings and a sense of self-coherence and readiness for new relationships; ability to experience positive states of mind	Failure to negotiate the process of mourning, which may be associated with inability to work or create, or to feel emotion or positive states of mind

From Horowitz, M. J. (1990). A model of mourning: change in schemas of self and other. *Journal of the American Psychoanalytic Association, 38*(2), 297–303.

symptomatic (e.g., profound depression or disorganization), other nursing diagnoses may come into play. *Ineffective coping, Compromised family coping, Disturbed sleep pattern, Risk for spiritual distress,* and *Social isolation* are examples.

EXPECTED OUTCOMES

Ideally, successful outcomes would include the following. An individual:

- Can tolerate intense emotions.
- Reports decreased preoccupation with the deceased (loss).
- Demonstrates increased periods of stability.
- Tends to previous responsibilities.
- Takes on new roles and responsibilities.
- Has energy to invest in new endeavors.
- Expresses positive expectations about the future.
- Remembers positive as well as negative aspects of the deceased loved one.

PLANNING

Nurses constantly encounter people and families who are faced with loss, although that loss might not be the reason they first entered the medical or psychiatric health care system. In hospital settings, grief is expressed when there is a loss besides death—for example, loss of a limb from amputation or loss of a breast after surgery for breast cancer. Sometimes simple active listening can go a long way in offering comfort and respite from loneliness, or perhaps a referral to a grieving support group is indicated. Still, at other times the nurse may realize that even though individuals present with a medical or emotional problem, they are also undergoing a profound loss; therefore the nurse might suggest the need for a referral for grief counseling, re-grief work, or psychotherapy. As mentioned, physical or emotional symptoms may be related to a complicated grief reaction.

IMPLEMENTATION

The nurse's focus when facilitating bereavement is on helping the bereaved deal with the most important issues emerging at a particular time. Often the nurse or other caregiver can best serve the grieving person simply by being present, listening with interest, and encouraging talking and the recounting of meaningful stories. Tables 25-3 and 25-4 provide guidelines for helping people grieve.

Psychotherapy

Grief is a process that most of us negotiate by receiving help from family and friends and by staying connected to community activities. Some people find comfort and support in grief counseling or support groups. A counselor with spiritual expertise may be helpful for some with existential or spiritual distress. For people at risk for complicated grief reactions (history of mental illness, loss by suicide or homicide, facing multiple simultaneous losses, loss of a child), brief and time-limited psychotherapy may be indicated. According to

TABLE 25-3 **Interventions for Helping People in Grief**	
Intervention	**Rationale**
1. Use methods that can facilitate the grieving process (Robinson, 1997). 　a. Give your full presence: use appropriate eye contact, attentive listening, and appropriate touch.	a. Talking is one of the most important ways of dealing with acute grief. Listening patiently helps the bereaved express all feelings, even ones he or she feels are "negative." Appropriate eye contact helps to convey the awareness that you are there and are sharing the person's sadness. Human touch can express warmth and nurture healing. Inappropriate touch can leave a person confused and uncomfortable.
b. Be patient with the bereaved in times of silence. Do not fill silence with empty chatter.	b. Sharing painful feelings during periods of silence is healing and conveys your concern.
2. Know about and share with the bereaved information about the phenomena that occur during the normal mourning process, because they may concern some people (intense anger at the deceased, guilt, symptoms the deceased had before death, unbidden floods of memories). Give the bereaved support during the occurrence of these phenomena and a written handout for reference.	2. Although the knowledge will not eliminate the emotions, it can greatly relieve a person who is thinking there is something wrong with having these feelings.
3. Encourage the support of family and friends. If no supports are available, refer the patient to a community bereavement group. (Bereavement groups are helpful even when a person has many friends or much family support.)	3. Friends can help with routine matters. For example: 　• Getting food into the house 　• Making phone calls 　• Driving to the mortuary 　• Taking care of children or other family members
4. Offer spiritual support and referrals when needed.	4. Dealing with an illness or catastrophic loss can cause the most profound spiritual anguish.
5. When intense emotions are in evidence, show understanding and support (see Table 25-4).	5. Empathic words that reflect acceptance of a bereaved individual's feelings are healing (Robinson, 1997).

Robinson, D. (1997). *Good intentions: the nine unconscious mistakes of nice people.* New York, NY: Warner Books.

TABLE 25-4   Guidelines for Communicating with a Bereaved Individual

Situation	Sample Response
When you sense an overwhelming *sorrow*	"This must hurt terribly."
When you hear *anger* in the bereaved person's voice	"I hear anger in your voice. Most people go through periods of anger when their loved one dies. Are you feeling angry now?"
If you discern *guilt*	"Are you feeling guilty? This is a common reaction many people have. What are some of your thoughts about this?"
If you sense a *fear* of the future	"It must be scary to go through this."
When the bereaved seems *confused*	"This can be a confusing time."
In almost any *painful situation*	"This must be very difficult for you."

Adapted from Robinson, D. (1997). *Good intentions: the nine unconscious mistakes of nice people* (p. 9). New York, NY: Warner Books.

Zisook and Zisook (2005), the following are essential components of effective short-term therapy:

1. **An educational component:** Helps people learn what to expect and how to normalize their confusing feelings and behaviors.
2. **Encouragement of full expression of emotions and affect:** May include writing letters to deceased, role-playing, and looking at pictures.
3. **An attempt to help bereaved come to peace with a new relationship to the deceased:** Involves the process of integrating the loss of the deceased into current reality (Box 25-6).

Box 25-7 offers guidelines that can help people and their families cope with loss. More complicated or pathological patterns of grief may require special techniques, such as re-grief work. When a major depression or other mental health illness is involved, psychotherapeutic techniques geared toward grief work as well as toward addressing the individual's mental health issues can help greatly in improving the person's quality of life. At times, psychobiological interventions may be needed (e.g., antidepressants).

BOX 25-6   Grief and Recovery: The Lived Experience

My husband died almost 4 years ago after 54 years of marriage, 12 children, and 29 grandchildren. Within 1 year of his death, our youngest child had her first baby. We all feel Bob had a hand in sending us Benjamin. When I lost Bob, it was very difficult. He died peacefully 5 days after he was diagnosed with pancreatic cancer. It was so sudden and unexpected that it left me feeling as though I had been ripped in half with bloody, jagged edges. The pain was so unbearable, I didn't know if I could survive. I could not imagine any way to get through this. With my deep faith in God's love, the unconditional love and support from my family and friends, I managed to cope. I had grief counselling

for 1 year. I learned that you heal in time but time does not heal. I put my whole self into the process of grieving and healing. It is the most difficult job a person can do and it takes all your energy. Now I live my life on a new level. Each day is a gift. I have grown to recognize it's important to just "be"—to be who I am; the integrated person of me and Bob, to be totally present to where I am and who I am with. My memories are laced with joy and gratitude as well as sadness. I am stronger; more resilient. I have peace. – Lois Kalafut, April 1, 2015 *(direct quote)*

BOX 25-7   Guidelines for Dealing with Loss

Take the time you need to grieve. The hard work of grief uses psychological energy. Resolution of the numb state that occurs after loss requires a few weeks at least. A minimum of one year, to cover all the birthdays, anniversaries, and other important dates without your loved one, is required before you can learn to live with your loss.

Express your feelings. Remember that anger, anxiety, loneliness, and even guilt are normal reactions and that everyone needs a safe place to express them. Tell your personal story of loss as many times as you need to—this repetition is a helpful and necessary part of the grieving process.

Establish a structure for each day and stick to it. Although it is hard to do, keeping to some semblance of structure makes the first few weeks after a loss easier. Getting through each day helps restore the confidence you need to accept the reality of loss.

Do not feel that you have to answer all the questions asked of you. Although most people try to be kind, they may be unaware of their insensitivity. Down the road you may want to read books about how others have dealt with similar circumstances. They often have helpful suggestions for a person in your situation.

As hard as it is, try to take good care of yourself. Eat well, talk with friends, get plenty of rest. Be sure to let your primary care clinician know if you are having trouble eating or sleeping. Make use of exercise. It can help you release pent-up frustrations. If you are losing weight, sleeping excessively or intermittently, or still experiencing deep depression after 3 months, be sure to seek professional assistance.

Expect the unexpected. You may begin to feel a bit better, only to have a brief emotional collapse. These are expected reactions. Moreover, you may find that you dream about, visualize, think about, or search for your loved one. This, too, is a part of the grieving process.

Give yourself time. Do not feel that you have to resume all of life's duties right away.

Make use of rituals. Those who take the time to say goodbye at a funeral or a viewing tend to find that it helps the bereavement process.

If you do not begin to feel better within a few weeks, at least for a few hours every day, be sure to tell your physician or primary care practitioner. If you had an emotional problem in the past (e.g., depression, substance abuse), be sure to get the additional support you need. Losing a loved one puts you at higher risk for a relapse of these disorders.

From Zerbe, K .J. (1999). *Women's mental health in primary care* (pp. 207–208). Philadelphia, PA: Saunders.

APPLYING EVIDENCE-BASED PRACTICE (EBP)

Problem A 76-year-old widow has become increasingly depressed after her husband of 53 years passed away 9 months ago. She has approached a physician in Oregon, where it is legal to prescribe medication for suicide via the Death With Dignity Act (one of five states that now have similar acts). She became aware of this option when a young woman with brain cancer was prominent in the news after choosing her death date rather than enduring prolonged suffering. The widow mentioned her thoughts to her husband's hospice nurse when she visited as part of follow-up care.

EBP Assessment

A. **What do you already know from experience?** Elderly patients who lose loved ones often become depressed and do not care for themselves. Thoughts of wanting to die and join their loved one are common. The grieving process takes considerable time, longer than many people recognize. The longer a couple has been together, the longer this process may take. Hospice programs often offer counseling for the surviving family member (National Institute on Aging, 2012).

B. **What does the literature say?** It can be difficult to differentiate between grief and depression in the elderly. Medications and other physical ailments can further complicate the scenario. Unfortunately, many people, including health care professionals, accept sadness and depressive symptoms as part of old age, but these can be treated (Phillips Lifeline, 2015). Assisted suicide is becoming more common and prominent in the news (Barone, 2014). Nurses will need to examine their feelings and positions on these issues and be

prepared to discuss them more often. Countries such as the Netherlands have had progressive suicide laws for many years, and offer a glimpse into the ethical dilemmas inherent in this issue (Fenigsen, 2011).

C. **What does the patient want?** Although this patient initially says she wants to die, through conversation it becomes evident that she really wants the emotional pain to end and is feeling very overwhelmed and lonely. She is in fairly good health, with the exception of decreased nutrition and hydration since her husband's death. She is willing to accept help and try other avenues rather than pursue assisted suicide.

Plan The hospice nurse arranges for the patient to see her primary care physician (PCP) and also for delivery of meals. The patient agrees to attend a grief support group. The hospice nurse helps the patient reach out to family and friends and increase her contacts and activities with them. One of the patient's children started leaving a family pet with her on the weekends, to see if that was something she would enjoy and could handle. The hospice nurse will continue to follow up with the patient for up to a year.

QSEN QSEN Prelicensure Knowledge, Skills, and Attitudes (KSAs) Addressed:

Patient-centered care was used in formulating goals and outcomes unique to this individual.

Evidence-based care was provided as tenets of grief and depression supported the care plan.

Barone, E. (2014). See which states allow assisted suicide. *Time*, November 4. Retrieved from Time.com/3551560/Brittany-maynard-right-to-die-laws/; Fenigsen, R. (2011). Other people's lives: reflections on medicine, ethics, and euthanasia, part two: medicine versus euthanasia. *Issues in Law & Medicine, 26*(3), 239–279; National Institute on Aging. (2012). *End of life: Helping with comfort and care.* NIH Publication no. 08-6036. Retrieved from http://tinyurl.com/o9fxv2o Phillips Lifeline. (2015). *Grief versus depression in the elderly: what's really going on?* Retrieved from http://www.lifelinesys-.com/content/blog/healthcare-professionals/acceptance-and-adherence/grief-vs-depression-in-the-elderly-whats-really-going-on

EVALUATION

Evaluation addresses whether the goals of care and outcomes have been met. The work of grief is over when the bereaved can realistically remember the pleasures and disappointments of the relationship with the lost loved one. Brief periods of intense emotions may still occur at significant times, such as holidays and anniversaries, but the person or family members have energy to reinvest in new relationships that bring shared joys, security, satisfaction, and comfort. If, after a normal period (12 to 24 months), a person has not been able to find pleasure, satisfaction, and comfort in his or her life, then reassessment and re-evaluation are indicated.

KEY POINTS TO REMEMBER

- The process of dying in the United States is undergoing transformation.
- Palliative care provides holistic interdisciplinary care for people with serious life-limiting illness. Palliative care includes hospice, which is a model of care designed to help patients and family members during the last 6 months of life.
- Grief is everything experienced inside a person in response to a loss, real or perceived, including the loss of a person, security, self-confidence, or a dream.
- Anticipatory grieving describes the complex experience of patients and families during the period following a serious diagnosis. Health care professionals can guide families through some of the tasks of anticipatory mourning, while providing much needed normalization and therapeutic presence.

- Mourning is the social expression of grief. Mourning is what enables people to move through the pain and trauma of major loss as part of the bereavement process.
- A spiritual and cultural assessment should be part of every nursing evaluation. It is crucial for health care professionals to avoid imposing their own views, faith, and beliefs on others, especially patients who are facing the vulnerabilities of serious illness and end of life.
- Compassion is a human quality and capacity that occurs and is nourished in relationships. It develops through a lifetime.
- Common phenomena are evident during the experience of grief, and people usually show similar patterns of grief and mourning within their cultural norms. Culture greatly affects the patterns of response to death and dying in patients as well as in nurses.
- Developing habits and practices of self-compassion is key to maintaining good self-care.
- Health care workers can use a number of communication skills to help comfort the bereaved and facilitate mourning. Actively listening to a grieving person's story without offering banal or philosophical responses can assist in healing. Short-term grief counseling and support groups are often helpful.
- Indicators of the potential for complicated or unresolved grief include social isolation, extensive dependency on the deceased person, unresolved interpersonal conflicts, loss of a child, violent and senseless death, or a catastrophic loss. A history will often reveal potential risks for complicated grieving.
- Grief work is successful when the relationship to the deceased person has been restructured and energy is available for new relationships and life pursuits. The work of mourning is complete when

the bereaved person or persons can remember realistically both the pleasures and the disappointments of the lost relationship. Outcomes for successful grief work have been identified.

- Grief, when experienced by health care workers, can reactivate distressing feelings related to previous losses. It is important to recognize that staff members need psychological support when they work with people who are grieving to avoid burnout or compassion fatigue.

APPLYING CRITICAL JUDGMENT

1. Mr. Hendrix's wife is now dying and she is ready to leave the hospital to go home with the aid of hospice. Mr. Hendrix asks you what hospice can do for his wife: "How can they help me care for her? Everything is so complicated and overwhelming. Who else will be there? I am so scared. I just don't know what to do."

   A. Since you know Mr. Hendrix is very anxious at this point, how would you explain to him clearly and concisely the services hospice can offer both him and his wife?

   B. Mr. Hendrix tells you he does not know what to say to his wife; he says that watching her die is too hard for him and it is very difficult to be with her, which makes him feel guilty. What guidelines can you give them in helping to say goodbye (consider the Four Gifts)?

   C. If you are the nurse on the hospice team, discuss ways in which you can provide therapeutic presences for Mr. and Mrs. Hendrix.

   D. If Mr. Hendrix has specific spiritual or religious beliefs that you believe might help him and his wife during this time, how could you assess these beliefs?

   E. Discuss the importance *to you* of how a person's spiritual beliefs or religious beliefs (e.g., What gives me strength? What is my purpose for being here? What brings me peace? How am I spiritually connected to other humans?) might help both the person who is dying and his or her loved ones.

2. What are some concrete ways in which you can help another person to cope with a loss? Identify specific components in the following areas:

   A. How can you let the person tell his or her story?

   B. What is the potential therapeutic value of doing so?

   C. Avoiding banal advice, what are some things you might say that could offer comfort? Use the guidelines in Tables 25-3 and 25-4 to describe how you would help a person who is suffering a profound loss.

CHAPTER REVIEW QUESTIONS

1. Sixteen years ago a toddler died in a tragic accident. Once a year, the parents place flowers at the accident site. How would the nurse characterize the parents' behavior?

   a. Mourning
   b. Bereavement
   c. Complicated grief
   d. Disenfranchised grief

2. A recently widowed adult says, "I've been calling my neighbors often but they act like they don't want to talk to me. I just need to talk about it, you know?" What is the nurse's best action?

   a. Say to the person, "You may call me anytime you need to talk."
   b. Ask the person, "What do you mean by 'I just need to talk about it'?"
   c. Educate the person about the importance of finding alternative activities.
   d. Tell the person the location and time of a local bereavement support group.

3. A physician informed an adult of the results of diagnostic tests that showed lung cancer. Later in the day the patient says to the nurse, "My doctor said I have breathing problems, right?" Which nursing diagnosis is applicable?

   a. *Denial* related to acceptance of new diagnosis
   b. *Chronic sorrow* related to unresolved life conflicts
   c. *Situational low self-esteem* related to stress of new diagnosis
   d. *Acute confusion* related to metastatic changes to cerebral function

4. A nurse leads a bereavement group. Which participant's comment best demonstrates that the work of grief has been successfully completed?

   a. "Our time together was too short. I only wish we had done more things together."
   b. "I know our life together was a blessing that I did not deserve. I wish I had said 'I love you' more often."
   c. "Other people knew my loved one as a good and helpful person. I hope people see me in the same way."
   d. "Our best vacations always involved water. When I see pictures of the ocean, those memories come flooding in."

5. A nurse who has worked for a community hospice organization for 8 years says, "My patients and their families experience overwhelming suffering. No matter how much I do, it's never enough." Which problem should the nursing supervisor suspect?

   a. The nurse is experiencing spiritual distress.
   b. The nurse is at risk for burnout and compassion fatigue.
   c. The nurse is not receiving adequate recognition from others.
   d. The nurse is at risk for overhelping, which creates dependency.

REFERENCES

American Nurses Association. (2015). *Code of ethics for nurses with interpretive statements*. Silver Spring, MD: ANA.

American Psychiatric Association (APA). (2013). *Diagnosis and statistical manual of mental disorders: DSM-5*. Washington, DC: APA.

Ayalon, L., & Green, V. (2012). Grief in the initial adjustment process to the continuing care retirement community. *Journal of Aging Studies, 26*(4), 394–400.

Baird, P. (2015). Spiritual care interventions. In B. R. Ferrell, N. Coyle, & J. Paice (Eds.), *Oxford textbook of palliative nursing* (4th ed.) (pp. 546–553). New York, NY: Oxford University Press.

Bonanno, G. A. (2009). *The other side of sadness: what the new science of bereavement tells us about life after a loss*. New York, NY: Basic Books.

Brown, H., & Johnston, B. (2011). Identifying care actions to conserve dignity in end of life care. *British Journal of Community Nursing, 16*(5), 238–245.

Byock, I. (2004). *Dying well: peace and possibilities at the end of life*. New York, NY: Riverhead Books.

Center to Advance Palliative Care (CAPC). (2014). *National Palliative Care Registry annual survey summary: results of the 2012 National Palliative Care Survey as of July, 2014*. Retrieved March 27, 2015, from https://registry.capc.org/cms/.

Clukey, L. (2007). "Just there": hospice caregivers' anticipatory mourning experience. *Journal of Hospice and Palliative Nursing, 9*(3), 150–158.

Corless, I. B. (2015). Bereavement. In B. R. Ferrell, N. Coyle, & J. Paice (Eds.), *Oxford textbook of palliative nursing* (4th ed.) (pp. 487–499). New York, NY: Oxford University Press.

Cotter, V. T., & Foxwell, A. M. (2015). The meaning of hope in the dying. In B. R. Ferrell, N. Coyle, & J. Paice (Eds.), *Oxford textbook of palliative nursing* (4th ed.) (pp. 475–486). New York, NY: Oxford University Press.

Dahlin, C. M., & Wittenberg, E. (2015). Communication in palliative care: an essential competency for nurses. In B. R. Ferrell, N. Coyle, & J. Paice (Eds.), *Oxford textbook of palliative nursing* (4th ed.) (pp. 81–109). New York, NY: Oxford University Press.

D'Antonio, J. (2014). Caregiver grief and anticipatory mourning. *Journal of Hospice and Palliative Nursing, 16*(2), 99–104.

Doka, K. (1989). *Disenfranchised grief: recognizing hidden sorrow.* New York, NY: Lexington Books.

Ferrell, B. R., & Coyle, N. (2008). *The nature of suffering and the goals of nursing.* New York, NY: Oxford University Press.

Gawande, A. (2014). *On being mortal: illness, medicine and what matters in the end.* London: Profile Books.

Institute of Medicine (IOM). (2014). *Dying in America: improving quality and honoring individual preferences near the end of life.* Washington, DC: National Academies Press. Retrieved February 13, 2015, from http://www.iom.edu/~/media/Files/Report%20Files/2014/EOL/Report%20Brief.pdf.

Jones, A. L., Moss, A. J., & Harris-Kojetin, L. D. (2011). *Use of advance directives in long-term care populations. NCHS Data Brief from the CDC.* No. 54. Hyattsville, MD: National Center for Health Statistics.

Kübler-Ross, E. (1969). *On death and dying.* New York, NY: Macmillan.

Lindemann, E. (1994). Symptomatology and management of acute grief. *American Journal of Psychiatry (Sesquicentennial Suppl), 151*(6), 156.

Long, C. O. (2011). Cultural and spiritual considerations in palliative care. *Journal of Pediatric Hematology/Oncology, 33*(Supp. 2), S96–S101.

National Consensus Project (NCP) for Quality Palliative Care. (2013). *Clinical practice guidelines for quality palliative care* (3rd ed.) Retrieved February 13, 2015, from. https://www.hpna.org/multimedia/NCP_Clinical_Practice_Guidelines_3rd_Edition.pdf.

National Hospice and Palliative Care Organization (NHPCO). (2014). *NHPCO's facts and figures: hospice care in America* (2014 ed.). Alexandria, VA: National Hospice and Palliative Care Organization. Retrieved from. http://www.nhpco.org.

Neimeyer, R. A., Burke, L. A., Mackay, M. M., et al. (2010). Grief therapy and the reconstruction of meanings from principles to practice. *Journal of Contemporary Psychotherapy, 40*(2), 73–83.

Prince-Paul, M. J., & Daly, B. (2015). Ethical considerations in palliative care. In B. R. Ferrell, N. Coyle, & J. Paice (Eds.), *Oxford textbook of palliative nursing* (4th ed.) (pp. 987–1000). New York, NY: Oxford University Press.

Puchalski, C., & Ferrell, B. R. (2010). *Making health care whole: integrating spirituality into palliative care.* West Conshohocken, PA: Templeton Press.

Puchalski, C., Ferrell, B. R., Virani, R., et al. (2009). Improving the quality of spiritual care as a dimension of palliative care: the report of the consensus conference. *Journal of Palliative Medicine, 12*(10), 885–904.

Reich, W. T. (1989). Speaking of suffering: a moral account of compassion. *Soundings, 72*, 83–108.

Robinson, D. (1997). *Good intentions: the nine unconscious mistakes of nice people.* New York, NY: Warner Books.

Steele, R., & Davies, B. (2015). Supporting families in palliative care. In B. R. Ferrell, N. Coyle, & J. Paice (Eds.), *Oxford textbook of palliative nursing* (4th ed.) (pp. 500–514). New York, NY: Oxford University Press.

Stroebe, M., & Schut, H. (1999). The dual process model of coping with bereavement: rationale and description. *Death Studies, 23*, 197–202.

Teno, J. M., Gozalo, P. L., Bynum, J. P. W., et al. (2013). Change in end of life care for Medicare beneficiaries: site of death, place of care, and health care transitions in 2000, 2005, and 2009. *Journal of the American Medical Association, 309*(5), 470–477.

Vachon, M., Huggard, P. K., & Huggard, J. (2015). Reflections on occupation stress in palliative care nursing: is it changing? In B. R. Ferrell, N. Coyle, & J. Paice (Eds.), *Oxford textbook of palliative nursing* (4th ed.) (pp. 969–986). New York, NY: Oxford University Press.

van Kessel, G. (2013). The ability of older people to overcome adversity: a review of the resilience concept. *Geriatric Nursing, 34*(2), 122–127.

Wittenberg-Lyles, E., Goldsmith, J., Ferrell, B., et al. (2013). *Communication in palliative nursing.* New York, NY: Oxford University Press.

Wittenberg-Lyles, E., Goldsmith, J., & Ragan, S. (2010). The COMFORT initiative: palliative nursing and the centrality of communication. *Journal of Hospice and Palliative Nursing, 12*(5), 282–292.

Worden, J. W. (2009). *Grief counseling and grief therapy: a handbook for the mental health professional* (4th ed.). New York, NY: Springer.

Zisook, S., & Zisook, S. A. (2005). Death, dying and bereavement. In B. J. Sadock & V. A. Sadock (Eds.), *Kaplan & Sadock's comprehensive textbook of psychiatry* (8th ed.) vol. 11. (pp. 2367–2392). Philadelphia, PA: Lippincott Williams & Wilkins.

UNIT V

Age-Related Mental Health Disorders

Shirley A. Smoyak, PhD, ScD, RN, FAAN
Author, Editor, Distinguished Professor, and Living Legend in the field of Psychiatric Mental Health Nursing

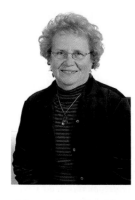

Dr. Shirley Smoyak is an icon in psychiatric mental health nursing. She has been a professor at Rutgers University for more than 50 years, teaching in the domains of mental health and illness, psychiatric nursing, family dynamics, health care administration, culture and health, and qualitative research methods. She was in the first class to finish the master's program for psychiatric nurses developed by Hildegard Peplau ("the Mother of Psychiatric Nursing"), whom Smoyak considered to be her professional mentor. Smoyak earned a PhD in sociology, with subspecialties in families, mental illness, and deviance, and received an Honorary Doctorate from Kingston University. The professor who nominated Dr. Smoyak described her as "an inspirational figure and role model for students. She has boundless energy and enthusiasm for her area of expertise and can explain complex concepts in a way that people can relate to... one of the figureheads of our profession." As a child of immigrants from Austria-Hungary, Smoyak developed a cultural sensitivity that has infused her work. A literature search for Dr. Smoyak's publications returns topics ranging from criminal stalking, to the future of psychiatric nursing, to writing well for publication, to the dangers of energy drinks. Since 1981, Smoyak has been editor of the *Journal of Psychosocial Nursing and Mental Health Services,* the only journal dedicated to psychiatric nursing practice, and she is an international lecturer. Additionally, Dr. Smoyak is the Founder and a Board member of the American Psychiatric Nurses Association, and has served on the Board of the New Jersey State Nurses Association. She is a Charter member of the New Jersey Society of Certified Clinical Specialists in Psychiatric and Mental Health Nursing and the American Academy of Nursing. She has received numerous awards, including the American Academy of Nursing Living Legend distinction, Excellence in Practice and Roll of Honor from the New Jersey State Nurses Association, and Distinguished Lifetime Professor from the Malta Psychiatric Nurses Association.

Children and Adolescents

Susan L. Frost, Chyllia D. Fosbre, Elizabeth M. Varcarolis

(e) http://evolve.elsevier.com/Varcarolis/essentials

KEY TERMS AND CONCEPTS

attention-deficit/hyperactivity disorder
 (ADHD), p. 409
autism spectrum disorder (ASD), p. 408
bibliotherapy, p. 415
conduct disorder (CD), p. 413
dramatic play therapy, p. 414
mental status assessment, p. 406

movement and dance therapy, p. 415
music therapy, p. 415
oppositional defiant disorder (ODD), p. 413
play therapy, p. 414
recreational therapy, p. 415
resilient child/adolescent, p. 406
separation anxiety disorder, p. 411

temperament, p. 406
therapeutic drawing, p. 415
therapeutic games, p. 415
therapeutic holding, p. 414
Tourette's disorder, p. 410

SELECTED CONCEPT: RESILIENCY

Many children and adolescents grow up with their childhoods threatened by poverty, homelessness, neglect, physical or sexual abuse, natural disasters, physical or mental illness of themselves or a parent, substance abuse, dangerous neighborhoods, or other traumas. These children are considered to be at higher risk of emotional or physical illness. Individuals with resiliency tend to survive the traumas or stressors more successfully. Resiliency is developed through the successful transition through a previous crisis, often with the guidance of parents and other supportive figures. Individuals who are resilient may also have better resources and parenting, and may be neurologically less vulnerable to stress. Most children can develop resiliency if provided with the necessary support (Henderson, 2012).

OBJECTIVES

1. Discuss the importance of understanding developmental theory when performing an assessment or providing care for children or adolescents. Give examples of developmental information you would gather.
2. **QSEN** **Using evidence-based practice** and considering holism, formulate a patient-centered care plan for a child or adolescent who is diagnosed with a mental health disorder.
3. **QSEN** When considering the disorders of children and adolescents discussed in this chapter, list the symptoms that would raise concern for the **patient's safety**.

4. **QSEN** Identify situations and opportunities requiring **teamwork and collaboration** with staff members, other departments, or parents and family when caring for minor patients.
5. **QSEN** Evaluate the emotional and physical needs of a child with either an autism spectrum disorder or attention-deficit/hyperactivity disorder, and identify **evidence-based behavioral interventions**.

INTRODUCTION

Children and adolescents are raised in diverse family and community environments, and they bring with them into these environments a variety of genetic and neurobiological traits, as well as widely differing talents and temperaments. Therefore no two children are exactly the same, and actually no one disorder is exactly the same in every child (USDHHS, 1999). Symptom clusters are assessed to make medical or psychiatric diagnoses, but nursing plans are most effective when they address the individuality of each child or adolescent. Obviously, the promotion of *safety* is the primary priority when working with children and adolescents who have mental health problems.

The *Diagnostic and Statistical Manual of Mental Disorders (DSM-5)* diagnoses that relate to children or adolescents will be listed in this

chapter. Some will be referenced only, the most common disorders will be discussed in more depth, and some that also occur in adults will include a reference to the appropriate chapter for further description and learning. Disorders are listed in the order that they appear in the *DSM-5*.

PREVALENCE AND COMORBIDITY

About half of all Americans will meet the criteria for a *DSM-5* disorder at some time during their lives. The first onset will most likely occur in early childhood or early adolescence (National Institute of Mental Health, 2011). About 4 million children and adolescents, or about 21% of 9- to 21-year-olds, in the United States suffer from a serious mental illness. In any given year, only about a fifth of young people receive the needed mental health care. Untreated mental illness leads to more serious complications later in life. One serious complication of mental illness is suicide, which is the third leading cause of death in 15- to 24-year-olds. More individuals in this age group die from suicide than from cancer, heart disease, acquired immunodeficiency syndrome (AIDS), birth defects, stroke, pneumonia, influenza, and chronic lung disease *combined* (National Alliance on Mental Illness [NAMI], 2016). Barriers to receiving care include stigma, lack of resources and funding, scarcity of providers, and poor coordination between systems (Corrigan, Druss, & Perlick, 2014).

Children with mental illness often meet the criteria for more than one diagnostic category. For example, attention-deficit/hyperactivity disorder (ADHD) has a 60% to 90% comorbidity in individuals with juvenile-onset bipolar disorder, a 60% to 70% comorbidity with oppositional defiant disorder, a 40% comorbidity with learning disorders, and a 20% to 25% comorbidity with conduct disorders. Conduct disorders are associated with later substance use disorders and elevated rates of mood disorders (Bostic & Prince, 2008; Brady, 2016).

THEORY

A child's vulnerability to psychopathological conditions is the result of complex interactions between biological, psychological, genetic, and environmental variables. Younger children are harder to diagnose than older children, because the boundaries between normal and abnormal behaviors are less distinct and children are less able to express themselves verbally. Intervention may be delayed until the child reaches school age and symptoms become more obvious.

Genetic Factors

Genetic factors have been implicated in a number of childhood mental disorders, including autism, bipolar disorders, schizophrenia, ADHD, and intellectual developmental disorders (mental retardation). Approximately 30% to 40% of children with ADHD have a family member with the disorder (Frank et al., 2012). Research studies have linked genetic mutations to autism spectrum disorder (ASD) although no one gene has been identified as causing autism (Autism Society, 2015). Researchers using new molecular biology techniques have discovered several sporadic genetic mutations in children with ASDs, similar to mutated genes that have been associated with schizophrenia and intellectual disability. A number of these mutated genes were located in regions of genomes that may have significant repercussions (Nauert, 2011).

Temperament, the style of behavior habitually used to cope with demands of the environment, is a constitutional factor thought to be genetically determined. It may be modified by the parent-infant relationship. In the case of the difficult-child temperament, if the caregiver is unable to respond positively to the child, there is an increased risk of insecure attachment, developmental problems, and mental disorders. Individuals, including children, react in differing ways to the same situation based on their unique temperament. For example, in a large, boisterous family, several children may flourish and enjoy the environment, while another child may isolate to avoid the excessive stimulation.

Biochemical Factors

Biochemical factors in childhood psychopathological conditions, as in adult conditions, include alterations in neurotransmitters. For example, inadequate norepinephrine and serotonin levels are related to depression and suicide. In ADHD, the neurotransmitter affected seems to relate to the subtype of ADHD symptoms. In inattentive type, the norepinephrine transporter gene is affected. Patients with predominantly hyperactive-impulsive type have a variation in their dopamine transporter gene. In combined type, the choline transporter gene is affected. This may explain why certain types of ADHD medications are more effective with certain subtypes. Stimulants tend to affect dopamine, while

nonstimulants such as atomoxetine (Strattera) affect norepinephrine. In addition, serotonin levels play a factor in impulse control and aggression. ADHD patients with normal serotonin levels seem to be more immune to the self-blame associated with ADHD symptoms (Gromisch, 2013).

Environmental Factors

Environmental factors cause stress to children and adolescents and shape their development. Any type of abuse or neglect increases a child's risk for developing psychopathological conditions (National Institute of Mental Health, 2012). The brain is plastic (moldable or malleable) during this critical developmental time frame of childhood, with neuronal chains being rapidly connected. These connections are based on environmental input telling the child that the world is good and safe, or scary and unpredictable. These early connections can guide thoughts and behaviors for the rest of a person's life without intervention to form more positive neuronal pathways. Traumatic events such as marital discord, overcrowding, parental mental illness, abuse, and foster care placement contribute to the development of mental illness. According to the Adverse Childhood Experiences (ACE) study, the greater the number of adverse events, the higher the probability that mental and physical issues will occur. These include anxiety, depression, oppositional defiant disorder, and ADHD (Greeson et al., 2014).

As discussed in Chapter 20 relating to crises, resiliency also plays a protective role. Children and adolescents who are resilient tend to have a strong relationship with a nurturing adult, an adaptive temperament, and problem-solving skills. Prior success in navigating stressful situations also builds resiliency (Masten, 2011).

MENTAL HEALTH ASSESSMENT

Although much of the data gathered for a mental health assessment with children and adolescents are similar to data elicited with an adult, there are unique differences as well. Important distinctions are the inclusion of developmental level, techniques used in the assessment, and involvement of parents. The amount and type of data collected to assess mental health depend on the setting and the presenting problem. The nurse is often the first health care professional to have contact with the young patient and often completes a holistic assessment including the presenting problem, medical and developmental issues, family history, physical examination, and a mental status assessment. In adolescents, it is also important to consider substance use, sexual activity, depression, and suicidal thoughts. Depending on the answers and presentation of the patient, additional details and areas of mental assessment may be explored. Assessing protective strengths and developmental maturity is helpful (Black & Andreasen, 2014). One popular assessment tool is the Denver II Developmental Screening Test, for infants and children up to 6 years of age.

Methods of collecting data include interviewing, screening, testing (neurological, psychological, intelligence), observing, and interacting with the child or adolescent. Histories are taken from parents or caregivers in young children, but the child or adolescent should be included as appropriate for his or her age and communication ability. Teachers can also provide insight or answer questionnaires. Drawing, games, and interactive play, such as with puppets or dollhouses, are helpful in eliciting information from children. It is important to keep in mind that children are concrete and literal in their thinking, and may also be afraid to directly disclose problems at home, at school, or within other activity groups. Play therapy can allow the nurse or care professional to gain information in a nonthreatening manner. Observing interactions with parents, siblings, or caregivers can provide insight as well. The child or adolescent should spend some time alone with the interviewer so the opportunity to disclose abuse is made available (Box 26-1).

BOX 26-1 Child-Adolescent Mental Status Assessment

General Appearance
Size: height and weight
General health and nutrition
Dress and grooming
Distinguishing characteristics
Gestures and mannerisms
Looks or acts younger or older than chronological age

Activity Level
Hyperactivity or hypoactivity
Tics, other body movements
Autoerotic and self-comforting movements (thumb sucking, ear or hair pulling, masturbation, rocking)

Speech
Rate, rhythm, intonation, pitch
Vocabulary and grammar appropriate to age
Mute, hesitant, talkative
Articulation problems
Unusual characteristics (pronoun reversal, echolalia, gender confusion, neologisms)

Coordination or Motor Function
Posture, gait, balance
Gross and fine motor movement
Writing and drawing skills
Unusual characteristics (bizarre postures, banging, biting self, tiptoe walking, hand flapping)

Affect
Predominant emotions expressed and facial expression
Feelings appropriate to the situation
Range and intensity of feelings
Unusual characteristics (apathy, sulking, oppositional behavior, overly emotional)

Manner of Relating
Eye contact
Ability to separate from caregiver, be independent
Attitude toward interviewer and others, social reciprocity
Behavior during interview (patience, impulsiveness, aggressive, ability to have fun or play, frustration level)

Intellectual Functions
Fund of general information
Ability to communicate (follow directions, answer questions)
Memory
Creativity, humor
Learning and problem solving
Conscience (sense of right and wrong, accepts limits)

Thought Processes and Content
Orientation
Attention span
Self-concept and body image
Fantasies and dreams
Ego-defense mechanisms
Perceptual distortions (hallucinations, illusions, unusual ideas)
Sex role, gender identity

Characteristics of Child's Play
Age-appropriate use of toys, and play with peers
Themes of play
Imagination and pretend play
Role and gender play
Relationships with peers (empathy, sharing, waiting for turns, best friends)

NEURODEVELOPMENTAL DISORDERS

Intellectual Disability (formerly called Mental Retardation)

Intellectual disability (ID) affects approximately 0.6% to 2% of the population (American Psychiatric Association [APA], 2013; Black & Andreasen, 2014). This disorder is categorized as mild, moderate, severe, or profound.

Causes may be hereditary factors (Tay-Sachs disease, fragile X syndrome, cerebral palsy), alterations in early embryonic development (Down syndrome, fetal alcohol syndrome, hydrocephalus), pregnancy and perinatal problems (fetal malnutrition, prematurity, maternal age, hypoxia, infections), and other factors such as trauma and poisoning (Krucik, 2015).

The mild form of intellectual disability constitutes 85% of cases. These children develop communication and social skills with minimal sensorimotor impairment, and are often indistinguishable from children with normal range intelligence quotients (IQs). They are able to perform self-care, and may be capable of vocational training and independent living. Conceptual domain is at a mid–elementary school level. More than half of these individuals will own a home, marry, and have children (APA, 2013; Pivalizza, 2015).

The moderate form of intellectual disability constitutes 10% of cases. These children develop communication, social, and academic skills slowly. Conceptual domain is at an elementary school level, with reading commonly at a first- to third-grade level. Although able to perform activities of daily living, ongoing assistance is needed for conceptual

tasks of daily life. They may have long-term intimate relationships and friends but may not interpret social cues accurately. Support is needed to obtain success in employment and in areas such as transportation and money management skills (APA, 2013; Pivalizza, 2015).

The severe form of intellectual disability constitutes 3% to 4% of cases. Speech developmental may be delayed or absent, and individuals often use single-word phrases and gestures. Most individuals in this category require assistance with daily living skills, may perform simple tasks with help, and require significant support and a supervised living environment. In general, these individuals do not marry or have children and have a shortened life span. Maladaptive behaviors such as self-harm may be present (APA, 2013; Pivalizza, 2015).

The profound form of intellectual disability constitutes 1% to 2% of cases. These individuals are mostly nonverbal and do not learn to read. Some individuals are able to learn simple tasks such as dressing themselves. They tend to have sensory and physical impairments, requiring medical equipment and constant supervision to support functioning. Life expectancy in this group is significantly reduced, usually between 4 and 20 years (APA, 2013; Pivalizza, 2015).

Assessment

In the past, severity of these disorders was delineated by IQ range (from <20 to 69). Beginning with the *DSM-5*, the ability to function within three domains—conceptual (academic learning, speech), social (interactions with others), and practical (ability for self-care, life management)—is used to identify the severity.

Diagnosis

In some severe cases of ID, physical traits such as short stature and almond-shaped eyes can be apparent, although in milder cases there may be no distinguishing physical features. ID would be assessed for when risk factors such as maternal age, exposure to substances, or poor fetal muscle tone are present. Blood and DNA testing, brain scans, and IQ testing can support diagnosis, as can failure to meet common developmental milestones (National Institutes of Health [NIH], 2015).

Implementation

The individual and family often need supportive counseling. Schools are required to provide "free and appropriate education," including an individualized education program (IEP), according to the federal Individuals with Disabilities Education Act (IDEA). To reach full academic and social potential, occupational and behavioral therapies as well as medication may be required.

VIGNETTE: INTELLECTUAL DISABILITY (ID)

An 8-year-old male is attending second grade. He was held back a year because of his poor reading comprehension and delayed social skills. Despite being with younger children, he is remarkably smaller than his classmates. He was initially diagnosed with ADHD and learning disabilities; however, after discussing his history with his adoptive parents, there was some suspicion that his intellectual disability was due to fetal alcohol syndrome. His physical characteristics, including small stature, wide-set eyes, and small head circumference, also support this diagnosis.

👤 COMMUNICATION DISORDERS

Language Disorders, Speech Sound Disorders, Childhood-Onset Fluency Disorder (Stuttering), and Social Communication Disorder

These disorders include deficits in language, speech, and communication. Assessment should take into account the child's cultural and language context (APA, 2013). Childhood-onset fluency disorder (stuttering) usually occurs before age 6 and is characterized by broken speech and word substitutions to avoid problematic words. Verbalization causes physical tension and anxiety for the child, which can then exacerbate the speech symptoms. Children who stutter may be teased or bullied and have difficulty performing in the classroom, contributing to self-esteem and socialization issues.

Assessment, Diagnosis, and Implementation

Delays or abnormalities in speech are noted by parents, by health care providers, or in school. Referral to a speech therapist or school psychologist may be made by the parent, health care provider, or teacher. These professionals are trained to differentiate the various types of communication disorders. Speech therapy, often for several years, is provided in the school or in private settings. Supportive counseling may be needed to address self-esteem issues caused by the communication disorder and resultant academic and social issues, including bullying.

👤 AUTISM SPECTRUM DISORDER (ASD)

Level 1, 2, or 3 (formerly called Autism, Asperger's Syndrome, and Pervasive Developmental Disorders)

Autism spectrum disorder (ASD) presents with deficits in social and communication interactions, as well as repetitive patterns of behavior, interests, or activities. Children may twirl, walk on tippy toes, flap their arms, or rock. Mannerisms may progress from self-stimulation to self-injurious, such as head banging and biting. Children and adults with this disorder tend to become focused on a particular subject and perseverate on it. They may gain a profound amount of knowledge about their preferred interest, but are delayed in most other academic and life domains. A lack of interest in social interaction is often the key symptom that is noticed initially. Children with this disorder are often loners and dislike physical affection and contact, except in limited amounts from a few close individuals such as parents. They tend to get very upset when routines are deviated from (CDC, 2010a).

The severity of autism spectrum disorder is categorized into levels based on functional ability. In Level 1 there is noticeable social deficit, but language and speech are normal. Individuals have difficulty switching between activities, and they struggle with organization and planning. In Level 2 there is noticeable deficit in both verbal and nonverbal social and communication skills. Social impairment and repetitive behaviors are obvious to others. These individuals do not tend to initiate social interactions, and change in routine causes distress. In Level 3 social deficits are severe, with communication being limited and needs-based. Individuals may be nonverbal, speak in few-word sentences, be difficult to understand, make odd noises, echo a word or sentence over and over, or use overly literal language. Repetitive and restrictive behaviors markedly interfere with functioning in all spheres. Changing focus, action, or routine causes great distress. Aggression toward self or others is more common at this level (Schoenstadt, 2006).

Assessment

The nurse will observe for social deficits, including bonding with parents, dislike of cuddling, poor eye contact, and lack of interaction with peers. In addition, communication delays, rigid routines, and ritualized behaviors and interests may be noted.

Diagnosis

Autism spectrum disorder is usually diagnosed around toddlerhood, when children begin to interact with one another, although if developmental delays are severe or the assessor is experienced it may be diagnosed in infancy (CDC, 2010b). About two thirds of individuals with autism spectrum disorder have a comorbid mental condition (APA, 2013). A new government survey finds that prevalence for children ages 3 through 17 is 1 in 45 children (Autism Speaks, 2015). Psychiatrists, psychiatric nurse practitioners, and psychologists use the *DSM-5* criteria, history from parents and teachers, and observation to make the diagnosis.

Implementation

According to the Swierzewski (2014), treatment for autism spectrum disorder can include behavioral management and cognitive therapies, early intervention, educational and school-based therapies, and joint therapy (improving ability to follow pointing, showing, and coordinating looks between a person and object, all of which are important in communication and language learning). Medications, including atypical antipsychotics such as risperidone (Risperdal) for aggression or self-harm and selective serotonin reuptake inhibitors (SSRIs) or beta blockers for obsessive or anxious symptoms, may be helpful. While milder levels can be managed in mainstreamed classrooms, severe levels require special classrooms environments. As individuals with severe ASD mature, their larger stature and impulsive behaviors may make continuing to live at home with aging parents impossible.

APPLYING EVIDENCE-BASED PRACTICE (EBP)

Problem A 16-year-old male in a motorized wheelchair arrives at the psychiatrist's office with his parents for a medication management visit. He is able to communicate positive and negative feelings through facial expressions and verbalizations, although he is unable to speak in full words or sentences. One of his primary diagnoses is autism spectrum disorder (ASD), Level 3 (American Psychiatric Association [APA], 2013). He displays repetitive actions and interests, which include wearing masks and hats. He is prone to lashing out at others and biting and hitting himself. As he has grown larger and stronger, it is becoming increasingly difficult for his supportive and loving, but elderly, parents to care for him.

EBP Assessment

A. **What do you already know from experience?** ASD appears in mild through severe presentations. Especially in severe cases, it becomes difficult for patients to remain at home as they mature. Size, strength, and hormones all contribute to additional challenges. Parents can be exhausted and even endangered, yet remain reluctant to place their children outside of the home. Communication can be especially difficult in severe cases of this disorder.

B. **What does the literature say?** Beliefs of elderly parents with autistic children affect their ability to cope. Some parents believe that autism is a punishment, while others see it as a manageable situation. Most parents have a positive outlook, and see their children as they could have been without the disorder, and that there is more to their children than most people see. They also experience guilt, and experience the judgment by others, for disruptive behaviors. Many parents do not realize that some features of autism can be improved (Hines et al., 2012).

C. **What does the patient want?** The patients in this example include the young man with ASD and his parents, as he cannot fully communicate and they are his guardians. His parents know him very well and are able in interpret a lot of his needs and interests for the provider. Both parents and the patient experience considerable frustration surrounding communication deficits and would like that to improve. All three parties are disappointed that their care aide has left and are displeased with their new aide, feeling there is not a good connection with the patient.

Plan The psychiatrist worked with the treatment team to arrange for a different caregiver. Medications were left the same, as the recent exacerbation in behaviors was situational to the previous aide leaving the position and was decreasing. The treatment team contacted disability services and arranged for the patient to receive an electronic communication device, as well as instruction in its use for patient and parents (National Autism Resources, 2015). The next time the psychiatrist saw this patient, he proudly showed her his progress using the device.

QSEN QSEN Prelicensure Knowledge, Skills, and Attitudes (KSAs) Addressed:

Safety was addressed through ensuring the aide was a good fit with the family, and evaluating medications.

Informatics played a role through use of an electronic communication device.

American Psychiatric Association (APA). (2013). *Diagnostic and statistical manual of mental disorders (DSM-5)* (5th ed.). Washington DC: APA.
Hines, M., Balandin, S., & Togher, L. (2012). Buried by autism: Older parents' perceptions of autism. *Autism, 16*(1), 15–26.
National Autism Resources. (2015). *Electronic communication and speech output devices*. Retrieved from http://www.nationalautismresources.com/assistive-technology.html

---

VIGNETTE: AUTISM SPECTRUM DISORDER (ASD)

Parents of a 4-year-old toddler notice their child prefers to play alone when they take her to the park. She spends most of her time in the sandbox spinning the wheels on the cars. When the toddler hears a word, she tends to repeat it over and over and is not using full sentences. She becomes easily overwhelmed in crowds and will start to flap her arms and cry. She resists hugs and physical affection. She is in preschool and teachers have suggested she be evaluated for autism by a developmental pediatrician.

ATTENTION-DEFICIT/HYPERACTIVITY DISORDER (ADHD)

Combined Presentation, Predominantly Inattentive Presentation (formerly called Attention-Deficit Disorder), and Predominantly Hyperactive or Impulsive Presentation

ADHD is further assessed as mild, moderate, or severe and symptoms present prior to age 12 (although they may not be recognized until later, including up to adulthood [see Chapter 27]).

Symptoms of attention-deficit/hyperactivity disorder (ADHD) include problems with concentration such as making careless mistakes, difficulty remaining focused, being easily distracted by things going on around the individual, appearing not to listen when spoken to, lack of follow-through, struggling with organizational and time management skills, and forgetfulness. Individuals with ADHD may also avoid tasks that require sustained mental effort, misplace items, and tend to be messy. Children may fidget, squirm, leave their seat at school, run or climb when not appropriate, blurt out answers or comments, interrupt, or talk excessively. As adults, this may present as an internal restlessness more than as physical impulsivity (APA, 2013). The symptoms of ADHD can cause children to be disciplined repeatedly in the classroom and at home, and peers may tease them, leading to problems with self-esteem. School work can fluctuate between excellent projects and poor assignments with multiple erasure marks. Students can be intelligent but performance is hindered by distractibility and other symptoms (Greenhill & Hechtman, 2010).

Assessment

The nurse may notice a high level of fidgeting activity in the child and behaviors such as running around the office or jumping on the furniture. Once children start school, teachers may notice difficulty paying attention in the classroom, fidgeting, jumping out of the seat, talking at inappropriate times, and inconsistent or messy assignments.

Diagnosis

Mayo (2016) states that a child should not be diagnosed until the age of 12 because possible signs or symptoms may come from another disorder. However, if the symptoms have been present early on and have been disruptive to the family/school environment, a diagnosis of ADHD may be made.

According to Mayo (2016) there is no specific test for ADHD, but making a diagnosis will likely include:

- **Medical exam**, to help rule out other possible causes of symptoms
- **Information gathering**, such as any current medical issues, personal and family medical history, and school records

- **Interviews or questionnaires** for family members, your child's teachers or other people who know your child well, such as baby sitters and coaches
- **ADHD criteria** from the Diagnostic and Statistical Manual of Mental Disorders DSM-5, published by the American Psychiatric Association
- **ADHD rating scales** to help collect and evaluate information about your child

Implementation

Behavior modification therapy, parent training, and school accommodations are successful in this population (CDC, 2015b). Nonstimulant (atomoxetine [Strattera], guanfacine [Tenex]) and stimulant medications (methylphenidate [Ritalin], dextroamphetamine/levoamphetamine [Adderall], lisdexamfetamine [Vyvanse]) may be needed during elementary and high school. Some individuals learn to compensate and no longer need medication in adulthood, while others continue to require it. Contrary to common belief, children with ADHD who are treated with medications are less likely to use illicit drugs later in life because their mental health symptoms have been addressed (Chang et al., 2013).

SPECIFIC LEARNING DISORDERS

Reading, Written Expression, Math

Onset of these disorders, which include dyslexia and dyscalculia, occurs during elementary school years. Symptoms include difficulty in learning and using academic skills. Learning disabilities are not related to developmental delays. It is estimated that 5% to 15% of school-age children have a learning disorder, which are more common in males. Learning disabilities are linked to higher rates of dropping out of school, depression, suicide, unemployment, underemployment, and lower income (APA, 2013).

Assessment, Diagnosis, and Implementation

Parents may report to the nurse that their child is having difficulty in school, receiving poor grades, or believe there is a vision problem. Diagnosis is normally made through testing with the school or a private psychologist, and learning accommodations such as tutoring can be made. Unfortunately, learning disabilities are often missed, causing lifetime academic and career difficulties.

MOTOR DISORDERS

Tourette's disorder, developmental coordination disorder, and several other motor or vocal tic disorders are listed in the *DSM-5* (APA, 2013; Sadock, Sadock, & Ruiz, 2015). Two are briefly discussed in this section.
- *Developmental coordination disorder.* Symptoms of this disorder include delayed coordinated motor skills presenting as clumsiness, slowness, and difficulty with handwriting or riding a bike (Nelson, 2015).
- *Tourette's disorder.* Symptoms of this disorder include motor as well as vocal tics, with an onset in early childhood. Tics can be mild, such as clearing the throat or jerking a limb, or as severe as loudly yelling out an animal noise or curse word, with spasms intense enough to cause the patient to be flung out of a chair. Tics can be very embarrassing to children and especially adolescents, as they attempt to navigate the social and dating scene.

Assessment, Diagnosis, and Implementation

Mild symptoms may be difficult to pinpoint, while severe symptoms such as jerking, cursing, or difficulty learning to write may be noticed by parents or nurses right away. Psychiatrists or psychiatric nurse practitioners diagnose the disorder using *DSM-5* criteria, history,

and observation. No treatment has proven to be globally successful, although children who receive physical and occupational therapy have better outcomes. Comprehensive Behavioral Intervention for Tics (CBIT) is a new treatment that includes habit reversal, insight, education, and relaxation techniques and has been shown to reduce tics (CDC, 2015a). Propranolol (Inderal) may be used for tremor, and haloperidol (Haldol) may be effective in decreasing tics (Duffy, 2013; Stahl, 2014).

SCHIZOPHRENIA AND PSYCHOTIC DISORDERS

There are several types of schizophrenia and other psychotic disorders, which are discussed in Chapter 17.

These disorders are characterized by symptoms of auditory or visual hallucinations, paranoia, delusional or bizarre thinking, diminished emotional expression, and social impairment. The psychotic features tend to emerge from the late teens to mid-30s, although prodromal symptoms can often be identified in hindsight (APA, 2013).

Assessment, Diagnosis, and Implementation

As symptoms emerge, the individual usually seeks assistance from a medical or psychiatric professional. Diagnosis is made by a psychiatrist or psychiatric nurse practitioner using the *DSM-5*, history, and observation. Treatment includes coping skills and antipsychotic medications. During acute phases, hospitalization may be necessary. Although rare in childhood, schizophrenia can occur and may be misdiagnosed as autism.

BIPOLAR AND RELATED DISORDERS

Bipolar I, Bipolar II, Cyclothymic Disorder

These disorders are discussed in Chapter 16. Symptoms include mood lability, vacillating from depression to elevated states called mania or the less severe hypomania. Individuals may speak very rapidly and be impulsive (spending money, promiscuity, substance use) during a manic or hypomanic state. During depression they are sad, tearful, and may isolate. Individuals are at risk for suicide in both manic and depressed phases (National Institute of Mental Health, 2016). The mean age for the first manic, hypomanic, or major depressive episode is 18 to 20, although it can occur as early as mid-childhood (APA, 2013).

Assessment, Diagnosis, and Implementation

Nurses should look for mood changes, and assess for suicidal thoughts, plans, or attempts using instruments such as the MODIFIED SAD PERSONS Scale (Warden et al., 2014) and the HEADSSS (Minnesota Department of Health, 2006). Diagnosis is made using the *DSM-5*, history, and observation. Treatment includes cognitive behavioral therapy and several categories of mood-stabilizing medications.

For information on the HEADSSS Adolescent Assessment, see www.health.state.mn.us/youth/providers/headssslong.html.

DEPRESSIVE DISORDERS AND DEPRESSION

Disruptive Mood Dysregulation Disorder, Major Depressive Disorder, Persistent Depressive Disorder (formerly called Dysthymia), and Premenstrual Dysphoric Disorder

These disorders are discussed in Chapter 15, with the exception of disruptive mood dysregulation disorder, which is reviewed here, as it must be diagnosed in childhood.

It is important to note that depression in children and adolescents can present in a similar manner as in adults, such as sadness, crying, lack of energy, change in appetite or sleep patterns, and negative or suicidal thoughts. However, depression can also present differently in this population. Children and adolescents may display anger, isolation, a change in dress (dark clothing, hair covering the face or eyes, poor grooming), a change in friends, use of drugs or alcohol, listening to music with sad or violent themes, sensitivity, poor school performance, physical complaints such as headaches or stomach aches, self-harm such as cutting, or other acting-out behaviors. Often symptoms of depression in younger age groups are seen to be behavioral problems, and the underlying depression goes unnoticed (APA, 2013; Mayo Clinic, 2015). Adolescents have a higher rate of suicide, so it is especially important to be aware of the typical and atypical presentations of depression (National Institute of Mental Health, 2016) (see Chapter 23).

- *Disruptive mood dysregulation disorder.* This mood disorder occurs only in childhood, with onset before age 10. Symptoms include severe, recurrent verbal or behavioral temper outbursts, inconsistent developmental level, and persistent irritability or anger for most of the day in various settings. Prevalence is 2% to 5% and it is more common in males.

Assessment, Diagnosis, and Implementation

As noted above, the nurse must be aware of typical and atypical presentation of depression in children and adolescents. Suicide is a risk, and instruments such as the MODIFIED SAD PERSONS Scale and HEADSSS are appropriate. Supportive therapy and behavior modification can be used. It will be important to involve the family to keep the patient supported and safe. Medications may include stimulants, antidepressants, or mood stabilizers (Child Mind Institute, 2015; Preston, et al., 2010).

ANXIETY DISORDERS

Separation Anxiety Disorder, Selective Mutism, Specific Phobias, Social Anxiety, Panic Disorder, Agoraphobia, and Generalized Anxiety Disorder

Separation anxiety disorder, selective mutism, and additional comments on specific phobias in childhood are discussed in this section. The remaining anxiety disorders are discussed in Chapter 11. The symptoms of anxiety are similar in all age groups, with the exception of separation anxiety disorder, which is only diagnosed in children.

- *Separation anxiety disorder.* Developmentally inappropriate fear or anxiety surrounding separation from the person to whom the child is most attached. The child may worry about losing important people to injury or death, or about being lost or kidnapped. The child may refuse to stay with grandparents or friends, and insist on sleeping near the parental figure. Nightmares with the theme of separation may occur, as well as somatic complaints such as stomach distress when separation is anticipated. The symptoms are considered normal up to age 1. The prevalence is 4% in children and 1.6% in adolescents.
- *Selective mutism.* Consistent failure to speak in situations where speaking is an expectation, although the child is able to speak at other times. Symptoms interfere with academic, social, or occupational achievement.
- *Specific phobias in childhood.* Phobias are discussed in Chapter 11. Some phobias often seen with children include fear of the dark, monsters, costumed characters, injections, water, and certain

animals. Phobias occur in 5% of children and 16% of adolescents (APA, 2013).

Assessment, Diagnosis, and Implementation

Nurses may ask questions about how a child reacts to spending the night with friends or when not around the parents. The nurse may observe overly clingy behaviors during appointments. The child may seem fearful and bite his or her fingernails or display fidgeting behavior. Instruments such as the Spence Children's Anxiety Scale (Spence, 1994) or the Hamilton Anxiety Rating Scale (Pomerantz, 2013) may be used. Supportive therapy, cognitive behavioral therapy (CBT), and family therapy may be appropriate. Relaxation and guided imagery are very helpful with anxiety, as are children's books that address separation anxiety such as *Growing Up Brave* by Donna Pincus, PhD. At times, medication such as SSRI antidepressants, beta blockers, or antihistamines may be used.

OBSESSIVE-COMPULSIVE AND RELATED DISORDERS

Obsessive-Compulsive Disorder (OCD), Body Dysmorphic Disorder, Hoarding Disorder, Trichotillomania, and Excoriation Disorder

Trichotillomania and excoriation disorder frequently begin in childhood, and are discussed in this section. The remaining obsessive-compulsive and related disorders are discussed in Chapter 11.

- *Trichotillomania.* Recurrent twisting or pulling out of one's hair, resulting in hair loss and sometimes damage. The individual attempts to stop without success, and the behavior causes distress. Prevalence in the adolescent and adult population is 1% to 2%, and it is more common in females.
- *Excoriation disorder.* Recurrent skin-picking, resulting in skin lesions, infection, and scarring. The individual attempts to stop without success, and the behavior causes distress. Lifetime prevalence is about 1%, and it is more common in females.

Assessment, Diagnosis, and Implementation

The nurse may notice bald patches or skin lesions on the patient, or may observe the actual behavior of twisting, pulling, or chewing the hair or picking the skin during an appointment. The patient may wear scarves or hats to hide thinning hair. Cognitive behavioral therapy, including techniques like snapping a rubber band on the wrist instead of pulling out hair, may help reduce the behavior. There is limited evidence to support the efficacy of medications, including SSRI or serotonin-norepinephrine reuptake inhibitor (SNRI) antidepressants, clomipramine (Anafranil), atypical antipsychotics such as olanzapine (Zyprexa) and aripiprazole (Abilify), and the opiate agonist naltrexone (Revia) (Franklin et al., 2011; Trichotillomania Learning Center, 2011; White & Koran, 2011).

TRAUMA AND STRESSOR-RELATED DISORDERS

Reactive Attachment Disorder

Reactive attachment disorder is discussed in this section. The remaining trauma and stressor-related disorders and other related topics are discussed in Chapter 10.

- *Reactive attachment disorder (RAD).* Consistent pattern of inhibited, emotionally withdrawn behavior. Children with RAD rarely seek comfort or respond to comforting. Symptoms include limited positive affect, irritability, sadness, fearfulness, and minimal social responsiveness. Causes of RAD include inconsistent care, frequent changes in caregivers, or living in foster homes or orphanages.

Assessment, Diagnosis, and Implementation

The nurse may observe a failure of the child to seek comfort and respond socially. This disorder may resemble autism spectrum disorder, depression, or disruptive mood dysregulation disorder in its presentation. Psychiatrists or psychiatric nurse practitioners diagnose the disorder using the *DSM-5*, history, and observation. Treatment includes individual and family therapy, and medication for any underlying depression or anxiety. Bibliotherapy, searching for books that relate to the individual child's situation such as living in foster care, can be very helpful.

DISSOCIATIVE DISORDERS

These disorders are discussed in Chapter 12. Dissociative disorders may present in childhood or adolescence as the result of abuse or trauma, or modeling of behavior in the family. If a child appears "spaced out" or withdrawn, abuse or trauma should be considered.

Assessment, Diagnosis, and Implementation

The nurse should be careful to watch for symptoms of abuse or of abusive parents, which will result in trauma to the child and potentially the development of a dissociative disorder. When assessing an abused child, drawing and play therapy are often used. Diagnosis and treatment of these disorders are covered in Chapter 12.

SOMATIC SYMPTOM DISORDER AND RELATED DISORDERS

This category of disorders is discussed thoroughly in Chapter 12. Children may suffer from somatic symptoms due to anxiety, stress, or modeling of behavior in the family. Common symptoms seen in children and adolescents with these disorders are headaches, stomach aches, fatigue, and frequent visits to the school nurse.

Assessment, Diagnosis, and Implementation

The nurse may notice frequent somatic symptoms, trips to the school nurse, missing a lot of school, and anxiety symptoms. There may be stressors in the home, a modeled pattern of focusing on physical sensations, or a pattern of being rewarded with attention when ill. The underlying impetus needs to be addressed, whether that be family dynamics, anxiety, or rewarding the behavior. Giving attention to nonsomatic topics is a good place to start.

VIGNETTE: SOMATIC SYMPTOM DISORDER (SSD)

A 12-year-old student has made daily trips to the school nurse for the past 3 days with complaints of an upset stomach. The school nurse suspects the student is having physical symptoms because of an increase in stress and gently assesses the situation. The student immediately bursts into tears when the nurse asks how things are going at home. The nurse learns the student heard her parents arguing about getting a divorce. She doesn't feel like she can talk to her parents and is embarrassed to talk about it with friends. The nurse helps the student realize her upset stomach is from the stress and anxiety and teaches her a simple guided imagery technique to help refocus her thoughts and calm her mind.

FEEDING AND EATING DISORDERS

Pica, Rumination Disorder, Avoidant/Restrictive Food Intake Disorder, Anorexia Nervosa, Bulimia Nervosa, and Binge-Eating Disorder

This category of disorders is partially covered in Chapter 14 (anorexia nervosa, bulimia nervosa, and binge-eating disorder). It is relevant to this chapter on children and adolescents to note that anorexia nervosa and bulimia nervosa often begin during adolescence.

The remaining three disorders (pica, rumination disorder, and avoidant/restrictive food intake disorder) will be presented briefly here.

- *Pica.* Persistent eating of nonfood substances, such as sand or dirt, chalk, paint chips, ice, cloth, or hair. It is not part of a culturally accepted ritual or practice, and onset is commonly in childhood. There is potential for harm or death depending on what is ingested.
- *Rumination disorder.* Repeated regurgitation of food, which is then re-chewed, re-swallowed, or spit out. The behavior may be self-soothing, and often corrects itself if it occurs in infancy.
- *Avoidant/restrictive food intake disorder.* Persistent failure to meet nutritional or energy needs. It results in weight loss or failure to gain weight, significant nutritional deficiency, or dependence on supplements. Eating disorders in children and teens can lead to a host of serious physical problems and even death. A child needs treatment right away since the best results occur when eating disorders are treated at the earliest stages.

Assessment, Diagnosis, and Implementation

The nurse may notice or it may be reported by parents that the child is eating unusual items, or the physical assessment may reveal weight loss, delayed growth, or nutritional deficit. Therapy to re-train behaviors and for individual and family support will likely be needed. Weight and nutrition should be monitored and documented. The child may need to be offered favorite foods or nutritional supplements. Medication such as the antihistamine cyproheptadine (Periactin) may help increase appetite. SSRI or SNRI antidepressants may help with stopping the compulsive aspect of the behavior, and a proton pump inhibitor may be needed in cases of esophageal damage. A collaborative approach by a gastroenterologist and a psychologist may be employed (Mayo Clinic, 2012).

ELIMINATION DISORDERS

Enuresis and Encopresis

- *Enuresis (nocturnal, diurnal, or both).* Repeated voiding of urine into bed or clothes; may be involuntary or intentional. It is considered normal until age 5.
- *Encopresis (with or without constipation and overflow incontinence).* Repeated passage of feces into inappropriate places such as clothing or the floor; may be involuntary or intentional. It is considered normal until age 4, and is further categorized into primary, secondary, retentive, and nonretentive, of which 80% to 90% of cases are retentive type (Tronshaw, 2012). If not treated, serious complications such as megalocolon can occur.

Assessment, Diagnosis, and Implementation

The parents report that bed-wetting or bed soiling has continued past a normal potty training age. A poor appetite or distended belly may be noted as well. In enuresis, a voiding schedule even during the night may be used, and fluids before bedtime may be limited. Positive reinforcement of success and avoiding shaming the child are important. The bell and pad method that triggers an alarm when urination occurs may have a 70% to 80% success rate (Tronshaw, 2012), and bladder training can be used. An IEP may be implemented at school. Pharmacological treatment includes imipramine (Tofranil), desmopressin (DDAVP), oxybutynin (Ditropan), various stimulants, indomethacin (Indocin), and SSRI antidepressants (Tronshaw, 2012). In encopresis, a referral to a gastroenterologist may be needed. Treatment includes dietary changes including an increase in fiber and fluids, using a positive approach, making the toilet accessible, and using a regular bathroom schedule. Cognitive behavioral therapy is aimed at reducing anxiety. Suppositories, enemas, stool softeners, and laxatives may be needed. There is limited evidence for using imipramine (Tronshaw, 2012).

SLEEP-WAKE DISORDERS

Numerous disorders are listed in the *DSM-5* (APA, 2013), including insomnia, narcolepsy, central sleep apnea, sleepwalking, sleep terror, nightmare disorder, and restless legs syndrome. Children and adolescents often experience sleepwalking, night terrors, and nightmares.

Assessment, Diagnosis, and Implementation

Identifying the underlying fear is important. Soothing music, nightlights, and books about fears can be helpful. Relaxation and guided imagery or hypnosis with a theme aimed at helping the child feel safe during the night, or addressing stress, can be used (Mayo Clinic, 2014). A regular sleep schedule, a calm and comfortable room, and good sleep hygiene are important. Scheduled awakening, where the child is awakened 15 minutes before the time of the usual night incident, may be used (Cleveland Clinic, 2014).

SEXUAL DYSFUNCTIONS

Several disorders related to problems with pain or arousal are listed in the *DSM-5* (APA, 2013). These are discussed in Chapters 22 and 27. Some of these symptoms may relate to the adolescent population in certain cases.

Gender Dysphoria

This disorder relates to the feeling that a person is in the wrong gender body and is discussed in Chapter 27.

This disorder is being discussed in a more open manner in our society. Caitlyn (formerly Bruce) Jenner, an Olympic medalist, is a recent example of an individual who underwent gender alignment procedures to physically appear like the woman she is inside. Some literature has found that young children can already report feeling like the opposite gender. Parents react in various ways to disclosures of this nature, with some showing acceptance in providing opposite-gender clothing and experiences, and others becoming distraught and rigid.

It is a good exercise for you as a student to think carefully about how you would react if your child were to tell you he or she is transgender. What behaviors would you allow or not allow, and why? How do you think other children at school or family members would react? What practical considerations exist, such as bathroom and locker room issues?

Assessment, Diagnosis, and Implementation

As nurses are trusted figures, a child or adolescent may disclose feelings of gender dysphoria. It is important to respond in a supportive and nonshaming way, and to provide a referral to a therapist who is a specialist in this area.

DISRUPTIVE, IMPULSE CONTROL, AND CONDUCT DISORDERS

Oppositional Defiant Disorder, Intermittent Explosive Disorder, Conduct Disorder, Antisocial Personality Disorder, Pyromania, and Kleptomania

Two disorders found in the child and adolescent populations are presented here. The remaining disorders are covered in Chapter 27.

- *Oppositional defiant disorder (ODD)*. While all children test limits or have tantrums, ODD goes beyond the normal scope of these behaviors. Symptoms must be displayed with at least one person who is not a sibling, and include at least four of these criteria: often loses temper, easily annoyed, angry, argues with authority figures, defies or refuses rules, deliberately annoys others, blames others for mistakes or misbehavior, vindictive (American Academy of Child & Adolescent Psychiatry, 2013; Mayo Clinic Staff, 2012).
- *Conduct disorder (CD)*. More severe than ODD. Must display at least three of these criteria: bullies or intimidates others; initiates physical fights; has used a weapon (bat, brick, knife); physically cruel to people or animals; has stolen while confronting a victim; has stolen nontrivial items; has forced someone into sexual activity; deliberate fire-setting to cause damage; deliberate destruction of property; has broken into a house, car, or building; lies to obtain favors or to avoid obligations; stays out at night despite parental rules; has run away overnight at least twice; often truant from school (Bernstein, et al., 2011; Mental Health America, 2012).

Assessment, Diagnosis, and Implementation

Parenting classes and parent management training, including limit setting, are necessary to deal with these disorders. For adolescents, the combination of individual therapy and parent management training has shown to be the most effective. Treatment is long term, usually several hours per week. Therapy includes problem-solving and social skills, controlling impulses, developing empathy, and medication to treat coexisting conditions such as ADHD, anxiety, or mood disorders (American Academy of Child & Adolescent Psychiatry, 2009). Behaviors may be a response to an unstable home environment. When parents are using substances or otherwise incapable of providing the needed structure to turn the child or adolescent's behavior around, out-of-home placement may be appropriate. Because of the aggressive behaviors seen in conduct disorder, law enforcement and Child Protective Services (CPS) are usually involved. Stronger medication such as mood stabilizers are frequently required, and hospitalization may be necessary to control aggressive behaviors. About 30% of patients with ODD develop CD, and CD is a precursor to antisocial personality disorder in adulthood.

SUBSTANCE-RELATED AND ADDICTIVE DISORDERS

This section of the *DSM-5* (APA, 2013) lists numerous, specific substance abuse disorders relating to alcohol and various drugs, including cannabis, opioids, and stimulants. This topic is discussed in detail in Chapter 19.

One study found that 9% of eighth graders and 37.4% of twelfth graders had used alcohol within the past month, and 27.2% of high school students had used illicit drugs within the past year (National Institute on Drug Abuse, 2014). It is important for nurses to be aware of the prevalence of substance abuse in child and adolescent populations.

Assessment, Diagnosis, and Implementation

The nurse can use structured questionnaires or an informal approach to ask about substance use. Whatever method is chosen, it is important to assess for substance use in all preteens and adolescents as a matter of course. Some drugs have permanent effects, including brain damage, when used just a few times; an example is huffing (inhaling substances such as paint or other aerosols). This age group does not have full development of the frontal lobe, affecting judgment and impulse control, and often feels invincible. The nurse can provide a lot of needed education and referrals.

NEUROCOGNITIVE DISORDERS

Dementia-related disorders are normally seen in older populations. See Chapters 18 and 28.

Personality Disorders
Cluster A – Paranoid, Schizoid, Schizotypal;
Cluster B – Antisocial, Borderline, Histrionic, Narcissistic;
Cluster C – Avoidant, Dependent, Obsessive-Compulsive

Personality disorders are discussed in Chapter 13. The symptoms must be present for more than 1 year if diagnosed prior to the age of 18. Antisocial personality disorder is the only exception and *cannot* be diagnosed before age 18.

Paraphillic Disorders
Voyeuristic Disorder, Exhibitionistic Disorder, Frotteuristic Disorder, Sexual Sadism Disorder, Sexual Masochism Disorder, Pedophilic Disorder, Fetishistic Disorder, and Transvestic Disorder

These disorders and related topics are discussed in Chapter 27. Pedophilic disorder is further touched on here. Symptoms include recurrent, intense, sexually arousing fantasies, urges, or behaviors involving sexual activity with a prepubescent child or children. The person has acted on the urges, or they have caused marked distress or interpersonal difficulty. The individual is at least 16 years old and at least 5 years older than the child (APA, 2013). A child can be the victim of pedophilia. An adolescent can be a victim or act out sexually on younger children.

Assessment, Diagnosis, and Implementation

A nurse may need to ask questions relating to being a victim or a perpetrator. A child may act sexually precocious, be secretive, or be fearful around an older child or adult. If abuse, either as victim or perpetrator, is disclosed or suspected, a CPS referral is in order, as well as a forensic examination and interview by a trained professional. Both victims and perpetrators will need therapy with a specialist.

OTHER CONDITIONS THAT MAY BE A FOCUS OF CLINICAL ATTENTION (FORMERLY AXIS IV IN THE *DSM-IV*, LISTING PSYCHOSOCIAL STRESSORS)

In addition to symptoms of diagnosable mental disorders, clinicians (including nurses) must be aware of various psychosocial stressors in the child's or adolescent's life. These include relational problems; abuse and neglect; educational and occupational problems; housing and economic problems; problems related to crime or interaction with the legal system; problems related to other psychosocial, personal, and environmental circumstances; or problems related to medical and other health care.

Assessment, Diagnosis, and Intervention

Assessment is through history and observation, and the nursing interventions will be individualized toward the specific psychosocial stressor, such as lack of housing.

THERAPEUTIC MODALITIES FOR CHILD AND ADOLESCENT DISORDERS

Parental involvement and support is recognized as a critical factor in the supportive and educational interventions for the child or adolescent. In addition to therapy with a single family, group therapy with several families facing similar challenges provides support and insight.

Group therapy for younger children takes the form of play. As children get older, more talk therapy can occur. Groups are effective for common issues such as bereavement, abuse, chronic illness, or addiction. One of the challenges of using groups when working with children and adolescents lies in the contagious effect of disruptive behavior.

Milieu therapy is a philosophical basis for structuring inpatient and other long-term treatment programs. The nurse and other team members collaborate to provide a therapeutic environment that facilitates growth, safety, and positive change.

Behavior modification and **cognitive behavioral therapy** are based on the principle that rewarded behavior is more likely to be repeated. Connections between thoughts, feelings, and behaviors are identified, and techniques help to develop rational thinking, better choices, and impulse control. Progress is rewarded with attention, praise, or other desired outcomes or privileges. Point systems or behavioral charts are examples. Rehearsing new behaviors and relaxation and guided imagery may be employed.

Removal and restraint are dangerous, controversial treatment modalities for children (as well as for adults). Injuries and even death have been associated with seclusion and restraint with children. In recent years, most facilities have become restraint-free in all but the most emergent of situations when a patient is in immediate danger of harming self or others. Seclusion and restraint are closely monitored and allowed only for short periods of time within prescribed and monitored guidelines. Gentle therapeutic holding, which is nonpunitive in nature, or helmets to protect a patient during head banging can be used.

Instead of seclusion, a unit may have an unlocked **quiet room** for a youth who needs to be removed from the situation for either self-control or control by the staff. **Time out** is a common method for intervening in disruptive or inappropriate behaviors, both by parents and in mental health settings. The child's individual behavioral goals, developmental stage, and age are considered in setting limits on behavior by using time-out periods. If they are overused or inconsistent, time outs lose their effectiveness.

Play therapy is based on the notion that play is the work of childhood and the way a child learns to master impulses and adapt to the environment. Play is also the language of childhood and the communication medium for assessing developmental and emotional status, determining diagnosis, and instituting therapeutic interventions. There are many forms of play therapy that can be used individually or in groups. Playrooms are equipped with art supplies and a variety of toys, including hand puppets, dolls, dollhouses, and action figures. These toys provide the child with opportunities to act out conflicts and stressful situations, to work through feelings, and with the help of the therapist to develop more adaptive ways of coping. Drawings can be evaluated for inner conflict, family relationships, and other stressors in the child's life.

Dramatic play therapy, also called **psychodrama**, is a treatment modality that uses dramatic techniques to act out emotional problems, examine the experience, develop new perspectives, and try out new behaviors. This modality may be used with groups of older children and adolescents. The dramas can be videotaped for reviewing the experience and facilitating new learning. This type of therapy is not recommended with psychotic youth.

Therapeutic games are an ideal assessment tool for children who may have difficulty talking about their feelings and problems, and also allow a nonthreatening way to develop rapport with health care workers. The game might be as simple as checkers, but therapeutic games are more effective in eliciting children's fears and fantasies. A well-known game is the *Talking, Feeling, and Doing Game* (Gardner, 2007). The player draws a talking, feeling, or doing card, which gives instructions or asks a question, such as "All the girls in the class were invited to a birthday party except one. How did she feel?" If this game is played with a group, additional responses can be elicited.

Bibliotherapy involves using children's books and literature to help the child express feelings in a supportive environment, gain insight into feelings and behavior, and learn new ways to cope with difficult situations. Children unconsciously identify with the characters in the story, so the books selected should reflect the situation or feeling that is problematic for the child (Pincus, 2012).

Therapeutic drawing allows children to spontaneously express themselves in artwork that captures thoughts, feelings, and tensions they may be unable to express verbally. When drawing any human figure, children leave an imprint of their inner self, including attitudes about the family. The following characteristics are general indicators of children's emotions or meanings found in a drawing. The normal presentation for age groups must be considered; for example, a toddler might not include arms in a drawing because he or she ran out of room on the paper, while missing arms in an older child would more likely indicate a feeling of powerlessness. It is recommended that the nurse working with children consult an authoritative book on interpreting children's drawings.

- Size of figures: very large (aggression, poor impulse control); very small (shyness, insecurity).
- Omission of body parts: hands (trauma, insecurity), arms (inadequacy, powerlessness), legs (lack of support), feet (insecure, helpless), mouth (difficulty expressing self, not having a voice).
- Facial expressions: personal mood and affect of child or others in the picture.
- Integration of body parts: scattered or disorganized parts indicate cognitive or psychological problems or both.
- Placement of the child in relation to other family members: is the child close to the father, with the mother in a distant corner of the page? This could indicate an emotional distance, or be an indication of living arrangements.
- Differences in facial expressions of family members: for example, is one person angry and the rest fearful?
- Colors can indicate a cheerful, angry, or sad mood.

Music therapy instigates changes in both the physiology of the nervous system and social interactions. Music therapy may incorporate recorded music, songs, songwriting, or use of a musical instrument. Children love to use simple noisemakers for the expression of feelings, for the development of coordination and rhythm, and as an opportunity for social interactions. Music on inpatient units is often used to create a relaxing mood for rest periods and bedtime.

Movement and dance therapy is a direct expression of the self that helps the youth become more aware of feelings and thoughts, dissipate tensions, develop greater body awareness, improve or correct a distorted body image, improve coordination, and increase social interactions. The type of movement used with children can be as simple as a game of "Follow the Leader" or it can be creative, free-form movements to the mood of the music. For older children and adolescents, more formal classes in exercise, karate, or the latest dance craze may be of interest.

Recreational therapy generally takes place off the unit and is often conducted by a recreational therapist with assistance from the nursing staff. Activities are often organized around a game that teaches psychomotor and social skills, such as volleyball or swimming. Special field trips give children the opportunity to be like other children and to act appropriately in public situations, leading to increased self-control and self-esteem.

KEY POINTS TO REMEMBER

- About 20% of children and adolescents are estimated to have mental health problems, and only a small percentage of these youths actually receive treatment.
- Risk factors known to contribute to the development of mental and emotional problems in children and adolescents include genetic, biochemical, developmental, environmental, and cultural factors.
- Resiliency helps protect children and adolescents in a stressful situation. Temperament, problem-solving skills, and the support of a nurturing adult contribute to resiliency and successful navigation of stressful events
- The most commonly diagnosed child psychiatric disorders are mood disorders, anxiety disorders, attention-deficit/hyperactivity disorder (ADHD), and conduct and oppositional disorders.
- Treatment of childhood and adolescent disorders requires a collaborative approach.
- In addition to individual, family, and group therapy, play therapy, art therapy, and bibliotherapy are helpful for children. The older the child, the more he or she should be involved in treatment decisions.
- The family is an integral part of the supportive and educational system for the child and adolescent.

APPLYING CRITICAL JUDGMENT

1. A 4-year-old boy has been diagnosed with an autism spectrum disorder (ASD).
   A. Describe the kinds of data you might find on assessment in terms of communication, socialization, behaviors, and activities.
   B. Name at least four realistic nursing interventions and outcomes for this child.
   C. Which treatment modalities and supports do you think would be the most effective for a child with ASD?
2. A 7-year-old girl in second grade has been diagnosed with attention-deficit/hyperactivity disorder (ADHD).
   A. What clinical behaviors might she be exhibiting at home and in the classroom, in the areas of inattention, hyperactivity, and impulsivity?
   B. Identify at least four nursing interventions that you might include in her treatment plan or suggest to the family.
   C. What type of medications might be considered for this client?
3. An 8-year-old boy has been diagnosed with conduct disorder.
   A. What are some of the behaviors you might expect to be reported about this child, in light of his diagnosis?
   B. What are the goals for this child? And what is the overall prognosis for children with this disorder? Do further research if necessary.
   C. What are at several ways you could support the child's parents in being more effective?
   D. Identify resources within your community to which you might refer this family for guidance.

CHAPTER REVIEW QUESTIONS

1. The nurse interviews the parent of a 7-year-old child diagnosed with moderate autism spectrum disorder. Which comment from the parent best describes autistic behavior?
    a. "My child occasionally has temper tantrums."
    b. "Sometimes my child wakes up with nightmares."
    c. "My child swings for hours on our backyard gym set."
    d. "Toilet training was more difficult for this child than my other children."

2. A nurse plans to lead a group in a residential facility for kindergarten-aged, abused children. Which strategy should the nurse incorporate?
    a. Building a house using blocks
    b. Telling a story about a child who felt sad
    c. Drawing pictures of fun activities at a park
    d. Reading and discussing a book about abused children

3. Which scenario presents the highest risk for a pregnancy resulting in offspring with an intellectual developmental disability (IDD)?
    a. 18-year-old mother who received no prenatal care
    b. 32-year-old woman diagnosed with anorexia nervosa
    c. 26-year-old father with a history of episodic alcohol abuse
    d. 38-year-old father diagnosed with generalized anxiety disorder

4. A community mental health nurse talks with a 6-year-old child whose divorced parents have shared custody. Which initial question will best help the nurse explore the child's perception of home life?
    a. "Is your life different from your friends' lives?"
    b. "Are you happiest at your mother's or your father's house?"
    c. "Do you find it hard to move back and forth between two homes?"
    d. "What are some of the good and bad things about living in two places?"

5. The parent of an adolescent recently diagnosed with schizophrenia says to the nurse, "This is entirely my fault. I should have spent more time with my child when he was a toddler." Which response by the nurse is correct?
    a. "Schizophrenia is genetically transmitted, so it was not in your control."
    b. "Your child's disorder is more likely the result of an undetected head injury."
    c. "Environmental toxins are directly implicated in the origins of schizophrenia."
    d. "Lack of prenatal care causes schizophrenia rather than early childhood events."

REFERENCES

American Academy of Child & Adolescent Psychiatry (AACAP). (2013). *Children with oppositional defiant disorder.* Retrieved from https://www.aacap.org/AACAP/Families_and_Youth/Facts_for_Families/Facts_for_Families_Pages/Children_With_Oppositional_Defiant_Disorder_72.aspx.

American Academy of Child & Adolescent Psychiatry (AACAP). (2009). *ODD: A guide for families by the American Academy of Child & Adolescent Psychiatry.* Retrieved from https://www.aacap.org/App_Themes/AACAP/docs/resource_centers/odd/odd_resource_center_odd_guide.pdf.

American Psychiatric Association. (2013). *Diagnostic and statistical manual of mental disorders (DSM-5)* (5th ed.). Washington, DC: APA.

Autism Speaks. (2015). *National Health Interview Survey underscores gap between the number of kids diagnosed with autism and the number receiving services.* Retrieved from https://www.autismspeaks.org/science/science-news/new-government-survey-pegs-autism-prevalence-1-45.

Autism Society. (2015). *Causes.* Retrieved from http://www.autism-society.org/what-is/causes.

Bernstein, B. E., Windle, M. L., Pataki, C., et al. (2011). *Conduct disorder.* Retrieved from http://emedicine.Medscape.com/article/918213-overview.

Black, D. W., & Andreasen, N. C. (2014). *Introductory textbook of psychiatry* (6th ed.). Washington, DC: American Psychiatric Publishing.

Bostic, J. Q., & Prince, J. B. (2008). Child and adolescent psychiatric disorders. In T. A. Stern, J. F. Rosenbaum, M. Fava, et al. (Eds.), *Massachusetts General Hospital comprehensive clinical psychiatry.* Philadelphia, PA: Mosby Elsevier.

Brady, K. T. (2016). Comorbidity with substance abuse. *Medscape Multispecialty.* Retrieved from http://www.medscape.org/viewarticle/457178.

Centers for Disease Control and Prevention (CDC). (2010b). *Autistic spectrum disorders.* Retrieved from http://www.cdc.gov/ncbddd/autism/data.html.

Centers for Disease Control and Prevention (CDC). (2010a). *Signs & symptoms, autism spectrum disorders.* Retrieved from http://www.cdc.gov/ncbddd/autism/signs.html.

Centers for Disease Control and Prevention (CDC). (2015b). *Attention-deficit/hyperactivity disorder (ADHD).* Retrieved from http://www.cdc.gov/ncbddd/adhd/treatment.html.

Centers for Disease Control and Prevention (CDC). (2015a). *Tourette syndrome (TS).* Retrieved from http://www.cdc.gov/ncbddd/tourette/treatments.html#CBIT.

Chang, Z., Lichtenstein, P., Halldner, L., et al. (2013). Stimulant ADHD medication and risk for substance abuse. *Journal of Child Psychology and Psychiatry, 55*(8), 878–885.

Child Mind Institute. (2015). *Disruptive mood dysregulation disorder.* Retrieved from http://www.childmind.org/en/health/disorder-guide/disruptive-mood-dysregulation-disorder.

Cleveland, Clinic (2014). *Sleepwalking: Symptoms, causes, & treatment options.* Retrieved from http://my.clevelandclinic.org/services/neurological_institute/sleep-disorders-center/disorders-conditions/hic-sleepwalking.

Corrigan, P. W., Druss, B. G., & Perlick, D. A. (2014). The impact of mental illness stigma on seeking and participating in mental health care. *Psychological Science in the Public Interest, 15*(2), 37–70.

Duffy, J. R. (2013). *Motor speech disorders: Substrates, differential diagnoses and management* (3rd ed.). St. Louis, MO: Elsevier.

Franke, B., Faraone, S. V., Asherson, P., Buitelaar, J., Bau, C. H. D., Ramos-Quiroga, J. A., & Reif, A. (2012). The genetics of attention deficit/hyperactivity disorder in adults, a review. *Molecular Psychiatry, 17*(10), 960–987.

Franklin, M. E., Zagrabbe, K., & Benavides, K. L. (2011). Trichotillomania and its treatment: A review and recommendations. *Expert Reviews in Neurotherapy, 11*(8), 1165–1174.

Gardner, R. A. (2007). *Psychotherapy of children with conduct disorders using games and stories.* Washington, DC: American Psychological Association. [DVD].

Greenhill, L. L., & Hechtman, L. I. (2010). Attention-deficit/hyperactivity disorder. In B. J. Sadock, V. A. Sadock, & P. Ruiz (Eds.), *Kaplan and Sadock's comprehensive textbook of psychiatry* (9th ed.) vol. 11. (pp. 3560–3572). Philadelphia, PA: Wolters Kluwer.

Greeson, J. K. P., Briggs, E. C., Layne, C. M., et al. (2014). Traumatic childhood experiences in the 21st century: Broadening and building on the ACE Studies with data from the National Child Traumatic Stress Network. *Journal of Interpersonal Violence, 29*(3), 536–556.

Gromisch, E. S. (2013). *Neurotransmitters involved in ADHD.* Retrieved from http://psychcentral.com/lib/neurotransmitters-involved-in-adhd/.

Henderson, N. (2012). *What is resiliency and why is it so important?* Retrieved from https://www.resiliency.com/what-is-resiliency/.

Krucik, G. (2015). *What causes mental retardation? 17 possible conditions.* Retrieved from http://www.healthline.com/symptom/mental-retardation.

Masten, A. S. (rev. 2011). *Resilience in children at-risk.* Retrieved from http://www.cchd.umn.edu/carei/reports/rpractice/Spring97/resilience.html.

Mayo Clinic. (2012). *Diseases and conditions: Rumination syndrome.* Retrieved from http://www.mayoclinic.org/diseases-conditions/rumination-syndrome/care-at-mayo-clinic/treatment/con-20037142.

Mayo Clinic. (2014). *Diseases and conditions: Sleep terrors (night terrors).* Retrieved from http://www.mayoclinic.org/diseases-conditions/night-terrors/basics/definition/con-20032552.

Mayo Clinic. (2015). *Teen depression.* Retrieved from http://www.mayoclinic.org/diseases-conditions/teen-depression/basics/symptoms/CON-20035222.

Mayo Clinic Staff. (2012). *Oppositional defiant disorder (ODD).* Retrieved from http://www.MayoClinic.com/health/oppositional-defiantdisorder/DS0063/DSECTION=s-.

Mayo Clinic Staff. (2016). *Attention-deficit/hyperactivity disorder (ADHD) in children.* Retrieved from http://www.mayoclinic.org/diseases-conditions/adhd/diagnosis-treatment/diagnosis/dxc-20196188?p=1.

Mental Health America. (2012). *Conduct disorder.* Retrieved from http://www.nmha.org/co-/conduct-disorder.

Minnesota Department of Health. (2006). *Sample HEADSSS questions.* Retrieved from http://www.health.state.mn.us/youth/providers/headssslong.html.

National Institute for Children's Health Quality and American Academy of Pediatrics. (2002). *NICHQ Vanderbilt Assessment Scales: Used for diagnosing ADHD.* Retrieved from http://www.nichq.org/childrens-health/adhd/resources/vanderbilt-assessment-scales.

National Institutes of Health (NIH), U.S. National Library of Medicine. (2015). *Intellectual disability.* Retrieved from https://www.nlm.nih.gov/medlineplus/ency/article/001523.htm.

National Institute of Mental Health. (2011). *Treatment of children with mental health.* Retrieved from http://www.nimh.nih.gov/health/publications/treatmentofchildrenwithmentalillnessfactsheet/index.shtml.

National Institute of Mental Health. (2012). *Attention deficit hyperactivity disorder.* Retrieved from http://www.nimh.nih.gov/health/publications/attention-deficit-hyperactivity-disorder/index.shtml.

National Institute of Mental Health. (2016). *Risk of suicide.* Retrieved from http://www.nami.org/Learn-More/Mental-Health-Conditions/Related-Conditions/Suicide.

National Institute on Drug Abuse. (2014). *Drug facts: High school and youth trends.* Retrieved from http://www.drugabuse.gov/publications/drugfacts/high-school-youth-trends.

Nauert, R. (2011). *Genetic mutations linked to autistic spectrum disorders.* Retrieved from http://psychcentral.com/news/2011/05/17/genetic-mutations-linked-to-autistic-spectrum-disorders/26248.htm.

Nelson, S. L. (2015). *Developmental coordination disorder treatment and management.* Retrieved from http://emedicine.medscape.com/article/915251-overview.

Pincus, D. B. (2012). *Growing up brave.* New York: Little, Brown and Company.

Pivalizza, P. (2015). *Intellectual disability (mental retardation) in children: Management; outcomes; and prevention.* Retrieved from http://www.uptodate.com/contents/intellectual-disability-mental-retardation-in-children-management-outcomes-and-prevention#references.

Pomerantz, J. M. (2013). *HAM-A Hamilton Anxiety Scale.* Retrieved from http://www.psychiatrictimes.

Preston, J. D., O'Neal, J. H., & Talaga, M. C. (2010). *Handbook of clinical psychopharmacology for therapists* (6th ed.). Oakland, CA: New Harbinger.

Sadock, B. J., Sadock, V. A., & Ruiz, P. (2015). *Child psychiatry. Kaplan & Sadock's Synopsis of Psychiatry: Behavioral Sciences/Clinical Psychiatry* (Ed. 11). Philadelphia: Lippincott Williams & Wilkins.

Schoenstadt, A. (2006). *Autism spectrum disorders symptoms.* Retrieved from http://autism.emedtv.com/autism-spectrum-disorders/autism-spectrum-disorder-symptoms.

Spence, S. H. (1994). *Spence Children's Anxiety Scale.* Retrieved from http://www.scaswebsite.com/.

Stahl, S. M. (2014). *Prescriber's guide: Stahl's essential psychopharmacology* (5th ed.). New York, NY: Cambridge University Press.

Swierzewski, S. J. (2014). *Autism.* Retrieved from http://www.healthcommunities.com/autism/children/overview-of-autism.shtml.

Trichotillomania Learning Center. (2011). *Expert consensus: Treatment guidelines for trichotillomania, skin picking and other body-focused repetitive behaviors.* Retrieved from http://www.trich.org/dnld/ExpertGuidelines_000.pdf.

Tronshaw, N. (2012). *Elimination disorders.* Retrieved from https://www.aacap.org/App_Themes/AACAP/docs/resources_for_primary_care/cap_resources_for_medical_student_educators/elimination_disorders.ppt.

U.S. Department of Health and Human Services (USDHHS). (1999). *Mental health: A report of the Surgeon General, executive summary.* Rockville, MD: USDHHS.

Warden, S., Spiwak, R., Sareen, J., et al. (2014). The SAD PERSONS Scale for suicide risk: A systematic review. *Archives of Suicide Research, 18*(4), 313–326.

White, M. P., & Koran, L. M. (2011). Open-label trial of aripiprazole in the treatment of trichotillomania. *Journal of Clinical Psychopharmacology, 31*(4), 503–506.

27

Adults

Edward A. Herzog

http://evolve.elsevier.com/Varcarolis/essentials

KEY TERMS AND CONCEPTS

cognitive behavioral therapy (CBT), p. 423
community mental health centers
   (CMHCs), p. 422
continuous positive airway pressure
   (CPAP), p. 433
deinstitutionalization, p. 421
impulse control disorders, p. 423
mental health courts, p. 421
National Alliance on Mental Illness
   (NAMI), p. 422

outpatient commitment, p. 420
paraphilias and paraphilic disorders, p. 426
peer specialist, p. 423
Programs of Assertive Community
   Treatment (PACT or ACT), p. 423
reality testing, p. 421
recidivism, p. 428
recovery model, p. 422
rehabilitation model, p. 422
severe mental illness (SMI), p. 418

sleep apnea and hypopnea, p. 431
sleep disorders, p. 431
sleep hygiene, p. 433
social skills training, p. 423
supported employment, p. 423
teletherapy, p. 423
transinstitutionalization, p. 421

SELECTED CONCEPT: IT TECHNOLOGIES TO FACILITATE AND INCREASE PATIENT FOLLOW-UP

Service providers in remote locations are using **"electronic technologies,"** such as speaking with patients by phone, computer-based video or Skype, email, or closed-circuit television, when patients cannot find transportation or travel to distant services.

The new communication technologies are increasingly being used to treat and follow up via chat messaging systems on the health care website, etc. These technologies have been especially effective in depression and anxiety disorders and are proving to be a needed and effective mode of communication for those who live in rural areas (Chan, Parish, & Yellowlees, 2015).

OBJECTIVES

1. Discuss ways in which severe mental illness affects individuals, families, and society.
2. **QSEN** Discuss the **safety** issues and problems experienced by those living with severe mental illness (SMI).
3. **QSEN** Describe **evidence-based treatments** for SMI.
4. Role-play a therapeutic interaction designed to improve treatment adherence for an individual with SMI.
5. Describe common sleep disorders, their treatment, and related nursing care.
6. Describe the core characteristics of impulse control disorders and their societal implications.
7. Role-play a therapeutic interaction with a person who is portraying impulse control disorders.
8. Describe sexual disorders and their implications for society.
9. Discuss the forms of treatment for pedophilia disorder.
10. Role-play a therapeutic interaction with a person who is portraying attention-deficit/hyperactivity disorder (ADHD).

INTRODUCTION

This chapter focuses on mental health issues and needs affecting primarily the adult population. We look at what it is like to have a severe mental illness (SMI), the issues and challenges faced by those diagnosed with these illnesses, and resources and treatment programs available for persons with SMIs. Other adult mental health issues examined in this chapter include disorders involving **impulse control and sexual functioning, sleep-related disorders,** and adult **attention-deficit/hyperactivity disorder (ADHD).**

UNDERSTANDING SEVERE MENTAL ILLNESS

Categorizing mental illness according to levels of severity has significant implications for setting mental health policy, determining insurance reimbursement, and facilitating access to appropriate care. The federal government classifies mental illness as "serious mental illness" (SMI, or mental disorders that significantly interfere with functioning). Each year in the United States, 4% of all adults experience a severe mental illness (Substance Abuse and Mental Health Services Administration [SAMHSA], 2014a). In this chapter, the focus is on severe mental illness, such as schizophrenia and bipolar disorder, which affects about half of the people in the SMI group. SMI involves significant continuous or reoccurring impairment of global functioning that creates disability in 30% to 50% of cases. Other SMIs include severe forms of depression, panic disorder, and obsessive-compulsive disorder.

VIGNETTE

You are a 19-year-old nursing student working as a nursing assistant. One night, while studying alone in your dorm, you hear someone call your name. No one is there, and you attribute it to lack of sleep. However, over the coming weeks this happens repeatedly, and the voices begin to comment on what you are doing, to criticize you, and to tell you what to do. You have trouble concentrating. Your schoolwork and grades suffer. It seems like people know what you're thinking, or hate you; now uncomfortable around others, you begin to avoid friends, skip classes, and quit work.

Distracted by ever-present voices, you step into the street and are struck by a car. A police officer comes to your aid, but you believe he wants to kill you and you run, only to be caught and restrained. The next few days are a confusing, frightening blur of doctors, nurses, injections, and restraints. You are on a psychiatric unit and told that you have something called schizophreniform disorder.

Medications push the voices into the background, but you feel disconnected, like you are wrapped in layers of cotton. Just as you begin to trust some of the staff, you are discharged with an appointment to see a new doctor in a mental health center far from your neighborhood. At the center people look and act strangely; some mumble to themselves, some get too close to you, and some pull away when you walk by. You think, "This can't be happening," and you wonder what your future will be like.

Individuals with SMI usually have difficulties in multiple areas, including activities of daily living (e.g., cooking, hygiene), relationships, social interaction, task completion, communication, leisure activities, safe movement about the community, finances and budgeting, health maintenance, vocational and academic activities, and coping with stressors. Associated issues for those with SMI include poverty, stigma, isolation, unemployment, poorer health outcomes, law enforcement encounters, victimization, and inadequate housing or homelessness.

Extent of the Problem
Effect on an Individual with Severe Mental Illness

Individuals with SMI often fall well short of their potential, experiencing significantly less academic, vocational, and relational success than they would have otherwise. They are often stigmatized and can experience rejection and discrimination. They are more likely to be victims of crime, have undertreated or untreated illnesses, die prematurely, be homeless, be incarcerated, be unemployed or underemployed, engage in substance abuse, live in poverty, and report a lower quality of life than those without such illnesses.

Effect on Families, Caregivers, and Significant Others

The burden on caregivers is significant and is affected by their own coping abilities, support systems, and financial and other resources. Caregivers may not understand the mental illness, may not know how to cope with it or how to help, and may not have access to their loved one's treatment team, leaving them feeling frustrated and powerless. Chronic caregiving demands can result in burnout, maladaptive coping, withdrawal from the patient, and even rejection or abuse (Settineri et al., 2014). Caregivers themselves can also be stigmatized simply by being associated with a person with SMI, leading them to keep the problem a secret and reducing access to social support.

Effect on Society

Historically, most treatment for severe mental illness has been financed with public dollars rather than private insurance; however, this is changing as a result of recent legislation (such as the Patient Protection and Affordable Care Act) pertaining to health care insurance and **parity** for mental illness coverage (e.g., requiring benefits for mental health and substance abuse treatment to be equal to those for medical illness) (Walker, 2014). Recent Medicaid expansion in a number of states represents a greater cost to taxpayers, but is expected to make more care available to persons with SMI. Such improved treatment is anticipated to help reduce costs such as lost economic output, which is expected to total $16.3 trillion worldwide between 2011 and 2030 (World Health Organization [WHO], 2013). Social Security Disability Income (SSDI), for disabled persons with a significant work history, and Supplemental Security Income (SSI), for indigents ineligible for SSDI, both provide income to assist people with SMIs who meet government criteria; income for an individual, however, is limited (for SSI the limit is $733 per month) and is reduced based on assets and non-SSI income (Social Security Administration, 2015). Persons with untreated or inadequately treated SMI are more likely to commit criminal offenses and be incarcerated. Finally, because these illnesses strike in the prime of life, they are among the top four causes of disability in those under 45 years of age (Murray et al., 2013).

Issues Facing Those with Severe Mental Illness

Even with successful treatment, people with SMI often experience **residual symptoms and relapse** (a reoccurring or worsening of one's illness), which can occur even when one adheres to treatment. These can lead to frustration and a fear that one will not get better, or that one's treatments are not effective. In turn, the patient may decide to discontinue treatment, ironically worsening the course of the illness and increasing the negative consequences to self and society.

Medication side effects can include a wide range of distressing effects, including sedation, visual blurring, involuntary movements, weight gain, sexual dysfunction, and medical conditions such as metabolic syndrome (hyperlipidemia, increased insulin resistance, increased abdominal fat deposits). Newer antipsychotic agents tend to have fewer and more tolerable side effects but can be more expensive and can cause metabolic syndrome, increasing the risk of cardiovascular disease and diabetes. Addressing side effects is essential because they may impair one's quality of life or lead to treatment nonadherence. Patient education is important because some side effects respond to treatment (e.g., antiparkinsonian drugs reducing involuntary movements) or can be counteracted by lifestyle or behavior changes (e.g., changing position slowly to prevent dizziness from orthostatic hypotension). Refer to Chapter 17 for a discussion of antipsychotics and patient and family teaching for these drugs.

Loss, hopelessness, and depression. Relapse may lead to feelings of guilt and helplessness. Persons with SMI may experience a profound sense of loss for the future they had anticipated, contributing to major depression or hopelessness. For example, one may have been a pre-med student with hopes of medical school, but a severe mental illness may leave the person unable to perform schoolwork, employed in a minimum wage job, and living in a group home. This loss of potential, along with the demands and effects of chronic illness on daily life, can lead to despair, substance abuse, or suicidality, especially if the individual has no family or outside supports (between 5% and 10% of those with SMI commit suicide).

Co-occurring medical illnesses, some a consequence of medication, frequently exist in severe mental illness. *Poverty* and lack of access to quality foods can cause poor nutrition. *Anhedonia* (inability to experience pleasure) and *anergia* (reduced spontaneous movement) lead to a sedentary lifestyle. People with SMI may not provide for their own health needs and may not receive adequate care because of costs, difficulty accessing health care, or ill will (e.g., emergency department personnel assuming that because a person is psychotic his chest pain is not real). Presenting complaints may be expressed bizarrely (e.g., describing pain as "demons sticking needles in me") and be misunderstood by staff. People with SMI may also make ill-advised choices regarding substance abuse or sexual activity, risking sexually transmitted infections (STIs) and unplanned pregnancies. The final result is that persons with SMI die 25 years earlier and have a risk of death that is 2.5 times that of the general population (Welsh & McEnany, 2015).

Unemployment and poverty contribute to poor self-esteem and lack of identity. Eighty-five percent of people with SMI are unemployed, and a person disabled by an SMI on SSI receives less than 25% of the median income (National Alliance on Mental Illness [NAMI], 2010). It can be difficult to find an employer open to hiring a person with an SMI, and laws to prevent discrimination do not guarantee a job.

Housing instability can contribute to stress for individuals with SMI. Persons who cannot afford a car need to live near public transportation, reducing their options. Limited affordable housing may require them to live where gunshots are common occurrences—not a good situation for anyone, let alone a person overwhelmed by mental illness. An episode of inappropriate behavior could lead to eviction and difficulty obtaining future housing.

Stigma about mental illness is a significant problem. Stigma is perpetuated by stereotypical images or language in the media, thoughtless comments by everyday people or celebrities, and misperceptions of mental illness. It can cause people to assume that those with SMI are less capable, responsible for their own illness, and even dangerous. It can leave the affected person feeling ashamed or angry, pushing one away from others and reducing access to potential support systems. Many people do not yet realize that calling a mentally ill person "crazy" is equivalent to calling someone with an intellectual disability a "retard." Mental health consumers and their advocates, such as the National Alliance on Mental Illness (NAMI) and other advocacy groups, work to reduce stigma, just as was once necessary for the stigma affecting intellectually disabled persons. Refer to Chapter 2 for more on stigma.

Social isolation and loneliness are significant issues for people with chronic illnesses, not just those with SMI. Stigma and social stratification reduce social contact with groups that are outside the mainstream, such as individuals with SMI. Poverty (which interferes with participation in social or recreational activities), impaired hygiene, gaps in social skills, and anxiety also reduce interaction and social support. Medication may reduce one's libido or sexual function and interfere with intimate physical relationships. Negative self-image and delusional thinking may create additional barriers to relationships. As a result, many people with SMI are socially isolated and experience significant amounts of loneliness.

Inadequate treatment and treatment nonadherence. Nearly half of all people with SMI may be receiving treatment that is dated, doesn't match guidelines, or is unsupported by current research (NAMI, 2010). Incorporating treatment innovations and changing practice standards can be a slow process. The newest medications or other treatments may be excluded from state hospital formularies or unapproved by third-party payers. Reduced public funding for health services during times of economic cutbacks intensifies problems with treatment access and

quality. Some medications can cost up to $20,000 per year, and even with Medicaid, co-pays or a spend-down (a need to exhaust one's own funds each month in order to reestablish Medicaid eligibility) may be required. Persons with very limited income may opt to spend it on personal needs instead of treatment. Stigma may lead a person to discontinue treatment so that he or she will not be labeled as mentally ill. Staff turnover and insufficient time to establish therapeutic relationships may reduce trust in staff and increase treatment resistance. Nonadherence increases the risk of relapse by 4 to 7 times.

Anosognosia, the inability of a person to recognize that he or she has an illness because of the illness itself, also contributes to nonadherence. With mental illness it is the brain itself, the same organ needed for self-awareness, that is sick. It is an extremely frustrating dilemma, and one that contributes significantly to treatment nonadherence and all its attendant problems (NAMI, 2015b). Consider: Would you take medicine for an illness you do not believe you have?

Substance use disorder co-occurs in 50% of those with an SMI. It may be maladaptive coping or self-medicating, a way of countering the dysphoria or other symptoms of one's illness or the side effects of one's medications (NAMI, 2015a). Substance abuse interferes with psychiatric treatment and contributes to relapse, physical health problems, incarceration, and reduced quality of life. Persons with concurrent psychiatric and substance abuse disorders are said to have a **dual diagnosis**. Persons with SMI are twice as likely to smoke, and less likely to reduce tobacco use, compared to the general population (Cook et al., 2014).

Victimization occurs more than twice as often among mentally ill people (Latalova et al., 2014). Impaired judgment; impaired interpersonal skills (e.g., unknowingly acting in ways that might provoke others, such as standing too close or not responding to commands); poor self-esteem; appearing more vulnerable to criminals; and living in high-crime, transient, and drug-infested neighborhoods all can contribute to victimization. Sexual victimization, such as sexual assault or coerced sexual activity, also occurs (e.g., a person whose boyfriend "loaned" her sexually to peers in return for drugs, compelling her to cooperate in return for housing).

Issues Affecting Society and the Individual

Some with SMI cannot be persuaded to accept treatment. **Involuntary treatment** involves treatment mandated by court order and delivered without the person's consent. Outpatient commitment requires that persons with SMI accept outpatient treatment and is designed to provide for mandatory continuing treatment in the least restrictive setting, typically after the patient leaves a hospital or prison. It is a form of assisted treatment that helps people with anosognosia and/or treatment resistance to maintain the best mental health status possible (Swanson & Swartz, 2014).

Criminalization of the mentally ill refers to persons with SMI being arrested for behavior caused by their illness instead of being treated as ill. Criminal actions may be the result of desperation, impaired judgment, psychotic thinking, or impulsivity. Those who are untreated have more symptoms and impairment and may become disruptive or commit (usually nonviolent) offenses such as trespassing. For example, during the winter a homeless man with SMI loiters in laundromats and libraries for warmth. He refuses traditional shelters and is at risk for hypothermia, so police who are not aware of other options may jail him for trespassing simply to protect him from hypothermia. Alternately, he might disrupt others at the library and be charged with disorderly conduct. Advocates for persons with SMI strongly support efforts to **decriminalize** behavior caused by mental illness. An important intervention is educating police and first responders (e.g., through crisis intervention training programs sponsored jointly by police and mental health agencies) to recognize mental illness, to safely de-escalate persons with SMI, and to connect mentally ill citizens with help and treatment instead of jailing them (Compton et al., 2014). Mental health courts are designed to intercept persons with SMI after arrest and divert them to treatment instead of incarceration.

Transinstitutionalization is the shifting of a person or population from one institution to another, such as from state hospitals to jails, prisons, nursing homes, or even the street. Although deinstitutionalization (moving persons from inpatient psychiatric care, such as state hospitals, to the community) was intended to provide care in less restrictive settings and reduce costs for state hospitals, in many cases the new setting is actually more restrictive, and the costs have simply been transferred to another provider (such as prisons or Medicare). Nearly one quarter of all persons under correctional control (imprisonment, probation, or parole) have an SMI, and about 15% of male inmates and 30% of female inmates suffer from SMI (Robertson et al., 2014). There are more persons with SMI in jails and prisons than in psychiatric hospitals, and less than half of those incarcerated were arrested for a violent offense (Kim et al., 2015). Settings such as jails, prisons, and nursing homes often lack the special programming and skilled staff needed to assist persons with SMI, and as a result their recovery and stability may be compromised.

APPLICATION OF THE NURSING PROCESS

ASSESSMENT

Assessment should focus especially on signs of risk to self or others (including unsafe behavior, suicide risk, and homicidal thinking); depression or hopelessness; substance use or abuse; sleep impairment; impulsivity; diminished reality testing (the ability to accurately determine what is or isn't real); delusional thinking; hallucinations; and inadequate attention to proper nutrition, clothing, or medical care. Impaired judgment, paranoia, and psychosis increase the risk of dangerous behavior; such persons may start fires by forgetting pots left on the stove, may hurt self or others in response to command hallucinations, or may hurt a person they perceive as a threat.

It is also essential to observe for signs of impending relapse and treatment nonadherence. Correcting nonadherence helps prevent relapse, and early detection and treatment of relapse reduces its severity and duration. It is also important to assess for physical health problems (e.g., tumors, metabolic disorders) that may cause psychiatric symptoms and be mistaken for mental illness. Monitoring co-occurring illnesses ensures that self-care and health care are satisfactory.

Areas that might need further investigation when planning long-term care for persons with SMI include:

- **Problems involving primary support groups** (death, illness, divorce, sexual or physical abuse, neglect of child, discord with siblings, birth of a sibling)
- **Problems related to the social environment** (death or loss of friends; inadequate social support; isolation; difficulty with acculturation, discrimination, adjustment to life changes [e.g., new housing])
- **Educational problems** (illiteracy, conflict with teachers or classmates, need for accommodation due to SMI symptoms)
- **Occupational problems** (unemployment, potential job loss, work stress, difficult work conditions, job dissatisfaction, unmet need for accommodations, conflict with others)
- **Economic problems** (income insufficient to meet essential needs, access to entitlements)
- **Problems with health care services or access** (inadequate care, lack of transportation to health care facilities, unable to afford treatment)
- **Problems involving crime or law enforcement** (arrest, incarceration, victim of crime)

DIAGNOSIS

Nursing diagnoses for persons who have an SMI include *Impaired adjustment, Compromised family coping, Ineffective individual coping, Ineffective health maintenance, Impaired impulse control, Risk for loneliness, Self-care deficit, Low self-esteem, Treatment non-adherence,* and *Chronic sorrow.* See Table 27-1 for selected interventions that are appropriate for helping persons who have an SMI.

OUTCOMES IDENTIFICATION

The following are examples of potential long-term outcome measures. The individual:

- Identifies "voices" as hallucinations.
- Distinguishes delusional thoughts from reality.
- Remains free from police involvement.
- Maintains stable housing.
- Remains free from harm.
- Demonstrates treatment adherence.

IMPLEMENTATION

Interventions to Promote Treatment Adherence

1. Monitor side effects and provide education and treatment to minimize resulting distress (e.g., for dry mouth, sugar-free lozenges to promote salivation; taking medications earlier in the evening to reduce morning grogginess at work or school).
2. Simplify treatment regimens to make them easier to follow (e.g., once-per-day dosing instead of twice daily).
3. Anosognosia (inability to recognize that one is ill) is a significant factor in nonadherence. Linking treatment adherence to achieving the patient's goals can bypass the patient's lack of insight by motivating with his or her own goals, not the goal of recovering from an illness that he or she cannot perceive (e.g., guide the patient to see that the medications will improve concentration and help the patient keep his or her job).
4. Emphasize and reinforce improvement, connecting this to the patient's treatment adherence.
5. Facilitate access to treatment providers and medication; inconvenient appointment times, inability to reach prescribers for refills, and similar issues are obstacles to adherence.
6. Facilitate referrals for assistance with treatment costs; some pharmaceutical companies have special low-cost options for low-income persons, and some persons may be eligible for Medicaid under Medicaid expansion legislation.
7. To improve insight and motivation, educate consumers about the nature of SMIs and the role of treatment in the person's recovery and quality of life.
8. Assign consistent, committed caregivers who have (or are skilled at building) therapeutic bonds with the patient; trusting one's providers is essential for treatment adherence.
9. Encourage involvement in support groups (e.g., National Alliance on Mental Illness [NAMI], www.NAMI.org); the patient may be more likely to accept support and information from peers who have more insight and experience with SMIs and treatment.
10. Provide culturally sensitive care. Appreciating a person's values and beliefs (such as suspicious attitudes toward authority figures or valuing of self-sufficiency) may be crucial to promoting treatment adherence.
11. When feasible, consider judicious use of medication decreases, changes, or discontinuation to control side effects and/or improve the therapeutic alliance.

TABLE 27-1 Interventions for Severe Mental Illness (SMI)

Intervention	Rationale
1. Mutually develop short- and long-term, consumer-centered goals and interventions that will help the consumer achieve the desired quality of life, rather than focus on symptom reduction.	1. Consumer involvement in goal setting and treatment selection builds the therapeutic alliance, increases the consumer's sense of control over his or her life, and increases the likelihood of treatment adherence and success.
2. Enhance and promote reality testing (e.g., teaching a consumer, when he or she hears voices, to scan the immediate environment to see if anyone else seems to be hearing the voices; if not, encourage the consumer to label it as a hallucination and to disregard it or distract self from it).	2. Impaired reality testing is common in SMI and contributes to hallucinations and delusional thinking. Training and encouraging the consumer to verify whether experiences are real can help the consumer meet his or her goals despite residual symptoms.
3. Provide psychoeducation, guidance, support, and reinforcement for actions that consumers can use to manage their symptoms of SMI (see Box 17-3). Include the family in psychoeducational activities as tolerated and possible.	3. Whistling or other simple auditory distractions can reduce auditory hallucinations; gaining mastery over symptoms improves function, reduces disruption, and provides one with a sense of control and confidence.
4. Reduce loneliness and isolation by interacting frequently with the consumer, supporting opportunities for interaction (e.g., day programs, social and recreational events), helping the consumer to manage social anxiety, helping the consumer who does not want to socialize to identify and use alternative means to achieve support or comfort (e.g., pets, stuffed animals, calling support phone lines), and involving the consumer in social skills training.	4. SMIs decrease sociability and predispose individuals to isolation as a result of stigma, loss of social skills, and social discomfort. Activities that increase skill and comfort with interaction, especially with supportive people and positive role models, such as other consumers who are farther along in recovery, contribute to improved functioning and a higher quality of life.
5. Encourage involvement of consumers and their loved ones in NAMI support meetings and peer-based services.	5. NAMI members and peers "have been there" and can provide support, socialization, and practical suggestions for issues and problems facing consumers and significant others; involvement in such groups also instills hope and empowers the consumer.
6. Provide education and support regarding making sound decisions about interpersonal relations, STI prevention, and family planning.	6. People with SMI may have impaired judgment, feel isolated, and feel vulnerable to victimization, STIs, and undesired pregnancies; consumers seeking to have families may benefit from genetic counseling.
7. Connect the consumer with case managers and other personnel who are likely to be able to work with him or her for extended periods and who are skilled at developing and maintaining therapeutic relationships.	7. Trusting and therapeutic relationships are key resources for achieving treatment adherence, and consumers with SMI often require extended periods of working with staff to form these connections.
8. Actively promote treatment adherence by tying adherence to the consumer's own goals and other motivational and educational approaches.	8. Treatment adherence reduces relapse and improves the long-term prognosis and quality of life.
9. Provide psychosocial support.	9. This aids in maintaining therapeutic rapport and helps the consumer to maintain a positive self-esteem and to cope effectively rather than maladaptively.
10. Provide regular and frequent contact with the consumer, but not so much that it overstimulates the consumer or contributes to paranoia.	10. Ongoing contact promotes therapeutic alliances and allows for monitoring so relapse or nonadherence can quickly be intercepted.
11. Educate, guide, support, and reinforce behaviors that prevent or control actual or potential medical comorbidities; act as an advocate as needed to ensure adequate health care for consumers with SMI.	11. Consumers with SMI have higher burdens of physical illness, poorer hygiene and health practices, less access to effective medical treatment, and more premature mortality than the general population.
12. Involve persons with co-occurring substance abuse or addiction with AA or NA and dual diagnosis SAMI services.	12. Substance abuse rates are high in SMI populations, increase relapse, and interfere with recovery; achieving sobriety is mostly associated with AA and integrated treatment programs.

AA, Alcoholics Anonymous; *NA*, Narcotics Anonymous; *NAMI*, National Alliance on Mental Illness; *SAMI*, substance abuse/mental illness; *STI*, sexually transmitted infection.

12. When medically appropriate, support the use of medication monitoring or long-acting forms of medication (depot injections or sustained-release formats) to maximize the benefits of medication.

13. Never reject, blame, or shame the patient when nonadherence occurs; instead, simply label it as an issue for continuing focus, and understand that adherence often requires numerous attempts.

Pharmacological, Biological, and Integrative Therapies

State hospitals and psychiatric units in general hospitals provide inpatient care. Outpatient care for SMI is provided by community mental health centers (CMHCs), private providers (primarily psychiatrists, psychologists, therapists, social workers, and advanced practice nurses), and private and governmental agencies. Community-based services vary with local needs and resources. Working the maze of multiple agencies and services can be challenging. See Chapter 5 for a full discussion of mental health treatment settings.

Rehabilitation versus Recovery

Until recently the rehabilitation model has been the dominant paradigm in mental health care. It focuses on deficits, symptoms, and stability rather than on quality of life and cure. It has been criticized for stabilization over growth and for producing dependence on health care providers, with staff relating to the patient as parents do to children. As a result, mental health consumers and advocates led a consumer movement that emphasizes choices and empowerment, culminating in the recovery model of care. It is promoted by the National Alliance on Mental Illness

(NAMI), a leading advocacy organization, along with many other mental health organizations and treatment providers. The recovery model stresses a partnership between care providers and the patient, both working together in planning and directing treatment. It emphasizes hope and empowerment and focuses on strengths rather than limitations, helping the consumer to use his or her strengths to achieve the highest quality of life possible. To reflect the emphasis on empowerment in the recovery model, those receiving care are called (mental health) **consumers,** and that term is used in lieu of "patient" hereafter for persons with SMI.

Evidence-Based Treatment Approaches and Services

The following evidence-based treatment approaches are recommended for use for SMI and are available in a variety of settings in many communities.

Programs of Assertive Community Treatment (PACT or ACT) use a treatment team approach and have been shown to improve symptom management and quality of life while reducing incarceration and homelessness (Center for Evidence-Based Practice, 2014). Instead of working with multiple departments or agencies, the consumer works solely with an established team of professionals who provide comprehensive services and 24/7 access to a team member.

Cognitive behavioral therapy (CBT), which helps persons to recognize and reduce unrealistic expectations and distorted thinking, has been effective in helping consumers with SMI to reduce and cope with symptoms such as auditory hallucinations (Zanello et al., 2014). CBT helps consumers perceive circumstances more accurately and positively by guiding them to reconsider their perceptions and restructure their thinking to be more in line with reality. The behavioral component uses natural consequences and positive reinforcers (rewards) to shape the person's behavior in a more positive or adaptive manner.

Promotion of family support and partnerships with providers is based on the premise that having sound support systems is one of the strongest predictors of recovery, and that treatment is enhanced when treatment providers work as empathic partners with consumers and significant others (NAMI, 2012). An example of this partnership is NAMI's Family-to-Family program, a psychoeducational program focusing on the skills families need to cope with their loved one's illness and to promote recovery (NAMI, 2012).

Social skills training focuses on teaching a wide variety of social skills. Social deficits cause both direct and indirect functional impairment; people unable to respond assertively, for example, may instead respond aggressively or may fail to meet their needs at all. Complex interpersonal skills (such as negotiating, or resolving a conflict) are broken down into subcomponents that are then taught in a concrete, stepwise fashion.

Vocational rehabilitation and supported employment enhances self-esteem, improves organizational abilities, and increases socialization and income. Vocational rehabilitation includes prevocational training (skills needed to obtain employment), initial employment in a sheltered setting (e.g., a consumer-managed business), building to competitive employment in the business world. Supported employment focuses on on-the-job training and support, often with job coaches at the employee's side, enabling rapid and continued employment (Waghorn et al., 2014).

Other Potentially Beneficial Approaches or Services

The following offer potential benefit to those living with severe mental illness:

- **Advance directives** give the consumer the opportunity to direct how future relapses and treatment needs should be managed. The directive is a document signed when the consumer's illness is under control and informed decisions are possible. For example, when well, a consumer can give consent to hospitalization or forced medications and specify when these responses may be used, maintaining control over treatment and avoiding involuntary admission and related court involvement.

- **Peer support and consumer-managed programming** range from informal "clubhouses" that offer socialization, recreation, and sometimes other services, to competitive businesses such as snack bars or janitorial services that provide needed services and consumer employment while encouraging independence and building vocational skills. Certified peer specialists are specially trained consumers who are further along in the recovery process and who provide supportive services to persons with SMIs; being in recovery themselves, they serve as role models and sources of hope, and their guidance may be perceived as more acceptable and valid than that provided by staff.

- **Advances in technology** help improve treatment access and outcomes, often while reducing costs. Electronic records available in multiple locations can improve treatment continuity anywhere the consumer may go. Service providers in remote locations are using technologies such as teletherapy—speaking with consumers by phone, computer-based video or Skype, or closed-circuit television—when consumers cannot travel to distant services; this can also save transit time for providers (Furber et al., 2014), freeing more time for providing care. Such technologies are also increasingly used for follow-up care via chat or messaging systems on health care websites. These technologies have been especially useful in depression and anxiety, and for keeping tabs on consumers with adherence issues (Cangelosi & Sorrell, 2014).

IMPULSE CONTROL DISORDERS

VIGNETTE

Kleptomania. Sarah, age 76, is shopping when she notices the lipstick display. She rarely wears lipstick, but is drawn to the display and feels an urge to take one. She suppresses the urge, but it grows harder to resist; ultimately she snatches the lipstick, putting it in her purse. She feels a sense of relief, almost an odd sort of pleasure. Over time this urge to steal things happens increasingly. Usually Sarah cannot resist, sometimes taking ridiculous chances in taking things that she doesn't even need. She feels ashamed and, consumed with remorse, sometimes returns the items or throws them away. Even having been caught and threatened with jail, the irresistible urge to steal continues.

Impulse control disorders involve a decreased ability to resist an impulse to perform certain acts. In most cases the pattern is one of increasing tension that builds until a particular action is taken, followed by a sense of relief. The actions may be impulsive (e.g., stealing) or involve considerable planning (e.g., fire setting), and range from benign or potentially harmful to self or others. The tension reduction reinforces the action and makes future resistance more difficult. Except for pathological gambling, these disorders are considered to be relatively rare (Table 27-2).

THEORY

Biological Factors

The causes underlying impulse control disorders are not clearly established. Certain disorders or abnormalities of the brain seem to increase impulsiveness or reduce one's ability to resist impulses.

Violent people often show electroencephalographic differences and may have higher serotonin metabolite levels in their cerebrospinal fluid (CSF) (Diaz, 2010). Frontotemporal dementia or tumors (especially those affecting the right hemisphere), Parkinson's disease, dementia, and multiple sclerosis can contribute to impulsivity, as can traumatic brain injury and substance abuse, but the link in these disorders is unclear. Dopamine receptor agonists (such as certain stimulants and antiparkinsonian medications) can also impair impulse control (Moore et al., 2014).

Genetic Factors

A gene associated with impulsive violence is suspected of weakening the brain's impulse control circuitry (Baum, 2013). Although the incidence of some impulse disorders is greater within families (e.g., trichotillomania), neither this gene nor others have been linked causally to these disorders.

Psychological Factors

Theories regarding psychological causes of these disorders include an impaired ability to manage anxiety, wherein the person might be defending against (coping with) anxiety by subconsciously choosing an action that gives a sense of control over the anxiety. This theory is supported by a pattern of increased impulsive acts during periods of high stress. Some of these disorders may be a variant, or an expression,

of disorders such as obsessive-compulsive disorder (OCD) or posttraumatic stress disorder (PTSD). Finally, a person may experience craving for the act and relief upon achieving it, suggesting an addictions-based etiology.

CLINICAL PICTURE

The person experiences a recurring and irresistible urge to enact a behavior despite its being illogical, distressing, or potentially harmful. Judgment is intact and psychotic elements are absent. Descriptions of each disorder can be found in Table 27-2.

Effect on Individuals, Families, and Society

People with impulse control disorders usually realize that the acts are illogical or wrong, but despite their best efforts, the urge to act overwhelms them. They are often confused and troubled by their urges, feeling embarrassment, shame, or guilt as a result of their behaviors; these responses can lead to depression and suicidality (Grant & Leppink, 2015). They may find themselves socially isolated or stigmatized.

Kleptomania can contribute to shoplifting losses. Gambling can cause tremendous personal financial losses and disrupt families, and cause loss of status, housing, possessions, jobs, and marriages. Intermittent explosive disorder and pyromania can cause property damage

TABLE 27-2	**Impulse Control Disorder**
Name	**Description**
Intermittent explosive disorder	Recurrent, unpremeditated episodes of marked verbal or behavioral aggression or rage. The acts are often severe enough to hurt people or destroy significant property and occur in otherwise normal individuals. The acts are disproportionate to the perceived provocation and can occur in response to ordinarily minor events such as traffic delays. The individual may feel depressed or remorseful afterward, and may face recrimination, arrest, civil actions, and loss of relationships and employment as a result of the acts. "Road rage" is sometimes a manifestation of this disorder.
Kleptomania	An uncontrollable and recurrent urge to steal. The thefts produce a sense of psychological gratification and often involve items of little value or use to the person who takes them. Persons often report a buildup of tension before stealing and a sense of relief afterward (APA, 2013). The objects taken may have a symbolic meaning (such as power or beauty), but often the person cannot explain the reason and usually perceives the thefts as illogical and wrong. Kleptomania may begin at any age, and two thirds of people affected are women. The behavior may occur at widely scattered intervals or be more regular and protracted. Prosecution may occur, though mental health advocates distinguish kleptomanic behavior from criminality.
Pyromania	A reoccurring compulsion to set fires and experiencing a sense of accomplishment or relief when setting fires, often accompanied by a sense of pleasure or release (APA, 2013). The fires are set for sexual or other emotional gratification, not arson for profit or revenge. The person has a fascination with fires and "gains great pleasure from starting them, watching them, helping to put them out, and watching what happened afterwards" (Francis 2013, p. 141), but has little regard for the life or property that may be destroyed in the fire. These individuals are known to cause false alarms or even become firefighters as part of the disorder, and may make elaborate preparations to start the fire. This disorder may result in criminal prosecution.
Gambling disorder	A preoccupation with gambling and an inability to resist the urge to gamble despite significant disruption of family, finances, work, and other aspects of one's life; sometimes known as pathological gambling. The individual feels aroused and positive when gambling and experiences a relief of tension. The gambler can't get enough and finds he or she needs to raise the stakes to feel the same high. When not gambling, the person experiences irritability, restlessness, anxiety, and sadness and can't wait to get back to the action (withdrawal) (Francis 2013, p. 139). Pathological gamblers may lie, rationalize, manipulate others, and conceal their behavior in order to maintain it. Work and social functioning may be disrupted. Most people with this disorder are men, and the lifetime prevalence of this disorder is about 0.5% to 1% (APA, 2013), but it may be higher in settings where gambling opportunities are more varied and easily accessed, and in families in which other members also have the disorder (refer to Chapter 19). The *DSM-5* categorizes this as an addictive disorder (APA, 2013).
Trichotillomania	Repetitively pulling out one's hair in order to relieve tension. The person may pull out hair only occasionally and for brief periods, or regularly and for hours at a time. It tends to worsen under stress but also occurs when the person is calm, sometimes in an almost absent-minded fashion. Occasionally the hair is ingested and can produce "hairballs" similar to those seen in animals. The hair loss is often noticeable and significantly affects the individual's social comfort and self-esteem, sometimes causing severe distress. It may be self-limited or continue for decades and can involve hair from any location.

Data from American Psychiatric Association. (2013). *Diagnostic and statistical manual of mental disease (DSM-5)* (5th ed.). Washington, DC: APA; Francis, A. (2013). *Essentials of psychiatric diagnoses: responding to the challenges of DSM-5.* New York, NY: Guilford Press.

and injury or death to others, and can place the person at risk of being sued or injured by the victim's defensive response. When criminal offenses are involved, society pays the costs of prosecution, incarceration, and forensic treatment, and the individual may subsequently lose civil rights (e.g., the right to vote) or access to private or governmental entitlements (e.g., eligibility for federal housing assistance, ability to hold a professional license or work in a particular field).

APPLICATION OF THE NURSING PROCESS

ASSESSMENT

The diagnosis of impulse control disorders first requires elimination of all other medical and psychiatric causes for the behavior (e.g., antisocial personality disorder, substance abuse), as well as ruling out other causes such as seeking profit or attaining revenge.

Information suggesting the presence of an impulse control disorder is often minimized, withheld, or concealed by the person or overlooked by staff; careful assessment is therefore important. Because the nurse's beliefs and attitudes about the behaviors in question may compromise his or her ability to perceive or remain objective about the disorder, self-awareness is essential. For example, if the nurse believes that setting fires is simply criminal behavior and not related to a mental disorder, the nurse may overlook the impulse control disorder or fail to help the person obtain care.

Because actions associated with impulse control disorders may be embarrassing or even criminal in nature, building trust and conveying empathy and acceptance are key to helping the person disclose these problems. Significant others who may be less reluctant to share information can also help identify concealed disorders. Nurses should look for patterns of recurrent loss of control in the consumer's responses and history, and should observe for signs such as fascination with fire, unusual familiarity with gambling terminology, patches where hair is thin, or pulling at one's hair.

It is helpful to ask about circumstances that increase tension, as well as ways in which the person reduces this tension. Empathic prompting can be helpful (e.g., "Sometimes people find themselves feeling tense and having urges to do things to release the tension. Can you tell me about times when this may have happened to you?"). Frank, direct questioning can set a tone for openness and prompt more candid responses (e.g., "Tell me about times when you've come close to losing control.").

A person's legal history may also suggest these disorders. Recurrent assaults or any episodes of fire setting merit further assessment. Further, the person may be dealing with concurrent depression or be sufficiently distressed to be considering self-harm. Assessment for these risks is essential. Finally, it is always important to assess how the disorder has affected the consumer and significant others, as well as the consumer's knowledge of the disorder and ways of reducing or coping with it.

DIAGNOSIS

A variety of nursing diagnoses may apply to people with impulse control disorders: *Impaired impulse control, Impaired adjustment, Anxiety, Compromised family coping, Ineffective coping, Risk for injury, Low self-esteem, Impaired social interaction,* and *Social isolation* (NANDA-I, 2012–2014). Nursing interventions for these disorders vary with the disorder, but some general interventions likely to fit most are listed in Table 27-3.

OUTCOMES IDENTIFICATION

Expected outcomes vary with the disorder but typically focus on reducing the problematic acts and substituting more adaptive means to reduce tension. Examples include: "(Person) does not set fires," "Hair loss is reduced by 20%," "(Person) demonstrates use of three or more tension reduction strategies," and "(Person) rates anxiety as 5 or less on a 0–10 scale."

TABLE 27-3 Interventions for Impulse Control Disorders	
Intervention	**Rationale**
1. Guide the person to understand and practice tension reduction and stress control strategies such as stress avoidance, correction of negative self-talk, and breathing control exercises.	1. Tension usually precedes and contributes to impulsive actions; tension reduction and adaptive tension management can reduce impulsive behavior.
2. Promote the progressive substitution of alternate, less maladaptive responses to tension, such as applying pressure to one's scalp with a thumb rather than pulling out one's hair.	2. Impulse control disorders involve maladaptive behaviors, some of which are criminal offenses; substitution of more adaptive responses can prevent negative consequences.
3. Assist the person to explore feelings associated with the impulses, such as shame, fear, or guilt, and to manage these feelings adaptively.	3. Negative emotions contribute to stress and tension, leading to maladaptive impulsive behaviors.
4. Assist the person to identify the consequences of his or her actions (e.g., "How do other people respond when you _____?" "Tell me what things are like the day after you've set a fire," "Imagine you set the fire: what do you think will happen in the days and weeks that follow?" [anticipatory fantasy])	4. Identifying consequences can help the person become more empathic to his or her effect on others, and increase motivation to refrain from problematic behaviors. Anticipatory fantasy guides the person to imagine the consequences of behavior and dampen urges to act on impulses.
5. Educate the person that drugs and alcohol may increase impulsiveness through disinhibition or impairment of judgment; educate the person regarding the effect of "triggers," that is, circumstances that evoke tension or impulses (e.g., going to bars).	5. Disinhibiting drugs and exposure to triggers that evoke impulsive behavior increase impulsive actions; reducing disinhibition and exposure to triggers reduces the frequency and intensity of the impulsive actions.
6. Pathological gamblers may respond well to group therapy; organizations such as Gamblers Anonymous (www.gamblersanonymous.org) provide significant assistance through support, education, and practical tips on managing gambling impulses and other concerns.	6. Twelve-step programs have been shown to be of significant help in reducing activities that have a compulsive or addictive component; peer support groups are effective for confronting defenses and rationalization used to support the gambling.
7. Persons with trichotillomania can benefit from special hair styling, hair weaves, or other cosmetology assistance; they may require considerable support in order to access such resources, however, because of embarrassment.	7. Hair loss can create a significant cosmetic defect, resulting in impaired self-esteem and further dysfunctional coping; compensating cosmetically for such defects can enhance the person's self-image and self-esteem.

IMPLEMENTATION

Pharmacological, Biological, and Integrative Therapies

Treatment for impulse control disorders may involve a combination of psychotherapy and medication. Because these disorders usually do not create an imminent risk to oneself or others, or present with emergent needs, treatment is usually provided on an outpatient basis.

Psychopharmacology

Selective serotonin reuptake inhibitors (SSRIs), the antidepressant bupropion, and opioid antagonists (e.g., naltrexone) are used in the treatment of kleptomania, trichotillomania, and pathological gambling (Tanwani et al., 2014). Lithium, a mood stabilizer; methylphenidate, a stimulant; and the antipsychotic risperidone may be helpful in the treatment of conduct disorder, a child/adolescent disorder with similarities to intermittent explosive disorder (Grant & Leppink, 2015).

Opioid antagonists (e.g., nalmefene) may be of particular benefit in pathological gambling (Grant et al., 2006). Anticonvulsants, lithium, SSRIs, and propranolol and similar β-adrenergic antagonists have shown possible efficacy for reducing aggression, particularly in individuals whose impulse control problems seem to stem from organic disorders such as dementia (Tanwani et al., 2014).

Nonpharmacological Treatments

Hypnotherapy may be of benefit in selected disorders, and cognitive behavioral approaches such as habit reversal (identifying and reducing thoughts that trigger undesired actions) and sensitization (imagining negative consequences such as getting caught when the urge occurs) are evidence-based practices in disorders such as trichotillomania (Garrett & Giddings, 2014). Biofeedback and behavioral conditioning (through the use of positive rewards and negative consequences) have been proposed for reducing habitual and impulsive behaviors (Howard et al., 2013). Group psychotherapy provides for therapeutic confrontation from peers and tends to be particularly helpful for people who have poor insight or difficulty accepting responsibility for their behavior.

SEXUAL DIFFERENCES AND SEXUAL DISORDERS

Sexual disorders involve sexual function and identity.

GENDER DYSPHORIA

Gender dysphoria, previously known as *gender identity disorder* (but now considered in the mental health field to be a *difference*, and **not a disorder or pathology**) is thought to be rather rare. It involves persistent, strong cross-gender identification wherein a person feels he or she is of a different gender than that indicated by his or her physiology (or that assigned by society in the case of ambiguous genitalia). It typically first becomes apparent in childhood or adolescence, and the cause is unknown; theories include abnormalities in sexual hormones and related neurodevelopment in utero or developmental differences in early life.

Often the person with gender dysphoria believes that he or she was born in the wrong body. People with gender dysphoria experience persistent discomfort with their present gender and their gender-related roles, and possess a strong and persistent desire to assume the characteristics (e.g., dress and mannerisms) and roles of the opposite gender, as well as a desire to have the primary and secondary sex characteristics of the other gender (American Psychiatric Association [APA], 2013). Persons with gender dysphoria may alter their dress, use hormonal medications, and pursue surgery in order to appear as, or become, their perceived gender.

People with gender dysphoria may experience significant embarrassment, shame, discrimination, and social isolation because many people in our society do not understand how one could believe that one is not of the gender that nature appeared to intend. There is considerable stigma about gender dysphoria, and others may react with repugnance. Gender dysphoria also raises practical issues: If you feel that you are female, you might prefer to use a restroom labeled for females; however, if you appear to others as a male, women might take exception to your presence in a restroom designated for females, and could even assume you are committing criminal behavior such as voyeurism.

Persons who choose sexual reassignment engage in specific steps to prepare for what lies ahead:

1. Counseling to assist the person in fully considering and preparing for this very involved and protracted (long-term) process.
2. Living for a period (e.g., 1 to 2 years) as a member of the desired gender (to ensure readiness). During this time the person is usually given hormonal therapy to suppress undesired physical characteristics and elicit desired sexual characteristics (e.g., to diminish facial hair and enlarge breasts, or to alter one's voice); this may be the last step for many people.
3. Surgical intervention to alter the person's genitalia to match those of the desired gender.

PARAPHILIAS AND PARAPHILIC DISORDERS

Paraphilias are sexual acts or fantasies that involve deviation from conventional, socially acceptable sexual behavior. They are not disorders per se; they are on a continuum with normal sexual interests and practices, and unless the person experiences distress about the sexual differences, they typically do not merit a need for treatment (Holoyda & Kellaher, 2016). The incidence of paraphilias is difficult to measure because stigma, potential for embarrassment, and other concerns cause reluctance to disclose this information. Divergent religious and cultural beliefs have created a conflict within our society about how to define appropriate sexual behavior. For example, opinions vary widely in terms of what is an appropriate age to begin sexual relations, or whom one should be able to choose as a sexual partner; conflict stemming from such beliefs can result in ostracism, hostility, and even aggression. Education, counseling, and support are helpful both for persons who come to perceive themselves as "perverted" or abnormal as a result of negative societal views and for family members and significant others who are hurt and confused.

In contrast, paraphilic disorders are defined in the *DSM-5* as paraphilias that cause distress, risk of harm, or actual harm to oneself or others (APA, 2013). Paraphilic disorders involve a preoccupation with sexual fantasies and related urges and behaviors that focus on nontraditional or socially unacceptable sexual "targets" such as children, animals, or objects. Persons with these disorders may or may not act on their fantasies and urges; enacting such fantasies can involve criminal acts.

THEORY

Biological Factors

The causes underlying paraphilic disorders have not yet been determined. As with impulse control disorders involving gambling or stealing, certain abnormalities of the brain can reduce one's ability to resist sexual impulses; examples include frontotemporal dementia, tumors, and Parkinson's disease, which have been documented as contributing to paraphilic disorders such as pedophilia (Rahman & Symeonides, 2008). Increased sympathetic activity and reduced serotonergic activity have been implicated in pedophilia. Traumatic brain injuries and cognitive impairment are also associated with impulsive behavior and behavioral dyscontrol generally (Rosenbloom et al., 2012).

Psychological Factors

A failure to develop appropriate attachments in early childhood, resulting in inadequate or inappropriate attachments at later developmental stages, may contribute to paraphilic disorders. Another theory is that the disorders are learned responses to inappropriate sexual role models. One's own sexual victimization may contribute to paraphilic disorders, particularly those associated with sexual offenses; 30% to 60% of pedophiles were themselves sexually abused as children. Funding entities and research institutions, perhaps because of the sometimes controversial aspects of these disorders, are sometimes reluctant to support research related to the causes and treatment of paraphilic disorders, limiting our understanding (Arehart-Treichel, 2006).

CLINICAL PICTURE

The *DSM-5* distinguishes multiple types of paraphilic disorders, described in Table 27-4. The diagnosis of these disorders first requires eliminating all other medical and psychiatric causes of the behavior in question (e.g., criminal intent, mania, dementia, substance abuse).

Paraphilic disorders do not involve psychotic features, and most have their onset during adolescence. Most people with paraphilic disorders are male, and diagnosis requires that the features must have been present for at least 6 months (i.e., occasional experiences of gratification through paraphilic-like experiences would not meet the diagnostic criteria for a paraphilia).

Although not paraphilic disorders, sexual addiction and other forms of distress or dysfunction related to sexuality can be diagnosed as *sexual disorders not otherwise specified* (NOS). Other disorders related to sexuality, although not covered in this chapter or classified as sexual disorders, include those relating to chromosomal abnormalities (e.g., Klinefelter's syndrome), head trauma or other organic disorder, compulsive use of pornography, and sexual aberrations arising from SMIs that affect impulse control and social and sexual interaction.

Effect on Individuals, Families, and Society

The effect of paraphilias may be relatively minor and limited to the individual with the diagnosis (e.g., a person with transvestic fetishism). When people with paraphilias engage sexually with unwilling partners (e.g., frotteurism or voyeurism), victims may feel violated and experience significant and protracted psychological distress.

TABLE 27-4 Paraphilic Disorders

Name	Description
Fetish	Any unusual preoccupation or desire for an object, body part, or activity that one needs in order to achieve sexual gratification. The object of the fetish is not one typically associated with sexual gratification by most persons within a given culture. It is a paraphilia (an unusual sexual interest), and not typically a sexual disorder in that it does not cause significant distress or harm.
Exhibitionistic disorder	The achievement of sexual arousal or pleasure by exposing one's genitals, usually to an unsuspecting stranger. Sufferers have strong, recurrent fantasies about exposing genitalia. Upon exhibiting genitalia, one may experience shame and embarrassment, and can face criminal charges and loss of relationships and employment. Exhibitionism usually starts in adolescence, and seems to taper off by age 40.
Fetishistic disorder (Fetishism)	Having difficult achieving sexual arousal except when using or thinking about an inanimate object or part of the body. The individual experiences significant distress and the fetish objects are not those usually associated with sexual arousal (e.g., feet, shoes).
Frottteuristic disorder (Frotteurism)	Obtaining sexual arousal and gratification from rubbing one's genitals against unsuspecting others in public places. It causes marked distress or interpersonal difficulties, and criminal prosecution can result.
Pedophilia	Pedophilia involves fantasized or actual sexual activity with a prepubescent child, wherein the person has either acted on the fantasies or has experienced significant distress or difficulties as a result of the fantasies (APA, 2013). Pedophiles may focus on children of the same, opposite, or both genders, although most are heterosexually focused. They may focus on children exclusively or may also have a sexual interest in adults. Some with pedophilia focus on relatives (incestual form), others on non–family members, and some on both. The disorder causes revulsion in most adults, and pedophilic actions are often considered the most intolerable of criminal offenses.
Sexual masochism and sexual sadism disorders	Deriving sexual gratification from having pain and/or humiliation inflicted upon oneself (masochism) or creating psychological and physical pain in others (sadism). Masochism can include bondage, verbal abuse, electrical shocks, whipping, being urinated on, or being forced to humiliate oneself. Sadism includes inflicting such acts on a (usually masochistic) partner, and often involves dominating one's partner physically and psychologically. The partner may be consenting or nonconsenting.
Transvestic disorder	Deriving sexual gratification by dressing as a person of the opposite gender. Unlike gender dysphoria, which involves a conflict between one's beliefs about true gender and biological gender (or the gender assigned by society), the transvestite does not perceive a conflict with gender, but enjoys dressing in a gender-incongruent manner.
Voyeuristic disorder	Also known as voyeurism, this disorder involves deriving sexual gratification from observing unsuspecting persons in sexually arousing situations (e.g., undressing or engaging in sexual activity).

American Psychiatric Association. (2013). *Diagnostic and statistical manual of mental disease (DSM-5)* (5th ed.). Washington, DC: APA.

Paraphilic, and especially pedophilic, *offenders* can harm or kill their victims, and even when the victim is physically uninjured, there is often significant, protracted, and sometimes disabling psychological damage. Survivors are at increased risk of disorders such as PTSD, depression, anxiety, and substance abuse disorders. Families, loved ones, and the general community are often traumatized and left unable to trust others or feel fully secure (refer to Chapter 22).

Sexual abuse is a significant problem in our society. However, only a portion of this abuse involves pedophilia. Parents and caregivers commit up to 90% or more of the sexual abuse of children in the United States, while strangers are believed to account for less than 5% of child sexual offenses (refer to Chapter 21). Family members may choose children not because of sexual attraction per se (as would most pedophiles) but because they are readily accessible, often unable to resist, and able to be controlled by the abuser through threat and intimidation. The recidivism (repeating of a previous offense) rates for untreated child sexual offenders (both pedophilic and nonpedophilic combined) range from 30% to 50% in offenders under 60 years of age (Harvard Health Publications, 2014).

Persons with these disorders may be distressed by their symptoms, overwhelmed with shame or guilt. Others display more antisocial tendencies and are indifferent or blasé about their sexual offenses, or may attempt to justify their actions through rationalization or other means. Some even lobby to decriminalize sexual acts involving children, claiming they are natural or will not harm children (viewpoints universally decried by child advocates). Conversely, some pedophiles seek to refrain from harming children directly, but may do so indirectly by accessing (and thus supporting) child pornography. Other sexual disorders such as compulsive sexual behavior (sometimes called sexual addiction) can contribute to guilt, relational discord, low self-esteem, and sexually transmitted infections.

Societal responses to sexual offenders include educating the public, warning potential victims (via sexual offender registries and notification of those residing nearby), correctional monitoring, and restricting access to potential victims (by prohibiting contact with children and restricting residences to areas away from schools and playgrounds). Although intended to prevent sexual offenses, these restrictions may ostracize possibly reformed offenders and create unintended consequences (e.g., isolation, unemployment, homelessness), which may in turn make it more difficult to track and treat offenders. Information on sexual offenses and sexual offender listings can typically be found on the web pages of local law enforcement agencies.

However, since reoffending after incarceration is not rare, some states now hold sexual offenders in inpatient psychiatric treatment settings (usually state forensic hospitals) for extended periods after they have completed their prison sentences. This "preventive psychiatric incarceration" is controversial within the mental health field; some believe it is an abuse of psychiatry to (1) hold a person who does not require inpatient psychiatric care in an inpatient setting, (2) incarcerate a person because of what he or she might do in the future, or (3) hold people in psychiatric settings when there may be no known (or further) psychiatric treatment available for their particular needs (Mental Health America, 2011).

APPLICATION OF THE NURSING PROCESS

SELF-CARE FOR NURSES

A nurse's beliefs and attitudes about these unusual (from the nurse's perspective) or sometimes abhorrent behaviors may compromise objectivity or create distress. If the nurse is a survivor of sexual abuse, treating perpetrators can be particularly difficult and even traumatic. Therefore self-care and self-awareness are essential when working with persons with these disorders (e.g., clinical supervision to help one recognize and deal with subjective responses to the patient; counseling

to help cope with reawakened memories of earlier abuse). If nurses believe they cannot work with the patient appropriately, perhaps reassignment, if possible, while working on reframing thoughts and feelings is best. Actions associated with paraphilias may be embarrassing or even criminal in nature, making building trust and conveying empathy and acceptance essential but sometimes challenging.

ASSESSMENT

People often conceal or deny paraphilic thoughts and behavior, making careful assessment and validation of the consumer's reports important. Written assessment questionnaires can elicit possibly embarrassing information without the tension of a face-to-face interview, forming the basis of a more focused interview thereafter. Significant others who are less reluctant to share information can also help identify concealed issues (e.g., it is not unusual for adult children of individuals with pedophilia to report inappropriate sexual contact during their childhood). In some cases, the person may be dealing with concurrent depression or be sufficiently distressed to be considering self-harm, making assessment for this risk essential; this is especially true for those who recently have been accused of (or publicly exposed in reference to) sexual offenses involving children, and who face considerable shame and even hostility within their families and communities as a result (such persons are at especially high risk of suicide in the first 24 to 48 hours after incarceration). Finally, it is always important to assess how the disorder has affected the person and significant others, as well as the person's knowledge of the disorder and ways of reducing or coping with it.

DIAGNOSIS

A variety of nursing diagnoses may apply to individuals with gender dysphoria, paraphilias, and paraphilic disorders, including *Impaired adjustment, Anxiety, Compromised family coping, Ineffective coping, Ineffective relationship, Risk for injury, Low self-esteem, Sexual dysfunction, Ineffective sexuality pattern, Risk for other-directed violence,* and *Social isolation* (NANDA, 2014). Nursing interventions for these disorders vary with the disorder and its expression in a particular person, and are affected by any comorbid mental health disorders. Some general interventions likely to fit most related circumstances are listed in Table 27-5.

OUTCOMES IDENTIFICATION

Expected outcomes vary with the disorder but typically focus on reducing the problematic acts and substituting more adaptive means to meet sexual needs. Examples of desired outcomes include "(Person) reports ability to fantasize about adults as well as children," "(Person) does not go to locations where children are likely to be found," and "(Person) rates urge to have contact with children a 5 or less on a 1 to 10 scale."

IMPLEMENTATION

Pharmacological and Therapeutic Interventions
Pedophilic Disorders

Pedophiles and other sexual offenders may seek treatment when sufficiently distressed by their disorder, when compelled to do so by courts, or when necessary to address the concerns of significant others. Except for criminal offenders with comorbid SMIs, treatment is usually on an outpatient basis and appears to be beneficial in some cases.

Treatment of pedophilia usually involves medications and psychotherapy. Pharmacological treatment typically involves medications that reduce impulsive or compulsive behavior, such as selected antidepressants or naloxone, or medications that interfere with the production of

TABLE 27-5   Interventions for Sexual Disorders

Intervention	Rationale
1. Use inclusive language, convey acceptance, normalize disclosure pertaining to sexuality, and provide active support.	1. These actions promote free and open discussion of the person's behavior and needs (Royal College of Psychiatrists, 2013).
2. Assist individuals with gender dysphoria to connect with peers and professionals who are supportive and receptive, and to access helpful resources such as www.wpath.org and www.transgenderlaw.org.	2. Stigma and discrimination can cause isolation and hopelessness; connecting with others and pursuing educational resources for the person and significant others can enhance understanding and acceptance.
3. Maintain and reinforce appropriate interpersonal boundaries with people with sexual disorders.	3. Role modeling of appropriate boundaries allows the person to identify and adopt more effective ways of relating to others, and maintains professional relationship.
4. Mutually set, track, revise, and reinforce incremental goals, along with related actions that will meet those goals.	4. Mutual goal setting enables the person to "own" the goal; incremental goals are easier to attain, reducing discouragement from unmet goals, and provide a series of successes that reinforce one's efforts.
5. Guide the person to practice tension reduction and stress control strategies such as avoidance of stress, correction of negative self-talk, and use of breathing control exercises.	5. High levels of stress and tension, especially when coupled with a limited or ineffective repertoire of coping strategies, increase the chance of maladaptive behaviors.
6. Educate the person (and any support persons and personnel from the criminal justice system) about the disorder: its causes, treatments, and ways to cope with and control symptoms and maladaptive behaviors.	6. Understanding one's disorder, as well as ways to cope with or reduce symptoms, can decrease guilt and powerlessness, instilling hope and improving the person's sense of control.
7. Assist the person to identify and explore feelings preceding or associated with the target behavior (e.g., excitement, shame, guilt).	7. Unresolved feelings can cause desperation and lead to acting-out or loss of control.
8. Assist the person to identify the consequences of his or her actions (e.g., ask "How do other people seem to feel about your behavior?" or "What tends to happen when you go where children play?").	8. Insight that develops from within tends to be more accepted than feedback provided externally; covert sensitization—guiding the person to connect an undesired behavior with negative consequences—diminishes unacceptable behaviors.
9. Address comorbid disorders and mental health needs (e.g., substance abuse, sexual victimization during one's youth).	9. Depression and other mental disorders impair problem-solving and coping abilities, draining the person's energy for addressing the target problems.

Royal College of Psychiatrists. (2013). *Good practice guidelines for the assessment and treatment of adults with gender dysphoria.* Retrieved May 5, 2015, from http://www.rcpsych.ac.uk/usefulresources/publications/collegereports/cr/cr181.aspx

sexual hormones in order to reduce sexual urges (Holoydi and Kellaher, 2016), in effect producing varying degrees of **chemical castration.** Patients typically receive a monthly injection and hormonal levels are monitored to ensure effectiveness. Side effects in men include feminization and weight gain. However, research suggests that testosterone plays a lesser role in sexual offenses than do gonadotropins such as luteinizing hormone (LH) and follicle-stimulating hormone (FSH); sexual offenders with higher LH and FSH levels were more likely to reoffend, while testosterone was not correlated with reoffending (Kingston et al., 2012). Gonadotropin-releasing hormone desensitizes gonadotropin-releasing receptors and has been shown to be efficacious in reducing sexual offenses (McManus et al., 2013). Psychotherapy typically involves individual and group therapy focused on improving impulse control.

Other Paraphilic Disorders and Sexual Differences

For people with gender dysphoria, counseling can help patients compare and choose various paths they might take, including sexual reassignment, and cope with their feelings and society's responses to this disorder. Hormonal agents to alter sexual characteristics may be used.

For paraphilic disorders, medications such as naltrexone, carbamazepine, clonazepam, and SSRI antidepressants may help reduce compulsive or impulsive behavior and are also used to treat paraphilias and sexually inappropriate behavior generally, particularly in neuropsychiatric conditions such as dementia and Parkinson's disease. They can have significant side effects, including weight gain, clotting disorders, thromboembolism, decreased fertility and sexual dysfunction, depression, and hypertension (Holoyda & Kellaher, 2016). Infrequently, agents used for chemical castration are used, and in rare cases, surgical castration may be pursued by the patient in lieu of drugs.

Psychotherapeutic treatments include group and one-to-one psychotherapy and psychoeducational interventions. Cognitive behavioral therapies in particular are believed to be helpful. Behavioral approaches

can include desensitization techniques to reduce sexual responsiveness to undesired stimuli. In some cases, patients are guided to fulfill their gratification needs in non–socially offensive ways, such as via masturbatory reconditioning. Twelve-step programs also have been effective for some, and treatment of comorbid disorders, particularly those that impair impulse control (e.g., substance abuse), can reduce the risk of recidivism or conversion to criminal behavior (Marshall, 2007).

ADULT ATTENTION-DEFICIT/HYPERACTIVITY DISORDER (ADHD)

VIGNETTE

Andrea, a 32-year-old graduate student in psychology, presents at the student health center concerned that she might have attention-deficit/hyperactivity disorder (ADHD). She reports that throughout her life teachers and others told her she was extremely bright, but that somehow this was not reflected in her grades, which were B's and C's. She notes that she has difficulty maintaining concentration, often "tuning out" during lectures and having to regularly reread parts of her assignments.

Andrea has difficulty sitting still and sometimes interrupts others impulsively, then apologizes. When distracted she has difficulty regaining her train of thought. Disorganization, worry, and irritability trouble her. She often loses track of belongings, spends much time looking for misplaced items, forgets appointments, and frequently overlooks tasks she had intended to do.

Other psychiatric and physical problems are ruled out. After treatment with methylphenidate and counseling, Andrea reports that she was able to finish a major written assignment in one third the time and with much less stress than before treatment. She is happy with the improvement and hopeful, and says that friends have commented that she seems more at ease and less scattered. She agrees to join an ADHD support group on campus to obtain support and practical suggestions for managing the disorder.

PREVALENCE AND COMORBIDITY

ADHD involves a persistent pattern of inattention, impaired ability to focus and concentrate, and hyperactivity and impulsivity that are more noticeable and more severe than would otherwise be seen at a given developmental level. **Attention deficit disorder (ADD)** involves a similar presentation but without the hyperactivity. ADHD and ADD are discussed in detail in Chapter 26; coverage here focuses only on aspects related to its presence in adults.

ADHD appears to have a lower prevalence in adulthood (2.5% versus 5% in children [APA, 2013]), though this may really reflect inadequate screening and the enhanced ability of adults to compensate or conceal their symptoms. Adult ADHD is associated with a wide variety of interpersonal and social problems, including relational discord and reduced academic and vocational performance. It can limit or disrupt a person's ability to function in any realm and can negatively affect health habits. Psychiatric comorbidity, particularly anxiety and mood disorders, is common in ADHD (Mayo Clinic, 2013). Co-occurring physical health disorders include Tourette's syndrome and other tic disorders, substance abuse, sexually transmitted infections, traumatic brain injuries, and general trauma.

THEORY

Genetic, Biological, and Psychological Factors

ADHD is believed to be a neurodevelopmental disorder with multiple contributing factors, including alterations in the neurotransmitters dopamine and serotonin and reduced levels of brain-derived neurotrophic factor (BDNF), which plays a role in neurogenesis (the development of new neurons) (Corominas-Roso et al., 2013). There appears to be a strong genetic and familial component, with an estimated heritability of approximately 60% (Corominas-Roso et al., 2013). Social and biological adversity (interpersonal and biological challenges) are possible factors; fetal distress, prematurity, and exposure to neurotoxins toxins such as lead, particularly in the prenatal and early postnatal period when brain development is rapid, are implicated, as are conflict and distress within one's family (Mayo Clinic, 2013).

CLINICAL PICTURE

ADHD tends to be underappreciated and underdiagnosed in adults. The diagnosis is complicated by the complexity and varied presentation of the disorder. Adult ADHD features are similar to those of children but affect adult roles such as postsecondary education, employment, and marriage. Common presentations include impaired focusing and concentration, disorganization, impulsiveness, impaired task completion, irritability and impaired frustration tolerance, labile mood, and impaired social/relational/educational/vocational functioning (Mayo Clinic, 2013). Because these features can occur for many reasons, it's not unusual for adults to be unaware that they have ADHD, or for clinicians to overlook this diagnosis in adults.

Effect on Individuals, Families, and Society

The effect of ADHD is significant. Adults diagnosed with ADHD as children tend to achieve lower socioeconomic status; complete fewer years of school; use nicotine, alcohol, and drugs at higher rates; have more traffic incidents (e.g., road rage, accidents, speeding offenses); have more contact with police; are at greater risk of sexually transmitted infections and trauma; change jobs more frequently; report more interpersonal and relational difficulties; and have higher rates of depression than people without ADHD (Mayo Clinic, 2013; Miranda et al., 2014). ADHD is also significantly more prevalent in incarcerated populations, suggesting ADHD may increase the propensity toward criminal activity.

The effect on society is less well established. ADHD inhibits academic achievement at all ages, and it is believed to reduce work productivity and increase criminal justice system costs significantly, but hard data do not yet exist.

APPLICATION OF THE NURSING PROCESS

ASSESSMENT

There is no laboratory test, scan, or other objective means for detecting ADHD. Instead, ADHD is diagnosed based on the characteristic patterns of behavior and organizational and attentional dysfunction that are the cardinal features of these disorders, using patient reports, nursing observation, and, when available, reports of employers, family members, and other third parties as assessment data. Assessment should also include the person's present knowledge of, and ability to cope with, the disorder. Support systems play a major role in the person achieving successful outcomes and should be assessed. ADHD can significantly impair parenting ability, so parental role functioning should be assessed as well. Because of the high percentage of co-occurring mental disorders and the complexity of ADHD, a complete mental health assessment (in complicated cases, by an ADHD specialist) is recommended.

Clinicians should use interview areas that are relatively quiet and free of distractions. It is usually helpful to keep comments and questioning concise and concrete. If needed, prompts can help the person organize responses and stay on track. Observe for disorganization; distractibility; irritability; lability; impulsive comments or actions; difficulty processing information or following instructions; difficulty achieving at the expected level in social, educational, and vocational settings; and hyperactivity (excess or nonpurposeful motor activity). Substance abuse, particularly of methamphetamine and other stimulants, can mimic ADHD and should be ruled out.

DIAGNOSIS

Nursing diagnoses for ADHD include *Impaired social interaction, Ineffective impulse control, Ineffective relationship, Defensive coping, Compromised family coping, Impaired adjustment, Anxiety,* and *Personal identity disturbance* (NANDA, 2015-2017). Nursing interventions focus on symptom management and coping with the illness (Table 27-6). Interventions for adults may be different from those for children.

OUTCOMES IDENTIFICATION

Examples of potential outcome measures include: "(Patient) demonstrates ability to stay on task by completing one task before starting another," "(Patient) discusses three techniques to reduce environmental distractions," and "(Patient) rates concentration as a 5 or greater on a 1 to 10 scale."

IMPLEMENTATION

Pharmacological, Biological, and Integrative Therapies

Medications are a well-established treatment for ADHD. In most cases the same drugs used to treat children are also used to treat adults. Stimulants are the most widely used medication for ADHD, and they show a high degree of efficacy, with 75% to 95% of patients reporting improvement. Examples include methylphenidate (e.g., Concerta, Metadate, Ritalin), dextroamphetamine (Dexedrine), dextroamphetamine-amphetamine

TABLE 27-6 Interventions for Adult Attention-Deficit/Hyperactivity Disorder (ADHD)

Intervention	Rationale
1. Educate the person and significant other(s) about ADHD: its causes, treatments, and especially ways to cope with and control its symptoms.	1. Understanding the psychological and psychiatric aspects of one's disorder, as well as ways to cope with or reduce symptoms, can decrease powerlessness, instill hope, and improve the person's sense of control.
2. Guide the person to understand and practice stimulation reduction strategies such as environmental structuring (reducing auditory and visual distractions).	2. Environmental distractions make already impaired concentration more difficult.
3. Mutually set, track, revise, and reinforce incremental goals, along with actions that will meet those goals.	3. Mutual goal setting increases person's "buy-in"; incremental goals are easier to attain, reducing discouragement from unmet goals and providing successes that reinforce the person's efforts.
4. Guide the person to identify and use enhanced organizational skills; many techniques exist to increase organization and efficiency in completing tasks, from reminder lists to using personal digital assistants (PDAs) to track appointments.	4. Enhancements in organization can improve functioning and promote a positive self-image as the person experiences increased task success; Internet resources and print publications can be accessed for this purpose.
5. Guide the person to identify and use enhanced time management skills (e.g., structured priority setting wherein the person asks self, "What will happen if I do not do this task next?" and then uses those responses to determine which task to tackle next).	5. Better time management can improve functioning and reduce stress; Internet resources and published materials on this topic can be readily accessed.
6. Assist the person to identify and explore feelings about ADHD and its effect on his or her life, and to correct any distorted self-talk pertaining to self-image.	6. ADHD may contribute to frustration or impaired self-esteem because of daily challenges and one's unmet potential; people with ADHD may be critical of themselves and use negative "self-talk" (e.g., "I am so stupid; why can't I do this? What is wrong with me!").
7. Encourage participation in ADHD support groups and vetted online support resources such as ADHD blogs.	7. Support groups and online resources can provide pragmatic "helpful hints" from peers and support from an "I've been there" perspective.
8. Address comorbid disorders and mental health needs such as substance abuse.	8. Depression and other disorders further impair problem-solving and coping abilities; substance abuse can significantly worsen impulsivity and concentration.

(Adderall XR), and lisdexamfetamine (Vyvanse); some are available in short- and long-acting forms, and some are available as dermal patches (Mayo Clinic, 2013). Longer-acting and timed-release forms allow persons to take the medicines only once or twice per day, before and after (rather than during) school or work, a popular feature that helps improves adherence (inattentiveness, disorganization, and distractibility contribute to decreased adherence in ADHD).

Stimulant medications are thought to augment dopamine and/or norepinephrine neurotransmission that regulates prefrontal cortex activities critical for modulation of behavior, attention, and cognition. It might seem counterintuitive for stimulants to help hyperactivity, but these medications all in some way promote enhanced dopamine and norepinephrine functioning and do not have the degree of classical stimulant effects seen when used by persons without ADHD. One concern noted in the use of such stimulants is sharing the medicine with others, or the medication being diverted by others; although this is a criminal offense, such sharing has been increasing, especially among college students, and should be addressed during patient education; ironically, research suggests that although stimulants may enhance learning in those with ADHD, its effects on learning in those without ADHD is negligible (Benson et al., 2015).

Other medications used to treat ADHD include antidepressants such as bupropion (Wellbutrin) and atomoxetine (Strattera). Antidepressants may take several weeks to take full effect, much longer than stimulants, but are useful for persons who have cardiovascular or other health problems that are contraindications for stimulants (Mayo Clinic, 2013). Also, unlike stimulants, antidepressants are not addictive and are unlikely to be abused.

Nonpharmacological Interventions

Psychotherapeutic treatments and symptom management skills are also important in managing ADHD. Cognitive therapy is helpful for correcting distortions in self-image and improving focus and concentration, and counseling can address co-occurring issues such as marital discord and coping with chronic illness. Psychoeducation about the disorder and its treatment, along with instruction in techniques for managing and coping with symptoms, is essential and may be done individually or in a group setting. Support groups, helpful for addressing self-esteem and anxiety issues, can be excellent sources of practical hints for managing the disorder and useful in adjusting to life with ADHD. One unusual treatment with preliminary research support is that of Whole Body Vibration, delivered by placing the person on a vibrating platform; the mechanism is unclear, but vibration stimulates muscle contraction that may in turn stimulate areas of the brain involved in concentration (Fuermaier et al., 2014). Micronutrient supplementation involving selected vitamins and minerals has also been shown to be of benefit (Rucklidge et al., 2014).

SLEEP-RELATED DISORDERS

Sleep-related disorders include a variety of alterations in sleep. They can involve physical illnesses or abnormalities (e.g., restless leg syndrome, obstructive sleep apnea) or psychological disorders or circumstances (e.g., anxiety, PTSD) that disrupt sleep. Sleep can also be affected by phenomena such as shift work (working rotating shifts or night shifts). Specific sleep-related disorders are described in Table 27-7. Medications and illness can increase or decrease sleep needs and abilities, and can disrupt its quality.

PREVALENCE AND COMORBIDITY

Temporary episodes of sleep disruption are universal experiences and often accompany stressful situations such as physical illness, surgery, work or school demands, and grief and loss situations. Some sleep disorders, such as insomnia (difficulty falling or staying asleep), are common, affecting about one third of all persons; others, such as sleep apnea and

TABLE 27-7   Sleep-Related Disorders

Name	Description
Insomnia disorder	Perceived insufficient sleep, or sleep that is perceived as not restful. Seven to nine hours of sleep per night is generally considered normal. Many physical, psychological, and social factors can contribute to insomnia (e.g., shift work, traumatic experiences, poor sleep hygiene).
Hypersomnolence disorder	Perceived excess sleep, either at night and/or falling asleep during the day.
Obstructive sleep apnea/hypopnea	A temporary cessation (**apnea**) or decrease (**hypopnea**) in breathing during sleep. Usually due to a mechanical obstruction that increases when prone or when muscles relax during sleep, it is more common in obese persons. It sometimes occurs for nonstructural reasons as well. It can impair cognitive function and increases many health risks, including cardiovascular disease and mortality risk.
Narcolepsy	Sudden, irresistible urges to sleep. One may suddenly fall asleep under any circumstances; some continue automatic behavior as if in a mental fog. Episodes are not recalled after awakening.
Circadian rhythm disorders	Dysregulation of the internal circadian rhythms relative to one's usual sleep cycle. The sleep-wake cycle can shift in various ways (e.g., sleeping during the day rather than at night). One variant stems from shift work and involves sleepiness at work and home.
Sleep arousal disorders	Abnormal experiences or behaviors occurring during sleep. In the rapid eye movement (REM) type the person experiences arousal during REM sleep and may vocalize or enact behaviors as if awake, often in response to what one is dreaming at the time. It can be dangerous (e.g., striking out if dreaming that one is being attacked). In the non-REM form the behavior is typically **sleepwalking**, and the abnormal experience is sleep terror, often accompanied by screaming. During sleepwalking the person is not consciously aware of his actions and is difficult to awaken; it can be dangerous depending on the environment in which it occurs.
Nightmare disorder	Recurrent experience of protracted, highly realistic, and very upsetting nightmares, often involving being in a threatening situation; the nightmares are readily recalled upon awakening.
Restless leg syndrome	An urge to move one's legs, usually in response to an irritating sensation in the legs that improves with movement. It can significantly disrupt sleep.

hypopnea (temporary absence or reduction of breathing during sleep) are less common and affect 2% to 20% of adults (APA, 2013). Other conditions, such as narcolepsy (inability to remain awake when needed) are rare, affecting less than 0.5% of persons (APA, 2013). Physical illnesses ranging from pulmonary insufficiency to restless leg syndrome commonly accompany and contribute to sleep disorders (Ohayon et al., 2014).

THEORY

Genetic, Biological, and Psychological Factors

Sleep is vital for life. It is believed to play a major role in memory, moving memories from short-term recall states to longer-term memory. Long known to provide a restorative function, sleep plays a key role in neurological health, increasing the circulation of cerebrofluid and removing damaging byproducts of neuronal activity such as beta-amyloid (Xie et al., 2013).

Sleep can be divided into two phases or types. **REM** (rapid eye movement) sleep is characterized by inhibition of voluntary movement, fluctuating periods of rapid eye movement, and dreaming. **Non-REM** sleep is further divided into four stages that are characterized by specific electroencephalogram (EEG) patterns, and one's ability to be aroused varies with each stage. Both REM and non-REM sleep can be disrupted in sleep disorders (Lubit, 2015).

The suprachiasmatic nucleus in the hypothalamus is believed to be the primary regulator of sleep cycles, affecting sleep cycles by stimulating the pineal gland to release melatonin. The neurotransmitters serotonin and norepinephrine play a role in promoting sleep, while dopamine affects wakefulness.

Disorders such as narcolepsy appear to have a genetic component, being more common in identical twins and first-degree relatives, while other sleep disorders do not yet have established genetic connections (Lubit, 2015). Mood disorders such as bipolar disorder are believed to involve abnormalities in a "clock" gene that result in sleep dysregulation (Sylvia et al., 2014).

Psychological states and disorders affect sleep in a variety of ways. Sleep disturbance and dysregulation can both contribute to and be caused by disorders such as depression (characterized by increased sleep, or hypersomnia, or insomnia) and mania (characterized by a decreased need for sleep) (Sylvia et al., 2014). Insomnia can signal or contribute to relapse in depression, mania, and schizophrenia. Anxiety and worry are common sources of insomnia. Traumatic experiences and related disorders such as PTSD feature sleep disruptions such as insomnia and nightmares.

CLINICAL PICTURE

Sleep disorders often begin in early adulthood and may worsen with age. Persons with sleep-related disorders typically complain of inadequate and/or low-quality sleep, or, conversely, excessive drowsiness. They may also report associated symptoms such as grogginess, increased accidents, and impaired concentration, or comorbidities such as anxiety, depressed mood, loss or grief, or physical illness. These features range from mildly to severely distressing and disruptive to normal functioning.

Effect on Individuals, Families, and Society

Sleep loss contributes to physical health problems such as obesity, diabetes, cardiovascular disease, and impaired immune system functioning (Schmid et al., 2015; Takahashi, 2014). Narcolepsy is associated with a 1.5-fold increase in mortality, though the mechanism is not understood (Ohayon et al., 2014). It is estimated that 15% to 30% of persons operate with insufficient sleep (less than 7 hours per night), leading to increased motor vehicle and other accidents; almost 30% of drivers report falling asleep at the wheel and almost 20% report having near misses due to driving while drowsy (Centers for Disease Control and Prevention [CDC], 2011; Inoue & Komada, 2014).

Daytime drowsiness can reduce alertness and vigilance, impair judgment, and interfere with memory; these are particular concerns for night shift workers in public safety health care fields who are at increased risk of accidents and making errors, endangering their patients (and themselves) because of occupational sleep disruptions (Hirsch-Allen et al., 2014; Takahashi, 2014). Such shift work is also disruptive to the employee's family and personal life.

APPLICATION OF THE NURSING PROCESS

ASSESSMENT

Screening for sleep disorders is very important due to their frequency, potential to affect health, and association with other physical and psychiatric disorders. Assessment is by interview pertaining to sleep habits and patterns, subjective quality of sleep, and associated features such as sleepwalking or nightmares. Sleep journals are used to determine actual sleep patterns and duration more objectively, and formal sleep studies (usually involving EEG and respiratory monitoring, along with direct observation during sleep, by specially trained technicians) can also be used for more accurate diagnosis. Respiratory function studies may be indicated as well. Interview the person and those he or she sleeps with for signs of nocturnal hypoxia (e.g., snoring, gasping, choking sensation, periods of apnea, restlessness, frequent arousal) or its later consequences (e.g., headaches, dry mouth in the morning, feeling unrested, daytime sleepiness or fatigue, morning confusion, irritability or depression).

DIAGNOSIS

The primary nursing diagnosis for sleep-related disorders is *Disturbed sleep pattern;* associated diagnoses include *Anxiety, Ineffective individual coping, Impaired gas exchange,* and *Risk for injury* (NANDA, 2012–2014).

OUTCOMES IDENTIFICATION

Examples of potential outcome measures include "Patient reports sleeping 7 to 9 hours per night," "Patient discusses three techniques to promote quality sleep," and "Patient rates quality of rest as a 6 or greater on a 1 to 10 scale."

IMPLEMENTATION

Nursing interventions for sleep disorder focus first on relieving underlying causes of sleep disturbance such as hospital noise, scheduling procedures during hours of sleep, and impaired sleep hygiene practices. Contributing emotional factors such as pain, grief, and anxiety are also addressed. Specific interventions related to sleep are discussed in Table 27-8.

Pharmacological, Biological, and Integrative Therapies

Insomnia is usually treated with sedative-hypnotic drugs. There are three benzodiazepine-like drugs that are the preferred medications for insomnia: zolpidem (Ambien), eszopiclone (Lunesta), zaleplon (Sonata). As well, suvorexant (Belsomra), a novel selective dual orexin receptor antagonist, may be prescribed. These drugs react quickly, reduce awakenings, increase total sleeping time, and are well tolerated (Burchum & Rosenthal, 2016).

As we already know, all benzodiazepine and benzodiazepine-like drugs can cause grogginess, impaired coordination and reflexes, dizziness, and fall risk in susceptible persons, and patients should be educated to use these with caution. Some are potentially addictive and because tolerance can develop, are encouraged to be used on a short-term basis.

Narcolepsy is treated with wake-promoting drugs such as methylphenidate (Ritalin) and modafinil (Provigil), which has fewer undesired effects on sleep; side effects include headache, irritability, and gastrointestinal complaints. Sodium oxybate (Xyrem), also known as gamma-hydroxybutyrate, or GHB, is an abusable drug (often sold and abused in group social settings such as nightclubs) that is also effective and approved for narcolepsy (Bozorg & Benbadis, 2015).

A sleep aid not approved by the U.S. Food and Drug Administration (FDA) and available over the counter that may be helpful for some is *melatonin* (appropriate doses are 0.3 to 1 mg about 2 hours before sleep). It appears safe for short-term use but long-term safety has not been confirmed. *Kava* products are used by some but have been linked with severe liver damage; persons using these products should consult their physician or nurse practitioner. *L-tryptophan supplements* are also used but should be used with caution due to an association with potentially dangerous eosinophilia-myalgia syndrome.

Nonpharmacological Interventions

Mechanical devices such as ventilation assistance devices (e.g., continuous positive airway pressure [CPAP] machines) may be necessary for obstructive sleep apnea (periods when breathing does not occur) and hypopnea (periods of inadequate ventilation). **Cognitive behavioral therapy (CBT)** focuses on changing patterns of thinking, especially negative thinking, to reduce stress and promote rest (Sylvia et al., 2014). Stress reduction and active relaxation reduce anxiety and promote rest. Environmental management (e.g., reducing distraction, exposure to stimulation) and normalizing sleep patterns are important interventions. Individual and family therapy to address underlying concerns may be needed.

APPLYING EVIDENCE-BASED PRACTICE (EBP)

Problem A 34-year-old transgender (female to male) patient approaches the nurse at his primary care physician's (PCP's) office after an appointment. He reveals that he has not had his male hormones for about 4 months since moving from a large city in California to a small rural town in Idaho, and that his current PCP has been unwilling to order them. At first, a slight elevation in liver enzymes was the reasoning, but as time has gone on the patient feels that the PCP does not understand or agree with his transgender transition. The patient is beginning to grow breasts again, and his mood has been irritable at home with the family.

EBP Assessment

A. **What do you already know from experience?** Transgender patients are becoming more common. There is still considerable stigma and lack of understanding in the general population and even among health care professionals. Transgender patients can cross-dress, take hormones, or have surgery as part of their transition.

B. **What does the literature say?** Lesbian, gay, bisexual, and transgender (LGBT) patients experience health care disparity and barriers, and may avoid treatment because of real or perceived discrimination (Zunner & Grace, 2012). Homophobia in medical practice is real; surveys found that about 10% of medical personnel "despised" lesbian and gay clients and about 40% felt they should "keep their sexuality private." Recommendations to improve care include providing a welcoming environment, using gender-neutral terminology, adding transgender to gender check boxes, screening for gender dysphoria, and addressing the patient using the preferred name or gender. Be open to discussing gender-related issues, and train staff in sensitivity. A gender-neutral or inclusive restroom is helpful (Bebinger, 2014; Gay and Lesbian Medical Association, n.d.).

C. **What does the patient want?** The patient wants to get back on his hormones as soon as possible, and wants to be supported by his health care team. He feels guilt for the stress his moodiness has inflicted on the family.

APPLYING EVIDENCE-BASED PRACTICE (EBP)—cont'd

Plan The nurse obtained contact information from the patient for his doctor in California. She recommended that the patient attempt to contact his former doctor for assistance in getting hormones in the interim. She also performed online research regarding transgender transitioning and issues in health care, and approached the PCP she works with to learn more information together. She also asked colleagues for recommendations for providers in the area with experience with transgender treatment. Her PCP appreciated her assistance, was open to consulting with these providers, and to possible referral if needed.

QSEN **QSEN Prelicensure Knowledge, Skills, and Attitudes (KSAs) Addressed:**

Patient-centered care was provided by additional learning and possible referral.

Team work and collaboration was addressed through contacting other providers, and the PCP and nurse learning together.

Bebinger, M. (2014). *12 tips for nurses and doctors treating transgender patients.* Retrieved from http://commonhealth.wbur.org/2014/11/treating-transgender-patients-tips; Gay and Lesbian Medical Association. (n.d.). *Guidelines for care of lesbian, gay, bisexual, and transgender patients.* Retrieved from http://www.glma.org/_data/n_0001/resources/live/GLMA%20guidelines%202006%20FINAL.pdf; Zunner, B. P., & Grace, P. J. (2012). The ethical nursing care of transgender patients: an exploration of bias in health care and how it affects this population. *American Journal of Nursing, 112*(12), 61–64.

TABLE 27-8 Interventions for Sleep Dysregulation

Intervention	Rationale
1. Educate the person and significant other(s) about proper sleep hygiene—practices that promote restful sleep such as those noted below.	1. Understanding one's disorder and the rationale for ways to cope with it can increase motivation and instill hope that the condition will improve.
2. Keep a sleep diary to track patterns related to sleep: time going to bed, time arising, awakenings during the night, and activities or anxieties occurring just before bed.	2. Tracking sleep and factors that affect it can help one recognize sleep disorders and identify causes that can then be addressed.
3. Mutually set concrete sleep-related goals and develop actions that will meet those goals (e.g., set a target time to be in bed and to wake). Tie these goals to other goals that the person is motivated to attain (e.g., note that adequate rest will promote healing and speed recovery, or improve concentration and help with success at work or school).	3. Mutual goal setting is motivating and increases the person's commitment to achieving the goals. Concrete goals are easier to target and measure, and provide a sense of success that reinforce the person's efforts and motivates adherence to the plan.
4. Engage in exercise or other physical activity in the evening, 2 hours prior to bedtime, to increase tiredness.	4. Exercise increases tiredness and promotes sleep, but is initially stimulating and should be avoided just before bedtime.
5. Guide the person to identify and use stress avoidance (e.g., assertive communication, time management), cognitive interventions (e.g., changing negative thoughts, distracting oneself from worries, making expectations of oneself more realistic), and relaxation techniques (e.g., deepening and slowing breathing, calming music, relaxing physical activity) to reduce anxiety.	5. Stress and worry contribute significantly toward insomnia.
6. Reduce stimulation such as background noise (e.g., use sound generators that produce white noise or calming environmental sounds) and exposure to bright light before sleep (e.g., dim lights and refrain from using any screen-based device for 1 hour before bed, or at least while trying to fall asleep). Use the bedroom only for sleep, not for TV viewing.	6. Stimulation promotes wakefulness and is useful for daytime drowsiness and narcolepsy, but interferes with sleep.
7. Establish a routine to stabilize sleep times wherever possible, finding and sticking to a consistent sleep pattern. Go to bed at least 8 hours prior to when one needs to awake. Maintain this pattern on days off.	7. A regular sleep pattern helps the body synchronize sleep with circadian rhythms and promotes sleep because the body does not have to adjust to a varying schedule.
8. If unable to sleep for more than 30 minutes, leave the bedroom and engage in relaxing and distracting activities, returning to bed again when feeling tired.	8. Sleep is unlikely if one is still awake after 30 minutes; getting up to engage in activities that promote sleep is more likely to cause sleep than staying in bed.
9. Adhere to treatment recommendations for any physical or emotional disorders that interfere with sleep.	9. Depression and other disorders further impair sleep dysregulation.
10. Minimize the use of all stimulants (e.g., caffeine, nicotine) and do not use these for at least 4 hours before bedtime. Also refrain from use of alcohol for sleep.	10. Stimulants are useful for narcolepsy but interfere with sleep; stopping them well before bedtime allows them to be at least somewhat metabolized before bedtime.
11. Neither go to bed hungry nor eat just before bedtime.	11. Hunger and digestive activity can both interfere with sleep.
12. If having trouble sleeping, consider refraining from napping, even if tired.	12. Naps can be helpful to promote alertness for shift workers or those who cannot get a full night's sleep, but can cause initial grogginess on awakening and can interfere with sleep at night.
13. Darken your sleeping space as much as possible.	13. Light can disturb sleep and disrupt sleep cycles.
14. Arrange your room and bedding for maximum comfort based on your personal preferences.	14. Uncomfortable bedding and room temperatures cause restlessness and interfere with sleep quality.
15. Persons doing night-shift work should expose themselves to bright light at night and keep all lighting dim during the day.	15. This lighting pattern simulates normal day-night light levels usually experienced and promotes better sleep during night-shift workers' sleep time.

KEY POINTS TO REMEMBER

- Severe mental illnesses (SMIs) are recurrent or long-lasting and often disruptive or disabling.
- Stigma and chronicity present many challenges to coping with an SMI and contribute to a variety of other social, physical health, and mental health problems: substance abuse, poverty and unemployment, comorbid physical illnesses and premature mortality, arrest and incarceration, homelessness, depression, powerlessness, and suicide risk.
- Assertive community treatment and peer-based services (e.g., clubhouses, certified peer specialists) are evidence-based practices shown to benefit persons with SMIs.
- Impulse control disorders involve impulsive behaviors that are disruptive and serve to relieve psychological tension. These disorders include impulsive thefts, setting fires, sudden assaults or property destruction, hair pulling, and pathological gambling.
- Impulse control disorders are treated primarily through psychotherapy and sometimes with antidepressant or anticonvulsant medications.
- Sexual disorders include gender dysphoria/gender identity disorders and the paraphilic disorders. A person with gender dysphoria believes his or her biological gender is incorrect, and that he or she should be the opposite gender.
- People with gender dysphoria may be subject to ridicule and harassment and may experience significant distress related to their gender dissatisfaction. One intervention is gender reassignment, which involves counseling, experiencing life for 1 or 2 years as the opposite gender, using hormones, and being surgically reassigned.
- Paraphilic disorders are disorders in which sexual gratification is obtained in atypical and often socially unacceptable ways.
- Pedophilia includes having sexual fantasies or contact with children. This disorder stirs strong feelings in staff and society.
- The causes of paraphilic disorders are not clearly established, but neurological dysfunction may be a contributing factor.
- Psychotherapy and medications that improve neurological dysfunction or reduce sexual drive can reduce offensive sexual behavior in pedophiles.
- ADHD is associated with childhood but may continue into or first be diagnosed in adulthood. In adults it is characterized by difficulty maintaining focus and organization, and can be disruptive to task completion, employment, relationships, and other areas of functioning.
- ADHD often goes undiagnosed in adults, who may try to compensate for its symptoms. It is treated with a combination of counseling and stimulants (or sometimes other drugs).
- Sleep disorders can have physical, psychological, or social causes. Physical and psychiatric disorders, stress, and shift work can disrupt sleep.
- Impaired sleep can affect one psychologically and physically, contributing to disorders such as depression, bipolar disorder, obesity, and immune system dysfunction.
- Sleep loss due to shift work (night and rotating shifts) can increase the risk of errors and accidents, a particular concern for health care and public safety workers.
- Sleep disorders are treated by correcting underlying conditions and promoting sound sleep hygiene practices.

APPLYING CRITICAL JUDGMENT

1. You are working with a person who has recently been diagnosed with adult ADHD. He is very impulsive and frequently makes comments to you and others that are inappropriate and rude. You find yourself avoiding him and feeling angry toward him. Describe or role-play what you would say in response to help reduce such comments.
2. The parents of a 37-year-old man with an SMI ask you for help; they are becoming frightened of their son, who is increasingly hostile in response to their efforts to get him to take showers, accept medication, and get a job. They report that they have not often been able to talk with those treating their son because of regulations restricting the sharing of private health care information. Discuss or enact how you might address both the issues of confidentiality and the conflicts experienced when the parents attempt to change their son's behavior.
3. Debate the pros and cons for the proposition that sexual offenders who harm children should be held indefinitely in preventive detention for the greater good of society.
4. A consumer with an SMI is about to begin outpatient services at your community mental health center after years of institutionalization in state hospitals and prisons. Discuss the major issues he will likely face, and the services that ideally would be available in your community.

CHAPTER REVIEW QUESTIONS

1. A nurse leads a milieu meeting in an outpatient program for adults diagnosed with serious mental illness. Four consumers complain that another consumer is "always begging us for money." Which comment by the nurse is therapeutic?
   a. "If you can afford to help each other, it is reasonable to do so."
   b. "Let's review what we have learned about being assertive with others."
   c. "No one needs to bring money to our program. Lunch is provided at no charge."
   d. "Let's show understanding of each other. Money management is a problem for everyone."
2. An outpatient nurse has lunch with a group of consumers diagnosed with severe mental illness. The nurse observes an obese adult ask a malnourished adult, "If you aren't going to eat your apple, will you give it to me?" What is the nurse's best action?
   a. Remind both adults that sharing food with each other is not permitted.
   b. Remind the malnourished adult of treatment goals related to weight gain.
   c. Reseat the consumers at two separate tables for the remainder of the meal.
   d. Overlook the remark. Both adults are permitted to make their own decisions.
3. A nurse plans a psychoeducational group about physical health in an outpatient program for consumers diagnosed with severe mental illness. Which topic has priority?
   a. Heart-healthy living
   b. Living with diabetes
   c. ABCDEs of skin cancer
   d. Breast and testicular self-examination
4. A nurse working in the county jail assesses four new inmates. The nurse should direct guards to place which inmate under suicide watch? An inmate charged with:
   a. Breaking and entering.
   b. Criminal solicitation (prostitution).
   c. Lewd and lascivious act on a minor.
   d. Assault and battery on an elderly person.

5. A person diagnosed with severe mental illness has been homeless for 8 years and says, "I don't have any money because I've never had a job. I can't afford a place to live." Which intervention should the outpatient mental health nurse add to the plan of care?
    a. Requisition the patient's legal record of arrests and convictions
    b. Help the patient to apply for Supplemental Security Income (SSI)
    c. Assist the patient to apply for Social Security Disability Income (SSDI)
    d. Seek to have the patient adjudicated *non compos mentis* (incompetent)

REFERENCES

American Psychiatric Association (APA). (2013). *Diagnostic and statistical manual of mental disorders* (5th ed.). Washington, DC: APA.

Arehart-Treichel, J. (2006). Pedophilia often in headlines, but not in research labs. *Psychiatric News, 41*(10), 37–39.

Baum, M. (2013). The monoamine oxidase A (MAOA) genetic predisposition to impulsive violence: Is it relevant to criminal trials? *Neuroethics, 6*(2), 287–306.

Benson, K., Flory, K., Humphries, K., et al. (2015). Misuse of stimulant medication among college students: A comprehensive review and meta-analysis. *Clinical Child and Family Psychology Review, 18*(1), 50–76.

Bozorg, A., & Benbadis, S. (2015). *Narcolepsy treatment & management.* Retrieved May 5, 2015, from http://emedicine.medscape.com/article/1188433-treatment.

Burchum, J., & Rosenthal, L. (2016). *Lehne's pharmacology for nursing care* (9th ed.). St Louis, MO: Elsevier.

Cangelosi, P., & Sorrell, J. (2014). Use of technology to enhance mental health for older adults. *Journal of Psychosocial Nursing, 52*(9), 17–20.

Center for Evidence-Based Practices. (2014). *Assertive community treatment: The evidence-based practice (monograph).* Retrieved May 7, 2015, from http://www.centerforebp.case.edu/client-files/pdf/actoverview.pdf.

Centers for Disease Control and Prevention (CDC). (2011). Unhealthy sleep-related behaviors. *Morbidity and Mortality Weekly Report, 60*(8), 234–266.

Chan, S., Parish, M., & Yellowlees, P. (2015). Telepsychiatry today. *Current Psychiatry Reports, 17,* 89.

Compton, M., Bakeman, R., Broussard, B., et al. (2014). The Police-Based Crisis Intervention Team (CIT) Model: I. Effects on Officers' Knowledge, Attitudes, and Skills. *Psychiatric Services, 65,* 517–522.

Cook, B. L., Wayne, G., Kafali, N., et al. (2014). Trends in smoking among adults with mental illness and association between mental health treatment and smoking cessation. *Journal of the American Medical Association, 311*(2), 172–182.

Corominas-Roso, M., Ramos-Quirogal, J., Ribases, M., et al. (2013). Decreased serum levels of brain-derived neurotrophic factor in adults with attention-deficit hyperactivity disorder. *International Journal of Neuropsychopharmacology, 16,* 1267–1275.

Diaz, J. (2010). The psychobiology of aggression and violence: Bioethical implications. *International Social Science Journal, 61*(200–201), 233–245.

Fuermaier, A., Tucha, L., Koerts, J., et al. (2014). Good vibrations—effects of whole body vibration on attention in healthy individuals and individuals with ADHD. *Plos One, 9*(2), 1–8.

Furber, G., Jones, G., Healey, D., et al. (2014). Comparison between phone-based psychotherapy with and without text messaging support in between sessions for crisis patients. *Journal of Medical Internet Research, 16*(10). Retrieved May 3, 2015, from http://www.ncbi.nlm.nih.gov/pmc/articles/PMC4210953/.

Grant, J. E., & Leppink, E. W. (2015). Impulse-control and conduct disorders: Limited evidence, no approved DRUGS to guide treatment. *Current Psychiatry, 14*(1), 29–35.

Grant, J. E., Potenza, M. N., Hollander, E., et al. (2006). Multicenter investigation of the opioid antagonist nalmefene in the treatment of pathological gambling. *American Journal of Psychiatry, 163,* 303–312.

Garrett, K., & Giddings, K. (2014). Improving impulse control: Using an evidence-based practice approach. *Journal of Evidence-Based Social Work, 11,* 73–83.

Harvard Health Publications. (2014). *Pessimism about pedophilia.* Retrieved April 30, 2015, from http://www.health.harvard.edu/newsletter_article/pessimism-about-pedophilia.

Hirsch Allen, A., Park, J., Adhami, N., et al. (2014). Impact of work schedules on sleep duration of critical care nurses. *American Journal of Critical Care, 23*(4), 290–295.

Holoyda, B., & Kellaher, D. (2016). The biological treatment of paraphilic disorders. *Current Psychiatry Reports, 18,* 19.

Howard, R., Schellhorn, K., & Lumsden, J. (2013). Complex case: A biofeedback intervention to control impulsiveness in a severely personality disordered forensic patient. *Personality and Mental Health, 7,* 168–173.

Inoue, Y., & Komada, Y. (2014). Sleep loss, sleep disorders and driving accidents. *Sleep and Biological Rhythms, 2014*(12), 96–105.

Kim, K., Becker-Cohen, M., & Serakos, M. (2015). *The processing and treatment of mentally ill persons in the criminal justice system.* Washington, DC: Urban Institute. Retrieved May 5, 2015, from http://www.urban.org/sites/default/files/alfresco/publication-pdfs/2000173-The-Processing-and-Treatment-of-Mentally-Ill-Persons-in-the-Criminal-Justice-System.pdf.

Kingston, D., Seto, M., & Ahmed, A. (2012). The role of central and peripheral hormones in sexual and violent recidivism in sex offenders. *Journal of the American Academy of Psychiatry and the Law, 40,* 476–485.

Latalova, K., Kamaradova, D., & Prasko, J. (2014). Violent victimization of adult patients with severe mental illness: A systematic review. *Neuropsychiatric Disease and Treatment, 10,* 1925–1940.

Lubit, R. (2015). *Sleep disorders.* Retrieved May 10, 2015, from http://emedicine.medscape.com/article/287104-overview.

Marshall, W. L. (2007). Diagnostic issues, multiple paraphilias, and comorbid disorders in sexual offenders: Their incidence and treatment. *Aggression and Violent Behavior, 12*(1), 16–35.

Mayo Clinic. (2013). *Adult attention-deficit/hyperactivity disorder.* Retrieved May 8, 2015, from http://www.mayoclinic.org/diseases-conditions/adult-adhd/basics/symptoms/con-20034552.

McManus, M., Hargreaves, P., Rainbow, L., et al. (2013). Paraphilias: Definition, diagnosis and treatment. *F1000Prime Reports, 5,* 36.

Mental Health America. (2011). *Position Statement 55: Confining sexual predators in the mental health system.* Retrieved May 8, 2015, from http://www.mentalhealthamerica.net/positions/sexual-predators.

Miranda, A., Berenguer, C., Colomer, C., et al. (2014). Influence of the symptoms of attention deficit hyperactivity disorder (ADHD) and comorbid disorders on functioning in adulthood. *Psicothema, 26*(4), 471–476.

Moore, T., Glenmullen, J., & Mattison, D. (2014). Reports of pathological gambling, hypersexuality, and compulsive shopping associated with dopamine receptor agonist drugs. *JAMA Internal Medicine, 174*(12), 1930–1933.

Murray, C. J., Atkinson, C., Bhalla, K., et al. (2013). The state of US health, 1990–2010: Burden of diseases, injuries, and risk factors. *Journal of the American Medical Association, 310*(6), 591–606.

NANDA International. (2014). *Nursing diagnoses: Definitions and classification 2015–2017.* Hoboken, NJ: Wiley.

National Alliance on Mental Illness (NAMI). (2010). *Creating the states 2009.* Retrieved September 4, 2013, from http://www2.nami.org/gtstemplate09.cfm?section=State_by_State09&Template=customsource/gts09StatebyState.cfm.

National Alliance on Mental Illness (NAMI). (2012). *Dual diagnosis.* Retrieved May 15, 2015, from http://www.nami.org/Learn-More/Mental-Health-Conditions/Related-Conditions/Dual-Diagnosis.

National Alliance on Mental Illness (NAMI). (2015b). *Anosognosia fact sheet.* Retrieved April 20, 2015, from http://www.nami.org/getattachment/Learn-More/Fact-Sheet-Library/Anosognosia-Fact-Sheet.pdf.

National Alliance on Mental Illness (NAMI). (2015a). *Dual diagnosis.* Retrieved April 25, 2015, from http://www.nami.org/Learn-More/Mental-Health-Conditions/Related-Conditions/Dual-Diagnosis.

Ohayon, M., Black, J., Lai, C., et al. (2014). Increased mortality in narcolepsy. *Sleep, 37*(3), 439–444.

Rahman, Q., & Symeonides, D. (2008). Neurodevelopmental correlates of paraphilic sexual interests in men. *Archives of Sexual Behaviour, 37*(1), 166–172.

Robertson, A., Lin, H., Frisman, L., et al. (2014). Mental health and re-offending outcomes of jail diversion participants with a brief incarceration after arraignment. *Psychiatric Services, 65*(9), 1113–1119.

Rosenbloom, M., Schmahmann, J., & Price, B. (2012). The functional neuroanatomy of decision-making. *Journal of Neuropsychiatry and Clinical Neurosciences, 24,* 266–277.

Royal College of Psychiatrists. (2013). *Good practice guidelines for the assessment and treatment of adults with gender dysphoria.* Retrieved May 5, 2015, from http://www.rcpsych.ac.uk/usefulresources/publications/collegereports/cr/cr181.aspx.

Rucklidge, J., Frampton, C., Gorman, B., et al. (2014). Vitamin-mineral treatment of attention-deficit hyperactivity disorder in adults: Double-blind randomised placebo-controlled trial. *British Journal of Psychiatry, 204,* 306–315.

Schmid, S., Hallschmid, M., & Schultes, B. (2015). The metabolic burden of sleep loss. *Lancet Diabetes and Endocrinology, 3*(1), 52–62.

Settineri, S., Rizzo, A., Liotta, M., et al. (2014). Caregiver's burden and quality of life: Caring for physical and mental illness. *International Journal of Psychological Research, 7*(1), 30–39.

Social Security Administration. (2015). *Understanding Supplemental Security Income SSI eligibility requirements, 2015 edition.* Retrieved April 30, 2015, from http://www.socialsecurity.gov/ssi/text-eligibility-ussi.htm.

Substance Abuse and Mental Health Services Administration (SAMHSA). (2014a). *Behavioral health barometer: United States, 2014.* Retrieved from http://www.samhsa.gov/data/sites/default/files/National_BHBarometer_2014/National_BHBarometer_2014.pdf.

Swanson, J., & Swartz, M. (2014). Why the evidence for outpatient commitment is good enough. *Psychiatric Services, 65*(6), 808–811.

Sylvia, L., Salcedo, S., Bianchi, M., et al. (2014). A novel home sleep monitoring device and brief sleep intervention for bipolar disorder: Feasibility, tolerability, and preliminary effectiveness. *Cognitive Therapy Research, 38,* 55–61.

Takahashi, M. (2014). Assisting shift workers through sleep and circadian research. *Sleep and Biological Rhythms, 12,* 85–95.

Tanwani, P., Fernie, B., Nikčević, A., et al. (2014). A systematic review of treatments for impulse control disorders and related behaviours in Parkinson's disease. *Psychiatry Research, 225,* 402–406.

Waghorn, G., Dias, S., Gladman, B., et al. (2014). A multi-site randomised controlled trial of evidence-based supported employment for adults with severe and persistent mental illness. *Australian Occupational Therapy Journal, 61*(6), 424–436.

Walker, C. (2014). The Affordable Care Act and mental health services. *Journal of Psychosocial Nursing, 52*(9), 3–4.

Welsh, E., & McEnany, G. (2015). Approaches to reduce physical comorbidity in individuals diagnosed with mental illness. *Journal of Psychosocial Nursing, 53*(2), 33–37.

World Health Organization (WHO). (2013). *Mental health action plan 2013–2020.* Retrieved April 24, 2015, from http://apps.who.int/iris/bitstream/10665/89966/1/9789241506021_eng.pdf.

Xie, L., Kang, H., Xu, Q., et al. (2013). Sleep drives metabolite clearance from the adult brain. *Science, 342,* 373–378.

Zanello, A., Mohr, S., Merlo, M., et al. (2014). Effectiveness of a brief group cognitive behavioral therapy for auditory verbal hallucinations. *Journal of Nervous and Mental Disease, 202*(2), 144–153.

Older Adults

Susan L. Frost, Chyllia D. Fosbre, Elizabeth M. Varcarolis

(e) http://evolve.elsevier.com/Varcarolis/essentials

KEY TERMS AND CONCEPTS

advance directive, p. 449
age discrimination, p. 439
ageism, p. 439
chemical restraints, p. 448
directive to physician, p. 449

durable power of attorney for health care, p. 449
elderspeak, p. 440
geropsychiatric nurses p. 440
living will, p. 449

Patient Self-Determination Act (PSDA), p. 449
physical restraints, p. 448

SELECTED CONCEPT: AGEISM

Ageism is stereotyping, prejudice, or discrimination against a person or group of people based on their age, typically toward the older adult but it can affect any age group. Ageism can be found at the individual, organizational, or systemic level. Interpersonal ageism occurs when an individual discriminates against another based on age. Organizational ageism can be written or unwritten business practices and policies. It may limit advancement opportunities based on the age of workers. Systemic ageism affects communities or runs in a culture and may be seen in how the elderly are treated by their families or within the health care system. It is a common belief in Western society that the elderly are less valuable. Rather than being respected for their accumulated wisdom, younger persons may yell at them for driving slowly, be irritated with them in the workplace, be impatient with hearing loss or slowed reactions, and believe that they are less of a person. Some other cultures such as Eastern and Native American, and some subgroups and subcultures within Western cultures, do revere the elderly and make sure they continue to have a useful place in the family and society.

OBJECTIVES

1. Identify facts and myths about aging.
2. Describe the negative effects that "ageism" and "elderspeak" can have on older adults.
3. Identify ways you can challenge ageism and increase the awareness of fellow students and others who care for older adults.
4. **QSEN** List group interventions commonly used with older adults and how implementing **teamwork and collaboration** plays a part.
5. Using a comprehensive geriatric assessment, identify guidelines for assessing an older adult including safety promotion.
6. Discuss how you might apply communication strategies during an interview or assessment with an older adult.
7. **QSEN** Identify differences between an older adult and younger adult in the approach to **patient-centered care** for a patient with depression and suicidal ideation, and identify risk factors for elder suicide.
8. **QSEN** Using **evidence-based research**, identify differences in the physiological effects of alcohol use on an older individual compared with those on a younger adult.
9. **QSEN** Identify **quality improvement methods** you can use to address the use of physical and/or chemical restraints.
10. Discuss institutional requirements related to the Patient Self-Determination Act of 1990.
11. **QSEN** Use **informatics** to determine laws and regulations in your state for the rights of older adults who are also lesbian, gay, bisexual, or transgender (LGBT).
12. Contrast and compare living wills, health care directives, and durable powers of attorney as used in health care settings.

INTRODUCTION

The older adult population is one of the most vulnerable populations in the United States. The baby boomer generation (individuals born between 1946 and 1964) is aging, and is predicted to strain the health care system with a rapid increase in the older adult population. The medical and mental health access of this population is an issue that will have to be addressed by all aspects of society (e.g.,

socioeconomic condition, legal system, and most profoundly, our health care system). This chapter discusses some of the concerns related to the growing numbers of older adults and health care issues unique to this population.

Several important considerations for promoting mental health in the older adult are presented in *Mental Health: A Report of the Surgeon General—Executive Summary* (U.S. Department of Health and Human

Services [USDHHS], 1999, p. 381). These include the need for older adults to continue to include social, intellectual, and physical activity in their routine. Older adults can continue to learn and contribute even when physiological changes occur. It is also important to recognize that mental and cognitive disorders are often not a normal part of aging but a sign of a disease process.

The increasing number of older adults is altering the socioeconomic condition and health care focus in the United States. By 2030, 20% of the U.S. population will consist of individuals older than 65 years of age, which translates into an increase in health care costs and a shrinking workforce. Among older adults, the fastest-growing subgroups are minorities, the poor, and those ages 85 years and older (Administration on Aging [AOA], 2014).

Older adults have been divided into the following age categories (Touhy & Jett, 2010):

- Young old: 65 to 74 years of age
- Middle old: 75 to 84 years of age
- Old old: 85 to 94 years of age
- Elite old: 94 years of age and older

About 65% of older adults have at least two chronic health conditions and over 40% have three or more (Health in Aging, 2016). After age 85, there is a one in three chance of developing dementia, immobility, incontinence, or another age-related disability.

Women generally outlive men by an average of 7 years. Husbands typically die before their spouses, so they benefit from the support of their wives to help with health-related issues. Older women are more likely to be widowed, to live alone, or to be institutionalized, and because they live longer than their spouse, they have more limited support. In Western society, families often live apart—in separate homes, states, or even countries. There is less of a community surrounding individuals as they age.

There are noticeable differences between individuals in their sixties and people in their eighties. Those in the younger group are relatively healthy, while those in the older group are much more vulnerable, frail, and at risk for visual problems, cognitive impairment, and falls. Persons in the older age group also have more limited economic resources and community supports and are more affected by the chronic diseases and disorders of aging (HealthyPeople2020, 2016; Touhy & Jett, 2010). Social Security constituted 90% or more of the income received by 35% of all Social Security beneficiaries, and about 9.7% of elderly persons are living below the poverty level (AOA, 2014).

A NOTE ON PHARMACOLOGY AND THE AGING ADULT

Pharmacology becomes increasingly complicated as adults age. One major factor is that the pharmacokinetics (absorption, distribution, metabolism, and excretion) of any drug change as we age. As the metabolism slows, drugs last longer and levels build up in the body. In addition to metabolism issues, older people frequently do not drink adequate fluids nor move as much. Approximately 50% of accidental drug-related deaths occur in the older population (HealthyPeople2020, 2016; Preston et al., 2013). Factors contributing to medication nonadherence include complicated directions in small print, hearing and visual impairments, cognitive and memory deficits, child-resistant packaging, and inability to pay for medication (Preston et al., 2013; Wick, 2011).

Previous studies have found that anticholinergic activity, which is a side effect of many commonly used drugs, has been linked with reduced brain function and early death in elder adults (Brooks, 2016). A recent neuroimaging study on the use of anticholinergic drugs between users and nonusers, demonstrated increased brain atrophy and hyper metabolism, thus explaining the increased risk for cognitive decline, poor memory, and diminish executive function (Brooks, 2016). Antihistamines and antidepressants are commonly prescribed medications with anticholinergic effects. This class also includes medications like nifedipine, codeine, hypertensive drugs, and drugs taken for congestive heart failure. Anticholinergics typically decrease saliva and cause sedation, leading to dry eyes, reduced fluid for body processes, and fall risk. The nurse needs to review all prescription and over-the-counter medications the patient is taking and be alert to the anticholinergic side effects, and keep in mind the delayed metabolism in elderly patients. It is best to avoid anticholinergic drugs in the elderly whenever possible. The physician needs to be notified if the patient is taking one or two medications that have this potential, since anticholinergic effects are cumulative.

AGEISM

Ageism refers to deeply rooted negative attitudes or bias toward people because of their age. In this text we are looking specifically at the bias toward the elderly. In American culture, there is a general dislike of the older adult by the younger generations (Bergman & Bodner, 2015). *Age prejudice* is based on the notion that aging makes people increasingly unattractive, unintelligent, asexual, unemployable, and senile. Age discrimination, on the other hand, includes actions and outcomes that reflect the bias toward the elderly. An example of this is hiring a younger, inexperienced person over an older, seasoned employee with years of experience.

Ageism is not limited to the way the young may look at the old. It can also be perpetrated by those in the older population when they become critical of themselves and their peers. The threat of social disgrace by association with the frail and infirm may prevent strong social groups. Age proximity raises feelings of vulnerability. This may explain why older adults often do not like to be referred to as "old." By seeing themselves as young, they adjust better to their advancing years (Gendron, et al., 2015).

Ageism differs from other forms of discrimination in that it cuts across gender, race, religion, sexual orientation, and national origin. In our culture, old age does not award a prestigious status recognizing the value of wisdom. Rather, it is a social category with negative connotations. Today, a new form of ageism puts the older adult in a no-win situation: those who are wealthy are envied for their economic success (even though it was earned), those who are middle class are blamed for straining the Social Security system, and those who are poor are resented for being tax burdens.

The results of ageism can be observed throughout every level of society. Even health care providers are not immune to its effects. Negative values can surface in myriad ways in the health care system: difficulty in obtaining insurance and support programs, caring for younger patient groups first, and personal beliefs and attitudes of the nurse that can infiltrate care.

Ageism among Health Care Workers

Health care personnel do not always share medical information, recommendations, and opportunities with the older adult. Studies show that older adults receive less information and sometimes less care than those who are younger. Ageism is also reflected in public policy, which leads to discrimination against older adults (American Society on Aging, 2012; Touhy & Jett, 2010).

Health care workers who deal on a daily basis with confused, ill, and frail older adults may tend to develop a somewhat negative and biased view of them. The negative attitudes of most health care workers are often a reflection of the stereotypical views of society. The rendering of medical care to older adults has been burdened with pessimism and professional aversion. In the Western culture there is an underlying belief that health care dollars should be spent on the younger and that the older adult has lived a good life and is no longer contributing financially to the pool (Kagan & Melendez-Torres, 2015). In Eastern or Native American cultures, the wisdom of the elderly is valued above the strength and stamina of the young, and past contributions are rewarded (North & Fiske, 2015).

Negative views of the older adult have significant implications for practice, education, and research. Positive attitudes toward older adults and their care need to be instilled as part of basic nursing education (Coleman, 2015). If the overall goal of nursing programs is to prepare students to practice in the future, then preparing students to care for older adults in a wide variety of settings is mandatory, because that *is* the future. The American Association of Colleges of Nursing (AACN) addresses this issue by calling for all nursing programs from diploma through doctoral level to "implement patient and family care around resolution of end-of-life and palliative care issues, such as symptom management, supportive rituals, and respect for patient and family preferences" (AACN, 2008). One of the ways institutional ageism is expressed is through length-of-stay averages that reflect a younger population's time frame and ability to heal (Kydd & Fleming, 2015). With the growing baby boomer population, there is an even greater need for health care professionals who can work with the older adult. The present health care system is unprepared to care adequately for the number of elderly persons with medical or mental health needs already in the system (Buckwalter et al., 2011). According to the literature, increased understanding of ageism leads to greater patient satisfaction (Ouchida & Lachs, 2015). To decrease this gap in care, suggestions have been made by the AACN (2008) for educational programs to adopt the following:

- Information about the aging process
- Discussion of attitudes relating to the care of the older adult
- Sensitization of participants to their patients' needs
- Use of valid and reliable assessment tools specific to the older adult
- Use of online guidelines to prevent, identify, and manage geriatric syndromes
- Exploration of the dynamics of nurse-patient and staff-patient interactions
  - Grief loss and bereavement
  - Ethical and legal issues
  - Communication

Box 28-1 lists some facts and myths about aging.

ASSESSMENT AND COMMUNICATION STRATEGIES

Nurses who work with older adults require specific knowledge about normal aging, drug interactions, chronic disease, treatment modalities, cultural influences, and the effect on loved ones. **Geropsychiatric nurses** work with older adult patients who have mental health problems and may be employed in a variety of settings, including nursing homes, assisted living facilities, community centers, inpatient units, prisons, and homeless shelters. One challenge is that this population still has medical issues in addition to psychiatric concerns, which must be ferreted out and addressed

The National Institutes of Health (NIH) recommends a comprehensive geriatric assessment to evaluate and manage the care and progress of all older adult patients. A comprehensive geriatric assessment takes into consideration the various aspects of functioning. These areas can include mental status, general physical health, ability to address health care needs, ability to manage finances, socialization, home maintenance and safety, nutrition and hydration, mobility, and a thorough review of medications and potentially negative interactions. Figure 28-1 provides an example of a comprehensive geriatric assessment. Younger patients may be

---

BOX 28-1   Facts and Myths about Aging

Facts

- The senses of vision, hearing, touch, taste, and smell decline with age.
- Muscular strength decreases with age. Muscle fibers atrophy and decrease in number.
- Regular sexual expressions are important to maintain sexual capacity and effective sexual performance.
- At least 50% of restorative sleep is lost as a result of the aging process.
- Older adults are major consumers of prescription drugs because of the high incidence of chronic diseases in this population.
- Older adults have a high incidence of depression.
- Many individuals experience difficulty when they retire.
- Older adults are prone to become victims of crime.
- Older widows appear to adjust better than younger ones.

Myths

- Most adults past the age of 65 years are demented.
- Sexual interest always declines with age.
- Older adults are not able to learn new tasks.
- As individuals age, they always become rigid in their thinking and resistant to change.
- Older adults are financially secure and no longer impoverished.
- Most older adults are infirm and require help with daily activities.
- Most older adults are socially isolated and lonely.
- All older adults are significantly hard of hearing and should be spoken to in a loud voice.

---

comfortable discussing personal issues such as family conflicts, feelings of sadness, sexual practices, finances, and bodily functions, while older adults may view these topics as private or taboo. Older generations were raised to keep personal matters private and were not taught to process emotions in the same way as younger generations have been. One of the gifts nurses can give their older patients is an understanding of this generational difference, and some gentle education guided by patient comfort level. A private and quiet setting is essential to a thorough assessment that touches on many personal topics, including sex and abuse. Additional measures include asking patients what they would like to be called, positioning self at the same level, using touch (per patient comfort level), body language, and eye contact to convey warmth and interest. Summarizing and inviting feedback are helpful.

Elderspeak is a term that refers to the unnecessary use of simple, childlike phrases; slow speech; high volume; and collective pronouns (do "we" want to take a bath?) when communicating with older adults. The intention behind it is typically aimed at creating a sense of caring; however, it can inadvertently imply that the older adult is incompetent. Studies are finding that these interactions can be perceived as insults, whether intentional or not, and contribute to poorer health outcomes. Adults who had a more positive outlook on becoming older had a slower rate of decline and better memory than those who had negative perceptions of aging (Oaklander, 2015).

Another related communication problem occurs when health care workers dismiss the presence of older adults in the room and speak *about* them rather than *to* them. Nursing students should consciously avoid using elderspeak. Address the older adult when asking a question, and when necessary, ask the family member or other health care worker(s) if they have anything to add. Box 28-2 provides helpful communication and interview techniques.

Comprehensive Geriatric Assessment

Name: _____ Date of birth: _____ Gender: _____

Physical Health

Chronic disorder

Vision	Adequate Inadequate Eyeglasses: Y N Needs evaluation

Hearing	Adequate Inadequate Hearing aids: Y N

Mobility   Ambulatory: Y N   Assistive device: _____
              Falls: Y N   Needs evaluation

Nutrition   Albumin: _____   TLC: _____   HCT: _____
               Weight: _____   Weight loss or gain: Y N   Needs evaluation

Incontinence   Y N   Treatment: Y N   Needs evaluation

Medications   Total number: _____   Reviewed & revised: Y N
                 Adverse effects/allergy: _____

Screening   Cholesterol: _____TSH: _____ B$_{12}$: _____ Folate: _____
               Mammogram: _____Date: _____ N/A
               Osteoporosis: _____Date: _____ N/A
               Pap smear: _____Date: _____ N/A
               PSA: _____Date: _____ N/A

Immunization   Influenza: _____Date: _____
                  Pneumonia: _____Date: _____
                  Tetanus: _____Date: _____ Booster: _____

Counseling   Diet   Exercise   Calcium   Vitamin D
                Smoking   Alcohol   Driving   Injury prevention

Mental Health

Dementia   Y N   MMSE score: _____Date: _____   Cause (if known):

Depression   Y N   GDS score: _____Date: _____   Treatment: Y N

Functional Status

ADL   Bathing: I   D   Dressing: I   D   Toileting: I   D
         Transferring: I   D   Feeding: I   D   Continence: I   D

KEY: *ADL*, Activities of daily living; *B$_{12}$*, vitamin B$_{12}$; *D*, dependent; *GDS*, Geriatric Depression Scale; *HCT*, hematocrit; *I*, independent; *MMSE*, Mini-Mental State Examination; *N*, no; *PSA*, prostate-specific antigen; *TLC*, total lymphocyte count; *TSH*, thyroid-stimulating hormone; *Y*, yes.

FIGURE 28-1 Comprehensive geriatric assessment.

APPLYING EVIDENCE-BASED PRACTICE (EBP)

Problem A parish nurse visits an elderly member of the church community after she had not attended church in a few weeks. The nurse finds her patient weak and confused. As part of her nursing assessment, she reviews all of the patient's medications. She finds some inconsistencies, including taking older prescriptions and newly ordered prescriptions together, taking similar class blood pressure medications from a primary care physician (PCP) for hypertension and from a psychiatric nurse practitioner for anxiety and sleep, and taking 3 units of insulin glargine (Lantus) instead of 30 units. The patient had become confused when changing from an insulin bottle and syringe to using an insulin pen several months previously. Her fluid intake was also inadequate.

EBP Assessment

A. **What do you already know from experience?** Elderly patients are vulnerable to medication interactions, polypharmacy, confusion, and dehydration. Many elderly patients resist drinking adequate fluids due to increased trips to the bathroom. Elderly patients may be hard of hearing and have memory impairments, which contribute to misunderstanding or forgetting provider instructions. This population may also lack a support system to help with these issues.

B. **What does the literature say?** Polypharmacy is a serious issue in the elderly, with daily pill burden of up to 60 pills per day. A "cascade" effect sometimes occurs when a medication is prescribed to treat side effects from the first medication. Most individuals over 65 years of age take between 5 and 10 medications, and the number is significantly higher in long-term residents.

Farrell and colleagues (2013) suggest a monitored medication taper, or even an inpatient stay during which medications are weaned over several weeks, to evaluate what is still needed. Being aware of pharmacological interactions and noncompliance in the elderly is imperative for nurses (Wooten, 2015).

C. **What does the patient want?** She wants to feel better so she can attend church again. She is confused about her medications and wants help organizing them.

Plan The parish nurse carefully reconciled the medications and disposed of older medications. She made the patient a chart of her current medications and times. She purchased four weekly medication sets, and loaded them with the morning and evening dosages. She spent time on patient education about the medication uses and side effects. She discussed the importance of hydration in metabolizing the medications safely. She made an appointment with the PCP and attended with the patient to discuss the incorrect medication usage, as well as to obtain a titration schedule for the insulin based on Accu-Chek readings. Once the patient was feeling better, she happily returned to her church activities and friends.

QSEN   **QSEN Prelicensure Knowledge, Skills, and Attitudes (KSAs) Addressed:**

Safety was addressed through medication reconciliation and patient education.

Team work and collaboration was apparent as the parish nurse worked with the PCP to assist the patient.

Farrell, B., Shamji, S., Monahan, A., et al. (2013). Reducing polypharmacy in the elderly. *Canadian Pharmacists Journal, 146* (5), 243–244; Wooten, J. M. (2015). Pharmacotherapy considerations in elderly adults. *Southern Medical Journal, 105*(8), 437–445.

BOX 28-2   Communication Guidelines for Interviewing the Older Adult

1. Gather preliminary data before the session and keep questionnaires relatively short.
2. Ask about often-overlooked problems, such as difficulty sleeping, incontinence, falling, depression, dizziness, sexual activity, alcohol or drug use, or loss of energy.
3. Pace the interview to allow the patient to formulate answers, resist the tendency to interrupt prematurely.
4. Use simple choice questions if the older patient has trouble coping with open-ended questions.
5. Begin with general questions such as, "How can I help you most at this visit?" or "What's been happening?"
6. Be alert for information on the patient's relationships with others, thoughts about family or co-workers, typical responses to stress, and attitudes toward aging, illness, occupation, and death.
7. Assess mental status for deficits in recent or remote memory, and determine if confusion exists.
8. Note all medications the patient is taking and assess for side effects, efficacy, possible drug interactions, and if the patient is taking them regularly and correctly.
9. Determine how fast the condition of the patient has been changing, and assess the extent of the patient's concerns.
10. Include the family or significant other in the interview process for added input, clarification, support, and reinforcement with patient's permission.

From National Institute on Aging. (2011). *Working with your older patient: A clinician's handbook.* Bethesda, MD.

PSYCHIATRIC DISORDERS IN OLDER ADULTS

Not only are older adults with mental disorders less likely to be accurately diagnosed, but they are also more likely to receive inappropriate or inadequate treatment compared with younger adults (McEnany, 2011). It is important to keep in mind that presentations of mental disorders vary substantially with age. This is especially true for individuals with depression and anxiety. Mental illness is sometimes misinterpreted as normal aging, and as a result patients are not provided with treatment that could improve quality of life. Solid evidence-based literature and studies dealing with geriatric anxiety disorder, bipolar disorders, geriatric schizophrenia, or geriatric alcohol use disorders are in short supply (Buckwalter et al., 2011). Common mental health issues affecting older adults discussed in this chapter are depression, suicide, memory impairment, and alcohol and drug use. In addition to mental health diagnoses, elder abuse and caregiver role strain are significant concerns in this population. These issues are discussed in Chapter 21. Cognitive symptoms affecting the elderly adult are discussed in Chapter 18.

Depression

Depression is the most common, the most debilitating, and also the most treatable psychiatric disorder in the older adult (Robinson et al., 2016). Depression in later life creates pain, suffering, poor quality of life, and spiritual anguish. Depression can be dangerous when the older person is also experiencing a chronic illness, loneliness, or losses (such as spouse, job, independence, home, finances, or health), and depression is the biggest risk factor for suicide (Robinson et al., 2016).

Health care providers frequently misinterpret clinical depression in older adults as a normal part of aging, especially if the older adult is experiencing neurological symptoms (dementia) or other physical illnesses (Robinson et al., 2016). Symptoms of depression such as memory loss, intellectual impairment, asocial behavior, or agitation may be misinterpreted as dementia or other cognitive disorders. As a result, older adults may miss out on treatment that would improve quality of life significantly.

A careful assessment is needed to distinguish among delirium, dementia, and depression because presenting symptoms can be similar, or two or more may co-occur. (See Table 28-1 for a comparison of delirium, dementia, and depression.) Chapter 18 gives thorough assessment guidelines and interventions for a patient experiencing delirium or dementia.

In making an assessment, the nurse needs to be familiar with the symptoms of depression in general, and how symptoms may differ in the elderly. Besides the core symptoms we recognize regarding depression (see Chapter 15), depression in the elderly may be expressed as physical symptoms or negative behaviors such as forgetfulness, agitation, combativeness, constant complaining, irritability and anger, treatment-resistant aches and pains, fatigue, apprehension, unwarranted suspicion or paranoia, and low self-esteem.

A variety of biological and psychosocial risk factors for depression have been identified. These include medical illness, functional disability, social isolation, accumulation of life stressors, losses, and genetic vulnerabilities. Depression can be caused by a wide variety of drugs, including steroids, beta blockers, weight loss medications, opioids, benzodiazepines, and varenicline (Chantix); and by medical disorders such as hepatitis, cardiac disease, cerebrovascular accident, and respiratory, endocrine, and thyroid disorders. Depression contributes to suicide potential. Thorough assessment for any medical- or drug-induced side effects should be performed in addition to the psychosocial assessment. (See Figure 28-2 for the Geriatric Depression Scale.)

Depression in later life increases the risk for medical comorbidities, suicide, disability, and family caregiving burden. Undiagnosed depression also increases the risk for unhealthy behaviors to compensate for mood, such as substance abuse or gambling, and contributes to the progression of other chronic illnesses (Andreescu & Reynolds, 2011; Byrd & Vito, 2011).

Depression in later life responds well to (1) *psychosocial treatments* that relieve loneliness, such as group aerobic exercise sessions; (2) *talk therapies* such as psychotherapy or cognitive behavioral therapy, which may be effective with or without the use of medications; and (3) *establishment of social support systems* such as group meals, scheduled visitors, and volunteer work (Robinson et al., 2016). These psychosocial and cognitive interventions can be critical in treating late-life depression since fewer than 50% of older adults on antidepressants achieve full symptom remission (Alexopoulos & Knosses, 2011).

In addition to the aforementioned therapies, antidepressants and electroconvulsive therapy (ECT) may be appropriate for more severe depressions, especially for those persons who have suffered a life-long battle with this disorder. Elderly persons with severe depression respond similarly to middle-aged adults with depression in terms of both psychopharmacology and ECT; however, the relapse rates are higher in older adults (Andreescu & Reynolds, 2011). Intractable depression may be treated with ECT, which is effective in 80% of cases (Kellner, 2015). However, this treatment is time consuming, usually requiring a course of around a dozen treatments, and carries unwanted side effects, including memory impairment and regular exposure to strong intravenous medications, including anesthesia. These untoward effects may be especially risky in elderly patients.

Antidepressant Therapy

In choosing a drug to treat depression in the older adult, primary emphasis is placed on avoidance of side effects rather than on efficacy. Lower dosages are initiated, often half of a usual adult dosage, and the medication is advanced gradually. Practitioners often remember the adage "start low, go slow" for young and elderly patients (Ruscin & Linnebur, 2014). The patient and caregivers must be aware that onset or increase of suicidal thoughts is a potential side effect of antidepressant medication. Although this does not occur in the majority of patients, it is important to provide patient education and monitoring for this serious potential side effect.

The choice of which class of antidepressants to use for older adults is complex. Selective serotonin reuptake inhibitors (SSRIs) have traditionally been the first-line antidepressants for older adults because of their more benign side effects and their lack of toxicity when taken in overdose. However, SSRIs may also cause increased risk of bone fractures and place older adults at risk for hip fractures

TABLE 28-1 Comparison of Delirium, Dementia, and Depression

	Delirium	Dementia	Depression
Onset	Sudden, over hours to days	Slowly, over months	May have been gradual with exacerbation during crisis or stress
Cause or contributing factors	Hypoglycemia, fever, dehydration, hypotension; infection, other conditions that disrupt body's homeostasis; adverse drug reaction; head injury; change in environment (e.g., hospitalization); pain; emotional stress	Alzheimer's disease, vascular disease, human immunodeficiency virus (HIV) infection, neurological disease, chronic alcoholism, head trauma	Lifelong history, losses, loneliness, crises, declining health, medical conditions
Cognition	Impaired memory, judgment, calculations, attention span; can fluctuate throughout the day	Impaired memory, judgment, calculations, attention span, abstract thinking; agnosia	Difficulty concentrating, forgetfulness, inattention
Level of consciousness	Altered	Not altered	Not altered
Activity level	Can be increased or reduced; restlessness, behaviors may worsen in evening (sundowning); sleep-wake cycle may be reversed	Not altered; behaviors may worsen in evening (sundowning)	Usually decreased; lethargy, fatigue, lack of motivation; may sleep poorly and awaken in early morning
Emotional state	Rapid swings; can be fearful, anxious, suspicious, aggressive, have hallucinations and delusions	Flat; delusions	Extreme sadness, apathy, irritability, anxiety, paranoid ideation

Geriatric Depression Scale (Short Form)

		Yes	No
1.	Are you basically satisfied with your life?	○	○
2.	Have you dropped many of your activities and interests?	○	○
3.	Do you feel that your life is empty?	○	○
4.	Do you often get bored?	○	○
5.	Are you in good spirits most of the time?	○	○
6.	Are you afraid that something bad is going to happen to you?	○	○
7.	Do you feel happy most of the time?	○	○
8.	Do you often feel helpless?	○	○
9.	Do you prefer to stay at home, rather than going out and doing new things?	○	○
10.	Do you feel you have more problems with memory than most?	○	○
11.	Do you think it is wonderful to be alive now?	○	○
12.	Do you feel pretty worthless the way you are now?	○	○
13.	Do you feel full of energy?	○	○
14.	Do you feel that your situation is hopeless?	○	○
15.	Do you think that most people are better off than you are?	○	○

FIGURE 28-2 Geriatric Depression Scale (Short Form). (From Sheikh, J. I., & Yesavage, J. A. (1986). Geriatric Depression Scale (GDS): Recent evidence and development of a shorter version. In T. L. Brink (Ed.), *Clinical gerontology: A guide to assessment and intervention* (pp. 165–173). New York, NY: Haworth Press.)

(Bakken et al., 2013) as well as increased bleeding. Some studies rate the risk of morbidity with SSRIs as higher than with tricyclic antidepressants. One study contends that SSRIs and "other" antidepressants resulted in increased adverse outcomes when compared with tricyclic antidepressants (Coupland et al., 2011). Fractures are twice as common when patients are using SSRIs, through falls or even minor activity such as walking. Tricyclic antidepressants have more cardiac and anticholinergic side effects, as well as more interactions with other medications. Studies have found a higher rate of stopping treatment with tricyclics due to the side effect profile (Espinoza & Unutzer, 2016). Although SSRIs followed by serotonin-norepinephrine reuptake inhibitors (SNRIs) are first-line treatment in the elderly due to tolerability (Espinoza & Unutzer, 2016), "low dose of a tricyclic (TCA) antidepressant may be more suitable in frail elderly patients [who are] at increased risk of falls and fractures" (Coupland & Hochhalter, 2011). The risks and benefits, medical profile, and medication list must be assessed carefully in choosing the best antidepressant for a particular patient. Discontinuation symptoms may occur when stopping a medication, with "shocky" feelings and moodiness. Antidepressants should be decreased slowly to prevent undue stress on the patient (Coupland & Hochhalter, 2011).

Psychotherapy

Clinicians, including nurses, nurse practitioners, therapists, and psychologists, may provide individual or group psychotherapy to the depressed patient. As previously mentioned, groups can diminish social isolation and loneliness and help the members understand that they are not alone in their situation. Mixed-age groups can be beneficial for a variety of energy and insights, while same-age groups can help provide support from others in similar situations. Group members can learn creative ways to raise their mood and increase quality of life within various types of groups (Table 28-2).

Cognitive behavioral therapy (CBT), problem-solving therapy (PST), interpersonal therapy (IPT), and supportive therapy are often used alone or as an adjunct to psychopharmacology. Most research shows a combination of therapy and medication to be the most effective approach.

Suicide

According to the CDC (2015), the suicide rate for those over 65 has dropped considerably, and now is the 17th leading causes of death among those 65 and over. That being said, nursing assessment and intervention for suicidal ideations and treatment of depression needs to be thorough in assessing elderly people. Early identification of risk factors needs to be made in all settings, especially the emergency department, primary care, and mental health settings. As many as 70% of elderly patients have visited their primary care provider within a month of committing suicide (American Psychological Association, 2016).

Even though the suicide rate among older adults has decreased from previous levels, it is likely underreported. Suicide is not always listed on the death certificate when suspected, and passive behaviors

TABLE 28-2 Useful Group Therapy Modalities for Older Adult Patients

Re-Motivation Therapy	Reminiscence Therapy (Life Review)	Psychotherapy
Purpose of Group		
Resocialize regressed and apathetic patients	Share memories of the past	Alleviate psychiatric symptoms
Reawaken interest in the environment	Increase self-esteem	Increase ability to interact with others in a group
	Increase socialization	Increase self-esteem
	Increase awareness of the uniqueness of each participant	Increase ability to make decisions and function more independently
Format		
Groups are made up of 10 to 15 people	Groups are made up of 6 to 8 people	Group size is 6 to 12 members
Meetings are held once or twice a week	Meetings are held once or twice weekly for 1 hour	Group members should share similar:
Meetings are highly structured in a classroom-like setting	Topics include holidays, major life events, birthdays, travel, and food	• Problems
Group uses props		• Mental status
Each session discusses a particular topic		• Needs
		• Sexual integration
		Group meets at regularly scheduled times (certain number of times a week, specific duration of session) and place
Desired Outcomes		
Increase participants' sense of reality	Alleviate depression in institutionalized older adult	Decrease sense of isolation
Offer practice of health roles	Through the process of reorganization and reintegration, provide avenue by members	Facilitate development of new roles and re-establish former roles
Realize more objective self-image than older adult can	Achieve a new sense of identity	Provide information for other group
	Achieve a positive self-concept	Provide group support for effecting changes and increasing self-esteem

From Matteson, M.A., & McConnell, E.S. (Eds.). (1988). *Gerontologic nursing: Concepts and practice* (p. 80). Philadelphia, PA: Saunders.

such as alcoholism, starvation, overmedicating, or losing the will to live may not be recognized as suicidal behaviors (CDC, 2016). The elderly have many risk factors that can lead to suicide such as feelings of hopelessness, uselessness, and despair; medical issues; functional loss and pain; financial distress; and a variety of losses. A history of suicide attempts is always a risk factor. Suicidal gestures in the elderly may be desperate cries for help or serious attempts at dying, as in other age groups. An inverse relationship between economic conditions and suicide rate has been identified.

Assessment of Suicide Risk

The assessment of elderly individuals must include attention to the high-risk factors that potentially contribute to suicide, such as widowhood, acute illnesses and intractable pain, status change, chronic illness, family history of suicide, chronic sleep problems, alcoholism, depression, and other losses (see Chapter 23). Losses may be personal (death of a family member or close friend), economic (loss of job or home), social (loss of prestige or position), or functional (loss of health or mobility). Multiple losses accompany the aging process, increasing stress at a time when the older adult may be the most vulnerable and least able to cope with stress, thus precipitating a depressive state. According to Erikson's Stages of Development, the elderly must find meaningful activities in their lives to replace the jobs and successes they have lost, in order to successfully transition to a fulfilling older life (Ego integrity versus Despair) (Heffner, 2015). Nurses can assist patients with this transition toward wisdom, reviewing their lives with a sense of completeness, and ultimately acceptance of death.

In assessing suicide risk, the health care provider must consider previous suicidal behavior, seriousness of the intent, presence of active plans, availability of the means to commit the act, and lethality of the method chosen. Compared to those in younger age groups, older adults are less likely or able to communicate their suicidal thoughts and plans.

Nurses play a vital role in the prevention of older adult suicide because of their presence in every care setting and the trust that patients place in them. Talking about suicide should not be avoided, but as with all age groups and even more so in the elderly due to generational differences in communication, the subject of suicide must be approached gently. Just the word "suicide" can be upsetting and stigmatizing, and people have differing definitions of that word. Examples of a beginning approach may be to ask the person if he or she is wishing to not be around, not be alive, be with deceased loves ones, or no longer experience all of the stressors. If the person answers affirmatively, the conversation can be continued. Helping the patient to remember and talk about what he or she has to live for, or what he or she would want to see in the future, is helpful in alleviating suicidal thoughts (Touhy & Jett, 2010; Yeates, Van Orden, & Caine, 2011). See Chapter 23 for more detailed information on this subject, including the newly MODIFIED SAD PERSONS Scale **and the Suicide Assessment Five-step Evaluation and Triage (SAFE-T) for Mental Health Professionals**. Attention must be focused on building awareness, routine screening, and use of community resources in the high-risk elderly population (USDHHS, 2016).

Right to Die

One ethical dilemma in nursing is the question of whether older adults have the right to end their lives themselves or by way of physician-assisted suicide (PAS). Suicide raises spiritual and moral issues. Some in society believe that older adults with terminal illnesses or those who suffer intractable pain should be able to control their own deaths. Others believe that suicide is never a correct option. If an alert older adult patient is confronted with an intractable, lingering, and painful illness, with no hope of relief except through death, is suicide justifiable?

According to the American Nurses Association (ANA), nurses are prohibited from participating in assisted suicide or euthanasia, as a direct violation of the ANA's *Code of Ethics for Nurses* and its covenant with society to provide humane, comprehensive, and compassionate care. The withholding or withdrawal of life-sustaining treatment (ventilation, cardiopulmonary support, chemotherapy, dialysis, medications, nutrition, and hydration) is ethically acceptable. This is considered allowing the patient to die from the underlying condition and does not involve direct action to end a life. Administering medications with the intent to promote comfort is not the same as the intent to end life. A common example is giving morphine with the intent to reduce pain in terminal illness, although this medication also depresses the respiratory center. Nurses are expected to care for their patients despite any philosophical differences with decisions regarding treatments and death (ANA, 2013). Assisted suicide is now legal in Oregon, Washington, California, and Vermont. If a nurse works in a state where assisted suicide in not legal and participates in helping a patient to end his or her life, the nurse is at risk for legal action and loss of licensure. The Oregon Nurses Association has developed guidelines for nurses, stating they can explain assisted suicide law, discuss options, and provide resources (ANA, 2013). Conversely, the American Public Health Association supports allowing a competent adult to obtain a prescription to self-administer, to control the time and manner of his or her own death (ANA, 2013). As the population ages, end-of-life discussions will become more common and pressing.

The Netherlands has historically been pro-PAS, with rates of PAS there progressively increasing through the years. The topic is explored by Richard Fenigsen, MD, PhD (2010, 2011). In one vignette, a lonely and depressed widow repeatedly asked her physician for a lethal dose of medication, and he finally complied. After the woman's death, when the physician was reviewing the case, a colleague queried, "Did you think of buying her a cat?" This scenario raises poignant questions and stimulates thought about the multiple aspects and concerns surrounding this issue.

Although suicide is discussed in Chapter 23, specific factors that concern older adults, such as retirement-related difficulties, physical illness, economic problems, loneliness, social isolation, multiple losses, and the concept of ageism, have been illuminated here. Education of the public and health care providers will become increasingly important as the general population ages.

Alcoholism and Substance Use and Addiction

The American Medical Association has called alcohol and substance abuse among older adults a hidden epidemic. Rates of alcoholism and prescription drug abuse may increase in the older population, as the baby boom generation who had greater lifetime rates of drug use is now aging. Identifying alcohol and substance abuse is often difficult because personality and behavioral changes may be unrecognized or attributed to medications, dementia, or medical issues. As with other generational communication differences previously discussed, such as processing emotions or discussing suicide, older patients may have a different definition or understanding of alcohol and substance use. Cocktail hours were common among older generations, as was the generous prescribing of benzodiazepines. Many older adults do not recognize their substance use patterns as a problem, until they go into withdrawal when their medication is left behind on vacation or they do not have access to alcohol while hospitalized.

Alcoholism

Elderly patients with substance use issues may have a long-term problem or a newly developed addiction in response to life stressors. The loss of a spouse and distance from family may contribute to alcoholism. The lack of structure from work or raising a family may be the impetus for a social drinker to advance to a problematic level of use.

Alcohol and Aging. Excessive consumption of alcohol can create particular problems for older adults. They have an increased biological sensitivity to (i.e., decreased tolerance for) the effects of alcohol. The decreased tolerance is related to a slower emptying of stomach contents; a slower metabolism, including hepatic function; and an increased sensitivity to alcohol in the brain. As people age there is a decline in lean muscle mass and an increase in fatty tissue that can contribute to increased blood alcohol levels (BALs) (USDHHS, 2014). Age-related changes such as decreased dexterity, balance, and flexibility can increase the likelihood of falls, burns, or other accidents when under the influence or alcohol or other substances. Injuries sustained while under the influence tend to heal more slowly than in younger years.

Some drinkers, as they get older, note changes in their response to alcohol, such as the occurrence of headaches, reduction in mental abilities with memory losses or lapses, and feelings of malaise rather than well-being. These problems start to occur at lower levels of consumption than was the case in earlier years, which can indicate liver damage or slowed metabolism in general. Older adults are likely to drink more frequently but in lesser quantities than younger individuals, who tend to drink larger amounts less often. Thus the possibility of alcohol use in cases of only moderate levels of use by older adults often is not recognized by friends or family as a problem.

Alcohol and Medication. The interaction of drugs and alcohol in the older adult can have serious consequences. Alcohol may prolong, potentiate, or accelerate the metabolism of various drugs. Some drugs, such as benzodiazepines or opiate pain medications, in combination with alcohol can be lethal or contribute to suicidal thoughts and suicide completion.

Older individuals can expect to reach higher blood alcohol levels than younger people with an equivalent intake of alcohol. Even a moderate intake of alcohol can impair the cognition and coordination skills that are already decreased with age. Extreme care is required when treating the older alcoholic with medication. Central nervous system toxicity from psychiatric drugs increases with aging. Ingestion of antidepressants or tranquilizers can be particularly harmful because their effect is further potentiated by alcohol, and the hepatotoxic effects of medications such as acetaminophen can be compounded.

Compared to younger individuals, older adults take longer to fall asleep and do not sleep as restfully. Although alcohol may help decrease the time it takes to fall asleep, this benefit is offset by frequent awakenings during the night caused by alcohol. Alcohol-related insomnia may encourage an older person to ask a health care provider for a sleeping medication, which can be dangerous in combination with alcohol or other medications. This is another example of why assessing substance use in the elderly population is important.

Symptoms of Elder Addiction. Health practitioners need to be concerned with, and sensitive to, possible alcohol abuse among their older patients. Signs of long-term alcohol abuse such as pancreatitis or liver disease, blackouts, or major trauma may not be present in adults who begin drinking later in life. Instead, the older alcoholic may display vague geriatric symptoms of contusions, malnutrition, self-neglect, impaired cognition, sleep disturbances, depression, and falls (USDHHS, 2014). Also present may be symptoms of diarrhea, urinary incontinence, a decrease in functional status, failure to thrive, and apparent dementia. Symptoms of poor coordination or visual changes may mimic the normal aging process, but actually may be a result of excessive drinking. Assessment is necessary to differentiate the normal physiological changes of aging from those attributable to excessive drinking.

Whenever there is a suspicion or indication that an older adult is abusing alcohol, the health care provider should conduct a screening test. The Short Michigan Alcohol Screening Test—Geriatric Version (SMAST-G; Figure 28-3) is commonly used to assess alcohol problems (Agency for Healthcare Research and Quality [AHRQ], 2012).

Short Michigan Alcoholism Screening Testing—Geriatric Version (S-MAST-G)

Please answer yes or no to each question by marking the line next to the question. When you finish answering the questions, please add up how many "yes" responses you checked and put that number in the space provided at the end.

	Yes	No
1. When talking to others, do you ever underestimate how much you actually drank?	☐	☐
2. After a few drinks, have you sometimes not eaten or been able to skip a meal because you didn't feel hungry?	☐	☐
3. Does having a few drinks help you decrease your shakiness or tremors?	☐	☐
4. Does alcohol sometimes make it hard for you to remember parts of the day or night?	☐	☐
5. Do you usually take a drink to relax or calm your nerves?	☐	☐
6. Do you drink to take your mind off your problems?	☐	☐
7. Have you ever increased your drinking after experiencing a loss in your life?	☐	☐
8. Has a doctor or nurse ever said they were worried or concerned about your drinking?	☐	☐
9. Have you ever made rules to manage your drinking?	☐	☐
10. When you feel lonely, does having a drink help?	☐	☐

Total:_____

Scoring: A score of 2 or higher is a positive screen for alcoholism.

FIGURE 28-3 Short Michigan Alcoholism Screening Testing—Geriatric Version (SMAST-G).

Treatment of the Older Adult Alcoholic. Because many older adults do not live in big families or have work-related contacts, they are less likely to be referred for treatment than are younger drinkers. Too often, by the time the older adult alcoholic is noticed by any treatment agencies, the patient's support systems and resources are severely decreased or depleted. Older patients may also hide their drinking out of shame, feeling sinful, or feeling that they can or should handle it themselves (Rogers & Weise, 2011; Touhy & Jett, 2010).

Treatment plans for the older patient with an addiction should emphasize social therapies. Older adult alcoholics tend to be more passive than younger alcoholics and may need more encouragement from health care professionals to participate in groups such as Alcoholics Anonymous and individual and family therapy. The prognosis for the patient who develops a drinking problem later in life is excellent, since the individual has lived most of his or her life without this habit. Brief treatment is often successful and nurses can be instrumental in educating the patient and encouraging the development of resources for the elderly. For those elderly adults with long histories of alcohol use who meet the criteria for alcohol dependence, a more rigorous treatment plan is required, including detoxification, often a few days in an inpatient unit (USDHHS, 2014). Medications to curb cravings such as naltrexone, an opiate agonist, may also play a part in longer-term treatment (Johnson, 2015). Recent studies show that gabapentin is very helpful in reducing cravings as patients become sober.

Substance USE

Illegal Drug Use. The number of older Americans seeking help for multiple substance abuse tripled from 13.7% to 39.7% between 1992 and 2008. During that same period, use of marijuana increased from 1% to 3%, cocaine from 3% to 11%, and heroin from 8% to 16% in the older population (Substance Abuse and Mental Health Services Administration [SAMHSA], 2010). The increasing numbers of older substance abusers will require expansion of age-specific services.

Prescription and Over-the-Counter Drug Use and Abuse. Because older adult patients use both prescription and over-the-counter drugs at a higher rate than the general population, it is difficult to accurately estimate the extent to which these drugs are abused or misused. The high use of medications coupled with age-related physiological changes raises the likelihood of medication-related adverse events such as increased sedation, delirium, confusion, and falls, resulting in hip fractures.

SAMHSA (2010) reported that prescription drug abuse increased from 0.7% to 3.5% from 1992 to 2008. Compounding these numbers is the fact that older adults often use multiple medications (polypharmacy), increasing the likelihood of severe medical, physical, and mental health complications.

Acquired Immunodeficiency Syndrome and AIDS-Related Dementia

Human immunodeficiency virus (HIV) infection and acquired immunodeficiency syndrome (AIDS) remain a growing problem among the elderly. People aged 55 and older accounted for one-quarter of all Americans living with HIV in 2012. Older Americans are more likely to be diagnosed with HIV infection later in the course of their disease (CDC, 2016). Of the 6955 deaths related to AIDS in 2013, 2588 (37%) were among people aged 55 and older (CDC, 2016).

Blood transfusions are no longer the main cause for the spread of AIDS in the older adult, unless the transfusion occurred before 1985. Research shows that older adults remain sexually active and thus are at risk for HIV and AIDS because of failure to understand and practice safe sex. Men who have been treated for erectile dysfunction are also considered at risk for HIV/AIDS. Diagnosis and treatment of HIV and AIDS in the older adult may be delayed because health care providers believe that this population is not sexually active, another aspect of ageism (Stein, 2011). Lack of adequate knowledge about HIV and AIDS, other sexually transmitted infections, and safe sex practices among older adults increases the risk for HIV infection and AIDS in this age group.

Older women who are sexually active are at higher risk for HIV and AIDS from an infected partner than are older men. Changes in vaginal tissue caused by the aging process can lead to tears in the vaginal mucosa during intercourse, which allow HIV to penetrate more easily. In addition, because pregnancy is no longer a threat, use of condoms in this age group is uncommon.

Dementia is often a sequela in people with HIV infection and AIDS. Dementia caused by AIDS and dementia caused by Alzheimer's disease can be easily confused. Therefore a careful assessment and workup are required, including testing for HIV/AIDS.

LEGAL AND ETHICAL ISSUES THAT AFFECT THE MENTAL HEALTH OF OLDER ADULTS

Among the most important of many legal and ethical issues for practicing nurses to be familiar with are the following:
1. Use of restraints
2. Decision making about health care
3. Elder abuse (a serious problem for the older adult discussed in Chapter 21)
4. End-of-life care (addressed in Chapter 25)

Use of Restraints

The use of restraints encompasses ethical, legal, and safety concerns. Restraints can be both physical and chemical. **Physical restraints** are any manual methods, materials, or equipment that inhibits free movement. Examples include tightening a bedsheet to limit movement, raising side rails, applying wrist or waist restraints, or positioning a wheelchair to restrict movement. Devices on clothing that trigger an alarm to notify staff that an older adult is leaving a room or an area are not considered restraints. **Chemical restraints** are drugs given for the specific purpose of inhibiting a certain behavior or movement and that are not part of the normal treatment plan. Although common in past decades, restraint use is becoming increasingly rare as facilities adopt restraint-free policies and train staff in advanced de-escalation and communication techniques (American Psychiatric Nurses Association [APNA], 2014; National Alliance on Mental Illness [NAMI], 2016).

Physical Restraints

Whether health care providers have the right to restrain another individual physically has always been debated (McCabe, et al., 2010). Surveys undertaken by the state and federal authorities in the United States in the 1970s and 1980s revealed levels of physical restraint use as high as 75% in some facilities (NAMI, 2016). Physical restraints were traditionally used with confused or medicated hospitalized patients primarily to prevent disruption of medical therapies and to prevent falls. Although meant to enhance safety, they are often perceived as abusive by patients and families.

Research beginning in the 1980s has shown more harm than benefit with the use of restraints (Minnesota Department of Health [MDH], 2010; NAMI, 2016). Physical restraints can pose a risk of death through strangulation or asphyxiation and lead to muscle loss, incontinence, pressure sores, agitation, and bone weakness when used for prolonged periods of time. In elderly patients, restraints can contribute to cognitive impairment, physical weakness, fall risk, anxiety, feelings of humiliation, and emotional withdrawal (MDH, 2010; Radziewicz et al., 2010).

More facilities are using electronic sensing systems to alert staff if a resident is about to stand up or try to get out of a bed or wheelchair, adjusting staffing patterns, and providing enhanced training of staff. Other efforts that replace the practice of restraint use include strength training for the patient, the use of mobility devices and hearing aids, lower beds, reduction of obstacles, improved lighting, and door alarms.

Physical restraints should be used for emergency purposes only when there is a threat to the safety of the resident or others, never as a means of controlling behavior or as punishment. According to The Joint Commission (Joint Commission on Accreditation of Healthcare Organizations [JCAHO], 2015), restraint use now has very specific and time-limited guidelines, requiring a provider order, constant monitoring, rotation of the restraints to rest the limbs, offering water and toileting, and documentation of alternative methods tried.

Nurses can avoid liability by knowing the laws in their state, adhering to the policies and procedures of the institution at which they work, and using good nursing judgment. All nursing homes and hospitals should have written restraint procedures and policies. If restraints are used, the nurse is responsible for the patient's safety, and creative nursing skills and interventions are frequently more beneficial.

Chemical Restraints

Unfortunately, with restrictions on physical restraints there has been an increase in off-label use of certain medications (particularly second-generation antipsychotics) as chemical restraints to control the behavior of elderly patients (Cassels, 2010; Gareri, Segura-Garcia, Graziella, & Manfredi, 2014). In 2008 the U.S. Food and Drug Administration (FDA) issued Black Box warnings for the use of antipsychotics in controlling behavioral symptoms in elderly patients with dementia (Cassels, 2010; Gareri et al., 2014). The FDA found that the dangers included increased risk for diabetes and cerebrovascular events as well as a doubled risk for mortality. Although the warning labels have decreased the use of antipsychotics in community and hospital elderly dementia patients, they have not appeared to decrease antipsychotic use in nursing homes across the country. A study by Chen and colleagues (2010) found that up to 29% of the study's residents in nursing homes received at least one antipsychotic medication, and nearly 32% were not psychotic and had no identified clinical indication for this therapy. Risk and benefits must be weighed carefully when using antipsychotics in the elderly population (Gareri et al., 2014; Mental Health Act, 2013).

CONTROL OF THE DECISION-MAKING PROCESS

Patient Self-Determination Act

Since the 1960s, the public's desire to participate in decision making about their own health care has increased. Congress passed the Patient Self-Determination Act (PSDA) in 1990, requiring that health care facilities provide clear, written information to every patient regarding his or her legal rights to make health care decisions, including the right to accept or refuse treatment. The PSDA also establishes the right of a person to provide written treatment directions for clinicians in the event of a serious illness. Increasing numbers of older adults are creating written directives.

An advance directive is a term used to describe living wills, durable powers of attorney for health care, and health care surrogate appointments. Health care institutions that receive federal funds are required to provide each patient with written information regarding his or her right to execute advance directives, and to inquire whether such directives have been made by the patient. The patient's admission records should state whether such directives exist.

Such a directive indicates preferences for the types of medical care desired. The directive comes into effect should physical or mental incapacitation prevent the patient from making health care decisions. These wishes can be communicated through one or more of the following: (1) a living will, (2) a directive to physician, and (3) a durable power of attorney for health care. These documents must be in writing and the patient's signature must be witnessed and in some states notarized.

Living Will

A living will is a personal statement of how and where one wishes to die, and can be changed at any time by the individual. It is activated only when the person is terminally ill and incapacitated. Executing a living will does not always guarantee its application.

Directive to Physician

In a directive to physician, a physician is appointed by the individual to serve as proxy. Many of the features of a directive to physician parallel those of a living will, and designating the physician as surrogate can be particularly useful in cases of terminal illness when an individual has no family. Unlike the living will, the directive to physician can be revoked orally at any time without regard to patient competency.

Durable Power of Attorney for Health Care

The durable power of attorney for health care differs from a living will in that a person is appointed to act as the patient's agent. Individuals do not have to be terminally ill or incompetent to allow the empowered individual to act on their behalf.

Older adults who are lesbian, gay, bisexual, or transgender (LGBT) often have many conflicts within state or federal facilities such as nursing homes. Many states have adopted laws that allow gay and lesbian couples to marry, and in 2013 the Supreme Court ruled that married same-sex couples were entitled to federal benefits, thereby allowing the rights of all spouses in a marriage. In states that have not adopted laws for gay and lesbian marriages, there is sometimes a cruel bias of not allowing visitation rights or power of attorney for LGBT patients' partners. These trends have been changing, and the recent Supreme Court ruling in favor of same-sex marriage should alleviate most of the prejudice and differential treatment between heterosexual and homosexual couples.

Nursing Role in the Decision-Making Process

The nurse explains the ethics and legal policies to both the patient and the family and helps them understand the concepts behind advance directives. The family need not feel morally obligated to provide for all possible medical care when such care will only extend the suffering of a loved one. This is especially true when such extraordinary measures *do not represent the person's values and beliefs*. The nurse serves as an *advocate* and a knowledgeable resource person for the older adult patient and family. The patient is encouraged to verbalize his or her feelings and thoughts during this sensitive time of decision making. Maintaining an open and continuing dialogue among patient, family, nurse, and primary care provider (physician or nurse practitioner) is important. The nurse supports the patient and person(s) appointed to act on the patient's behalf and seeks consultation for any ethical issues the nurse feels unprepared to handle.

The law does not specify who should talk with patients about treatment decisions, but in many facilities nurses are being asked to discuss this issue with the patient. If the advance directive of a patient is not being followed, the nurse intervenes on the patient's behalf. Although nurses, especially in nursing homes, may discuss options with their patients, they may not assist patients in writing advance directives because this is considered a conflict of interest. The existence of an advance directive serves as a guide for the older adult patient's rightful wishes in this process.

KEY POINTS TO REMEMBER

- The older adult population continues to increase as the baby boomers start reaching 65 years of age.
- The increase in the number of older adults poses a challenge to the entire health care system. There is much to be done to prepare and respond to the special needs of this population.
- Attitudes toward the older adult are often negative and stereotypical, reflecting an ageism bias common in our society. Health care providers can hold biased views of the elderly that affect caregiving.
- Nurses should be knowledgeable about the process of aging, including the differences between normal and abnormal aging changes.
- Older adults face increasing problems of alcoholism, illicit drug use, abuse and misuse of prescription and over-the-counter drugs, and suicide.
- Current philosophy of care mandates that patients be free from unnecessary use of drugs and physical restraints (Gareri et al., 2014; JCAHO, 2015; Mental Health Act, 2013).
- Nurses working with mentally ill patients should study psychotherapeutic approaches relevant for older adults, such as remotivation and reminiscence therapy, and offer psychotherapy groups geared toward the special needs of this population.
- When it comes to dying and death, older adults' wishes and those of their families may differ, and are frequently ignored. The implementation of the Patient Self-Determination Act (PSDA), passed in 1990, can afford patients autonomy, choice, and dignity in their death process.

APPLYING CRITICAL JUDGMENT

1. A 70-year-old male has been admitted to the intensive care unit with a diagnosis of alcohol withdrawal delirium. He is confused and combative, and threatens to strike the nurse who is trying to render care to him unless he is allowed to leave the unit. The nurse applies wrist restraints to prevent him from striking her and from leaving the room.
   A. What are the mandates of The Joint Commission regarding the use of restraints? What were the reasons restraints were found to be dangerous?
   B. What other actions besides applying restraints could the nurse employ in this situation, consistent with a restraint-free philosophy?
   C. What are the possible legal repercussions for the nurse?
   D. What potential harmful consequences, physical and psychological, could occur with this patient?
2. The same patient as above has received treatment for alcohol withdrawal. He appears very quiet, refuses to eat, does not sleep at night, and admits to thoughts of desperation and wishes that he could die. He also confides that he started drinking heavily and attempted suicide when his wife died 5 years earlier.
   A. Choose specific assessment tools to use in assessing the patient's depression, suicide risk, and alcohol use.
   B. What kinds of supports would you suggest be available to the patient upon discharge? What types of information might

you need to know about this patient to best plan his discharge care?
3. A 57-year-old woman is admitted to the hospital after a heart attack exacerbated by the chemotherapy used to treat metastasized liver cancer. Her son says that she does not want anyone to resuscitate her. Acting both as a nurse and as a patient advocate, explain to the patient and her son what an advance directive is and what needs to be done to make the patient's wishes known.
4. Think about an example of ageism you may have noticed in your family or in your role as a nursing student, or that you may have participated in yourself toward an elderly person without recognizing it. Discuss your example with a classmate, and listen to his or her example.
5. Briefly interview someone older than 70 years of age about the changes he or she has noticed in his or her own life and health, and the world. Also, ask for examples of ageism the person has noticed.

CHAPTER REVIEW QUESTIONS

1. An 85-year-old woman says to the nurse, "I raised three children, but now two of them barely speak to me. I did not do a good job of instilling a family spirit." Which response should the nurse provide?
   a. "Do you think this situation is likely to change?"
   b. "If you could relive those earlier years, what would you do differently?"
   c. "There's no guidebook for parenting. Your children have made their own choices."
   d. "Your children are likely to regret their behavior. I hope you can find it in your heart to forgive them."
2. The nurse asks an 87-year-old, "How are you doing?" The patient replies, "I have good days and bad days." Select the nurse's therapeutic response.
   a. "How is your sleep?"
   b. "Tell me more about that."
   c. "Are you feeling depressed?"
   d. "We expect that from people your age."
3. A 92-year-old lives alone but family members assist with transportation and home maintenance. This adult tells the nurse, "They mean well but sometimes my family treats me like a child." What is the nurse's best action?
   a. Encourage the adult to overlook these behaviors from family members.
   b. Role-play with the adult ways to share these feelings with family members.
   c. Contact family members privately and educate them about the harmful effects of ageism.
   d. Reinforce family members' good intentions and say, "It's fortunate your family is so helpful."
4. A nurse assesses a 78-year-old patient who lives alone at home and is beginning three new prescriptions. Which question by the nurse will provide best for the patient's safety?
   a. "How do you store your medications at home?"
   b. "What is your usual bowel elimination pattern?"
   c. "Who usually helps you with your medications?"
   d. "How much alcohol do you drink on a normal day?"
5. Which scenario presents the most risk factors for suicide?
   a. 64-year-old black female whose husband died 3 months ago
   b. 72-year-old white female scheduled for hip replacement in 2 weeks

c. 82-year-old widowed white male recently diagnosed with pancreatic cancer

d. 92-year-old black male who recently moved into the home of his adult children

REFERENCES

Administration on Aging, U.S. Department of Health and Human Services. (2014). *A profile of older Americans: 2014.* Retrieved from http://www.aoa.acl.gov/Aging_Statistics/Profile/2014/docs/2014-Profile.pdf.

Agency for Healthcare Research and Quality (AHRQ). (2012). *Screening, behavioral counseling, and referral in primary care to reduce alcohol misuse. Comparative Effectiveness Review, No. 64.* Retrieved from http://www.ncbi.nlm.nih.gov/books/NBK99199/pdf/Bookshelf_NBK99199.pdf.

Alexopoulos, G. S., & Knosses, D. N. (2011). *Geriatric psychiatry: Advances and directions.* Retrieved from http://www.psych.theclinics.com/article/S0193-953X(11)00031-1/fulltext.

American Association of Colleges of Nursing (AACN). (2008). *The essentials of baccalaureate education for professional nursing practice (3rd revision).* Washington, DC: AACN. Retrieved from http://www.aacn.nche.edu/Education/pdf/BaccEssentials08.pdf.

American Nurses Association (ANA). (2013). *Euthanasia, assisted suicide, and aid in dying.* Retrieved from http://www.nursingworld.org/MainMenuCategories/EthicsStandards/Ethics-Position-Statements/Euthanasia-Assisted-Suicide-and-Aid-in-Dying.pdf.

American Psychiatric Nurses Association. (2014). *APNA position statement on the use of seclusion and restraint.* Retrieved from http://www.apna.org/i4a/pages/index.cfm?pageid=3730.

American Psychological Association (APA). (2016). *Mental and behavioral health and older Americans.* Retrieved from http://www.apa.org/about/gr/issues/aging/mental-health.aspx.

American Society on Aging (ASA). (2012). Entrenched ageism in healthcare isolates, ignores and imperils elders. *Aging Today.* Retrieved from http://www.asaging.org/blog/entrenched-ageism-healthcare-isolates-ignores-and-imperils-elders.

Andreescu, C., & Reynolds, C. F. (2011). Late-life depression: Evidence-based treatment and promising new directions for research and clinical practice. *Psychiatric Clinics of North America, 34*(2), 335–355.

Bakken, M. S., Engeland, A., Engesaeter, L. B., et al. (2013). Increased risk of hip fracture among older people using antidepressant drugs: Data from the Norwegian Prescription Database and the Norwegian Hip Fracture Registry. *Age Aging, 42*(4), 514–520.

Bergman, Y. S., & Bodner, E. (2015). Ageist attitudes block young adults' ability for compassion toward incapacitated older adults. *International Psychogeriatrics, 27*(9), 1541–1550.

Brooks, M. (2016). *Imaging shows basis for anticholinergic harm in elderly.* Retrieved from http://www.medscape.com/viewarticle/862299.

Buckwalter, K. C., Beck, C., & Evens, L. K. (2011). Envisioning the future of geropsychiatric nursing. In K. D. Melillo & S. C. Houde (Eds.), *Geropsychiatric and mental health nursing* (2nd ed.) (pp. 465–475). Sudbury, MA: Jones and Bartlett Learning.

Cassels, C. (2010). *Inappropriate use of antipsychotics in the elderly continued use despite FDA warnings.* Retrieved from http://www.medscape.com/viewarticle/715257_print.

Centers for Disease Control and Prevention (CDC). (2016). *Study looks at suicide rates from 1928–2007.* Retrieved from http://www.cdc.gov/ViolencePrevention/suicide/index.html.

Centers for Disease Control and Prevention (CDC). (2015). *Suicide facts at a glance, 2015.* Retrieved from http://www.cdc.gov/violenceprevention/pdf/suicide-datasheet-a.pdf.

Centers for Disease Control and Prevention (CDC). (2016). *HIV among people 50 or over.* Retrieved from http://www.cdc.gov/hiv/group/age/olderamericans/index.html.

Chen, W., Briesacher, B. A., Field, T. S., et al. (2010). *Unexplained variation across U.S. nursing homes in antipsychotic prescribing rates.* Retrieved from http://archinte.ama-assn.org/cgi/content/abstract/170/1/89.

Coleman, D. (2015). Does ageism still exist in nursing education? *Nursing and Older People, 27*(5), 16–21.

Conwell, Y., Van Orden, K., & Caine, E. D. (2011). Suicide in older adults. *Psychiatric Clinic of North America, 42*(2), 451–468.

Coupland, C., Dhiman, P., Morriss, R., et al. (2011). *Antidepressant use and risk of adverse outcomes in older people.* Retrieved from http://www.medscape.com/viewarticle/748441.

Coupland, C., & Hochhalter, A. (2011). *Popular antidepressants not always best choice for seniors.* Retrieved from http://www.nlm.nih.gov/medlineplus/news/fullstory_114940.html.

Espinoza, R. T., & Unutzer, J. (2016). *Diagnosis and management of late-life unipolar depression.* Retrieved from http://www.uptodate.com/contents/diagnosis-and-management-of-late-life-unipolar-depression.

Fenigsen, R. (2010). Other people's lives: Reflections on medicine, ethics, and euthanasia. *Issues in Law & Medicine, 26*(1), 33–76.

Fenigsen, R. (2011). Other people's lives: Reflections on medicine, ethics, and euthanasia, part two: Medicine versus euthanasia. *Issues in Law & Medicine, 26*(3), 239–279.

Fox, C., Richardson, K., Maidment, I. D., et al. (2011). Anticholinergic medication use and cognitive impairment in the older population: The Medical Research Council Cognitive Function and Ageing Study. *Journal of the American Geriatrics Society, 59*(8), 1477–1483.

Gareri, P., Segura-Garcia, C., Graziella, V., et al. (2014). Use of atypical antipsychotics in the elderly: A clinical review. *Clinical Interventions in Aging, 9,* 1363–1373.

Gendron, T. L., Welleford, E. A., Inker, J., et al. (2015). The language of ageism: Why we need to use words carefully. *Gerontologist [online],* 1–10.

Health in Aging. (2016). *Many older adults have both chronic illness and "geriatric syndromes."* Retrieved from http://www.healthinaging.org/resources/resource:many-older-adults-have-both-chronic-illnesses-and-geriatric-syndromes/.

HealthyPeople2020. (2016). *Older adults.* Retrieved from https://www.healthypeople.gov/2020/topics-objectives/topic/older-adults.

Heffner, C. (2015). *Erikson's stages of psychosocial development.* Retrieved from http://allpsych.com/psychology101/social_development/#.Vdo5E_lVikp.

Johnson, B. A. (2015). *Pharmacotherapy for alcohol use disorder.* Retrieved from http://www.uptodate.com.

Joint Commission on Accreditation of Healthcare Organizations (JCAHO). (1999). *Standards for behavioral health care.* Oakbrook, IL: JCAHO.

Kagan, S. H., & Melendez-Torres, G. J. (2015). Ageism in nursing. *Journal of Nursing Management, 23*(5), 644–650.

Kelland, K. (2011). *Anti-cholinergic drug effects boosts elderly death risk.* Retrieved from http://www.medscape.com/viewarticle/745256_print.

Kellner, C. (2015). *Unipolar major depression in adults: Indications for and efficacy of electroconvulsive therapy (ECT).* Retrieved from http://www.uptodate.com.

Kydd, A., & Fleming, A. (2015). Ageism and age discrimination in healthcare: Fact or fiction? A narrative review of literature. *Maturitas, 81*(4), 432–438.

McCabe, D. E., Alvarez, C. D., McNulty, S. R., et al. (2010). Perceptions of physical restraints use in the elderly among registered nurses and nurse assistants in a single acute care hospital. *Geriatric Nursing, 32*(1), 39–45.

McEnany, J. P. (2011). Psychopharmacology. In K. D. Melillo & S. C. Houde (Eds.), *Geropsychiatric and mental health nursing* (2nd ed.). Sudbury, MA: Jones and Bartlett Learning.

Mental Health Act. (2013). *Chemical restraint.* Retrieved from http://www.dhhs.tas.gov.au/__data/assets/pdf_file/0004/148261/24_CFP_Clinical_Guideline_10_-_Chemical_Restraint.pdf.

Minnesota Department of Health (MDH). (2010). *Minnesota Department of Health safety without restraints: A new practice standard for safe care.* Retrieved from http://www.health.state.mn.us/divs/fpc/safety.htm.

National Alliance on Mental Illness (NAMI). (2016). *NAMI calls for major reforms in use of physical restraints in psychiatric facilities.* Retrieved from http://www.nami.org/Press-Media/Press-Releases/1998/NAMI-Calls-For-Major-Reforms-In-Use-Of-Physical-Re.

North, M. S., & Fiske, S. T. (2015). Modern attitudes toward older adults in the aging world: A cross-cultural meta-analysis. *Psychological Bulletin, 141*(5), 993–1021.

Oaklander, M. (2015). Your attitude about aging may impact how you age. *Time.* Retrieved from http://time.com/4138476/aging-alzheimers-disease/.

Ortman, J. M., Velkoff, V. A., & Hogan, H. (2014). A*n aging nation: the older population in the united states population estimates and projections current population reports issued may 2014 p25-1140.* Retrieved from https://www.census.gov/prod/2014pubs/p25-1140.pdf.

Ouchida, K. M., & Lachs, M. S. (2015). *Not for doctors only: Ageism in healthcare.* Retrieved from http://www.asaging.org/blog/not-doctors-only-ageism-healthcare.

Preston, J. D., O'Neal, J. H., & Talaga, M. C. (2013). *Handbook of clinical psychopharmacology for therapists* (7th ed.). Oakland, CA: New Harbinger Publications.

Radziewicz, R. M., Amoto, S., & Bradas, C. (2010). *Use of physical restraints with elderly patients.* Retrieved from http://www.gerin.org/topics/physicalrestraints/want_toknowmore__.

Robinson, L., Smith, M., & Segal, J. (2016). *Depression in older adults and the elderly.* Retrieved from http://www.helpguide.org/articles/depression/depression-in-older-adults-and-the-elderly.htm.

Rogers, J., & Wiese, B. S. (2011). Geriatric drinkers: Evaluation and treatment for alcohol overuse. *British Columbia Medical Journal, 53*(7), 353–356.

Ruscin, J. M., & Linnebur, S. A. (2014). Drug-related problems in the elderly. *Merck Manual Professional Version.* Retrieved from http://www.merckmanuals.com/professional/geriatrics/drug-therapy-in-the-elderly/drug-related-problems-in-the-elderly.

Sadock, B. J., & Sadock, V. A. (2014). *Kaplan and Sadock's synopsis of psychiatry: Behavioral sciences/Clinical psychiatry* (11th ed.). Philadelphia, PA: Wolters-Kluwer/Lippincott Williams & Wilkins.

Stein, J. (2011). *High-risk older patients are not screened for HIV.* Retrieved from http://www.medscape.com/viewarticle/743632.

Substance Abuse and Mental Health Services Administration (SAMHSA), Office of Applied Studies. (2010). *The TEDS report: Changing substance abuse patterns among older admissions: 1992 and 2008.* Rockville, MD: SAMHSA.

Touhy, T. A., & Jett, K. (2010). *Ebersole and Hess' gerontological nursing & healthy aging.* St Louis, MO: Mosby/Elsevier.

U.S. Department of Health and Human Services. (2016). *2020 topics and objectives: Older adults.* Retrieved from https://www.healthypeople.gov/2020/topics-objectives/topic/older-adults.

U.S. Department of Health and Human Services. (2014). *NIH SeniorHealth: Prescription and illicit drug abuse.* Retrieved from http://nihseniorhealth.gov/drugabuse/treatingsubstanceabuse/01.html.

U.S. Department of Health and Human Services (USDHHS). (1999). *Mental health: A report of the Surgeon General, executive summary.* Rockville, MD: USDHHS.

U.S. Food and Drug Administration (FDA). (2008). *Antipsychotics are not indicated for the treatment of dementia-related psychoses.* Retrieved from http://www.fda.gov/drugs/drugsafety/postsmarketdrugsafetyinformationforpatientsandprovider.

Wick, J. Y. (2011). Adherence issues in elderly patients. *Pharmacy Times.* Retrieved from http://www.pharmacytimes.com/publications/issue/2011/January2011/RxFocus-0111.

Wooten, J. M. (2015). Pharmacotherapy considerations in elderly adults. *Southern Medical Journal, 105*(8), 437–445. Retrieved from http://www.medscape.com/viewarticle/769412_1.

DSM-5 Classification

Before each disorder name, ICD-9-CM codes are provided, followed by ICD-10-CM codes in parentheses. Blank lines indicate that either the ICD-9-CM or the ICD-10-CM code is not applicable. For some disorders, the code can be indicated only according to the subtype or specifier.

ICD-9-CM codes were used for coding purposes in the United States through September 30, 2014. ICD-10-CM codes are to be used starting October 1, 2014.

Following chapter titles and disorder names, page numbers for the corresponding text or criteria are included in parentheses.

Note for all mental disorders due to another medical condition: Indicate the name of the other medical condition in the name of the mental disorder due to [the medical condition]. The code and name for the other medical condition should be listed first, immediately before the mental disorder due to the medical condition.

NEURODEVELOPMENTAL DISORDERS (31)

Intellectual Disabilities (33)

319	(—.—)	Intellectual Disability (Intellectual Developmental Disorder) (33)
		Specify current severity:
	(F70)	Mild
	(F71)	Moderate
	(F72)	Severe
	(F73)	Profound
315.8	(F88)	Global Developmental Delay (41)
319	(F79)	Unspecified Intellectual Disability (Intellectual Developmental Disorder) (41)

Communication Disorders (41)

315.39	(F80.9)	Language Disorder (42)
315.39	(F80.0)	Speech Sound Disorder (44)
315.35	(F80.81)	Childhood-Onset Fluency Disorder (Stuttering) (45)
		Note: Later-onset cases are diagnosed as 307.0 (F98.5) adult-onset fluency disorder.
315.39	(F80.98)	Social (Pragmatic) Communication Disorder (47)
307.9	(F80.9)	Unspecified Communication Disorder (49)

Autism Spectrum Disorder (50)

299.00	(F84.0)	Autism Spectrum Disorder (50)

Specify if: Associated with a known medical or genetic condition or environmental factor; Associated with another neurodevelopmental, mental or behavioral disorder

Specify current severity for Criterion A and Criterion B: Requiring very substantial support, Requiring substantial support, Requiring support

Specify if: With or without accompanying intellectual impairment, With or without accompanying language impairment, With catatonia (use additional code 293.89 [F06.1])

Attention-Deficit/Hyperactivity Disorder (59)

—.—	(—.—)	Attention-Deficit/Hyperactivity Disorder (59)
		Specify whether:
314.01	(F90.2)	Combined presentation
314.00	(F90.0)	Predominantly inattentive presentation
314.01	(F90.1)	Predominantly hyperactive/impulsive presentation
		Specify if: In partial remission
		Specify current severity: Mild, Moderate, Severe
314.01	(F90.8)	Other Specified Attention-Deficit/Hyperactivity Disorder (65)
314.01	(F90.9)	Unspecified Attention-Deficit/Hyperactivity Disorder (66)

Specific Learning Disorder (66)

—.—	(—.—)	Specific Learning Disorder (66)
		Specify if:
315.00	(F81.0)	With impairment in reading (*specify* if with word reading accuracy, reading rate or fluency, reading comprehension)
315.2	(F81.81)	With impairment in written expression (*specify* if with spelling accuracy, grammar and punctuation accuracy, clarity or organization of written expression)
315.1	(F81.2)	With impairment in mathematics (*specify* if with number sense, memorization or arithmetic facts, accurate or fluent calculation, accurate math reasoning)
		Specify current severity: Mild, Moderate, Severe

Motor Disorders (74)

315.4	(F82)	Developmental Coordination Disorder (74)
307.3	(F98.4)	Stereotypic Movement Disorder (77)

Specify if: With self-injurious behavior, Without self-injurious behavior

Specify if: Associated with a known medical or genetic condition, neurodevelopmental disorder, or environmental factor

Specify current severity: Mild, Moderate, Severe

Tic Disorders

307.23	**(F95.2)**	Tourette's Disorder (81)
307.22	**(F95.1)**	Persistent (Chronic) Motor or Vocal Tic Disorder (81)
		Specify if: With motor tics only, With vocal tics only
307.21	**(F95.0)**	Provisional Tic Disorder (81)
307.20	**(F95.8)**	Other Specified Tic Disorder (85)
307.20	**(F95.9)**	Unspecified Tic Disorder (85)

Other Neurodevelopmental Disorders (86)

315.8	**(F88)**	Other Specified Neurodevelopmental Disorder (86)
315.9	**(F89)**	Unspecified Neurodevelopmental Disorder (86)

SCHIZOPHRENIA SPECTRUM AND OTHER PSYCHOTIC DISORDERS (87)

The following specifiers apply to Schizophrenia Spectrum and Other Psychotic Disorders where indicated:

[a]*Specify* if: The following course specifiers are only to be used after a 1-year duration of the disorder: First episode, currently in acute episode; First episode, currently in partial remission; First episode, currently in full remission; Multiple episodes, currently in acute episode; Multiple episodes, currently in parital remission; Multiple episodes, currently in full remission; Continuous; Unspecified

[b]*Specify* if: With catatonia (use additional code 293.89 [F06.1])

[c]*Specify* current severity of delusions, hallucinations, disorganized speech, abnormal psychomotor behavior, negative symptoms, impaired cognition, depression, and mania symptoms

301.22	**(F21)**	Schizotypal (Personality) Disorder (90)
297.1	**(F22)**	Delusional Disorder[a,c] (90)
		Specify whether: Erotomanic type, Grandiose type, Jealous type, Persecutory type, Somatic type, Mixed type, Unspecified type
		Specify if: With bizarre content
298.8	**(F23)**	Brief Psychotic Disorder[b,c] (94)
		Specify if: With marked stressor(s), Without marked stressor(s), With postpartum onset
295.40	**(F20.81)**	Schizophreniform Disorder[b,c] (96)
		Specify if: With good prognostic features, Without good prognostic features
295.90	**(F20.9)**	Schizophrenia[a,b,c] (99)
—.—	(—.—)	Schizoaffective Disorder[a,b,c] (105)
		Specify whether:
295.70	**(F25.0)**	Bipolar type
295.70	**(F25.1)**	Depressive type
—.—	(—.—)	Substance/Medication-Induced Psychotic Disorder[c] (110)
		Note: See the criteria set and corresponding recording procedures for substance-specific codes and ICD-9-CM and ICD-10-CM coding.
		Specify if: With onset during intoxication, With onset during withdrawal

—.—	(—.—)	Psychotic Disorder Due to Another Medical Condition[c] (115)
		Specify whether:
293.81	**(F06.2)**	With delusions
293.82	**(F06.0)**	With hallucinations
293.89	**(F06.1)**	Catatonia Associated With Another Mental Disorder (Catatonia Specifier) (119)
293.89	**(F06.1)**	Catatonic Disorder Due to Another Medical Condition (120)
293.89	**(F06.1)**	Unspecified Catatonia (121)
		Note: Code first 781.99 (R29.818) other symptoms involving nervous and musculoskeletal systems.
298.8	**(F28)**	Other Specified Schizophrenia Spectrum and Other Psychotic Disorder (122)
298.9	**(F29)**	Unspecified Schizophrenia Spectrum and Other Psychotic Disorder (122)

BIPOLAR AND RELATED DISORDERS (123)

The following specifiers apply to Bipolar and Related Disorders where indicated:

[a]*Specify:* With anxious distress (*specify* current severity: mild, moderate, moderate-severe, severe); With mixed features; With rapid cycling; With melancholic features; With atypical features; With mood-congruent psychotic features; With mood-incongruent psychotic features; With catatonia (use additional code 293.89 [F06.1]); With peripartum onset; With seasonal pattern

—.—	(—.—)	Bipolar I Disorder[a] (123)
—.—	(—.—)	Current or most recent episode manic
296.41	**(F31.11)**	Mild
296.42	**(F31.12)**	Moderate
296.43	**(F31.13)**	Severe
296.44	**(F31.2)**	With psychotic features
296.45	**(F31.73)**	In partial remission
296.46	**(F31.74)**	In full remission
296.40	**(F31.9)**	Unspecified
296.40	**(F31.0)**	Current or most recent episode hypomanic
296.45	**(F31.73)**	In partial remission
296.46	**(F31.74)**	In full remission
296.40	**(F31.9)**	Unspecified
—.—	(—.—)	Current or most recent episode depressed
296.51	**(F31.31)**	Mild
296.52	**(F31.32)**	Moderate
296.53	**(F31.4)**	Severe
296.54	**(F31.5)**	With psychotic features
296.55	**(F31.75)**	In partial remission
296.56	**(F31.76)**	In full remission
296.50	**(F31.9)**	Unspecified
296.7	**(F31.9)**	Current or most recent episode unspecified
296.89	**(F31.81)**	Bipolar II Disorder[a] (132)
		Specify current or most recent episode: Hypomanic, Depressed
		Specify course if full criteria for a mood episode are not currently met: In partial remission, In full remission
		Specify severity if full criteria for a mood episode are not currently met: Mild, Moderate, Severe

301.13	**(F34.0)**	Cyclothymic Disorder (139)
		Specify if: With anxious distress
—.—	(—.—)	Substance/Medication-Induced Bipolar and Related Disorder (142)
		Note: See the criteria set and corresponding recording procedures for substance-specific codes and ICD-9-CM and ICD-10-CM coding.
		Specify if: With onset during intoxication, With onset during withdrawal
293.83	(—.—)	Bipolar and Related Disorder Due to Another Medical Condition (145)
		Specify if:
	(F06.33)	With manic features
	(F06.33)	With manic- or hypomanic-like episode
	(F06.33)	With mixed features
296.89	**(F31.89)**	Other Specified Bipolar and Related Disorder (148)
296.80	**(F31.9)**	Unspecified Bipolar and Related Disorder (149)

DEPRESSIVE DISORDERS (155)

The following specifiers apply to Depressive Disorders where indicated:
[a]*Specify*: With anxious distress (*specify* current severity: mild, moderate, moderate-severe, severe); With mixed features; With melancholic features; With atypical features; With mood-congruent psychotic features; With mood-incongruent psychotic features; With catatonia (use additional code 293.89 [F06.1]); With peripartum onset; With seasonal pattern

296.99	**[F34.8]**	Disruptive Mood Dysregulation Disorder (156)
—.—	(—.—)	Major Depressive Disorder[a] (160)
—.—	(—.—)	Single episode
296.21	**(F32.0)**	Mild
296.22	**(F32.1)**	Moderate
296.23	**(F32.2)**	Severe
296.24	**(F32.3)**	With psychotic features
296.25	**(F32.4)**	In partial remission
296.26	**(F32.5)**	In full remission
296.20	**(F32.9)**	Unspecified
—.—	(—.—)	Recurrent episode
296.31	**(F33.0)**	Mild
296.32	**(F33.1)**	Moderate
296.33	**(F33.2)**	Severe
296.34	**(F33.3)**	With psychotic features
296.35	**(F33.41)**	In partial remission
296.36	**(F33.42)**	In full remission
296.30	**(F33.9)**	Unspecified
300.4	**(F34.1)**	Persistent Depressive Disorder (Dysthymia)[a] (168)
		Specify if: In partial remission, In full remission
		Specify if: Early onset, Late onset
		Specify if: With pure dysthymic syndrome; With persistent major depressive episode; With intermittent major depressive episodes, with current episode; With intermittent major depressive episodes, without current episode

		Specify current severity: Mild, Moderate, Severe
625.4	**(N94.3)**	Premenstrual Dysphoric Disorder (171)
—.—	(—.—)	Substance/Medication-Induced Depressive Disorder (175)
		Note: See the criteria set and corresponding recording procedures for substance-specific codes and ICD-9-CM and ICD-10-CM coding.
		Specify if: With onset during intoxication, With onset during withdrawal
293.83	(—.—)	Depressive Disorder Due to Another Medical Condition (180)
		Specify if:
	(F06.31)	With depressive features
	(F06.32)	With major depressive-like episode
	(F06.34)	With mixed features
311	**(F32.8)**	Other Specified Depressive Disorder (183)
311	**(F32.9)**	Unspecified Depressive Disorder (184)

ANXIETY DISORDERS (189)

309.21	**(F93.0)**	Separation Anxiety Disorder (190)
312.23	**(F94.0)**	Selective Mutism (195)
300.29	(—.—)	Specific Phobia (197)
		Specify if:
	(F40.218)	Animal
	(F40.228)	Natural environmental
	(—.—)	Blood-injection-injury
	(F40.230)	Fear of blood
	(F40.231)	Fear of injections and transfusions
	(F40.232)	Fear of other medical care
	(F40.233)	Fear of injury
	(F40.248)	Situational
	(F40.298)	Other
300.23	**(F40.10)**	Social Anxiety Disorder (Social Phobia) (202)
		Specify if: Performance only
300.01	**(F41.0)**	Panic Disorder (208)
—.—	(—.—)	Panic Attack Specifier (214)
300.22	**(F40.00)**	Agoraphobia (217)
300.02	**(F41.1)**	Generalized Anxiety Disorder (222)
—.—	(—.—)	Substance/Medication-Induced Anxiety Disorder (226)
		Note: See the criteria set and corresponding recording procedures for substance-specific codes and ICD-9-CM and ICD-10-CM coding.
		Specify if: With onset during intoxication, With onset during withdrawal, With onset after medication use
293.84	**(F06.4)**	Anxiety Disorder Due to Another Medical Condition (230)
300.09	**(F41.8)**	Other Specified Anxiety Disorder (233)
300.00	**(F41.9)**	Unspecified Anxiety Disorder (233)

OBSESSIVE-COMPULSIVE AND RELATED DISORDERS (235)

The following specifiers apply to Obsessive-Compulsive and Related Disorders where indicated:
[a]*Specify* if: With good or fair insight, With poor insight, With absent insight/delusional beliefs

300.3	**(F42)**	Obsessive-Compulsive Disorder[a] (237)
		Specify if: Tic-related
300.7	**(F45.22)**	Body Dysmorphic Disorder[a] (242)
		Specify if: With muscle dysmorphia
300.3	**(F42)**	Hoarding Disorder[a] (247)
		Specify if: With excessive acquisition
312.39	**(F63.2)**	Trichotillomania (Hair-Pulling Disorder) (251)
698.4	**(L98.1)**	Excoriation (Skin-Picking) Disorder (254)
—.—	**(—.—)**	Substance/Medication-Induced Obsessive-Compulsive and Related Disorder (257)
		Note: See the criteria set and corresponding recording procedures for substance-specific codes and ICD-9-CM and ICD-10-CM coding.
		Specify if: With onset during intoxication, With onset during withdrawal, With onset after medication use
294.8	**(F06.8)**	Obsessive-Compulsive and Related Disorder Due to Another Medical Condition (260)
		Specify if: With obsessive-compulsive disorder–like symptoms, With appearance preoccupations, With hoarding symptoms, With hair-pulling symptoms, With skin-picking symptoms
300.3	**(F42)**	Other Specified Obsessive-Compulsive and Related Disorder (263)
300.3	**(F42)**	Unspecified Obsessive-Compulsive and Related Disorder (264)

TRAUMA- AND STRESSOR-RELATED DISORDERS (265)

313.89	**(F94.1)**	Reactive Attachment Disorder (265)
		Specify if: Persistent
		Specify current severity: Severe
313.89	**(F94.2)**	Disinhibited Social Engagement Disorder (268)
		Specify if: Persistent
		Specify current severity: Severe
309.81	**(F43.10)**	Posttraumatic Stress Disorder (includes Posttraumatic Stress Disorder for Children 6 Years and Younger) (271)
		Specify whether: With dissociative symptoms
		Specify if: With delayed expression
308.3	**(F43.0)**	Acute Stress Disorder (280)
—.—	**(—.—)**	Adjustment Disorder (286)
		Specify whether:
309.0	**(F43.21)**	With depressed mood
309.24	**(F43.22)**	With anxiety
309.28	**(F43.23)**	With mixed anxiety and depressed mood
309.3	**(F43.24)**	With disturbance of conduct
309.4	**(F43.25)**	With mixed disturbance of emotions and conduct
309.9	**(F43.20)**	Unspecified
309.89	**(F43.8)**	Other Specified Trauma- and Stressor-Related Disorder (289)
309.9	**(F43.9)**	Unspecified Trauma- and Stressor-Related Disorder (290)

DISSOCIATIVE DISORDERS (291)

300.14	**(F44.81)**	Dissociative Identity Disorder (292)
300.12	**(F44.0)**	Dissociative Amnesia (298)
		Specify if:
300.13	**(F44.1)**	With dissociative fugue
300.6	**(F48.1)**	Depersonalization/Derealization Disorder (302)
300.15	**(F44.89)**	Other Specified Dissociative Disorder (306)
300.15	**(F44.9)**	Unspecified Dissociative Disorder (307)

SOMATIC SYMPTOM AND RELATED DISORDERS (309)

300.82	**(F45.1)**	Somatic Symptom Disorder (311)
		Specify if: With predominant pain
		Specify if: Persistent
		Specify current severity: Mild, Moderate, Severe
300.7	**(F45.21)**	Illness Anxiety Disorder (315)
		Specify whether: Care seeking type, Care avoidant type
300.11	**(—.—)**	Conversion Disorder (Functional Neurological Symptom Disorder) (318)
		Specify symptom type:
	(F44.4)	With weakness or paralysis
	(F44.4)	With abnormal movement
	(F44.4)	With swallowing symptoms
	(F44.4)	With speech symptom
	(F44.5)	With attacks or seizures
	(F44.6)	With anesthesia or sensory loss
	(F44.6)	With special sensory symptom
	(F44.7)	With mixed symptoms
		Specify if: Acute episode, Persistent
		Specify if: With psychological stressor (specify stressor), Without psychological stressor
316	**(F54)**	Psychological Factors Affecting Other Medical Conditions (322)
		Specify current severity: Mild, Moderate, Severe, Extreme
300.19	**(F68.10)**	Factitious Disorder (includes Factitious Disorder Imposed on Self, Factitious Disorder Imposed on Another) (324)
		Specify: Single episode, Recurrent episodes
300.89	**(F45.8)**	Other Specified Somatic Symptom and Related Disorder (327)
300.82	**(F45.9)**	Unspecified Somatic Symptom and Related Disorder (327)

FEEDING AND EATING DISORDERS (329)

The following specifiers apply to Feeding and Eating Disorders where indicated:

[a]*Specify* if: In remission

[b]*Specify* if: In partial remission, In full remission

[c]*Specify* current severity: Mild, Moderate, Severe, Extreme

307.52	**(—.—)**	Pica[a] (329)
	(F98.3)	In children

	(F50.8)	In adults
307.53	(F98.21)	Rumination Disorder[a] (332)
307.59	(F50.8)	Avoidant/Restrictive Food Intake Disorder[a] (334)
307.1	(—.—)	Anorexia Nervosa[b,c] (338)
		Specify whether:
	(F50.01)	Restricting type
	(F50.02)	Binge-eating/purging type
307.51	(F50.2)	Bulimia Nervosa[b,c] (345)
307.51	(F50.8)	Binge-Eating Disorder[b,c] (350)
307.59	(F50.8)	Other Specified Feeding or Eating Disorder (353)
307.50	(F50.9)	Unspecified Feeding or Eating Disorder (354)

ELIMINATION DISORDERS (355)

307.6	(F98.0)	Enuresis (355)
		Specify whether: Nocturnal only, Diurnal only, Nocturnal and diurnal
307.7	(F98.1)	Encopresis (357)
		Specify whether: With constipation and overflow incontinence, Without constipation and overflow incontinence
—.—	(—.—)	Other Specified Elimination Disorder (359)
788.39	(N39.498)	With urinary symptoms
787.60	(R15.9)	With fecal symptoms
—.—	(—.—)	Unspecified Elimination Disorder (360)
788.30	(R32)	With urinary symptoms
787.60	(R15.9)	With fecal symptoms

SLEEP-WAKE DISORDERS (361)

The following specifiers apply to Sleep-Wake Disorders where indicated:
[a]*Specify* if: Episodic, Persistent, Recurrent
[b]*Specify* if: Acute, Subacute, Persistent
[c]*Specify* current severity: Mild, Moderate, Severe

780.52	(G47.00)	Insomnia Disorder[a] (362)
		Specify if: With non-sleep disorder mental comorbidity, With other medical comorbidity, With other sleep disorder
780.54	(G47.10)	Hypersomnolence Disorder[b,c] (368)
		Specify if: With mental disorder, With medical condition, With another sleep disorder
—.—	(—.—)	Narcolepsy[c] (372)
		Specify whether:
347.00	(G47.419)	Narcolepsy without cataplexy but with hypocretin deficiency
347.01	(G47.411)	Narcolepsy with cataplexy but without hypocretin deficiency
347.00	(G47.419)	Autosomal dominant cerebellar ataxia, deafness, and narcolepsy
347.00	(G47.419)	Autosomal dominant narcolepsy, obesity, and type 2 diabetes
347.10	(G47.429)	Narcolepsy secondary to another medical condition

Breathing-Related Sleep Disorders (378)

327.23	(G47.33)	Obstructive Sleep Apnea Hypopnea[c] (378)
—.—	(—.—)	Central Sleep Apnea (383)
		Specify whether:
327.21	(G47.31)	Idiopathic central sleep apnea
786.04	(R06.3)	Cheyne-Stokes breathing
780.57	(G47.37)	Central sleep apnea comorbid with opioid use
		Note: First code opioid use disorder, if present.
		Specify current severity
—.—	(—.—)	Sleep-Related Hypoventilation (387)
		Specify whether:
327.24	(G473.34)	Idiopathic hypoventilation
327.25	(G47.35)	Congenital central alveolar hypoventilation
327.26	(G47.36)	Comorbid sleep-related hypoventilation
		Specify current severity
—.—	(—.—)	Circadian Rhythm Sleep-Wake Disorders[a] (390)
		Specify whether:
307.45	(G47.21)	Delayed sleep phase type (391)
		Specify if: Familial, Overlapping with non-24-hour sleep-wake type
307.45	(G47.22)	Advanced sleep phase type (393)
		Specify if: Familial
307.45	(G47.23)	Irregular sleep-wake type (394)
307.45	(G47.24)	Non-24-hour sleep-wake type (396)
307.45	(G47.26)	Shift work type (397)
307.45	(G47.20)	Unspecified type

Parasomnias (399)

—.—	(—.—)	Non–Rapid Eye Movement Sleep Arousal Disorders (399)
		Specify whether:
307.46	(F51.3)	Sleepwalking type
		Specify if: With sleep-related eating, With sleep-related sexual behavior (sexsomnia)
307.46	(F51.4)	Sleep terror type
307.47	(F51.5)	Nightmare Disorder[b,c] (404)
		Specify if: During sleep onset
		Specify if: With associated non–sleep disorder, With associated other medical condition, With associated other sleep disorder
327.42	(G473.52)	Rapid Eye Movement Sleep Behavior Disorder (407)
333.94	(G25.81)	Restless Legs Syndrome (410)
—.—	(—.—)	Substance/Medication-Induced Sleep Disorder (413)
		Note: See the criteria set and corresponding recording procedures for substance-specific codes and ICD-9-CM and ICD-10-CM coding.
		Specify whether: Insomnia type, Daytime sleepiness type, Parasomnia type, Mixed type
		Specify if: With onset during intoxication, With onset during discontinuation/withdrawal

780.52	(G47.09)	Other Specified Insomnia Disorder (420)
780.52	(G47.00)	Unspecified Insomnia Disorder (420)
780.54	(G47.19)	Other Specified Hypersomnolence Disorder (421)
780.54	(G47.10)	Unspecified Hypersomnolence Disorder (421)
780.59	(G47.8)	Other Specified Sleep-Wake Disorder (421)
780.59	(G47.9)	Unspecified Sleep-Wake Disorder (422)

SEXUAL DYSFUNCTIONS (423)

The following specifiers apply to Sexual Dysfunctions where indicated:
[a]*Specify* whether: Lifelong, Acquired
[b]*Specify* whether: Generalized, Situational
[c]*Specify* current severity: Mild, Moderate, Severe

302.74	(F52.32)	Delayed Ejaculation[a,b,c] (424)
302.72	(F52.21)	Erectile Disorder[a,b,c] (426)
302.73	(F52.31)	Female Orgasmic Disorder[a,b,c] (429)
		Specify if: Never experienced an orgasm under any situation
302.72	(F52.22)	Female Sexual Interest/Arousal Disorder[a,b,c] (433)
302.76	(F52.6)	Genito-Pelvic Pain/Penetration Disorder[a,c] (437)
302.71	(F52.0)	Male Hypoactive Sexual Desire Disorder[a,b,c] (440)
302.75	(F52.4)	Premature (Early) Ejaculation[a,b,c] (443)
—.—	(—.—)	Substance/Medication-Induced Sexual Dysfunction[c] (446)
		Note: See the criteria and corresponding recording procedures for substance-specific codes and ICD-9-CM and ICD-10-CM coding.
		Specify if: With onset during intoxication, With onset during withdrawal, With onset after medication use
302.79	(F52.8)	Other Specified Sexual Dysfunction (450)
302.70	(F52.9)	Unspecified Sexual Dysfunction (450)

GENDER DYSPHORIA (451)

—.—	(—.—)	Gender Dysphoria (452)
302.6	(F64.2)	Gender Dysphoria in Children
		Specify if: With a disorder of sex development
302.85	(F64.1)	Gender Dysphoria in Adolescents and Adults
		Specify if: With a disorder of sex development
		Specify if: Posttransition
		Note: Code the disorder of sex development if present, in addition to gender dysphoria.
302.6	(F64.8)	Other Specified Gender Dysphoria (459)
302.6	(F64.)	Unspecified Gender Dysphoria (459)

DISRUPTIVE, IMPULSE-CONTROL, AND CONDUCT DISORDERS (461)

313.81	(F91.3)	Oppositional Defiant Disorder (462)
		Specify current severity: Mild, Moderate, Severe
312.34	(F63.81)	Intermittent Explosive Disorder (466)
—.—	(—.—)	Conduct Disorder (469)
		Specify whether:
312.81	(F91.1)	Childhood-onset type
312.32	(F91.2)	Adolescent-onset type
312.89	(F91.9)	Unspecified onset
		Specify if: With limited prosocial emotions
		Specify current severity: Mild, Moderate, Severe
301.7	(F60.2)	Antisocial Personality Disorder (476)
312.33	(F63.1)	Pyromania (476)
312.32	(F63.3)	Kleptomania (478)
312.89	(F91.8)	Other Specified Disruptive, Impulse-Control, and Conduct Disorder (479)
312.9	(F91.9)	Unspecified Disruptive, Impulse-Control, and Conduct Disorder (480)

SUBSTANCE-RELATED AND ADDICTIVE DISORDERS (481)

The following specifiers and note apply to Substance-Related and Addictive Disorders where indicated:
[a]*Specify* if: In early remission, In sustained remission
[b]*Specify* if: In a controlled environment
[c]*Specify* if: With perceptual disturbances
[d]The ICD-10-CM code indicated the comorbid presence of a moderate or severe substance use disorder, which must be present in order to apply the code for substance withdrawal.

Substance-Related Disorders (483)
Alcohol-Related Disorders (490)

—.—	(—.—)	Alcohol Use Disorder[a,b] (490)
		Specify current severity:
305.00	(F10.10)	Mild
303.90	(F10.20)	Moderate
303.90	(F10.20)	Severe
303.00	(—.—)	Alcohol Intoxication (497)
	(F10.129)	With use disorder, mild
	(F10.229)	With use disorder, moderate or severe
	(F10.929)	Without use disorder
291.81	(—.—)	Alcohol Withdrawal[c,d] (499)
	(F10.239)	Without perceptual disturbances
	(F10.232)	With perceptual disturbances
—.—	(—.—)	Other Alcohol-Induced Disorder (502)
291.9	(F10.99)	Unspecified Alcohol-Related Disorder (503)

Caffeine-Related Disorders (503)

305.90	(F15.929)	Caffeine Intoxication (503)
292.0	(F15.93)	Caffeine Withdrawal (506)
—.—	(—.—)	Other Caffeine-Induced Disorder (508)
292.9	(F15.99)	Unspecified Caffeine-Related Disorder (509)

Cannabis-Related Disorders (509)

—.—	(—.—)	Cannabis Use Disorder[a,b] (509)
		Specify current severity:
305.20	(F12.10)	Mild
304.30	(F12.20)	Moderate
304.30	(F12.20)	Severe
292.89	(—.—)	Cannabis Intoxication[c] (516)
		Without perceptual disturbances
	(F12.129)	With use disorder, mild
	(F12.229)	With use disorder, moderate or severe
	(F12.929)	Without use disorder
		With perceptual disturbances
	(F12.122)	With use disorder, mild
	(F12.222)	With use disorder, moderate or severe
	(F12.922)	Without use disorder
292.0	(F12.288)	Cannabis Withdrawal[d] (517)
—.—	(—.—)	Other Cannabis-Induced Disorder (519)
292.9	(F12.99)	Unspecified Cannabis-Related Disorder (519)

Hallucinogen-Related Disorders (520)

—.—	(—.—)	Phencyclidine Use Disorder[a,b] (520)
		Specify current severity:
305.90	(F16.10)	Mild
304.60	(F16.20)	Moderate
304.60	(F16.20)	Severe
—.—	(—.—)	Other Hallucinogen Use Disorder[a,b] (523)
		Specify the particular hallucinogen
		Specify current severity:
305.30	(F16.10)	Mild
304.50	(F16.20)	Moderate
304.50	(F16.20)	Severe
292.89	(—.—)	Phencyclidine Intoxication (527)
	(F16.129)	With use disorder, mild
	(F16.229)	With use disorder, moderate or severe
	(F16.292)	Without use disorder
292.89	(—.—)	Other Hallucinogen Intoxication (529)
	(F16.129)	With use disorder, mild
	(F16.229)	With use disorder, moderate or severe
	(F16.929)	Without use disorder
292.89	(F16.983)	Hallucinogen Persisting Perception Disorder (531)
—.—	(—.—)	Other Phencyclidine-Induced Disorder (532)
—.—	(—.—)	Other Hallucinogen-Induced Disorder (532)
292.9	(F16.99)	Unspecified Phencyclidine-Related Disorder (533)
292.9	(F16.99)	Unspecified Hallucinogen-Related Disorder (533)

Inhalant-Related Disorder (533)

—.—	(—.—)	Inhalant Use Disorder[a,b] (533)
		Specify the particular inhalant
		Specify current severity:
305.90	(F18.10)	Mild
304.60	(F18.20)	Moderate
304.60	(F18.20)	Severe
292.89	(—.—)	Inhalant Intoxication (538)
	(F18.129)	With use disorder, mild
	(F18.229)	With use disorder, moderate or severe
	(F18.929)	Without use disorder
—.—	(—.—)	Other Inhalant-Induced Disorder (540)
292.9	(F18.99)	Unspecified Inhalant-Related Disorder (540)

Opioid-Related Disorders (540)

—.—	(—.—)	Opioid Use Disorder[a] (541)
		Specify if: On maintenance therapy, In a controlled environment
		Specify current severity:
305.50	(F11.10)	Mild
304.00	(F11.20)	Moderate
304.00	(F11.20)	Severe
292.89	(—.—)	Opioid Intoxication[c] (546)
		Without perceptual disturbances
	(F11.129)	With use disorder, mild
	(F11.229)	With use disorder, moderate or severe
	(F11.929)	Without use disorder
		With perceptual disturbances
	(F11.122)	With use disorder, mild
	(F11.222)	With use disorder, moderate or severe
	(F11.922)	Without use disorder
292.0	(F11.23)	Opioid Withdrawal[d] (547)
—.—	(—.—)	Other Opioid-Induced Disorder (549)
292.9	(F11.99)	Unspecified Opioid-Related Disorder (550)

Sedative-, Hynotic-, or Anxiolytic-Related Disorders (550)

—.—	(—.—)	Sedative, Hypnotic, or Anxiolytic Use Disorder[a,b] (550)
		Specify current severity:
305.40	(F13.10)	Mild
304.10	(F13.20)	Moderate
304.10	(F13.20)	Severe
292.89	(—.—)	Sedative, Hypnotic, or Anxiolytic Intoxication (556)
	(F13.129)	With use disorder, mild
	(F13.229)	With use disorder, moderate or severe
	(F13.929)	Without use disorder
292.0	(—.—)	Sedative, Hypnotic, or Anxiolytic Withdrawal[c,d] (557)
	(F13.229)	Without perceptual disturbances
	(F13.232)	With perceptual disturbances
—.—	(—.—)	Other Sedative-, Hypnotic-, or Anxiolytic-Induced Disorder (560)
292.9	(F13.99)	Unspecified Sedative-, Hypnotic-, or Anxiolytic-Related Disorder (560)

Stimulant-Related Disorders (561)

—.—	(—.—)	Stimulant Use Disorder[a,b] (561)
		Specify current severity:
—.—	(—.—)	Mild
305.70	(F15.10)	Amphetamine-type substance
305.60	(F14.10)	Cocaine
305.70	(F15.10)	Other or unspecified stimulant
—.—	(—.—)	Moderate
304.40	(F15.20)	Amphetamine-type substance
304.20	(F14.20)	Cocaine
304.40	(F15.20)	Other or unspecified stimulant
—.—	(—.—)	Severe
304.40	(F15.20)	Amphetamine-type substance
304.20	(F14.20)	Cocaine

304.40	**(F15.20)**	Other or unspecified stimulant
292.89	**(—.—)**	Stimulant Intoxication[c] (567)
		Specify the specific intoxicant
292.89	**(—.—)**	Amphetamine or other stimulant, Without perceptual disturbances
	(F15.129)	With use disorder, mild
	(F15.229)	With use disorder, moderate or severe
	(F15.929)	Without use disorder
292.89	**(—.—)**	Cocaine, Without perceptual disturbances
	(F14.129)	With use disorder, mild
	(F14.229)	With use disorder, moderate or severe
	(F14.929)	Without use disorder
292.89	**(—.—)**	Amphetamine or other stimulant, With perceptual disturbances
	(F15.122)	With use disorder, mild
	(F15.222)	With use disorder, moderate or severe
	(F15.922)	Without use disorder
292.89	**(—.—)**	Cocaine, With perceptual disturbances
	(F14.122)	With use disorder, mild
	(F14.222)	Without use disorder, moderate or severe
	(F14.922)	Without use disorder
292.0	**(—.—)**	Stimulant Withdrawal[d] (569)
		Specify the specific substance causing the withdrawal syndrome
	(F15.23)	Amphetamine or other stimulant
	(F14.23)	Cocaine
—.—	**(—.—)**	Other Stimulant-Induced Disorder (570)
292.9	**(—.—)**	Unspecified Stimulant-Related Disorder (570)
	(F15.99)	Amphetamine or other stimulant
	(F14.99)	Cocaine

Tobacco-Related Disorders (571)

—.—	**(—.—)**	Tobacco Use Disorder[a] (571)
		Specify if: On maintenance therapy, In a controlled environment
		Specify current severity:
305.1	**(Z72.0)**	Mild
305.1	**(F17.200)**	Moderate
305.1	**(F17.200)**	Severe
292.0	**(F17.203)**	Tobacco Withdrawal[d] (575)
—.—	**(—.—)**	Other Tobacco-Induced Disorder (576)
292.9	**(F17.209)**	Unspecified Tobacco-Related Disorder (577)

Other (or Unknown) Substance-Related Disorders (577)

—.—	**(—.—)**	Other (or Unknown) Substance Use Disorder[a,b] (577)
		Specify current severity:
305.90	**(F19.10)**	Mild
304.90	**(F19.20)**	Moderate
304.90	**(F19.20)**	Severe
292.89	**(—.—)**	Other (or Unknown) Substance Intoxication (581)
	(F19.129)	With use disorder, mild
	(F19.229)	With use disorder, moderate or severe
	(F19.229)	Without use disorder
292.0	**(F19.23)**	Other (or Unknown) Substance Withdrawal[d] (583)

—.—	**(—.—)**	Other (or Unknown) Substance-Induced Disorder (584)
292.2	**(F19.99)**	Unspecified Other (or Unknown) Substance-Related Disorder (585)

Non-Substance-Related Disorders (585)

312.31	**(F63.0)**	Gambling Disorder[a] (585)
		Specify if: Episodic, Persistent
		Specify current severity: Mild, Moderate, Severe

NEUROCOGNITIVE DISORDERS (591)

—.—	**(—.—)**	Delirium (596)
		[a]**Note:** See the criteria set and corresponding recording procedures for substance-specific codes and ICD-9-CM and ICD-10-CM coding.
		Specify whether:
—.—	**(—.—)**	Substance intoxication delirium[a]
—.—	**(—.—)**	Substance withdrawal delirium[a]
292.81	**(—.—)**	Medication-induced delirium[a]
293.0	**(F05)**	Delirium due to another medical condition
293.0	**(F05)**	Delirium due to multiple etiologies
		Specify if: Acute, Persistent
		Specify if: Hyperactive, Hypoactive, Mixed level of activity
780.09	**(R41.0)**	Other Specified Delirium (602)
780.09	**(R41.0)**	Unspecified Delirium (602)

Major and Mild Neurocognitive Disorders (602)

Specify whether due to: Alzheimer's disease, Frontotemporal lobar degeneration, Lewy body disease, Vascular disease, Traumatic brain injury, Substance/medication use, HIV infection, Prion disease, Parkinson's disease, Huntington's disease, Another medical condition, Multiple etiologies, Unspecified

[a]*Specify:* Without behavioral disturbance, With behavioral disturbance. *For possible major neurocognitive disorder and for mild neurocognitive disorder, behavioral disturbance cannot be coded but should still be indicated in writing.*

[b]*Specify* current severity: Mild, Moderate, Severe. *This specifier applies only to major neurocognitive disorder (including probable and possible).*

Note: As indicated for each subtype, an additional medical code is needed for probable major neurocognitive disorder or major neurocognitive disorder. An additional medical code should *not* be used for possible major neurocognitive disorder or mild neurocognitive disorder.

Major or Mild Neurocognitive Disorder Due to Alzheimer's Disease (611)

—.—	**(—.—)**	Probable Major Neurocognitive Disorder Due to Alzheimer's Disease[b]
		Note: Code first **331.0 (G30.9)** Alzheimer's disease
294.11	**(F02.81)**	With behavioral disturbance
294.10	**(F02.80)**	Without behavioral disturbance
331.9	**(G31.9)**	Possible Major Neurocognitive Disorder Due to Alzheimer's Disease[a,b]
331.83	**(G31.84)**	Mild Neurocognitive Disorder Due to Alzheimer's Disease[a]

Major or Mild Frontotemporal Neurocognitive Disorder (614)

—.—	(—.—)	Probable Major Neurocognitive Disorder Due to Frontotemporal Lobar Degeneration[b]
		Note: Code first **331.19 (G31.09)** frontotemporal disease.
294.11	(F02.81)	With behavioral disturbance
294.10	(F02.80)	Without behavioral disturbance
331.9	(G31.9)	Possible Major Neurocognitive Disorder Due to Frontotemporal Lobar Degeneration[a,b]
331.83	(G31.84)	Mild Neurocognitive Disorder Due to Frontotemporal Lobar Degeneration[a]

Major or Mild Neurocognitive Disorder with Lewy Bodies (618)

—.—	(—.—)	Probable Major Neurocognitive Disorder With Lewy Bodies[b]
		Note: Code first **331.82 (G31.83)** Lewy body disease.
294.11	(F02.81)	With behavioral disturbance
294.10	(F02.80)	Without behavioral disturbance
331.9	(G31.9)	Possible Major Neurocognitive Disorder With Lewy Bodies[a,b]
331.83	(G31.84)	Mild Neurocognitive Disorder With Lewy Bodies[a]

Major or Mild Vascular Neurocognitive Disorder (621)

—.—	(—.—)	Probable Major Vascular Neurocognitive Disorder[b]
		Note: No additional medical code for vascular disease.
290.40	(F01.51)	With behavioral disturbance
290.40	(F01.50)	Without behavioral disturbance
331.9	(G31.9)	Possible Major Vascular Neurocognitive Disorder[a,b]
331.83	(G31.84)	Mild Vascular Neurocognitive Disorder[a]

Major or Mild Neurocognitive Disorder Due to Traumatic Brain Injury (624)

—.—	(—.—)	Major Neurocognitive Disorder Due to Traumatic Brain Injury[b]
		Note: For ICD-9-CM, code first **907.0** late effect of intracranial injury without skull fracture. For ICD-10-CM, code first **S06.2X9S** diffuse traumatic brain injury with loss of consciousness of unspecified duration, sequela.
294.11	(F02.81)	With behavioral disturbance
294.10	(F02.80)	Without behavioral disturbance
331.83	(G31.84)	Mild Neurocognitive Disorder Due to Traumatic Brain Injury[a]

Substance/Medication-Induced Major or Mild Neurocognitive Disorder[a] (627)

Note: No additional medical code. See the criteria set and corresponding recording procedures for substance-specific codes and ICD-9-CM and ICD-10-CM coding.

Specify if: Persistent

Major or Mild Neurocognitive Disorder Due to HIV Infection (632)

—.—	(—.—)	Major Neurocognitive Disorder Due to HIV Infection[b]
		Note: Code first **042 (B20)** HIV infection.
294.11	(F02.81)	With behavioral disturbance
294.10	(F02.80)	Without behavioral disturbance
331.83	(G31.84)	Mild Neurocognitive Disorder Due to HIV Infection[a]

Major or Mild Neurocognitive Disorder Due to Prion Disease (634)

—.—	(—.—)	Major Neurocognitive Disorder Due to Prion Disease[b]
		Note: Code first **046.79 (A81.9)** prion disease.
294.11	(F02.81)	With behavioral disturbance
294.10	(F02.80)	Without behavioral disturbance
331.83	(G31.84)	Mild Neurocognitive Disorder Due to Prion Disease[a]

Major or Mild Neurocognitive Disorder Due to Parkinson's Disease (636)

—.—	(—.—)	Major Neurocognitive Disorder Probably Due to Parkinson's Disease[b]
		Note: Code first **332.0 (G20)** Parkinson's disease.
294.11	(F02.81)	With behavioral disturbance
294.10	(F02.80)	Without behavioral disturbance
331.9	(G31.9)	Major Neurocognitive Disorder Possibly Due to Parkinson's Disease[a,b]
331.83	(G31.84)	Mild Neurocognitive Disorder Due to Parkinson's Disease[a]

Major or Mild Neurocognitive Disorder Due to Huntington's Disease (638)

—.—	(—.—)	Major Neurocognitive Disorder Due to Huntington's Disease[b]
		Note: Code first **333.4 (G10)** Huntington's disease.
294.11	(F02.81)	With behavioral disturbance
294.10	(F02.80)	Without behavioral disturbance
331.83	(G31.84)	Mild Neurocognitive Disorder Due to Huntington's Disease[a]

Major or Mild Neurocognitive Disorder Due to Another Medical Condition[a] (641)

—.—	(—.—)	Major Neurocognitive Disorder Due to Another Medical Condition[b]
		Note: Code first the other medical condition.
294.11	(F02.81)	With behavioral disturbance
294.10	(F02.80)	Without behavioral disturbance
331.83	(G31.84)	Mild Neurocognitive Disorder Due to Another Medical Condition[a]

Major or Mild Neurocognitive Disorder Due to Multiple Etiologies (642)

—.—	(—.—)	Major Neurocognitive Disorder Due to Multiple Etiologies[b]

Note: Code first all the etiological medical conditions (with the exception of vascular disease).

294.11	(F02.81)	With behavioral disturbance
294.10	(F02.80)	Without behavioral disturbance
331.83	(G31.84)	Mild Neurocognitive Disorder Due to Multiple Etiologies[a]

Unspecified Neurocognitive Disorder (643)

799.59	(R41.9)	Unspecified Neurocognitive Disorder[a]

PERSONALITY DISORDERS (645)

Cluster A Personality Disorders

301.0	(F60.0)	Paranoid Personality Disorder (649)
301.20	(F60.1)	Schizoid Personality Disorder (652)
301.22	(F21)	Schizotypal Personality Disorder (655)

Cluster B Personality Disorders

301.7	(F60.2)	Antisocial Personality Disorder (659)
301.83	(F60.3)	Borderline Personality Disorder (663)
301.50	(F60.4)	Histrionic Personality Disorder (667)
301.81	(F60.81)	Narcissistic Personality Disorder (669)

Cluster C Personality Disorders

301.82	(F60.6)	Avoidant Personality Disorder (672)
301.6	(F60.7)	Dependent Personality Disorder (675)
301.4	(F60.5)	Obsessive-Compulsive Personality Disorder (678)

Other Personality Disorders

310.1	(F07.0)	Personality Change Due to Another Medical Condition (682)
		Specify whether: Labile type, Disinhibited type, Aggressive type, Apathetic type, Paranoid type, Other type, Combined type, Unspecified type
301.89	(F60.89)	Other Specified Personality Disorder (684)
301.9	(F60.9)	Unspecified Personality Disorder (684)

PARAPHILIC DISORDERS (685)

The following specifier applies to Paraphilic Disorders where indicated:
[a]*Specify* if: In a controlled environment, In full remission

302.82	(F65.3)	Voyeuristic Disorder[a] (686)
302.4	(F65.2)	Exhibitionistic Disorder[a] (689)
		Specify whether: Sexuallly aroused by exposing genitals to prepubertal children, Sexually aroused by exposing genitals to physically mature individuals, Sexually aroused by exposing genitals to prepubertal children and to physically mature individuals
302.89	(F65.81)	Frotteuristic Disorder[a] (691)
302.83	(F65.51)	Sexual Masochism Disorder[a] (694)
		Specify if: With asphyxiophilia
302.84	(F65.52)	Sexual Sadism Disorder[a] (695)
302.2	(F65.4)	Pedophilic Disorder (697)

Specify whether: Exclusive type, Non-exclusive type
Specify if: Sexually attracted to males, Sexually attracted to females, Sexually attracted to both
Specify if: Limited to incest

302.81	(F65.0)	Fetishistic Disorder[a] (700)
		Specify: Body part(s), Nonliving object(s), Other
302.3	(F65.1)	Transvestic Disorder[a] (702)
		Specify if: With fetishism, With autogynephilia
302.89	(F65.89)	Other Specified Paraphilic Disorder (705)
302.9	(F65.9)	Unspecified Paraphilic Disorder (705)

OTHER MENTAL DISORDERS (707)

294.8	(F06.8)	Other Specified Mental Disorder Due to Another Medical Condition (707)
294.9	(F09)	Unspecified Mental Disorder Due to Another Medical Condition (708)
300.9	(F99)	Other Specified Mental Disorder (708)
300.9	(F99)	Unspecified Mental Disorder (708)

MEDICATION-INDUCED MOVEMENT DISORDERS AND OTHER ADVERSE EFFECTS OF MEDICATION (709)

332.1	(G21.11)	Neuroleptic-Induced Parkinsonism (709)
332.1	(G21.19)	Other Medication-Induced Parkinsonism (709)
333.92	(G21.0)	Neuroleptic Malignant Syndrome (709)
333.72	(G24.02)	Medication-Induced Acute Dystonia (711)
333.99	(G25.71)	Medication-Induced Acute Akathisia (711)
333.85	(G24.01)	Tardive Dyskinesia (712)
333.72	(G24.09)	Tardive Dystonia (712)
333.99	(G25.71)	Tardive Akathisia (712)
333.1	(G25.1)	Medication-Induced Postural Tremor (712)
333.99	(G25.79)	Other Medication-Induced Movement Disorder (712)
—.—	(—.—)	Antidepressant Discontinuation Syndrome (712)
995.29	(T43.205A)	Initial encounter
995.29	(T43.205D)	Subsequent encounter
995.29	(T43.205S)	Sequelae
—.—	(—.—)	Other Adverse Effect of Medication (714)
995.20	(T50.905A)	Initial encounter
995.20	(T50.905D)	Subsequent encounter
995.20	(T50.905S)	Sequelae

OTHER CONDITIONS THAT MAY BE A FOCUS OF CLINICAL ATTENTION (715)

Relational Problems (715)
Problems Related to Family Upbringing (715)

V61.20	(Z62.820)	Parent-Child Relational Problem (715)
V61.8	(Z62.891)	Sibling Relational Problem (716)

V61.8	**(Z62.29)**	Upbringing Away From Parents (716)
V61.29	**(Z62.898)**	Child Affected by Parental Relationship Distress (716)

Other Problems Related to Primary Support Group (716)

V61.10	**(Z63.0)**	Relationship Distress With Spouse or Intimate Partner (716)
V61.03	**(Z63.5)**	Disruption of Family by Separation or Divorce (716)
V61.8	**(Z63.8)**	High Expressed Emotion Level Within Family (716)
V62.82	**(Z63.4)**	Uncomplicated Bereavement (716)

Abuse and Neglect (717)
Child Maltreatment and Neglect Problems (717)
Child Physical Abuse (717)
Child Physical Abuse, Confirmed (717)

995.54	**(T743.12XA)**	Initial encounter
995.54	**(T74.12XD)**	Subsequent encounter

Child Physical Abuse, Suspected (717)

995.54	**(T76.12XA)**	Initial encounter
995.54	**(T76.12XD)**	Subsequent encounter

Other Circumstances Related to Child Physical Abuse (718)

V61.21	**(Z69.010)**	Encounter for mental health services for victim of child abuse by parent
V61.21	**(Z69.020)**	Encounter for mental health services for victim of nonparental child abuse
V15.41	**(Z62.810)**	Personal history (past history) of physical abuse in childhood
V61.22	**(Z69.011)**	Encounter for mental health services for perpetrator of parental child abuse
V62.83	**(Z69.021)**	Encounter for mental health services for perpetrator of nonparental child abuse

Child Sexual Abuse (718)
Child Sexual Abuse, Confirmed (718)

995.53	**(T74.22XA)**	Initial encounter
995.53	**(T74.22XD)**	Subsequent encounter

Child Sexual Abuse, Suspected (718)

995.53	**(T76.22XA)**	Initial encounter
995.53	**(T76.22XD)**	Subsequent encounter

Other Circumstances Related to Child Sexual Abuse (718)

V61.21	**(Z69.010)**	Encounter for mental health services for victim of child sexual abuse by parent
V61.21	**(Z69.020)**	Encounter for mental health services for victim of nonparental child sexual abuse
V15.21	**(Z62.810)**	Personal history (past history) of sexual abuse in childhood
V61.22	**(Z69.011)**	Encounter for mental health services for perpetrator of parental child sexual abuse
V62.83	**(Z69.021)**	Encounter for mental health services for perpetrator of nonparental child sexual abuse

Child Neglect (718)
Child Neglect, Confirmed (718)

995.52	**(T74.02ZA)**	Initial encounter
995.52	**(T74.02XD)**	Subsequent encounter

Child Neglect, Suspected (719)

995.52	**(T76.02XA)**	Initial encounter
995.52	**(T76.02XD)**	Subsequent encounter

Other Circumstances Related to Child Neglect (719)

V61.21	**(Z69.010)**	Encounter for mental health services for victim of child neglect by parent
V61.21	**(Z69.020)**	Encounter for mental health services for victim of nonparental child neglect
V15.42	**(Z62.812)**	Personal history (past history) of neglect in childhood
V61.22	**(Z69.011)**	Encounter for mental health services for perpetrator of parental child neglect
V62.83	**(Z69.021)**	Encounter for mental health services for perpetrator of nonparental child neglect

Child Psychological Abuse (719)
Child Psychological Abuse, Confirmed (719)

995.51	**(T74.32XA)**	Initial encounter
995.51	**(T74.32XD)**	Subsequent encounter

Child Psychological Abuse, Suspected (719)

995.51	**(T76.32XA)**	Initial encounter
995.51	**(T76.32XD)**	Subsequent encounter

Other Circumstances Related to Child Psychological Abuse (719)

V61.21	**(Z69.010)**	Encounter for mental health services for victim of child psychological abuse by parent
V61.21	**(Z69.020)**	Encounter for mental health services for victim of nonparental child psychological abuse
V15.42	**(Z62.811)**	Personal history (past history) of psychological abuse in childhood
V61.22	**(Z69.011)**	Encounter for mental health services for perpetrator of parental child psychological abuse
V62.83	**(Z69.021)**	Encounter for mental health services for perpetrator of nonparental child psychological abuse

Adult Maltreatment and Neglect Problems (720)
Spouse or Partner Violence, Physical (720)
Spouse or Partner Violence, Physical, Confirmed (720)

995.81	**(T74.11XA)**	Initial encounter
995.81	**(T74.11XD)**	Subsequent encounter

Spouse or Partner Violence, Physical, Suspected (720)

995.81	**(T76.11XA)**	Initial encounter
995.81	**(T76.11XD)**	Subsequent encounter

Other Circumstances Related to Spouse or Partner Violence, Physical (720)

V61.11	**(Z96.11)**	Encounter for mental health services for victim of spouse or partner violence, physical
V15.41	**(Z91.410)**	Personal history (past history) of spouse or partner violence, physical
V61.12	**(Z69.12)**	Encounter for mental health services for perpetrator of spouse or partner violence, physical

Spouse or Partner Violence, Sexual (720)

Spouse or Partner Violence, Sexual, Confirmed (720)

995.83 **(T74.21XA)**   Initial encounter
995.83 **(T74.21XD)**   Subsequent encounter

Spouse or Partner Violence, Sexual, Suspected (720)

995.83 **(T76.21XA)**   Initial encounter
995.83 **(T76.21XD)**   Subsequent encounter

Other Circumstances Related to Spouse or Partner Violence, Sexual (720)

V61.11   **(Z69.81)**   Encounter for mental health services for victim of spouse or partner violence, sexual

V15.41   **(Z91.410)**   Personal history (past history) of spouse or partner violence, sexual

V61.12   **(Z69.12)**   Encounter for mental health services for perpetrator of spouse or partner violence, sexual

Spouse or Partner Neglect (721)

Spouse or Partner Neglect, Confirmed (721)

995.85 **(T47.01XA)**   Initial encounter
995.85 **(T74.01XD)**   Subsequent encounter

Spouse or Partner Neglect, Suspected (721)

995.85 **(T76.01XA)**   Initial encounter
995.85 **(T76.01XD)**   Subsequent encounter

Other Circumstances Related to Spouse or Partner Neglect (721)

V61.11   **(Z69.11)**   Encounter for mental health services for victim of spouse or partner neglect

V15.42   **(Z91.412)**   Personal history (past history) of spouse or partner neglect

V61.12   **(Z69.12)**   Encounter for mental health services for perpetrator of spouse or partner neglect

Spouse or Partner Abuse, Psychological (721)

Spouse or Partner Abuse, Psychological, Confirmed (721)

995.82 **(T74.31XA)**   Initial encounter
995.82 **(T74.31XD)**   Subsequent encounter

Spouse or Partner Abuse, Psychological, Suspected (721)

995.82 **(T76.31XA)**   Initial encounter
995.82 **(T76.31XD)**   Subsequent encounter

Other Circumstances Related to Spouse or Partner Abuse, Psychological (721)

V61.11   **(Z69.11)**   Encounter for mental health services for victim of spouse or partner psychological abuse

V15.42   **(Z91.411)**   Personal history (past history) of spouse or partner psychological abuse

V61.12   **(Z69.12)**   Encounter for mental health services for perpetrator of spouse or partner psychological abuse

Adult Abuse by Nonspouse or Nonpartner (722)

Adult Physical Abuse by Nonspouse or Nonpartner, Confirmed (722)

995.81 **(T74.11XA)**   Initial encounter
995.81 **(T74.11XD)**   Subsequent encounter

Adult Physical Abuse by Nonspouse or Nonpartner, Suspected (722)

995.81 **(T76.11XA)**   Initial encounter
995.81 **(T76.11XD)**   Subsequent encounter

Adult Sexual Abuse by Nonspouse or Nonpartner, Confirmed (722)

995.83 **(T74.21XA)**   Initial encounter
995.83 **(T74.21XD)**   Subsequent encounter

Adult Sexual Abuse by Nonspouse or Nonpartner, Suspected (722)

995.83 **(T76.21XA)**   Initial encounter
995.83 **(T76.21XD)**   Subsequent encounter

Adult Psychological Abuse by Nonspouse or Nonpartner, Confirmed (722)

995.82 **(T74.31XA)**   Initial encounter
995.82 **(T74.31XD)**   Subsequent encounter

Adult Psychological Abuse by Nonspouse or Nonpartner, Suspected (722)

995.82 **(T76.31XA)**   Initial encounter
995.82 **(T76.31XD)**   Subsequent encounter

Other Circumstances Related to Adult Abuse by Nonspouse or Nonpartner (722)

V65.49   **(Z69.81)**   Encounter for mental health services for victim of nonspousal adult abuse

V62.83   **(Z69.82)**   Encounter for mental health services for perpetrator of nonspousal adult abuse

Educational and Occupational Problems (723)
Educational Problems (723)

V62.3   **(Z55.9)**   Academic or Educational Problem (723)

Occupational Problems (723)

V62.21   **(Z56.82)**   Problem Related to Current Military Deployment Status (723)

V62.29   **(Z56.9)**   Other Problem Related to Employment (723)

Housing and Economic Problems (723)
Housing Problems (723)

V60.0   **(Z59.0)**   Homelessness (723)
V60.1   **(Z59.1)**   Inadequate Housing (723)
V60.89   **(Z59.2)**   Discord With Neighbor, Lodger, or Landlord (723)
V60.6   **(Z59.3)**   Problem Related to Living in a Residential Institution (724)

Economic Problems (724)

V60.2   **(Z59.4)**   Lack of Adequate Food or Safe Drinking Water (724)
V60.2   **(Z59.5)**   Extreme Poverty (724)
V60.2   **(Z59.6)**   Low Income (724)
V60.2   **(Z59.7)**   Insufficient Social Insurance or Welfare Support (724)
V60.9   **(Z59.9)**   Unspecified Housing or Economic Problem (724)

Other Problems Related to the Social Environment (724)

V62.89   **(Z60.0)**   Phase of Life Problem (724)
V60.3   **(Z60.2)**   Problem Related to Living Alone (724)
V62.4   **(Z60.3)**   Acculturation Difficulty (724)
V62.4   **(Z60.4)**   Social Exclusion or Rejection (724)
V62.4   **(Z60.5)**   Target of (Perceived) Adverse Discrimination or Persecution (724)
V62.9   **(Z60.9)**   Unspecified Problem Related to Social Environment (725)

Problems Related to Crime or Interaction With the Legal System (725)

V62.879	**(Z65.4)**	Victim of Crime (725)
V62.5	**(Z65.0)**	Conviction in Civil or Criminal Proceedings Without Imprisonment (725)
V62.5	**(Z65.1)**	Imprisonment or Other Incarceration (725)
V62.5	**(Z65.2)**	Problems Related to Release From Prison (725)
V62.5	**(Z65.3)**	Problems Related to Other Legal Circumstances (725)

Other Health Service Encounters for Counseling and Medical Advice (725)

V65.4	**(Z70.9)**	Sex Counseling (725)
V65.40	**(Z71.9)**	Other Counseling or Consultation (725)

Problems Related to Other Psychosocial, Personal, and Environmental Circumstances (725)

V62.89	**(Z65.8)**	Religious or Spiritual Problem (725)
V61.7	**(Z64.0)**	Problems Related to Unwanted Pregnancy (725)
V61.5	**(Z64.1)**	Problems Related to Multiparity (725)
V62.89	**(Z64.4)**	Discord With Social Service Provider, Including Probation Officer, Case Manager, or Social Service Worker (725)
V62.89	**(Z65.4)**	Victim of Terrorism or Torture (725)
V62.22	**(Z65.5)**	Exposure to Disaster, War, or Other Hostilities (725)
V62.89	**(Z65.8)**	Other Problem Related to Psychosocial Circumstances (725)
V62.9	**(Z65.9)**	Unspecified Problem Related to Unspecified Psychosocial Circumstances (725)

Other Circumstances of Personal History (726)

V15.49	**(Z91.49)**	Other Personal History of Psychological Trauma (726)
V15.59	**(Z91.5)**	Personal History of Self-Harm (726)
V62.22	**(Z91.82)**	Personal History of Military Deployment (726)
V15.89	**(Z91.89)**	Other Personal Risk Factors (726)
V69.9	**(Z72.9)**	Problem Related to Lifestyle (726)
V71.01	**(Z72.811)**	Adult Antisocial Behavior (726)
V71.02	**(Z72.810)**	Child or Adolescent Antisocial Behavior (726)

Problems Related to Access to Medical and Other Health Care (726)

V63.9	**(Z75.3)**	Unavailability or Inaccessibility of Health Care Facilities (726)
V63.8	**(Z75.4)**	Unavailability or Inaccessibility of Other Helping Agencies (726)

Nonadherence to Medical Treatment (726)

V15.81	**(Z91.19)**	Nonadherence to Medical Treatment (726)
278.00	**(E66.9)**	Overweight or Obesity (726)
V65.2	**(Z76.5)**	Malingering (726)
V40.31	**(Z91.83)**	Wandering Associated With a Mental Disorder (727)
V62.89	**(R41.83)**	Borderline Intellectual Functioning (727)

From American Psychiatric Association. (2013). *Diagnostic and statistical manual of disorders* (5th ed.). Washington, DC: Author.

NANDA-Approved Nursing Diagnoses 2015–2017

Indicates new diagnosis for 2015–2017—25 total

Indicates revised diagnosis for 2015–2017—14 total

1. Activity Intolerance
2. Activity Intolerance, Risk for
3. Activity Planning, Ineffective
4. Activity Planning, Risk for Ineffective
5. Adaptive Capacity, Decreased Intracranial
6. Airway Clearance, Ineffective
7. Allergy Response, Risk for
8. Anxiety
9. Aspiration, Risk for
10. Attachment, Risk for Impaired
11. Autonomic Dysreflexia
12. Autonomic Dysreflexia, Risk for
13. Behavior, Disorganized Infant
14. Behavior, Readiness for Enhanced Organized Infant
15. Behavior, Risk for Disorganized Infant
16. Bleeding, Risk for
17. Blood Glucose Level, Risk for Unstable
18. Body Image, Disturbed
19. Body Temperature, Risk for Imbalanced
20. Breastfeeding, Readiness for Enhanced
21. Breastfeeding, Ineffective
22. Breastfeeding, Interrupted
23. Breast Milk, Insufficient
24. Breathing Pattern, Ineffective
25. Cardiac Output, Decreased
26. Cardiac Output, Risk for Decreased
27. Cardiovascular Function, Risk for Impaired
28. Childbearing Process, Ineffective
29. Childbearing Process, Readiness for Enhanced
30. Childbearing Process, Risk for Ineffective
31. Comfort, Impaired
32. Comfort, Readiness for Enhanced
33. Communication, Readiness for Enhanced
34. Confusion, Acute
35. Confusion, Chronic
36. Confusion, Risk for Acute
37. Constipation
38. Constipation, Perceived
39. Constipation, Risk for
40. Constipation, Chronic Functional
41. Constipation, Risk for Chronic Functional
42. Contamination
43. Contamination, Risk for
44. Coping, Compromised Family
45. Coping, Defensive
46. Coping, Disabled Family
47. Coping, Ineffective
48. Coping, Ineffective Community
49. Coping, Readiness for Enhanced
50. Coping, Readiness for Enhanced Community
51. Coping, Readiness for Enhanced Family
52. Death Anxiety
53. Decision-Making, Readiness for Enhanced
54. Decisional Conflict
55. Denial, Ineffective
56. Dentition, Impaired
57. Development, Risk for Delayed
58. Diarrhea
59. Disuse Syndrome, Risk for
60. Diversional Activity, Deficient
61. Dry Eye, Risk for
62. Electrolyte Imbalance, Risk for
63. Elimination, Impaired Urinary
64. Elimination, Readiness for Enhanced Urinary
65. Emancipated Decision Making, Impaired
66. Emancipated Decision Making, Readiness for Enhanced
67. Emancipated Decision Making, Risk for Impaired
68. Emotional Control, Labile
69. Falls, Risk for
70. Family Processes, Dysfunctional
71. Family Processes, Interrupted
72. Family Processes, Readiness for Enhanced
73. Fatigue
74. Fear
75. Feeding Pattern, Ineffective Infant
76. Fluid Balance, Readiness for Enhanced
77. Fluid Volume, Deficient
78. Fluid Volume, Excess
79. Fluid Volume, Risk for Deficient
80. Fluid Volume, Risk for Imbalanced
81. Frail Elderly Syndrome
82. Frail Elderly Syndrome, Risk for
83. Gas Exchange, Impaired
84. Gastrointestinal Motility, Dysfunctional
85. Gastrointestinal Motility, Risk for Dysfunctional
86. Gastrointestinal Perfusion, Risk for Ineffective
87. Grieving
88. Grieving, Complicated
89. Grieving, Risk for Complicated
90. Growth, Risk for Disproportionate
91. Health, Deficient Community
92. Health Behavior, Risk-Prone
93. Health Maintenance, Ineffective
94. Health Management, Ineffective
95. Health Management, Readiness for Enhanced
96. Health Management, Ineffective Family
97. Home Maintenance, Impaired
98. Hope, Readiness for Enhanced

99. Hopelessness
100. Human Dignity, Risk for Compromised
101. Hyperthermia
102. Hypothermia
103. Hypothermia, Risk for
104. Hypothermia, Risk for Perioperative
105. Impulse Control, Ineffective
106. Incontinence, Functional Urinary
107. Incontinence, Overflow Urinary
108. Incontinence, Reflex Urinary
109. Incontinence, Risk for Urge Urinary
110. Incontinence, Stress Urinary
111. Incontinence, Urge Urinary
112. Incontinence, Bowel
113. Infection, Risk for
114. Injury, Risk for
115. Injury, Risk for Corneal
116. Injury, Risk for Perioperative-Positioning
117. Injury, Risk for Thermal
118. Injury, Risk for Urinary Tract
119. Insomnia
120. Jaundice, Neonatal
121. Jaundice, Risk for Neonatal
122. Knowledge, Deficient
123. Knowledge, Readiness for Enhanced
124. Latex Allergy Response
125. Latex Allergy Response, Risk for
126. Lifestyle, Sedentary
127. Liver Function, Risk for Impaired
128. Loneliness, Risk for
129. Maternal/Fetal Dyad, Risk for Disturbed
130. Memory, Impaired
131. Mobility, Impaired Bed
132. Mobility, Impaired Physical
133. Mobility, Impaired Wheelchair
134. Mood Regulation, Impaired
135. Moral Distress
136. Nausea
137. Noncompliance
138. Nutrition, Imbalanced: Less Than Body Requirements
139. Nutrition, Readiness for Enhanced
140. Obesity
141. Oral Mucous Membrane, Impaired
142. Oral Mucous Membrane, Risk for Impaired
143. Other-Directed Violence, Risk for
144. Overweight
145. Overweight, Risk for
146. Pain, Acute
147. Pain, Chronic
148. Pain, Labor
149. Pain Syndrome, Chronic
150. Parenting, Impaired
151. Parenting, Readiness for Enhanced
152. Parenting, Risk for Impaired
153. Peripheral Neurovascular Dysfunction, Risk for
154. Personal Identity, Disturbed
155. Personal Identity, Risk for Disturbed
156. Poisoning, Risk for
157. Post-Trauma Syndrome
158. Post-Trauma Syndrome, Risk for
159. Power, Readiness for Enhanced
160. Powerlessness
161. Powerlessness, Risk for
162. Pressure Ulcer, Risk for
163. Protection, Ineffective
164. Rape-Trauma Syndrome
165. Reaction to Iodinated Contrast Media, Risk for
166. Relationship, Ineffective
167. Relationship, Risk for Ineffective
168. Relationship, Readiness for Enhanced
169. Religiosity, Impaired
170. Religiosity, Readiness for Enhanced
171. Religiosity, Risk for Impaired
172. Relocation Stress Syndrome
173. Relocation Stress Syndrome, Risk for
174. Renal Perfusion, Risk for Ineffective
175. Resilience, Impaired
176. Resilience, Readiness for Enhanced
177. Resilience, Risk for Impaired
178. Role Conflict, Parental
179. Role Performance, Ineffective
180. Role Strain, Caregiver
181. Role Strain, Risk for Caregiver
182. Self-Care, Readiness for Enhanced
183. Self-Care Deficit, Bathing
184. Self-Care Deficit, Dressing
185. Self-Care Deficit, Feeding
186. Self-Care Deficit, Toileting
187. Self-Concept, Readiness for Enhanced
188. Self-Directed Violence, Risk for
189. Self-Esteem, Chronic Low
190. Self-Esteem, Risk for Chronic Low
191. Self-Esteem, Situational Low
192. Self-Esteem, Risk for Situational Low
193. Self-Mutilation
194. Self-Mutilation, Risk for
195. Self-Neglect
196. Sexual Dysfunction
197. Sexuality Pattern, Ineffective
198. Shock, Risk for
199. Sitting, Impaired
200. Skin Integrity, Impaired
201. Skin Integrity, Risk for Impaired
202. Sleep, Readiness for Enhanced
203. Sleep Deprivation
204. Sleep Pattern, Disturbed
205. Social Interaction, Impaired
206. Social Isolation
207. Sorrow, Chronic
208. Spiritual Distress
209. Spiritual Distress, Risk for
210. Spiritual Well-Being, Readiness for Enhanced
211. Spontaneous Ventilation, Impaired
212. Standing, Impaired
213. Stress Overload
214. Sudden Infant Death Syndrome, Risk for
215. Suffocation, Risk for
216. Suicide, Risk for
217. Surgical Recovery, Delayed
218. Surgical Recovery, Risk for Delayed
219. Swallowing, Impaired
220. Thermoregulation, Ineffective
221. Tissue Integrity, Impaired
222. Tissue Integrity, Risk for Impaired

223. Tissue Perfusion, Ineffective Peripheral
224. Tissue Perfusion, Risk for Ineffective Peripheral
225. Tissue Perfusion, Risk for Decreased Cardiac
226. Tissue Perfusion, Risk for Ineffective Cerebral
227. Transfer Ability, Impaired
228. Trauma, Risk for
229. Vascular Trauma, Risk for

230. Unilateral Neglect
231. Urinary Retention
232. Ventilatory Weaning Response, Dysfunctional
233. Verbal Communication, Impaired
234. Walking, Impaired
235. Wandering

From NANDA International, Inc. (2014). *Nursing diagnoses: Definitions & classifications 2015–2017* (10th ed.). Hoboken, NJ: John Wiley & Sons, Ltd. http://www.wiley.com/go/nursingdiagnoses

Answers to Chapter Review Questions

Chapter 1

1. Answer – b. Pages 6–7. While all of the scenarios present opportunities for a nurse to intervene, the correct response presents an imminent danger to the patient's safety and well-being.
2. Answer – c. Pages 5–6. Trauma occurs in many forms, including physical, sexual, and emotional abuse; war; natural disasters; and other harmful experiences. Trauma-informed care provides guidelines for integrating an understanding of how trauma affects patients into clinical programming.
3. Answer – d. Page 4. The patient's report suggests that depression is occurring. With the increased understanding of the biology of psychiatric illnesses, treatment approaches have evolved rapidly into more scientifically grounded methods, particularly psychopharmacology.
4. Answer – d. Page 5. The correct response recognizes the recovery model, which has the following tenets: Mental health care is consumer and family driven, with patients being partners in all aspects of care; care must focus on increasing the consumer's success in coping with life's challenges and building resilience; and an individualized care plan is at the core of consumer-centered recovery.
5. Answer – a. Page 6. Caring is evidenced by empathic understanding, actions, and patience on another's behalf; actions, words, and presence that lead to happiness and touch the heart; and giving of self while preserving the importance of self. Comforting is a part of caring, which includes social, emotional, physical, and spiritual support.

Chapter 2

1. Answer – c. Pages 8–9. Stigma refers to the array of negative attitudes and beliefs regarding mental illness. Bias, prejudice, fear, and misinformation contribute to stigma.
2. Answer – c. Pages 13–14. In the correct response, the nurse answers rather than evades the question, provides accurate information, and uses terminology a 9- or 10-year-old child can understand. Many of the most prevalent and disabling mental disorders have been found to have strong biological influences, including genetic transmission.
3. Answer – d. Page 12. Resiliency is the ability to recover from or adjust successfully to trauma or change. A successful transition through a crisis builds resiliency for the next difficult trial. In the correct response, the person demonstrates acceptance of the paralysis and a focus on his or her abilities and assets.
4. Answer – a. Page 14. Diagnoses classify disorders that people have, not the person. For this reason, it is important to avoid use of expressions such as "a schizophrenic" or "an alcoholic." The nurse has a responsibility to educate the coworker.
5. Answer – c. Page 10. Many biological, cultural, and environmental factors influence mental health. Persons who are normal also may experience dysfunction during their lives. The death of a spouse is a difficult experience, so crying is expected.

Chapter 3

1. Answer – b. Page 31. A therapeutic milieu provides a healthy social structure within an inpatient setting or structured outpatient clinic. Groups aim to help increase patients' self-esteem, decrease social isolation, encourage appropriate social behaviors, and educate patients in basic living skills, such as good hand washing.
2. Answer – b. Page 24 (Figure 3-2). Maslow's hierarchy of needs are placed conceptually on a pyramid, with the most basic and important needs on the lower level. The higher levels, the more distinctly human needs, occupy the top sections of the pyramid. When lower-level needs are met, higher-level needs are able to emerge. Self-actualization and esthetics are the highest-level needs.
3. Answer – c. Page 25. The goal of cognitive behavioral therapy (CBT) is to identify the negative patterns of thought that lead to negative emotions. Once the maladaptive patterns are identified, they can be replaced with rational thoughts. A person must be able to engage in meaningful dialogue to benefit from CBT.
4. Answer – c. Page 25 (Table 3-3). Rapid, unthinking responses are known as automatic thoughts. Often these automatic thoughts, or cognitive distortions, are irrational because people make false assumptions and misinterpretations. Once the negative patterns of thought that lead to negative emotions are identified, they can be replaced with rational thoughts.
5. Answer – a. Page 31 (Box 3-2). Rigid or disengaged boundaries are those in which the rules and roles are followed despite the consequences.

Chapter 4

1. Answer – a. Page 37 (Figure 4-2). The cerebellum is critical in both motor and cognitive functions. Alterations in cerebello-thalamo-cortical circuits may manifest as disturbances of coordination, balance, and gait. Safety is the nurse's first concern.
2. Answer – c. Page 48. Risperidone blocks α_1- and H_1 receptors. It can cause orthostatic hypotension and sedation, which can lead to falls.
3. Answer – b. Page 48. Olanzapine (Zyprexa) has metabolic side effects, particularly weight gain. Metabolic monitoring for all patients receiving atypicals is recommended, although risperidone (Risperdal) and quetiapine (Seroquel) have a lower weight gain. Ziprasidone (Geodon) and aripiprazole (Abilify) are considered weight neutral. Metabolic monitoring usually includes measurements of body weight, body mass index (BMI), waist circumference, fasting plasma glucose level, and fasting lipid profile.
4. Answer – c. Page 45. At lower doses, trazodone loses its antidepressant action while retaining hypnotic effects through histamine receptor antagonism; therefore it is useful for insomnia. Fifty milligrams is a low dose. High doses of trazodone are required for the serotonergic action to relieve depression.
5. Answer – d. Page 35. Executive functions occur in the cerebrum. Loss of cortical tissue has been associated with schizophrenia as

well as with treatment involving haloperidol and other typical antipsychotics. In contrast, newer atypical antipsychotics and antidepressants have been found to increase brain volume and structural synaptic/neuronal plasticity.

Chapter 5

1. Answer – a. Page 55 (Box 5-1). The patient's comments indicate problems with use of leisure time. Recreational activities improve emotional, physical, cognitive, and social well-being. A recreational therapist is the best member of the treatment team to provide these services.
2. Answer – c. Page 56. Begins with a medical assessment to rule out or consider co-occurring/comorbid conditions.
3. Answer – d. Page 56. Safety is a key consideration in selection of activities. The correct response identifies an activity likely to appeal to the population but without physical contact between patients or equipment, which may be associated with injury.
4. Answer – a. Page 58. Mental health parity refers to third-party (insurance) coverage of care for mental illness and addictions similarly to care of physical illness. Federal and state legislation apply, but coverage varies by state. Some states offer full parity for mental illness insurance coverage.
5. Answer – c. Page 59. The nurse's skills from the medical unit will be valuable, but this nurse will need to expand his or her skill set to effectively care for a psychiatric population. Working with an experienced psychiatric nurse will provide opportunities for learning.

Chapter 6

1. Answer – d. Page 66. Despite personal misgivings, the nurse must maintain the fiancé's confidentiality.
2. Answer – c. Pages 65–66. The scenario offers no indication that the patient is dangerous or out of control; therefore less restrictive interventions should be employed. The nurse has a responsibility to provide guidance to the certified nursing assistant (CNA).
3. Answer – a. Page 62. Fidelity is an ethical principle that involves maintaining loyalty and commitment to patients.
4. Answer – d. Page 69. Institutional policies and practices do not absolve an individual nurse of responsibility to practice on the basis of professional standards of nursing care. State nurse practice acts specify that unlicensed assistive personnel (UAP) work under a nurse's supervision.
5. Answer – d. Page 70. Sleep deprivation causes impaired practice, which jeopardizes patient safety. The colleague's comments indicate that impairment is likely. The nurse should confer with the supervisor to determine the appropriate action.

Chapter 7

1. Answer – c. Pages 79–80. The patient's thyroid problems may have reemerged and can mimic depression.
2. Answer – d. Page 83. The focus of the question is the caregiver. Demands associated with the care of three elderly persons who live at a distance have the potential of overwhelming the caregiver. Because there is no evidence of role strain, a risk diagnosis is formulated.
3. Answer – b. Pages 76, 86. Hypnosis is not within the scope of practice of a staff level registered nurse. The state nurse practice act details regulations regarding scope of practice. Hypnosis is an advanced practice intervention.
4. Answer – c. Pages 84–85. Outcomes, as well as interventions, must always be individualized to the patient and should reflect the patient's multidimensional needs. While it is important to confer with the patient about which outcomes are desirable, a patient

experiencing panic is unable to engage in decision making or learning activities.
5. Answer – b. Page 89 (Box 7-7). It is important to document the events and actions taken in both patients' records; however, confidentiality must be maintained. Using the initials of patients involved is one way to ensure that confidentiality is maintained.

Chapter 8

1. Answer – b. Page 97 (Table 8-2). The correct response encourages description and helps the patient to express feelings related to this experience.
2. Answer – d. Page 97 (Table 8-2). The correct response demonstrates the therapeutic technique of presenting reality. Giving advice, disagreeing, and changing the subject are nontherapeutic communication techniques.
3. Answer – a. Page 97 (Table 8-2). The correct response demonstrates the therapeutic technique of reflection.
4. Answer – c. Page 101. Therapeutic use of touch is a basic aspect of the nurse-patient relationship and often perceived as a gesture of warmth and friendship, but the response to touch is culturally defined. Many Hispanic Americans are accustomed to frequent physical contact and perceive it in a positive way.
5. Answer – a. Page 91. Telehealth is a live interactive mechanism used to track clinical progress and provide access to people who otherwise might not receive good medical or psychosocial help. The nurse should accurately provide education about this mechanism as well as ensure the patient's rights to privacy.

Chapter 9

1. Answer – d. Pages 110, 114. The correct response is respectful and recognizes that trust between the nurse and patient needs to be developed. The correct response is also open ended, which is an appropriate communication technique to begin a new relationship.
2. Answer – b. Pages 114, 118. The nurse has a responsibility for self-care and must set limits on the neighbor's intrusive calls. Specifying the frequency and time allotment for calls shows compassion for the neighbor while preventing infringement on the nurse's personal life.
3. Answer – d. Page 121. Preparing and analyzing a process recording provides an opportunity for clinical supervision of the experienced nurse. The nurse and the supervisor examine the nurse's feelings and reactions to the patient and the way in which they affect the relationship.
4. Answer – c. Page 118. It's important for the nurse to continue to assess the adult, respect the adult's individuality, and delay judgment regarding whether the person is experiencing illness. Avoiding crowds may be an effective coping technique for this patient.
5. Answer – c. Page 112. Countertransference refers to the tendency of the nurse to displace onto the patient feelings related to people in his or her past. Frequently, the patient's transference to the nurse evokes countertransference feelings in the nurse.

Chapter 10

1. Answer – b. Page 120. Eustress is beneficial stress that will help the couple to focus, problem solve, and successfully plan their wedding.
2. Answer – a. Page 123 (Box 10-1). Yoga and other physical activities can be effective ways to manage stress. These activities deepen breathing, relieve muscle tension, and can elevate levels of the body's own endorphins, which induces a sense of well-being.
3. Answer – d. Page 122 (Figure 10-2). The scenario suggests that the spouse has experienced the effects of long-term stress. When stress is prolonged, the body stays alert. Chemicals produced by the stress

response can have damaging effects on the body, causing physical diseases. While all of the actions may be indicated, obtaining a health assessment from the primary care provider has the first priority.

4. Answer – a. Pages 122–123. The veteran had high risk for posttraumatic stress disorder (PTSD). When PTSD is untreated or undertreated, painful repercussions often occur, particularly marital problems, unemployment, heavy substance abuse, and suicide. The highest priority is an assessment of suicide risk.

5. Answer – b. Pages 121, (Figure 10-1), 123 (Box 10-1). Stress can be psychological (e.g., anxiety, guilt, or joy) or physical (e.g., stressful environment, such as loud noises, extreme heat or cold, or other disturbing physical condition). Stress is a part of everyday life for everyone. Skills in stress reduction will assist the individual to cope with the jet noise. Later, the individual may consider the other options.

Chapter 11

1. Answer – b. Page 135. Rationalization refers to justifying an action to satisfy the listener.

2. Answer – c. Page 131. While all of these situations may produce some level of fear or anxiety, the correct response presents a scenario of imminent, specific danger.

3. Answer – d. Pages 136–137. The student is demonstrating projection, as evidenced by not taking responsibility for his or her own behavior and blaming the instructor for a perception of failing. In the correct answer, the instructor avoids a defensive response and reinforces that responsibility belongs to the student.

4. Answer – d. Pages 133–134. Altruism is a health defense mechanism in which emotional conflicts and stressors are addressed by meeting the needs of others. With altruism, the person receives gratification either vicariously or from the response of others.

5. Answer – d. Page 142. Safety is the nurse's first priority. Individuals diagnosed with hoarding disorder often live in unsafe conditions. A home visit will help to identify whether safety is the primary concern.

Chapter 12

1. Answer – a. Pages 153, 156, 158. Safety is the nurse's first concern. One serious risk associated with doctor-shopping is medication interactions and duplicate medications.

2. Answer – d. Page 160. War is a traumatic experience for anyone. The veteran's comments about his peers and hearing deficit clearly indicate that he was exposed to explosives. Some studies show that between 5% and 20% of veterans are amnesic for their combat experiences.

3. Answer – c. Pages 153, 157. Working with people who have somatic symptom disorders can be frustrating as well as fascinating. The correct response presents a comment indicating that the nurse may have lost objectivity regarding the patient. Guidance from the nursing supervisor is needed.

4. Answer – b. Page 158. It's important for the nurse to convey compassion and support to the patient but without reinforcing the symptoms. Case management can help to limit health care costs. Seeing the patient at regular intervals can instill security and avoid frantic and frequent demands. The patient who establishes a relationship with the case manager often feels less anxiety because he or she has an advocate and feels that someone is managing and aware of his or her care.

5. Answer – b. Pages 154–155, 158 (Table 12-2). A paresthesia is a tingling or pricking sensation. Conversion disorder (functional neurobiological symptom disorder) usually involves weakness or paralysis, abnormal movement, swallowing or speech difficulties, seizures or attacks, and sensory problems. Patients may be distressed or show *la belle indifference* (a lack of emotional concern).

Despite the diagnosis, the patient's complaints must be taken seriously. Further evaluation is needed.

Chapter 13

1. Answer – a. Pages 167–168. The correct response shows callousness, entitlement, lack of remorse, and disregard for the rights of others. These characteristics are common in persons diagnosed with antisocial personality disorder.

2. Answer – c. Page 170. People diagnosed with narcissistic personality disorder consider themselves special and expect special treatment. Their demeanor is arrogant and haughty. They have a sense of entitlement.

3. Answer – a. Pages 169–170. People diagnosed with borderline personality disorder frequently use the defense of splitting, which strains personal relationships. Splitting is the inability to integrate both the positive and the negative qualities of an individual into one person.

4. Answer – c. Page 168. Genetics seem to play a significant role in the development of schizotypal personality disorder, which is more common in families with a history of schizophrenia.

5. Answer – b. Page 169. Alcohol abuse is a commonly occurring problem in persons diagnosed with antisocial personality disorder.

Chapter 14

1. Answer – b. Pages 184, 186. Body mass index (BMI) is used to gauge the level of severity, degree of functional disability, and need for supervision for persons diagnosed with anorexia nervosa. BMI is calculated as weight in kilograms divided by height in meters squared. Ideal BMIs are between 19 and 25. A person whose BMI is over or equal to 17 kg/m^2 meets one criterion for anorexia nervosa with mild severity. The BMI for the correct response is 17.2.

2. Answer – c. Page 187 (Table 14-1). Thought processes that accompany anorexia nervosa include a terror of gaining weight, viewing oneself as fat even when emaciated, and judging one's self-worth by one's weight or size.

3. Answer – c. Pages 183–184, 186. The comment by the psychiatric technician trivializes the patients' problems. Low self-esteem and self-doubts about personal worth are characteristic features of persons who have eating disorders. The comment contributes to these aspects of self-perception.

4. Answer – c. Page 187 (Box 14-4). Cognitive distortions with underlying emotions of anxiety, dysphoria, low self-esteem, and feeling lack of control are often present in persons suffering with eating disorders. In this instance, the adolescent is catastrophizing. The nurse should first help the patient to identify the fears. Cognitive distortions are consistently confronted by all members of the interdisciplinary team in preparation for carefully planned challenges to the patient later in treatment.

5. Answer – d. Page 185 (Box 14-2). The laboratory results show hypokalemia and hypocalcemia, which is likely to affect cardiac function, producing bradycardia, arrhythmias, and/or murmurs.

Chapter 15

1. Answer – c. Pages 199–200. The stress-diathesis model explains depression from an environmental, interpersonal, and life events perspective combined with biological vulnerability or predisposition (diathesis). Psychosocial stressors and interpersonal events, such as abuse, trigger certain neurophysical and neurochemical changes in the brain. Early life trauma is a significant component in the stress reaction.

2. Answer – d. Page 198 (Table 15-1). The correct response accomplishes two results: the nurse can further assess the patient's complaint and the nurse uses clarification, a therapeutic communication technique.

3. Answer – c. Pages 200–201. Helplessness is sometimes a finding in major depressive disorder. The nurse has a responsibility for patient advocacy. Helping the patient to advocate for self is empowering.

4. Answer – c. Page 211. The possibility that antidepressant medication might contribute to suicidal behavior, especially in children and adolescents, has been a long-time concern and all antidepressants include a black box warning; however, there is no conclusive evidence to support this concern. Use of selective serotonin reuptake inhibitors shows a strong association with a reduction in suicide. All treatments have potential risks; each patient should be considered individually when antidepressants are prescribed. All consumers of antidepressants should be observed carefully for worsening of depression and suicidal thoughts.

5. Answer – d. Page 218. Electroconvulsive therapy (ECT) is safe and effective and can achieve a 70% to 90% remission rate in depressed patients within 1 to 2 weeks. ECT is especially indicated when there is a need for a rapid, definitive response when a patient is suicidal or homicidal as well as in selected other circumstances.

Chapter 16

1. Answer – c. Pages 227, 230–232. The nurse has responsibility for advocacy. In view of the patient's long history of problems, a legal guardian should be considered.

2. Answer – b. Page 229. Numerous posts on a social network page indicate hyperactivity, which is a hallmark of mania.

3. Answer – a. Page 236 (Box 16-1). Patients should stop taking lithium if excessive diarrhea, vomiting, or sweating occurs. These problems can lead to dehydration, which can raise serum lithium to toxic levels.

4. Answer – d. Page 239 (Box 16-2). The correct response shows use of the therapeutic communication technique of verbalizing the implied. Gaining insight contributes to relapse prevention.

5. Answer – a. Pages 230–231. Safety is a priority. Mania impairs the person's judgment and impulse control, which may result in harm to self. The correct response identifies potential dangers and shows care for the patient.

Chapter 17

1. Answer – b. Page 248. Concrete thinking refers to the literal interpretation, with an inability to comprehend abstract concepts.

2. Answer – a. Page 245. The daily experience of negativity creates a scenario in which the risk for suicide is high. Depressive symptoms occur frequently in schizophrenia. Suicide is the leading cause of premature death in this population.

3. Answer – c. Page 268 (Table 17-10). Neuroleptic malignant syndrome (NMS) occurs in persons who have taken antipsychotic agents and usually begins early in the course of therapy. It is characterized by a decreased level of consciousness, greatly increased muscle tone, and autonomic dysfunction, including hyperpyrexia, labile hypertension, tachycardia, tachypnea, diaphoresis, and drooling. Treatment consists of early detection, discontinuation of the antipsychotic agent, management of fluid balance, reduction of temperature, and monitoring for complications. Treatment of this problem should occur in a medical unit.

4. Answer – b. Page 268 (Table 17-10). The patient's comments suggest that akathisia, which is an extrapyramidal symptom, is occurring. The nurse should assess the patient for other indicators of this side effect of antipsychotic medication.

5. Answer – c. Pages 252–253. Paranoia causes an inability to trust the actions of others. Therapeutic strategies should focus on lowering the patient's anxiety and decreasing defensive patterns. Application

of principles for dealing with paranoia is helpful for establishing trust and rapport.

Chapter 18

1. Answer – c. Page 291. Silence is a therapeutic communication technique. It is respectful and provides an opportunity for the adult to compose responses.

2. Answer – d. Page 290. Side effects of rivastigmine (Exelon) include nausea, vomiting, diarrhea, weight loss, loss of appetite, and muscle weakness.

3. Answer – a. Page 274 (Box 18-1). Withdrawal from alcohol, anxiolytics, opioids, and central nervous system stimulants presents a significant risk for development of delirium. The correct response identifies a patient who is likely to have tolerance to alcohol and is thus at risk for alcohol withdrawal delirium.

4. Answer – b. Pages 282, 292. Important considerations for promoting mental health in the older adult include the need for older adults to continue to include social, intellectual, and physical activity in their routine. Older adults can continue to learn and contribute even when physiological changes occur.

5. Answer – c. Pages 281–282. Memantine (Namenda), an N-methyl-D-aspartate (NMDA) antagonist, and some cholinesterase inhibitors may be prescribed to treat symptoms of moderate to severe Alzheimer's disease.

Chapter 19

1. Answer – d. Pages 296, 300, 305, 310, 312. The correct response recognizes the power of addiction but presents the reality of the consequences of continued use.

2. Answer – c. Page 301 (Table 19-2). Lorazepam is a benzodiazepine. Sudden withdrawal from this class of medications has medical complications, including the possibility of death; hence this refill request has priority.

3. Answer – b. Page 297. The nurse should educate the patient. E-cigarettes are advertised as safe; however, they contain nicotine as well as other hazardous chemicals.

4. Answer – c. Page 297. All of the options are correct, but safety is the nurse's first concern. Marijuana is a psychoactive substance. Effects include euphoria, sedation, perceptual distortions, and hallucinations; therefore driving or operating machinery may be hazardous.

5. Answer – c. Page 304 (Table 19-5). Naltrexone (ReVia, Vivitrol) reduces the desired pleasant feelings related to alcohol or opioid intake and helps to reduce drug cravings. It is part of a total program for maintaining sobriety.

Chapter 20

1. Answer – a. Page 325 (Figure 20-1). This scenario presents a potential adventitious crisis in phase one. The nurse must first consider safety. After moving to a secure location, the nurse can activate the school's code for an intruder and describe the intruder to law enforcement.

2. Answer – c. Page 326. The scenario presents a maturational crisis. Helping the spouse to consider other options is the nurse's most therapeutic action.

3. Answer – b. Page 327. In phase 1 of a crisis, a person faces a conflict or problem that threatens the self-concept and responds with increased feelings of anxiety. The nurse should first assure students that they are safe and then specify the reason for the session.

4. Answer – d. Page 330 (Table 20-2). After addressing safety concerns, the nurse should take steps to help patients feel safe and lower anxiety, such as providing a quiet environment, building

rapport, and acknowledging their crisis experience. A group session will allow patients who are unable to articulate their feelings to hear from patients who are able to discuss it.

5. Answer – a. Page 327. Nurses need to monitor their thoughts and feelings and learn to recognize when they need self-care, support, or professional help. This is especially true in the aftermath of violence. Nurses often suppress their own feelings in order to effectively handle the immediate situation and react later with anxiety.

Chapter 21

1. Answer – b. Page 325 (Box 21-1). The majority of the victims of reported intimate partner violence are women. Intimate partner violence is the number one cause of emergency department visits by women. Patterns of damage are often in locations that cannot be noticed easily, such as the torso, back, upper arms, upper legs, inside body orifices, and under the hair.

2. Answer – b. Page 344 (Box 21-3). The acute injury, coupled with bruises of different ages, suggest that the child may be abused. Abusive parents may perceive the child as bad or evil or project blame. The nurse is required to report suspicions of abuse to child protective services.

3. Answer – b. Page 340 (Figure 21-1). The cycle of violence consists of three phases: (1) tension-building phase, (2) acute battering phase, and (3) honeymoon phase. The question scenario shows acute battering, so a period of loving calm is likely to follow.

4. Answer – d. Page 342. Nurses must be self-aware, particularly in highly charged situations. Wishing harm on an abuser may be understandable, but it is an indicator of the nurse's need for guidance.

5. Answer – a. Page 338. While the nurse may include any of the topics, appropriate behaviors with intimate partners has priority. Characteristics of the game of football, the physical power required to be a player, and the risk for drug or alcohol misuse among this age group are factors that increase the risk for intimate partner violence.

Chapter 22

1. Answer – c. Pages 350, 353. The scenario presents the risk for sexual assault. Many people are sensitive about sexual matters, so the nurse should first give recognition to the widow for her willingness to share the problem. The most common drug used to facilitate the crime of rape is alcohol. Sexual violence occurs across all ages to men, women, and children. Cultural and societal factors play a part in forming attitudes about sexual violence.

2. Answer – a. Page 354. A sexual assault victim who arrives at the emergency department needs compassionate, supportive care and should not be left alone.

3. Answer – a. Pages 354–355. The correct response demonstrates use of reflection, a therapeutic communication technique. Consequences of rape can cause serious, long-term psychological trauma. Rape-trauma syndrome is a common sequela. Later in this interaction, the nurse should encourage the patient to consider professional counseling.

4. Answer – c. Pages 355–336 (Table 22-2). Prior to leaving the emergency department, the patient should have a scheduled follow-up appointment with a rape counselor or crisis counselor.

5. Answer – d. Pages 355–356 (Table 22-2). Common emotional reactions after a sexual assault include anger, fear, anxiety, guilt, humiliation, embarrassment, self-blame, and mood swings. Compassionate care involves approaching the person who has been sexually assaulted in a nonjudgmental and empathic manner. Patients need to hear and understand that the rape is not their fault. It is important to help survivors separate the issues of vulnerability from blame.

Chapter 23

1. Answer – b. Page 366. The correct response represents a covert message and suggests possible suicidal thinking by the parent. The nurse should further assess the meaning of the comment.

2. Answer – b. Page 365 (Box 23-1). All health care members who provided care for a suicide victim, including medical staff, nursing staff, and ancillary staff, are at risk for being traumatized by suicide. Staff also may experience symptoms of posttraumatic stress disorder with guilt, shock, anger, shame, and decreased self-esteem. To reduce the trauma associated with the sudden loss, posttrauma loss debriefing can help to initiate an adaptive grief process and prevent self-defeating behaviors.

3. Answer – a. Pages 362–363. The nurse should always take an individual very seriously if he or she mentions some form of suicidal ideation and ask directly about suicide.

4. Answer – a. Page 369 (Table 23-1). The patient's comment suggests hopelessness, helplessness, and worthlessness. Physical illnesses play a role in increasing suicide risk. Suicide precautions should be initiated.

5. Answer – d. Page 366 (Box 23-2). Referrals need to be made available to family members and friends to assist them in dealing with and addressing the many emotional reactions and problems that easily may develop after suicide of a family member or friend. Self-help groups are extremely beneficial for survivors.

Chapter 24

1. Answer – c. Pages 375, 384. Talking about one's feelings is healthier than violence or avoidance.

2. Answer – c. Pages 375, 379. The patient's behavior is aggressive. Aggressive behaviors reflect rage, hostility, and potential for physical assault or verbal destructiveness and can be directed at others or oneself. Aggression is a hostile reaction that occurs when control over anger is lost. It is used in an attempt to regain control over the stressor or flee the situation. By suggesting an appropriate behavior, the nurse offers an opportunity for the patient to regain control.

3. Answer – b. Pages 375, 379. In the original response, the nurse personalized the request and responded in an aggressive manner. The correct answer demonstrates an assertive response, which would have been more effective.

4. Answer – c. Pages 375, 379. Bullying is an intentional display and a use of violence, though it may appear mild in some instances. Bullying can be defined as an offensive, intimidating, malicious, condescending behavior designed to humiliate. The scenario identifies an instance of lateral bullying. All kinds of bullying behaviors create a toxic environment. Those who are bullied are prone to negative feelings about self, humiliation, poor self-concept, and great emotional pain, and many can suffer severe, long-term reactions. After educating the parents about bullying, the nurse should assist them in setting limits with the child.

5. Answer – b. Page 375. Sarcasm is a veiled form of anger.

Chapter 25

1. Answer – a. Page 390. Mourning refers to all of the ways in which a person outwardly expresses grief and the efforts taken to manage grief. It does not have a designated time frame and may continue for many years. A once-a-year ritual is an adaptive coping technique to recognize the parents' loss.

2. Answer – d. Page 397 (Table 25-3). This person is mourning. A grief or bereavement support group is indicated and can provide comfort.

3. Answer – a. Pages 390–391. While emotional responses to grief vary from one individual to the next, a common first response is

that of denial. The person is emotionally unable to accept his or her painful loss. Denial functions as a buffer against intolerable pain and allows the person to acknowledge the reality of a loss slowly.

4. Answer – d. Pages 390–391. The work of grief is over when the bereaved can realistically remember the pleasures and the disappointments of the relationship with the lost loved one. Brief periods of intense emotions may still occur at significant times, but the person or family members have energy to reinvest in new relationships that bring shared joys, security, satisfaction, and comfort.

5. Answer – b. Page 395. The nurse's comment suggests a negative self-judgment. Burnout, decreased work performance, and compassion fatigue (the emotional pain or cost of working with traumatized persons) may result in stress responses for nurses.

Chapter 26

1. Answer – c. Page 408. Prominent behavioral characteristics of autism spectrum disorder (ASD) include motions repeated over and over (flaps hands, rocks body, spins self in circles, repeatedly turns light on and off), playing with toys the same way every time, getting upset by minor changes (changes furniture around, changes route going someplace familiar), and obsessive interests.

2. Answer – b. Page 414. Therapeutic interventions should be matched to the developmental level of the child. Abused children are likely to have problems with anxiety or depression. Storytelling is a form of bibliotherapy likely to appeal to kindergarten-aged children. Children unconsciously identify with the characters in the story, allowing self-expression in a safe environment to occur.

3. Answer – b. Page 407. Causes of intellectual developmental disability may be a result of hereditary factors, alterations in early embryonic development, pregnancy and perinatal problems, and other factors such as trauma and poisoning.

4. Answer – d. Pages 406–407. Developmental level is an important part of the assessment with children, so the nurse should select terms the child will understand. A semistructured interview provides an opportunity for the child to express perceptions about life at home and life at school with teachers and peers. Severe marital discord is a factor that may contribute to mental illness in children.

5. Answer – a. Page 406. Genetic factors have been implicated in a number of childhood mental disorders, including autism, bipolar disorders, schizophrenia, attention-deficit/hyperactivity disorder (ADHD), intellectual developmental disorders, and some others.

Chapter 27

1. Answer – b. Page 419. Individuals with severe mental illness (SMI) usually have difficulties in multiple areas, including finances and budgeting. Psychoeducational programming builds interpersonal skills, including assertiveness.

2. Answer – b. Pages 422–423. The consumer has an active role in treatment and quality of life. Poverty and lack of access to quality foods can cause poor nutrition. The recovery model stresses a partnership between care providers and the patient, both working together to plan and direct treatment. Empowering the consumer and focusing on strengths rather than limitations helps the consumer to use his or her strengths to achieve the highest quality of life possible.

3. Answer – a. Page 429. While all of the topics are important, heart-healthy living encompasses diet, exercise, lifestyle or behavior changes, and management of hypertension. Persons who take antipsychotic medications are particularly at risk for heart disease and metabolic syndrome as a result of weight gain and hyperlipidemia.

4. Answer – c. Pages 427–428. Pedophilia involves lewd or lascivious (sexual) acts on a minor. These persons are at especially high risk of suicide, especially in the first 24 to 48 hours after incarceration.

5. Answer – b. Page 419. Issues for those with severe mental illness (SMI) include poverty, stigma, isolation, unemployment, poorer health outcomes, law enforcement encounters, victimization, and inadequate housing or homelessness. Supplemental Security Income (SSI) provides a modest income for indigent persons ineligible for Social Security Disability Income (SSDI).

Chapter 28

1. Answer – b. Page 445. The developmental task of late life is integrity vs. despair. The patient's comment shows feelings of hopelessness and loss, which contributes to despair. The correct response assists the patient to find meaning in life.

2. Answer – b. Page 445. The patient's comment may relate to physical or mental concerns. The nurse should first clarify and explore the meaning of the comment.

3. Answer – b. Page 449. As an advocate, the nurse can help to empower the patient to address the problem. Role-playing provides an opportunity to safely practice different responses.

4. Answer – d. Pages 445–446. The interaction of drugs and alcohol in the older adult can have serious consequences. Alcohol may prolong, potentiate, or accelerate the metabolism of various drugs.

5. Answer – c. Page 444. The highest suicide rate is among white males age 65 and older. Depression can be dangerous when the older person is also experiencing illness, loneliness, or other life losses.

INDEX

Note: Page numbers followed by "b", "f", and "t" indicate boxes, figures, and tables, respectively.